ELSEVIER

evolve

W9-BZL-768

∴ For additional resources, visit:
http://evolve.elsevier.com/DrugConsult/hp/

Evolve ® Learning Resources for *Mosby's Drug Consult for Health Professions,* 1st Edition offer the following features:

Resources

- **Biannual Updates**
  Check here for abbreviated monographs for recently released drugs, alerts regarding drug withdrawals, and up-to-date drug safety information.

- **Color Pill Atlas**
  See how common drugs appear in full color!

- **Immunization Schedules**
  Recommended childhood and adult immunization schedules are compiled in these tables for easy reference.

- **Drugs by Disorder**
  A handy reference of over 65 disorders, with the drugs that treat those disorders listed below them by generic and trade name.

- **Herbal Therapies/Interactions**
  Provides a quick reference for health professionals with patients and clients who take herbal therapies.

- **Weapons of Mass Destruction Guidelines**
  At-a-glance tables provide information on this timely topic!

- **Weblinks**
  Access links to places of interest on the web.

First Edition

Mosby's
DRUG CONSULT
for HEALTH
PROFESSIONS

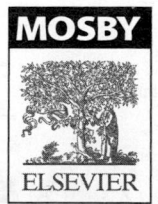

MOSBY

ELSEVIER

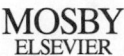

MOSBY
ELSEVIER

11830 Westline Industrial Drive
St. Louis, Missouri 63146

MOSBY'S DRUG CONSULT   ISBN-13: 978-0-323-03463-0
FOR HEALTH PROFESSIONS   ISBN-10: 0-323-03463-2
Copyright © 2006 by Mosby Inc., an affiliate of Elsevier Inc.

Notice

Knowledge and best practice in this field are constantly changing. As new research
and experience broaden our knowledge, changes in practice, treatment and drug
therapy may become necessary or appropriate. Readers are advised to check the
most current information provided (i) on procedures featured or (ii) by the
manufacturer of each product to be administered, to verify the recommended dose
or formula, the method and duration of administration, and contraindications. It is
the responsibility of the practitioner, relying on their own experience and knowledge
of the patient, to make diagnoses, to determine dosages and the best treatment for
each individual patient, and to take all appropriate safety precautions. To the fullest
extent of the law, neither the Publisher nor the Editors assumes any liability for any
injury and/or damage to persons or property arising out or related to any use of the
material contained in this book.

ISBN-13: 978-0-323-03463-0
ISBN-10: 0-323-03463-2

Publishing Director: Linda Duncan
Acquisitions Editor: Kellie Fitzpatrick
Developmental Editor: Jennifer Watrous
Editorial Assistant: Elizabeth Clark
Publishing Services Manager: Julie Eddy
Project Manager: Kelly E.M. Steinmann
Designer: Jyotika Shroff

Printed in the United States of America

Last digit is the print number: 9 8 7 6 5 4 3 2 1

Working together to grow
libraries in developing countries
www.elsevier.com | www.bookaid.org | www.sabre.org

ELSEVIER   BOOK AID International   Sabre Foundation

Reviewers

John Albrecht, BA, CPhT
Director of Education
Education
Olympia College
North Aurora, Illinois

Lynn Augenstern, CMA, MA
Program Director
Medical Assisting Program
Ridley-Lowell Business & Technical
    Institute
Binghamton, New York

Deborah J. Bedford
Program Coordinator/Instructor
Medical Assisting Department
North Seattle Community College
Seattle, Washington

Bhaswati Bhattacharya, MA, MPH, MD
Assistant Professor of Family
    Practice in Medicine,
    Weill/Cornell Medical College
Director, Division of Complementary
    and Alternative Medicines,
    Wyckoff Heights Medical Center
New York, New York

Heather Davis, MS, NREMT-P
Education Program Director
Los Angeles County Fire Department
Valencia, California

Deborah A. DeLuca, MS ChE, JD
Assistant Professor, Health Law,
    Biomedical Ethics and Medical
    Sciences
Health Professions Leadership
Seton Hall University School of
    Graduate Medical Education
South Orange, New Jersey

Ronald De Vera Barredo, PT, EdD, GCS
Associate Professor
Graduate Program in Physical
    Therapy
Arkansas State University
State University, Arkansas

Gautam J. Desai, DO
Physician Educator
Department of Medical Affairs
Associate Professor
Department of Family Medicine/OPP
Kansas City University of Medicine
    and Biosciences
College of Osteopathic Medicine
Kansas City, Missouri

Karen Drummond, CPC, CMC
National Presenter for the American
    Academy of Professional Coders
Instructor
Medical Billing/Coding
Stark State College
Canton City Schools Adult Education
Canton, Ohio

Ruth Ann Ehrlich, RT(R)
Instructor
Diagnostic Imaging
Radiology
Western States Chiropractic College
Adjunct Faculty
Portland Community College
Portland, Oregon

George Fakhoury, MD, DORCP, CMA
Academic Program Manager
Healthcare Programs
Heald College
San Francisco, California

Foreword

INTRODUCTION

Health care professionals face many challenges in today's environment, not the least of which is familiarity with the large number of medications available. New medications are being introduced, and new applications, dosage forms, and different routes of administration for existing medications are increasing at a rapid rate. This voluminous amount of drug information must be quickly integrated into the patient care environment. *Mosby's Drug Consult for Health Professions* is designed as an easy-to-use source of the current drug information needed by the busy health care provider.

This guide contains:

1. *Practice-oriented precautions and considerations.* Every drug entry provides extensive, practice-oriented precautions and considerations, putting essential drug facts directly into the context of your care.
2. *Vital lifespan considerations.* Throughout its pages, the book highlights key points related to drug therapy in pregnant, breast-feeding, pediatric, and elderly patients.
3. *Comprehensive appendices.* Thirteen ready-reference appendices give you easy access to additional vital drug-related information, such as the English-Spanish Drug Phrase Translator and an insulin table for a quick reference when working with diabetic clients and patients.

4. *Prioritized side effects.* Each drug entry ranks side effects by frequency of occurrence, from most common to least common. Entries also include the percentage of frequency, when known. This information helps you focus your care by knowing which effects to monitor more closely.
5. *Highlights on serious adverse reactions.* In each drug entry, the book calls attention to dangerous or life-threatening reactions so that you can identify them easily and act on them promptly.
6. *Alert icons.* Alert icons are used to spotlight critical health professions considerations that require special attention.
8. *Free updates.* A companion website, http://evolve.elsevier.com/DrugConsult/hp/, provides biannual updates to drug information to keep you current on new drugs and indications, recent warnings, withdrawals from the market, and more.

A detailed guide to *Mosby's Drug Consult for Health Professions*:

Mosby's Drug Consult for Health Professions provides essential drug information in a user-friendly format. The bulk of the handbook contains an alphabetical listing of drug entries by generic name. Drug entries include the following:

Generic and Brand Names. Drug entries begin with the generic drug name, followed by its pronunciation and U.S. and Canadian brand names.

Classification. Each entry highlights this important information for easy identification.

Category and schedule. This section lists the drug's pregnancy risk category and, when appropriate, its controlled substance schedule or over-the-counter (OTC) status.

Mechanism of action. This section clearly and concisely details the drug's mechanism of action and therapeutic effects.

Pharmacokinetics. Under this heading, a quick-reference chart outlines the drug's route, onset, peak, and duration, when known. This information is followed by a discussion of the drug's absorption, distribution, metabolism, excretion, and half-life.

Availability. This section identifies the forms that the drug comes in, such as tablets, sustained-release capsules, or an injectable solution. Available doses and concentrations are also listed.

Indications and dosages. Here, you'll find the approved indications and routes, along with the dosage information for all age groups and populations, including adults, elderly patients, children, neonates, and those with pre-existing conditions such as liver or kidney disease.

Contraindications. Each entry lists conditions in which use of the generic drug is contraindicated and should not be used.

Interactions. For drugs, herbal supplements, and food, this section supplies vital information about interactions with the topic drug.

Diagnostic test effects. Under this heading, you'll see a brief description of the drug's effects on laboratory and diagnostic test results, such as liver enzyme levels and electrocardiogram tracings.

IV incompatibilities and IV compatibilities. These twin sections let you know which IV drugs can and cannot be given with the featured drug, whether by IV push, Y-site, or IV piggyback administration.

Side effects. Unlike other handbooks that mix common, deadly effects with rare, minor ones in a long, undifferentiated list, this book ranks side effects by frequency of occurrence by indicating: expected, frequent, occasional, and rare. Within each frequency, effects are listed by highest to lowest percentage of occurrence, when known.

Serious adverse reactions. Because serious adverse reactions are life-threatening responses that require prompt intervention, this section highlights them, apart from other side effects, for easy identification.

Precautions and considerations. Using a practice-oriented format and written specifically for health professions, this section presents precautions and considerations for each drug entry.

Mosby's Drug Consult for Health Professions is an easy-to-use source of the current drug information for a wide spectrum of health care providers. When it comes to providing quality patient care, you'll need no other drug reference.

Contents

Abarelix
a-ba-rel′iks
(Plenaxis)

CATEGORY AND SCHEDULE
Pregnancy Risk Category: X

CLASSIFICATION
Antineoplastics, hormones/
hormone modifiers, gonadotropin-
releasing hormone analogs

MECHANISM OF ACTION
A luteinizing hormone-releasing
hormone (LHRH) antagonist that
inhibits gonadotropin and androgen
production by blocking gonadotropin
releasing-hormone receptors in the
pituitary. *Therapeutic Effect:*
Suppresses luteinizing hormone,
follicle stimulating hormone
secretion, reducing the secretion of
testosterone by the testes.

PHARMACOKINETICS
Slowly absorbed following
intramuscular administration.
Distributed extensively. Protein
binding: 96%-99%. **Half-life:**
13.2 days.

AVAILABILITY
Powder for Injection: 113 mg kit
containing 10 ml 0.9% NaCl,
18-gauge needle, 22-gauge needle.

INDICATIONS AND DOSAGES
▸ **Prostate cancer**
IM
Adults, Elderly. 100 mg on days 1,
15, 29, and every 4 weeks thereafter.
Treatment failure can be detected by
obtaining serum testosterone concentration prior to abarelix administration, day 19 and every 8 weeks
thereafter.

CONTRAINDICATIONS
This drug should not be used in
women and children.

INTERACTIONS
Drug
None known.
Herbal
None known.
Food
None known.

DIAGNOSTIC TEST EFFECTS
May increase serum transaminase,
serum SGOT (AST), SGPT (ALT),
and serum triglyceride levels. May
slightly decrease blood hemoglobin
concentrations. May decrease bone
mineral density.

SIDE EFFECTS
Frequent (79%-30%)
Hot flashes, sleep disturbances,
breast enlargement
Occasional (20%-11%)
Breast pain, nipple tenderness, back
pain, constipation, peripheral edema,
dizziness, upper respiratory tract
infection, diarrhea
Rare (10%)
Fatigue, nausea, dysuria, micturition
frequency, urinary retention, urinary
tract infection

SERIOUS REACTIONS
• Immediate-onset systemic allergic
reaction characterized by hypotension,
urticaria, pruritus, periorbital and/or
circumoral edema, shortness of breath,
wheezing, and syncope may occur.
• Prolongation of the QT interval
may occur tightening of throat,
tongue swelling, wheezing, shortness
of breath, and low blood pressure
occur rarely.

PRECAUTIONS & CONSIDERATIONS
Caution is warranted with prolonged
QT interval or who weigh more than

225 lbs (103 kg). Be aware that this drug is not for use in women or children. Be aware that there are no age-related precautions noted in the elderly.

Potential side effects, including hot flashes, sleep disturbances, breast enlargement, and nipple tenderness, may occur. Notify the physician if rash, hives, itching, tingling, or flushing develops; the skin reaction may occur immediately after injection or several days later. Serum testosterone concentration should be measured prior to administration beginning on day 29 and every 8 weeks thereafter. Serum PSA and serum transaminase levels should be periodically monitored.

Storage
Store at room temperature. Shake abarelix vial gently before reconstituting.

Administration
Withdraw 2.2 ml of 0.9% NaCl using 18-gauge needle and a 3-ml syringe. Insert the needle into the abarelix vial and inject the diluent quickly. Shake immediately for 15 seconds. Allow vial to stand for 2 minutes. Tap the vial to reduce foaming and swirl the vial. Shake the vial again for 15 seconds and allow to stand again for 2 minutes. Insert 18-gauge needle, invert the vial, and draw up some of the suspension into the syringe. Without removing the needle from the vial, re-inject it at any remaining solids in the vial. Repeat this process until all solids are dispersed. Swirl the vial before withdrawal, then withdraw the entire contents, about 2.2 ml. Reconstitution will provide a concentration of 50 mg/ml and should be used within 1 hour of reconstitution. Exchange the 18-gauge needle with the 22-gauge needle and give entire suspension IM into the dorsogluteal

or vetrogluteal region of the buttock. Monitor the patient for 30 minutes. The cumulative risk for allergic reaction increases with each injection.

Abciximab
ab-six'ih-mab
(c7E3 Fab, ReoPro)

CATEGORY AND SCHEDULE
Pregnancy Risk Category: C

CLASSIFICATION
Monoclonal antibodies, platelet inhibitors, recombinant DNA origin

MECHANISM OF ACTION
A glycoprotein IIb/IIIa receptor inhibitor that rapidly inhibits platelet aggregation by preventing the binding of fibrinogen to GP IIb/IIIa receptor sites on platelets.
Therapeutic Effect: Prevents closure of treated coronary arteries. Prevents acute cardiac ischemic complications.

PHARMACOKINETICS
Rapidly cleared from plasma. Initial-phase half-life is less than 10 min; second-phase half-life is 30 min. Platelet function generally returns within 48 hr.

AVAILABILITY
Injection: 2 mg/ml (5-ml vial).

INDICATIONS AND DOSAGES
▸ **Percutaneous coronary intervention (PCI)**
IV BOLUS
Adults. 0.25 mg/kg 10-60 min before angioplasty or atherectomy,

then 12-hr IV infusion of
0.125 mcg/kg/min. Maximum:
10 mcg/min.
▸ **PCI (unstable angina)**
IV BOLUS
Adults. 0.25 mg/kg, followed by
18- to 24-hr infusion of 10 mcg/min,
ending 1 hr after procedure.

CONTRAINDICATIONS
Active internal bleeding, arteriovenous malformation or aneurysm,
cerebrovascular accident (CVA) with
residual neurologic defect, history of
CVA (within the past 2 years) or oral
anticoagulant use within the past
7 days unless PT is less than 1.2 ×
control, history of vasculitis,
intracranial neoplasm, prior IV
dextran use before or during PTCA,
recent surgery or trauma (within the
past 6 weeks), recent (within the past
6 weeks or less) GI or GU bleeding,
thrombocytopenia (less than 100,000
cells/mcl), and severe uncontrolled
hypertension

INTERACTIONS
Drug
Anticoagulants, including heparin:
May increase risk of hemorrhage.
**Platelet aggregation inhibitors
(such as aspirin, dextran, thrombo-
lytic agents):** May increase risk of
bleeding.
Herbal
None known.
Food
None known.

DIAGNOSTIC TEST EFFECTS
Increases activated clotting time
(ACT), aPTT, and PT. Decreases
platelet count.

▓ IV INCOMPATIBILITIES
Administer in separate line; no other
medication should be added to
infusion solution.

SIDE EFFECTS
Frequent
Nausea (16%), hypotension (12%)
Occasional (9%)
Vomiting
Rare (3%)
Bradycardia, confusion, dizziness,
pain, peripheral edema, urinary tract
infection

SERIOUS REACTIONS
• Major bleeding complications
may occur. If complications occur,
stop the infusion immediately.
• Hypersensitivity reaction may
occur.
• Atrial fibrillation or flutter,
pulmonary edema, and complete
atrioventricular block occur
occasionally.

PRECAUTIONS & CONSIDERATIONS
Caution is warranted with persons
who weigh less than 75 kg, those
who are over age 65, those who have
a history of GI disease, and those
who are receiving aspirin, heparin, or
thrombolytics. Also use abciximab
cautiously in those who've had a
PTCA within 12 hours of the onset
of signs and symptoms of acute MI,
who've had a prolonged PTCA
(greater than 70 minutes), or who've
had a failed PTCA, because they are
at increased risk for bleeding. It is
unknown if abciximab is distributed
in breast milk. Safety and efficacy
have not been established in children.
There is an increased risk of
bleeding in the elderly. An electric
razor and soft toothbrush should be
used to prevent bleeding.
    Notify the physician of signs of
bleeding, including black or red
stool, coffee-ground emesis, red or
dark urine, or red-speckled mucus
from cough. To assess for preexisting
blood abnormalities, aPTT, platelet
count, and PT before abciximab

infusion, 2 to 4 hours after treatment, and 24 hours after treatment or before discharge, whichever is first. Signs and symptoms of hemorrhage, including a decrease in B/P, increase in pulse rate, abdominal or back pain, and severe headache, should be monitored. Laboratory test results, including ACT, aPTT, platelet count, and PT, should also be assessed. Female's menstrual discharge should be determined and monitored for increase.

Storage
Store vials in refrigerator.

Administration
Solution for injection normally appears clear and colorless. Do not shake. Discard any unused portion or any preparation that contains opaque particles. Avoid IM injections and venipunctures; also avoid using indwelling urinary catheters and nasogastric tubes. Expect to discontinue heparin 4 hours before the arterial sheath is removed. Stop abciximab and heparin infusion if serious bleeding uncontrolled by pressure occurs.

For bolus injection and continuous infusion, use a sterile, nonpyrogenic, low protein binding 0.2- or 0.22-micron filter. The continuous infusion may be filtered either during drug preparation or at the time of administration. Withdraw the desired dose and dilute in 250 ml of 0.9% NaCl or D_5W (for example, 10 mg in 250 ml equals a concentration of 40 mcg/ml). The bolus dose may be given undiluted. Give in separate IV line; do not add other medications to infusion. While femoral artery sheath is in position, maintain patient on complete bed rest with head of bed elevated at 30 degrees. Maintain affected limb in straight position. After the sheath has

been removed, apply femoral pressure for 30 minutes, either manually or mechanically; then apply a pressure dressing. Bed rest should be maintained for 6 to 8 hours after the sheath is removed or the drug is discontinued, whichever is later.

Acamprosate
ah-cam'pro-sate
(Campral)

CATEGORY AND SCHEDULE
Pregnancy Risk Category: C

CLASSIFICATION
Antialcoholics

MECHANISM OF ACTION
An alcohol abuse deterrent that appears to interact with glutamate and gamma-aminobutyric acid neurotransmitter systems centrally, restoring their balance.
Therapeutic Effect: Reduces alcohol dependence.

PHARMACOKINETICS
Slowly absorbed from the GI tract. Steady-state plasma concentrations are reached within 5 days. Does not undergo metabolism. Excreted in urine.
Half-life: 20-33 hr.

AVAILABILITY
Tablets: 333 mg.

INDICATIONS AND DOSAGES
▶ **Maintenance of alcohol abstinence in alcohol-dependent patients who are abstinent at initiation of treatment.**

PO
Adults, Elderly: Two tablets 3 times
a day.
▶ **Dosage in renal impairment**
For patients with creatinine clearance of 30-49 ml/min, dosage is
decreased to one tablet 3 times a day.

CONTRAINDICATIONS
Severe renal impairment (creatinine
clearance of 30 ml/min or less)

INTERACTIONS
Drug
Antidepressants: May cause weight
gain or loss.
Naltrexone: May increase acam-
prosate blood concentration.
Herbal
None known.
Food
None known.

DIAGNOSTIC TEST EFFECTS
None known.

SIDE EFFECTS
Frequent (17%)
Diarrhea
Occasional (6%-4%)
Insomnia, asthenia, fatigue, anxiety,
flatulence, nausea, depression,
pruritus
Rare (3%-1%)
Dizziness, anorexia, paresthesia,
diaphoresis, dry mouth

SERIOUS REACTIONS
• None known.

PRECAUTIONS & CONSIDERATIONS
It is unknown if acamprosate is
distributed in breast milk. The safety
and efficacy of acamprosate have
not been established in children.
Age-related renal impairment may
require a dosage adjustment in the
elderly. Be aware that acamprosate

does not eliminate or diminish
withdrawal symptoms. Acamprosate
helps maintain abstinence only when
used as part of a treatment program
that includes counseling and support.
Avoid tasks that require mental
alertness or motor skills until
response to the drug has been
established.
   Dizziness may occur. BUN and
serum creatinine levels should be
obtained before beginning treatment.
Know that acamprosate use is
contraindicated with severe renal
impairment (creatinine clearance of
30 ml/min or less). Pattern of daily
bowel activity should be assessed
during therapy.
Administration
❗ Expect to decrease the dosage with
moderate renal impairment (creatinine clearance of 30-50 ml/minute).
Don't crush or break enteric-coated
tablets. Take acamprosate without
regard to food. However, persons
who regularly eat three meals a day
may be more compliant with the
drug regimen if instructed to take
acamprosate with food.

Acarbose

a-car´bose
(α-amylase inhibitor,
α-glucosidase inhibitor,
antidiabetic, hypoglycemic)
(Glucobay [AUS], Prandase [CAN],
Precose)
**Do not confuse Precose with
PreCare.**

CATEGORY AND SCHEDULE
Pregnancy Risk Category: B

CLASSIFICATION
Alpha glucosidase inhibitors,
antidiabetic agents

MECHANISM OF ACTION
An alpha glucosidase inhibitor that
delays glucose absorption and
digestion of carbohydrates, resulting
in a smaller rise in blood glucose
concentration after meals.
Therapeutic Effect: Lowers postpran-
dial hyperglycemia.

AVAILABILITY
Tablets: 25 mg, 50 mg, 100 mg.

INDICATIONS AND DOSAGES
▶ **Diabetes mellitus**
PO
Adults, Elderly. Initially, 25 mg
3 times a day with first bite of each
main meal. Increase at 4- to 8-wk
intervals. Maximum: For patients
weighing more than 60 kg, 100 mg
3 times a day; for patients weighing
60 kg or less, 50 mg 3 times a day.

CONTRAINDICATIONS
Chronic intestinal diseases
associated with marked disorders of
digestion or absorption, cirrhosis,
colonic ulceration, conditions that
may deteriorate as a result of
increased gas formation in the
intestine, diabetic ketoacidosis,
hypersensitivity to acarbose, inflammatory bowel disease, partial intestinal obstruction or predisposition to
intestinal obstruction, significant
renal dysfunction (serum creatinine
level greater than 2 mg/dl)

INTERACTIONS
Drug
**Digestive enzymes, intestinal
absorbents (such as charcoal):**
Reduces effects of acarbose.
Herbal
None known.
Food
None known.

DIAGNOSTIC TEST EFFECTS
May increase AST(SGOT) levels.

SIDE EFFECTS
Side effects diminish in frequency
and intensity over time.
Frequent
Transient GI disturbances: flatulence
(77%), diarrhea (33%), abdominal
pain (21%)

SERIOUS REACTIONS
• Elevated liver transaminases may
occur.

PRECAUTIONS & CONSIDERATIONS
Caution is warranted with fever or
infection and in those who've had
surgery or trauma because these
states may cause loss of glycemic
control. Acarbose use is not recommended during pregnancy. It is
unknown if acarbose is distributed in
breast milk. Safety and efficacy have
not been established in children.
Hypoglycemia may be difficult to
recognize in the elderly. Also,
age-related renal impairment may
increase sensitivity to the glucose-
lowering effect of acarbose. Avoid
alcoholic beverages.

Food intake and blood glucose should be monitored before and during therapy. Glycosylated hemoglobin, and AST (SGOT) levels should also be assessed. Consult the physician when glucose demands are altered (such as with fever, heavy physical activity, infection, stress, trauma). Excrcise, good personal hygiene (including foot care), not smoking, and weight control are essential parts of therapy.

Administration

Take acarbose with the first bite of each main meal.

Do not skip or delay meals.

Acebutolol

a-se-byoo'toe-lole
(Monitan [CAN],
Novo-Acebutolol [CAN],
Rhotral [CAN], Sectral)
Do not confuse with Sectral, Factrel, or Septra.

CATEGORY AND SCHEDULE

Pregnancy Risk Category: B
(D if used in second or third trimester)

CLASSIFICATION

Antiadrenergics, beta blocking, antiarrhythmics, class II

MECHANISM OF ACTION

A beta$_1$-adrenergic blocker that competitively blocks beta$_1$-adrenergic receptors in cardiac tissue. Reduces the rate of spontaneous firing of the sinus pacemaker and delays AV conduction.

Therapeutic Effect: Slows heart rate, decreases cardiac output, decreases BP, and exhibits antiarrhythmic activity.

PHARMACOKINETICS

Route	Onset	Peak	Duration
PO (hypotensive)	1-1.5 hr	2-8 hr	24 hr
PO (antiarrhythmic)	1 hr	4-6 hr	10 hr

Well absorbed from the GI tract. Protein binding: 26%. Undergoes extensive first-pass liver metabolism to active metabolite. Eliminated via bile, secreted into GI tract via intestine, and excreted in urine. Removed by hemodialysis. **Half-life:** 3-4 hr; metabolite, 8-13 hr.

AVAILABILITY

Capsules: 200 mg, 400 mg.

INDICATIONS AND DOSAGES

▸ **Mild to moderate hypertension**

PO

Adults. Initially, 400 mg/day in 12 divided doses. Range: Up to 1200 mg/day in 2 divided doses. Maintenance: 400-800 mg/day.

▸ **Ventricular arrhythmias**

PO

Adults. Initially, 200 mg q12hr. Increase gradually to 600-1200 mg/day in 2 divided doses. *Elderly.* Initially, 200-400 mg/day. Maximum: 800 mg/day.

▸ **Dosage in renal impairment**

Dosage is modified based on creatinine clearance.

Creatinine Clearance	% of Usual Dosage
Less than 50 ml/min	50
Less than 25 ml/min	25

OFF-LABEL USES
Treatment of anxiety, chronic angina pectoris, hypertrophic cardiomyopathy, MI, pheochromocytoma, syndrome of mitral valve prolapse, thyrotoxicosis, tremors

CONTRAINDICATIONS
Cardiogenic shock, heart block greater than first degree, overt heart failure, severe bradycardia

INTERACTIONS
Drug
Diuretics, other antihypertensives: May increase hypotensive effect of acebutolol.
Sympathomimetics, xanthines: May mutually inhibit effects of acebutolol; may mask symptoms of hypoglycemia and prolong hypoglycemic effect of insulin and oral hypoglycemics.
Herbal
None known.
Food
None known.

DIAGNOSTIC TEST EFFECTS
May increase antinuclear antibody titer and serum alkaline phosphatase, serum bilirubin, BUN, serum creatinine, HDL, lipoproteins, serum potassium, AST (SGOT), ALT (SGPT), triglyceride, and uric acid levels.

SIDE EFFECTS
Frequent
Hypotension manifested as dizziness, nausea, diaphoresis, headache, cold extremities, fatigue, constipation, or diarrhea
Occasional
Insomnia, urinary frequency, impotence or decreased libido
Rare
Rash, arthralgia, myalgia, confusion (especially in the elderly), altered taste

SERIOUS REACTIONS
• Overdose may produce profound bradycardia and hypotension.
• Abrupt withdrawal may result in diaphoresis, palpitations, headache, and tremors.
• Acebutolol administration may precipitate CHF or MI in patients with heart disease; thyroid storm in those with thyrotoxicosis; or peripheral ischemia in those with existing peripheral vascular disease.
• Hypoglycemia may occur in patients with previously controlled diabetes.
• Signs of thrombocytopenia, such as unusual bleeding or bruising, occur rarely.

PRECAUTIONS & CONSIDERATIONS
Caution is warranted with bronchospastic disease, diabetes, hyperthyroidism, impaired renal or hepatic function, inadequate cardiac function, and peripheral vascular disease. Acebutolol readily crosses the placenta and is distributed in breast milk. Acebutolol use should be avoided in pregnant women after the first trimester because it may result in low-birth-weight infants. The drug may also produce apnea, bradycardia, hypoglycemia, or hypothermia during childbirth. No age-related precautions have been noted in children and dosages have not been established. Use cautiously in the elderly, who may have age-related peripheral vascular disease. Be aware that salt and alcohol intake should be restricted. Nasal decongestants or OTC cold preparations (stimulants) should not be used without physician approval.
Notify the physician of excessive fatigue, headache, prolonged dizziness, shortness of breath, or weight gain. B/P for hypotension, respiratory status for shortness of

breath, pattern of daily bowel activity and stool consistency, EKG for arrhythmias, and pulse for quality, rate and rhythm should be monitored during treatment. If pulse rate is 60 beats/minute or lower or systolic B/P is less than 90 mm Hg, withhold the medication and contact the physician. Signs and symptoms CHF, such as decreased urine output, distended neck veins, dyspnea (particularly on exertion or lying down), night cough, peripheral edema, and weight gain should also be assessed.

Administration
Acebutolol may be taken without regard to meals. Do not abruptly discontinue the drug.

Acetaminophen
ah-seet′ah-min-oh-fen
(Abenol [CAN],
Apo-Acetaminophen [CAN],
Atasol [CAN], Dymadon [AUS],
Feverall, Panadol [AUS], Panamax
[AUS], Paralgin [AUS], Setamol
[AUS], Tempra, Tylenol)
Do not confuse with Fiorinal, Hycodan, Indocin, Percodan, or Tuinal.

CATEGORY AND SCHEDULE
Pregnancy Risk Category: B
OTC

CLASSIFICATION
Analgesics, non-narcotic, antipyretics

MECHANISM OF ACTION
A central analgesic whose exact mechanism is unknown, but appears to inhibit prostaglandin synthesis in the central nervous system (CNS) and, to a lesser extent, block pain impulses through peripheral action. Acetaminophen acts centrally on hypothalamic heat-regulating center, producing peripheral vasodilation (heat loss, skin erythema, sweating). *Therapeutic Effect:* Results in antipyresis. Produces analgesic effect. Results in antipyresis.

PHARMACOKINETICS

Route	Onset	Peak	Duration
PO	15-30 min	1-1.5 hr	4-6 hr

Rapidly, completely absorbed from gastrointestinal (GI) tract; rectal absorption variable. Protein binding: 20%-50%. Widely distributed to most body tissues. Metabolized in liver; excreted in urine. Removed by hemodialysis. **Half-life:** 1-4 hr (half-life is increased in those with liver disease, elderly, neonates; decreased in children).

AVAILABILITY
Caplet (Genapap, Tylenol): 500 mg.
Caplet, extended release (Mapap, Tylenol Arthritis Pain): 650 mg.
Capsule (Mapap): 500 mg.
Elixir: 160 mg/5 ml.
Liquid, oral (Tylenol Extra Strength): 500 mg/15 ml.
Solution, oral drops (Genapap Infant): 80 mg/0.8 ml.
Suppository, rectal (Feverall): 80 mg, *(Acephen, Feverall):* 120 mg, 325 mg, 650 mg.
Tablet (Genapap, Mapap, Tylenol): 325 mg, 500 mg.
Tablet, chewable (Genapap, Mapap, Tylenol): 80 mg.

INDICATIONS AND DOSAGES
▸ **Analgesia and antipyresis**
PO
Adults, Elderly. 325-650 mg q4-6hr
or 1 g 3-4 times/day. Maximum:
4 g/day.
Children. 10-15 mg/kg/dose
q4-6hr as needed. Maximum:
5 doses/24 hr.
Neonates. 10-15 mg/kg/dose q6-8hr
as needed.
RECTAL
Adults. 650 mg q4-6hr. Maximum:
6 doses/24 hr.
Children. 10-20 mg/kg/dose q4-6hr
as needed.
Neonates. 10-15 mg/kg/dose q6-8hr
as needed.
▸ **Dosage in renal impairment**

Creatinine Clearance	Frequency
10-50 ml/min	q6hr
Less than 10 ml/min	q8hr

CONTRAINDICATIONS
Active alcoholism, liver disease, or
viral hepatitis, all of which increase
the risk of hepatotoxicity

INTERACTIONS
Drug
**Alcohol (chronic use), hepatotoxic
medications (e.g., phenytoin), liver
enzyme inducers (e.g., cimetidine):**
May increase risk of hepatotoxicity
with prolonged high dose or single
toxic dose.
Warfarin: May increase the risk of
bleeding with regular use.
Herbal
None known.
Food
None known.

DIAGNOSTIC TEST EFFECTS
May increase serum bilirubin,
prothrombin time (may indicate

hepatotoxicity), SGOT (AST), and
SGPT (ALT). Therapeutic serum
level: 10-30 mcg/ml; toxic serum
level: greater than 200 mcg/ml.

SIDE EFFECTS
Rare
Hypersensitivity reaction

SERIOUS REACTIONS
• Acetaminophen toxicity is the
primary serious reaction.
• Early signs and symptoms of
acetaminophen toxicity include
anorexia, nausea, diaphoresis, and
generalized weakness within the first
12 to 24 hr.
• Later signs of acetaminophen
toxicity include vomiting, right
upper quadrant tenderness, and
elevated liver function tests within
48 to 72 hr after ingestion.
• The antidote to acetaminophen
toxicity is acetylcysteine.

PRECAUTIONS & CONSIDERATIONS
Caution is warranted with G6PD
deficiency, phenylketonuria,
sensitivity to acetaminophen and
severe impaired renal function.
Acetaminophen crosses the placenta
and is distributed in breast milk.
Acetaminophen is routinely used in
all stages of pregnancy and appears
safe for short term use. There are no
age-related precautions noted in
children or the elderly. Be aware
children may receive repeat doses
4 to 5 times a day to a maximum of
5 doses in 24 hours. Withhold the
drug and contact the physician if
respirations are 12 per minute or
lower (20 per minute or lower in
children).
    Consult with the physician before
using acetaminophen in children
under 2 years of age; oral use for
more than 5 days in children, more

than 10 days in adults, or fever lasting more than 3 days. Severe or recurrent pain or high, continuous fever, which may indicate a serious illness, should be monitored. Be aware the therapeutic serum level is 10 to 30 mcg/ml and a toxic serum level is greater than 200 mcg/ml.

Administration

Take oral acetaminophen without regard to meals. Tablets may be crushed.

For rectal use, moisten suppository with cold water before inserting well up into the rectum.

A

Acetazolamide

ah-seat-ah-zole-ah-myd
(Apo-Acetazolamide [CAN], Dazamide, Diamox, Diamox Sequels)
Do not confuse with acetohexamide.

CATEGORY AND SCHEDULE

Pregnancy Risk Category: C

CLASSIFICATION

Carbonic anhydrase inhibitors

MECHANISM OF ACTION

A carbonic anhydrase inhibitor that reduces formation of hydrogen and bicarbonate ions from carbon dioxide and water by inhibiting, in proximal renal tubule, the enzyme carbonic anhydrase, thereby promoting renal excretion of sodium, potassium, bicarbonate, water. Ocular: Reduces rate of aqueous humor formation, lowers intraocular pressure. *Therapeutic Effect:* Produces anticonvulsant activity.

PHARMACOKINETICS

Rapidly absorbed. Protein binding: 95%. Widely distributed throughout body tissues including erythrocytes, kidneys, and blood brain barrier. Not metabolized. Excreted unchanged in urine. Removed by hemodialysis.
Half-life: 2.4-5.8 hr.

AVAILABILITY

Capsules, sustained release: 500 mg (Diamox Sequels).
Powder for reconstitution: 500 mg.
Tablets: 125 mg, 250 mg (Diamox).

INDICATIONS AND DOSAGES
▸ **Glaucoma**
PO
Adults. 250 mg 1-4 times/day.
Extended-Release: 500 mg
1-2 times/day usually given in morning and evening.
▸ **Secondary glaucoma, preop treatment of acute congestive glaucoma**
PO/IV
Adults. 250 mg q4hr, 250 mg q12hr; or 500 mg, then 125-250 mg q4hr.
PO
Children. 10-15 mg/kg/day in divided doses.
IV
Children. 5-10 mg/kg q6hr.
▸ **Edema**
IV
Adults. 25-375 mg once daily.
Children. 5 mg/kg or 150 mg/m^2 once daily.
▸ **Epilepsy**
ORAL
Adults, Children. 375-1000 mg/day in 1-4 divided doses.
▸ **Acute mountain sickness**
PO
Adults. 500-1000 mg/day in divided doses. If possible, begin 24-48 hr before ascent; continue at least 48 hr at high altitude.
Usual elderly dosage
PO
Initially, 250 mg 2 times/day; use lowest effective dose.
Dosage in renal impairment

Creatinine Clearance	Dosage Interval
10-50 ml/min	q12hr
Less than 10 ml/min	Avoid use

OFF-LABEL USES
Urine alkalinization, respiratory stimulant in COPD

CONTRAINDICATIONS
Severe renal disease, adrenal insufficiency, hypochloremic acidosis, hypersensitivity to acetazolamide, to any component of the formulation, or to sulfonamides.

INTERACTIONS
Drug
Amphetamines: May increase effects and toxicity of amphetamines.
Cyclosporine: May increase cyclosporine trough concentrations and possible neprotoxicity and neurotoxicity.
Digoxin: May increase the risk of digoxin toxicity caused by hypokalemia.
Lithium: May increase lithium excretion and decrease serum levels.
Methenamine: May decrease effects of methenamine.
Phenytoin: May increase serum concentrations of phenytoin.
Primidone: May decrease serum concentrations of primidone.
Quinidine: May decrease urinary excretion of quinidine and increase effects.
Salicylates: May increase risk of acetazolamide accumulation and toxicity including CNS depression and metabolic acidosis.
Herbal
None known.
Food
None known.

DIAGNOSTIC TEST EFFECTS
May increase ammonia, bilirubin, glucose, chloride, uric acid, calcium. May decrease bicarbonate, potassium.

▓ IV INCOMPATIBILITIES
No drug incompatibilities reported.

IV compatibilities
Cimetidine (Tagament), procaine,
ranitidine (Zantac)

SIDE EFFECTS
Frequent
Unusually tired/weak, diarrhea,
increased urination/frequency,
decreased appetite/weight, altered
taste (metallic), nausea, vomiting,
numbness in extremities, lips, mouth
Occasional
Depression, drowsiness
Rare
Headache, photosensitivity, confusion, tinnitus, severe muscle weakness, loss of taste

SERIOUS REACTIONS
• Long-term therapy may result in
acidotic state.
• Nephrotoxicity/hepatotoxicity
occurs occasionally, manifested as
dark urine/stools, pain in lower back,
jaundice, dysuria, crystalluria, renal
colic/calculi.
• Bone marrow depression may be
manifested as aplastic anemia,
thrombocytopenia, thrombocytopenic purpura, leukopenia, agranulocytosis, hemolytic anemia.

PRECAUTIONS & CONSIDERATIONS
Caution is warranted with a history
of hypercalcemia, diabetes mellitus,
gout, digitalized patients, obstructive
pulmonary disease, debilitated, and
the elderly. It is unknown if acetazolamide crosses the placenta or is
distributed in the breast milk. Safety
and efficacy has not be established
in children.
    Acetazolamide may cause drowsi-
ness. Avoid alcohol and performing
tasks that require mental alertness or
motor skills.
Storage
Reconstituted solution for injection
may be stored up to 12 hours at room
temperature and for 3 days
under refrigeration. Stability of
IVPB solution is 5 days at room
temperature and 44 days under
refrigeration.
Administration
IM administration is not
recommended because of pain
secondary to the alkaline pH.
    Standard diluent is 500 mg/50 ml
D_5W. Minimum volume is 50 ml
D_5W. Reconstitute with at least 5 ml
of sterile water to provide a solution
containing not more than 100 mg/ml.
Further dilute in 50 ml of either
D_5W or 0.9% NaCl for IV
infusion administration.
Recommended rate of administration
is 100-500 mg/minute for IV push
and 4 8 hr for IV infusions.
Maximum concentration is
100 mg/ml. Maximum rate of IV
infusion is 500 mg/ml.
    Give oral acetazolamide with
regard to food. Do not crush,
chew, or swallow contents of
long-acting capsule. Capsules
may be opened and sprinkled
on soft food.

Acetic Acid
a-cee'tik as'id
(Acetasol; Acidic Vaginal Jelly;
Acid Jelly; Aci-Jel; Borofair;
Fem pH; Relagard; Vasotate;
Vosol; Aquaear [AUS])
**Do not confuse with salicylic
acid.**

CLASSIFICATION
Anti-infectives, otics

MECHANISM OF ACTION
The mechanism by which acetic acid exerts its antibacterial and antifungal actions is unknown.
Therapeutic effect: Antibacterial and antifungal.

PHARMACOKINETICS
Unknown.

AVAILABILITY
Solution (irrigation): 0.25%
Solution (otic): 2%
Gel (vaginal): 0.92%
Solution (compounding): 36%

INDICATIONS AND DOSAGES
▶ **Superficial infections of the external auditory canal**
TOPICAL
Adults, Elderly, Children. Carefully remove all cerumen and debris to allow acetic acid to contact infected surfaces directly. To promote continuous contact, insert a wick saturated with acetic acid into the ear canal; the wick may also be saturated after insertion. Instruct the patient to keep the wick in for at least 24 hours and to keep it moist by adding 3-5 drops of acetic acid every 4-6 hours. The wick may be removed after 24 hours but the patient should continue to instill 5 drops of acetic acid 3 or 4 times daily thereafter, for as long as indicated. Dosing should be tapered gradually after apparent response to avoid relapse.

CONTRAINDICATIONS
Hypersensitivity to acetic acid or any of the ingredients. Perforated tympanic membrane is frequently considered a contraindication to the use of any medication in the external ear canal.

INTERACTIONS
Drug
None known.
Herbal
None known.
Food
None known.

DIAGNOSTIC TEST EFFECTS
None known.

SIDE EFFECTS
Occasional
Stinging or burning
Rare
Local irritation, superinfection

SERIOUS REACTIONS
• Super infection with prolonged use
❗ Discontinue promptly if sensitization or irritation occurs.

PRECAUTIONS & CONSIDERATIONS
It is unknown if acetic acid crosses the placenta or is distributed into breast milk. There are no age-related precautions noted in children or the elderly. Discontinue otic solution if sensitization or irritation occurs.

Transient burning or stinging may be noted when otic solution is first instilled into acutely inflamed ear.
Administration
Insert saturated wick of cotton into the ear canal and leave for at least 24 hours, keeping moist by adding 3-5 drops every 4-6 hours. For maintenance, instill drops as long as indicated.

To restore and maintain vaginal acidity, use 1 applicatorful intravaginally in morning and evening and determine duration of treatment based on the individual's response.

Acetylcysteine
a-see-til-sis'tay-een
(Acetadote, Mucomyst, Parvolex
[CAN])
**Do not confuse acetylcysteine
with acetylcholine.**

CATEGORY AND SCHEDULE
Pregnancy Risk Category: B

CLASSIFICATION
Antidotes, mucolytics

MECHANISM OF ACTION
An intratracheal respiratory
inhalant that splits the linkage
of mucoproteins, reducing the
viscosity of pulmonary secretions.
Therapeutic Effect: Facilitates the
removal of pulmonary secretions
by coughing, postural drainage,
mechanical means. Protects against
acetaminophen overdose-induced
hepatotoxicity.

AVAILABILITY
Injection (Acedote): 20%
(200 mg/ml).
Inhalation Solution (Mucomyst): 10%
(100 mg/ml), 20% (200 mg/ml).

INDICATIONS AND DOSAGES
▸ **Adjunctive treatment of
viscid mucus secretions
from chronic bronchopulmonary
disease and for pulmonary
complications of cystic
fibrosis**
NEBULIZATION
Adults, Elderly, Children. 3-5 ml
(20% solution) 3-4 times a day or
6-10 ml (10% solution) 3-4 times a
day. Range: 1-10 ml (20% solution)
q2-6hr or 2-20 ml (10% solution)
q2-6hr.

Infants. 1-2 ml (20%) or 2-4 ml
(10%) 3-4 times a day.
▸ **Treatment of viscid mucus secretions in patients with a tracheostomy**
INTRATRACHEAL
Adults, Children. 1-2 ml of 10% or
20% solution instilled into
tracheostomy q1-4hr.
▸ **Acetaminophen overdose**
PO (ORAL SOLUTION 5%)
Adults, Elderly, Children.
Loading dose of 140 mg/kg,
followed in 4 hr by maintenance
dose of 70 mg/kg q4hr for 17 additional doses (unless acetaminophen
assay reveals nontoxic level).
IV
Adults, Elderly, Children. 150 mg/kg
infused over 15 minutes, then
50 mg/kg infused over 4 hr, then
100 mg/kg infused over 16 hr. See
administration and handling. Repeat
dose if emesis occurs within 1 hr of
administration. Continue until all
doses are given, even if acetaminophen plasma level drops below
toxic range.
▸ **Prevention of renal damage
from dyes used during certain
diagnostic tests**
PO (ORAL SOLUTION 5%)
Adults, Elderly. 600 mg twice a day
for 4 doses starting the day before
the procedure.

OFF-LABEL USES
Prevention of renal damage from
dyes given during certain diagnostic
tests (such as CT scans)

CONTRAINDICATIONS
None known.

INTERACTIONS
Drug
None known.
Herbal
None known.

Food
None known.

DIAGNOSTIC TEST EFFECTS
None known.

SIDE EFFECTS
Frequent
Inhalation: Stickiness on face, transient unpleasant odor
Occasional
Inhalation: Increased bronchial secretions, throat irritation, nausea, vomiting, rhinorrhea
Rare
Inhalation: Rash
Oral: Facial edema, bronchospasm, wheezing

SERIOUS REACTIONS
- Large doses may produce severe nausea and vomiting.

PRECAUTIONS & CONSIDERATIONS
Caution is warranted with bronchial asthma and in the elderly or debilitated with severe respiratory insufficiency. Maintain adequate hydration. Be aware a disagreeable color may emanate from the solution during initial administration but it disappears quickly.

If bronchospasm occurs, discontinue treatment, notify the physician, and a bronchodilator may be needed. Respiratory rate, depth, rhythm, and type (such as abdominal or thoracic) and color, consistency, and amount of sputum should be assessed.

Administration
To create the oral solution, dilute 20% solution with water or soft drinks to create a 5% concentration. Use within 1 hour. When administering the solution by nebulizer, avoid using equipment that contains copper, iron, or rubber because the drug will react with these materials on contact.

For IV use, give 3 infusions of different strengths: first dose (150 mg/kg) in 200 ml D_5W and infused over 15 minutes, second dose (50 mg/kg) in 500 ml D_5W and infused over 4 hours, third dose (100 mg/kg) in 1000 ml D_5W and infused over 16 hours.

For inhalation, may administer either undiluted or diluted with 0.9% NaCl.

Acitretin
a-si-tre'tin
(Soriatane)

CATEGORY AND SCHEDULE
Pregnancy Risk Category: X

CLASSIFICATION
Antipsoriatics, dermatologics, retinoids

MECHANISM OF ACTION
A second-generation retinoid that adjusts factors influencing epidermal proliferation, RNA/DNA synthesis, controls glycoprotein, and governs immune response. *Therapeutic Effect:* Regulates keratinocyte growth and differentiation.

PHARMACOKINETICS
Well absorbed from the gastro-intestinal (GI) tract. Food increases rate of absorption. Protein binding: greater than 99%. Metabolized in liver. Excreted in bile and urine. Not removed by hemodialysis.
Half-life: 49 hrs.

AVAILABILITY
Capsules: 10 mg, 25 mg (Soriatane).

INDICATIONS AND DOSAGES
▸ **Psoriasis**
PO
Adults, Elderly. 25-50 mg/day as a single dose with main meal. May increase to 75 mg/day if necessary and dose tolerated. Maintenance: 25-50 mg/day after the initial response is noted. Continue until lesions have resolved.

OFF-LABEL USES
Treatment of Darier's disease, palmoplantar pustulosis, lichen planus; children with lameliar ichthyosis, nonbullous and bullous ichthyosiform erythroderma, Sjogren-Larsson syndrome

CONTRAINDICATIONS
Pregnancy or those who intend to become pregnant within 3 years following discontinuation of therapy, severely impaired liver or kidney function, chronic abnormal elevated lipid levels, concomitant use of methotrexate or tetracyclines, ingestion of alcohol (in females of reproductive potential), hypersensitivity to acitretin, etretinate or other retinoids, sensitivity to parabens (used as preservative in gelatin capsule)

INTERACTIONS
Drug
Alcohol: May prevent elimination of acitretin.
'Minipill' oral contraceptive: May interfere with contraceptive effect.
Methotrexate: May increase risk of hepatotoxicity.
Tetracyclines: May increase risk of increased intracranial pressure.
Herbal
St. John's Wort: May increase risk of unplanned pregnancy and birth defects.
Vitamin A: May increase risk of vitamin A toxicity.

Food
None known.

DIAGNOSTIC TEST EFFECTS
May increase triglycerides, SGOT (AST), SGPT (ALT). May decrease HDL (high density lipoprotein).

SIDE EFFECTS
Frequent
Lip inflammation, alopecia, skin peeling, shakiness, dry eyes, rash, hyperesthesia, paresthesia, sticky skin, dry mouth, epistaxis, dryness/thickening of conjunctiva
Occasional
Eye irritation, brow and lash loss, sweating, chills, sensation of cold, flushing, edema, blurred vision, diarrhea, nausea, thirst

SERIOUS REACTIONS
* Benign intracranial hypertension (pseudotumor cerebri) occurs rarely.

PRECAUTIONS & CONSIDERATIONS
Caution is warranted with impaired hepatic/renal function, those with elevated cholesterol/triglycerides. Triglycerides should be monitored at 1-2 week intervals until response to drug is established. Safety and efficacy have not been established in children. Be aware that acitretin should be avoided in the elderly with renal impairment. Decreased tolerance to contact lenses may develop. Follow a cholesterol-free diet for best results.

Be aware that acitretin is contraindicated in pregnant women. Women should not take acitretin if pregnant or planning to become pregnant within the next 3 years. Two pregnancy tests with negative results must be obtained before starting treatment. Two forms of birth control must be used for 1 month before beginning with acitretin,

during treatment, and 3 years after treatment. Acitretin has teratogenic effects. An agreement/informed consent must be signed before treatment begins.
Storage
Store at room temperature.
Administration
Give with main meal of the day or milk.

Acyclovir
ay-sye′kloe-ver
(Aciclovir-BC IV [AUS], Acihexal [AUS], Acyclo-V [AUS], Avirax [CAN], Lovir [AUS], Zovirax, Zyclir [AUS])
Do not confuse with Zostrix, Zyvox.

CATEGORY AND SCHEDULE
Pregnancy Risk Category: B

CLASSIFICATION
Antivirals

MECHANISM OF ACTION
A synthetic nucleoside that converts to acyclovir triphosphate, becoming part of the DNA chain. *Therapeutic Effect:* Interferes with DNA synthesis and viral replication. Virustatic.

PHARMACOKINETICS
Poorly absorbed from the GI tract; minimal absorption following topical application. Protein binding: 9%-36%. Widely distributed. Partially metabolized in liver. Excreted primarily in urine. Removed by hemodialysis.
Half-life: 2.5 hr (increased in impaired renal function).

AVAILABILITY
Capsules: 200 mg.
Tablets: 400 mg, 800 mg.
Injection, solution: 50 mg/ml.
Oral Suspension: 200 mg/5 ml.
Powder for Injection: 500 mg, 1000 mg.
Ointment: 5%/50 mg.

INDICATIONS AND DOSAGES
▸ **Genital herpes (initial episode)**
IV
Adults, Elderly, Children 12 yr and older. 5 mg/kg q8hr for 5 days.
PO
Adults, Elderly, Children 12 yr and older. 200 mg q4hr 5 times a day.
▸ **Genital herpes (recurrent)**
Less than 6 episodes per year:
PO
Adults, Elderly, Children 12 yr and older. 200 mg q4hr 5 times a day for 5 days.
6 episodes or more per year:
PO
Adults, Elderly, Children 12 yr and older. 400 mg 2 times a day or 200 mg 3-5 times a day for up to 12 months.
▸ **Herpes simplex mucocutaneous**
IV
Adults, Elderly, Children 12 yr and older. 5 mg/kg/dose q8hr for 7 days.
Children younger than 12 yr. 10 mg/kg q8hr for 7 days.
▸ **Herpes simplex neonatal**
IV
Children younger than 4 mo. 10 mg/kg q8hr for 10 days.
▸ **Herpes simplex encephalitis**
IV
Adults, Elderly, Children 12 yr and older. 10 mg/kg q8hr for 10 days.
Children 3 mo - younger than 12 yr. 20 mg/kg q8hr for 10 days.
▸ **Herpes zoster (caused by varicella)**
IV
Adults, Elderly, Children 12 yr and older. 10 mg/kg q8hr for 7 days.

Children younger than 12 yr.
20 mg/kg q8hr for 7 days.
▶ **Herpes zoster (shingles)**
PO
*Adults, Elderly, Children 12 yr and
older.* 800 mg q4hr 5 times a day for
7-10 days.
TOPICAL
Adults, Elderly. Apply to affected
area 3-6 times a day for 7 days.
▶ **Varicella (chickenpox)**
PO
*Adults, Elderly, Children older than
12 yr or children 2-12 yr, weighing
40 kg or more.* 800 mg 4 times a
day for 5 days.
*Children 2-12 yr, weighing less than
40 kg.* 20 mg/kg 4 times a day for
5 days. Maximum: 800 mg/dose.
Children younger than 2 yr.
80 mg/kg/day.
▶ **Dosage in renal impairment**
Dosage and frequency are modified
based on severity of infection and
degree of renal impairment.
PO
For creatinine clearance of
10 ml/min or less, dosage is 200 mg
q12hr.
IV

Creatinine Clearance	Dosage Percent	Dosage Interval
Greater than 50 ml/min	100	8 hr
25-50 ml/min	100	12 hr
10-25 ml/min	100	24 hr
Less than 10 ml/min	50	24 hr

OFF-LABEL USES
Treatment of herpes simplex ocular
infections, infectious mononucleosis

CONTRAINDICATIONS
Use in neonates when acyclovir is
reconstituted with bacteriostatic
water containing benzyl alcohol.

INTERACTIONS
Drug
**Nephrotoxic medications (such as
aminoglycosides):** May increase the
nephrotoxicity of acyclovir.
Probenecid: May increase acyclovir
half-life.
Herbal
None known.
Food
None known.

DIAGNOSTIC TEST EFFECTS
May increase BUN and serum creatinine concentrations.

🖾 IV INCOMPATIBILITIES
Aztreonam (Azactam), cefepime
(Maxipime), diltiazem (Cardizem),
dobutamine (Dobutrex), dopamine
(Intropin), levofloxacin
(Levaquin), meropenem (Merrem
IV), ondansetron (Zofran),
piperacillin and tazobactam
(Zosyn)
🖾 IV compatibilities
Allopurinol (Alloprim), amikacin
(Amikin), ampicillin, cefazolin
(Ancef), cefotaxime (Claforan),
ceftazidime (Fortaz), ceftriaxone
(Rocephin), cimetidine (Tagamet),
clindamycin (Cleocin), famotidine
(Pepcid), fluconazole (Diflucan),
gentamicin, heparin, hydromorphone
(Dilaudid), imipenem (Primaxin),
lorazepam (Ativan), magnesium
sulfate, methylprednisolone
(SoluMedrol), metoclopramide
(Reglan), metronidazole (Flagyl),
morphine, multivitamins, potassium
chloride, propofol (Diprivan), ranitidine (Zantac), vancomycin

SIDE EFFECTS
Frequent
Parenteral (9%-7%): Phlebitis or
inflammation at IV site, nausea,
vomiting
Topical (28%): Burning, stinging

Occasional

Parenteral (3%): Pruritus, rash, urticaria

Oral (12%-6%): Malaise, nausea

Topical (4%): Pruritus

Rare

Oral (3%-1%): Vomiting, rash, diarrhea, headache

Parenteral (2%-1%): Confusion, hallucinations, seizures, tremors

Topical (less than 1%): Rash

SERIOUS REACTIONS

• Rapid parenteral administration, excessively high doses, or fluid and electrolyte imbalance may produce renal failure exhibited by such signs and symptoms as abdominal pain, decreased urination, decreased appetite, increased thirst, nausea, and vomiting.

• Toxicity has not been reported with oral or topical use.

PRECAUTIONS & CONSIDERATIONS

Caution is warranted with concurrent use of nephrotoxic agents, dehydration, fluid and electrolyte imbalance, neurologic abnormalities or renal or hepatic impairment. Acyclovir crosses the placenta and is distributed in breast milk. Be aware that safety and efficacy have not been established in children less than 2 years of age or less than 1 year of age for IV use. In the elderly, age-related renal impairment may require dosage adjustment. Analgesics and comfort measures should be provided, especially to the elderly. Females should have a pap smear at least annually because of the increased risk of cervix cancer in women with genital herpes. Avoid touching lesions with fingers to prevent spreading infection to new sites.

History of allergies, particularly to acyclovir should be obtained before treatment. Herpes simplex lesions should be assessed before treatment to compare baseline with treatment effect. IV site should be assessed for signs and symptoms of phlebitis, including heat, pain, or red streaking over the vein. Cutaneous lesions should be evaluated for signs of effective drug treatment. Adequate ventilation as well as hydration should be maintained. Appropriate isolation precautions should be maintained in persons with chickenpox and disseminated herpes zoster.

Storage

Store capsules at room temperature. Store vials at room temperature. Solutions of 50 mg/ml will remain stable for 12 hours at room temperature; may form precipitate when refrigerated. Potency not affected by precipitate and redissolution. IV infusion (piggyback) is stable for 24 hours at room temperature. Yellow discoloration does not affect potency.

Administration

Take without regard to food. Do not crush or break capsules.

Use finger cot or rubber glove to prevent autoinoculation to apply topical acyclovir. Avoid eye contact.

Add 10 ml sterile water for injection to each 500-mg vial (50 mg/ml). Do not use bacteriostatic water for injection containing benzyl alcohol or parabens because this will cause a precipitate to form. Shake well until solution is clear. Further dilute with at least 100 ml D_5W or 0.9% NaCl. Final concentration should be less than or equal to 7 mg/ml.

Infuse over at least 1 hour because renal tubular damage may occur with too rapid administration. Maintain adequate hydration during infusion and for 2 hours following IV administration.

Adalimumab
(Humira)

CATEGORY AND SCHEDULE
Pregnancy Risk Category: B

CLASSIFICATION
Disease modifying antirheumatic drugs, immunomodulators, monoclonal antibodies, tumor necrosis factor modulators

MECHANISM OF ACTION
A monoclonal antibody that binds specifically to tumor necrosis factor (TNF) alpha, blocking its interaction with cell surface TNF receptors. *Therapeutic Effect:* Reduces inflammation, tenderness, and swelling of joints; slows or prevents progressive destruction of joints in rheumatoid arthritis.

PHARMACOKINETICS
Half-life: 10-20 days.

AVAILABILITY
Injection: 40 mg/0.8 ml in prefilled syringes.

INDICATIONS AND DOSAGES
▶ **Rheumatoid arthritis**
SUBCUTANEOUS
Adults, Elderly. 40 mg every other week. Dose may be increased to 40 mg/wk in those not taking methotrexate.

CONTRAINDICATIONS
Active infections

INTERACTIONS
Drug
Methotrexate: Reduces the absorption of adalimumab by 29%-40%, but dosage adjustment is unnecessary if given concurrently.
Herbal
None known.
Food
None known.

DIAGNOSTIC TEST EFFECTS
May increase levels of blood cholesterol, other lipids, and serum alkaline phosphatase

SIDE EFFECTS
Frequent (20%)
Injection site, erythema, pruritus, pain, and swelling
Occasional (12%-9%)
Headache, rash, sinusitis, nausea
Rare (7%-5%)
Abdominal or back pain, hypertension

SERIOUS REACTIONS
• Rare reactions include hypersensitivity reactions, malignancies, respiratory tract infections, bronchitis, UTIs, and more serious infections (such as pneumonia, tuberculosis, cellulitus, pyelonephritis, and septic arthritis).

PRECAUTIONS & CONSIDERATIONS
Caution is warranted with cardiovascular disease, demyelinating disorders, history of sensitivity to monoclonal antibodies, pre-existing or recent onset of CNS disturbances, in the elderly, and pregnant women. It is unknown if adalimumab is excreted in breast milk. The safety and efficacy of adalimumab have not been established in children.

Cautious use in the elderly is necessary because they're at increased risk for serious infection and malignancy. Avoid receiving live-vaccines during adalimumab treatment.

Laboratory values, particularly serum alkaline phosphatase levels, should be monitored before and during therapy. Therapeutic response, such as improved grip strength, increased joint mobility, reduced joint tenderness, and relief of pain, stiffness, and swelling, should also be assessed.

Storage
Refrigerate adalimumab. Do not freeze it.

Administration
For subcutaneous use, rotate injection sites. Administer each injection at least 1 inch from previous site. Never inject drug into bruised, hard, red, or tender areas. Discard any unused portion. Injection site reactions generally occur in the first month of treatment and decrease with continued therapy.

Adapalene
a-dap′a-leen
(Differin)

CATEGORY AND SCHEDULE
Pregnancy Risk category: C

CLASSIFICATION
Dermatologics, retinoids

MECHANISM OF ACTION
Binds to retinoic acid receptors in cell nuclei modulating cell differentiation, keratinization. Possesses anti-inflammatory properties.
Therapeutic effect: Normalizes differentiation of follicular epithelial cells.

PHARMACOKINETICS
Absorption through the skin is low. Trace amount found in plasma following topical application. Excreted primarily by biliary route.

AVAILABILITY
Gel: 0.1%
Cream: 0.1%
Pledget (solution): 0.1%

INDICATIONS AND DOSAGES
▸ **Acne vulgaris**
TOPICAL
*Adults, elderly, children
>12 years.* Apply to affected area once daily at bedtime after washing.

CONTRAINDICATIONS
Hypersensitivity to adapalene, vitamin A or any one of its components.

INTERACTIONS
Drug
Quinolones (particularly sparfloxacin), phenothiazines, sulfonamides, sulfonylureas, tetra-cyclines, thiazide diuretics: Adapalene may increase the effects of these photosensitizing agents.
Benzoyl peroxide, salicylic acid, sulfur, resorcinol, alcohol: Additive local irritation when used with adapalene.
Herbal
None known.
Food
None known.

DIAGNOSTIC TEST EFFECTS
None known.

SIDE EFFECTS
Frequent
Erythema, scaling, dryness, pruritis, burning (likely to occur first 2-4 weeks, lessens with continued use)
Occasional
Skin irritation, stinging, sunburn, acne flares, erythema, photosensitivity, pruritis, xerosis

SERIOUS REACTIONS
• Concurrent use of other potential irritating topical products (soaps, cleansers, aftershave, cosmetics) may produce severe topical irritation.

PRECAUTIONS & CONSIDERATIONS
Caution is warranted with eczema and seborrheic dermatitis.
Adapalene has not been studied in pregnant women. It is unknown if adapalene enters the breast milk. Safety and efficacy has not been established in children younger than 12 years or the elderly.

A burning sensation, stinging, dryness, itching, or redness of the skin may occur especially during the first month of use. Other skin products such as hair removal products, shaving creams with a large amount of alcohol, other acne medications, as well as certain soaps and cleansers may irritate the skin while using adapalene.
Storage
Store at room temperature.
Administration
Apply a small amount as a thin film once a day, at least one hour before bedtime. Apply the medicine to dry, clean areas affected by acne. Rub in gently and well.

A

Adefovir
ah-deh'foh-veer
(Hepsera)

CATEGORY AND SCHEDULE
Pregnancy Risk Category: C

CLASSIFICATION
Antivirals

MECHANISM OF ACTION
An antiviral that inhibits the enzyme DNA polymerase, causing DNA chain termination after its incorporation into viral DNA. *Therapeutic Effect:* Prevents cell replication of viral DNA.

PHARMACOKINETICS
Binds to proteins after PO administration. Excreted in urine. **Half-life:** 7 hr (increased in impaired renal function).

AVAILABILITY
Tablets: 10 mg.

INDICATIONS AND DOSAGES
▸ **Chronic hepatitis B in patients with normal renal function**
PO
Adults, Elderly. 10 mg once a day.
▸ **Chronic hepatitis B in patients with impaired renal function**
Adults, Elderly with creatinine clearance 20-49 ml/min. 10 mg q48hr.
Adults, Elderly with creatinine clearance 10-19 ml/min. 10 mg q72hr.
Adults, Elderly on hemodialysis. 10 mg every 7 days following dialysis.

CONTRAINDICATIONS
None known.

INTERACTIONS
Drug
Ibuprofen: Increases adefovir plasma concentration.
Herbal
None known.
Food
None known.

DIAGNOSTIC TEST EFFECTS
May increase serum amylase, creatinine, AST (SGOT) and ALT (SGPT) levels.

SIDE EFFECTS
Frequent (13%)
Asthenia
Occasional (9%-4%)
Headache, abdominal pain, nausea, flatulence
Rare (3%)
Diarrhea, dyspepsia

SERIOUS REACTIONS
• Nephrotoxicity (characterized by increased serum creatinine and decreased serum phosphorus levels) is a treatment-limiting toxicity of adefovir therapy.
• Lactic acidosis and severe hepatomegaly occur rarely, particularly in female patients.

PRECAUTIONS & CONSIDERATIONS
Caution is warranted with impaired renal function and known risk factors for liver disease and in the elderly. Baseline renal function laboratory values should be obtained before therapy begins and routinely thereafter. Adjust adefovir dosage with pre-existing renal insufficiency. Blood specimen should be obtained for HIV antibody testing before therapy begins because unrecognized or untreated HIV infection may result in an emergence of HIV resistance.
! Notify the physician immediately if unusual muscle pain, stomach pain with nausea and vomiting, cold feeling in arms and legs, or dizziness occurs. These signs and symptoms may signal the onset of lactic acidosis. Continue to take adefovir as prescribed because there is a risk for developing a worse or very serious hepatitis if the drug is stopped. Notify physician if yellow skin color or yellowing of the whites of the eyes or other unusual signs or symptoms occur. Reliable forms of contraception should be used.
Administration
Give adefovir without regard to food.

Adenosine
ah-den'oh-seen
(Adenocard, Adenocor [AUS], Adenoscan)

CATEGORY AND SCHEDULE
Pregnancy Risk Category: C

CLASSIFICATION
Antiarrhythmics, diagnostics, nonradioactive

MECHANISM OF ACTION
A cardiac agent that slows impulse formation in the SA node and conduction time through the AV node. Adenosine also acts as a diagnostic aid in myocardial perfusion imaging or stress echocardiography. *Therapeutic Effect:* Depresses left ventricular function and restores normal sinus rhythm.

AVAILABILITY
Injection (Adenocard): 3 mg/ml in 2-ml, 4-ml syringes.

than 0.9% NaCl, flush the line first before administering adenosine. Follow the rapid bolus injection with a rapid 0.9% NaCl flush.

Agalsidase Beta
a-gal′si-daze
(Fabrazyme)

CATEGORY AND SCHEDULE
Pregnancy Risk Category: B

CLASSIFICATION
Enzymes, metabolic

MECHANISM OF ACTION
An enzyme that treats Fabry disease, an X-linked genetic disorder by catalyzing the hydrolysis of glycosphingolipids, reducing their accumulation in the kidneys' capillary endothelium and other body tissues. *Therapeutic Effect:* Provides an exogenous source of alpha-galactosidase A, an enzyme, missing in those with Fabry disease.

AVAILABILITY
Powder for Injection: 37 mg (5 mg/ml when reconstituted).

INDICATIONS AND DOSAGES
▸ **Fabry disease**
IV
Adults, Elderly. 1 mg/kg q2wk. Give no more than 0.25 mg/min (15 mg/hr). May slow infusion rate if infusion-related reaction occurs. If no reaction occurs, infusion rate may be increased in increments of 0.05 to 0.08 mg/min (3 to 5 mg/hr).

CONTRAINDICATIONS
None known.

INTERACTIONS
Drug
None known.
Herbal
None known.
Food
None known.

DIAGNOSTIC TEST EFFECTS
None known.

▨ IV INCOMPATIBILITIES
Don't mix any other medications with agalsidase beta.

SIDE EFFECTS
Expected (52%-45%)
Infusion reactions (rigors, fever, headache)
Frequent (38%-21%)
Rhinitis, nausea, anxiety, pharyngitis, edema, skeletal pain
Occasional (17%-14%)
Temperature change sensation, hypotension, pallor, paresthesia, pruritus, urticaria, bronchitis
Rare (10%-7%)
Depression, arthralgia, dyspepsia, laryngitis, sinusitis

SERIOUS REACTIONS
• Serious infusion reactions, such as tachycardia, hypertension, throat tightness, chest pain, dyspnea, vomiting, lip edema, and rash occur frequently.
• Other serious reactions include bradycardia, arrhythmias, vertigo, nephrotic syndrome, CVA, and cardiac arrest.

PRECAUTIONS & CONSIDERATIONS
Caution is warranted with fever, compromised cardiac function, moderate to severe hypertension, and renal impairment.
Storage
Store vials in the refrigerator. Allow them to reach room temperature

Injection (Adenoscan): 3 mg/ml in 20-ml, 30-ml vials.

INDICATIONS AND DOSAGES
▸ **Paroxysmal supraventricular tachycardia (PSVT)**
RAPID IV BOLUS
Adults, Elderly. Initially, 6 mg given over 1-2 sec. If first dose does not convert within 1-2 min, give 12 mg; may repeat 12-mg dose in 1-2 min if no response has occurred.
Children. Initially 0.1 mg/kg (maximum: 6 mg). If ineffective, may give 0.2 mg/kg (maximum: 12 mg).
▸ **Diagnostic testing**
IV INFUSION
Adults. 140 mcg/kg/min for 6 min.

CONTRAINDICATIONS
Atrial fibrillation or flutter, second- or third-degree AV block or sick sinus syndrome (with functioning pacemaker), ventricular tachycardia

INTERACTIONS
Drug
Carbamazepine: May increase degree of heart block caused by adenosine.
Dipyridamole: May increase effect of adenosine.
Methylxanthines (e.g., caffeine, theophylline): May decrease effect of adenosine.
Herbal
None known.
Food
None known.

DIAGNOSTIC TEST EFFECTS
None known.

▨ IV INCOMPATIBILITIES
Any drug or solution other than 0.9% NaCl or D_5W.

SIDE EFFECTS
Frequent (18%-12%)
Facial flushing, dyspnea
Occasional (7%-2%)
Headache, nausea, light-headedness, chest pressure
Rare (less than or equal to 1%)
Numbness or tingling in arms; dizziness; diaphoresis; hypotension; palpitations; chest, jaw, or neck pain

SERIOUS REACTIONS
• May produce short-lasting heart block.

PRECAUTIONS & CONSIDERATIONS
Caution is warranted with arrhythmias at time of conversion, asthma, heart block, and hepatic and renal failure.
    Facial flushing, headache, and nausea may occur but these symptoms will resolve. Notify the physician if chest pain, pounding or palpitations or difficultly breathing or shortness of breath occurs. Before administering adenosine, the arrhythmia should be identified on a 12-lead EKG. Heart rate and rhythm on a continuous cardiac monitor and the apical pulse rate, rhythm, and quality should be assessed. B/P, respirations, intake and output, and electrolytes should also be monitored.
Storage
Solution may be stored at room temperature and normally appears clear. Crystallization occurs if solution is refrigerated. If crystallization occurs, dissolve crystals by warming to room temperature. Discard unused portion.
Administration
Administer undiluted very rapidly, over 1 to 2 seconds, directly into vein, or if using an IV line, use the port closest to the insertion site. If the IV line is infusing fluid other

before reconstitution, which takes about 30 minutes. The reconstituted and diluted solution should be used immediately; if this is not possible, the solution may be stored in the refrigerator for 24 hours.

Administration

Reconstitute each vial by slowly injecting 7.2 ml sterile water for injection. Roll and tilt gently. Before adding the reconstituted solution to 500 ml 0.9% NaCl, remove an equal volume from the 500-ml infusion bag, and then add it to the 500-ml 0.9% NaCl infusion bag. Administer at a rate of no more than 0.25 mg/minute (15 mg/hour). Expect to decrease the infusion rate if an infusion reaction occurs. If no reaction occurs, the infusion rate may be increased in increments of 0.05 to 0.08 mg/minute (3 to 5 mg/hour). Plan to decrease the infusion rate or temporarily stop the infusion if a reaction occurs. As prescribed, give additional antipyretics, antihistamines, or steroids to alleviate these symptoms. Patients with compromised cardiac function should be closely monitored because they're at increased risk for severe complications from infusion reactions.

Albendazole
all-ben'dah-zole
(Albenza)

CATEGORY AND SCHEDULE
Pregnancy Risk Category: C

CLASSIFICATION
Anthelmintic

MECHANISM OF ACTION

A benzimidazole carbamate anthelmintic that degrades parasite cytoplasmic microtubules, irreversibly blocks cholinesterase secretion, glucose uptake in helminth and larvae (depletes glycogen, decreases ATP production, depletes energy). Vermicidal.
Therapeutic Effect: Immobilizes and kills worms.

PHARMACOKINETICS

Poorly and variable absorbed gastrointestinal (GI) tract. Widely distributed, cyst fluid and including cerebrospinal fluid (CSF). Protein binding: 70%. Extensively metabolized in liver. Primarily excreted in urine and bile. Not removed by hemodialysis. **Half-life:** 8-12 hr.

AVAILABILITY

Tablets: 200 mg (Albenza).

INDICATIONS AND DOSAGES

▸ **Neurocysticercosis**
PO
Adults, Elderly more than 60 kg.
400 mg 2 times/day. Continue for 28 days, rest 14 days, repeat cycle 3 times.
Adults, Elderly less than 60 kg.
15 mg/kg/day. Continue for 28 days, rest 14 days, repeat cycle 3 times.

▸ **Cystic hydatid**
PO
Adults, Elderly more than 60 kg.
400 mg 2 times/day. Continue for 8-30 days.
Adults, Elderly less than 60 kg.
15 mg/kg/day. Continue for 8-30 days.

OFF-LABEL USES

Angiostrongyliasis, cysticercosis, gnathostomiasis, liver flukes, trichuriasis

CONTRAINDICATIONS
Hypersensitivity to albendazole or any component of the formulation, pregnancy

INTERACTIONS
Drug
Dexamethasone, praziquantel: May increase albendazole concentration.
Theophylline: May increase risk of theophylline toxicity.
Herbal
Ginseng: May decrease intestinal concentration of active drug.
Food
Grapefruit juice: May increase risk of albendazole adverse effects.

DIAGNOSTIC TEST EFFECTS
May decrease total white blood cell (WBC) count.

SIDE EFFECTS
Frequent
Neurocysticerosis: Nausea, vomiting, headache
Hydatid: Abnormal liver function tests, abdominal pain, nausea, vomiting
Occasional
Neurocysticerosis: Increased intracranial pressure, meningeal signs
Hydatid: Headache, dizziness, alopecia, fever

SERIOUS REACTIONS
• Pancytopenia occurs rarely.
• In presence of cysticercosis, drug may produce retinal damage in presence of retinal lesions.

PRECAUTIONS & CONSIDERATIONS
Caution is warranted with liver or renal impairment, hypersensitivity to other triazoles, such as itraconazole or terconazole, or hypersensitivity to imidazoles, such as butoconazole and ketoconazole. It is unknown if albendazole is excreted in breast milk. Safety and efficacy of albendazole have not been established in children. Therefore, expect to use the smallest dose necessary to achieve optimal results. There are no age-related precautions noted in the elderly. Fecal specimens should be obtained 3 weeks after treatment.

If fever, chills, sore throat, unusual bleeding or bruising, rash, or hives occurs, notify the physician.
Administration
Take albendazole with meals.

Albumin, Human
al-byew'min
(Albumex [AUS], Albuminar, Albutein, Buminate, Plasbumin)
Do not confuse with albuterol.

CATEGORY AND SCHEDULE
Pregnancy Risk Category: C

CLASSIFICATION
Plasma expanders

MECHANISM OF ACTION
A plasma protein fraction that acts as a blood volume expander. *Therapeutic Effect:* Provides temporary increase in blood volume; reduces hemoconcentration and blood viscosity.

PHARMACOKINETICS

Route	Onset	Peak	Duration
IV	15 min (in well-hydrated patient)	N/A	N/A

Distributed throughout extracellular fluid. **Half-life:** 15-20 days.

AVAILABILITY
Injection: 5%, 25%.

INDICATIONS AND DOSAGES
▶ **Hypovolemia**
IV
Adults, Elderly. Initially, 25 g; may repeat in 15-30 min. Maximum: 250 g within 48 hr.
Children. 0.5-1 g/kg/dose (10-20 ml/kg/dose of 5% albumin) Maximum: 6 g/kg/day.
▶ **Hypoproteinemia**
IV
Adults, Elderly, Children. 0.5-1 g/kg/dose (10-20 ml/kg/dose of 5% albumin). Repeat in 1-2 days.
▶ **Burns**
IV
Adults, Elderly, Children. Initially, give large volumes of crystalloid infusion to maintain plasma volume. After 24 hr, give 25 g, then adjust dosage to maintain plasma albumin concentration of 2-2.5 g/100 ml.
▶ **Cardiopulmonary bypass**
IV
Adults, Elderly. 5% or 25% albumine with crystalloid to maintain plasma albumin concentration of 2.5 g/100 ml.
▶ **Acute nephrosis, nephrotic syndrome**
IV
Adults, Elderly. 25 g of 25% injection, with diuretic once a day for 7-10 days.
▶ **Hemodialysis**
IV
Adults, Elderly. 100 ml (25 g) of 25% albumin.
▶ **Hyperbilirubinemia, Erythroblastosis fetalis**
IV

Infants. 1 g/kg 1-2 hr before transfusion.

CONTRAINDICATIONS
Heart failure, history of allergic reaction to albumin level, hypervolemia, normal serum albumin, pulmonary edema, severe anemia

INTERACTIONS
Drug
None known.
Herbal
None known.
Food
None known.

DIAGNOSTIC TEST EFFECTS
May increase serum alkaline phosphatase concentration.

▦ IV INCOMPATIBILITIES
Midazolam (Versed), vancomycin (Vancocin), verapamil (Isoptin)
▦ **IV compatibilities**
Diltiazem (Cardizem), lorazepam (Ativan)

SIDE EFFECTS
Occasional
Hypotension
Rare
High dose in repeated therapy: altered vital signs, chills, fever, increased salivation, nausea, vomiting, urticaria, tachycardia

SERIOUS REACTIONS
• Fluid overload may occur, marked by increased BP, and distended neck veins. Neurologic changes that may occur include headache, weakness, blurred vision, behavioral changes, incoordination, and isolated muscle twitching. Pulmonary edema may also occur, evidenced by rapid breathing, rales, wheezing, and coughing.

PRECAUTIONS & CONSIDERATIONS

Caution is warranted with hepatic or renal impairment, hypertension, normal serum albumin level, poor heart function, and pulmonary disease. It is unknown if albumin crosses the placenta or is distributed in breast milk. No age-related precautions have been noted in children or the elderly.

Notify the physician of difficulty breathing, itching, or rash. B/P for hypertension or hypotension, intake and output, and skin for flushing and urticaria should be monitored. Signs and symptoms of fluid overload and pulmonary edema should be assessed frequently.

Storage

Store at room temperature. Albumin normally appears as a clear, brownish, odorless, and moderately viscous fluid. Do not use if the solution has been frozen, appears turbid, or contains sediment, or if the vial has been open 4 hours or more.

Administration

! Dosage is based on the condition; duration of administration is based on the response. Make a 5% solution from 25% solution by adding 1 volume 25% solution to 4 volumes 0.9% NaCl (preferred) or D_5W. Do not use sterile water for injection because life threatening acute renal failure and hemolysis can occur. Give by IV infusion. Rate varies depending on therapeutic use, blood volume, and concentration of the solute. Give 5% solution at 5 to 10 ml/minute. Give 25% at a usual rate of 2 to 3 ml/minute. Administer 5% solution undiluted; administer 25% solution undiluted or diluted with 0.9% NaCl (preferred) or D_5W. May give without regard to patient's blood group or Rh factor.

Albuterol

al-byoo′ter-ole
(AccuNeb, Airomir [AUS], Asmol CFC-Free [AUS], Epaq Inhaler [AUS], Novosalmol [CAN], Proventil, Proventil Repetabs, Respax [AUS], Ventolin, Ventolin CFC-Free [AUS], Volmax, Vospire ER)
Do not confuse albuterol with Albutein or atenolol, or Proventil with Prinivil.

CATEGORY AND SCHEDULE

Pregnancy Risk Category: C

CLASSIFICATION

Adrenergic agonists, bronchodilators

MECHANISM OF ACTION

A sympathomimetic that stimulates beta₂-adrenergic receptors in the lungs, resulting in relaxation of bronchial smooth muscle. *Therapeutic Effect:* Relieves bronchospasm and reduces airway resistance.

PHARMACOKINETICS

Route	Onset	Peak	Duration
PO	15-30 min	2-3 hr	4-6 hr
PO (extended-release)	30 min	2-4 hr	12 hr
Inhalation	5-15 min	0.5-2 hr	2-5 hr

Rapidly, well absorbed from the GI tract; gradually absorbed from the bronchi after inhalation. Metabolized in the liver. Primarily excreted in urine.
Half-life: 2.7-5 hr (PO); 3.8 hr (inhalation).

AVAILABILITY
Syrup: 2 mg/5ml.
Tablet: 2 mg, 4 mg.
Tablet (Extended-Release [Proventil Repetabs]): 4 mg.
Tablets (Extended-Release [Volmax, VoSpire ER]): 4 mg, 8 mg.
Inhalation (Aerosol [Proventil, Ventolin]): 90 mcg/spray.
Inhalation (Solution [AccuNeb]): 0.75 mg/3 ml, 1.5 mg/3 ml.
Inhalation (Solution [Proventil]): 0.083%, 0.5%.

INDICATIONS AND DOSAGES
▸ **Bronchospasm**
PO
Adults, Children older than 12 yr. 2-4 mg 3-4 times a day. Maximum: 8 mg 4 times/day.
Elderly. 2 mg 3-4 times a day. Maximum: 8 mg 4 times a day.
Children 6-12 yr. 2 mg 3-4 times a day. Maximum: 24 mg/day.
PO (EXTENDED-RELEASE)
Adults, Children older than 12 yr. 4-8 mg q12hr.
INHALATION
Adults, Elderly, Children older than 12 yr. 1-2 puffs by metered dose inhaler q4-6hr as needed.
Children 4-12 yr. 1-2 puffs 4 times a day.
NEBULIZATION
Adults, Elderly, Children older than 12 yr. 2.5 mg 3-4 times a day.
Children 2-12 yr. 0.63-1.25 mg 3-4 times a day.
▸ **Exercise-induced bronchospasm**
INHALATION
Adults, Elderly, Children 4 yr and older. 2 puffs 15-30 min before exercise.

CONTRAINDICATIONS
History of hypersensitivity to sympathomimetics

INTERACTIONS
Drug
Beta blockers: Antagonize effects of albuterol.
Digoxin: May increase the risk of arrhythmias.
MAOIs, tricyclic antidepressants: May potentiate cardiovascular effects.
Herbal
None known.
Food
None known.

DIAGNOSTIC TEST EFFECTS
May increase blood glucose level. May decrease serum potassium level.

SIDE EFFECTS
Frequent
Headache (27%); nausea (15%); restlessness, nervousness, tremors (20%); dizziness (less than 7%); throat dryness and irritation, pharyngitis (less than 6%); BP changes, including hypertension (5%-3%); heartburn, transient wheezing (less than 5%)
Occasional (3%-2%)
Insomnia, asthenia, altered taste Inhalation: Dry, irritated mouth or throat; cough; bronchial irritation
Rare
Somnolence, diarrhea, dry mouth, flushing, diaphoresis, anorexia

SERIOUS REACTIONS
• Excessive sympathomimetic stimulation may produce palpitations, extrasystole, tachycardia, chest pain, a slight increase in BP followed by a substantial decrease, chills, diaphoresis, and blanching of skin.
• Too-frequent or excessive use may lead to decreased bronchodilating effectiveness and severe, paradoxical bronchoconstriction.

PRECAUTIONS & CONSIDERATIONS

Caution is warranted with cardiovascular disease, diabetes mellitus, hypertension, and hyperthyroidism. Albuterol appears to cross the placenta; it is unknown if albuterol is distributed in breast milk. Albuterol may inhibit uterine contractility. The safety and efficacy of this drug have not been established in children less than 2 years (syrup) or less than 6 years (tablets). The elderly may be more prone to tremors and tachycardia because of increased sensitivity to sympathomimetics. Drink plenty of fluids to decrease the thickness of lung secretions. Avoid excessive use of caffeinated products, such as chocolate, cocoa, cola, coffee, and tea.

Pulse rate and quality, 12-lead EKG, respiratory rate, depth, rhythm and type, ABG, and serum potassium levels should be monitored.

Administration

Don't crush or break extended-release tablets. Take albuterol without regard to food.

For inhalation, shake the container well before inhalation. Wait 2 minutes before inhaling the second dose to allow for deeper bronchial penetration. Rinse mouth with water immediately after inhalation to prevent mouth and throat dryness. Take no more than 2 inhalations at any one time because excessive use may decrease the drug's effectiveness or produce paradoxical bronchoconstriction.

For nebulizer use, dilute 0.5 ml of 0.5% solution to a final volume of 3 ml with 0.9% NaCl to provide 2.5 mg. Administer over 5 to 15 minutes. The nebulizer should be used with compressed air or oxygen (O_2) at a rate of 6 to 10 L/minute.

Alclometasone
al-kloe-met′a-sone
(Aclovate)

CATEGORY AND SCHEDULE
Pregnancy Risk Category: C

CLASSIFICATION
Corticosteroids, topical, dermatologics

MECHANISM OF ACTION
Topical corticosteroids exhibit anti-inflammatory, antipruritic, and vasoconstrictive properties. Clinically, these actions correspond to decreased edema, erythema, pruritus, plaque formation, and scaling of the affected skin.

PHARMACOKINETICS
Approximately 3% is absorbed during an 8-hour period. Metabolized in the liver. Excreted in the urine.

AVAILABILITY
Cream, as dipropionate: 0.05% (Aclovate)
Ointment, as diproprionate: 0.05% (Aclovate)

INDICATIONS AND DOSAGES
▸ **Atopic dermatitis, contact dermatitis, dermatitis, discoid lupus erythematosus, eczema, exfoliative dermatitis, granuloma annulare, lichen planus, lichen simplex, polymorphous light eruption, pruritus, psoriasis, Rhus dermatitis, seborrheic dermatitis, xerosis**
TOPICAL
Adults, adolescents, children 1 year and older. Apply a thin film to the affected area 2-3 times a day.

CONTRAINDICATIONS
Hypersensitivity to alclometasone, other corticosteroids, or any of its components.

INTERACTIONS
Drug
None known.
Herbal
None known.
Food
None known.

DIAGNOSTIC TEST EFFECTS
None known.

SIDE EFFECTS
Frequent
Burning, erythema, maculopapular rash, pruritis, skin irritation, xerosis
Occasional
Acneiform rash, contact dermatitis, folliculitis, glycosuria, growth inhibition, headache, hyperglycemia, infection, miliaria, papilledema, skin atrophy, skin hypopigmentation, skin ulcer, striae, telangiectasia
Rare
Adrenalcortical insufficiency, increased intracranial pressure, pseudotumor cerebri, impaired wound healing, Cushing's syndrome, HPA suppression, skin ulcers, tolerance, withdrawal, visual impairment, ocular hypertension, cataracts

PRECAUTIONS & CONSIDERATIONS
Caution is warranted with pregnancy. It is unknown if alclometasone is distributed in the breast milk. Alclometasone should not be used for diaper dermatitis. Children are more susceptible to HPA axis suppression than adults. There are no age-related precautions noted in the elderly.
The most common side effect is transient mild skin irritation consisting of burning, pruritus, or erythema.

Storage
Store at room temperature.
Administration
Do not use occlusive dressings unless directed by physician. Apply a thin film topically to affected area 2-3 times/day. Massage gently until medication disappears.

Alefacept
ale'fah-cept
(Amevive)

CATEGORY AND SCHEDULE
Pregnancy Risk Category: B

CLASSIFICATION
Immunosuppressives

MECHANISM OF ACTION
An immunologic agent that interferes with the activation of T lymphocytes by binding to the lymphocyte antigen, thus reducing the number of circulating T lymphocytes. *Therapeutic Effect:* Prevents T cells from becoming overactive, which may help reduce symptoms of chronic plaque psoriasis.

PHARMACOKINETICS
Half-life: 270 hr.

AVAILABILITY
Powder for Injection: 7.5 mg, 15 mg.

INDICATIONS AND DOSAGES
▸ **Plaque psoriasis**
IV
Adults, Elderly. 7.5 mg once weekly for 12 wk.
IM
Adults, Elderly. 15 mg once weekly for 12 wk.

CONTRAINDICATIONS
History of systemic malignancy, concurrent use of immunosuppressive agents or phototherapy

INTERACTIONS
Drug
None known.
Herbal
None known.
Food
None known.

DIAGNOSTIC TEST EFFECTS
Decreases serum T-lymphocyte levels. May increase serum AST (SGOT) and ALT (SGPT) levels.

▓ IV INCOMPATIBILITIES
Don't mix alefacept with any other medications. Don't reconstitute it with any diluent other than that supplied by the manufacturer.

SIDE EFFECTS
Frequent (16%)
Injection site pain and inflammation (with IM administration)
Occasional (5%)
Chills
Rare (2% or less)
Pharyngitis, dizziness, cough, nausea, myalgia

SERIOUS REACTIONS
• Rare reactions include hypersensitivity reactions, lymphopenia, malignancies, and serious infections requiring hospitalization (such as abscess, pneumonia, and postoperative wound infection).
• Coronary artery disease and MI occur in fewer than 1% of patients.

PRECAUTIONS & CONSIDERATIONS
Caution is warranted with chronic infections, history of recurrent infections, high risk for malignancy, and in the elderly. It is unknown if alefacept crosses the placenta or is distributed in breast milk. The safety and efficacy of this drug have not been established in children. Cautious use is necessary in the elderly because they're at increased risk for infections and certain malignancies. Avoid contact with infected individuals and situations that might increase risk for infection.

Notify the physician of any signs of infection or malignancy. CD4₊ T-lymphocyte counts should be monitored before and weekly during the 12-week treatment period. Withhold the dose if the CD4₊ count is less than 250 cells/microliter. Discontinue treatment if the count remains below 250 cells/microliter.

Storage
Store unopened vials at room temperature. Use the drug immediately after reconstitution or within 4 hours if refrigerated. Discard unused portion within 4 hours of reconstitution.

Administration
! The patient may be re-treated for an additional 12 weeks, as prescribed, if at least 12 weeks have elapsed since the previous course of therapy and the patient's CD4₊ T-lymphocyte count is within normal limits. For both IV and IM administration, withdraw 0.6 ml of the supplied diluent and, with the needle pointed at the sidewall of the vial, slowly inject the diluent into the vial of alefacept. Swirl the vial gently to dissolve the contents; don't shake or vigorously agitate the vial to avoid excessive foaming. The reconstituted solution should be clear and colorless to slightly yellow. Don't use it if it becomes discolored or cloudy or contains undissolved material.

For IV use, reconstitute the 7.5-mg vial with 0.6 ml of the supplied diluent (sterile water for injection);

0.5 ml of the reconstituted solution contains 7.5 mg alefacept. Prepare two syringes with 3 ml 0.9% NaCl for a pre- and post-administration flush. Prime the winged infusion set with 3 ml 0.9% NaCl and insert the set into the vein. Attach the drug-filled syringe to the infusion set, and administer the solution over no more than 5 seconds. Flush the infusion set with 3 ml 0.9% NaCl.

For IM use, reconstitute 15-mg vial with 0.6 ml of the supplied diluent (sterile water for injection); 0.5 ml of reconstituted solution contains 15 mg alefacept. Inject the full 0.5 ml of solution. Use a different IM site for each new IM injection.

Administer each injection at least 1 inch from an old site, avoiding tender, bruised, red, or hard areas.

Alemtuzumab
uh-lem-tooz′uh-mab
(Campath)

CATEGORY AND SCHEDULE
Pregnancy Risk Category: C

CLASSIFICATION
Antineoplastics, monoclonal antibodies

MECHANISM OF ACTION
Binds to CD52, a cell surface glyco-protein, found on the surface of all B and T lymphocytes, most monocytes, macrophages, natural killer cells, and granulocytes. *Therapeutic Effect:* Produces cytotoxicity reducing tumor size.

PHARMACOKINETICS
Half-life: About 12 days. Peak and trough levels rise during first few weeks of therapy and approach steady state by about week 6.

AVAILABILITY
Solution for Injection: 30 mg/3 ml.

INDICATIONS AND DOSAGES
▸ **Chronic lymphocytic leukemia**
IV
Adults, Elderly. Initially, 3 mg/day as a 2-hr infusion. When the 3-mg daily dose is tolerated (with only low-grade or no infusion-related toxicities), increase daily dose to 10 mg. When the 10 mg/day dose is tolerated, maintenance dose may be initiated. Maintenance: 30 mg/day 3 times a week on alternate days (such as Monday, Wednesday, and Friday or Tuesday, Thursday, and Saturday) for up to 12 wk. The increase to 30 mg/day is usually achieved in 3-7 days.

CONTRAINDICATIONS
Active systemic infections, history of hypersensitivity or anaphylactic reaction to the drug, immunosuppression

INTERACTIONS
Drug
Live virus vaccines: May potentiate viral replication, increase side effects, and decrease the patient's antibody response to the vaccine.
Herbal
None known.
Food
None known.

DIAGNOSTIC TEST EFFECTS
May decrease Hgb level, platelet count, and WBC count.

▨ IV INCOMPATIBILITIES
Don't mix alemtuzumab with any other medications.

SIDE EFFECTS

Frequent

Rigors, tremors (86%), fever (85%), nausea (54%), vomiting (41%), rash (40%), fatigue (34%), hypotension (32%), urticaria (30%), pruritus, skeletal pain, headache (24%), diarrhea (22%), anorexia (20%)

Occasional (less than 10%)

Myalgia, dizziness, abdominal pain, throat irritation, vomiting, neutropenia, rhinitis, bronchospasm, urticaria

SERIOUS REACTIONS

- Neutropenia occurs in 85% of patients, anemia occurs in 80% of patients, and thrombocytopenia occurs in 72% of patients.
- A rash occurs in 40% of patients.
- Respiratory toxicity, manifested as dyspnea, cough, bronchitis, pneumonitis, and pneumonia, occurs in 26%-16% of patients.

PRECAUTIONS & CONSIDERATIONS

Alemtuzumab has the potential to cause depletion of B- and T-lymphocytes in the fetus. Discontinue breast-feeding during treatment and for at least 3 months after the last dose. The safety and efficacy of alemtuzumab have not been established in children. No age-related precautions have been noted in the elderly. Vaccinations and contact with anyone who has recently received a live-virus vaccine should be avoided. Crowds and those with known infection should also be avoided.

Infusion-related reactions, including chills, fever, hypotension, and rigors, should be monitored which usually occur 30 minutes to 2 hours after starting the first infusion; these reactions may resolve by slowing the drip rate. Signs and symptoms for hematologic toxicity, including excessive fatigue or weakness, ecchymosis, fever, signs of local infection, sore throat or unusual bleeding from any site, should be assessed. CBC should be monitored frequently during and after therapy to assess for anemia, neutropenia, and thrombocytopenia.

Storage

Refrigerate ampoules before dilution. Don't freeze them. Use the solution within 8 hours after dilution. The diluted solution may be stored at room temperature or refrigerated. Discard the solution if it becomes discolored or contains particulate matter.

Administration

! Expect to pretreat with 650 mg acetaminophen and 50 mg diphenhydramine before each infusion to prevent infusion-related side effects.

Withdraw the needed amount from the ampoule into a syringe. Inject it into 100-ml 0.9% NaCl or D_5W, using a low-protein binding, nonfiber-releasing 5-micron filter. Invert the bag to mix the contents; don't shake it. Give the 100-ml solution as a 2-hour IV infusion. Do not give alemtuzumab by IV push or bolus.

Alendronate

a-len'dro-nate

(Fosamax)

Do not confuse Fosamax with Flomax.

CATEGORY AND SCHEDULE

Pregnancy Risk Category: C

CLASSIFICATION

Bisphosphonates

MECHANISM OF ACTION
A bisphosphonate that inhibits normal and abnormal bone resorption, without retarding mineralization. *Therapeutic Effect:* Leads to significantly increased bone mineral density; reverses the progression of osteoporosis.

PHARMACOKINETICS
Poorly absorbed after oral administration. Protein binding: 78%. After oral administration, rapidly taken into bone, with uptake greatest at sites of active bone turnover. Excreted in urine. **Terminal half-life:** Greater than 10 yr (reflects release from skeleton as bone is resorbed).

AVAILABILITY
Tablets: 5 mg, 10 mg, 35 mg, 40 mg, 70 mg.
Oral Solution: 70 mg/75 ml.

INDICATIONS AND DOSAGES
▸ **Osteoporosis (in men)**
PO
Adults, Elderly. 10 mg once a day in the morning.
▸ **Glucocorticoid-induced osteoporosis**
PO
Adults, Elderly. 5 mg once a day in the morning.
Post-menopausal women not receiving estrogen. 10 mg once a day in the morning.
▸ **Post menopausal osteoporosis**
PO (TREATMENT)
Adults, Elderly. 10 mg once a day in the morning or 70 mg weekly.
PO (PREVENTION)
Adults, Elderly. 5 mg once a day in the morning or 35 mg weekly.
▸ **Paget's disease**
PO
Adults, Elderly. 40 mg once a day in the morning.

OFF-LABEL USES
Treatment of breast cancer

CONTRAINDICATIONS
GI disease, including dysphagia, frequent heartburn, gastrointestinal reflux disease, hiatal hernia, and ulcers, inability to stand or sit upright for at least 30 minutes; renal impairment; sensitivity to alendronate

INTERACTIONS
Drug
Aspirin: May increase GI disturbances.
IV ranitidine: May double the bioavailability of alendronate.
Herbal
None known.
Food
Beverages other than plain water, dietary supplements, food: May interfere with absorption of alendronate.

DIAGNOSTIC TEST EFFECTS
Reduces serum calcium and serum phosphate concentrations. Significantly decreases serum alkaline phosphatase level in patients with Paget's disease.

SIDE EFFECTS
Frequent (8%-7%)
Back pain, abdominal pain
Occasional (3%-2%)
Nausea, abdominal distention, constipation, diarrhea, flatulence
Rare (Less than 2%)
Rash

SERIOUS REACTIONS
• Overdose causes hypocalcemia, hypophosphatemia, and significant GI disturbances.
• Esophageal irritation occurs if alendronate is not given with 6-8 ounces of plain water or if the

patient lies down within 30 minutes of drug administration.

PRECAUTIONS & CONSIDERATIONS

Caution is warranted with hypocalcemia or vitamin D deficiency. Alendronate may cause decreased maternal weight gain and incomplete fetal ossification and delay delivery. It is unknown if alendronate is excreted in breast milk. Do not give to women who are breast feeding. Safety and efficacy of alendronate have not been established in children. No age-related precautions have been noted in the elderly.

Consider beginning weight-bearing exercises and modifying behavioral factors, such as reducing alcohol consumption and stopping cigarette smoking. Plan to correct hypocalcemia and vitamin D deficiency, if present, before starting alendronate therapy. Serum electrolytes, including serum alkaline phosphatase and serum calcium levels, should be monitored.

Administration

! Give at least 30 minutes before the first food, beverage, or medication of the day.

Expected benefits occur only when alendronate is taken with a full glass (6-8 ounces) of plain water first thing in the morning and at least 30 minutes before the first food, beverage, or medication of the day. Taking alendronate with beverages other than plain water, including mineral water, orange juice, and coffee, significantly reduces absorption of the medication. Lie down for at least 30 minutes after taking the medication. Remaining upright helps the drug move quickly to the stomach and reduces the risk of esophageal irritation.

Alfuzosin
ale-few-zoe'sin
(Uroxatral)

CATEGORY AND SCHEDULE

Pregnancy Risk Category: This drug is not indicated for use in women.

CLASSIFICATION

Antiadrenergics, alpha blocking, peripheral

MECHANISM OF ACTION

An $alpha_1$ antagonist that targets receptors around bladder neck and prostate capsule. *Therapeutic Effect:* Relaxes smooth muscle and improves urinary flow and symptoms of prostatic hyperplasia.

PHARMACOKINETICS

Rapidly absorbed and widely distributed. Protein binding: 90%. Extensively metabolized in the liver. Primarily excreted in urine. **Half-life:** 3-9 hr.

AVAILABILITY

Tablets (Extended-Release): 10 mg.

INDICATIONS AND DOSAGES
▸ **Benign prostatic hyperplasia**
PO
Adults. 10 mg once a day, approximately 30 min after same meal each day.

CONTRAINDICATIONS

History of hypersensitivity to alfuzosin

INTERACTIONS
Drug
Cimetidine: May increase alfuzosin blood concentration.

Other alpha blockers, such as doxazosin, prazosin, tamsulosin, and terazosin: May increase the alpha-blockade effects of both drugs.
Herbal
None known.
Food
None known.

DIAGNOSTIC TEST EFFECTS
None known.

SIDE EFFECTS
Frequent (7%-6%)
Dizziness, headache, malaise
Occasional (4%)
Dry mouth
Rare (3%-2%)
Nausea, dyspepsia (such as heartburn, and epigastric discomfort), diarrhea, orthostatic hypotension, tachycardia, drowsiness

SERIOUS REACTIONS
• Ischemia-related chest pain may occur rarely.

PRECAUTIONS & CONSIDERATIONS
Caution is warranted with coronary artery disease, hepatic impairment, orthostatic hypotension, and those under general anesthesia. Alfuzosin is not indicated for use in women and children. No age-related precautions have been noted in the elderly.
Dizziness and lightheadedness may occur. Tasks that require mental alertness or motor skills should be avoided until response to the drug is established.
Notify the physician if headache occurs.
Administration
Take after the same meal each day. The extended-release tablet should not be crushed or chewed.

Allopurinol
al-oh-pure'i-nole
(Aloprim, Allohexal [AUS], Allosig [AUS], Apo-Allopurinol [CAN], Capurate [AUS], Progout [AUS], Purinol [CAN], Zyloprim)
Do not confuse with ZORprin.

CATEGORY AND SCHEDULE
Pregnancy Risk Category: C

CLASSIFICATION
Antigout agents, purine analogs

MECHANISM OF ACTION
A xanthine oxidase inhibitor that decreases uric acid production by inhibiting xanthine oxidase, an enzyme. *Therapeutic Effect:* Reduces uric acid concentrations in both serum and urine.

PHARMACOKINETICS

Route	Onset	Peak	Duration
PO/IV	2-3 days	1-3 wk	1-2 wk

Well absorbed from the GI tract. Widely distributed. Metabolized in the liver to active metabolite. Excreted primarily in urine. Removed by hemodialysis.
Half-life: 1-3 hr; metabolite, 12-30 hr.

AVAILABILITY
Tablets (Zyloprim): 100 mg, 300 mg.
Powder for Injection (Aloprim): 500 mg.

INDICATIONS AND DOSAGES
▶ **Chronic gouty arthritis**
PO
Adults, Children older than 10 yr.
Initially, 100 mg/day; may increase

by 100 mg/day at weekly intervals.
Maximum: 800 mg/day.
Maintenance: 100-200 mg 2-3 times
a day or 300 mg/day.
▶ **To prevent uric acid nephropathy
during chemotherapy**
PO
Adults: Initially, 600-800 mg/day
starting 2-3 days before initiation
of chemotherapy or radiation
therapy.
Children 6-10 yr. 100 mg 3 times a
day or 300 mg once a day.
Children less than 6 yr. 50 mg
3 times a day.
IV
Adults. 200-400 mg/m^2/day begin-
ning 24-48 hr before initiation of
chemotherapy.
Children. 200 mg/m^2/day.
Maximum: 600 mg/day.
▶ **Prevention of uric acid calculi**
PO
Adults. 100-200 mg 1-4 times a day
or 300 mg once a day.
▶ **Recurrent calcium oxalate calculi**
PO
Adults. 200-300 mg/day.
Elderly. Initially, 100 mg/day, gradu-
ally increased until optimal uric acid
level is reached.
▶ **Dosage in renal impairment**
Dosage is modified based on creati-
nine clearance.

Creatinine Clearance	Dosage Adjustment
10-20 ml/min	200 mg/day
3-9 ml/min	100 mg/day
Less than 3 ml/min	100 mg at extended intervals

OFF-LABEL USES
In mouthwash following fluorouracil
therapy to prevent stomatitis

CONTRAINDICATIONS
Asymptomatic hyperuricemia

INTERACTIONS
Drug
Amoxicillin, ampicillin: May
increase incidence of rash.
Azathioprine, mercaptopurine:
May increase therapeutic effect and
toxicity of azathioprine and mercap-
topurine.
Oral anticoagulants: May increase
anticoagulant effect.
Thiazide diuretics: May decrease
the effect of allopurinol.
Herbal
None known.
Food
None known.

DIAGNOSTIC TEST EFFECTS
May increase BUN, serum
creatinine, serum alkaline phosphatase, AST (SGOT), and ALT
(SGPT) levels.

▩ IV INCOMPATIBILITIES
Amikacin (Amikin), carmustine
(BiCNU), cefotaxime (Claforan),
chlorpromazine (Thorazine),
cimetidine (Tagamet), clindamycin
(Cleocin), cytarabine (Ara-C),
dacarbazine (DTIC), diphenhydramine (Benadryl), doxorubicin
(Adriamycin), doxycycline
(Vibramycin), droperidol (Inapsine),
fludarabine (Fludara), gentamicin
(Garamycin), haloperidol (Haldol),
hydroxyzine (Vistaril), idarubicin
(Idamycin), imipenem-cilastatin
(Primaxin), meperidine (Demerol),
methylprednisolone (Solu-Medrol),
metoclopramide (Reglan),
ondansetron (Zofran), prochlorperazine (Compazine), promethazine
(Phenergan), streptozocin (Zanosar),
tobramycin (Nebcin), vinorelbine
(Navelbine)
▩ IV compatibilities
Bumetanide (Bumex), calcium
gluconate, furosemide (Lasix),

heparin, hydromorphone (Dilaudid),
lorazepam (Ativan), morphine,
potassium chloride

SIDE EFFECTS
Occasional
Oral: Somnolence, unusual hair loss
IV: Rash, nausea, vomiting
Rare
Diarrhea, headache

SERIOUS REACTIONS
• Pruritic maculopapular rash
possibly accompanied by malaise,
fever, chills, joint pain, nausea, and
vomiting should be considered a
toxic reaction.
• Severe hypersensitivity may
follow appearance of rash.
• Bone marrow depression, hepatic
toxicity, peripheral neuritis, and
acute renal failure occur rarely.

PRECAUTIONS & CONSIDERATIONS
Caution is warranted with CHF,
diabetes mellitus, hypertension, and
impaired renal or hepatic function. It
is unknown if allopurinol crosses
placenta or is distributed in breast
milk. No age-related precautions
have been noted in children or the
elderly. The drug should be discontinued if rash or other evidence of
allergic reaction appears. Avoid tasks
that require mental alertness or
motor skills until response to the
drug has been established.

High fluid intake (3000 ml/day)
should be encouraged; intake and
output should be monitored; output
should be at least 2000 ml/day, urine
for cloudiness and unusual color and
odor, CBC, hepatic enzyme test
results, and serum uric acid levels
should also be assessed. Signs and
symptoms of a therapeutic response,
including improved joint range of
motion and reduced redness,
swelling, and tenderness, should be
evaluated.

Storage
Store unreconstituted vials at room
temperature. May store reconstituted
solution at room temperature; give
within 10 hours. Do not use if
precipitate forms or solution is
discolored.

Administration
May take with or immediately after
meals or milk. Drink 10 to 12 eight-
ounce glasses of fluid daily while
taking allopurinol. Administer
dosages greater than 300 mg/day in
divided doses. It may take 1 week or
more or the full therapeutic effect of
the drug to be evident.

For IV use, reconstitute 500-mg
vial with 25 ml sterile water for
injection, which produces a clear,
almost colorless solution (concentration of 20 mg/ml). Further dilute
with 0.9% NaCl or D_5W (19 ml of
added diluent yields 1 mg/ml, 9 ml
yields 2 mg/ml, and 2.3 ml
yields maximum concentration of
6 mg/ml). Infuse over 30 to
60 minutes.

Almotriptan
al-moe-trip'tan
(Axert)
Do not confuse with Antivert.

CATEGORY AND SCHEDULE
Pregnancy Risk Category: C

CLASSIFICATION
Serotonin receptor agonists

MECHANISM OF ACTION
A serotonin receptor agonist that
binds selectively to vascular

receptors, producing a vaso-constrictive effect on cranial blood vessels. *Therapeutic Effect:* Produces relief of migraine headache.

PHARMACOKINETICS
Well absorbed after PO administration. Metabolized by the liver, excreted in urine. **Half-life:** 3-4 hr.

AVAILABILITY
Tablets: 6.5 mg, 12.5 mg.

INDICATIONS AND DOSAGES
▶ **Migraine headache**
PO
Adults, Elderly. 6.25-12.5 mg. If headache improves but then returns, dose may be repeated after 2 hr. Maximum: 2 doses/24 hr.
▶ **Dosage in renal impairment**
For adult and elderly patients, recommended initial dose is 6.25 mg and maximum daily dose is 12.5 mg.

CONTRAINDICATIONS
Arrhythmias associated with conduction disorders, hemiplegic or basilar migraine, ischemic heart disease (including angina pectoris, history of MI, silent ischemia, and Prinzmetal's angina), uncontrolled hypertension, use within 24 hours of ergotamine-containing preparation or another serotonin receptor antagonist, use within 14 days of MAOIs, Wolff-Parkinson-White syndrome

INTERACTIONS
Drug
Ergotamine-containing medications: May produce a vasospastic reaction.
Erythromycin, itraconazole, ketoconazole, MAOIs, ritonavir: May increase the almotriptan plasma level.
Fluoxetine, fluvoxamine, paroxetine, sertraline: May produce

weakness, hyperreflexia, and incoordination.
Herbal
None known.
Food
None known.

DIAGNOSTIC TEST EFFECTS
None known.

SIDE EFFECTS
Frequent
Nausea, dry mouth, paresthesia, flushing
Occasional
Changes in temperature sensation, asthenia, dizziness

SERIOUS REACTIONS
• Excessive dosage may produce tremor, red extremities, reduced respirations, cyanosis, seizures, and chest pain.
• Serious arrhythmias occur rarely, particularly in patients with hypertension or diabetes, obese patients, smokers, and those with a strong family history of coronary artery disease.

PRECAUTIONS & CONSIDERATIONS
Caution is warranted with controlled hypertension, a history of CVA, mild to moderate hepatic or renal impairment, and cardiovascular risk factors. It is unknown if almotriptan is distributed in breast milk. The safety and efficacy of almotriptan have not been established in children younger than 12 years. No age-related precautions have been noted in the elderly. Tasks that require mental alertness or motor skills should be avoided.

Notify the physician immediately if palpitations, pain or tightness in the chest or throat, or pain or weakness in the extremities occurs. Migraines and associated symptoms, including nausea and vomiting, photophobia, and phonophobia (sound sensitivity) should be assessed before and during treatment.

Administration

! Don't administer erythromycin, itraconazole, ketoconazole, or ritonavir during the last 7 days of almotriptan therapy.

Swallow tablets whole with a full glass of water.

Alosetron
a-loe'se-tron
(Lotronex)

CATEGORY AND SCHEDULE
Pregnancy Risk Category: B

CLASSIFICATION
Antidiarrheals, gastrointestinals, serotonin receptor antagonists

MECHANISM OF ACTION
A serotonin (5-HT$_3$) receptor antagonist that mediates abdominal pain, bloating, nausea, vomiting, peristalsis, and secretory reflexes.
Therapeutic Effect: Alleviates diarrhea, reduces gastric pain.

PHARMACOKINETICS
Rapidly absorbed after PO administration. Extensively metabolized in liver. Excreted primarily in urine and, to a lesser extent, in feces.
Half-life: 1.5 hr.

AVAILABILITY
Tablets: 1 mg.

INDICATIONS AND DOSAGES
▸ **Irritable bowel syndrome**
PO
Adults (Women older than 18 yr). 1 mg twice a day. Maximum: 2 mg/day.

OFF-LABEL USES
Treatment of carcinoid diarrhea, irritable bowel syndrome in men

CONTRAINDICATIONS
Breast-feeding; constipation; diverticulitis (active or history of); GI bleeding, obstruction, or perforation; history ischemic colitis, ulcerative colitis, or Crohn's disease; thrombophlebitis

INTERACTIONS
Drug
Hydralazine, isoniazid, procainamide: May alter the effects of these drugs.
Herbal
St. John's wort: May increase alosetron blood concentration.
Food
All foods: May decrease the absorption or delay the peak blood concentration of alosetron.

DIAGNOSTIC TEST EFFECTS
May increase serum alkaline phosphatase, bilirubin, ALT (SGPT) and AST (SGOT) levels.

SIDE EFFECTS
Frequent (28%)
Constipation
Occasional (10%-2%)
Nausea, GI or abdominal discomfort or pain, dyspepsia, flatulence, hypertension, clinical depression
Rare
Sedation, abnormal dreams, anxiety

SERIOUS REACTIONS
• Acute ischemic colitis and serious complications of constipation have resulted in the need for blood transfusions and surgery.

PRECAUTIONS & CONSIDERATIONS
Caution is warranted with hepatic function impairment. Be aware

alosetron is indicated for use in women only. The safety and efficacy of this drug have not been established in men. It is unknown if alosetron is excreted in breast milk. The safety and efficacy of alosetron have not been established in children. No age-related precautions have been noted in the elderly.

Urgency and diarrhea may be reduced within 1 week of treatment but the drug's full therapeutic effects may not occur for up to 4 weeks. Persistent constipation may require interruption of treatment or drug management. Notify the physician or nurse if bloody diarrhea, severe constipation, or a sudden worsening of stomach pain occurs. Pattern of daily bowel activity and stool consistency should be monitored. Adequate hydration should be maintained.

Administration

Take alosetron without regard to food.

Alprazolam

al-pray'zoe-lam

(Apo-Alpraz [CAN], Kalma [AUS], Novo-Alprazol [CAN], Xanax, Xanax XR)

Do not confuse alprazolam with lorazepam, or Xanax with Tenex or Zantac.

CATEGORY AND SCHEDULE

Pregnancy Risk Category: D
Controlled Substance: Schedule IV

CLASSIFICATION

Anxiolytics, benzodiazepines, sedatives/hypnotics

MECHANISM OF ACTION

A benzodiazepine that enhances the action of the inhibitory neurotransmitter gamma-aminobutyric acid in the brain. *Therapeutic Effect*: Produces anxiolytic effect from its CNS depressant action.

PHARMACOKINETICS

Well absorbed from GI tract. Protein binding: 80%. Metabolized in the liver. Primarily excreted in urine. Minimal removal by hemodialysis. **Half-life:** 11-16 hr.

AVAILABILITY

Oral Solution: 1 mg/ml.
Tablets: 0.25 mg (Xanax), 0.5 mg (Xanax), 1 mg (Xanax), 2 mg (Xanax).
Tablets (Extended-Release): 0.5 mg (Xanax XR), 1 mg (Xanax XR), 2 mg (Xanax XR), 3 mg (Xanax XR).

INDICATIONS AND DOSAGES

▸ **Anxiety disorders**
PO
Adults (immediate release). Initially, 0.25-0.5 mg 3 times a day. May titrate q3-4 days. Maximum: 4 mg/day in divided doses.
Elderly, Debilitated patients, Patients with hepatic disease or low serum albumin. Initially, 0.25 mg 2-3 times a day. Gradually increase to optimum therapeutic response.
▸ **Panic disorder**
PO, IMMEDIATE RELEASE
Adults. Initially, 0.5 mg 3 times a day. May increase at 3- to 4-day intervals. Range: 5-6 mg/day. Maximum: 10 mg/day.
PO, EXTENDED RELEASE
Adults. Initially, 0.5-1 mg once a day. May titrate at 3- to 4-day

intervals. Range: 3-6 mg/day.
Maximum: 10 mg/day.
Elderly. Initially, 0.125-0.25 mg
2 times a day; may increase in
0.125-mg increments until desired
effect attained.
▸ **Premenstrual syndrome**
PO
Adults. 0.25 mg 3 times a day.

OFF-LABEL USES
Management of premenstrual
syndrome symptoms (mood
disturbances, insomnia, and cramps),
irritable bowel syndrome

CONTRAINDICATIONS
Acute alcohol intoxication with
depressed vital signs, acute angle-
closure glaucoma, concurrent use of
itraconazole or ketoconazole, myasthenia gravis, severe COPD

INTERACTIONS
Drug
Alcohol, other CNS depressants:
Potentiate effects of alprazolam and
may increase sedation.
**Fluvoxamine, itraconazole,
ketoconazole, nefazodone:**
May inhibit metabolism and
increase serum concentrations of
alprazolam.
Herbal
Kava kava, valerian: May increase
CNS depressant effect of
alprazolam.
Food
Grapefruit, grapefruit juice:
May inhibit alprazolam's metabo-
lism.

DIAGNOSTIC TEST EFFECTS
None known.

SIDE EFFECTS
Frequent
Ataxia; lightheadedness; transient,
mild somnolence; slurred speech

(particularly in elderly or debilitated
patients)
Occasional
Confusion, depression,
blurred vision, constipation,
diarrhea, dry mouth, headache,
nausea
Rare
Behavioral problems such as anger,
impaired memory, paradoxical reactions such as insomnia, nervousness,
or irritability

SERIOUS REACTIONS
• Abrupt or too rapid withdrawal
may result in pronounced restlessness, irritability, insomnia, hand
tremors, abdominal and muscle
cramps, diaphoresis, vomiting, and
seizures.
• Overdose results in somnolence,
confusion, diminished reflexes, and
coma.
• Blood dyscrasias have been
reported rarely.

PRECAUTIONS & CONSIDERATIONS
Caution is warranted with impaired
renal or hepatic function.
Dizziness and drowsiness may occur.
Change positions slowly from
recumbent, to sitting, before standing to prevent dizziness. Alcohol,
tasks that require mental alertness
or motor skills, and smoking should
also be avoided. Female on long-
term therapy should use effective
contraception during therapy
and notify the physician
immediately if she becomes or may
be pregnant.
Administration
Take alprazolam without
regard to food. Crush tablets as
needed.
Take extended-release once a
day; swallow tablets whole and
do not break, chew, or crush
tablets.

Alprostadil
al-pros'ta-dil
(Caverject, Edex, Muse, Prostin VR Pediatric)

CATEGORY AND SCHEDULE
Pregnancy Risk Category: C

CLASSIFICATION
Impotence agents, prostaglandins, vasodilators

MECHANISM OF ACTION
A prostaglandin that directly affects vascular and ductus arteriosus smooth muscle and relaxes trabecular smooth muscle. *Therapeutic Effect:* Causes vasodilation; dilates cavernosal arteries, allowing blood flow to and entrapment in the lacunar spaces of the penis.

AVAILABILITY
Injection (Prostin VR Pediatric): 500 mcg/ml.
Powder for Injection (Caverject, Edex): 10 mcg, 20 mcg, 40 mcg.
Urethral Pellet (Muse): 125 mcg, 250 mcg, 500 mcg, 1000 mcg.

INDICATIONS AND DOSAGES
▸ **Maintain patency of ductus arteriosus**
IV INFUSION
Neonates. Initially, 0.05-0.1 mcg/kg/min. Maintenance: 0.01-0.4 mcg/kg/min. Maximum: 0.4 mcg/kg/min.
▸ **Impotence**
PELLET, INTRACAVERNOSAL
Adults. Dosage is individualized.

OFF-LABEL USES
Treatment of atherosclerosis, gangrene, pain due to severe peripheral arterial occlusive disease

CONTRAINDICATIONS
Conditions predisposing to anatomic deformation of penis, hyaline membrane disease, penile implants, priapism, respiratory distress syndrome

INTERACTIONS
Drug
Anticoagulants, including heparin, thrombolytics: May increase risk of bleeding.
Sympathomimetics: May decrease effect of alprostadil.
Vasodilators: May increase risk of hypotension.
Herbal
None known.
Food
None known.

DIAGNOSTIC TEST EFFECTS
May increase blood bilirubin levels. May decrease glucose, serum calcium, and serum potassium levels.

▓ IV INCOMPATIBILITIES
No information available.

SIDE EFFECTS
Frequent
Intracavernosal (4%-1%):
Penile pain (37%), prolonged erection, hypertension, localized pain, penile fibrosis, injection site hematoma or ecchymosis, headache, respiratory infection, flu-like symptoms
Intraurethral (3%): Penile pain (36%), urethral pain or burning, testicular pain, urethral bleeding,

headache, dizziness, respiratory infection, flu-like symptoms
Systemic (greater than 1%): Fever, seizures, flushing, bradycardia, hypotension, tachycardia, apnea, diarrhea, sepsis

Occasional

Intracavernosal (less than 1%): Hypotension, pelvic pain, back pain, dizziness, cough, nasal congestion
Intraurethral (less than 3%): Fainting, sinusitis, back and pelvic pain
Systemic (less than 1%): Anxiety, lethargy, myalgia, arrhythmias, respiratory depression, anemia, bleeding, thrombocytopenia, hematuria

SERIOUS REACTIONS

• Overdose is manifested as apnea, flushing of the face and arms, and bradycardia.
• Cardiac arrest and sepsis occur rarely.

PRECAUTIONS & CONSIDERATIONS

Caution is warranted with coagulation defects, leukemia, multiple myeloma, polycythemia, severe hepatic disease, sickle cell disease, and thrombocythemia. Be aware that erection should occur within 2 to 5 minutes of administration. Alprostadil should not be used if sexual partner is pregnant, unless a condom barrier is being used. Notify the physician if erection lasts for longer than 4 hours or becomes painful.

Arterial pressure by auscultation, Doppler transducer, or umbilical artery catheter should be monitored with ductus arteriosus. Infusion rate should be decreased immediately if a significant decrease in arterial pressure occurs. Continuous

cardiac monitoring should be performed. Heart sounds, femoral pulse (to monitor lower extremity circulation), and respiratory status should be assessed. In addition, signs and symptoms of hypotension should be monitored and B/P, ABG values, and temperature should be assessed. If apnea or bradycardia occurs, infusion should be discontinued immediately and the physician should be notified.

Storage

Refrigerate pellet unless used within 14 days. Store the parenteral form in refrigerator. Dilute drug before administration. Prepare fresh dose every 24 hours and discard unused portions.

Administration

! Doses greater than 40 mcg (Edex) or 60 mcg (Caverject) are not recommended.

! Give by continuous IV infusion or through umbilical artery catheter placed at ductal opening.

Prepare continuous IV infusion by diluting 1 ml alprostadil, containing 500-mcg, with D_5W or 0.9% NaCl to yield a solution containing 2 to 20 mcg/ml. Diluting volumes can range from 25 to 250 ml, depending on the patient and the available infusion device. Infuse the lowest possible dose over the shortest possible time. Decrease the infusion rate immediately if a significant decrease in arterial pressure is noted via auscultation, Doppler transducer, or umbilical artery catheter. Discontinue the infusion immediately if signs and symptoms of overdose, such as apnea and bradycardia, occur.

Alteplase
al-teep′lase
(Activase, Actilyse [AUS], Cathflo Activase)
Do not confuse alteplase or Activase with Altace.

CATEGORY AND SCHEDULE
Pregnancy Risk Category: C

CLASSIFICATION
Thrombolytics

MECHANISM OF ACTION
A tissue plasminogen activator that acts as a thrombolytic by binding to the fibrin in a thrombus and converting entrapped plasminogen to plasmin. This process initiates fibrinolysis. *Therapeutic Effect:* Degrades fibrin clots, fibrinogen, and other plasma proteins.

PHARMACOKINETICS
Rapidly metabolized in the liver. Primarily excreted in urine.
Half-life: 35 min.

AVAILABILITY
Powder for Injection (Cathflo Activase): 2 mg.
Powder for Injection(Activase): 50 mg, 100 mg.

INDICATIONS AND DOSAGES
▸ **Acute MI**
IV INFUSION
Adults weighing greater than 67 kg. 100 mg over 90 min, starting with 15-mg bolus over 1-2 min, then 50 mg over 30 min, then 35 mg over 60 min. Or a 3-hour infusion, giving 60 mg over first hr (6-10 mg as bolus over 1-2 min), 20 mg over second hr, and 20 mg over third hr.

Adults weighing 67 kg or less. 100 mg over 90 min, starting with 15-mg bolus, then 0.75 mg/kg over 30 min (maximum: 50 mg), then 0.5 mg/kg over 60 min (maximum: 35 mg). Or 3-hour infusion of 1.25 mg/kg giving 60% of dose over first hr (6%-10% as 1- to 2-min bolus), 20% over second hr, and 20% over third hr.
▸ **Acute pulmonary emboli**
IV INFUSION
Adults. 100 mg over 2 hr. Institute or reinstitute heparin near end or immediately after infusion when aPTT or thrombin time (TT) returns to twice normal or less.
▸ **Acute ischemic stroke**
IV INFUSION
Adults. 0.9 mg/kg over 60 min (10% total dose as initial IV bolus over 1 min).
▸ **Central venous catheter clearance**
IV
Adults, Elderly. 2 mg; may repeat after 2 hr.

OFF-LABEL USES
Coronary thrombolysis, to decrease ischemic events in unstable angina

CONTRAINDICATIONS
Active internal bleeding, AV malformation or aneurysm, bleeding diathesis, intracranial neoplasm, intracranial or intraspinal surgery or trauma, recent (within past 2 months) cerebrovascular accident, severe uncontrolled hypertension

INTERACTIONS
Drug
Anticoagulants, including cefotetan, heparin, plicamycin, valproic acid: May increase risk of hemorrhage.
Platelet aggregation inhibitors, including aspirin, NSAIDs, ticlopidine: May increase risk of bleeding.

Herbal
None known.
Food
None known.

DIAGNOSTIC TEST EFFECTS
Decreases plasminogen and fibrinogen levels during infusion, which decreases clotting time (and confirms the presence of lysis). Decreases Hgb and Hct.

▓ IV INCOMPATIBILITIES
Do not add other medications to the container of alteplase solution or administer other medications through the same IV line.

🖫 IV compatibilities
Lidocaine, metoprolol (Lopressor), morphine, nitroglycerin, propranolol (Inderal)

SIDE EFFECTS
Frequent
Superficial bleeding at puncture sites, decreased BP
Occasional
Allergic reaction, such as rash or wheezing; bruising

SERIOUS REACTIONS
• Severe internal hemorrhage may occur.
• Lysis of coronary thrombi may produce atrial or ventricular arrhythmias or stroke.

PRECAUTIONS & CONSIDERATIONS
Caution is warranted with recent (within past 10 days) major surgery or GI bleeding, organ biopsy, trauma, cerebrovascular disease, cardiopulmonary resuscitation, diabetic retinopathy, endocarditis, left heart thrombus, occluded AV cannula at infected site, severe hepatic or renal disease, thrombophlebitis, in the elderly, and pregnant women or within the first

10 postpartum days. Alteplase is used only when the benefit to the mother outweighs the risk to a fetus. Also, it is unknown if alteplase crosses the placenta or is distributed in breast milk. Safety and efficacy have not been established in children. In the elderly, there is an increased risk of bleeding. Patients must be carefully selected and monitored. An electric razor and a soft toothbrush should be used to reduce the risk of bleeding.

Immediately report signs of bleeding, such as oozing from cuts or gums. Serum creatine kinase (CK), and CK-MB concentrations, 12-lead EKG, electrolyte levels, Hct, platelet count, TT, aPTT, PT, and fibrinogen level should be evaluated before therapy starts. B/P and pulse and respiration rates should be checked every 15 minutes until stable; then check hourly. Continuous cardiac monitoring should be performed.
Storage
Store vials at room temperature. Solution is stable for 8 hours after reconstitution. Discard unused portion.
Administration
Reconstitute immediately before use with sterile water for injection. Reconstitute 100-mg vial with 100 ml sterile water for injection (50-mg vial with 50 ml sterile water for injection) without preservative to provide a concentration of 1 mg/ml. May dilute further with equal volume D_5W or 0.9% NaCl to provide a concentration of 0.5 mg/ml. Gently swirl or slowly invert vial; avoid excessive agitation. After reconstitution, solution normally appears colorless to pale yellow. Give by IV infusion via infusion pump. (See individual dosages above.) If minor bleeding occurs at puncture site, apply pressure for 30 seconds; if unrelieved, apply a pressure dressing. If uncontrolled

hemorrhage occurs, discontinue the infusion immediately. Slowing the rate of infusion may worsen the hemorrhage. Avoid undue pressure when injecting the drug into the catheter because the catheter can rupture or expel a clot into circulation.

Aluminum Chloride Hexahydrate
a-loo′mi-num
(Drysol, Xerac AC)
(powder, solution)

CATEGORY AND SCHEDULE
Pregnancy Risk Category: C

CLASSIFICATION
Antiperspirants

MECHANISM OF ACTION
Aluminum salts cause an obstruction of the distal sweat gland. This obstruction causes metal ions to precipitate with mucopolysaccharides, damaging epithelial cells along the lumen of the duct, and forming a plug to block sweat output. *Therapeutic Effect:* Results in decreased secretion of the sweat glands.

PHARMACOKINETICS
Not known.

AVAILABILITY
Topical Solution: 6.25% (Xerac AC), 20% (Drysol).

INDICATIONS AND DOSAGES
▸ **Antiperspirant**
TOPICAL
Adults, Elderly, Children 12 yr and older. Apply to each underarm once a day, at bedtime.

▸ **Hyperhidrosis**
TOPICAL
Adults, Elderly, Children 12 yr and older. Apply to affected areas once a day, at bedtime.

CONTRAINDICATIONS
Hypersensitivity to aluminum chloride or any one of its components.

INTERACTIONS
Drug
None known.
Herbal
None known.
Food
None known.

DIAGNOSTIC TEST EFFECTS
None known.

▨ IV INCOMPATIBILITIES
None known.
▨ IV compatibilities
None known.

SIDE EFFECTS
Frequent
Itching, burning, tingling sensation
Occasional
Rash

SERIOUS REACTIONS
• Hypersensitivity reaction, such as rash may occur.

PRECAUTIONS & CONSIDERATIONS
It is unknown if aluminum chloride hexahydrate crosses the placenta or is distributed in breast milk. Deodorants or antiperspirants should be avoided during treatment. It may be harmful to cotton fibers and certain metals.
    Skin may become irritated during use. Aluminum chloride hexahydrate should not be applied to

broken, irritated, or recently shaved skin.

Administration

Aluminum chloride hexahydrate is for external use only. It should be applied to dry skin. The treated area should be wrapped with a sheet of saran wrap to avoid aluminum chloride hexahydrate rubbing off at night. The next morning, discard the saran wrap if used and wash the skin with a mild soap.

Aluminum Hydroxide

a-loo'mi-num hye-drox'ide
(Alternagel, Alu-Tab, Amphojel [CAN], Basaljel [CAN])

CATEGORY AND SCHEDULE

Pregnancy Risk Category: C (Considered safe except for chronic, high-dose use).
OTC

CLASSIFICATION

Gastrointestinals,
vitamins/minerals

MECHANISM OF ACTION

An antacid that reduces gastric acid by binding with phosphate in the intestine and is then excreted as aluminum carbonate in feces; decreased serum phosphate levels may result in increased absorption of calcium. The drug also has astringent and adsorbent properties. *Therapeutic Effect:* Neutralizes or increases gastric pH; reduces phosphate levels in urine, preventing formation of phosphate urinary calculi; reduces the serum phosphate level; decreases the fluidity of stools.

AVAILABILITY

Capsules: 475 mg.
Suspension: 320 mg/5 ml, 600 mg/5 ml.

INDICATIONS AND DOSAGES

▶ **Antacid**
PO
Adults, Elderly. 600-1200 mg between meals and at bedtime.
▶ **Hyperphosphatemia**
PO
Adults, Elderly. Initially, 300-600 mg 3 times a day with meals.
Children. 50-150 mg/kg/day in divided doses q4-6hr.

CONTRAINDICATIONS

Children age 6 years or younger, intestinal obstruction

INTERACTIONS

Drug
Anticholinergics, quinidine: May decrease excretion of aluminum hydroxide.
Iron preparations, isoniazid, ketoconazole, quinolones, tetracyclines: May decrease absorption of aluminum hydroxide.
Methenamine: May decrease effects of the methenamine.
Salicylate: May increase salicylate excretion.
Herbal
None known.
Food
None known.

DIAGNOSTIC TEST EFFECTS

May increase the serum gastrin level and systemic and urinary pH. May decrease the serum phosphate level.

SIDE EFFECTS

Frequent
Chalky taste, mild constipation, abdominal cramps

Occasional
Nausea, vomiting, speckling or whitish discoloration of stools

SERIOUS REACTIONS
• Prolonged constipation may result in intestinal obstruction.
• Excessive or chronic use may produce hypophosphatemia manifested as anorexia, malaise, muscle weakness, or bone pain, which may result in osteomalacia and osteoporosis.
• Prolonged use may produce urinary calculi.

PRECAUTIONS & CONSIDERATIONS
Caution is warranted with Alzheimer's disease, chronic diarrhea, constipation, dehydration, fecal impaction, fluid restrictions, gastric outlet obstruction, GI or rectal bleeding, impaired renal function, symptoms of appendicitis, and in the elderly. Aluminum hydroxide is contraindicated for children 6 years or younger.

Stool discoloration may occur but will resolve when the drug is discontinued. Adequate hydration should be maintained. Pattern of daily bowel activity and stool consistency and serum aluminum, calcium, phosphate, and uric acid levels should be monitored.

Administration
The usual dose of aluminum hydroxide is 30 to 60 ml. Take aluminum hydroxide 1 to 3 hours after meals and at bedtime. Expect the dosage to be individualized based on the antacid's neutralizing capacity. Thoroughly chew chewable tablets (combination forms) before swallowing and then to drink a glass of water or milk. Shake the suspension well before use. Don't take other oral drugs within 1 to 2 hours of antacid administration.

Aluminum Salts
a-loo′min-um
Aluminum acetate & acetic acid (Otic Domeboro); aluminum hydroxide & magnesium carbonate (Gaviscon Extra Strength, Gaviscon Liquid); aluminum hydroxide & magnesium hydroxide (Diovol [CAN], Diovol EX [CAN], Gelusil [CAN], Gelusil Extra Strength [CAN], Maalox, Maalox TC, Mylanta [CAN], Univol [CAN]); aluminum hydroxide and magnesium trisillicate (Gaviscon); aluminum hydroxide, magnesium hydroxide, & simethicone (Diovol Plus [CAN], Maalox Fast Release Liquid, Maalox Max, Mylanta Extra Strength Liquid, Mylanta Liquid, Mylanta Double Strength [CAN], Mylanta Extra Strength [CAN], Mylanta Regular Strength [CAN]); aluminum sulfate & calcium acetate (Bluboro, Domeboro, Pedi-Boro)

CATEGORY AND SCHEDULE
Pregnancy Risk Category: C

CLASSIFICATION
Antacid

MECHANISM OF ACTION
An antacid that reduces gastric acid by binding with phosphate in the intestine, and then is excreted as aluminum carbonate in feces. Aluminum carbonate may increase the absorption of calcium due to decreased serum phosphate levels. The drug also has astringent and adsorbent properties. *Therapeutic Effect:* Neutralizes or increases gastric pH; reduces phosphates in urine, preventing formation of

phosphate urinary stones; reduces serum phosphate levels; decreases fluidity of stools.

PHARMACOKINETICS
Varies in each formulation.

AVAILABILITY
Aluminum hydroxide
Capsules: 400 mg (Alu-Cap), 500 mg (Dialume).
Liquid: 600 mg/5 mg (ALternagel).
Suspension: 320 mg/5 ml (Amphojel), 450 mg/5 ml, 675 mg/ 5 ml.
Tablets: 300 mg (Amphojel), 500 mg (Alu-Tab), 600 mg (Amphojel).
Aluminum acetate & acetic acid (Otic Domeboro)
Otic solution: 2% acetic acid and aluminum acetate (Otic Domeboro).
Aluminum hydroxide and magnesium carbonate
Liquid: 31.7 mg aluminum hydroxide and 119.3 mg magnesium carbonate/5 ml (Gaviscon Liquid), 84.6 mg aluminum hydroxide and 79.1 mg magnesium carbonate/5 ml (Gaviscon Extra Strength).
Tablets, chewable: 160 mg aluminum hydroxide and 1.5 mg magnesium carbonate (Gaviscon Extra Strength Relief).
Aluminum hydroxide & magnesium hydroxide
Suspension: 225 mg aluminum hydroxide and 200 mg magnesium hydroxide/5 ml (Maalox).
Suspension: 600 mg aluminum hydroxide and 300 mg magnesium hydroxide/5 ml (Maalox TC).
Aluminum hydroxide & magnesium trisillicate
Tablets, chewable: 80 mg aluminum hydroxide and 20 mg magnesium hydroxide (Gaviscon).
Aluminum hydroxide, magnesium hydroxide, & simethicone
Liquid: 200 mg aluminum hydroxide, 200 mg magnesium hydroxide, and 20 mg simethicone/5 ml (Mylanta), 400 mg aluminum hydroxide, 400 mg magnesium hydroxide, and 40 mg simethicone/5 ml (Maalox Max), 500 mg aluminum hydroxide, 450 mg magnesium hydroxide, and 20 mg simethicone/5 ml (Maalox Fast Release), 400 mg aluminum hydroxide, 400 mg magnesium hydroxide, and 40 mg simethicone/5 ml (Mylanta Extra Strength).
Aluminum sulfate & calcium acetate
Powder, for topical solution: packets (Bluboro, Domeboro, Pedi-Boro).
Tablets, effervescent, for topical solution: effervescent tablets (Domeboro).

INDICATIONS AND DOSAGES
Aluminum hydroxide
▸ **Peptic ulcer disease**
PO
Adults, Elderly. Children. 5-15 ml as above.
15-45 ml q3-6hr or 1 and 3 hr after meals and at bedtime.
▸ **Antacid**
PO
Adults, Elderly. 30 ml 1 and 3 hr after meals and at bedtime.
▸ **Gastrointestinal (GI) bleeding prevention**
PO
Adults, Elderly. 30-60 ml/hr.
Children. 5-15 ml. q1-2hr.
▸ **Hyperphosphatemia**
PO
Adults, Elderly. 500-1800 mg 1 and 3 hr after meals and at bedtime.
Children. 50-150 mg/kg/24 hr q4-6hr.
Aluminum acetate & acetic acid
Superficial infections of the external auditory canal
OTIC

Adults, Elderly. Instill 4-6 drops in ear(s) q2-3hr.

Aluminum hydroxide & magnesium carbonate

▸ **Antacid**

PO

Adults, Elderly. 15-30 ml 4 times/day of the liquid; chew 2-4 tablets 4 times/day.

Aluminum hydroxide & magnesium hydroxide

▸ **Antacid**

PO

Adults, Elderly. 5-10 ml 4-6 times/day.

Aluminum hydroxide & magnesium trisillicate

▸ **Antacid**

PO

Adults, Elderly. Chew 2-4 tablets 4 times/day or as directed.

Aluminum hydroxide, magnesium hydroxide, and simethicone

▸ **Antacid (with flatulence)**

PO

Adults, Elderly. 10-20 ml or 2-4 tablets 4-6 times/day.

Aluminum sulfate & calcium acetate

Inflammtory skin conditions with weeping that occurs in dermatitis

TOPICAL

Adults, Elderly. Soak affected area in solution 2-4 times/day for 15-30 min or apply wet dressing soaked in solution 2-4 times/day for 30 min treatment periods. Domeboro: Saturate dressing and apply to affected area and saturate every 15-30 min; or soak for 15-30 min 3 times/day.

CONTRAINDICATIONS

Children age 6 yrs or younger, intestinal obstruction, hypersensitivity to aluminum or any component of the formulation

INTERACTIONS

Drug

Anticholinergics, quinidine: May decrease excretion of aluminum salts.

Iron preparations, isoniazid, ketoconazole, quinolones, tetracyclines: May decrease absorption of aluminum salts.

Methenamine: May decrease effects of methenamine.

Salicylate: May increase salicylate excretion.

Herbal

None known.

Food

None known.

DIAGNOSTIC TEST EFFECTS

May increase serum gastrin levels and systemic and urinary pH. May decrease serum phosphate levels.

SIDE EFFECTS

Frequent

PO: Chalky taste, mild constipation, stomach cramps

Topical: Burning, itching

Occasional

PO: Nausea, vomiting, speckling or whitish discoloration of stools

Otic: Burning or stinging in ear

Topical: New or continued redness, skin dryness

Rare

Otic: Skin rash, redness, swelling, or pain in ear

SERIOUS REACTIONS

• Prolonged constipation may result in intestinal obstruction.

• Excessive or chronic use may produce hypophosphatemia manifested as anorexia, malaise, muscle weakness or bone pain and resulting in osteomalacia and osteoporosis.

• Prolonged use may produce urinary calculi.

PRECAUTIONS & CONSIDERATIONS

Caution is warranted with Alzheimer's disease, advanced age, chronic diarrhea, constipation, dehydration, fecal impaction, fluid

prevent insomnia. Continue therapy for the full length of treatment and evenly space drug doses around the clock.

Ambenonium
am-be-noe′nee-um
(Mytelase)

CATEGORY AND SCHEDULE
Pregnancy Risk Category: C

CLASSIFICATION
Cholinesterase inhibitors, musculoskeletal agents, stimulants, muscle

MECHANISM OF ACTION
A cholinesterase inhibitor that enhances and prolongs cholinergic function by increasing the concentration of acetylcholine through inhibition of the hydrolysis of acetylcholine. *Therapeutic Effect:* Increases muscle strength in myasthenia gravis.

PHARMACOKINETICS
Poorly absorbed after PO administration.

AVAILABILITY
Tablets: 10 mg (Mytelase).

INDICATIONS AND DOSAGES
▶ Myasthenia gravis
PO
Adults. 5-25 mg 3 or 4 times a day. If well tolerated, after 1 or 2 days, may increase to 50-75 mg 3 times a day. Range: 5-200 mg/day in divided doses.

CONTRAINDICATIONS
Not recommended in patients receiving routine administration of atropine or other belladonna derivatives. Not recommended in patients receiving mecamylamine.

INTERACTIONS
Drug
Atropine: Suppresses the symptoms of ambenonium overdose.
Herbal
None known.
Food
None known.

DIAGNOSTIC TEST EFFECTS
None known.

SIDE EFFECTS
Frequent
Abdominal pain, diarrhea, increased salivation, miosis, sweating, and vomiting
Occasional
Anxiety, blurred vision, and urinary urgency
Rare
Trembling, difficulty moving or controlling movement of the tongue, neck, or arms

SERIOUS REACTIONS
• Overdosage may result in cholinergic crisis, characterized by severe nausea, vomiting, diarrhea, increased salivation, diaphoresis, bradycardia, hypotension, flushed skin, stomach pain, respiratory depression, seizures, and paralysis of muscles.
• Increasing muscle weakness of myasthenia gravis may occur.
Antidote: 0.5-1 mg IV atropine sulfate with other supportive treatment.

PRECAUTIONS & CONSIDERATIONS
Caution is warranted with asthma, bladder outflow obstruction, COPD, and history of peptic ulcer disease.

It is unknown if ambenonium crosses the placenta or is excreted in breast milk. Safety and efficacy of ambenonium has not been established. Cholinergic reaction, such as diaphoresis, dizziness, excessive salivation, feeling of facial warmth, gastrointestinal (GI) cramping or discomfort, lacrimation, pallor, trembling or difficulty moving or controlling movement of the tongue, neck, or arms, and urinary urgency should be reported.

Administration

Ambenonium should be given after food in divided doses at the same time each day.

Amcinonide
am-sin'oh-nide
(Cylocort)

CATEGORY AND SCHEDULE
Pregnancy Risk Category: C

CLASSIFICATION
Corticosteroids, topical, dermatologics

MECHANISM OF ACTION
Topical corticosteroids have anti-inflammatory, antipruritic, and vasoconstrictive properties. The exact mechanism of the anti-inflammatory process is unclear. *Therapeutic Effect:* Reduces or prevents tissue response to inflammatory process.

PHARMACOKINETICS
Well absorbed systemically. Large variation in absorption among sites: forearm 1%; scalp 4%, forehead 7%, scrotum 36%. Greatest penetration occurs at groin, axillae, and face.

Protein binding in varying degrees. Metabolized in liver. Primarily excreted in urine.

AVAILABILITY
Lotion: 0.1% (Cylocort).
Cream: 0.1% (Cylocort).
Ointment: 0.1% (Cylocort).

INDICATIONS AND DOSAGES
▸ **Dermatoses**
TOPICAL
Adults, Elderly. Apply sparingly 2-3 times/day.

CONTRAINDICATIONS
History of hypersensitivity to amcinonide or other corticosteroids.

INTERACTIONS
Drug
None known.
Herbal
None known.
Food
None known.

DIAGNOSTIC TEST EFFECTS
None known.

SIDE EFFECTS
Frequent
Itching, redness, irritation, burning
Occasional
Dryness, folliculitis, hypertrichosis, acneiform eruptions, hypopigmentation, perioral dermatitis
Rare
Allergic contact dermatitis, maceration of the skin, secondary infection, skin atrophy.
Systemic: Absorption more likely with occlusive dressings or extensive application in young children.

SERIOUS REACTIONS
• The serious reactions of long-term therapy and the addition of occlusive dressings are reversible

hypothalamic-pituitary-adrenal (HPA) axis suppression, manifestations of Cushing's syndrome, hyperglycemia and glucosuria.
• Abruptly withdrawing the drug after long-term therapy may require supplemental systemic corticosteroids.

PRECAUTIONS & CONSIDERATIONS

Caution is necessary when using amcinonide over large surface areas, prolonged use, and the addition of occlusive dressings. Long-term therapy and the addition of occlusive dressings can lead to reversible hypothalamic-pituitary-adrenal (HPA) axis suppression, manifestations of Cushing's syndrome, hyperglycemia and glucosuria. Children may absorb larger amounts and may be more susceptible to toxicity. It is unknown if amcinonide is distributed in breast milk.

Signs of a rash in addition to fever and sore throat should be reported. Sunlight should be avoided.

Administration

Amcinonide should be applied sparingly to the skin and rubbed gently into affected area. Apply after bath or shower for best absorption and do not cover the area with any coverings, plastic pants, or tight diapers unless instructed. Avoid contact with eyes.

Amikacin
am-i-kay'sin
(Amikin)
Do not confuse with Amicar.

CATEGORY AND SCHEDULE
Pregnancy Risk Category: C

CLASSIFICATION
Antibiotics, aminoglycosides

MECHANISM OF ACTION
An aminoglycoside antibiotic that irreversibly binds to protein on bacterial ribosomes. *Therapeutic Effect:* Interferes with protein synthesis of susceptible microorganisms.

PHARMACOKINETICS
Rapid, complete absorption after IM administration. Protein binding: 0%-10%. Widely distributed (doesn't cross blood-brain barrier, low concentrations in CSF). Excreted unchanged in urine. Removed by hemodialysis. **Half-life:** 2-4 hr (increased in impaired renal function and neonates; decreased in cystic fibrosis and burn or febrile patients).

AVAILABILITY
Injection. 50 mg/ml, 250 mg/ml.

INDICATIONS AND DOSAGES
▸ **UTIs**
IV, IM
Adults, Elderly. 250 mg q12hr.
▸ **Moderate to severe infections**
IV, IM
Adults, Elderly. 15 mg/kg/day in divided doses q8-12hr. Maximum 1.5 g/day.
Children, Infants. 15-22.5 mg/kg/day in divided doses q8hr.
Neonates. 7.5-10 mg/kg/dose q8-24hr.
▸ **Dosage in Renal Impairment**
Dosage and frequency are modified based on the degree of renal impairment and serum drug concentration. After a loading dose of 5-7.5 mg/kg, the maintenance dose and frequency are based on serum creatinine levels and creatinine clearance.

CONTRAINDICATIONS
Hypersensitivity to amikacin, or other aminoglycosides (cross-sensitivity), or their components.

INTERACTIONS
Drug
Nephrotoxic medications, other aminoglycosides, ototoxic medications: May increase the risk of nephrotoxicity or ototoxicity and neuromuscular blockers: May enhance neuromuscular blockade.
Herbal
None known.
Food
None known.

DIAGNOSTIC TEST EFFECTS
May increase serum bilirubin, BUN, serum creatinine, serum LDH, SGOT (AST) and SGPT (ALT) levels. May decrease serum calcium, magnesium, potassium, and sodium concentrations. Therapeutic peak serum level is greater than 30 mcg/ml; toxic trough serum level is greater than 10 mcg/ml.

▒ IV INCOMPATIBILITIES
Amphotericin, ampicillin, cefazolin (Ancef), heparin, propofol (Diprivan)
▒ IV compatibilities
Amiodarone (Cordarone), aztreonam (Azactam), calcium gluconate, cefepime (Maxipime), cimetidine (Tagamet), ciprofloxacin (Cipro), clindamycin (Cleocin), diltiazem (Cardizem), enalapril (Vasotec), esmolol (BreviBloc), fluconazole (Diflucan), furosemide (Lasix), levofloxacin (Levaquin), lorazepam (Ativan), magnesium sulfate, midazolam (Versed), morphine, ondansetron (Zofran), potassium chloride, ranitidine (Zantac), vancomycin

SIDE EFFECTS
Frequent
IM: Pain, induration
IV: Phlebitis, thrombophlebitis
Occasional
Hypersensitivity reactions (rash, fever, urticaria, pruritus)

Rare
Neuromuscular blockade (difficulty breathing, drowsiness, weakness)

SERIOUS REACTIONS
• Serious reactions may include nephrotoxicity (as evidenced by increased thirst, decreased appetite, nausea, vomiting, increased BUN and serum creatinine levels, and decreased creatinine clearance); neurotoxicity (manifested as muscle twitching, visual disturbances, seizures, and tingling); and ototoxicity (as evidenced by tinnitus, dizziness, and loss of hearing).

PRECAUTIONS & CONSIDERATIONS
Caution is warranted with patients with 8th cranial nerve (vestibulo-cochlear nerve) impairment, decreased renal function, myasthenia gravis, and Parkinson's disease. Amikacin readily crosses the placenta, and small amounts are distributed in breast milk. It may produce fetal nephrotoxicity. Neonates and premature infants may be more susceptible to amikacin toxicity because of their immature renal function. The elderly are at increased risk for amikacin toxicity because of age-related renal impairment as well as an increased risk for hearing loss. Signs and symptoms of superinfection, particularly changes in the oral mucosa, diarrhea, and genital or anal pruritus, should be monitored.

Determine the history of allergies, especially to aminoglycosides and sulfites. Expect to correct dehydration before beginning aminoglycoside therapy. Establish the baseline hearing acuity before beginning therapy. Obtain a specimen for culture and sensitivity testing before giving the first dose. Therapy may begin before test results are known. Urinalysis results to detect casts,

RBCs, WBCs, and decreased specific gravity should be monitored. Expect to monitor peak and trough serum amikacin levels. Be alert for ototoxic and neurotoxic side effects.

Storage
Store vials at room temperature. Solutions normally appear clear but may become pale yellow; the yellow color does not affect the drug's potency. Discard the solution if a precipitate forms or dark discoloration occurs. Intermittent IV infusion (piggyback) is stable for 24 hours at room temperature.

Administration
For intermittent IV infusion (piggyback), dilute each 500 mg with 100 ml of 0.9% NaCl or D5W. Infuse over 30 to 60 minutes for adults and older children. Infuse over 60 to 120 minutes for infants and young children.

For IM injection, administer slowly to minimize patient discomfort. Injections administered into the gluteus maximus are less painful than those given in the lateral aspect of the thigh.

Amiloride
a-mill'oh-ride
(Kaluril [AUS], Midamor)
Do not confuse with amiodarone or amlodipine.

CATEGORY AND SCHEDULE
Pregnancy Risk Category: B (D if used in pregnancy-induced hypertension)

CLASSIFICATION
Diuretics, potassium sparing

MECHANISM OF ACTION
A guanidine derivative that acts as a potassium-sparing diuretic, antihypertensive, and antihypokalemic by directly interfering with sodium reabsorption in the distal tubule. *Therapeutic Effect:* Increases sodium and water excretion and decreases potassium excretion.

PHARMACOKINETICS

Route	Onset	Peak	Duration
PO	2 hrs	6-10 hrs	24 hrs

Incompletely absorbed from gastrointestinal (GI) tract. Protein binding: Minimal. Primarily excreted in urine; partially eliminated in feces. **Half-life:** 6-9 hr.

AVAILABILITY
Tablets: 5 mg.

INDICATIONS AND DOSAGES
▸ **To counteract potassium loss induced by other diuretics**
PO
Adults, Children weighing more than 20 kg. 5-10 mg/day up to 20 mg.
Elderly. Initially, 5 mg/day or every other day.
Children weighing 6-20 kg. 0.625 mg/kg/day. Maximum: 10 mg/day.
▸ **Dosage in renal impairment**

Creatinine Clearance	Dosage
10-50 ml/min	50% of normal
Less than 10 ml/min	Avoid use

OFF-LABEL USES
Treatment of edema associated with congestive heart failure (CHF), liver cirrhosis, and nephrotic syndrome; treatment of hypertension, reduces lithium-induced polyuria, slows pulmonary function reduction in cystic fibrosis

CONTRAINDICATIONS

Acute or chronic renal insufficiency, anuria, diabetic nephropathy, patients on other potassium-sparing diuretics, serum potassium greater than 5.5 mEq/L

INTERACTIONS

Drug

ACE inhibitors, including captopril, and potassium-containing diuretics: May increase potassium levels.

Anticoagulants, including heparin: May decrease effect of anticoagulants, including heparin.

Lithium: May decrease lithium clearance and increase risk of amiloride toxicity.

NSAIDs: May decrease antihypertensive effect.

Herbal

None known.

Food

None known.

DIAGNOSTIC TEST EFFECTS

May increase BUN, calcium excretion, and glucose, serum creatinine, serum magnesium, serum potassium, and uric acid levels. May decrease serum sodium levels.

SIDE EFFECTS

Frequent (8%-3%)

Headache, nausea, diarrhea, vomiting, decreased appetite

Occasional (3%-1%)

Dizziness, constipation, abdominal pain, weakness, fatigue, cough, impotence

Rare (less than 1%)

Tremors, vertigo, confusion, nervousness, insomnia, thirst, dry mouth, heartburn, shortness of breath, increased urination, hypotension, rash

SERIOUS REACTIONS

• Severe hyperkalemia may produce irritability, anxiety, a feeling of heaviness in the legs, paresthesia of hands, face, and lips, hypotension, bradycardia, tented T waves, widening of QRS, and ST depression.

PRECAUTIONS & CONSIDERATIONS

Caution is warranted with cardiopulmonary disease, diabetes mellitus, or liver insufficiency, BUN greater than 30 mg/dl or serum creatinine greater than 1.5 mg/dl, and in the elderly and debilitated. Be aware that it is unknown if amiloride crosses the placenta or is distributed in breast milk. There are no age-related precautions noted in children.

In the elderly, age-related decreased renal function increases the risk of hyperkalemia and may require caution. Be aware a high-potassium diet and potassium supplements can be dangerous, especially with liver or kidney problems; avoid foods high in potassium such as apricots, bananas, legumes, meat, orange juice, raisins, whole grains, including cereals, and white and sweet potatoes.

Notify the physician of signs and symptoms of hyperkalemia: confusion, difficulty breathing, irregular heartbeat, nervousness, numbness of the hands, feet, or lips, unusual tiredness, and weakness in the legs. Blood pressure (B/P), vital signs, electrolytes, intake and output, weight, and potassium level should be monitored before and during treatment. A baseline 12-lead EKG should also be obtained.

Administration

Take with food to avoid GI distress. Therapeutic effect of the drug takes several days to begin and can last for several days after the drug is discontinued.

Aminocaproic Acid
a-mee-noe-ka-proe'ik
(Amicar)
Do not confuse Amicar with amikacin or Amikin.

CATEGORY AND SCHEDULE
Pregnancy Risk Category: C

CLASSIFICATION
Hemostatics

MECHANISM OF ACTION
A systemic hemostatic that acts as an antifibrinolytic and antihemorrhagic by inhibiting the activation of plasminogen activator substances. *Therapeutic Effect:* Prevents formation of fibrin clots.

AVAILABILITY
Syrup: 250 mg/ml.
Tablets: 500 mg.
Injection: 250 mg/ml.

INDICATIONS AND DOSAGES
▸ **Acute bleeding**
PO, IV INFUSION
Adults, Elderly. 4-5 g over first hr; then 1-1.25 g/hr. Continue for 8 hr or until bleeding is controlled. Maximum: 30 g/24 hr.
Children. 3 g/m^2 over first hr; then 1 g/m^2/hr. Maximum: 18 g/m^2/24 hr.
▸ **Dosage in renal impairment**
Decrease dose to 25% of normal.

OFF-LABEL USES
Prevention of recurrence of subarachnoid hemorrhage, prevention of hemorrhage in hemophiliacs following dental surgery

CONTRAINDICATIONS
Evidence of active intravascular clotting process, disseminated intravascular coagulation without concurrent heparin therapy, hematuria of upper urinary tract origin (unless benefit outweighs risk); newborns (parenteral form).

INTERACTIONS
Drug
None known.
Herbal
None known.
Food
None known.

DIAGNOSTIC TEST EFFECTS
May elevate serum potassium level.

IV INCOMPATIBILITIES
Sodium lactate. Do not mix with other medications.

SIDE EFFECTS
Occasional
Nausea, diarrhea, cramps, decreased urination, decreased B/P, dizziness, headache, muscle fatigue and weakness, myopathy, bloodshot eyes

SERIOUS REACTIONS
• Too rapid IV administration produces tinnitus, rash, arrhythmias, unusual fatigue, and weakness.
• Rarely, a grand mal seizure occurs, generally preceded by weakness, dizziness, and headache.

PRECAUTIONS & CONSIDERATIONS
Caution is warranted with hyperfibrinolysis and impaired cardiac, hepatic, or renal function. No information is available

concerning the distribution of aminocaproic acid in breast milk. There is no documented evidence of adverse effects in children. Although no elderly-related problems have been noted, cautious use is advised because of the risk of age-related renal impairment, which may require dosage reduction. Females may experience an increase in menstrual flow.

Notify the physician of red or dark urine, muscular pain or weakness, abdominal or back pain, gingival bleeding, black or red stool, coffee-ground vomitus, or blood-tinged mucus from cough. B/P, heart rate and rhythm, and pulse rate, serum creatine kinase and AST (SGOT) levels should be monitored.

Storage
Store tablets in a tight container. Protect syrup from freezing.

Administration
! Expect to administer a reduced dose if the patient has cardiac, renal, or hepatic impairment. The syrup may be given as an oral rinse for the control of bleeding during dental and oral surgery in hemophilic patients.

For IV use, dilute each 1 g in up to 50 ml 0.9% NaCl, D_5W, Ringer's solution, or sterile water for injection. Do not use sterile water for injection in those with subarachnoid hemorrhage. Do not give by direct injection. Give only by IV infusion. Infuse 5 g or less over the first hour in 250 ml of solution. Give each succeeding 1 g over 1 hour in 50 to 100 ml of solution. Monitor for hypotension during the infusion. Be aware that rapid infusion may produce arrhythmias, including bradycardia.

Aminophylline
am-in-off'i-lin
(Phyllocontin)
(Elixophyllin, Quibron-T, Quibron-T/SR, Slo-Bid Gyrocaps, Theo-24, Thoechron, Theodur, Theolair, T-Phyl, Uniphyl).
Do not confuse aminophylline with amitriptyline or ampicillin or Slo-Bid with Dolobid.

CATEGORY AND SCHEDULE
Pregnancy Risk Category: C

CLASSIFICATION
Bronchodilators, xanthine derivatives

MECHANISM OF ACTION
A xanthine derivative that acts as a bronchodilator by directly relaxing smooth muscle of the bronchial airways and pulmonary blood vessels. *Therapeutic Effect:* Relieves bronchospasm and increases vital capacity.

AVAILABILITY
Capsules (Extended-Release [Theo-24]): 100 mg, 200 mg, 300 mg, 400 mg.
Elixir (Elixophyllin): 80 mg/15 ml.
Oral Solution: 80 mg/15 ml.
Tablets (Controlled-Release [Quibron-T/SR]): 300 mg.
Tablets (Controlled-Release [Theochron]): 100 mg, 200 mg, 300 mg.
Tablets (Controlled-Release [Theolair-SR]): 300 mg, 500 mg.
Tablets (Controlled-Release [T-Phyl]): 200 mg.

Tablets (Controlled-Release [Uniphyl]): 400 mg, 600 mg.
Infusion (theophylline): 0.8 mg/ml, 1.6 mg/ml, 2 mg/ml, 3.2 mg/ml, 4 mg/ml.
Injection (Aminophylline): 25 mg/ml.

INDICATIONS AND DOSAGES
▸ **Chronic bronchospasm**
PO
Adults, Elderly, Children. 16 mg/kg or 400 mg/day (whichever is less) in 3-4 divided doses (8-hr intervals); may increase by 25% every 2-3 days. Maximum: 13 mg/kg/day (children 13-16 yr); 18 mg/kg/day (children 9-12 yr); 20 mg/kg/day (children 1-8 yr). Maximum dosages are based on serum theophylline concentrations, clinical condition, and presence of toxicity.
▸ **Acute bronchospasm in patients not currently taking theophylline**
PO
Adults, children older than 1 yr. Initially, loading dose of 5 mg/kg (theophylline); then maintenance dosage of theophylline based on patient group (shown below).

Patient Group	Maintenance Theophylline Dosage
Healthy, nonsmoking adults	3 mg/kg q8hr
Elderly patients, patients with cor pulmonale	2 mg/kg q8hr
Patients with CHF or hepatic disease	1-2 mg/kg q12hr
Children 9-16 yr, young adult smokers	3 mg/kg q6hr
Children 1-8 yr	4 mg/kg q6hr

IV
Adults, Children older than 1 yr. Initially, loading dose of 6 mg/kg (aminophylline); maintenance dosage of aminophylline based on patient group (shown below).

Patient Group	Maintenance Aminophylline Dosage
Healthy, nonsmoking adults	0.7 mg/kg/hr
Elderly patients, patients with cor pulmonale, CHF, or hepatic impairment	0.25 mg/kg/hr
Children 13-16 yr	0.7 mg/kg/hr
Children 9-12 yr, young adult smokers	0.9 mg/kg/hr
Children 1-8 yr	1-1.2 mg/kg/hr
Children 6 mo-1 yr	0.6-0.7 mg/kg/hr
Children 6 wk-6 mo	0.5 mg/kg/hr
Neonates	5 mg/kg q12hr

▸ **Acute bronchospasm in patients currently taking theophylline**
PO, IV
Adults, children older than 1 yr. Obtain serum theophylline level. If not possible and patient is in respiratory distress and not experiencing toxic effects, may give 2.5 mg/kg dose. Maintenance: Dosage based on peak serum theophylline concentration, clinical condition, and presence of toxicity.

OFF-LABEL USES
Treatment of apnea in neonates

CONTRAINDICATIONS
History of hypersensitivity to caffeine or xanthine

INTERACTIONS
Drug
Beta blockers: May decrease the effects of aminophylline.
Cimetidine, ciprofloxacin, erythromycin, norfloxacin: May increase aminophylline blood concentration and risk of aminophylline toxicity.

Glucocorticoids: May produce hypernatremia.
Phenytoin, primidone, rifampin: May increase aminophylline metabolism.
Smoking: May decrease amino-phylline blood concentration.
Herbal
None known.
Food
Charcoal-broiled foods; high-protein, low-carbohydrate diet: May decrease the theophylline blood level.

DIAGNOSTIC TEST EFFECTS
None known.

🔲 IV INCOMPATIBILITIES
Amiodarone (Cordarone), ciprofloxacin (Cipro), dobutamine (Dobutrex), ondansetron (Zofran)

🔲 IV compatibilities
Aztreonam (Azactam), ceftazidime (Fortaz), fluconazole (Diflucan), heparin, morphine, potassium chloride

SIDE EFFECTS
Frequent
Altered smell (during IV administration), restlessness, tachycardia, tremor
Occasional
Heartburn, vomiting, headache, mild diuresis, insomnia, nausea

SERIOUS REACTIONS
• Too-rapid IV administration may produce marked hypotension with accompanying faintness, light-headedness, palpitations, tachycardia, hyperventilation, nausea, vomiting, angina-like pain, seizures, ventricular fibrillation, and cardiac standstill.

PRECAUTIONS & CONSIDERATIONS
Caution is warranted with diabetes mellitus, glaucoma, hypertension,

hyperthyroidism, cardiac, renal or hepatic impairment, peptic ulcer disease, and seizure disorder. Aminophylline crosses the placenta and small amounts of the drug may be distributed in breast milk and cause irritability in the breast-feeding infant. Use the drug cautiously in children less than 1 year. Drink plenty of fluids to decrease the thickness of lung secretions. Avoid excessive use of caffeinated products, such as chocolate, cocoa, cola, coffee, and tea. Smoking, charcoal-broiled foods, and a high-protein, low carbohydrate diet may decrease the theophylline level.

Pulse rate and quality, respiratory rate, depth, rhythm and type, ABG levels, and serum potassium levels should be monitored. Peak serum concentration should be obtained 1 hour after an IV dose, 1 to 2 hours after an immediate-release dose, and 3 to 8 hours after a sustained-release dose. Serum trough level should be obtained just before the next dose. Lips and fingernails for signs of hypoxemia, such as a blue or gray color in light-skinned patients and a gray color in dark-skinned patients, should be assessed.

Storage
Store vials at room temperature.
Administration
! Aminophylline dosage is calculated based on lean body weight. It's also based on peak serum theophylline concentrations, the clinical condition, and the absence of theophylline toxicity. The therapeutic serum level range is 10 to 20 mcg/ml.

Take oral aminophylline with food to avoid GI distress. Don't crush or break sustained-release forms.

Discard the solution for injection if it contains a precipitate. For IV use, give loading dose diluted in 100 to

200 ml of D₅W or 0.9% NaCl. Prepare maintenance dose in larger volume parenteral infusion. Don't exceed a flow rate of 1 ml/minute (25 mg/minute) for either piggyback or infusion. Administer loading dose over 20 to 30 minutes. Use an infusion pump or microdrip to regulate IV administration.

Aminosalicylic Acid
a-mee-noe-sal-i-sil-ik as-id
(Nemasol [CAN], Paser)

CATEGORY AND SCHEDULE
Pregnancy Risk Category: C

CLASSIFICATION
Antimycobacterials, salicylates

MECHANISM OF ACTION
An antitubercular agent active against M. tuberculosis. Thought to exhibit competitive antagonism of folic acid synthesis.
Therapeutic Effect: Bacteriostatic activity in susceptible microorganisms.

PHARMACOKINETICS
Readily absorbed from the gastrointestinal (GI) tract. Protein binding: 50%-60%. Widely distributed (including cerebrospinal fluid [CSF]). Metabolized in liver. Primarily excreted in urine. Removed by hemodialysis.
Half-life: 1.1-1.62 hr.

AVAILABILITY
Packet granules: 4 g/packet granules (Paser).
Tablets, enteric-coated: 7.7 grains (Paser).

Tablets, sustained-release: 500 mg (Paser).

INDICATIONS AND DOSAGES
▶ **Tuberculosis**
PO
Adults, Elderly. 4 g in divided doses 3 times/day.
Children. 150 mg/kg/day in divided doses 3 times/day. Maximum: 12 g/day.

OFF-LABEL USES
Crohn's disease, hyperlipidemia, ulcerative colitis

CONTRAINDICATIONS
End-stage renal disease, hypersensitivity to aminosalicylic acid products

INTERACTIONS
Drug
Cyanocobalamin: May decrease cyanocobalamin absorption.
Isoniazid: May increase isoniazid serum levels.
Herbal
None known.
Food
None known.

DIAGNOSTIC TEST EFFECTS
May alter bilirubin levels in urinalysis.

SIDE EFFECTS
Occasional
Abdominal pain, diarrhea, nausea, vomiting
Rare
Hypersensitivity reactions, hepatotoxicity, thrombocytopenia

SERIOUS REACTIONS
• Liver toxicity and hepatitis, blood dyscrasias occur rarely.
• Agranulocytosis, methemoglobinemia, thrombocytopenia have been reported.

PRECAUTIONS & CONSIDERATIONS
Precaution is necessary with liver insufficiency, peptic ulcer disease, impaired renal function, and congestive heart failure. It is unknown if aminosalicylic acid crosses the placenta or is excreted in breast milk. There are no age-related precautions noted in children or the elderly. Be aware that skeleton of the granules may appear in the stool.

Liver function should be monitored during therapy. Symptoms of hepatitis as evidenced by anorexia, dark urine, fatigue, jaundice, nausea, vomiting, and weakness should be assessed. If hepatitis is suspected, withhold the drug and notify the physician promptly.

Administration
May sprinkle granules on applesauce or yogurt or mix with juice. Discard medication if the package is swollen or the granules are dark brown or purple.

Amiodarone
a-mee′oh-da-rone
(Aratac [AUS], Cordarone, Cordarone X [AUS], Pacerone)
Do not confuse amiodarone with amiloride or Cordarone with Cardura.

CATEGORY AND SCHEDULE
Pregnancy Risk Category: D

CLASSIFICATION
Antiarrhythmics, class III

MECHANISM OF ACTION
A cardiac agent that prolongs duration of myocardial cell action potential and refractory period by acting directly on all cardiac tissue. Decreases AV and sinus node function. *Therapeutic Effect:* Suppresses arrhythmias.

PHARMACOKINETICS

Route	Onset	Peak	Duration
PO	3 days-3 wk	1 wk-5 mo	7-50 days after discontinuation

Slowly, variably absorbed from GI tract. Protein binding: 96%. Extensively metabolized in the liver to active metabolite. Excreted via bile; not removed by hemodialysis. **Half-life:** 26-107 days; metabolite, 61 days.

AVAILABILITY
Tablets (Cordarone): 200 mg.
Tablets (Pacerone): 100 mg, 200 mg, 400 mg.
Injection (Cordarone): 50 mg/ml.

INDICATIONS AND DOSAGES
▸ **Life-threatening recurrent ventricular fibrillation or hemodynamically unstable ventricular tachycardia**
PO
Adults, Elderly. Initially, 800-1600 mg/day in 2-4 divided doses for 1-3 wk. After arrhythmia is controlled or side effects occur, reduce to 600-800 mg/day for about 4 wk. Maintenance: 200-600 mg/day. *Children.* Initially, 10-15 mg/kg/day for 4-14 days, then 5 mg/kg/day for several wk. Maintenance: 2.5 mg/kg or lowest effective maintenance dose for 5 of 7 days/wk.
IV INFUSION
Adults. Initially, 1050 mg over 24 hr; 150 mg over 10 min, then 360 mg over 6 hr; then 540 mg over 18 hr.

May continue at 0.5 mg/min for up to 2-3 wk regardless of age or renal or left ventricular function.

OFF-LABEL USES
Treatment and prevention of supraventricular arrhythmias and symptomatic atrial flutter refractory to conventional treatment

CONTRAINDICATIONS
Bradycardia-induced syncope (except in the presence of a pacemaker), second- and third-degree AV block, severe hepatic disease, severe sinus-node dysfunction

INTERACTIONS
Drug
Antiarrhythmics: May increase cardiac effects.
Beta blockers, oral anticoagulants: May increase effect of beta blockers and oral anticoagulants.
Digoxin, phenytoin: May increase drug concentration and risk of toxicity of digoxin and phenytoin.
Herbal
None known.
Food
None known.

DIAGNOSTIC TEST EFFECTS
May increase antinuclear antibody titers and AST (SGOT), ALT (SGPT), and serum alkaline phosphatase levels. May cause changes in EKG and thyroid function test results. Therapeutic serum level is 0.5-2.5 mcg/ml; toxic serum level has not been established.

▓ IV INCOMPATIBILITIES
Aminophylline (theophylline), cefazolin (Ancef), heparin, sodium bicarbonate
▽ IV compatibilities
Dobutamine (Dobutrex), dopamine (Intropin), furosemide (Lasix), insulin (regular), labetalol (Normodyne), lidocaine, midazolam (Versed), morphine, nitroglycerin, norepinephrine (Levophed), phenylephrine (Neo-Synephrine), potassium chloride, vancomycin

SIDE EFFECTS
Expected
Corneal microdeposits are noted in almost all patients treated for more than 6 months (can lead to blurry vision).
Frequent (greater than 3%)
Parenteral: Hypotension, nausea, fever, bradycardia.
Oral: Constipation, headache, decreased appetite, nausea, vomiting, paresthesias, photosensitivity, muscular incoordination.
Occasional (less than 3%)
Oral: Bitter or metallic taste; decreased libido; dizziness; facial flushing; blue-gray coloring of skin (face, arms, and neck); blurred vision; bradycardia; asymptomatic corneal deposits.
Rare (less than 1%)
Oral: Rash, vision loss, blindness.

SERIOUS REACTIONS
• Serious, potentially fatal pulmonary toxicity (alveolitis, pulmonary fibrosis, pneumonitis, acute respiratory distress syndrome) may begin with progressive dyspnea and cough with crackles, decreased breath sounds, pleurisy, CHF or hepatotoxicity.
• Amiodarone may worsen existing arrhythmias or produce new arrhythmias (called proarrhythmias).

PRECAUTIONS & CONSIDERATIONS
Caution is warranted with thyroid disease. Amiodarone crosses the placenta and is distributed in breast milk; it adversely affects fetal development. Safety and efficacy of

amiodarone have not been established in children. The elderly may be more sensitive to amiodarone's effects on thyroid function and may experience increased incidence of ataxia or other neurotoxic effects.
! Signs and symptoms of pulmonary toxicity, including progressively worsening cough and dyspnea, should be assessed. Dosage should be discontinued or reduced if toxicity occurs. The drug's therapeutic blood level is 0.5 to 2.5 mcg/ml; the drug's toxic level has not been established.

Chest X-ray, EKG, pulmonary function tests, liver enzyme tests, AST, ALT, and serum alkaline phosphatase level should be obtained at baseline and during therapy. Apical pulse and B/P should be assessed immediately before giving amiodarone. Withhold the medication and notify the physician if the pulse rate is 60 beats/minute or lower or the systolic B/P is less than 90 mm Hg. Pulse rate for bradycardia, an irregular rhythm, and quality should be monitored. EKG for changes such as widening of the QRS complex and prolonged PR and QT intervals should be assessed; notify the physician of significant interval changes. Signs and symptoms of hyperthyroidism, such as difficulty breathing, bulging eyes (exophthalmos), eyelid edema, frequent urination, hot and dry skin, and weight loss, and signs and symptoms of hypothyroidism, such as cool and pale skin, lethargy, night cramps, periorbital edema, and pudgy hands and feet should also be monitored.

Storage
Store at room temperature.
Administration
For oral use, take with meals to reduce GI distress. Tablets may be crushed if necessary.

! Solution concentrations greater than 3 mg/ml can cause peripheral vein phlebitis.

For IV administration, use glass or polyolefin containers for dilution. Dilute the loading dose of 150 mg in 100 ml D₅W to yield a solution of 1.5 mg/ml. Dilute the maintenance dose of 900 mg in 500 ml D₅W to yield a solution of 1.8 mg/ml.

Amitriptyline
a-mee-trip'ti-leen
(Apo-Amitriptyline [CAN], Elavil, Endep [AUS], Levate [CAN], Novo-Triptyn [CAN], Tryptanol [AUS])
Do not confuse amitriptyline with aminophylline or nortriptyline, or Elavil with Equanil or Mellaril.

CATEGORY AND SCHEDULE
Pregnancy Risk Category: C

CLASSIFICATION
Antidepressants, tricyclic

MECHANISM OF ACTION
A tricyclic antidepressant that blocks the reuptake of neurotransmitters, including norepinephrine and serotonin, at presynaptic membranes, thus increasing their availability at postsynaptic receptor sites. Also has strong anticholinergic activity. *Therapeutic Effect:* Relieves depression.

PHARMACOKINETICS
Rapidly and well absorbed from the GI tract. Protein binding: 90%.

Undergoes first-pass metabolism in the liver. Primarily excreted in urine. Minimal removal by hemodialysis.
Half-life: 10-26 hr.

AVAILABILITY
Tablets: 10 mg, 25 mg, 50 mg, 75 mg, 100 mg, 150 mg.
Injection: 10 mg/ml.

INDICATIONS AND DOSAGES
▶ **Depression**
PO
Adults. 30-100 mg/day as a single dose at bedtime or in divided doses. May gradually increase up to 300 mg/day. Titrate to lowest effective dosage.
Elderly. Initially, 10-25 mg at bedtime. May increase by 10-25 mg at weekly intervals. Range: 25-150 mg/day.
Children 6-12 yr. 1-5 mg/kg/day in 2 divided doses.
IM
Adults. 20-30 mg 4 times a day.
▶ **Pain management**
PO
Adults, Elderly. 25-100 mg at bedtime.

OFF-LABEL USES
Relief of neuropathic pain, such as that experienced by patients with diabetic neuropathy or postherpetic neuralgia; treatment of bulimia nervosa

CONTRAINDICATIONS
Acute recovery period after MI, use within 14 days of MAOIs

INTERACTIONS
Drug
Antithyroid agents: May increase the risk of agranulocytosis.
Cimetidine, valproic acid: May increase amitriptyline blood concentration and risk of toxicity.

Clonidine, guanadrel: May decrease the effects of these drugs.
CNS depressants (including alcohol, anticonvulsants, barbiturates, phenothiazines, and sedative-hypnotics): May increase CNS and respiratory depression and the hypotensive effects of amitriptyline.
MAOIs: May increase the risk of neuroleptic malignant syndrome, seizures, hypertensive crisis, and hyperpyrexia.
Phenothiazines: May increase the sedative and anticholinergic effects of amitriptyline.
Sympathomimetics: May increase the risk of cardiac effects.
Herbal
None known.
Food
None known.

DIAGNOSTIC TEST EFFECTS
May alter blood glucose levels and EKG readings. Therapeutic serum drug level is 120-250 ng/ml; toxic serum drug level is greater than 500 ng/ml.

SIDE EFFECTS
Frequent
Dizziness, somnolence, dry mouth, orthostatic hypotension, headache, increased appetite, weight gain, nausea, unusual fatigue, unpleasant taste
Occasional
Blurred vision, confusion, constipation, hallucinations, delayed micturition, eye pain, arrhythmias, fine muscle tremors, parkinsonian syndrome, anxiety, diarrhea, diaphoresis, heartburn, insomnia
Rare
Hypersensitivity, alopecia, tinnitus, breast enlargement, photosensitivity

SERIOUS REACTIONS

• Overdose may produce confusion, seizures, severe somnolence, arrhythmias, fever, hallucinations, agitation, dyspnea, vomiting, and unusual fatigue or weakness.

• Abrupt discontinuation after prolonged therapy may produce headache, malaise, nausea, vomiting, and vivid dreams.

• Blood dyscrasias and cholestatic jaundice occur rarely.

PRECAUTIONS & CONSIDERATIONS

Caution is warranted with cardiovascular disease, diabetes mellitus, glaucoma, hiatal hernia, history of seizures, history of urine retention or urinary obstruction, hyperthyroidism, increased IOP, hepatic or renal disease, benign prostatic hyperplasia, and schizophrenia. Amitriptyline crosses the placenta and is minimally distributed in breast milk. Children are more sensitive to an acute overdose and are at increased risk for amitriptyline toxicity. The elderly are more sensitive to the drug's anticholinergic effects and are at increased risk for amitriptyline toxicity.

Anticholinergic, sedative, and hypotensive effects may occur but tolerance usually develops to these effects. Since dizziness may occur, change positions slowly, avoid alcohol and tasks that require alertness or motor skills. CBC and blood chemistry profile should be obtained before and periodically during therapy, especially with long-term use. B/P and pulse rate should be monitored to detect for arrhythmias and hypotension.

Administration

! Make sure at least 14 days elapse between the use of MAOIs and amitriptyline.

Take oral amitriptyline tablets with food or milk if GI distress occurs. Do not abruptly discontinue the drug. Full therapeutic effect may be noted in 2 to 4 weeks.

Give the drug by IM injection only if oral administration is not feasible. If crystals form in the ampoule, immerse it in hot water for 1 minute. Slowly inject drug deep into a large muscle, such as the gluteus maximus, to minimize pain at the injection site. Avoid the lateral aspect of the thigh.

Amlexanox
am-lecks-ah-knocks
(Apthasol)
Do not confuse with Ambesol.

CATEGORY AND SCHEDULE
Pregnancy Risk Category: B

CLASSIFICATION
Dermatologics

MECHANISM OF ACTION
A mouth agent that has anti-allergic and anti-inflammatory properties. Appears to inhibit formation and/or release of inflammatory mediators (e.g., histamine) from mast cells, neutrophils, mononuclear cells. *Therapeutic Effect:* Alleviates signs and symptoms of ahpthous ulcers.

PHARMACOKINETICS
After topical application, most systemic absorption occurs from the gastrointestinal (GI) tract. Metabolized to inactive metabolite. Excreted in urine. **Half-life:** 3.5 hrs.

AVAILABILITY
Paste: 5% (Apthasol).

INDICATIONS AND DOSAGES
▸ **Aphthous ulcers**
TOPICAL
Adults, Elderly. Administer ¼ inch directly to ulcers 4 times/day (after meals and at bedtime) following oral hygiene.

CONTRAINDICATIONS
Hypersensitivity to amlexanox or any component of the formulation

INTERACTIONS
Drug
None known.
Herbal
None known.
Food
None known.

DIAGNOSTIC TEST EFFECTS
None known.

SIDE EFFECTS
Rare
Stinging, burning at administration site, transient pain, rash

SERIOUS REACTIONS
• Ingestion of a full tube would result in nausea, vomiting, and diarrhea.

PRECAUTIONS & CONSIDERATIONS
Be aware that amlexanox should be discontinued if rash or contact mucositis develops. It is unknown if amlexanox crosses the placenta or is distributed in breast milk. There are no age-related precautions noted in children or the elderly.
Storage
Store at room temperature.
Administration
Apply as soon as possible after noticing symptoms. Apply directly on ulcers following oral hygiene, after meals, and at bedtime.

Amlodipine
am-low'di-peen
(Norvasc)
Do not confuse amlodipine with amiloride, or Norvasc with Navane or Vascor.

CATEGORY AND SCHEDULE
Pregnancy Risk Category: C

CLASSIFICATION
Calcium channel blockers

MECHANISM OF ACTION
A calcium channel blocker that inhibits calcium movement across cardiac and vascular smooth-muscle cell membranes. *Therapeutic Effect:* Relieves angina by dilating coronary arteries, peripheral arteries, and arterioles. Decreases total peripheral vascular resistance and B/P by vasodilation.

PHARMACOKINETICS
Route	Onset	Peak	Duration
PO	0.5-1 hr	6-12 hr	24 hr

Slowly absorbed from the GI tract. Protein binding: 93%. Undergoes first-pass metabolism in the liver. Excreted primarily in urine. Not removed by hemodialysis. **Half-life:** 30-50 hr (increased in the elderly and those with liver cirrhosis).

AVAILABILITY
Tablets: 2.5 mg, 5 mg, 10 mg.

INDICATIONS AND DOSAGES
▸ **Hypertension**
PO
Adults. Initially, 5 mg/day as a
single dose. Maximum: 10 mg/day.
Small-Frame, Fragile, Elderly.
Initially, 2.5 mg/day as a single dose.
▸ **Angina (chronic stable or
vasospastic)**
PO
Adults. 5-10 mg/day as a single
dose.
*Elderly, Patients with hepatic insuffi-
ciency:* 5 mg/day as a single dose.
▸ **Dosage in renal impairment**
For adults and elderly patients, give
2.5 mg/day.

CONTRAINDICATIONS
Severe hypotension

INTERACTIONS
Drug
None known.
Herbal
None known.
Food
Grapefruit, grapefruit juice: May
increase amlodipine blood concen-
tration and hypotensive effects.

DIAGNOSTIC TEST EFFECTS
None known.

SIDE EFFECTS
Frequent (greater than 5%)
Peripheral edema, headache, flushing
Occasional (less than 5%)
Dizziness, palpitations, nausea,
unusual fatigue or weakness
(asthenia)
Rare (less than 1%)
Chest pain, bradycardia, orthostatic
hypotension

SERIOUS REACTIONS
• Overdose may produce excessive
peripheral vasodilation and marked
hypotension with reflex tachycardia.

PRECAUTIONS & CONSIDERATIONS
Caution is warranted with aortic
stenosis, CHF, and impaired hepatic
function. It is unknown if amlodipine crosses the placenta or is
distributed in breast milk. The safety
and efficacy of amlodipine have not
been established in children. The
elderly are more sensitive to
amlodipine's hypotensive effects and
its half-life may be increased in the
elderly. Grapefruit juice, which may
increase amlodipine blood concentration, should be avoided. Tasks that
require alertness and motor skills
should also be avoided.
    Asthenia or headache may occur.
Apical pulse, B/P, and renal and
hepatic function test results should
be monitored before and during
therapy. Skin should be assessed for
flushing and peripheral edema, especially behind the medial malleolus
and the sacral area.
Administration
! Expect to increase amlodipine
dosage slowly over 7 to 14 days
based on response. Amlodipine
may be taken without regard to
food. Do not abruptly discontinue
amlodipine.

Ammonium Lactate
ah-moe′nee-um lack′tate
(Amlactin, Lac-Hydrin,
Lac-Hydrin Five, LAClotion)

CATEGORY AND SCHEDULE
Pregnancy Risk Category: C

CLASSIFICATION
Dermatologics

MECHANISM OF ACTION
Lactic acid is an alpha-hydroxy acid
that influences hydration, decreases

corneocyte cohesion, reduces excessive epidermal keratinization in hyperkeratotic conditions, and induces synthesis of mucopolysaccharides and collagen in photodamaged skin. The exact mechanism is not known. *Therapeutic Effect:* Increases hydration of the skin.

PHARMACOKINETICS
Not known.

AVAILABILITY
Cream: 12% (Amlactin).
Lotion: 5% (Lac-Hydrin Five), 12% (Amlactin, Lac-Hydrin. LAClotion).

INDICATIONS AND DOSAGES
▶ **Treatment of ichthyosis vulgaris and xerosis**
PO
Adults, Elderly. Apply sparingly and rub into area thoroughly q12hr.

CONTRAINDICATIONS
Hypersensitivity to ammonium lactate.

INTERACTIONS
Drug
Calcipotriene: May decrease the effects calcipotriene.
Herbal
None known.
Food
None known.

DIAGNOSTIC TEST EFFECTS
None known.

SIDE EFFECTS
Occasional (15%-2%)
Burning, stinging, rash, dry skin

PRECAUTIONS & CONSIDERATIONS
Caution is warranted in patients who are exposed to sunlight. Ammonium lactate should not be used on broken skin or in areas of infection and do not apply to the face, inguinal areas, or abraded skin. It is not known if ammonium lactate is distributed in breast milk. Safety and efficacy has not been established in children younger than 2 years of age.

Administration
Gently cleanse area prior to application. Use occlusive dressings only as ordered.
Apply sparingly and rub into area thoroughly.

Amobarbital
am-oh-bar'bi-tal
(Amytal sodium, Neur-Amyl [AUS])

CATEGORY AND SCHEDULE
Pregnancy Risk Category: D
Controlled substance: Schedule II

CLASSIFICATION
Barbiturates, preanesthetics, sedatives/hypnotics

MECHANISM OF ACTION
A barbiturate that depresses the sensory cortex, decreases motor activity, and alters cerebellar function. *Therapeutic Effect:* Produces drowsiness, sedation, and hypnosis.

PHARMACOKINETICS
Readily absorbed from the gastrointestinal (GI) tract and distributed. Protein binding: 60%. Metabolized in liver primarily by the hepatic microsomal enzyme system. Primarily excreted in urine.
Half-life: 16-40 hr.

AVAILABILITY
Powder for injection: 500 mg
(Amytal sodium).

INDICATIONS AND DOSAGES
▸ **Hypnotic**
IM/IV
Adults, Children older than 6 yrs.
65 to 200 mg at bedtime.
IM: Administer deeply into a large
muscle. Do not use more than 5 ml
at any single site (may cause tissue
damage). Maximum: 500 mg.
IV: Use only when IM administra-
tion is not feasible. Administer by
slow IV injection. Maximum:
50 mg/min in adults.
Children younger than 6 yrs. 2 to
3 mg/kg/dose.
▸ **Preanesthetic**
IM/IV
Adults, Children older than 6 yrs.
65 to 500 mg at bedtime.
▸ **Sedative**
IV
Adults. 30 to 50 mg given 2 or
3 times/day.

OFF-LABEL USES
Anticonvulsant

CONTRAINDICATIONS
History of manifest or latent
porphyria, marked liver dysfunction,
marked respiratory disease in which
dyspnea or obstruction is evident,
and hypersensitivity to amobarbital
products.

INTERACTIONS
Drug
Anticoagulants, steroids: May
decrease the effects of anticoagulants and steroids.
**Anticonvulsants, barbiturates,
benzodiazepines, valproic acid:**
May increase the metabolism of
anticonvulsants, barbiturates, benzodiazepines, and valproic acid.

**Central nervous system (CNS)
depressants:** May increase respiratory depression and hypotension.
**Corticosteroids, doxycycline,
griseofulvin:** May decrease the
effect of corticosteroids, doxycycline,
and griseofulvin.
MAOIs: May cause convulsions
and hypertensive crises.
Herbal
Valerian: May increase central
nervous system (CNS) depression.
St. John's wort: May decrease the
effects of amobarbital sodium.
Food
Ethanol: May increase central
nervous system (CNS) depression.
Food may decrease the rate of
absorption.

DIAGNOSTIC TEST EFFECTS
May falsely elevate phenobarbital
levels when measured with EMIT(R)
system.

▒ IV INCOMPATIBILITIES
Anileridine [CAN], atracurium
(Tacrium), cefazolin (Ancef),
cephalothin (Ceporacin [CAN]),
chlorpromazine (Thorazine), cimetidine (Tagamet), clindamycin
(Cleocin), codeine, dimenhydrinate
(Dramamine), diphenhydramine
(Benadryl), droperidol (Inapsine),
hydrocortisone, hydroxyzine
(Atarax, Vistaril), insulin, isopro-
terenol (Isuprel), levorphanol (Levo-
Dromaron), meperidine (Demerol),
metaraminol (Aramine), methadone
(Dolophine, Methadose), methyl-
dopa (Aldomet), methylphenidate
(Concerta, Ritalin), morphine
(Avinza, Kadian, Roxanol),
norepinephrine (Levophed),
oxytetracycline (Terramycin),
pancuronium (Pavulon), penicillin G
(Bicillin), pentazocine (Talwin),
phytonadione (AquaMEPHYTON,
Mephyton), procaine (Novocain),

prochlorperazine (Compazine), propiomazine (Largon), streptomycin, succinylcholine (Anectine), tetracycline (Sumycin), vancomycin (Vancocin)

🝳 IV compatibilities
Amikacin, aminophylline, sodium bicarbonate

SIDE EFFECTS
Frequent
Somnolence, headache, confusion, dizziness
Occasional
Nausea, vomiting, visual abnormalities, such as spots before eyes, difficulty focusing, blurred vision, dry mouth or pharynx, tongue irritation, water retention, increased sweating, constipation, or diarrhea

SERIOUS REACTIONS
• Overdosage results in severe respiratory depression, skeletal muscle flaccidity, bronchospasm, cardiovascular disturbances, such as congestive heart failure (CHF), hypotension or hypertension, arrhythmias, cold and clammy skin, cyanosis, and coma.
• Tolerance may occur with repeated use.

PRECAUTIONS & CONSIDERATIONS
Caution is necessary in patients with impaired cardiac, liver, or renal function. Amobarbital crosses the placenta and is distributed in breast milk. Behavioral changes are more likely to occur in children and the elderly. Blood pressure (B/P) for hypotension, level of sedation, and pulse for bradycardia as well as respiratory rate and rhythm should be monitored. Change positions slowly to avoid orthostatic hypotension. Tasks that require mental alertness or motor skills should be avoided.

Storage
Store at room temperature.
Administration
Each 125 mg must be diluted with a maximum of 1.25 ml of sterile water for injection to make a 10% solution. Vial should not be left opened for more than 30 minutes until it is injected. The rate of IV injection should not exceed 50 mg/min to prevent sleep or sudden respiratory depression.

Amoxapine
a-moks-a-peen
(Ascendin)
Do not confuse with atomoxetine or atropine.

CATEGORY AND SCHEDULE
Pregnancy Risk Category: C

CLASSIFICATION
Antidepressants, tricyclic

MECHANISM OF ACTION
A tricyclic antidepressant that blocks the reuptake of neurotransmitters, such as norepinephrine and serotonin, at central nervous system (CNS) presynaptic membranes, increasing their availability at postsynaptic receptor sites. The metabolite, 7-OH-amoxapine has significant dopamine receptor blocking activity similar to haloperidol. *Therapeutic Effect:* Produces antidepressant effects.

PHARMACOKINETICS
Rapidly, well absorbed from the gastrointestinal (GI) tract. Protein binding: 90%. Metabolized in liver.

Excreted in urine and feces.
Half-life: 8 hr.

AVAILABILITY
Tablets: 25 mg, 50 mg, 100 mg,
150 mg (Ascendin).

INDICATIONS AND DOSAGES
▶ **Depression**
PO
Adults. 25 mg 2-3 times/day. May
increase to 100 mg 2-3 times/day.
Adolescents. Initially, 25-50 mg/day
as single or divided doses. May
increase to 100 mg/day.
Elderly. Initially, 25 mg at bedtime.
May increase by 25 mg/day q3-
7 days. Maximum: 400 mg/day
(outpatient), 600 mg/day (inpatient).

OFF-LABEL USES
Panic disorder

CONTRAINDICATIONS
Acute recovery period following
myocardial infarction (MI), within
14 days of MAOI ingestion, hypersensitivity to dibenzoxazepine
compounds

INTERACTIONS
Drug
Alcohol, CNS depressants: May
increase CNS and respiratory
depression and amoxapine's
hypotensive effects.
Antithyroid agents: May increase
risk of agranulocytosis.
Cimetidine: May increase amoxapine blood concentration and risk of
toxicity.
Clonidine, guanadrel: May
decrease the effects of clonidine and
guanadrel
Estrogens, SSRIs: May increase
risk of amoxapine toxicity.
**Fluoroquinolones, sympa-
thomimetics:** May increase cardiac
effects.

MAOIs: May increase the risk of
convulsions, hyperpyresis, and
hypertensive crisis.
Nefopam: May increase risk of
seizures.
Phenothiazines: May increase the
anticholinergic and sedative effects
of clomipramine.
Herbal
St. John's Wort: May increase risk
of serotonin syndrome.
Food
None known.

DIAGNOSTIC TEST EFFECTS
None known.

SIDE EFFECTS
Frequent
Drowsiness, fatigue, xerostomia,
constipation, weight gain
Occasional
Nausea, dizziness, headache, confusion, nervousness, restlessness, insomnia, edema, tremor, blurred vision,
aggressiveness, muscle weakness
Rare
Paradoxical reactions (agitation, restlessness, nightmares, insomnia,
extrapyramidal symptoms, particularly
fine hand tremor), laryngitis, seizures

SERIOUS REACTIONS
• High dosage may produce cardiovascular effects, including severe
postural hypotension, dizziness,
tachycardia, palpitations, and
arrhythmias, and seizures. High
dosage may also result in altered
temperature regulation, such as
hyperpyrexia or hypothermia.
• Abrupt withdrawal from
prolonged therapy may produce
headache, malaise, nausea, vomiting,
and vivid dreams.

PRECAUTIONS & CONSIDERATIONS
Caution is warranted with cardiac
conduction disturbances,

cardiovascular disease, hyperthy-roidism, seizure disorders, and urinary retention, and in persons taking thyroid replacement therapy. Be aware that amoxapine is distrib-uted in breast milk. There are no age-related precautions noted in children older than 16 years of age. Expect to use lower dosages in the elderly. Higher dosages are not tolerated well, and increase the risk of toxicity in the elderly. Blurred vision, drowsiness, constipation, and dry mouth may occur during therapy. Change positions slowly to avoid postural hypotension. Avoid alcohol and tasks that require mental alertness or motor skills. Tolerance usually develops to amoxapine's anticholinergic effects, postural hypotension, and sedative effects.

Administration
May be taken as a single dose usually at bedtime, usually without food. Doses greater than 300 mg/day should be taken in divided doses.

Amoxicillin
a-mox′i-sill-in
(Alphamox [AUS], Amohexal [AUS], Amoxil, Apo-Amoxi [CAN], Cilamox [AUS], Clamoxyl [AUS], DisperMox, Fisamox [AUS], Moxamox [AUS], Moxacin [AUS], Novamoxin [CAN], Polymox, Trimox, Wymox)
Do not confuse amoxicillin with amoxapine, Diamox, Trimox, or Tylox.

CATEGORY AND SCHEDULE
Pregnancy Risk Category: B

CLASSIFICATION
Antibiotics, penicillins

MECHANISM OF ACTION
A penicillin that inhibits bacterial cell wall synthesis. *Therapeutic Effect:* Bactericidal in susceptible microorganisms.

PHARMACOKINETICS
Well absorbed from the GI tract. Protein binding: 20%. Partially metabolized in the liver. Primarily excreted in urine. Removed by hemodialysis. **Half-life:** 1-1.3 hr (increased in impaired renal function).

AVAILABILITY
Capsules (Amoxil, Moxillin, Trimox): 250 mg, 500 mg.
Oral drops (Amoxil): 125 mg/5 ml, 200 mg/5 ml, 250 mg/5 ml, 400 mg/5 ml.
Tablets (Amoxil): 500 mg, 875 mg.
Tablets, chewable (Amoxil): 200 mg, 250 mg, 400 mg.
Tablets for Oral Suspension (DisperMox): 200 mg, 400 mg.

INDICATIONS AND DOSAGES
▸ **Ear, nose, throat, GU, skin, and skin-structure infections**
PO
Adults, Elderly, Children weighing more than 20 kg. 250-500 mg q8hr or 500-875 mg (tablets) twice a day
Children weighing less than 20 kg. 20-40 mg/kg/day in divided doses q8-12hr.
▸ **Lower respiratory tract infections**
PO
Adults, Elderly, Children weighing more than 20 kg. 500 mg q8hr or 875 mg (tablets) twice a day.
Children weighing less than 20 kg. 40 mg/kg/day in divided doses q8-12hr.
▸ **Acute, uncomplicated gonorrhea**
PO
Adults. 3 g one time with 1 g probenecid. Follow with tetracycline or erythromycin therapy.

Children 2 yr and older. 50 mg/kg plus probenecid 25 mg/kg as a single dose.

▶ **Acute otitis media**
PO
Children. 80-90 mg/kg/day in divided doses q12hr.

▶ ***Helicobacter pylori* infection**
PO
Adults, Elderly. 1 g twice a day for 10 days (in combination with other antibiotics).

▶ **Prevention of endocarditis**
PO
Adults, Elderly. 2 g 1 hr before procedure.
Children. 50 mg/kg 1 hr before procedure.

▶ **Usual pediatric dosage**
Children younger than 3 mo, Neonates. 20-30 mg/kg/day in divided doses q12hr.

▶ **Dosage in renal impairment**
Dosage interval is modified based on creatinine clearance.
Creatinine clearance 10-30 ml/min. Usual dose q12hr.
Creatinine clearance less than 10 ml/min. Usual dose q24hr.

OFF-LABEL USES
Treatment of Lyme disease and typhoid fever

CONTRAINDICATIONS
Hypersensitivity to any penicillin, infectious mononucleosis

INTERACTIONS
Drug
Allopurinol: May increase incidence of rash.
Oral contraceptives: May decrease effectiveness of oral contraceptives.
Probenecid: May increase amoxicillin blood concentration and risk of toxicity.
Herbal
None known.

Food
None known.

DIAGNOSTIC TEST EFFECTS
May increase BUN and serum LDH, bilirubin, creatinine, AST (SGOT), and ALT (SGPT) levels. May cause a positive Coombs' test.

SIDE EFFECTS
Frequent
GI disturbances (mild diarrhea, nausea, or vomiting), headache, oral or vaginal candidiasis
Occasional
Generalized rash, urticaria

SERIOUS REACTIONS
• Antibiotic-associated colitis and other superinfections may result from altered bacterial balance.
• Severe hypersensitivity reactions, including anaphylaxis and acute interstitial nephritis occur rarely.

PRECAUTIONS & CONSIDERATIONS
Caution is warranted with antibiotic-associated colitis or a history of allergies, especially to cephalosporins. Amoxicillin crosses the placenta, appears in cord blood and amniotic fluid, and is distributed in breast milk in low concentrations. Amoxicillin administration may lead to allergic sensitization, candidiasis, diarrhea, and skin rash in infants. Immature renal function in neonates and young infants may delay renal excretion of amoxicillin. Age-related renal impairment may require dosage adjustment in the elderly.

History of allergies, especially to cephalosporins or penicillins, should be determined before giving the drug. Withhold amoxicillin and promptly notify the physician if rash or diarrhea occurs. Severe diarrhea with abdominal pain, blood or mucus in stool, and fever may indicate antibiotic-associated colitis. Signs and symptoms of superinfection, including anal or genital pruritus, black hairy tongue, diarrhea, increased fever, sore throat, ulceration or changes of oral mucosa, and vomiting should be monitored.

Storage
Store capsules or tablets at room temperature. After reconstitution, the oral solution is stable for 14 days either at room temperature or refrigerated.

Administration
Chew or crush chewable tablets thoroughly before swallowing. Take amoxicillin without regard to food. Take evenly around the clock and continue for the full course of treatment.

Amoxicillin/ Clavulanate

a-mox′i-sill-in clav-u-lan′ate
(Augmentin, Augmentin ES 600, Augmentin XR, Ausclav [AUS], Ausclav Duo Forte [AUS], Ausclav Duo 400 [AUS], Clamoxyl [AUS], Clamoxyl Duo 400 [AUS], Clamoxyl Duo Forte [AUS], Clavulin [CAN], Clavulin Duo Forte [AUS])
Do not confuse with amoxapine.

CATEGORY AND SCHEDULE
Pregnancy Risk Category: B

CLASSIFICATION
Antibiotics, penicillins

MECHANISM OF ACTION
Amoxicillin inhibits bacterial cell wall synthesis, while clavulanate inhibits bacterial beta-lactamase. *Therapeutic Effect:* Amoxicillin is bactericidal in susceptible microorganisms. Clavulanate protects amoxicillin from enzymatic degradation.

PHARMACOKINETICS
Well absorbed from the GI tract. Protein binding: 20%. Partially metabolized in the liver. Primarily excreted in urine. Removed by hemodialysis. **Half-life**: 1-1.3 hr (increased in impaired renal function).

AVAILABILITY
Powder for Oral Suspension:
125 mg/5 ml, 200 mg/5 ml, 250 mg/5 ml, 400 mg/5 ml, 600 mg/5 ml.
Tablets: 250 mg, 500 mg, 875 mg.
Tablets (Extended-Release):
1000 mg.
Tablets (Chewable): 125 mg, 200 mg, 250 mg, 400 mg.

INDICATIONS AND DOSAGES
▸ **Mild to moderate infections**
PO
Adults, Elderly, Children weighing more than 40 kg. 250 mg q8hr or 500 mg q12hr.
Children weighing less than 40 kg. 20 mg/kg/day in divided doses q8hr.
▸ **Respiratory tract and other severe infections**
PO
Adults, Elderly, Children weighing more than 40 kg. 500 mg q8hr or 875 mg q12hr.
Children weighing less than 40 kg. 40 mg/kg/day in divided doses q8hr.
▸ **Otitis media**
PO
Children. 90 mg/kg/day in divided doses q12hr for 10 days.

▸ **Sinusitis, lower respiratory tract infections**

PO

Children. 40 mg/kg/day in divided doses q8hr or 45 mg/kg/day in divided doses q12hr.

▸ **Usual neonate dosage**

PO

Neonates, Children younger than 3 mos. 30 mg/kg/day in divided doses q12hr.

▸ **Dosage in renal impairment**

Dosage and frequency are modified based on creatinine clearance.

Creatinine clearance 10-30 ml/min: 250-500 mg q12hr.

Creatinine clearance less than 10 ml/min: 250-500 mg q24hr.

OFF-LABEL USES

Treatment of bronchitis and chancroid

CONTRAINDICATIONS

Hypersensitivity to any penicillins, infectious mononucleosis

INTERACTIONS

Drug

Allopurinol: May increase incidence of rash.

Oral contraceptives: May decrease effects of oral contraceptives.

Probenecid: May increase amoxicillin and clavulanate blood concentration and risk of toxicity.

Herbal

None known.

Food

None known.

DIAGNOSTIC TEST EFFECTS

May increase serum AST (SGOT) and ALT (SGPT) levels. May cause a positive Coombs' test.

SIDE EFFECTS

Frequent

GI disturbances (mild diarrhea, nausea, vomiting), headache, oral or vaginal candidiasis

Occasional

Generalized rash, urticaria

SERIOUS REACTIONS

• Antibiotic-associated colitis and other superinfections may result from altered bacterial balance.

• Severe hypersensitivity reactions, including anaphylaxis and acute interstitial nephritis occur rarely.

PRECAUTIONS & CONSIDERATIONS

Caution is warranted with antibiotic-associated colitis or a history of allergies, especially to cephalosporins. Amoxicillin and clavulanate crosses the placenta, appears in cord blood and amniotic fluid, and is distributed in breast milk in low concentrations. Amoxicillin and clavulanate may lead to allergic sensitization, candidiasis, diarrhea, and skin rash in infants. Immature renal function in neonates and young infants may delay renal excretion of amoxicillin and clavulanate. Age-related renal impairment may require dosage adjustment in the elderly.

History of allergies, especially to cephalosporins or penicillins, should be determined before giving the drug. Withhold and promptly notify the physician if rash or diarrhea occurs. Severe diarrhea with abdominal pain, blood or mucus in stool, and fever may indicate antibiotic-associated colitis. Signs and symptoms of superinfection, including anal or genital pruritus, black hairy tongue, diarrhea, increased fever, sore throat, ulceration or changes of oral mucosa, and vomiting should be monitored.

Storage
Store capsules or tablets at room
temperature. After reconstitution, the
oral solution is stable for 14 days
either at room temperature or refrigerated.
Administration
! Drug dosage is expressed in
terms of amoxicillin. Be aware
that an alternative dosage is
500 to 875 mg twice a day
for adults and 200 to 400 mg
twice a day for children.
Take the drug without regard
to meals. Chew or crush
chewable tablets thoroughly
before swallowing. Space doses
evenly around the clock and
continue for the full course of
treatment.

Amphetamine
am-fet′ah-meen

CATEGORY AND SCHEDULE
Pregnancy Risk Category: C
Controlled substance:
Schedule II

CLASSIFICATION
Adrenergic agonists, amphetamines, anorexiants, stimulants,
central nervous system

MECHANISM OF ACTION
A sympathomimetic amine that
produces central nervous system
(CNS) and respiratory stimulation,
mydriasis, bronchodilation, a pressor
response, and contraction of the
urinary sphincter. Directly affects
alpha and beta receptor sites in
peripheral system. Enhances release
of norepinephrine by blocking reuptake, inhibiting monoamine oxidase.

Therapeutic Effect: Increases motor
activity, mental alertness; decreases
drowsiness, fatigue.

PHARMACOKINETICS
Well absorbed from the gastrointestinal (GI) tract. Protein binding: 20%.
Widely distributed (including CSF).
Metabolized in liver. Excreted in
urine. Unknown if removed by
hemodialysis. **Half-life:** 7-31 hr.

AVAILABILITY
Tablets: 5 mg, 10 mg.

INDICATIONS AND DOSAGES
▶ **Attention-deficit hyperactivity
disorder (ADHD)**
PO
Adults. 5-20 mg 1-3 times/day.
Adults, Children older than 12 yr.
Initially, 5 mg twice a day.
Increase by 10 mg at weekly inter-
vals until therapeutic response
achieved.
Children 6-12 yr. Initially, 2.5 mg
twice a day. Increase by 5 mg/day at
weekly intervals until therapeutic
response achieved.
Children 3-6 yr. Initially, 2.5 mg
twice a day. Increase by 2.5 mg/day
at weekly intervals until therapeutic
response achieved.
▶ **Narcolepsy**
PO
Adults. 5-20 mg 1-3 times/day.
*Adults, Children older than
12 yr.* Initially, 5 mg twice a day.
Increase by 10 mg at weekly intervals until therapeutic response
achieved.
Children 6-12 yr. Initially, 2.5 mg
twice a day. Increase by 5 mg/day at
weekly intervals until therapeutic
response achieved.

OFF-LABEL USES
Depression, obsessive-compulsive
disorder

CONTRAINDICATIONS

Advanced arteriosclerosis, agitated states, glaucoma, history of drug abuse, history of hypersensitivity to sympathomimetic amines, hyperthyroidism, moderate to severe hypertension, symptomatic cardiovascular disease, within 14 days following discontinuation of an MAOI

INTERACTIONS
Drug

Beta-blockers: May increase risk of bradycardia, heart block, and hypertension.

Central nervous system (CNS) stimulants: May increase the effects of amphetamine.

Digoxin: May increase the risk of arrhythmias with this drug.

MAOIs: May prolong and intensify the effects of amphetamine.

Meperidine: May increase the risk of hypotension, respiratory depression, seizures, and vascular collapse.

Tricyclic antidepressants: May increase cardiovascular effects.

Herbal

None known.

Food

None known.

DIAGNOSTIC TEST EFFECTS

May increase plasma corticosteroid concentrations.

SIDE EFFECTS
Frequent

Irregular pulse, increased motor activity, talkativeness, nervousness, mild euphoria, insomnia

Occasional

Headache, chills, dry mouth, gastrointestinal (GI) distress, worsening depression in patients who are clinically depressed, tachycardia, palpitations, chest pain

SERIOUS REACTIONS

• Overdose may produce skin pallor or flushing, arrhythmias, and psychosis.
• Abrupt withdrawal following prolonged administration of high dosage may produce lethargy (may last for weeks).
• Prolonged administration to children with ADHD may produce a temporary suppression of normal weight and height patterns.

PRECAUTIONS & CONSIDERATIONS

Precaution is necessary with acute stress reaction, emotional instability, history of drug dependence, hypertension, seizures as well as the elderly and debilitated and those who are tartrazine-sensitive. It is unknown if amphetamine crosses the placenta or is distributed in breast milk. Children may be more susceptible to develop abdominal pain, anorexia, decreased weight, and insomnia. There are no age-related precautions noted in the elderly.

Decreased appetite, dizziness, dry mouth, or pronounced nervousness may be experienced. Tasks that require mental alertness or motor skills should be avoided until the effects of the drug are determined.

Administration

Take dose 30 to 45 minutes before meals. Do not take in afternoon or evening because the drug can cause insomnia.

Amphotericin B

am-foe-ter'i-sin bee
(Abelcet, AmBisome, Amphocin,
Amphotec, Fungizone)

CATEGORY AND SCHEDULE

Pregnancy Risk Category: B

CLASSIFICATION

Antifungals

MECHANISM OF ACTION

An antifungal and antiprotozoal that
is generally fungistatic but may
become fungicidal with high dosages
or very susceptible microorganisms.
This drug binds to sterols in the
fungal cell membrane. *Therapeutic
Effect:* Increases fungal cell-membrane
permeability, allowing loss of potassium and other cellular components.

PHARMACOKINETICS

Protein binding: 90%. Widely
distributed. Metabolic fate unknown.
Cleared by nonrenal pathways.
Minimal removal by hemodialysis.
Amphotec and Abelcet are not
dialyzable. **Half-life:** Fungizone,
24 hr (increased in neonates and children); Amphotec, 26-28 hr; Abelcet,
7.2 days; AmBisome, 100-153 hr.

AVAILABILITY

Cream (Fungizone): 3%.
*Injection, powder for reconstitution:
(Amphotec):* 50 mg, 100 mg.
*Injection, powder for reconstitution
(AmBisome, Amphocin, Fungizone):*
50 mg.
Injection, suspension (Abelcet):
5 mg/ml.

INDICATIONS AND DOSAGES

▶ **Cryptococcosis; blastomycosis;
systemic candidiasis; disseminated**
forms of moniliasis, coccidioidomycosis, and histoplasmosis; zygomycosis; sporotrichosis; aspergillosis
IV INFUSION (FUNGIZONE)
Adults, Elderly. Dosage based on
patient tolerance and severity of
infection. Initially, 1-mg test dose is
given over 20-30 min. If test dose is
tolerated, 5-mg dose may be given
the same day. Subsequently, dosage
is increased by 5 mg q12-24hr until
desired daily dose is reached.
Alternatively, if test dose is tolerated,
0.25 mg/kg is given on same day and
0.5 mg/kg on second day; then
dosage is increased until desired
daily dose reached. Total daily dose:
1 mg/kg/day up to 1.5 mg/kg every
other day. Maximum: 1.5 mg/kg/day.
Children. Test dose of
0.1 mg/kg/dose (maximum 1 mg) is
infused over 20-60 min. If test dose
is tolerated, initial dose of 0.4 mg/kg
may be given on same day; dosage is
then increased in 0.25-mg/kg increments as needed. Maintenance dose:
0.25-1 mg/kg/day.
Invasive fungal infections unresponsive to or intolerant of Fungizone
IV INFUSION (ABELCET)
Adults, Children. 5 mg/kg at rate of
2.5 mg/kg/hr.
▶ **Empiric treatment of fungal infections in patients with febrile
neutropenia; aspergillosis, candidiasis, or cryptococcosis in patients
with renal impairment and those
who have experienced toxicity or
treatment failure with Fungizone**
IV INFUSION (AMBISOME)
Adults, Children. 3-5 mg/kg over 1 hr.
▶ **Invasive aspergillosis in patients
with renal impairment and those
who have experienced toxicity or
treatment failure with Fungizone**
IV INFUSION (AMPHOTEC)
Adults, Children. 3-4 mg/kg over
2-4 hr.

▸ **Cutaneous and mucocutaneous infections caused by Candida albicans, such as paronychia, oral thrush, perléche, diaper rash, and intertriginous candidiasis**
TOPICAL
Adults, Elderly, Children. Apply liberally to affected area and rub in 2-4 times a day.

CONTRAINDICATIONS
Hypersensitivity to amphotericin B or sulfites

INTERACTIONS
Drug
Bone marrow depressants: May increase the risk of anemia.
Digoxin: May increase the risk of digoxin toxicity from hypokalemia.
Nephrotoxic medications: May increase the risk of nephrotoxicity.
Steroids: May cause severe hypokalemia.
Herbal
None known.
Food
None known.

DIAGNOSTIC TEST EFFECTS
May increase BUN, serum alkaline phosphatase, serum creatinine, serum SGOT (AST), and SGPT (ALT) levels. May decrease serum calcium, magnesium, and potassium levels.

▨ IV INCOMPATIBILITIES
Abelcet, AmBisome, Amphotec: Don't mix with any other drug, diluent, or solution. Fungizone: Allopurinol (Aloprim), amifostine (Ethyol), aztreonam (Azactam), calcium gluconate, cefepime (Maxipime), cimetidine (Tagamet), ciprofloxacin (Cipro), docetaxel (Taxotere), dopamine (Intropin), doxorubicin (Adriamycin), enalapril (Vasotec), etoposide (VP-16),

filgrastim (Neupogen), fluconazole (Diflucan), fludarabine (Fludara), foscarnet (Foscavir), gemcitabine (Gemzar), magnesium sulfate, meropenem (Merrem IV), ondansetron (Zofran), paclitaxel (Taxol), piperacillin and tazobactam (Zosyn), potassium chloride, propofol (Diprivan), vinorelbine (Navelbine)

▨ IV compatibilities
None known; don't mix with other medications or electrolytes.

SIDE EFFECTS
Frequent (greater than 10%)
Abelcet: Chills, fever, increased serum creatinine level, multiple organ failure
AmBisome: Hypokalemia, hypomagnesemia, hyperglycemia, hypocalcemia, edema, abdominal pain, back pain, chills, chest pain, hypotension, diarrhea, nausea, vomiting, headache, fever, rigors, insomnia, dyspnea, epistaxis, increased hepatic or renal function test results
Amphotec: Chills, fever, hypotension, tachycardia, increased serum creatinine level, hypokalemia, bilirubinemia
Fungizone: Fever, chills, headache, anemia, hypokalemia, hypomagnesemia, anorexia, malaise, generalized pain, nephrotoxicity
Topical: Local irritation, dry skin
Rare
Topical: Rash

SERIOUS REACTIONS
• Cardiovascular toxicity (as evidenced by hypotension, ventricular fibrillation, and anaphylaxis) occurs rarely.
• Altered vision and hearing, seizures, hepatic failure, coagulation defects, multiple organ failure, and sepsis may be noted.

PRECAUTIONS & CONSIDERATIONS

Caution is warranted with renal impairment and in combination with antineoplastic therapy. Drug is prescribed only for progressive, potentially fatal fungal infection. Keep in mind that conventional amphotericin, Fungizone, is more nephrotoxic than the alternative formulations of amphotericin B, including Albecet, AmBisome, and Amphotec. Amphotericin B crosses the placenta, and it is unknown if amphotericin B is distributed in breast milk. Safety and efficacy of amphotericin B have not been established in children. Therefore, expect to use the smallest dose necessary to achieve optimal results. There are no age-related precautions noted in the elderly.

History of allergies, especially to amphotericin B and sulfites, should be determined before giving the drug. Be aware that other nephrotoxic medications should be avoided, if possible. Antiemetics, antihistamines, antipyretics, or small doses of corticosteroids may be given before or during amphotericin administration to help control adverse reactions.

Blood pressure (B/P), pulse, respirations, and temperature should be monitored twice every 15 minutes, then every 30 minutes for the initial 4 hours of the infusion to assess for adverse reactions. Adverse reactions include abdominal pain, anorexia, chills, fever, nausea, shaking, and vomiting. If signs and symptoms of adverse reactions occur, slow the infusion and give prescribed drugs to provide symptomatic relief. For a severe reaction or for patients without orders for symptomatic relief, stop the infusion and notify the physician.

Storage

Refrigerate Albecet as unreconstituted solution. Albecet reconstituted solution is stable for 48 hours if refrigerated and 6 hours at room temperature.

Refrigerate AmBisome as unreconstituted solution. AmBisome reconstituted solution of 4 mg/ml is stable for 24 hours. AmBisome reconstituted solution concentration of 1-2 mg/ml is stable for 6 hours.

Store Amphotec as unreconstituted solution at room temperature. Amphotec reconstituted solution is stable for 24 hours.

Refrigerate Fungizone as unreconstituted solution. Fungizone reconstituted solution is stable for 24 hours at room temperature or 7 days if refrigerated. Diluted solution less than or equal to 0.1 mg/ml should be used promptly. Do not use the solution if it is cloudy or contains a precipitate.

Administration

For IV use, observe strict aseptic technique because no bacteriostatic agent or preservative is present in the diluent.

Shake Abelcet 20-ml (100-mg) vial gently until contents are dissolved. Withdraw required Abelcet dose using a 5-micron filter needle supplied by manufacturer. Inject Abelcet dose into D_5W; 4 ml D_5W is required for each 1 ml (5 mg) to final concentration of 1 mg/ml. Reduce dose by half for pediatric, fluid-restricted patients (2 mg/ml). Infuse Abelcet over 2 hours by slow IV infusion. Shake the contents if the infusion is greater than 2 hours. Reconstitute each 50-mg AmBisome vial with 12 ml sterile water for injection to provide concentration of 4 mg/ml. Shake AmBisome vial vigorously for 30 seconds. Then, withdraw the required AmBisome dose and empty the syringe contents through a 5-micron filter into an infusion of D_5W to provide final concentration of 1 to 2 mg/ml. Infuse AmBisome over 1 to 2 hours by slow IV infusion.

Add 10 ml sterile water for injection to each 50-mg Amphotec vial to provide a concentration of 5 mg/ml. Shake the Amphotec vial gently. Further dilute Amphotec vial only with D_5W using specific amount recommended by manufacturer to provide concentration of 0.16 to 0.83 mg/ml. Infuse Amphotec over 2 to 4 hours by slow IV infusion.

Rapidly inject 10 ml Sterile Water for Injection to each 50-mg Fungizone vial to provide concentration of 5 mg/ml. Immediately shake Fungizone vial until the solution is clear. Further dilute each 1 mg Fungizone in at least 10 ml D_5W to provide a concentration of 0.1 mg/ml. Be aware that the potential for thrombophlebitis may be less with the use of pediatric scalp vein needles or by adding dilute heparin solution, as prescribed. Infuse conventional amphotericin, Fungizone, over 2 to 6 hours by slow IV infusion.

Amphotericin B/ Amphotericin B Cholesteryl/ Amphotericin B Lipid Complex/ Liposomal Amphotericin B

(Abelcet, AmBisome, Amphotec, Fungizone)

CATEGORY AND SCHEDULE
Pregnancy Risk Category: B

CLASSIFICATION
Antifungal agent

MECHANISM OF ACTION
The amphotericin B group is antifungal and antiprotozoal and generally fungistatic but may become fungicidal with high dosages or very susceptible microorganisms. This drug binds to sterols in the fungal cell membrane. *Therapeutic Effect:* Increases fungal cell-membrane permeability, allowing loss of potassium, and other cellular components.

PHARMACOKINETICS
Protein binding: 90%. Widely distributed. Metabolic fate unknown. Cleared by nonrenal pathways. Minimal removal by hemodialysis. Amphotec and Abelcet are not dialyzable. **Half-life:** 24 hr (half-life increased in neonates, children). Amphotec **half-life:** 26-28 hr. Abelcet **half-life:** 7.2 days. AmBisome **half-life:** 100-153 hr.

AVAILABILITY
Injection: 50 mg, 50 mg (Fungizone), 100 mg (Amphotec), 50 mg (AmBisome).
Suspension for Injection: 5 mg/ml (Amphotericin B lipid complex, Abelcet).
Cream, Lotion, Ointment: 3% (Fungizone).

INDICATIONS AND DOSAGES
▶ **Invasive fungal infections unresponsive or intolerant to Fungizone (Abelcet)**
IV INFUSION
Adults, Children. 5 mg/kg at rate of 2.5 mg/kg/hr.
▶ **Empiric treatment for fungal infection in patients with febrile neutropenia; for aspergillus, candida, or cryptococcus infections unresponsive to Fungizone; or for patients with renal impairment or toxicity from Fungizone (AmBisome)**
IV INFUSION

Adults, Children. 3-5 mg/kg over 1 hr.
▶ **Invasive aspergillus in patients with renal impairment, renal toxicity, or treatment failure with Fungizone.(Amphotec)**
IV INFUSION
Adults, Children. 3-4 mg/kg over 2-4 hrs.
▶ **Cutaneous and mucocutaneous infections caused by *Candida albicans*, such as paronychia, oral thrush, perléche, diaper rash, and intertriginous candidiasis (Topical)**
Adults, Elderly, Children. Apply liberally to the affected area and rub in 2-4 times/day.
▶ **Cryptococcosis; blastomycosis; systemic candidiasis; disseminated forms of moniliasis, coccidioidomycosis, and histoplasmosis; zygomycosis; sporotrichosis; and aspergillosis (Fungizone)**
IV INFUSION
Adults, Elderly. Dosage based on pt tolerance, severity of infection. Initially, 1-mg test dose is given over 20-30 min. If test dose is tolerated, 5-mg dose may be given the same day. Subsequently, increases of 5 mg/dose are made q12-24hr until desired daily dose is reached. Alternatively, if test dose is tolerated, a dose of 0.25 mg/kg is given same day; increased to 0.5 mg/kg the second day. Dose increased until desired daily dose reached. Total daily dose: 1 mg/kg/day up to 1.5 mg/kg every other day. Do not exceed maximum total daily dose of 1.5 mg/kg.
Children. Test dose: 0.1 mg/kg/dose (maximum 1 mg) infused over 20-60 min. If tolerated, then initial dose: 0.4 mg/kg same day; dose may be increased in 0.25 mg/kg increments. Maintenance dose: 0.25-1 mg/kg/day.

CONTRAINDICATIONS
Hypersensitivity to amphotericin B, sulfite

INTERACTIONS
Drug
Bone marrow depressants: May increase risk for anemia.
Digoxin: May increase risk of digoxin toxicity from hypokalemia.
Nephrotoxic medications: May increase risk of nephrotoxicity.
Steroids: May cause severe hypokalemia.
Herbal
None known.
Food
None known.

DIAGNOSTIC TEST EFFECTS
May increase BUN, serum alkaline phosphatase, serum creatinine, SGOT (AST), and SGPT (ALT) levels. May decrease serum calcium, magnesium, and potassium levels.

▓ IV INCOMPATIBILITIES
Abelcet/Amphotec/AmBisome: Do not mix with any other drug, diluent, or solution. Fungizone: Allopurinol (Aloprim), amifostine (Ethyol), aztreonam (Azactam), calcium gluconate, cefepime (Maxipime), cimetidine (Tagamet), ciprofloxacin (Cipro), docetaxel (Taxotere), dopamine (Intropin), doxorubicin (Adriamycin), enalapril (Vasotec), etoposide (VP-16), filgrastim (Neupogen), fluconazole (Diflucan), fludarabine (Fludara), foscarnet (Foscavir), gemcitabine (Gemzar), magnesium sulfate, meropenem (Merrem IV), ondansetron (Zofran), paclitaxel (Taxol), piperacillin/ tazobactam (Zosyn), potassium chloride, propofol (Diprivan), vinorelbine (Navelbine)

📖 **IV compatibilities**
None known; do not mix with other medications or electrolytes.

SIDE EFFECTS

Frequent (greater than 10%)
Abelcet: Chills, fever, increased serum creatinine, multiple organ failure
AmBisome: Hypokalemia, hypomagnesemia, hyperglycemia, hypocalcemia, edema, abdominal pain, back pain, chills, chest pain, hypotension, diarrhea, nausea, vomiting, headache, fever, rigors, insomnia, dyspnea, epistaxis, increased liver/renal function test results
Amphotec: Chills, fever, hypotension, tachycardia, increased creatinine, hypokalemia, bilirubinemia
Fungizone: Fever, chills, headache, anemia, hypokalemia, hypomagnesemia, anorexia, malaise, generalized pain, nephrotoxicity
Topical: Local irritation, dry skin
Rare
Topical: Skin rash

SERIOUS REACTIONS

• Cardiovascular toxicity as evidenced by hypotension and ventricular fibrillation and anaphylaxis occur rarely.
• Vision and hearing alterations, seizures, liver failure, coagulation defects, multiple organ failure, and sepsis may be noted.

PRECAUTIONS & CONSIDERATIONS

Caution is warranted with renal impairment and in combination with antineoplastic therapy. Drug is prescribed only for progressive, potentially fatal fungal infection. Keep in mind that conventional amphotericin, Fungizone, is more nephrotoxic than the alternative formulations of amphotericin B,

including Albecet, AmBisome, and Amphotec. Amphotericin B crosses the placenta, and it is unknown if amphotericin B is distributed in breast milk. Safety and efficacy of amphotericin B have not been established in children. Therefore, expect to use the smallest dose necessary to achieve optimal results. There are no age-related precautions noted in the elderly.

History of allergies, especially to amphotericin B and sulfites, should be determined before giving the drug. Be aware that other nephrotoxic medications should be avoided, if possible. Antiemetics, antihistamines, antipyretics, or small doses of corticosteroids may be given before or during amphotericin administration to help control adverse reactions.

Blood pressure (B/P), pulse, respirations, and temperature should be monitored twice every 15 minutes, then every 30 minutes for the initial 4 hours of the infusion to assess for adverse reactions. Adverse reactions include abdominal pain, anorexia, chills, fever, nausea, shaking, and vomiting. If signs and symptoms of adverse reactions occur, slow the infusion and give prescribed drugs to provide symptomatic relief. For a severe reaction or for patients without orders for symptomatic relief, stop the infusion and notify the physician.

Storage
Refrigerate Albecet as unreconstituted solution. Albecet reconstituted solution is stable for 48 hours if refrigerated and 6 hours at room temperature.

Refrigerate AmBisome as unreconstituted solution. AmBisome reconstituted solution of 4 mg/ml is stable for 24 hours. AmBisome reconstituted solution concentration of 1-2 mg/ml is stable for 6 hours. Store Amphotec as unreconstituted solution at room temperature. Amphotec reconstituted solution is stable for 24 hours.

Refrigerate Fungizone as unreconstituted solution. Fungizone reconstituted solution is stable for 24 hours at room temperature or 7 days if refrigerated. Diluted solution less than or equal to 0.1 mg/ml should be used promptly. Do not use the solution if it is cloudy or contains a precipitate.

Administration
For IV use, observe strict aseptic technique because no bacteriostatic agent or preservative is present in the diluent.

Shake Abelcet 20-ml (100-mg) vial gently until contents are dissolved. Withdraw required Abelcet dose using a 5-micron filter needle supplied by manufacturer. Inject Abelcet dose into D_5W; 4 ml D_5W is required for each 1 ml (5 mg) to final concentration of 1 mg/ml. Reduce dose by half for pediatric, fluid-restricted patients (2 mg/ml). Infuse Abelcet over 2 hours by slow IV infusion. Shake the contents if the infusion is greater than 2 hours.

Reconstitute each 50-mg AmBisome vial with 12 ml sterile water for injection to provide concentration of 4 mg/ml. Shake AmBisome vial vigorously for 30 seconds. Then, withdraw the required AmBisome dose and empty the syringe contents through a 5-micron filter into an infusion of D_5W to provide final concentration of 1 to 2 mg/ml. Infuse AmBisome over 1 to 2 hours by slow IV infusion.

Add 10 ml sterile water for injection to each 50-mg Amphotec vial to provide a concentration of 5 mg/ml. Shake the Amphotec vial gently.

Further dilute Amphotec vial only with D_5W using specific amount recommended by manufacturer to provide concentration of 0.16 to 0.83 mg/ml. Infuse Amphotec over 2 to 4 hours by slow IV infusion.

Rapidly inject 10 ml sterile water for injection to each 50-mg Fungizone vial to provide concentration of 5 mg/ml. Immediately shake Fungizone vial until the solution is clear.

Further dilute each 1 mg Fungizone in at least 10 ml D_5W to provide a concentration of 0.1 mg/ml. Be aware that the potential for thrombophlebitis may be less with the use of pediatric scalp vein needles or by adding dilute heparin solution, as prescribed. Infuse conventional amphotericin, Fungizone, over 2 to 6 hours by slow IV infusion.

Ampicillin
am′pi-sill-in
(Alpovex [AUS], Amficot, Apo-Ampi [CAN], Novo-Ampicillin [CAN], Nu-Ampi [CAN], Omnipen, Omnipen-N, Polycillin, Polycillin-N, Principen, Totacillin, Totacillin-N)
Do not confuse with aminophylline, Imipenem, or Unipen.

CATEGORY AND SCHEDULE
Pregnancy Risk Category: B

CLASSIFICATION
Antibiotics, penicillins

MECHANISM OF ACTION
A penicillin that inhibits cell wall synthesis in susceptible

microorganisms. *Therapeutic Effect:* Produces bactericidal effect.

PHARMACOKINETICS
Moderately absorbed from the gastrointestinal (GI) tract. Protein binding: 28%. Widely distributed. Partially metabolized in liver. Primarily excreted in urine. Removed by hemodialysis.
Half-life: 1-1.9 hrs (half-life increased in impaired renal function).

AVAILABILITY
Capsules: 250 mg (Amficot), 500 mg (Omnipen, Principen, Totacillin).
Powder for PO Suspension: 100/ml (Polycillin), 125 mg/5 ml (Omnipen, Polycillin, Principen, Totacillin), 250 mg/5 ml (Omnipen, Polycillin, Principen, Totacillin), 500 mg/5 ml (Polycillin).
Powder for Injection: 125 mg (Omnipen-N, Polycillin-N), 250 mg (Omnipen-N, Polycillin-N, Totacillin-N), 500 mg (Omnipen-N, Polycillin-N, Totacillin-N), 1 g (Omnipen-N, Polycillin-N, Totacillin-N), 2 g (Omnipen-N, Polycillin-N, Totacillin-N), 10 g (Omnipen-N, Polycillin-N).

INDICATIONS AND DOSAGES
▶ **Respiratory tract, skin/skin-structure infections**
PO
Adults, Elderly, Children weighing more than 20 kg. 250-500 mg q6hr.
Children weighing less than 20 kg. 50 mg/kg/day in divided doses q6hr.
IM/IV
Adults, Elderly, Children weighing more than 40 kg. 250-500 mg q6hr.
Children weighing less than 40 kg. 25-50 mg/kg/day in divided doses q6-8hr. Bacterial meningitis, septicemia

IM/IV
Adults, Elderly. 2 g q4hr or 3 g q6hr.
Children. 100-200 mg/kg/day in divided doses q4hr. Gonococcal infections
PO
Adults. 3.5 g one time with 1 g probenecid. Perioperative prophylaxis
IM/IV
Adults, Elderly. 2 g 30 min before procedure. May repeat in 8 hrs.
Children. 50 mg/kg using same dosage regimen. Usual neonate dosage
IM/IV
Neonates 7-28 days old. 75 mg/kg/day in divided doses q8hr up to 200 mg/kg/day in divided doses q6hr.
Neonates 0-7 days old. 50 mg/kg/day in divided doses q12hr up to 150 mg/kg/day in divided doses q8hr.

CONTRAINDICATIONS
Hypersensitivity to any penicillin, infectious mononucleosis

INTERACTIONS
Drug
Allopurinol: May increase incidence of rash.
Oral contraceptives: May decrease effectiveness of oral contraceptives.
Probenecid: May increase ampicillin blood concentration and risk of ampicillin toxicity.
Herbal
None known.
Food
None known.

DIAGNOSTIC TEST EFFECTS
May increase SGOT (AST) and SGPT (ALT) levels. May cause positive Coombs' test.

A

⬛ IV INCOMPATIBILITIES
Amikacin (Amikin), gentamicin, diltiazem (Cardizem), midazolam (Versed)

⬛ IV compatibilities
Calcium gluconate, cefepime (Maxipime), dopamine (Inotropin), famotidine (Pepcid), furosemide (Lasix), heparin, hydromorphone (Dilaudid), insulin (regular), levofloxacin (Levaquin), magnesium sulfate, morphine, multivitamins, potassium chloride, propofol (Diprivan)

SIDE EFFECTS
Frequent
Pain at IM injection site, GI disturbances, including mild diarrhea, nausea, or vomiting, oral or vaginal candidiasis
Occasional
Generalized rash, urticaria, phlebitis, thrombophlebitis with IV administration, headache
Rare
Dizziness, seizures, especially with IV therapy

SERIOUS REACTIONS
• Altered bacterial balance may result in potentially fatal superinfections and antibiotic-associated colitis as evidenced by abdominal cramps, watery or severe diarrhea, and fever.
• Severe hypersensitivity reactions, including anaphylaxis and acute interstitial nephritis occur rarely.

PRECAUTIONS & CONSIDERATIONS
History of allergies especially to cephalosporins and penicillins should be determined before giving ampicillin. Ampicillin may lead to allergic sensitization, candidiasis, diarrhea, and skin rash in infants. Immature renal function in neonates and young infants may delay renal excretion of ampicillin. Higher dosages may be needed for neonatal meningitis. Signs and symptoms of superinfection such as anal or genital pruritus, black hairy tongue, oral ulcerations or pain, diarrhea, increased fever, sore throat, and vomiting should be monitored.

Since hypersensitivity can occur evaluate the IV site for phlebitis as evidenced by heat, pain, and red streaking over the vein. Check the IM injection site for pain and swelling.

Storage
Store capsules at room temperature. Oral suspension, after reconstituted, is stable for 7 days at room temperature, 14 days if refrigerated.

Reconstituted solution for IM injection is stable for 1 hour.

An IV solution, diluted with 0.9% NaCl, is stable for 2 to 8 hours at room temperature or 3 days if refrigerated. An IV solution diluted with D_5W is stable for 2 hours at room temperature or 3 hours if refrigerated. Discard the IV solution if a precipitate forms.

Administration
Capsules should be taken 1 hour before or 2 hours after meals for maximum absorption.

Reconstitute each vial for IM injection with sterile water for injection or bacteriostatic water for injection. Consult individual ampicillin vials for specific volumes of diluent. Give injection deeply in a large muscle mass.

For IV injection, dilute each vial with 5 ml sterile water for injection or 10 ml for 1- and 2-g vials. For intermittent IV infusion or piggyback, further dilute with 50 to 100 ml 0.9% NaCl or D_5W. For IV injection, give over 3 to 5 minutes or 10 to 15 minutes for a 1- to 2-g dose. For intermittent IV infusion

or piggyback, infuse over 20 to
30 minutes. Because of the potential
for hypersensitivity and anaphylaxis,
start the initial dose at a few drops/
minute, increase the dosage slowly
to the prescribed rate. Assess for signs
and symptoms of hypersensitivity or
anaphylaxis. Expect to switch to the
oral route as soon as possible.

Ampicillin Sodium
am-pi-sill'in soe'dee-um
(Alphacin [AUS], Apo-Ampi
[CAN], Novo-Ampicillin [CAN],
Nu-Ampi [CAN], Polycillin)
**Do not confuse ampicillin with
aminophylline, Imipenem, or
Unipen.**

CATEGORY AND SCHEDULE
Pregnancy Risk Category: B

CLASSIFICATION
Antibiotics, penicillins

MECHANISM OF ACTION
A penicillin that inhibits cell wall
synthesis in susceptible microorganisms. *Therapeutic Effect:* Bactericidal.

PHARMACOKINETICS
Moderately absorbed from the GI
tract. Protein binding: 28%. Widely
distributed. Partially metabolized in
the liver. Primarily excreted in urine.
Removed by hemodialysis. **Half-life:**
1-1.5 hr (increased in impaired renal
function).

AVAILABILITY
Capsules: 250 mg, 500 mg.
Powder for Oral Suspension:
125 mg/5 ml, 250 mg/5 ml,
500 mg/5 ml.

Powder for Injection: 125 mg,
250 mg, 500 mg, 1 g, 2 g.

INDICATIONS AND DOSAGES
▸ **Respiratory tract, skin and skin-
structure infections**
PO
Adults, Elderly. 250-500 mg q6hr.
Children. 50-100 mg/kg/day in
divided doses q6hr. Maximum:
3 g/day.
IV, IM
Adults, Elderly. 500 mg to 3 g q6hr.
Maximum: 14 g/day.
Children. 100-200 mg/kg/day in
divided doses q6hr
Neonates. 50-100 mg/kg/day in
divided doses q6-12hr.
▸ **Meningitis**
IV
Children. 200-400 mg/kg/day in
divided doses q6hr. Maximum:
12 g/day
Neonates. 100-200 mg/kg/day in
divided doses q6-12hr.
▸ **Gonococcal infections**
PO
Adults. 3.5 g one time with 1 g
probenecid.
▸ **Perioperative prophylaxis**
IV, IM
Adults, Elderly. 2 g 30 min
before procedure. May repeat
in 8 hr.
Children. 50 mg/kg 30 min
before procedure. May repeat
in 8 hr.
▸ **Dosage in renal impairment**

Creatinine Clearance	% of Normal Dosage
10-30 ml/min	Give q6-12hr
Less than 10 ml/min	Give q12hr

CONTRAINDICATIONS
Hypersensitivity to any
penicillin, infectious mononucleosis

INTERACTIONS
Drug
Allopurinol: May increase incidence of rash.
Oral contraceptives: May decrease effectiveness of oral contraceptives.
Probenecid: May increase ampicillin blood concentration and risk of ampicillin toxicity.
Herbal
None known.
Food
None known.

DIAGNOSTIC TEST EFFECTS
May increase AST (SGOT) and ALT (SGPT) levels. May cause a positive Coombs' test.

IV INCOMPATIBILITIES
Amikacin (Amikin), diltiazem (Cardizem), gentamicin, midazolam (Versed)
IV compatibilities
Calcium gluconate, cefepime (Maxipime), dopamine (Intropin), famotidine (Pepcid), furosemide (Lasix), heparin, hydromorphone (Dilaudid), insulin (regular), levofloxacin (Levaquin), magnesium sulfate, morphine, multivitamins, potassium chloride, propofol (Diprivan)

SIDE EFFECTS
Frequent
Pain at IM injection site, GI disturbances (mild diarrhea, nausea, vomiting), oral or vaginal candidiasis
Occasional
Generalized rash, urticaria, phlebitis or thrombophlebitis (with IV administration), headache
Rare
Dizziness, seizures (especially with IV therapy)

SERIOUS REACTIONS
• Antibiotic-associated colitis and other superinfections may result from altered bacterial balance.
• Severe hypersensitivity reactions, including anaphylaxis and acute interstitial nephritis, occur rarely.

PRECAUTIONS & CONSIDERATIONS
Caution is warranted with antibiotic-associated colitis or a history of allergies, especially to cephalosporins. Ampicillin readily crosses the placenta, appears in cord blood and amniotic fluid, and is distributed in breast milk in low concentrations. Ampicillin may lead to allergic sensitization, candidiasis, diarrhea, and skin rash in infants. Immature renal function in neonates and young infants may delay renal excretion of ampicillin. Keep in mind that high dosages may be needed for neonatal meningitis. Age-related renal impairment may require dosage adjustment in the elderly.

History of allergies, especially to cephalosporins or penicillins, should be determined before giving the drug. Withhold and promptly notify the physician if rash or diarrhea occurs. Severe diarrhea with abdominal pain, blood or mucus in stool, and fever may indicate antibiotic-associated colitis. Signs and symptoms of superinfection, including anal or genital pruritus, black hairy tongue, diarrhea, increased fever, sore throat, ulceration or changes of oral mucosa, and vomiting should be monitored. Intake and output, renal function tests, urinalysis, and the injection sites should be assessed.
Storage
Store capsules or tablets at room temperature. After reconstitution, the oral solution is stable for 7 days either at room temperature or

14 days if refrigerated. An IV solution diluted with 0.9% NaCl is stable for 2 to 8 hours at room temperature or 3 days if refrigerated. An IV solution diluted with D_5W is stable for 2 hours at room temperature or 3 hours if refrigerated. Discard the IV solution if a precipitate forms. The reconstituted solution for IM injection is stable for 1 hour.

Administration
Give oral forms 1 hour before or 2 hours after meals for maximum absorption.

For IV injection, dilute each 125-, 250-, or 500-mg vial with 5 ml sterile water for injection and each 1- or 2-g vial with 10 ml. For intermittent IV infusion (piggyback), further dilute with 50 to 100 ml 0.9% NaCl or D_5W. Administer each 125-, 250-, or 500-mg dose over 3 to 5 minutes and each 1- to 2-g dose over 10 to 15 minutes. Infuse intermittent IV infusion (piggyback) over 20 to 30 minutes. Because of the potential for hypersensitivity and anaphylaxis, start the initial dose at a few drops per minute, increase the dosage slowly to the prescribed rate, and stay with the patient for the first 10 to 15 minutes. Then assess every 10 minutes during the infusion for signs and symptoms of hypersensitivity or anaphylaxis. Expect to switch to the oral route as soon as possible.

For IM use, reconstitute each vial with sterile water for injection or bacteriostatic water for injection. Consult individual ampicillin vials or package insert for specific volumes of diluent. Inject the drug deep into a large muscle mass.

Ampicillin/ Sulbactam
am′pi-sill-in/sul-bac′tam
(Unasyn)

CATEGORY AND SCHEDULE
Pregnancy Risk Category: B

CLASSIFICATION
Antibiotics, penicillins

MECHANISM OF ACTION
Ampicillin inhibits bacterial cell wall synthesis, while sulbactam inhibits bacterial beta-lactamase. *Therapeutic Effect:* Ampicillin is bactericidal in susceptible microorganisms. Sulbactam protects ampicillin from enzymatic degradation.

PHARMACOKINETICS
Protein binding: 28%-38%. Widely distributed. Partially metabolized in the liver. Primarily excreted in urine. Removed by hemodialysis. **Half-life:** 1 hr (increased in impaired renal function).

AVAILABILITY
Powder for Injection: 1.5 g (ampicillin 1 g/sulbactam 500 g), 3 g (ampicillin 2 g/sulbactam 1 g).

INDICATIONS AND DOSAGES
▶ **Skin/skin-structure, intra-abdominal, and gynecologic infections**
IV, IM
Adults, Elderly. 1.5 g (1 g ampicillin/500 mg sulbactam) to 3 g (2 g ampicillin/1 g sulbactam) q6hr.

> **Skin and skin-structure infections**
IV
Children 1-12 yr. 150-300 mg/kg/day in divided doses q6hr.
> **Dosage in renal impairment**
Dosage and frequency are modified based on creatinine clearance and the severity of the infection.

Creatinine Clearance	Dosage
Greater than 30 ml/min	0.5-3 g q6-8hr
15-29 ml/min	1.5-3 g q12hr
5-14 ml/min	1.5-3 g q24hr
Less than 5 ml/min	Not recommended

CONTRAINDICATIONS
Hypersensitivity to any penicillin, infectious mononucleosis

INTERACTIONS
Drug
Allopurinol: May increase incidence of rash.
Oral contraceptives: May decrease effectiveness of oral contraceptives.
Probenecid: May increase ampicillin blood concentration and risk of ampicillin toxicity.
Herbal
None known.
Food
None known.

DIAGNOSTIC TEST EFFECTS
May increase serum LDH, alkaline phosphatase, creatinine, AST (SGOT), and ALT (SGPT) levels. May cause a positive Coombs' test.

IV INCOMPATIBILITIES
Diltiazem (Cardizem), idarubicin (Idamycin), ondansetron (Zofran), sargramostim (Leukine)

IV compatibilities
Famotidine (Pepcid), heparin, insulin (regular), morphine

SIDE EFFECTS
Frequent
Diarrhea and rash (most common), urticaria, pain at IM injection site, thrombophlebitis with IV administration, oral or vaginal candidiasis
Occasional
Nausea, vomiting, headache, malaise, urine retention

SERIOUS REACTIONS
• Severe hypersensitivity reactions, including anaphylaxis, acute interstitial nephritis, and blood dyscrasias may occur.
• Antibiotic-associated colitis and other superinfections may result from altered bacterial balance.
• Overdose may produce seizures.

PRECAUTIONS & CONSIDERATIONS
Caution is warranted with antibiotic-associated colitis or a history of allergies, especially to cephalosporins. Ampicillin and sulbactam readily crosses the placenta, appears in cord blood and amniotic fluid, and is distributed in breast milk in low concentrations. Ampicillin and sulbactam may lead to allergic sensitization, candidiasis, diarrhea, and skin rash in infants. The safety and efficacy of ampicillin and sulbactam have not been established in children younger than 1 year. Age-related renal impairment may require dosage adjustment in the elderly.
History of allergies, especially to cephalosporins or penicillins, should be determined before giving the drug. Withhold and promptly notify the physician if rash or diarrhea occurs. Severe diarrhea with

abdominal pain, blood or mucus in stool, and fever may indicate antibiotic-associated colitis. Signs and symptoms of superinfection, including anal or genital pruritus, black hairy tongue, diarrhea, increased fever, sore throat, ulceration or changes of oral mucosa, and vomiting should be monitored. Intake and output, renal function tests, urinalysis, and the injection sites should be assessed.

Storage

When reconstituted with 0.9% NaCl, the IV solution is stable for 8 hours at room temperature or 48 hours if refrigerated. Stability may differ with other diluents. Discard the IV solution if a precipitate forms.

Administration

For IV injection, dilute with 10 to 20 ml sterile water for injection. For intermittent IV infusion (piggyback), further dilute with 50 to 100 ml D_5W or 0.9% NaCl. Administer IV injection slowly, over 10 to 15 minutes. Administer intermittent IV infusion (piggyback) over 15 to 30 minutes. Because of the potential for hypersensitivity and anaphylaxis, start the initial dose at a few drops per minute, and then increase the dose slowly to the ordered rate. Stay with the patient for the first 10 to 15 minutes; then check every 10 minutes during the infusion for signs and symptoms of hypersensitivity or anaphylaxis. Expect to switch to an oral antibiotic as soon as possible.

For IM use, reconstitute each 1.5-g vial with 3.2 ml or each 3-g vial with 6.4 ml of sterile water for injection to provide a concentration of 250 mg ampicillin/125 mg sulbactam per milliliter. Administer the injection deep into a large muscle mass within 1 hour of preparation.

Amyl Nitrite

am′il

(Amyl Nitrite)

Do not confuse with Nicobid, Nicoderm, Nilstat, nitroprusside, Nizoral, or Nystatin.

CATEGORY AND SCHEDULE

Pregnancy Risk Category: C

CLASSIFICATION

Nitrates, vasodilators

MECHANISM OF ACTION

A nitrite vasodilator that relaxes smooth muscles. Reduces afterload and improves vascular supply to the myocardium. *Therapeutic Effect:* Dilates coronary arteries, improves blood flow to ischemic areas within myocardium. Following inhalation, systemic vasodilation occurs.

PHARMACOKINETICS

The vapors are absorbed rapidly through the pulmonary alveoli and metabolized rapidly. Partially excreted in the urine.

AVAILABILITY

Solution: 0.3 ml (Amyl Nitrite).

INDICATIONS AND DOSAGES
▶ **Acute relief of angina pectoris**
NASAL INHALATION
Adults, Elderly. Place crushed capsule to nostrils for 0.18-0.3 ml inhalation of vapors. Repeat at 5-10 min intervals. No more than 3 doses in 15-30 min period.

OFF-LABEL USES

Cyanide toxicity

CONTRAINDICATIONS
Closed-angle glaucoma, severe anemia, head injury, postural hypotension, pregnancy, hypersensitivity to nitrates

INTERACTIONS
Drug
Sildenafil: May increase hypotensive effects.
Herbal
None known.
Food
Ethanol: May increase hypotensive effects.

DIAGNOSTIC TEST EFFECTS
None known.

SIDE EFFECTS
Frequent
Headache (may be severe) occurs mostly in early therapy, diminishes rapidly in intensity, usually disappears during continued treatment; transient flushing of face and neck; dizziness (especially if patient is standing immobile or is in a warm environment); weakness; postural hypotension
Occasional
Nausea, rash vomiting
Rare
Involuntary passage of urine and feces, restlessness, weakness

SERIOUS REACTIONS
• Large doses may produce hemolytic anemia or methemoglobinemia.
• Severe postural hypotension manifested by fainting, pulselessness, cold or clammy skin, and profuse sweating may occur.
• Tolerance may occur with repeated, prolonged therapy.
• High dose tends to produce severe headache.

PRECAUTIONS & CONSIDERATIONS
A

Caution is warranted in patients with acute MI, blood volume depletion from diuretic therapy, glaucoma (contraindicated in closed-angle glaucoma), liver or renal disease, and systolic B/P less than 90 mm Hg. Apical pulse and blood pressure before amyl nitrate is administered and periodically after dose. Facial or neck flushing should be reported.

It is unknown if amyl nitrite crosses the placenta or is distributed in breast milk. Safety and efficacy of amyl nitrite has not been established in children. The elderly are more susceptible to the hypotensive effects of amyl nitrite, and age-related renal impairment may require cautious use.

Storage
Store at room temperature and protect from light. Keep the drug container away from heat and moisture.

Administration
Capsules for inhalation should be used at the first sign of angina. Crush amyl nitrite capsule with fingers and hold to the nostrils for inhalation of vapors. Wave under the nose; patient should inhale 1 to 6 times. May repeat in 3 to 5 minutes.

Anagrelide
ah-na′greh-lide
(Agrylin)

CATEGORY AND SCHEDULE
Pregnancy Risk Category: C

CLASSIFICATION
Platelet inhibitors

MECHANISM OF ACTION

A hematologic agent that reduces platelet production and prevents platelet shape changes caused by platelet aggregating agents. *Therapeutic Effect:* Inhibits platelet aggregation.

PHARMACOKINETICS

After oral administration, plasma concentration peak within 1 hr. Extensively metabolized. Primarily excreted in urine. **Half-life:** About 3 days.

AVAILABILITY

Capsules: 0.5 mg, 1 mg.

INDICATIONS AND DOSAGES

▸ **Thrombocythemia**
PO
Adults, Elderly. Initially, 0.5 mg 4 times a day or 1 mg twice a day. Adjust to lowest effective dosage, increasing by up to 0.5 mg/day or less in any 1 wk. Maximum: 10 mg/day or 2.5 mg/dose.

CONTRAINDICATIONS

None known.

INTERACTIONS

Drug
None known.
Herbal
None known.
Food
None known.

DIAGNOSTIC TEST EFFECTS

May increase hepatic enzyme levels (rare).

SIDE EFFECTS

Frequent (5% or more)
Headache, palpitations, diarrhea, abdominal pain, nausea, flatulence, bloating, asthenia, pain, dizziness

Occasional (less than 5%)
Tachycardia, chest pain, vomiting, paresthesia, peripheral edema, anorexia, dyspepsia, rash
Rare
Confusion, insomnia

SERIOUS REACTIONS

• Angina, heart failure, and arrhythmias occur rarely.

PRECAUTIONS & CONSIDERATIONS

Caution is warranted with cardiac disease and hepatic or renal impairment. It is unknown if anagrelide crosses the placenta or is distributed in breast milk. Anagrelide may cause fetal harm; it is not recommended in pregnant women. Strongly urge females to use contraceptives while taking anagrelide. Safety and efficacy of anagrelide have not been established in children younger than 16 years. Use anagrelide cautiously in the elderly, who may have age-related cardiac disease and decreased renal and hepatic function.

Hgb, Hct, and platelet and WBC counts should be obtained before treatment, every 2 days during the first week of treatment, and weekly thereafter until therapeutic range is achieved. Skin should be monitored for bruises or petechiae and catheter and needle sites should be inspected for bleeding. Persons with suspected heart disease should be assessed for tachycardia, palpitations, and signs and symptoms of CHF, such as dypsnea.

Administration
Take without regard to food. Platelet count should respond within 7 to 14 days of beginning therapy.

Anakinra
an-a-kin′ra
(Kineret)

CATEGORY AND SCHEDULE
Pregnancy Risk Category: B

CLASSIFICATION
Disease modifying antirheumatic drugs, interleukin receptor antagonists

MECHANISM OF ACTION
An interleukin-1 (IL-1) receptor antagonist that blocks the binding of IL-1, a protein that is a major mediator of joint disease and is present in excess amounts in patients with rheumatoid arthritis. *Therapeutic Effect:* Inhibits the inflammatory response.

PHARMACOKINETICS
No accumulation of anakinra in tissues or organs was observed after daily subcutaneous doses. Excreted in urine.
Half-life: 4-6 hr.

AVAILABILITY
Solution: 100-mg syringe.

INDICATIONS AND DOSAGES
▸ **Rheumatoid arthritis**
SUBCUTANEOUS
Adults, Children older than 18 yr, Elderly. 100 mg/day, given at same time each day.

CONTRAINDICATIONS
Known hypersensitivity to *Escherichia coli*-derived proteins, serious infection

INTERACTIONS
Drug
Live-virus vaccines: May cause the vaccines to be ineffective.
Herbal
None known.
Food
None known.

DIAGNOSTIC TEST EFFECTS
May increase the eosinophil count. May decrease WBC, platelet, and absolute neutrophil counts.

SIDE EFFECTS
Occasional
Injection site ecchymosis, erythema, and inflammation
Rare
Headache, nausea, diarrhea, abdominal pain

SERIOUS REACTIONS
• Infections, including upper respiratory tract infection, sinusitis, flu-like symptoms, and cellulitis, have been noted.
• Neutropenia may occur, particularly when anakinra is used in combination with tumor necrosis factor-blocking agents.

PRECAUTIONS & CONSIDERATIONS
Caution is warranted with asthma and renal impairment. Asthmatics are at increased risk for serious infection, and those with renal impairment are at increased risk for a toxic reaction. It is unknown if anakinra is distributed in breast milk. The safety and efficacy of anakinra have not been established in children. Use anakinra cautiously in the elderly, who may experience age-related renal impairment. Avoid contact with infected individuals and situations that might increase risk for infection. Neutrophil count should be monitored before therapy begins, monthly

for 3 months during therapy, and then quarterly for up to 1 year. Evaluate for inflammatory reactions, especially during the first 4 weeks of therapy. Inflammation is uncommon after the first month of therapy.

Storage

Keep the drug refrigerated. Don't freeze or shake it.

Administration

Don't use the drug if it becomes discolored or contains particles. Give the drug by subcutaneous injection. Don't administer live-virus vaccines concurrently with anakinra because the vaccines may not be effective.

Anastrozole

(Arimidex)

Do not confuse Arimidex with Imitrex.

CATEGORY AND SCHEDULE

Pregnancy Risk Category: D

CLASSIFICATION

Antineoplastics, aromatase inhibitors, hormones/hormone modifiers

---

MECHANISM OF ACTION

Decreases the circulating estrogen level by inhibiting aromatase, the enzyme that catalyzes the final step in estrogen production. *Therapeutic Effect:* Inhibits the growth of breast cancers that are stimulated by estrogens.

PHARMACOKINETICS

Well absorbed into systemic circulation (absorption not affected by food). Protein binding: 40%. Extensively metabolized in the liver. Eliminated by biliary system and, to a lesser extent, kidneys. **Mean half-life:** 50 hr in

postmenopausal women. Steady-state plasma levels reached in about 7 days.

AVAILABILITY

Tablets: 1 mg.

INDICATIONS AND DOSAGES

▶ **Breast cancer**

PO

Adults, Elderly. 1 mg once a day.

CONTRAINDICATIONS

None known

INTERACTIONS

Drug

None known.

Herbal

None known.

Food

None known.

DIAGNOSTIC TEST EFFECTS

May elevate serum GGT level in patients with liver metastasis. May increase serum LDL, serum alkaline phosphate, AST (SGOT), ALT (SGPT), and total cholesterol levels.

SIDE EFFECTS

Frequent (16%-8%)

Asthenia, nausea, headache, hot flashes, back pain, vomiting, cough, diarrhea

Occasional (6%-4%)

Constipation, abdominal pain, anorexia, bone pain, pharyngitis, dizziness, rash, dry mouth, peripheral edema, pelvic pain, depression, chest pain, paresthesia

Rare (2%-1%)

Weight gain, diaphoresis

SERIOUS REACTIONS

• Thrombophlebitis, anemia, leukopenia, and vaginal hemorrhage occur rarely.
• Vaginal hemorrhage occurs rarely (2%).

PRECAUTIONS & CONSIDERATIONS

Anastrozole is indicated only for postmenopausal women. Women who are or may be pregnant should not use anastrozole because the drug crosses the placenta and may cause fetal harm. Pregnancy should be determined before therapy begins. It is unknown if anastrozole is excreted in breast milk. The safety and efficacy of anastrozole have not been established in children. No age-related precautions have been noted in the elderly.

Potential side effects, including dizziness and weakness, may occur. Notify the physician if asthenia, hot flashes, and nausea become unmanageable. If diarrhea occurs, an antidiarrheal should be given; if nausea or vomiting occurs, an antiemetic should be prescribed.

Administration

Take oral anastrozole without regard to food.

Anthralin

anth-rah′lin
(A-Fil, Anthra-Derm, Anthraforte [CAN], Anthranol [CAN], Anthrascalp [CAN], Dithrocream [AUS], Drithocreme, Dritho-Scalp, Micanol, Psoriatec)
(capsules, tablets, chewable tablets, syrup, elixir, cream, spray)
Do not confuse with Antagon, Antabuse, or Andriol.

CATEGORY AND SCHEDULE

Pregnancy Risk Category: C

CLASSIFICATION

Dermatologics

MECHANISM OF ACTION

A topical agent that binds DNA, inhibiting synthesis of nucleic protein, and reduces mitotic activity. *Therapeutic Effect:* Results in damage to DNA sugar and enhances membrane lipid peroxidation, which may play a critical role in the antipsoriatic action.

PHARMACOKINETICS

Poorly absorbed systemically, but excellent epidermal absorption. Autooxidized to inactive metabolites — danthrone and dianthrone. Rapid urinary excretion, so significant levels do not accumulate in the blood or other tissues. **Half-life:** 6 hr.

AVAILABILITY

Cream: 0.1% (Drithocreme), 0.25% (Drithocreme, Dritho-Scalp), 0.5% (Drithocreme, Dritho-Scalp), 1% (Anthra-Derm).
Ointment: 0.1% (Anthra-Derm), 0.25% (Anthra-Derm), 0.5 % (Anthra-Derm), 1% (Micanol, Psoriatec).

INDICATIONS AND DOSAGES

▸ **Psoriasis**

TOPICAL

Adults, Elderly. Apply in a thin layer to affected areas q12hr or q24hr.

OFF-LABEL USES

Inflammatory linear verrucous epidermal nevus

CONTRAINDICATIONS

Acute psoriasis where inflammation is present, erythroderma, hypersensitivity to anthralin

INTERACTIONS

Drug
None known.
Herbal
None known.
Food
None known.

SIDE EFFECTS
Frequent
Irritation
Rare
Neutrophilia, proteinuria, staining of
the skin

SERIOUS REACTIONS
• Patients with renal disease should
have routine urine tests for albuminuria.
• Hypersensitivity reaction, such as
burning, erythema, and dermatitis,
may occur.

PRECAUTIONS & CONSIDERATIONS
Caution should be used in renal
disease. Patch test should be obtained
to rule out the possibility of allergy
versus an irritation reaction. It is
unknown if anthralin crosses the
placenta and is detected in breast
milk. Safety and effectiveness has not
been determined in children. Severe
irritation or edema should be reported.
Administration
For external use only. Apply only to
the skin affected with psoriasis. Do
not apply to face, or genitalia areas.
Wash hands thoroughly after using
because anthralin may stain skin,
hair, and fabric.

Antihemophilic Factor (Factor VIII, AHF)
(Alphanate, Hemofil M,
Humanate P, Koate DVI, Monarc
M, Monoclate-P)
Do not confuse with Alfenta.

CATEGORY AND SCHEDULE
Pregnancy Risk Category: C

CLASSIFICATION
Antihemophilic agents, blood
clotting factors

MECHANISM OF ACTION
An antihemophilic agent that assists
in conversion of prothrombin to
thrombin, essential for blood coagulation. Replaces missing clotting
factor. *Therapeutic Effect:* Produces
hemostasis; corrects or prevents
bleeding episodes.

AVAILABILITY
Injection: Actual number of AHF
units is listed on each vial.

INDICATIONS AND DOSAGES
▸ **Treatment and prevention of bleeding in patients with hemophilia A
factor VIII deficiency, hypofibrino-
genemia, von Willebrand's disease**
Adults, Elderly, Children. Dosage is
highly individualized and is based on
patient's weight, severity of bleeding,
and coagulation studies.

OFF-LABEL USES
Treatment of disseminated intravascular coagulation

CONTRAINDICATIONS
None known

INTERACTIONS
Drug
None known.
Herbal
None known.
Food
None known.

DIAGNOSTIC TEST EFFECTS
None known.

🔲 IV INCOMPATIBILITIES
Do not mix with other IV solutions
or medications.

SIDE EFFECTS
Occasional
Allergic reaction, including fever,
chills, urticaria, wheezing,

hypotension, nausea, feeling of chest tightness; stinging at injection site; dizziness; dry mouth; headache; altered taste

SERIOUS REACTIONS
• There is a risk of transmitting viral hepatitis.
• Intravascular hemolysis may occur if large or frequent doses are used with blood group A, B, or AB.

PRECAUTIONS & CONSIDERATIONS
Caution is warranted with hepatic disease and in those with blood type A, B, or AB. If large doses are given with these blood types, expect to monitor Hct and direct Coombs test to check for hemolytic anemia. If hemolytic anemia occurs, expect to give transfusions with type O blood. Avoid over-inflating cuff when monitoring B/P. Take B/P manually, avoiding automatic B/P cuffs. Electric razor and soft toothbrush should be used to prevent bleeding.

Notify the physician of abdominal or back pain, gingival bleeding, black or red stool, coffee-ground emesis, dark or red urine, or red-speckled mucus from cough. IV site should be monitored for oozing. Vital signs should also be monitored throughout therapy.
Administration
For IV use, refer to individual vials for specific storage requirements. Warm concentrate and diluent to room temperature. Gently agitate or rotate to dissolve. Do not shake vigorously. Complete dissolution may take 5 to 10 minutes. Filter before administering. Administer IV at a rate of approximately 2 ml/minute. Can give up to 10 ml/minute.

Apomorphine
aye-poe-more'feen
(Apokyn)

CATEGORY AND SCHEDULE
Pregnancy Risk Category: C

CLASSIFICATION
Antiparkinson agents, dopaminergics

MECHANISM OF ACTION
An antiparkinson agent that stimulates postsynaptic dopamine receptors in the brain. *Therapeutic Effect:* Relieves signs and symptoms of Parkinson's disease and improves motor function.

PHARMACOKINETICS
Rapidly absorbed after subcutaneous administration. Protein binding: 99.9%. Widely distributed. Rapidly eliminated from plasma. Not detected in urine or secretions. **Half-life:** 41-45 min.

AVAILABILITY
Injection: 10 mg/ml.

INDICATIONS AND DOSAGES
▶ **Acute, intermittent treatment of hypomobility ('off' episodes) associated with advanced Parkinson's disease**
SUBCUTANEOUS
Adults, Elderly. Initially, 0.2 ml (2 mg); may be increased in 0.1-ml (1-mg) increments every few days. Maximum: 0.6 ml (6 mg).

CONTRAINDICATIONS
Concurrent use of alosetron, dolasetron, granisetron, ondansetron, or palonosetron

INTERACTIONS
Drug
Alosetron, dolasetron, granisetron, ondansetron, palonosetron: May

produce profound hypotension and loss of consciousness.

Butyrophenones, metoclopramide, phenothiazines, thioxanthenes: Decrease the effectiveness of apomorphine.

CNS depressants: May increase CNS depressant effects.

Herbal
None known.

Food
None known.

DIAGNOSTIC TEST EFFECTS
May increase serum alkaline phosphatase level.

SIDE EFFECTS
Occasional (4%-3%)
Injection site discomfort, arthralgia, somnolence, hypersalivation, pallor, yawning, headache, dizziness, diaphoresis, vomiting, orthostatic hypotension

Rare (less than 2%)
Psychosis, stomatitis, altered taste, hallucinations

SERIOUS REACTIONS
• Respiratory depression or CNS stimulation (characterized by tachypnea, bradycardia, or persistent vomiting) may occur.
• Apomorphine use may cause or exacerbate preexisting dyskinesia.

PRECAUTIONS & CONSIDERATIONS
Caution is warranted with asthma, cardiac decompensation, cardiovascular or cerebrovascular disease, concomitant use of alcohol, antihypertensives or vasodilators, hypotension, sleep disorders, and renal impairment. Caution should also be used in persons prone to nausea and vomiting and those susceptible to QT/QTc prolongation such as persons with hypokalemia,

hypomagnesemia, bradycardia, genetic predisposition or concomitant use of drugs that prolong the QTc interval. It is unknown if apomorphine is distributed in breast milk. The safety and efficacy of apomorphine have not been established in children. No age-related precautions have been noted in the elderly; however, they may be more prone to develop hallucinations. Nausea, vomiting, headache, hallucinations, somnolence, sedation, dizziness, bradycardia, and hypotension may occur. Chronic subcutaneous administration produces painful nodules. Rarely, syncope has occurred during use of sublingual apomorphine. Prolonged QT intervals have been reported with apomorphine.

Storage
Store at room temperature.

Administration
! Do not use intravenously. The manufacturer recommends expressing the dose of apomorphine in milliliters (ml) not milligrams (mg) to avoid confusion. Apomorphine should be given with an anti-nauseant but not a serotonin 5-HT3 antagonist. 5-HT3 antagonists are contraindicated due to reports of profound hypotension when used with apomorphine.

For Parkinson's disease, apomorphine is dosed from 0.2 ml (2 mg) to 0.6 ml (6 mg) subcutaneously as needed and titrated upwards in 0.1 ml (1 mg) increments every few days if necessary. Initial doses are determined by administering test doses in-clinic where a medical professional can closely monitor blood pressure pre-dose and at 20, 40, and 60 minutes post dose. No more than 1 dose per "off" episode should be administered. Doses greater than 0.6 ml (6 mg), total daily doses greater than 2 ml (20 mg) and dosing more than 5 times per day are not recommended.

Aprepitant
ap-re′pi-tant
(Emend)

CATEGORY AND SCHEDULE
Pregnancy Risk Category: B

CLASSIFICATION
Antiemetics/antivertigo, substance P antagonists

MECHANISM OF ACTION
A selective human substance P and neurokinin-1 (NK_1) receptor antagonist that inhibits chemotherapy-induced nausea and vomiting centrally in the chemoreceptor trigger zone. *Therapeutic Effect:* Prevents the acute and delayed phases of chemotherapy-induced emesis, including vomiting caused by high-dose cisplatin.

PHARMACOKINETICS
Crosses the blood-brain barrier. Extensively metabolized in the liver. Eliminated primarily by liver metabolism (not excreted renally). **Half-life:** 9-13 hr.

AVAILABILITY
Capsules: 80 mg, 125 mg.

INDICATIONS AND DOSAGES
▸ **Prevention of chemotherapy-induced nausea and vomiting**
PO
Adults, Elderly. 125 mg 1 hr before chemotherapy on day 1 and 80 mg once a day in the morning on days 2 and 3.

CONTRAINDICATIONS
Breast-feeding, concurrent use of pimozide (Orap)

INTERACTIONS
Drug
Alprazolam, docetaxel, etoposide, ifosfamide, imatinib, irinotecan, midazolam, paclitaxel, triazolam, vinblastine, vincristine, vinorelbine: May increase the plasma concentrations of these drugs.
Antifungals, clarithromycin, diltiazem, nefazodone, nelfinavir, ritonavir: Increase aprepitant plasma concentration.
Carbamazepine, phenytoin, rifampin: Decrease aprepitant plasma concentration.
Contraceptives: May decrease the effectiveness of contraceptives.
Paroxetine: May decrease the effectiveness of either drug.
Steroids: Increases the blood levels and effects of steroids.
Warfarin: May decrease the effectiveness of warfarin.
Herbal
None known.
Food
None known.

DIAGNOSTIC TEST EFFECTS
May increase BUN level and serum creatinine, AST (SGOT), and ALT (SGPT) levels. May produce proteinuria.

SIDE EFFECTS
Frequent (17%-10%)
Fatigue, nausea, hiccups, diarrhea, constipation, anorexia
Occasional (8%-4%)
Headache, vomiting, dizziness, dehydration, heartburn
Rare (3% or less)
Abdominal pain, epigastric discomfort, gastritis, tinnitus, insomnia

SERIOUS REACTIONS
- Neutropenia and mucous membrane disorders occur rarely.

PRECAUTIONS & CONSIDERATIONS
It is unknown if aprepitant crosses the placenta or is distributed in breast milk. The safety and efficacy of aprepitant have not been established in children. No age-related precautions have been noted in the elderly.

Nausea and vomiting should be relieved shortly after drug administration. Notify the physician if headache or persistent vomiting occurs. Pattern of daily bowel activity and stool consistency should be assessed.

Administration
! As prescribed, give aprepitant with 12 mg dexamethasone PO and 32 mg ondansetron IV on day 1, and with 8 mg dexamethasone PO on days 2 to 4.

Take aprepitant orally without regard to food. If the patient is also receiving a steroid, expect to reduce the IV steroid dose by 25% and the oral dose by 50%.

Argatroban
ar-gat'tro-ban
(Acova)
Do not confuse with Aggrestat or Orgaran.

CATEGORY AND SCHEDULE
Pregnancy Risk Category: B

CLASSIFICATION
Anticoagulants, thrombin inhibitors

MECHANISM OF ACTION
A direct thrombin inhibitor that reversibly binds to thrombin-active sites. Inhibits thrombin-catalyzed or thrombin-induced reactions, including fibrin formation, activation of coagulant factors V, VIII, and XIII; also inhibits protein C formation; and platelet aggregation. *Therapeutic Effect:* Produces anticoagulation.

PHARMACOKINETICS
Following IV administration, distributed primarily in extracellular fluid. Protein binding: 54%. Metabolized in the liver. Primarily excreted in the feces, presumably through biliary secretion. **Half-life:** 39-51 min.

AVAILABILITY
Injection: 100 mg/ml.

INDICATIONS AND DOSAGES
▸ **To prevent and treat heparin-induced thrombocytopenia**
IV INFUSION
Adults, Elderly. Initially, 2 mcg/kg/min administered as a continuous infusion. After initial infusion, dose may be adjusted until steady state aPTT is 1.5-3 times initial baseline value, not to exceed 100 sec.
▸ **Percutaneous coronary intervention**
IV INFUSION
Adults, Elderly. Initially, 25 mcg/kg/min and administer bolus of 350 mcg/kg over 3-5 min. ACT checked in 5-10 min following bolus. If ACT is less than 300 sec, give additional bolus 150 mcg/kg, increase infusion to 30 mcg/kg/min. If ACT is greater than 450 sec, decrease infusion to 15 mcg/kg/min. Once ACT of 300-450 sec achieved, proceed with procedure.
▸ **Dosage in hepatic impairment**
Adults, Elderly. Initially, 0.5 mcg/kg/min.

CONTRAINDICATIONS
Overt major bleeding

INTERACTIONS
Drug
Antiplatelet agents, thrombolytics, other anticoagulants: May increase the risk of bleeding.
Herbal
None known.
Food
None known.

DIAGNOSTIC TEST EFFECTS
Increases aPTT, International Normalized Ratio, and PT

▓ IV INCOMPATIBILITIES
Do not mix with other medications or solutions.

SIDE EFFECTS
Frequent (8%-3%)
Dyspnea, hypotension, fever, diarrhea, nausea, pain, vomiting, infection, cough

SERIOUS REACTIONS
• Ventricular tachycardia and atrial fibrillation occur occasionally.
• Major bleeding and sepsis occur rarely.

PRECAUTIONS & CONSIDERATIONS
Caution is warranted with congenital or acquired bleeding disorders, hepatic impairment, severe hypertension, and ulcerations. Also, use argatroban cautiously immediately following administration of spinal anesthesia, lumbar puncture, and major surgery. It is unknown if argatroban is excreted in breast milk. Safety and efficacy of argatroban have not been established in children younger than 18 years of age. No age-related precautions have been noted in the elderly. An electric razor and soft toothbrush should be used to prevent bleeding.

Notify the physician of abdominal pain, bleeding at surgical site, black or red stool, coffee-ground vomitus, red or dark urine, or blood-tinged mucus from cough. Activated coagulation time, aPTT, PT, platelet count, B/P, pulse rate, and menstrual flow should be monitored.

Storage
Following reconstitution, the solution is stable for 24 hours at room temperature and for 48 hours if refrigerated. Avoid exposing the solution to direct sunlight. Discard the solution if it appears cloudy or has an insoluble precipitate.

Administration
Before infusion, dilute the solution 100 fold in 0.9% NaCl, D_5W, or lactated Ringer's solution to provide a final concentration of 1 mg/ml. Mix the solution by repeatedly inverting the diluent bag for 1 minute. Following reconstitution, the solution may briefly appear hazy because of formation of microprecipitates. These rapidly dissolve when the solution is mixed. Rate of administration is based on body weight at 2 mcg/kg/min; (for example, for a 50-kg person, infuse at rate of 6 ml/hr).

Aripiprazole
ara-pip′rah-zole
(Abilify)

CATEGORY AND SCHEDULE
Pregnancy Risk Category: C

CLASSIFICATION
Antipsychotics

MECHANISM OF ACTION

An antipsychotic agent that provides partial agonist activity at dopamine and serotonin (5-HT$_{1A}$) receptors and antagonist activity at serotonin (5-HT$_{2A}$) receptors. *Therapeutic Effect:* Diminishes schizophrenic behavior.

PHARMACOKINETICS

Well absorbed through the GI tract. Protein binding: 99% (primarily albumin). Reaches steady levels in 2 wks. Metabolized in the liver. Eliminated primarily in feces and, to a lesser extent, in urine. Not removed by hemodialysis. **Half-life:** 75 hr.

AVAILABILITY

Tablets: 5 mg, 10 mg, 15 mg, 20 mg, 30 mg.

INDICATIONS AND DOSAGES

▸ **Schizophrenia**
PO
Adults, Elderly. Initially, 10-15 mg once a day. May increase up to 30 mg/day.

OFF-LABEL USES

Schizoaffective disorder

CONTRAINDICATIONS

None known.

INTERACTIONS

Drug
Carbamazepine: May decrease the aripiprazole blood concentration.
Fluoxetine, ketoconazole, quinidine, paroxetine: May increase the aripiprazole blood concentration.
Herbal
None known.
Food
None known.

DIAGNOSTIC TEST EFFECTS

None known.

SIDE EFFECTS

Frequent (11%-5%)
Weight gain, headache, insomnia, vomiting
Occasional (4%-3%)
Light-headedness, nausea, akathisia, somnolence
Rare (2% or less)
Blurred vision, constipation, asthenia or loss of energy and strength, anxiety, fever, rash, cough, rhinitis, orthostatic hypotension

SERIOUS REACTIONS

• Extrapyramidal symptoms and neuroleptic malignant syndrome occur rarely.

PRECAUTIONS & CONSIDERATIONS

Caution is warranted with cardiovascular or cerebrovascular diseases (because it may induce hypotension), history of seizures or conditions that may lower the seizure threshold (such as Alzheimer's disease), hepatic or renal impairment, and Parkinson's disease (because of potential for exacerbation). CNS depressants and alcohol should be avoided during therapy. It is unknown if aripiprazole crosses the placenta. Because this drug may be distributed in breast milk, female patients should avoid breast-feeding during therapy. The safety and efficacy of aripiprazole have not been established in children. No age-related precautions have been noted in the elderly. Extrapyramidal symptoms and tardive dyskinesia, manifested as chewing or puckering of the mouth, puffing of the cheeks, or tongue protrusion should be monitored. B/P, pulse rate, weight, and therapeutic response should also be monitored. Hydration and hypovolemia should be corrected before beginning therapy.

Administration
! Keep in mind that at least 2 weeks should elapse between dosage adjustments. Take aripiprazole without regard to food.

Arsenic Trioxide
ar´sen-ik try-ox´ide
(Trisenox)
Do not confuse with Trimox.

CATEGORY AND SCHEDULE
Pregnancy Risk Category: D

CLASSIFICATION
Antineoplastics, miscellaneous

MECHANISM OF ACTION
An antineoplastic that produces morphologic changes and DNA fragmentation in promyelocytic leukemia cells. *Therapeutic Effect:* Produces cell death.

AVAILABILITY
Injection: 1 mg/ml.

INDICATIONS AND DOSAGES
▶ **Acute promyelocytic leukemia**
IV
Adults, Elderly. Induction: 0.15 mg/kg/day until myelosuppression occurs. Do not exceed 60 induction doses. Beginning 3-6 wk after completion of induction therapy, 0.15 mg/kg/day for 25 doses over a period of up to 5 wk.

CONTRAINDICATIONS
None known.

INTERACTIONS
Drug
Amphotericin B, diuretics: May produce electrolyte imbalances.

Antiarrhythmics, thioridazine: May prolong QT interval.
Herbal
None known.
Food
None known.

DIAGNOSTIC TEST EFFECTS
May decrease Hgb levels, serum calcium and magnesium levels, and platelet and WBC counts. May increase AST (SGOT) and ALT (SGPT) levels.

▓ IV INCOMPATIBILITIES
Don't mix arsenic trioxide with any other medications.

SIDE EFFECTS
Expected (75%-50%)
Nausea, cough, fatigue, fever, headache, vomiting, abdominal pain, tachycardia, diarrhea, dyspnea
Frequent (43%-30%)
Dermatitis, insomnia, edema, rigors, prolonged QT interval, sore throat, pruritus, arthralgia, paresthesia, anxiety
Occasional (28%-20%)
Constipation, myalgia, hypotension, epistaxis, anorexia, dizziness, sinusitis
Occasional (15%-8%)
Ecchymosis, nonspecific pain, weight gain, herpes simplex, wheezing, flushing, diaphoresis, tremor, hypertension, palpitations, dyspepsia, eye irritation, blurred vision, asthenia, diminished breath sounds, crackles
Rare
Confusion, petechiae, dry mouth, oral candidiasis, incontinence, rhonchi

SERIOUS REACTIONS
• Seizures, GI hemorrhage, renal impairment or failure, pleural or pericardial effusion, hemoptysis, and sepsis occur rarely.

• Prolonged QT interval, complete AV block, unexplained fever, dyspnea, weight gain, and effusion are evidence of arsenic toxicity. If arsenic toxicity is apparent, stop arsenic trioxide treatment and begin steroid treatment as ordered.

PRECAUTIONS & CONSIDERATIONS
Caution is warranted with cardiac abnormalities and renal impairment. Arsenic trioxide is distributed in breast milk and may cause fetal harm. It should not be used by pregnant or breast-feeding women.

Notify the physician if confusion, muscle weakness, fever, vomiting, difficulty breathing, or rapid pulse rate occurs. CBC, hepatic function test results, blood chemistry values, serum potassium levels (hypokalemia is more common than hyperkalemia) and blood glucose levels (hyperglycemia is more common than hypoglycemia) should be assessed before and during therapy.

Storage
Store the drug at room temperature. The diluted solution is stable for 24 hours at room temperature and 48 hours if refrigerated.

Administration
! A central venous line is not required for administration of arsenic; the drug may be infused through a peripheral line.

After withdrawing the drug from ampoule, dilute it with 100 to 250 ml D_5W or 0.9% NaCl. Infuse the solution over 1 to 2 hours. The duration of the infusion may be extended up to 4 hours.

Ascorbic Acid (Vitamin C)
a-skor´bic
(Apo-C [CAN], Cecon, Cenolate, Pro-C [AUS], Redoxon [CAN])

CATEGORY AND SCHEDULE
Pregnancy Risk Category: A (C if used in doses above recommended daily allowance)
OTC

CLASSIFICATION:
Vitamins/minerals

MECHANISM OF ACTION
Assists in collagen formation and tissue repair and is involved in oxidation reduction reactions and other metabolic reactions. *Therapeutic Effect:* Involved in carbohydrate use and metabolism, as well as synthesis of carnitine, lipids, and proteins. Preserves blood vessel integrity.

PHARMACOKINETICS
Readily absorbed from the GI tract. Protein binding: 25%. Metabolized in the liver. Excreted in urine. Removed by hemodialysis.

AVAILABILITY
Capsules (Controlled-Release): 500 mg.
Liquid: 500 mg/5 ml.
Oral Solution: 500 mg/5 ml.
Tablets: 100 mg, 250 mg, 500 mg, 1 g.
Tablets (Chewable): 100 mg, 250 mg, 500 mg.
Tablets (Controlled-Release): 500 mg, 1 g, 1,500 mg.
Injection: 250 mg/ml, 500 mg/ml.

INDICATIONS AND DOSAGES
▸ **Dietary supplement**
PO
Adults, Elderly. 50-200 mg/day.
Children. 35-100 mg/day.
▸ **Acidification of urine**
PO
Adults, Elderly. 4-12 g/day in 3-4
divided doses.
Children. 500 mg q6-8hr.
▸ **Scurvy**
PO
Adults, Elderly. 100-250 mg
1-2 times a day.
Children. 100-300 mg/day in
divided doses.
▸ **Prevention and reduction of
severity of colds**
PO
Adults, Elderly. 1-3 g/day in divided
doses.

OFF-LABEL USES
Prevention of common cold, control
of idiopathic methemoglobinemia,
urine acidifier

CONTRAINDICATIONS
None known.

INTERACTIONS
Drug
Deferoxamine: May increase iron
toxicity.
Herbal
None known.
Food
None known.

DIAGNOSTIC TEST EFFECTS
May decrease serum bilirubin level
and urinary pH. May increase urine,
uric acid, and urine oxalate levels.

🔲 IV INCOMPATIBILITIES
No information available for Y-site
administration.
📙 IV compatibilities
Calcium gluconate, heparin

SIDE EFFECTS
Rare
Abdominal cramps, nausea, vomiting, diarrhea, increased urination
with doses exceeding 1 g
Parenteral: Flushing, headache,
dizziness, sleepiness or insomnia,
soreness at injection site.

SERIOUS REACTIONS
• Ascorbic acid may acidify urine,
leading to crystalluria.
• Large doses of IV ascorbic acid
may lead to deep vein thrombosis.
• Abrupt discontinuation after
prolonged use of large doses may
produce rebound ascorbic acid deficiency.

PRECAUTIONS & CONSIDERATIONS
Caution is warranted with diabetes
mellitus, history of renal scalculi,
persons on sodium restricted diet,
and those receiving warfarin or daily
doses of salicylate. Ascorbic acid
crosses the placenta and is excreted
in breast milk. Large doses of ascorbic acid taken during pregnancy may
produce scurvy in neonates. No age-
related precautions have been noted
in children or the elderly. Eating
foods rich in vitamin C, including
citrus fruits, green peppers, brussel
sprouts, rose hips, spinach, strawber-
ries, and watercress, is encouraged.
Clinical improvement, such as
improved wound healing, should be
assessed. Signs and symptoms of
recurring vitamin C deficiency,
including bleeding gums, digestive
difficulties, gingivitis, poor wound
healing, and arthralgia, should also
be monitored.
Storage
Refrigerate vials and protect them
from freezing and sunlight.
Administration
Take oral ascorbic acid without
regard to food. Reduce the dosage

gradually because abrupt discontinuation may produce rebound deficiency.

Ascorbic acid may be given undiluted or may be diluted in D₅W, 0.9% NaCl, or lactated Ringer's solution. For IV push, dilute with an equal volume of D₅W or 0.9% NaCl and infuse over 10 minutes. For IV solution, infuse over 4 to 12 hours.

Asparaginase
a-spare′a-gi-nase
(Elspar, Kidrolase [CAN], Leunase [AUS])
Do not confuse with pegaspargase.

CATEGORY AND SCHEDULE
Pregnancy Risk Category: C

CLASSIFICATION
Antineoplastics, enzymes

MECHANISM OF ACTION
An enzyme that inhibits DNA, RNA, and protein synthesis by breaking down asparagine, thus depriving tumor cells of this essential amino acid. Cell cycle-specific for G_1 phase of cell division. *Therapeutic Effect:* Kills leukemic cells.

PHARMACOKINETICS
Metabolized by the reticuloendothelial system through slow sequestration.
Half-life: 39-49 hr IM; 8-30 hr IV.

AVAILABILITY
Powder for Injection: 10,000 international units.

INDICATIONS AND DOSAGES
▸ **Acute lymphocytic leukemia**
IV

Adults, Elderly, Children.
1000 units/kg/day for 10 days as combination therapy or 200 units/kg/day for 28 days as monotherapy.
IM
Adults, Elderly, Children. 6 to 6000 units/m²/dose 3 times/wk for 3 wk as combination therapy.

OFF-LABEL USES
Treatment of acute myelocytic leukemia, acute myelomonocytic leukemia, chronic lymphocytic leukemia, Hodgkin's disease, lymphosarcoma, melanosarcoma, and reticulum cell sarcoma

CONTRAINDICATIONS
History of hypersensitivity to asparaginase, pancreatitis

INTERACTIONS
Drug
Antigout medications: May decrease the effects of these drugs.
Live-virus vaccines: May potentiate virus replication, increase vaccine side effects, and decrease the patient's antibody response to the vaccine.
Methotrexate: May block effects of methotrexate.
Steroids, vincristine: May increase the risk of neuropathy and disturbances of erythropoiesis; may enhance hyperglycemic effect of asparaginase.
Herbal
None known.
Food
None known.

DIAGNOSTIC TEST EFFECTS
May increase BUN, blood ammonia, and blood glucose levels; serum alkaline phosphatase, bilirubin, uric acid AST (SGOT), and ALT (SGPT) levels; platelet count, PT; activated partial thromboplastin time; and

thrombin time. May decrease blood-clotting factors, (including antithrombin, plasma fibrinogen, and plasminogen) as well as serum albumin, calcium, and cholesterol levels.

☷ IV INCOMPATIBILITIES
None known. Consult pharmacy.

SIDE EFFECTS
Frequent
Allergic reaction (rash, urticaria, arthralgia, facial edema, hypotension, respiratory distress) pancreatitis (severe stomach pain, nausea, and vomiting).
Occasional
CNS effects (confusion, drowsiness, depression, anxiety, and fatigue), stomatitis, hypoalbuminemia or uric acid nephropathy, (manifested as edema of feet or lower legs), hyperglycemia
Rare
Hyperthermia (including fever or chills), thrombosis, seizures

SERIOUS REACTIONS
- Hepatotoxicity usually occurs within 2 weeks of initial treatment.
- The risk of an allergic reaction, including anaphylaxis, increases after repeated therapy.
- Myelosuppression may be severe.

PRECAUTIONS & CONSIDERATIONS
Caution is warranted with diabetes mellitus, current or recent chickenpox, gout, herpes zoster, infection, hepatic or renal impairment, and in those who have recently had cytotoxic or radiation therapy. Asparaginase use should be avoided during pregnancy, especially during the first trimester, and breast-feeding. No age-related precautions have been noted in children or the elderly. Immunizations and coming in contact with those who have recently received a live-virus vaccine should be avoided.
! Expect to discontinue asparaginase at the first sign or symptom of renal failure (oliguria, anuria) or pancreatitis (abdominal pain, nausea and vomiting, elevated serum amylase and lipase levels). Adequate hydration should be maintained to help prevent kidney problems.

Signs and symptoms of hematologic toxicity, such as excessive fatigue and weakness, ecchymosis, fever, signs of local infection, sore throat, and unusual bleeding from any site should be assessed. Baseline CNS function should be assessed and a comprehensive blood chemistry should be obtained before therapy begins and whenever more than 1 week has elapsed between doses.
Storage
Refrigerate the powder for the injected form. Reconstituted solutions are stable for 8 hours if refrigerated.
Administration
! Asparaginase dosage is individualized based on clinical response and the tolerance of the drug's adverse effects. When administering this drug in combination therapy, consult specific protocols for optimum dosage and sequence of drug administration. Asparaginase may be carcinogenic, mutagenic, or teratogenic. Handle with extreme care during preparation and administration. Treat urine as infectious waste. Asparaginase powder or solution may irritate the skin on contact. Wash the affected area for 15 minutes if contact occurs.
! Administer an intradermal test dose (2 international units) before beginning asparaginase therapy and when more than 1 week has elapsed between doses. To prepare the test

solution, reconstitute 10,000-units vial with 5 ml sterile water for injection or 0.9% NaCl and shake to dissolve. Withdraw 0.1 ml and inject it into another vial containing 9.9 ml of the same diluent to produce a concentration of 20 international units/ml. After injecting the test dose, observe the site for 1 hour for the appearance of erythema or a wheal. Keep antihistamines, epinephrine, IV corticosteroid, and oxygen equipment readily available before administering asparaginase. If gelatinous, fiber-like particles develop in the solution, remove them by using a 5 micron filter during administration. For IV use, reconstitute the 10,000-units vial with 5 ml sterile water for injection or 0.9% NaCl to provide a concentration of 2000 international units/ml. Shake gently to ensure complete dissolution. Vigorous shaking will produce foam and cause some loss of potency. For IV injection, administer asparaginase solution into the tubing of free-flowing IV solution of D₅W or 0.9% NaCl over at least 30 minutes. For IV infusion, further dilute with up to 1000 ml D₅W or 0.9% NaCl.

For IM use, add 2 ml 0.9% NaCl to 10,000-units vial to provide a concentration of 5000 international units/ml. Administer no more than 2 ml at any one site.

Aspirin
as´pir-in
(Ascriptin, Aspro [AUS], Bayer, Bex [AUS], Bufferin, Disprin [AUS], Ecotrin, Entrophen [CAN], Halfprin, Novasen [CAN], Solprin [AUS], Spren [AUS])
Do not confuse with Aricept, Afrin, Asendin, or Edecrin.

CATEGORY AND SCHEDULE
Pregnancy Risk Category: C (D if full dose used in third trimester of pregnancy)
OTC

CLASSIFICATION
Analgesics, non-narcotic, antipyretics, salicylates

MECHANISM OF ACTION
A nonsteroidal salicylate that inhibits prostaglandin synthesis, acts on the hypothalamus heat-regulating center, and interferes with the production of thromboxane A, a substance that stimulates platelet aggregation. *Therapeutic Effect:* Reduces inflammatory response and intensity of pain; decreases fever; inhibits platelet aggregation.

PHARMACOKINETICS

Route	Onset	Peak	Duration
PO	1 hr	2-4 hr	24 hr

Rapidly and completely absorbed from GI tract; enteric-coated absorption delayed; rectal absorption delayed and incomplete. Protein binding: High. Widely distributed. Rapidly hydrolyzed to salicylate.

Half-life: 15-20 min (aspirin); 2-3 hr (salicylate at low dose); more than 20 hr (salicylate at high dose).

AVAILABILITY
Tablets (Bayer): 325 mg, 500 mg.
Tablets (Chewable [Bayer and St. Joseph]): 81 mg.
Tablets (Enteric-Coated [Bayer, Ecotrin, St. Joseph]): 81 mg, 325 mg, 500 mg, 650 mg.
Tablets (Hafprin): 162 mg.
Caplet (Bayer): 81 mg, 325 mg, 500 mg.
Gelcap (Bayer): 325 mg, 500 mg.
Suppository: 60 mg, 120 mg, 125 mg, 200 mg, 325 mg, 600 mg, 650 mg.

INDICATIONS AND DOSAGES
▶ **Analgesia, fever**
PO, RECTAL
Adults, Elderly. 325-1000 mg q4-6hr
Children. 10-15 mg/kg/dose q4-6hr.
Maximum: 4 g/day.
▶ **Anti-inflammatory**
PO
Adults, Elderly. Initially, 2.4-3.6 g/day in divided doses; then 3.6-5.4 g/day.
Children. Initially, 60-90 mg/kg/day in divided doses; then 80-100 mg/kg/day.
▶ **Suspected MI**
PO
Adults, Elderly. 162 mg as soon as the MI is suspected, then daily for 30 days after the MI.
▶ **Prevention of MI**
PO
Adults, Elderly. 75-325 mg/day.
▶ **Prevention of stroke after transient ischemic attack**
PO
Adults, Elderly. 50-325 mg/day.
▶ **Kawasaki disease**
PO
Children. 80-100 mg/kg/day in divided doses.

OFF-LABEL USES
Prevention of thromboembolism, treatment of Kawasaki disease

CONTRAINDICATIONS
Allergy to tartrazine dye, bleeding disorders, chickenpox or flu in children and teenagers, GI bleeding or ulceration, hepatic impairment, history of hypersensitivity to aspirin or NSAIDs

INTERACTIONS
Drug
Alcohol, NSAIDs: May increase the risk of adverse GI effects, including ulceration.
Antacids, urinary alkalinizers: Increase the excretion of aspirin.
Anticoagulants, heparin, thrombolytics: Increase the risk of bleeding.
Insulin, oral antidiabetics: May increase the effects of these drugs (with large doses of aspirin).
Methotrexate, zidovudine: May increase the risk of toxicity of these drugs.
Ototoxic medications, vancomycin: May increase the risk of ototoxicity.
Platelet aggregation inhibitors, valproic acid: May increase the risk of bleeding.
Probenecid, sulfinpyrazone: May decrease the effects of these drugs.
Herbal
None known.
Food
None known.

DIAGNOSTIC TEST EFFECTS
May alter serum alkaline phosphatase, uric acid, AST (SGOT), and ALT (SGPT) levels. May prolong PT and bleeding time. May decrease serum cholesterol, serum potassium, and T_3 and T_4 levels.

SIDE EFFECTS
Occasional
GI distress (including abdominal distention, cramping, heartburn, and mild nausea); allergic reaction (including bronchospasm, pruritus, and urticaria)

SERIOUS REACTIONS
• High doses of aspirin may produce GI bleeding and gastric mucosal lesions.
• Dehydrated, febrile children may experience aspirin toxicity quickly. Reye's syndrome may occur in children with the chickenpox or the flu.
• Low-grade toxicity characterized by tinnitus, generalized pruritus (possibly severe), headache, dizziness, flushing, tachycardia, hyperventilation, diaphoresis, and thirst.
• Market toxicity is characterized by hyperthermia, restlessness, seizures, abnormal breathing patterns, respiratory failure, and coma.

PRECAUTIONS & CONSIDERATIONS
Caution is warranted with chronic renal insufficiency, vitamin K deficiency and the "aspirin triad" of asthma, nasal polyps, and rhinitis. Aspirin readily crosses the placenta and is distributed in breast milk. Pregnant women should not take aspirin during the last trimester of pregnancy because the drug may prolong gestation and labor and cause adverse effects in the fetus such as premature closure of the ductus arteriosus, low birth weight, hemorrhage, stillbirth, and death. Caution should be used giving aspirin to children with acute febrile illness. Don't give aspirin to children with chickenpox or the flu because this increases their risk of developing Reye's syndrome. Know that behavioral changes and vomiting may be early signs of Reye's syndrome. Lower aspirin dosages are recommended for the elderly because they're more susceptible to aspirin toxicity. Withhold the drug and contact the physician if respirations are 12 per minute or lower (20 per minute or lower in children). Alcohol and NSAIDs should be avoided because of increased risk of GI bleeding.

Notify the physician if ringing in the ears (tinnitus) or persistent abdominal or GI pain occurs. Temperature should be taken just before and 1 hour after giving the drug. Urine pH should be monitored for signs of sudden acidification, indicated by a pH of 6.5 to 5.5; sudden acidification may cause the serum salicyalte level to greatly increase, leading to toxicity. Be aware the therapeutic serum aspirin level for antiarthritic effect is 20 to 30 mg/dl; the toxic serum level is over 30 mg/dl. Be aware the anti-inflammatory effect should occur within 1 to 3 weeks.

Storage
Refrigerate suppositories.
Administration
Don't give aspirin to children or teenagers with chickenpox or the flu because this increases their risk of developing Reye's syndrome. Do not use aspirin that smells of vinegar because this odor indicates chemical breakdown of the drug. Don't crush or break enteric-coated or extended-release tablets. Take aspirin with water, milk, or meals if GI distress occurs.

For rectal use, if the suppository is too soft, refrigerate it for 30 minutes or run cold water over the foil wrapper. Moisten the suppository with cold water before inserting it well into the rectum.

Atenolol

a-ten′oh-lol

(Apo-Atenol [CAN], AteHexal [AUS], Noten [AUS], Tenolin [CAN], Tenormin, Tensig [AUS])
Do not confuse atenolol with albuterol or timolol.

CATEGORY AND SCHEDULE
Pregnancy Risk Category: D

CLASSIFICATION
Antiadrenergics, beta blocking

MECHANISM OF ACTION
A beta$_1$-adrenergic blocker that acts as an antianginal, antiarrhythmic, and antihypertensive agent by blocking beta$_1$-adrenergic receptors in cardiac tissue. *Therapeutic Effect:* Slows sinus node heart rate, decreasing cardiac output and blood pressure (B/P). Decreases myocardial oxygen demand.

PHARMACOKINETICS

Route	Onset	Peak	Duration
PO	1 hr	2-4 hr	24 hr

Incompletely absorbed from the GI tract. Protein binding: 6%-16%. Minimal liver metabolism. Primarily excreted unchanged in urine. Removed by hemodialysis. **Half-life:** 6-7 hr (increased in impaired renal function).

AVAILABILITY
Tablets: 25 mg, 50 mg, 100 mg.
Injection: 5 mg/10 ml.

INDICATIONS AND DOSAGES
▸ **Hypertension**
PO
Adults. Initially, 25-50 mg once a day. May increase dose up to 100 mg once a day.
Elderly. Usual initial dose, 25 mg a day.
Children. Initially, 0.8-1 mg/kg/dose given once a day. Range: 0.8-1.5 mg/kg/day. **Maximum:** 2 mg/kg/day or 100 mg/day.
▸ **Angina pectoris**
PO
Adults. Initially, 50 mg once a day. May increase dose up to 200 mg once a day.
Elderly. Usual initial dose, 25 mg a day.
▸ **Acute MI**
IV
Adults. Give 5 mg over 5 min; may repeat in 10 min. In those who tolerate full 10-mg IV dose, begin 50-mg tablets 10 min after last IV dose followed by another 50-mg oral dose 12 hr later. Thereafter, give 100 mg once a day or 50 mg twice a day for 6-9 days. Or, for those who do not tolerate full IV dose, give 50 mg orally twice a day or 100 mg once a day for at least 7 days.
▸ **Dosage in renal impairment**
Dosage interval is modified based on creatinine clearance.

Creatinine Clearance	Dosage Interval
15-35 ml/min	50 mg a day
Less than 15 ml/min	50 mg every other day

OFF-LABEL USES
Improved survival in diabetics with heart disease; treatment of hypertrophic cardiomyopathy, pheochromocytoma, and syndrome of mitral valve prolapse; prevention of migraine, thyrotoxicosis, tremors

CONTRAINDICATIONS
Cardiogenic shock, overt heart failure, second- or third-degree heart block, severe bradycardia

INTERACTIONS
Drug
Cimetidine: May increase atenolol blood concentration.
Diuretics, other antihypertensives: May increase hypotensive effect of atenolol.
Insulin, oral hypoglycemics: May mask symptoms of hypoglycemia and prolong hypoglycemic effect of insulin and oral hypoglycemics.
NSAIDs: May decrease antihypertensive effect of atenolol.
Sympathomimetics, xanthines: May mutually inhibit effects.
Herbal
None known.
Food
None known.

DIAGNOSTIC TEST EFFECTS
May increase serum antinuclear antibody titer and BUN, serum creatinine, potassium, lipoprotein, triglyceride, and uric acid levels.

🖳 IV INCOMPATIBILITIES
Amphotericin complex (Abelcet, AmBisome, Amphotec)

SIDE EFFECTS
Atenolol is generally well tolerated, with mild and transient side effects.
Frequent
Hypotension manifested as cold extremities, constipation or diarrhea, diaphoresis, dizziness, fatigue, headache, and nausea
Occasional
Insomnia, flatulence, urinary frequency, impotence or decreased libido, mental depression

Rare
Rash, arthralgia, myalgia, confusion (especially in the elderly), altered taste

SERIOUS REACTIONS
• Overdose may produce profound bradycardia and hypotension.
• Abrupt atenolol withdrawal may result in diaphoresis, palpitations, headache, and tremors.
• Atenolol administration may precipitate CHF or MI in patients with cardiac disease; thyroid storm in those with thyrotoxicosis; and peripheral ischemia in those with existing peripheral vascular disease.
• Hypoglycemia may occur in patients with previously controlled diabetes.
• Thrombocytopenia, manifested as unusual bruising or bleeding, occurs rarely.

PRECAUTIONS & CONSIDERATIONS
Caution is warranted with bronchospastic disease, diabetes, hyperthyroidism, impaired renal or hepatic function, inadequate cardiac function, and peripheral vascular disease. Atenolol readily crosses the placenta and is distributed in breast milk. Atenolol use should be avoided in pregnant women after the first trimester because it may result in low-birth-weight infants. The drug may also produce apnea, bradycardia, hypoglycemia, or hypothermia during childbirth. No age-related precautions have been noted in children. Use cautiously in the elderly, who may have age-related peripheral vascular disease and impaired renal function. Be aware that salt and alcohol intake should be restricted.

Nasal decongestants or OTC cold preparations (stimulants) should not be used without physician approval.

Orthostatic hypotension may occur, so rise slowly from a lying to sitting position and dangle the legs from the bed momentarily before standing. Notify the physician of confusion, depression, dizziness, rash, or unusual bruising or bleeding. B/P for hypotension, respiratory status for shortness of breath, and pulse for quality, rate and rhythm should be monitored during treatment. If pulse rate is 60 beats/minute or lower or systolic B/P is less than 90 mm Hg, withhold the medication and contact the physician. Signs and symptoms of CHF, such as decreased urine output, distended neck veins, dyspnea (particularly on exertion or lying down), night cough, peripheral edema, and weight gain should also be assessed.

Storage

Store at room temperature. After reconstitution, store parenteral form for up to 48 hours at room temperature.

Administration

Take oral atenolol without regard to meals. Crush tablets if necessary. Do not abruptly discontinue the drug. Compliance is essential to control angina and hypertension.

For IV use, give undiluted or dilute in 10 to 50 ml 0.9% NaCl or D₅W. Give IV push over 5 minutes and IV infusion over 15 minutes.

A

Atomoxetine
auto-mox′eh-teen
(Strattera)

CATEGORY AND SCHEDULE
Pregnancy Risk Category: C

CLASSIFICATION
Selective norepinephrine reuptake inhibitor

MECHANISM OF ACTION
A norepinephrine reuptake inhibitor that enhances noradrenergic function by selective inhibition of the presynaptic norepinephrine transporter. *Therapeutic Effect:* Improves symptoms of attention-deficit hyperactivity disorder (ADHD).

PHARMACOKINETICS
Rapidly absorbed after PO administration. Protein binding: 98% (primarily to albumin). Eliminated primarily in urine and, to a lesser extent, in feces. Not removed by hemodialysis.
Half-life: 4-5 hr in general population, 22 hr in 7% of Caucasians and 2% of African-Americans; (increased in moderate to severe hepatic insufficiency).

AVAILABILITY
Capsules: 10 mg, 18 mg, 25 mg, 40 mg, 60 mg.

INDICATIONS AND DOSAGES
▸ **ADHD**
PO
Adults, Children weighing 70 kg and more. 40 mg once a day. May increase after at least 3 days to 80 mg as a single daily dose or

in divided doses. Maximum:
100 mg.
Children weighing less than 70 kg.
Initially, 0.5 mg/kg/day. May
increase after at least 3 days to
1.2 mg/kg/day. Maximum:
1.4 mg/kg/day or 100 mg.
▸ **Dosage in hepatic impairment**
Expect to administer 50% of
normal atomoxetine dosage to
patients with moderate hepatic
impairment and 25% of normal
dosage to those with severe hepatic
impairment.

OFF-LABEL USES
Treatment of depression.

CONTRAINDICATIONS
Angle-closure glaucoma, use within
14 days of MAOIs

INTERACTIONS
Drug
Fluoxetine, paroxetine, quinidine:
May increase atomoxetine blood
concentration.
MAOIs: May increase the risk of
toxic effects.
Herbal
None known.
Food
None known.

DIAGNOSTIC TEST EFFECTS
None known.

SIDE EFFECTS
Frequent
Headache, dyspepsia, nausea, vomit-
ing, fatigue, decreased appetite,
dizziness, altered mood
Occasional
Tachycardia, hypertension, weight
loss, delayed growth in children,
irritability
Rare
Insomnia, sexual dysfunction in
adults, fever

SERIOUS REACTIONS
• Urine retention or urinary hesi-
tance may occur.
• In overdose, gastric emptying
and repeated use of activated
charcoal may prevent systemic
absorption.

PRECAUTIONS & CONSIDERATIONS
Caution is warranted with cardiovascular disease, tachycardia, hypertension, moderate or severe hepatic
impairment, and a risk of urine
retention. Be aware concurrent use
of medications that can increase
heart rate or blood pressure should
be avoided. It is unknown if
atomoxetine is excreted in breast
milk. The safety and efficacy of
atomoxetine have not been established in children younger than 6
years. Age-related cardiovascular or
cerebrovascular disease and hepatic
or renal impairment may increase
the risk of side effects in the
elderly.
   Dizziness may occur, so avoid
tasks that require mental alertness and
motor skills. Notify the physician if
fever, irritability, palpitations, or
vomiting occurs. B/P, pulse rate,
mood changes, urine output, and fluid
and electrolyte status should be monitored.
Administration
Take atomoxetine without
regard to food. Take the last
daily dose of atomoxetine early
in the evening to avoid
insomnia.

Atorvastatin
a-tor'va-sta-tin
(Lipitor)
Do not confuse Lipitor with Levatol.

CATEGORY AND SCHEDULE
Pregnancy Risk Category: X

CLASSIFICATION
Antihyperlipidemics, HMG CoA reductase inhibitors

MECHANISM OF ACTION
An antihyperlipidemic that inhibits HMG-CoA reductase, the enzyme that catalyzes the early step in cholesterol synthesis. *Therapeutic Effect:* Decreases LDL and VLDL cholesterol, and plasma triglyceride levels; increases HDL cholesterol concentration.

PHARMACOKINETICS
Poorly absorbed from the GI tract. Protein binding: greater than 98%. Metabolized in the liver. Minimally eliminated in urine. Plasma levels are markedly increased in chronic alcoholic hepatic disease, but are unaffected by renal disease. **Half-life:** 14 hr.

AVAILABILITY
Tablets: 10 mg, 20 mg, 40 mg, 80 mg.

INDICATIONS AND DOSAGES
▶ **Hyperlipidemia, reduction of risk of myocardial infarction (MI), angina revascularization procedures**
PO
Adults, Elderly. Initially, 10-40 mg a day given as a single dose.

Dose range: Increase at 2- to 4-wk intervals to maximum of 80 mg/day.
Children 10-17 yr. Initially, 10 mg/day, may increase to 20 mg/day.
▶ **Familial hypercholesterolemia**
PO
Children 10-17 yr. Initially, 10 mg/day. May increase to 20 mg/day.

CONTRAINDICATIONS
Active hepatic disease, lactation, pregnancy, unexplained elevated hepatic function test results

INTERACTIONS
Drug
Antacids, colestipol, propranolol: Decreases atorvastatin activity.
Cyclosporine, erythromycin, gemfibrozil, nicotinic acid: Increases the risk of acute renal failure and rhabdomyolysis with these drugs.
Digoxin, itraconazole, oral contraceptives, warfarin: May increase atorvastatin blood concentration, producing severe muscle inflammation, pain, and weakness.
Herbal
None known.
Food
Grapefruit juice may increase the bioavailability of atorvastatin resulting in an increased risk of myopathy or rhabdomyolysis.

DIAGNOSTIC TEST EFFECTS
May increase serum CK and transaminase concentrations.

SIDE EFFECTS
Atorvastatin is generally well tolerated. Side effects are usually mild and transient.
Frequent (16%)
Headache

Occasional (5%-2%)
Myalgia, rash or pruritus, allergy
Rare (2%-1%)
Flatulence, dyspepsia

SERIOUS REACTIONS
• Cataracts may develop, and
photosensitivity may occur.
Hepatotoxicity or rhabdomyolysis
occur rarely.

PRECAUTIONS & CONSIDERATIONS
Caution is warranted with a history
of hepatic disease, hypotension,
major surgery, severe acute infection, substantial alcohol consumption, trauma, those receiving
anticoagulant therapy, and those with
severe acute infection, uncontrolled
seizures, or severe endocrine, electrolyte, or metabolic disorders.
Atorvastatin is distributed in breast
milk. It is contraindicated during
pregnancy because it may produce
skeletal malformation. Pregnancy
should be determined before beginning therapy. Safety and efficacy of
atorvastatin have not been established in children. No age-related
precautions have been noted in the
elderly.
 Notify the physician of headache,
malaise, pruritus, or rash.
Laboratory results and serum cholesterol and triglyceride levels and
hepatic function test results should
be documented before therapy.
Serum cholesterol and triglyceride
levels should be monitored
periodically during therapy. Be
aware that diet is an important part
of treatment.
Administration
May be taken without regard to
food. Do not break film-coated
tablets.

Atovaquone
a-toe′va-kwone
(Mepron, Wellvone [AUS])

CATEGORY AND SCHEDULE
Pregnancy Risk Category: C

CLASSIFICATION
Antiprotozoals

MECHANISM OF ACTION
A systemic anti-infective that
inhibits the mitochondrial electron-
transport system at the cytochrome
bc1 complex (Complex III), which
interrupts nucleic acid and adenosine
triphosphate synthesis. *Therapeutic
Effect:* Antiprotozoal and antipneu-
mocystic activity.

PHARMACOKINETICS
Absorption increased with a high-fat
meal. Protein binding: greater than
99%. Metabolized in liver.
Primarily excreted in feces. **Half-
life:** 2-3 days.

AVAILABILITY
Oral suspension: 750 mg/5 ml.

INDICATIONS AND DOSAGES
▸ *Pneumocystis carinii* pneumonia
(PCP)
PO
Adults. 750 mg twice a day with
food for 21 days.
Children. 40 mg/kg/day in
2 divided doses. Maximum:
1500 mg/day.
▸ Prevention of PCP
PO
Adults. 1500 mg once a day with
food.
Children 4-24 mos. 45 mg/kg/day as
single dose. Maximum:
1500 mg/day.

Atropine   125

A

Children 1-3 mo and older than 24 mo. 30 mg/kg/day as single dose. Maximum: 1500 mg/day.
▸ **Usual pediatric dosage**
PO
Children. 40 mg/kg/day with food.

CONTRAINDICATIONS
Development or history of potentially life-threatening allergic reaction to the drug

INTERACTIONS
Drug
Rifampin: May decrease atovaquone blood concentration and increase rifampin blood concentration.
Herbal
None known.
Food
None known.

DIAGNOSTIC TEST EFFECTS
May increase serum alkaline phosphatase, amylase, AST (SGOT), and ALT (SGPT) levels. May decrease serum sodium levels.

SIDE EFFECTS
Frequent (greater than 10%)
Rash, nausea, diarrhea, headache, vomiting, fever, insomnia, cough
Occasional (less than 10%)
Abdominal discomfort, thrush, asthenia, anemia, neutropenia

SERIOUS REACTIONS
• Anemia occurs rarely.

PRECAUTIONS & CONSIDERATIONS
Caution is warranted with chronic diarrhea, malabsorption syndromes, severe PCP and in the elderly. Elderly patients require close monitoring because of age-related cardiac, hepatic, and renal impairment.

Notify the physician if diarrhea, rash, or other new symptoms occur. Pattern of daily bowel activity and stool consistency and skin for rash should be monitored. Hgb levels, intake and output, and renal function should be assessed. Medical history for problems that may interfere with the drug's absorption, such as GI disorders, should be determined before beginning therapy.
Administration
Take atovaquone for the full course of treatment.

Atropine
a′troe-peen
(Atropine Sulfate, Atropt [AUS])
Do not confuse with Akarpine or Aplisol.

CATEGORY AND SCHEDULE
Pregnancy Risk Category: C

CLASSIFICATION
Antiarrhythmics, anticholinergics, antidotes, cycloplegics, mydriatics, ophthalmics, preanesthetics

MECHANISM OF ACTION
An acetylcholine antagonist that inhibits the action of acetylcholine by competing with acetylcholine for common binding sites on muscarinic receptors, which are located on exocrine glands, cardiac and smooth-muscle ganglia, and intramural neurons. This action blocks all muscarinic effects. *Therapeutic Effect:* Decreases GI motility and secretory activity, and GU muscle tone (ureter, bladder); produces

ophthalmic cycloplegia, and mydriasis.

AVAILABILITY
Injection: 0.05 mg/ml, 0.1 mg/ml, 0.4 mg/0.5 ml, 0.4 mg/ml, 0.5 mg/ml, 1 mg/ml.

INDICATIONS AND DOSAGES
▸ **Asystole, slow pulseless electrical activity**
IV
Adults, Elderly. 1 mg; may repeat q3-5min up to total dose of 0.04 mg/kg.
▸ **Pre-anesthetic**
IV/IM/SUBCUTANEOUS
Adults, Elderly. 0.4-0.6 mg 30-60 min pre-op.
Children weighing 5 kg or more. 0.01-0.02 mg/kg/dose to maximum of 0.4 mg/dose.
Children weighing less than 5 kg. 0.02 mg/kg/dose 30-60 min pre-op.
▸ **Bradycardia**
IV
Adults, Elderly. 0.5-1 mg q5min not to exceed 2 mg or 0.04 mg/kg.
Children. 0.02 mg/kg with a minimum of 0.1 mg to a maximum of 0.5 mg in children and 1 mg in adolescents. May repeat in 5 min. Maximum total dose: 1 mg in children, 2 mg in adolescents.

CONTRAINDICATIONS
Bladder neck obstruction due to prostatic hypertrophy, cardiospasm, intestinal atony, myasthenia gravis in those not treated with neostigmine, narrow-angle glaucoma, obstructive disease of the GI tract, paralytic ileus, severe ulcerative colitis, tachycardia secondary to cardiac insufficiency or thyrotoxicosis, toxic megacolon, unstable cardiovascular status in acute hemorrhage

INTERACTIONS
Drug
Antacids, antidiarrheals: May decrease absorption of atropine.
Anticholinergics: May increase effects of atropine.
Ketoconazole: May decrease absorption of ketoconazole.
Potassium chloride: May increase severity of GI lesions (wax matrix).
Herbal
None known.
Food
None known.

DIAGNOSTIC TEST EFFECTS
None known.

▦ IV INCOMPATIBILITIES
Pentothal (Thiopental)
▯ **IV compatibilities**
Diphenhydramine (Benadryl), droperidol (Inapsine), fentanyl (Sublimaze), glycopyrrolate (Robinul), heparin, hydromorphone (Dilaudid), midazolam (Versed), morphine, potassium chloride, propofol (Diprivan)

SIDE EFFECTS
Frequent
Dry mouth, nose, and throat that may be severe; decreased sweating, constipation, irritation at subcutaneous or IM injection site
Occasional
Swallowing difficulty, blurred vision, bloated feeling, impotence, urinary hesitancy
Rare
Allergic reaction, including rash and urticaria; mental confusion or excitement, particularly in children, fatigue

SERIOUS REACTIONS
• Overdosage may produce tachycardia, palpitations, hot, dry or

flushed skin, absence of bowel sounds, increased respiratory rate, nausea, vomiting, confusion, somnolence, slurred speech, dizziness and CNS stimulation.
• Overdosage may also produce psychosis as evidenced by agitation, restlessness, rambling speech, visual hallucinations, paranoid behavior, and delusions, followed by depression.

PRECAUTIONS & CONSIDERATIONS
Extreme caution should be used with autonomic neuropathy, diarrhea, known and suspected GI infections, and mild to moderate ulcerative colitis. Caution is also warranted with CHF, COPD, coronary artery disease, esophageal reflux or hiatal hernia associated with reflux esophagitis, gastric ulcer, hepatic or renal disease, hypertension, hyperthyroidism, and tachyarrhythmias. Use atropine cautiously in the elderly and in infants.

Warm, dry, flushing feeling may occur upon administration. The patient should urinate before giving this drug to reduce the risk of urine retention. B/P, pulse rate, temperature, pattern of daily bowel activity and stool consistency, intake and output, and skin turgor and mucous membranes should be assessed.

Administration
! Notify physician and expect to discontinue atropine immediately if blurred vision, dizziness, or increased pulse rate occurs.

For IV use, give the drug rapidly, to prevent paradoxical slowing of the heart rate. Atropine may be given by IM or subcutaneous injection.

Auranofin
ah-ran′oh-fin
(Ridaura)
(Gold-50 [AUS], Solganal)
Do not confuse Ridaura with Cardura.

CATEGORY AND SCHEDULE
Pregnancy Risk Category: C

CLASSIFICATION
Disease modifying antirheumatic drugs, gold compounds

MECHANISM OF ACTION
Gold compounds that alter cellular mechanisms, collagen biosynthesis, enzyme systems, and immune responses. *Therapeutic Effect:* Suppress synovitis in the active stage of rheumatoid arthritis.

PHARMACOKINETICS
Auranofin (29% gold): Moderately absorbed from the GI tract. Protein binding: 60%. Rapidly metabolized. Primarily excreted in urine. **Half-life:** 21-31 days. Aurothioglucose (50% gold): Slowly and erraticly absorbed after IM administration. Protein binding: 95%-99%. Primarily excreted in urine. **Half-life:** 3-27 days (increased with increased number of doses).

AVAILABILITY
Capsules (Ridaura): 3 mg.
Injection (Solganal): 50-mg/ml suspension.

INDICATIONS AND DOSAGES
▶ **Rheumatoid arthritis**
PO

Adults, Elderly. 6 mg/day as a single or 2 divided doses. If there is no response in 6 mo, may increase to 9 mg/day in 3 divided doses. If response is still inadequate, discontinue.
Children. 0.1 mg/kg/day as a single or 2 divided doses. Maintenance: 0.15 mg/kg/day. Maximum: 0.2 mg/kg/day.
IM
Adults, Elderly. Initially, 10 mg, followed by 25 mg for 2 doses, then 50 mg weekly until total dose of 0.8-1 g has been given. If patient has improved and shows no signs of toxicity, may give 50 mg q3-4wk for many months.
Children. 0.25 mg/kg; may increase by 0.25 mg/kg each week. Maintenance: 0.75-1 mg/kg/dose. Maximum: 25 mg/dose for 20 doses, then repeated q2-4wk.

OFF-LABEL USES
Treatment of pemphigus, psoriatic arthritis

CONTRAINDICATIONS
Bone marrow aplasia, history of gold-induced pathologies (including blood dyscrasias, exfoliative dermatitis, necrotizing enterocolitis, and pulmonary fibrosis), severe blood dyscrasias

INTERACTIONS
Drug
Bone marrow depressants; hepatotoxic and nephrotoxic medications: May increase the risk of aurothioglucose toxicity.
Penicillamine: May increase the risk of hematologic or renal adverse effects.
Herbal
None known.
Food
None known.

DIAGNOSTIC TEST EFFECTS
May decrease Hgb level, Hct, and WBC and platelet counts.
May increase urine protein level.
May alter hepatic function test results.

SIDE EFFECTS
Frequent
Auranofin: Diarrhea (50%), pruritic rash (26%), abdominal pain (14%), stomatitis (13%), nausea (10%)
Aurothioglucose: Rash (39%), stomatitis (19%), diarrhea (13%).
Occasional
Aurothioglucose: Nausea, vomiting, anorexia, abdominal cramps

SERIOUS REACTIONS
• Signs and symptoms of gold toxicity, the primary serious reaction, include decreased Hgb level, decreased granulocyte count (less than 150,000/mm^3), proteinuria, hematuria, stomatitis, blood dyscrasias (anemia, leukopenia [WBC count less than 4000/mm^3], thrombocytopenia, and eosinophilia), glomerulonephritis, nephrotic syndrome, and cholestatic jaundice.

PRECAUTIONS & CONSIDERATIONS
Caution is warranted with blood dyscrasias, compromised cerebral or cardiovascular circulation, eczema, a history of sensitivity to gold compounds, marked hypertension, renal or liver impairment, severe debilitation, Sjögren's syndrome in rheumatoid arthritis, and systemic lupus erythematosus. Auranofin and aurothioglucose cross the placenta and are distributed in breast milk. These drugs should be used only when their benefits outweigh the possible risks to the fetus.

No age-related precautions have been noted in children. Use these drugs cautiously in the elderly, who may have age-related renal impairment. Avoid exposure to sunlight, which may turn skin gray or blue. Oral hygiene should be diligently maintained to help prevent stomatitis.

Notify the physician if GI symptoms (nausea, vomiting, or abdominal cramps), metallic taste, sore mouth, pruritus, or rash occurs. Pattern of daily bowel activity and stool consistency, urine for hematuria and proteinuria, CBC (particularly Hgb level, Hct, and WBC and platelet counts), renal and liver function tests (especially BUN level and serum alkaline phosphatase, creatinine, AST [SGOT], and ALT [SGPT] levels), skin for rash, and oral mucous membranes for stomatitis should be monitored. Therapeutic response, including improved grip strength, increased joint mobility, reduced joint tenderness, and relief of pain, stiffness, and swelling, should also be assessed.

Administration
Take these drugs without regard to food. Therapeutic response to the drug may occur in 3 to 6 months.
! Give auranofin or aurothioglucose as weekly injections.

Inject the drug in the upper outer quadrant of the gluteus maximus.

Aurothioglucose/ Gold Sodium Thiomalate
ah-row-thigh-oh-glue′cose
(Gold-50 [AUS], Solganal);
(Myochrysine, Myocrisin [AUS])

A

CATEGORY AND SCHEDULE
Pregnancy Risk Category: C

CLASSIFICATION
Antirheumatic agents

MECHANISM OF ACTION
Aurothioglucose: A gold compound that alters cellular mechanisms, collagen biosynthesis, enzyme systems, and immune responses. *Therapeutic Effect:* Suppresses synovitis of the active stage of rheumatoid arthritis.
Gold sodium thiomalate: A gold compound whose mechanism of action is unknown. May decrease prostaglandin synthesis or alter cellular mechanisms by inhibiting sulfhydryl systems. *Therapeutic Effect:* Decreases synovial inflammation, retards cartilage and bone destruction, suppresses or prevents but does not cure, arthritis, synovitis.

PHARMACOKINETICS
Aurothioglucose (50% gold): Slow, erratic absorption after IM administration. Protein binding: 95%-99%. Primarily excreted in urine.
Half-life: 3- 27 days (half-life increased with increased number of doses).
Gold sodium thiomalate: Well absorbed. Protein binding: 95%. Widely distributed. Metabolized in liver. Excreted in urine and feces. Not removed by hemodialysis. **Half-life:** 5 days.

AVAILABILITY

Aurothioglucose
Injection: 50 mg/ml suspension
(Solganal).
Gold sodium thiomalate
Injection: 50 mg/ml
(Myochrysine).

INDICATIONS AND DOSAGES

▸ **Rheumatoid arthritis**
Aurothioglucose
IM
Adults, Elderly. Initially, 10 mg,
then 25 mg for 2 doses, then
50 mg weekly thereafter until total
dose of 0.8-1 g given. If patient is
improved and there are no signs
of toxicity, may give 50 mg at 3-
to 4-wk intervals for many
months.
Children. 0. 25 mg/kg, may increase
by 0. 25 mg/kg each week.
Maintenance: 0.75-1 mg/kg/dose.
Maximum: 25-mg dose for total of
20 doses, then q2-4wks.
▸ **Gold sodium thiomalate**
IM
Adults, Elderly. Initially, 10 mg,
then 25 mg for second dose.
Follow with 25- 50 mg/wk until
improvement noted or total of
1 g administered. Maintenance:
25-50 mg q2wks for 2-20 wks;
if stable, may increase to q3-4wk
intervals.
Children. Initially, 10 mg, then
1 mg/kg/wk. Maximum single dose:
50 mg. Maintenance: 1 mg/kg/dose
at 2- to 4-wk intervals.
▸ **Dosage in renal impairment**

Creatinine Clearance	Dosage
50-80 ml/min less than 50 ml/min	50% of usual dosage not recommended

OFF-LABEL USES

Treatment of pemphigus, psoriatic
arthritis

CONTRAINDICATIONS

Aurothioglucose
Bone marrow aplasia, history of
gold-induced pathologies, including
blood dyscrasias, exfoliative
dermatitis, necrotizing enterocolitis,
and pulmonary fibrosis, serious
adverse effects with previous gold
therapy, severe blood dyscrasias
Gold sodium thiomalate
Colitis, concurrent use of antimalarials, immunosuppressive agents,
penicillamine, or phenylbutazone,
congestive heart failure (CHF), exfoliative dermatitis, history of blood
dyscrasias, severe liver or renal
impairment, systemic lupus erythematosus

INTERACTIONS

Drug
Bone marrow depressants;
hepatotoxic, nephrotoxic medica-
tions: May increase risk of auroth-
ioglucose toxicity.
Penicillamine: May increase risk of
hematologic or renal adverse effects
of aurothioglucose.
Herbal
None known.
Food
None known.

DIAGNOSTIC TEST EFFECTS

May decrease Hgb, Hct, platelets,
white blood cell (WBC) count. May
alter liver function tests. May
increase urine protein.

SIDE EFFECTS

Frequent
Aurothioglucose: Rash, stomatitis,
diarrhea
Gold sodium thiomalate: Pruritic
dermatitis, stomatitis, marked by
erythema, redness, shallow ulcers of
oral mucous membranes, sore throat,
and difficulty swallowing, diarrhea or
loose stools, abdominal pain, nausea

Occasional
Aurothioglucose: Nausea, vomiting, anorexia, abdominal cramps
Gold sodium thiomalate: Vomiting, anorexia, flatulence, dyspepsia, conjunctivitis, photosensitivity
Rare
Gold sodium thiomalate: Constipation, urticaria, rash

SERIOUS REACTIONS
• Gold toxicity is the primary serious reaction. Signs and symptoms of gold toxicity include decreased hemoglobin, leukopenia (WBC count less than 4000/mm^3), reduced granulocyte counts (less than 150,000/mm^3), proteinuria, hematuria, stomatitis (sores, ulcers and white spots in the mouth and throat), blood dyscrasias (anemia, leukopenia, thrombocytopenia, and eosinophilia), glomerulonephritis, nephritic syndrome, and cholestatic jaundice.

PRECAUTIONS & CONSIDERATIONS
Caution is warranted with blood dyscrasias, compromised cerebral or cardiovascular circulation, eczema, a history of sensitivity to gold compounds, marked hypertension, renal or liver impairment, severe debilitation, Sjögren's syndrome in rheumatoid arthritis, and systemic lupus erythematosus. Gold salts have been considered to cross the placenta and be distributed in the breast milk. There are no age-related precautions noted in children. Use cautiously in the elderly, who may have decreased renal function. Maintain diligent oral hygiene to prevent stomatitis. Avoid exposure to sunlight because it may cause a gray to blue pigment to appear on the skin.
   Determine if the patient is pregnant before beginning treatment. Check the results of complete blood count (CBC), particularly BUN, Hct, Hgb,

platelet count, serum alkaline phosphatase, creatinine, SGOT (AST), and SGPT (ALT) levels to assess renal and liver function and urinalysis, before and during therapy. If indigestion, metallic taste, pruritus, rash, or sore mouth occurs, notify the physician.
Storage
Store at room temperature and protect from light.
Administration
Be aware to give as weekly injections. Give in upper outer quadrant of gluteus maximus. Therapeutic response of the drug may be expected in 3 to 6 months.

Azacitidine
ay-zah-sigh'tih-deen
(Vidaza)

CATEGORY AND SCHEDULE
Pregnancy Risk Category: D

CLASSIFICATION
Antineoplastics, antimetabolites

MECHANISM OF ACTION
An antineoplastic agent that exerts a cytotoxic effect on rapidly dividing cells by causing demethylation of DNA in abnormal hematopoietic cells in the bone marrow.
Therapeutic Effect: Restores normal function to tumor-suppressor genes regulating cellular differentiation and proliferation.

PHARMACOKINETICS
Rapidly absorbed after subcutaneous administration. Metabolized by the liver. Eliminated in urine. **Half-life:** 4 hr.

AVAILABILITY
Powder for Injection: 100 mg.

INDICATIONS AND DOSAGES
▶ **Refractory anemia, chronic myelomonocytic leukemia**
SUBCUTANEOUS
Adults, Elderly. 75 mg/m²/day for 7 days every 4 wk. Dosage may be increased to 100 mg/m² if initial dose is insufficient and toxicity is manageable.

CONTRAINDICATIONS
Advanced malignant hepatic tumors, hypersensitivity to mannitol

INTERACTIONS
Drug
Bone marrow suppressants: May increase myelosuppression.
Herbal
None known.
Food
None known.

DIAGNOSTIC TEST EFFECTS
May decrease hemoglobin level, hematocrit, and WBC, RBC, and platelet counts. May increase serum creatinine and potassium levels.

SIDE EFFECTS
Frequent (71%-29%)
Nausea, vomiting, fever, diarrhea, fatigue, injection site erythema, constipation, ecchymosis, cough, dyspnea, weakness
Occasional (26%-16%)
Rigors, petechiae, injection site pain, pharyngitis, arthralgia, headache, limb pain, dizziness, peripheral edema, back pain, erythema, epistaxis, weight loss, myalgia
Rare (13%-8%)
Anxiety, abdominal pain, rash, depression, tachycardia, insomnia, night sweats, stomatitis

SERIOUS REACTIONS
• Hematologic toxicity, manifested most commonly as anemia, leukopenia, neutropenia, and thrombocytopenia, is a common adverse effect.

PRECAUTIONS & CONSIDERATIONS
Caution is warranted with hepatic or renal impairment. Azacitidine may be embryotoxic, causing developmental abnormalities in the fetus. Barrier contraception should be used while receiving azacitidine. Women of childbearing age should avoid becoming pregnant while taking azacitidine. Breast-feeding while taking azacitidine should be avoided. The safety and efficacy of azacitidine have not been established in children. Age-related renal impairment may increase the risk of renal toxicity in the elderly.

Notify the physician of nausea and vomiting, bleeding, and any signs of infection, including fever and flu-like symptoms. Blood counts should be obtained before each dosing cycle to monitor the response and assess for drug toxicity.
Storage
Store vials at room temperature. The reconstituted solution may be stored for up to 1 hour at room temperature or up to 8 hours if refrigerated. After removing from refrigeration, allow the drug suspension to return to room temperature and use it within 30 minutes.
Administration
For subcutaneous administration, use strict aseptic technique when preparing the drug. Reconstitute azacitidine with 4 ml sterile water for injection. The reconstituted solution will appear cloudy. Use the solution within 1 hour after reconstitution. Divide doses greater than 4 ml equally into two syringes. To resuspend the contents, invert the syringe 2 or 3 times and roll it between your palms for 30 seconds

immediately before administration. Rotate injection sites among the abdomen, upper arm, and thigh for each injection. Administer each new injection at least 1 inch from a previous injection site.

Azathioprine
ay-za-thye′oh-preen
(Alti-Azathioprine [CAN], Azasan, Imuran, Thioprine [AUS])
Do not confuse azathioprine with Azulfidine or azatadine, or Imuran with Elmiron or Imferon.

CATEGORY AND SCHEDULE
Pregnancy Risk Category: D

CLASSIFICATION
Disease modifying antirheumatic drugs, immunosuppressives

MECHANISM OF ACTION
An immunologic agent that antagonizes purine metabolism and inhibits DNA, protein, and RNA synthesis. *Therapeutic Effect:* Suppresses cell-mediated hypersensitivities; alters antibody production and immune response in transplant recipients; reduces the severity of arthritis symptoms.

AVAILABILITY
Tablets (Azasan): 25 mg, 50 mg, 75 mg, 100 mg.
Tablets (Imuran): 50 mg.
Injection: 100-mg vial.

INDICATIONS AND DOSAGES
▸ **Adjunct in prevention of renal allograft rejection**

PO, IV
Adults, Elderly, Children.
2-5 mg/kg/day on day of transplant, then 1-3 mg/kg/day as maintenance dose.
▸ **Rheumatoid arthritis**
PO
Adults. Initially, 1 mg/kg/day as a single dose or in 2 divided doses. May increase by 0.5 mg/kg/day after 6-8 wk at 4-wk intervals up to maximum of 2.5 mg/kg/day. Maintenance: Lowest effective dosage. May decrease dose by 0.5 mg/kg or 25 mg/day q4wk (while other therapies, such as rest, physiotherapy, and salicylates, are maintained).
Elderly. Initially, 1 mg/kg/day (50-100 mg); may increase by 25 mg/day until response or toxicity.
▸ **Dosage in renal impairment**
Dosage is modified based on creatinine clearance.

Creatinine Clearance	Dose
10-50 ml/min	75% of usual dose
Less than 10 ml/min	50% of usual dose

OFF-LABEL USES
Treatment of biliary cirrhosis, chronic active hepatitis, glomerulonephritis, inflammatory bowel disease, inflammatory myopathy, multiple sclerosis, myasthenia gravis, nephrotic syndrome, pemphigoid, pemphigus, polymyositis, systemic lupus erythematosus

CONTRAINDICATIONS
Pregnant patients with rheumatoid arthritis

INTERACTIONS
Drug
Allopurinol: May increase activity and risk of toxicity of azathioprine.

Bone marrow depressants: May increase myelosuppression.

Live-virus vaccines: May potentiate virus replication, increase the vaccine's side effects, and decrease the patient's antibody response to the vaccine.

Other immunosuppressants: May increase the risk of infection or neoplasms.

Herbal
None known.

Food
None known.

DIAGNOSTIC TEST EFFECTS
May decrease serum albumin, Hgb, and serum uric acid levels. May increase serum alkaline phosphatase, amylase, bilirubin, AST (SGOT), and ALT (SGPT) levels.

▒ IV INCOMPATIBILITIES
Methyl and propyl parabens, phenol

SIDE EFFECTS
Frequent
Nausea, vomiting, anorexia (particularly during early treatment and with large doses)

Occasional
Rash

Rare
Severe nausea and vomiting with diarrhea, abdominal pain, hypersensitivity reaction

SERIOUS REACTIONS
• Azathioprine use increases the risk of developing neoplasia (new abnormal-growth tumors).
• Significant leukopenia and thrombocytopenia may occur, particularly in those undergoing kidney transplant rejection.
• Hepatotoxicity occurs rarely.

PRECAUTIONS & CONSIDERATIONS
Azathioprine should be used cautiously in immunosuppressed patients, previous treatment for rheumatoid arthritis with alkylating agents (such as chlorambucil, cyclophosphamide, and melphalan), and current or recent chickenpox. Avoid pregnancy during treatment.

Notify the physician if abdominal pain, fever, mouth sores, sore throat, or unusual bleeding occurs. CBC (especially platelet count) and serum hepatic enzyme levels should be monitored weekly during the first month of therapy, twice monthly during the second and third months of treatment, and monthly thereafter. The dosage should be reduced or discontinued if the WBC count falls rapidly. Therapeutic response, including improved grip strength, increased joint mobility, reduced joint tenderness, and relief of pain, stiffness, and swelling, should be assessed.

Storage
Store the tablets at room temperature. Store the parenteral form at room temperature. After reconstitution, the IV solution is stable for 24 hours at room temperature.

Administration
Take oral azathioprine during or after meals to reduce the risk of GI disturbances. The drug's therapeutic response may take up to 12 weeks to appear.

For IV use, reconstitute the 100-mg vial with 10 ml sterile water for injection to provide a concentration of 10 mg/ml. Swirl the vial gently to dissolve the solution. The solution may be further diluted in 50 ml D_5W or 0.9% NaCl. Infuse the solution over 30 to 60 minutes (range is 5 minutes to 8 hours).

Azelastine
a′zel-ah-steen
(Astelin, Optivar)
Do not confuse Optivar with Optiray.

CATEGORY AND SCHEDULE
Pregnancy Risk Category: C

CLASSIFICATION
Antihistamines, H1, inhalation, ophthalmics

MECHANISM OF ACTION
An antihistamine that competes with histamine for histamine receptor sites on cells in the blood vessels, GI tract, and respiratory tract. *Therapeutic Effect:* Relieves symptoms associated with seasonal allergic rhinitis such as increased mucus production and sneezing and symptoms associated with allergic conjunctivitis, such as redness, itching, and excessive tearing.

PHARMACOKINETICS

Route	Onset	Peak	Duration
Nasal spray	0.5-1 hr	2-3 hr	12 hr
Ophthalmic	N/A	3 min	8 hr

Well absorbed through nasal mucosa. Primarily excreted in feces.
Half-life: 22 hrs

AVAILABILITY
Nasal Spray (Astelin): 137 mcg.
Ophthalmic Solution (Optivar): 0.05%.

INDICATIONS AND DOSAGES
▶ **Allergic rhinitis**
NASAL
Adults, Elderly, Children 12 yr and older. 2 sprays in each nostril twice a day.
Children 5-11 yr. 1 spray in each nostril twice a day.
▶ **Allergic conjunctivitis**
OPHTHALMIC
Adults, Elderly, Children 3 yr or older. 1 drop into affected eye twice a day.

CONTRAINDICATIONS
Breast-feeding women, history of hypersensitivity to antihistamines, neonates or premature infants, third trimester of pregnancy

INTERACTIONS
Drug
Alcohol, other CNS depressants: May increase CNS depression.
Cimetidine: May increase azelastine blood concentration.
Herbal
None known.
Food
None known.

DIAGNOSTIC TEST EFFECTS
May increase ALT (SGPT) levels. May suppress flare and wheal reactions to antigen skin testing unless drug is discontinued 4 days before testing.

SIDE EFFECTS
Frequent (20%-15%)
Headache, bitter taste
Rare
Nasal burning, paroxysmal sneezing
Ophthalmic: Transient eye burning or stinging, bitter taste, headache

SERIOUS REACTIONS
• Epistaxis occurs rarely.

PRECAUTIONS & CONSIDERATIONS

Caution is warranted with renal impairment. It is unknown if azelastine crosses the placenta or is distributed in breast milk. Don't use azelastine during the third trimester of pregnancy. The safety and efficacy of azelastine have not been established in children younger than 12 years. No age-related precautions have been noted in the elderly. Avoid drinking alcoholic beverages during therapy.

Administration

For intranasal use, prime the pump with 4 sprays or until a fine mist appears before using the nasal spray the first time. After the first use and if the pump hasn't been used for 3 or more days, prime the pump with 2 sprays or until a fine mist appears. To administer the spray, clear nasal passages as much as possible before use. Tilt head slightly forward. Insert the applicator tip into one nostril, pointing the tip toward the nasal passage and away from the nasal septum. While holding the other nostril closed, spray into the nostril and inhale at the same time to deliver the drug as high into the nasal passages as possible. Repeat in the other nostril. Wipe the applicator tip with a clean, damp tissue and replace cap immediately after use. Avoid spraying nasal drug into the eyes.

For ophthalmic use, tilt head back and instill the solution in the conjunctival sac of the affected eye. Close the eye; then press gently on the lacrimal sac for 1 minute.

Azithromycin

ay-zi-thro-mye'sin
(Zithromax, Zithromax TRI-PAK, Zithromax Z-PAK)
Do not confuse azithromycin with erythromycin.

CATEGORY AND SCHEDULE

Pregnancy Risk Category: B

CLASSIFICATION

Antibiotics, macrolides

MECHANISM OF ACTION

A macrolide antibiotic that binds to ribosomal receptor sites of susceptible organisms, inhibiting RNA-dependent protein synthesis. *Therapeutic Effect:* Bacteriostatic or bactericidal, depending on the drug dosage.

PHARMACOKINETICS

Rapidly absorbed from the GI tract. Protein binding: 7%-50%. Widely distributed. Eliminated primarily unchanged by biliary excretion.
Half-life: 68 hr.

AVAILABILITY

Oral Suspension: 100 mg/5 ml, 200 mg/5 ml.
Tablets: 250 mg, 500 mg, 600 mg. Tri-Pak: 500 mg (3s). Z-Pak: 250 mg (6s).
Injection: 500 mg.

INDICATIONS AND DOSAGES

▸ **Respiratory tract, skin, and skin-structure infections**
PO
Adults, Elderly. 500 mg once, then 250 mg/day for 4 days.
Children 6 mo and older. 10 mg/kg once (maximum 500 mg) then

5 mg/kg/day for 4 days (maximum 250 mg).

▸ **Acute bacterial exacerbations of COPD**
PO
Adults. 500 mg/day for 3 days.

▸ **Otitis media**
PO
Children 6 mo and older. 10 mg/kg once (maximum 500 mg) then 5 mg/kg/day for 4 days (maximum 250 mg). Single dose: 30 mg/kg. Maximum: 1500 mg. Three day regimen: 10 mg/kg/day as single daily dose. Maximum: 500 mg/day.

▸ **Pharyngitis, tonsillitis**
PO
Children older than 2 yr.
12 mg/kg/day (maximum 500 mg) for 5 days.

▸ **Chancroid**
PO
Adults, Elderly. 1 g as single dose.
Children. 20 mg/kg as single dose.
Maximum: 1 g.

▸ **Treatment of *Mycobacterium avium* complex (MAC)**
PO
Adults, Elderly. 500 mg/day in combination.
Children. 5 mg/kg/day (maximum 250 mg) in combination.

▸ **Prevention of MAC**
PO
Adults, Elderly. 1200 mg/wk alone or with rifabutin.
Children. 5 mg/kg/day (maximum 250 mg) or 20 mg/kg/wk (maximum 1200 mg) alone or with rifabutin.

▸ **Nongonococcal urethritis and cervicitis due to *Chlamydia trachomatis***
PO
Adults. 1 g as a single dose.

▸ **Usual pediatric dosage**
PO
Children older than 6 mo. 10 mg/kg once (maximum: 500 mg) then

5 mg/kg/day for 4 days (maximum 250 mg).

▸ **Usual parenteral dosage (Community Acquired Pneumonia, PID)**
IV
Adults. 500 mg/day, followed by oral therapy.

OFF-LABEL USES
Chlamydial infections, gonococcal pharyngitis, uncomplicated gonococcal infections of the cervix, urethra, and rectum

CONTRAINDICATIONS
Hypersensitivity to azithromycin or other macrolide antibiotics

INTERACTIONS
Drug
Aluminum- or magnesium-containing antacids: May decrease azithromycin blood concentration.
Carbamazepine, cyclosporine, theophylline, warfarin: May increase the serum concentrations of these drugs.
Herbal
None known.
Food
None known.

DIAGNOSTIC TEST EFFECTS
May increase serum CK, AST (SGOT), and ALT (SGPT) levels.

▓ IV INCOMPATIBILITIES
Information is not available.
▓ **IV compatibilities**
None known; don't mix with other medications.

SIDE EFFECTS
Occasional
Nausea, vomiting, diarrhea, abdominal pain

Rare
Headache, dizziness, allergic reaction

SERIOUS REACTIONS
• Antibiotic-associated colitis and other superinfections may result from altered bacterial balance.
• Acute interstitial nephritis and hepatotoxicity occur rarely.

PRECAUTIONS & CONSIDERATIONS
Caution is warranted with hepatic or renal dysfunction. Determine if there is a history of hepatitis or allergies to azithromycin or other macrolides before beginning therapy. It is unknown if azithromycin is distributed in breast milk. The safety and efficacy of azithromycin have not been established in children younger than 16 years for IV use and younger than 6 months for oral use. No age-related precautions have been noted in elderly patients with normal renal function.

GI discomfort, nausea, or vomiting should be assessed. Evaluate for signs and symptoms of superinfection, including genital or anal pruritus, sore mouth or tongue, and moderate to severe diarrhea. Assess for signs and symptoms of hepatotoxicity, such as abdominal pain, fever, GI disturbances, and malaise. Liver function tests should be monitored.

Storage
Store the oral suspension at room temperature. The suspension is stable for 10 days after reconstitution. Store vials at room temperature. After reconstitution, the solution is stable for 24 hours at room temperature or 7 days if refrigerated.

Administration
Give tablets without regard to food. Don't administer the oral suspension with food. Give it at least 1 hour before or 2 hours after a meal. Take the oral suspension with 8 oz of water at least 1 hour before or 2 hours after consuming any food or beverages. Azithromycin should be taken 1 hour before or 2 hours after antacids. Space doses evenly around the clock and continue taking for the full course of treatment.

For IV use, reconstitute each 500-mg vial with 4.8 ml sterile water for injection to provide a concentration of 100 mg/ml. Shake well to ensure dissolution. Further dilute the solution with 250 or 500 ml 0.9% NaCl or D_5W to provide a final concentration of 2 mg/ml or 1 mg/ml, respectively. Infuse the drug over 60 minutes.

Aztreonam
az-tree'oo-nam
(Azactam)

CATEGORY AND SCHEDULE
Pregnancy Risk Category: B

CLASSIFICATION
Antibiotics, monobactams

MECHANISM OF ACTION
A monobactam antibiotic that inhibits bacterial cell wall synthesis. *Therapeutic Effect:* Bactericidal.

PHARMACOKINETICS
Completely absorbed after IM administration. Protein binding: 56%-60%. Partially metabolized by hydrolysis. Primarily excreted unchanged in urine. Removed by hemodialysis. **Half-life:** 1.4-2.2 hr

(increased in impaired renal or hepatic function).

AVAILABILITY
Injection Powder for Reconstitution:
500 mg, 1 g, 2 g.

INDICATIONS AND DOSAGES
▶ **UTIs**
IV, IM
Adults, Elderly. 500 mg-1 g q8-12hr.
▶ **Moderate to severe systemic infections**
IV, IM
Adults, Elderly. 1-2 g q8-12hr.
▶ **Severe or life-threatening infections**
IV
Adults, Elderly. 2 g q6-8hr.
▶ **Cystic Fibrosis**
IV
Children. 50 mg/kg/dose q6-8hr up to 200 mg/kg/day. Maximum: 8g/d.
▶ **Mild to severe infections in children**
IV
Children. 30 mg/kg q6-8hr. Maximum: 120 mg/kg/day.
Neonates. 60-120 mg/kg/day q6-12hr.
▶ **Dosage in renal impairment**
Dosage and frequency are modified based on creatinine clearance and the severity of the infection:

Creatinine Clearance	Dosage
10-30 ml/min	1-2 g initially, then $\frac{1}{2}$ usual dose at usual intervals
Less than 10 ml/min	1-2 g initially; then $\frac{1}{4}$ usual dose at usual intervals

OFF-LABEL USES
Treatment of bone and joint infections

CONTRAINDICATIONS
None known.

INTERACTIONS
Drug
None known.
Herbal
None known.
Food
None known.

DIAGNOSTIC TEST EFFECTS
May increase serum alkaline phosphatase, creatinine, LDH, AST (SGOT), and ALT (SGPT) levels. Produces a positive Coombs' test.

▓ IV INCOMPATIBILITIES
Acyclovir (Zovirax), amphotericin (Fungizone), daunorubicin (Cerubidine), ganciclovir (Cytovene), lorazepam (Ativan), metronidazole (Flagyl), vancomycin (Vancocin)
▓ IV compatibilities
Aminophylline, bumetanide (Bumex), calcium gluconate, cimetidine (Tagamet), diltiazem (Cardizem), dobutamine (Dobutrex), dopamine (Intropin), famotidine (Pepcid), furosemide (Lasix), heparin, hydromorphone (Dilaudid), insulin (regular), magnesium sulfate, morphine, potassium chloride, propofol (Diprivan)

SIDE EFFECTS
Occasional (less than 3%)
Discomfort and swelling at IM injection site, nausea, vomiting, diarrhea, rash
Rare (less than 1%)
Phlebitis or thrombophlebitis at IV injection site, abdominal cramps, headache, hypotension

SERIOUS REACTIONS
• Antibiotic-associated colitis and other superinfections may result from altered bacterial balance.

- Severe hypersensitivity reactions, including anaphylaxis, occur rarely.

PRECAUTIONS & CONSIDERATIONS

Caution is warranted with hepatic or renal impairment or a history of allergies, especially to antibiotics. Aztreonam crosses the placenta, and is distributed in amniotic fluid and in low concentrations in breast milk. The safety and efficacy of aztreonam have not been established in children less than 9 months old. Age-related renal impairment may require a dosage adjustment in the elderly. History of allergies, especially to antibiotics, should be determined before giving aztreonam.

GI discomfort, nausea, and vomiting may occur. Pattern of daily bowel activity and stool consistency and skin for rash should be assessed. Signs and symptoms of phlebitis, such as heat, pain, and red streaking over the vein and pain at the IM injection site should also be assessed. Be alert for signs and symptoms of superinfection, including anal or genital pruritus, black hairy tongue, vomiting, diarrhea, fever, sore throat, and ulceration or changes of oral mucosa.

Storage

Store vials at room temperature. The solution normally appears colorless to light yellow. After reconstitution, the solution is stable for 48 hours at room temperature and 7 days if refrigerated. Discard the solution if a precipitate forms. Discard unused portions of solution. After reconstitution for IM injection, the solution is stable for 48 hours at room temperature and 7 days if refrigerated.

Administration

For IV push, dilute each gram with 6-10 ml of sterile water for injection. For intermittent IV infusion, further dilute with 50 to 100 ml of D5W or 0.9% NaCl. Administer IV push, over 3 to 5 minutes. Administer IV infusion, over 20 to 60 minutes. For IM use, shake the vial immediately and vigorously after adding the diluent. Inject the drug deep into a large muscle mass.

Bacitracin
bass-i-tray'sin
(Baciguent, Baci-IM, Bacitracin)
Do not confuse bacitracin with Bactrim or Bactroban.

CATEGORY AND SCHEDULE
Pregnancy Risk Category: C
OTC

CLASSIFICATION
Anti-infectives, ophthalmics, topical, antibiotics, miscellaneous, dermatologics

MECHANISM OF ACTION
An antibiotic that interferes with plasma membrane permeability and inhibits bacterial cell wall synthesis in susceptible bacteria. *Therapeutic Effect:* Bacteriostatic.

AVAILABILITY
Powder for Irrigation:
50,000 units.
Ophthalmic Ointment: 500 units/g.
Topical Ointment: 500 units/g.

INDICATIONS AND DOSAGES
▸ **Superficial ocular infections**
OPHTHALMIC
Adults: ½-inch ribbon in conjunctival sac q3-4hr.
▸ **Skin abrasions, superficial skin infections**
TOPICAL
Adults, Children. Apply to affected area 1-5 times a day.
▸ **Surgical treatment and prophylaxis**
IRRIGATION
Adults, Elderly. 50,000-150,000 units, as needed.

CONTRAINDICATIONS
None known

INTERACTIONS
Drug
None known.
Herbal
None known.
Food
None known.

DIAGNOSTIC TEST EFFECTS
None known.

SIDE EFFECTS
Rare
Ophthalmic: Burning, itching, redness, swelling, pain
Topical: Hypersensitivity reaction (allergic contact dermatitis, burning, inflammation, pruritus)

SERIOUS REACTIONS
• Severe hypersensitivity reactions, including apnea and hypotension, occur rarely.

PRECAUTIONS & CONSIDERATIONS
! When administering a fixed-combination product containing bacitracin, be familiar with the side effects of each of the product's drug components. History of allergies, especially to bacitracin, should be determined before giving the drug.

Burning, itching, increased irritation, and rash should be reported immediately. Be alert for signs and symptoms of hypersensitivity, such as burning, inflammation and pruritus. When using preparations containing corticosteroids, closely monitor the patient for any unusual signs or symptoms because corticosteroids may mask clinical signs.

Administration
For ophthalmic use, place a gloved finger on the lower eyelid and pull it out until a pocket is formed between the eye and lower lid. Place ¼ to ½ inch of the ointment in the pocket.

Close the eye gently for 1 to 2 minutes and roll the eyeball to increase the drug's contact with the eye. Remove excess ointment around the eye with a tissue.

Baclofen
bak'loe-fen
(Apo-Baclofen [CAN], Baclo [AUS], Clofen [AUS], Lioresal, Liotec [CAN], Stelax [AUS])
Do not confuse baclofen with Bactroban or Beclovent.

CATEGORY AND SCHEDULE
Pregnancy Risk Category: C

CLASSIFICATION
Musculoskeletal agents, relaxants, skeletal muscle

MECHANISM OF ACTION
A direct-acting skeletal muscle relaxant that inhibits transmission of reflexes at the spinal cord level.
Therapeutic Effect: Relieves muscle spasticity.

PHARMACOKINETICS
Well absorbed from the GI tract. Protein binding: 30%. Partially metabolized in the liver. Primarily excreted in urine. **Half-life:** 2.5-4 hr; intrathecal: 1.5 hr.

AVAILABILITY
Tablets: 10 mg, 20 mg.
Intrathecal Injection: 500 mcg/ml.

INDICATIONS AND DOSAGES
▸ **Spasticity**
PO
Adults. Initially, 5 mg 3 times a day. May increase by 15 mg/day at

3-day intervals. Range: 40-80 mg/day. Maximum: 80 mg/day.
Elderly. Initially, 5 mg 2-3 times a day. May gradually increase dosage.
Children. Initially, 10-15 mg/day in divided doses q8hr. May increase by 5-15 mg/day at 3-day intervals. Maximum: 40 mg/day (children 2-7 yr); 60 mg/day (children 8 yr and older).
Usual intrathecal dosage
Adults, Elderly, Children older than 12 yr. 300-800 mcg/day.
Children 12 yr and younger. 100-300 mcg/day.

OFF-LABEL USES
Treatment of trigeminal neuralgia

CONTRAINDICATIONS
Skeletal muscle spasm due to cerebral palsy, Parkinson's disease, rheumatic disorders, CVA

INTERACTIONS
Drug
Alcohol, other CNS depressants: May increase CNS depression.
Herbal
None known.
Food
None known.

DIAGNOSTIC TEST EFFECTS
May increase blood glucose level and serum alkaline phosphatase, AST (SGOT), and ALT (SGPT) levels.

SIDE EFFECTS
Frequent (greater than 10%)
Transient somnolence, asthenia, dizziness, light-headedness, nausea, vomiting
Occasional (10%-2%)
Headache, paresthesia, constipation, anorexia, hypotension, confusion, nasal congestion

Rare (less than 1%)
Paradoxical CNS excitement or rest-lessness, slurred speech, tremor, dry mouth, diarrhea, nocturia, impotence

SERIOUS REACTIONS
• Abrupt discontinuation of baclofen may produce hallucinations and seizures.
• Overdose results in blurred vision, seizures, myosis, mydriasis, severe muscle weakness, strabismus, respiratory depression, and vomiting.

PRECAUTIONS & CONSIDERATIONS
Caution is warranted with diabetes mellitus, epilepsy, impaired renal function, pre-existing psychiatric disorders, and a history of CVA. It is unknown if baclofen crosses the placenta or is distributed in breast milk. The safety and efficacy of baclofen have not been established in children younger than 12 years. The elderly may require decreased dosage because of age-related renal impairment. They're also at increased risk for CNS toxicity, manifested as confusion, hallucina-tions, depression, and sedation.

Drowsiness may occur but usually diminished with continued therapy. Avoid alcohol, CNS depressants, and tasks that require mental alertness or motor skills. Blood counts and liver and renal function tests should be obtained periodically for those on long-term therapy. Therapeutic response, such as decreased intensity of skeletal muscle pain, should be assessed.

Administration
Take baclofen without regard to food. Crush tablets as needed. Do not abruptly discontinue the drug after long-term therapy.

Balsalazide
ball-sal'a-zide
(Colazal)

B

CATEGORY AND SCHEDULE
Pregnancy Risk Category: B

CLASSIFICATION
Gastrointestinals, salicylates

MECHANISM OF ACTION
A 5-aminosalicylic acid derivative that changes intestinal microflora, altering prostaglandin production and inhibiting function of natural killer cells, mast cells, neutrophils, and macrophages. *Therapeutic Effect:* Diminishes inflammatory effect in colon.

AVAILABILITY
Capsules: 750 mg.

INDICATIONS AND DOSAGES
▶ **Ulcerative colitis**
PO
Adults, Elderly. Three 750-mg capsules 3 times a day for 8 wk.

CONTRAINDICATIONS
Hypersensitivity to salicylates

SIDE EFFECTS
Frequent (8%-6%)
Headache, abdominal pain, nausea, diarrhea
Occasional (4%-2%)
Vomiting, arthralgia, rhinitis, insom-nia, fatigue, flatulence, coughing, dyspepsia

SERIOUS REACTIONS
• Liver toxicity occurs rarely.

Caution is warranted with hepatic
or renal impairment. Notify the
physician if abdominal pain,
severe headache or chest pain,
or unresolved diarrhea occurs.
Serum chemistry laboratory values,
including BUN, alkaline phosphatase, bilirubin, creatinine,
AST (SGOT), and ALT (SGPT)
levels, should be obtained before
treatment.
Administration
Take capsules whole; don't open or
crush them. Take as directed.

Basiliximab
bay-zul-ix'ah-mab
(Simulect)
**Do not confuse with
daclizumab.**

CATEGORY AND SCHEDULE
Pregnancy Risk Category: B

CLASSIFICATION
Immunosuppressives, mono-
clonal antibodies

MECHANISM OF ACTION
A monoclonal antibody that
binds to and blocks the receptor
of interleukin-2, a protein that
stimulates the proliferation of
T lymphocytes, which play a major
role in organ transplant rejection.
Therapeutic Effect: Prevents
lymphocytic activity and impairs
response of the immune system to
antigens, which prevents acute renal
transplant rejection.

PHARMACOKINETICS
Half-life: Adults, 4-10 days; children,
5-17 days.

AVAILABILITY
Powder for Injection: 10 mg, 20 mg.

INDICATIONS AND DOSAGES
▸ **Prevention of acute organ
rejection in patients receiving
a kidney transplant**
IV
*Adults, Elderly, Children weighing
35 kg or more.* 20 mg within 2 hr
before transplant surgery and 20 mg
4 days after transplant.
Children weighing less than 35 kg.
10 mg within 2 hr before transplant
surgery and 10 mg 4 days after
transplant.

CONTRAINDICATIONS
Hypersensitivity to basiliximab,
murine proteins, or any component
of the formulation.

INTERACTIONS
Drug
None known.
Herbal
None known.
Food
None known.

DIAGNOSTIC TEST EFFECTS
May increase BUN and serum
cholesterol, creatinine, and uric acid
levels. May decrease platelet count
and serum magnesium and phosphate levels. May increase or
decrease blood glucose, Hct, Hgb
level, and serum calcium and potassium levels.

▧ IV INCOMPATIBILITIES
Specific information is not available.
Don't infuse other drugs through the
same IV line.

B

SIDE EFFECTS
Frequent (greater than 10%)
GI disturbances (constipation, diarrhea, dyspepsia), CNS effects (dizziness, headache, insomnia, tremor), respiratory tract infection, dysuria, acne, leg or back pain, peripheral edema, hypertension
Occasional (10%-3%)
Angina, neuropathy, abdominal distention, tachycardia, rash, hypotension, urinary disturbances (urinary frequency, genital edema, hematuria), arthralgia, hirsutism, myalgia

SERIOUS REACTIONS
* None known.

PRECAUTIONS & CONSIDERATIONS
Caution is warranted with infection and history of malignancy. It is unknown if basiliximab crosses the placenta or is distributed in breast milk. Basiliximab is not recommended for breast-feeding or pregnant women; avoid pregnancy. No age-related precautions have been noted in children or the elderly.

Notify the physician of fever, sore throat, unusual bleeding or bruising, difficulty breathing or swallowing, itching, rapid heartbeat, rash, swelling of lower extremities, or weakness. BUN, blood glucose, serum calcium, creatinine, alkaline phosphatase, potassium, uric acid levels, vital signs, particularly B/P and pulse rate, should be assessed before and during therapy.
Storage
Refrigerate unopened vials. Use drug within 4 hours after reconstitution (within 24 hours if refrigerated).
Administration
Discard the solution if a precipitate forms. Reconstitute with 5 ml sterile water for injection. Shake gently to dissolve. Further dilute with 50 ml 0.9% NaCl or D_5W. Gently invert to avoid foaming. Infuse over 20 to 30 minutes.

BCG, Intravesical
(TheraCys, Tice BCG)

CATEGORY AND SCHEDULE
Pregnancy Risk Category: D

CLASSIFICATION
Antineoplastics, biological response modifiers, vaccines

MECHANISM OF ACTION
An antineoplastic that produces a local inflammatory reaction with histiocytic and leukocytic infiltration in the urinary bladder. *Therapeutic Effect:* Decreases superficial cancerous lesions in the urinary bladder.

AVAILABILITY
Parenteral Vials: 50 mg, 81 mg

INDICATIONS AND DOSAGES
▶ **Treatment and prevention of bladder carcinoma in situ**
INTRAVESICAL (THERACYS)
Adults, Elderly. One dose in 50 ml 0.9% NaCl once weekly for 6 wk, then repeated 3, 6, 12, 18, and 24 months after initial treatment. Begin 7-14 days after biopsy or transurethral resection.
INTRAVESICAL (TICE BCG)
Adults, Elderly. One dose in 50 ml 0.9% NaCl once weekly for 6 wk; may repeat once. Thereafter, continue monthly for 6-12 mo.

CONTRAINDICATIONS

Compromised immune system, concurrent corticosteroid or immunosuppressive therapy, fever due to infection or undetermined cause, HIV infection, positive Mantoux test, UTI

INTERACTIONS
Drug

Bone marrow depressants, immunosuppressants: May decrease the immune response and increase the risk of osteomyelitis and disseminated BCG infection.
Live-virus vaccines: May potentiate virus replication, increase vaccine side effects, and decrease the patient's antibody response to the vaccine.
Herbal
None known.
Food
None known.

DIAGNOSTIC TEST EFFECTS
None known.

SIDE EFFECTS
Frequent
Dysuria, urinary frequency, hematuria, hypersensitivity reaction (manifested as malaise, fever, chills)
Occasional
Cystitis, urinary urgency, nausea, vomiting, anorexia, diarrhea, myalgia, arthralgia

SERIOUS REACTIONS

• Disseminated BCG infection is usually characterized by a fever higher than 103° F (or persistently higher than 101° F for more than 2 days), chills and severe malaise.

PRECAUTIONS & CONSIDERATIONS

Before beginning treatment, establish renal status; obtain a urine specimen for culture and sensitivity tests to rule out a UTI; determine medications the person is taking concurrently, especially corticosteroids and immunosuppressants; and determine if the person has compromised immune system, has a fever, or is HIV positive. Immunizations and coming in contact with those who have recently received a live-virus vaccine should be avoided during BCG treatment.

Notify the physician if blood in urine, chills, fever, frequent or painful urination, joint pain, and nausea or vomiting occurs. Adequate hydration should be maintained within 4 hours of administration. The patient should void immediately before the drug is given. During the first hour of drug administration, the patient should lie in different positions (supine, prone, and both sides) for 15 minutes each to allow the drug to come in contact with all parts of the bladder. The patient should try to retain the solution for 2 hours. The patient should sit while voiding after instillation to avoid spraying or splashing the infected urine. All urine should be disinfected when expelled within 6 hours of drug instillation with an equal volume of 5% hypochlorite solution (undiluted household bleach), before flushing. Renal status should be diligently monitored. Dysuria, hematuria, urinary frequency, and urinalysis should be assessed to check for UTI.

Storage
Store vials at room temperature. The reconstituted solution may be stored for up to 1 hour at room temperature or up to 8 hours if refrigerated. After removing from refrigeration, allow the drug suspension to return to room temperature and use it within 30 minutes.

Administration
! Be aware that BCG contains live, attenuated mycobacteria. Treat the

drug as infectious material, and use protective gear when reconstituting it. Avoid contact with the drug if immunocompromised.

For intravesical use, reconstitute the powder immediately before administration. Discard any unused portion within 2 hours of reconstitution. After adding diluent to the powder, gently swirl the solution, or repeatedly inject and withdraw the solution from the vial until the solution is mixed. Avoid vigorous shaking, which could cause foaming. Don't give BCG intravenously or subcutaneously; plan to deliver the drug by urethral catheter.

Becaplermin
beh-cap-lear-min
(Regranex)

CATEGORY AND SCHEDULE
Pregnancy Risk Category: C

CLASSIFICATION
Dermatologics

MECHANISM OF ACTION
A platelet-derived growth factor that heals open wounds. *Therapeutic Effect:* Stimulates body to grow new tissue.

PHARMACOKINETICS
None reported.

AVAILABILITY
Gel: 0.01% (Regranex).

INDICATIONS AND DOSAGES
▸ **Ulcers**
TOPICAL
Adults, Elderly. Apply once daily (spread evenly; cover with saline-moistened gauze dressing). After 12 hrs, rinse ulcer, re-cover with saline gauze.

CONTRAINDICATIONS
Neoplasms at site of application, hypersensitivity to becaplermin or any component of the formulation.

INTERACTIONS
Drug
None known.
Herbal
None known.
Food
None known.

DIAGNOSTIC TEST EFFECTS
None known.

SIDE EFFECTS
Occasional
Local rash near ulcer.

SERIOUS REACTIONS
• None reported.

PRECAUTIONS & CONSIDERATIONS
Caution should be used on wounds showing exposed joints, tendons, ligaments, or bones. It is unknown if becaplermin crosses the placenta or is distributed in breast milk. Safety and efficacy have not been established in children less than 16 years of age. There are no age-related precautions noted in the elderly.
Storage
Refrigerate gel.
Administration
Measure gel on a clean, nonabsorbable surface. Transfer to ulcer and spread as a thin, continuous layer onto the ulcer. Cover site with saline-moistened dressing for approx. 12 hours. Remove and wash any residual gel from ulcer and replace

with new gauze pad moistened with 0.9% NaCl until time of next application. Dose requires recalculation weekly or bi-weekly, depending on rate of change in the width and length of ulcer.

Beclomethasone
be-kloe-meth′a-sone
(Aldecin [AUS], Aldecin Hayfever Aqueous Nasal Spray [AUS], Beclodisk [CAN], Becloforte inhaler [CAN], Beconase AQ, Becotide [AUS], Qvar)
Do not confuse Becloforte or Beconase with baclofen.

CATEGORY AND SCHEDULE
Pregnancy Risk Category: C

CLASSIFICATION
Corticosteroids, inhalation

MECHANISM OF ACTION
An adrenocorticosteroid that prevents or controls inflammation by controlling the rate of protein synthesis; decreasing migration of polymorphonuclear leukocytes and fibroblasts; and reversing capillary permeability. *Therapeutic Effect:* Inhalation: Inhibits bronchoconstriction, produces smooth muscle relaxation, decreases mucus secretion. Intranasal: Decreases response to seasonal and perennial rhinitis.

PHARMACOKINETICS
Rapidly absorbed from pulmonary, nasal, and GI tissue. Undergoes extensive first-pass metabolism in the liver. Protein binding: 87%. Primarily eliminated in feces. **Half-life:** 15 hr.

AVAILABILITY
Oral Inhalation (QVAR). 40 mcg per inhalation, 80 mcg/inhalation.
Nasal spray (Beconase AQ). 42 mcg/inhalation.

INDICATIONS AND DOSAGES
▸ **Long-term control of bronchial asthma, reduces need for oral corticosteroid therapy for asthma**
ORAL INHALATION
Adults, Elderly Children 12 yr and older. 40-160 mcg twice a day. Maximum: 320 mcg twice a day.
Children 5-11 yr. 40 mcg twice a day. Maximum: 80 mcg twice a day.
▸ **Relief of seasonal or perennial rhinitis, prevention of nasal polyp recurrence after surgical removal, treatment of nonallergic rhinitis**
NASAL INHALATION
Adults, Children older than 12 yr. 1-2 sprays in each nostril twice a day.
Children 6-12 yr. 1 spray in each nostril twice a day. May increase up to 2 sprays in each nostril twice a day.

OFF-LABEL USES
Prevention of seasonal rhinitis (nasal form)

CONTRAINDICATIONS
Hypersensitivity to beclomethasone, status asthmaticus

INTERACTIONS
Drug
None known.
Herbal
None known.

Food
None known.

DIAGNOSTIC TEST EFFECTS
None known.

SIDE EFFECTS
Frequent
Inhalation (14%-4%): Throat irritation, dry mouth, hoarseness, cough
Intranasal: Nasal burning, mucosal dryness
Occasional
Inhalation (3%-2%): Localized fungal infection (thrush)
Intranasal: Nasal-crusting epistaxis, sore throat, ulceration of nasal mucosa
Rare
Inhalation: Transient bronchospasm, esophageal candidiasis
Intranasal: Nasal and pharyngeal candidiasis, eye pain

SERIOUS REACTIONS
• An acute hypersensitivity reaction, as evidenced by urticaria, angioedema, and severe bronchospasm, occurs rarely.
• A transfer from systemic to local steroid therapy may unmask previously suppressed bronchial asthma condition.

PRECAUTIONS & CONSIDERATIONS

Caution is warranted with cirrhosis, glaucoma, hypothyroidism, osteoporosis, tuberculosis, and untreated systemic infections. It is unknown if beclomethasone crosses the placenta or is distributed in breast milk. In children, prolonged treatment and high doses may decrease cortisol secretion and the short-term growth rate. No age-related precautions have been noted in the elderly.

Those receiving beclomethasone by inhalation should maintain fastidious oral hygiene; notify the physician or nurse if sore throat or mouth develops. If using a bronchodilator inhaler concomitantly with a steroid inhaler, use the bronchodilator several minutes before using the corticosteroid to help the steroid penetrate into the bronchial tree. Those using beclomethasone intranasally should notify the physician if nasal irritation occurs or if symptoms, such as sneezing, fail to improve. Persons who are using drugs that suppress the immune system are more susceptible to infections than healthy individuals.

Administration
For inhalation, first shake the container well. Exhale completely and place the mouthpiece between the lips. Inhale and hold breath for as long as possible before exhaling. Allow at least 1 minute between inhalations. Rinse mouth after each use to decrease dry mouth and hoarseness and prevent fungal infection of the mouth. Do not change the beclomethasone dosage schedule or stop taking the drug abruptly; taper dosage gradually under medical supervision.

For intranasal use, clear nasal passages as much as possible. Insert the spray tip into the nostril, pointing toward the nasal passages, away from the nasal septum. Spray beclomethasone into the nostril while holding the other nostril closed, and at the same time, inhale through the nose to deliver the medication as high into the nasal passages as possible. Do not change the beclomethasone dosage schedule or stop taking the drug abruptly; taper dosage gradually under medical supervision.

Belladonna Alkaloids

bell-a-don-a al-kuh-loydz
(Antispas, Antispasmodic,
Barbidonna, Barophen,
Bellalphen, Bellatal,
Chardonna-2, Donnapine,
Donnatal, Donnatal Extentabs,
D-Tal, Haponal, Spacol,
Spasmolin, Spasquid)

CATEGORY AND SCHEDULE
Pregnancy risk category: C

CLASSIFICATION
Anticholinergic, antispasmodic,
gastrointestinal

MECHANISM OF ACTION
Competitive inhibitors of the
muscarinic actions of acetylcholine,
acting at receptors located in
exocrine glands, smooth and cardiac
muscle and intramural neurons.
Composed of 3 main constituents
atropine, scopolamine, and
hyoscyamine. Scopolamine exerts
greater effects on the CNS, eye, and
secretory glands than the
constituents atropine and
hyoscyamine. Atropine exerts more
activity on the heart, intestine, and
bronchial muscle and exhibits a
more prolonged duration of action
compared to scopolamine.
Hyoscyamine exerts similar actions
to atropine but has more potent
central and peripheral nervous
system effects. *Therapeutic effect:*
Peripheral anticholinergic and
antispasmodic action, mild
sedation.

PHARMACOKINETICS
None known.

AVAILABILITY
Tablet: 40 mg phenobarbital, 0.6 mg
ergotamine tartrate, 0.2 mg levorota-
tory alkaloids of belladonna
(Bellergal, Bellergal-S, Bellergal-R,
Spasmolin, Bellalphen, Antispas,
Spacol, Chardonna-2, Barbidonna)
Tablet, extended release:
0.0582 mg–48.6 mg–
0.0195 mg (Donnatal Extendtabs)
Elixir: 0.0194 mg–0.1037 mg–
16.2 mg–0.0065 mg/5 ml (Barophen,
Donnapine, Antispasmodic, Spacol,
Donnatal, D-Tal, Spasquid)

INDICATIONS AND DOSAGES
▸ **Irritable bowel syndrome, acute
enterocolitis**
PO
Adults. 1-2 tablets or capsules
3-4 times daily or 1-2 teaspoonfuls
of elixir 3-4 times daily according
to conditions and severity of
symptoms.
Children. Dosage varies depending
on body weight and may be dosed
every 4 or 6 hours.

CONTRAINDICATIONS
Glaucoma, obstructive uropathy,
obstructive disease of gastrointestinal tract, paralytic ileus, intestinal
atony of the elderly or debilitated
patient, unstable cardiovascular
status in acute hemorrhage, severe
ulcerative colitis especially if
complicated by toxic megacolon,
myasthenia gravis, hiatal hernia
associated with reflux esophagitis,
hypersensitivity to any component of
the formulation, acute intermittent
porphyria.

INTERACTIONS
Drug
Oral medications: Belladonna
decreases gastric emptying time
therefore affecting absorption of
orally administered agents.

B

Anticholinergic drugs: May enhance anticholinergic effect.
Ambenonium, arbutamine, belladonna, cisapride, cromolyn, halothane, methacholine, procainamide: May enhance effects of atropine constituent of belladonna alkaloids.
Tricyclic antidepressants: May enhance anticholinergic effect.
Cisapride: Atropine may decrease effects of cisapride.
Antiarrhythmics: May result in additive anti-vagal effects on atrioventricular nodal conduction.
Alcohol: May result in additive CNS depression.
Tacrine: May attenuate cognitive deficits of belladonna alkaloids.
Herbal
Anticholinergic herbs: May enhance anticholinergic effect.
Food
None known.

DIAGNOSTIC TEST EFFECTS
None known.

SIDE EFFECTS
Frequent
Dry mouth, urinary retention, flushing, pupillary dilation, constipation, confusion, redness of the skin, flushing, dry skin, allergic contact dermatitis, headache, excitement, agitation, dizziness, lightheadedness, drowsiness, unsteadiness, confusion, slurred speech, sedation, hyperreflexia, convulsions, vertigo, coma, mydriasis, photophobia, blurred vision, dilation of pupils
Rare
Hallucinations, acute psychosis, Stevens-Johnson Syndrome, photosensitivity

SERIOUS REACTIONS
• Signs and symptoms of overdose include headache, nausea, vomiting, blurred vision, dilated pupils, hot and dry skin, dizziness, dryness of the mouth, difficulty in swallowing and CNS stimulation.
• Treatment should consist of gastric lavage, emetics, and activated charcoal. If indicated, parenteral cholinergic agents such as physostigmine or bethanechol chloride should be added.

PRECAUTIONS & CONSIDERATIONS
Caution is warranted with ulcerative colitis or intestinal disease, coronary artery disease, dehydration, diarrhea caused by poisoning, Down's syndrome, acute dysentery, glaucoma, hepatic and renal function impairment, hiatal hernia, prostatic hyperplasia, urinary retention, asthma, COPD, and brain damage. Belladonna alkaloids cross the placenta and are distributed into breast milk. Safety and efficacy has not been established in children younger than 6 years. Infants and young children may be more susceptible to adverse effects of belladonna alkaloids. The elderly may be more susceptible to fluid and electrolyte loss as well as memory impairment. Constipation, difficulty urinating, decreased sweating, drowsiness, dry mouth, increased heart rate, headache, orthostatic hypotension may occur. Change positions slowly to avoid lightheadedness. Avoid alcohol, CNS depressants, and tasks that require mental alertness.
Administration
Dose should be adjusted to the needs of the individual to assume symptomatic control with minimum adverse effects.

Belladonna and Opium

bell-a-don′a
(B&O Supprettes 15-A, B&O
Supprettes 16-A, PMS-Opium
& Beladonna [CAN])

CATEGORY AND SCHEDULE
Pregnancy Risk Category: C
Controlled Substance:
Schedule II

CLASSIFICATION
Analgesics, narcotic, anticholinergics

MECHANISM OF ACTION
Anticholinergic alkaloids that
inhibits the action of acetylcholine
at post-ganglionic (muscarinic)
receptor sites. Morphine (10% of
opium) depresses cerebral cortex,
hypothalamus, and medullary
centers. *Therapeutic Effect:*
Decreases digestive secretions,
increases GI muscle tone, reduces
GI force, alters pain perception and
emotional response to pain.

PHARMACOKINETICS
Onset of action occurs within
30 minutes. Absorption is dependent
on body hydration. Metabolized
in liver to form glucuronide
metabolites.

AVAILABILITY
Suppository: 16.2 mg belladonna
extract/30 mg opium (B&O
Supprettes 15-A), 16.2 mg
belladonna extract/60 mg opium
(B&O Supprettes 16-A).

INDICATIONS AND DOSAGES
▸ **Analgesic, antispasmodic**

RECTAL
Adults, Elderly. 1 suppository
1-2 times/day. Maximum: 4 doses/day.

OFF-LABEL USES
Glaucoma, severe renal or hepatic
disease, bronchial asthma, respiratory
depression, convulsive disorders,
acute alcoholism, premature labor,
hypersensitivity to belladonna or
opium or its components

CONTRAINDICATIONS
None known.

INTERACTIONS
Drug
Alcohol, CNS depressants: May
increase CNS or respiratory depres-
sion, hypotension.
Anticholinergics: May increase the
effects of belladonna and opium.
Phenothiazines: May decrease
the antipsychotic effects of these
drugs.
Herbal
None known.
Food
None known.

DIAGNOSTIC TEST EFFECTS
May increase serum SGOT (AST)
and SGPT (ALT) levels

▨ IV INCOMPATIBILITIES
None known.
▯ **IV Compatibilities**
None known.

SIDE EFFECTS
Frequent
Dry mouth, nose, skin and throat,
decreased sweating, constipation,
irritation at site of administration,
drowsiness, urinary retention,
dizziness
Occasional
Blurred vision, decreased flow
of breast milk, bloated feeling,

drowsiness, headache, intolerance to light, nervousness, flushing

Rare

Dizziness, faintness, pruritis, urticaria

SERIOUS REACTIONS

• Respiratory depression, increased intraocular pain, loss of memory, orthostatic hypotension, tachycardia, and ventricular fibrillation rarely occur.

• Tolerance to the drug's analgesic effect and physical dependence may occur with repeated use.

PRECAUTIONS & CONSIDERATIONS

Extreme caution should be used with acute alcoholism, anoxia, CNS depression, hypercapnia, respiratory depression or dysfunction, seizures, shock, and untreated myxedema. Caution is also warranted with acute abdominal conditions, Addison's disease, chronic obstructive pulmonary disease (COPD), hypothyroidism, impaired liver function, increased intracranial pressure, prostatic hypertrophy, and urethral stricture. It is unknown if belladonna and opium crosses the placenta or is distributed in breast milk. Children may be more susceptible to respiratory depression. The elderly may also be more susceptible to respiratory depression, and the drug may cause paradoxical excitement. Age-related prostatic hypertrophy or obstruction and renal impairment may increase the risk of urinary retention, and dosage adjustment is recommended in the elderly. Alcohol, tasks that require mental alertness and motor skills, hot baths, and saunas should be avoided.

Storage

Store at room temperature.

Administration

Moisten finger and suppository before rectal insertion.

Benazepril

be-naze'a-pril

(Lotensin)

Do not confuse benazepril with Benadryl, or Lotensin with Loniten or lovastatin.

CATEGORY AND SCHEDULE

Pregnancy Risk Category: C (D if used in second or third trimester)

CLASSIFICATION

Angiotensin converting enzyme inhibitors

MECHANISM OF ACTION

An ACE inhibitor that decreases the rate of conversion of angiotensin I to angiotensin II, a potent vasoconstrictor. Reduces peripheral arterial resistance. *Therapeutic Effect:* Lowers blood pressure (B/P).

PHARMACOKINETICS

Route	Onset	Peak	Duration
PO	1 hr	2-4 hr	24 hr

Partially absorbed from the GI tract. Protein binding: 97%. Metabolized in the liver to active metabolite. Primarily excreted in urine. Minimal removal by hemodialysis. **Half-life:** 35 min; metabolite 10-11 hr.

AVAILABILITY

Tablets: 5 mg, 10 mg, 20 mg, 40 mg.

INDICATIONS AND DOSAGES

▸ **Hypertension (monotherapy)**

PO

Adults. Initially, 10 mg/day. Maintenance: 20-40 mg/day as

single in 2 divided doses. Maximum: 80 mg/day.
Elderly. Initially, 5-10 mg/day. Range: 20-40 mg/day.
▶ **Hypertension (combination therapy)**
PO
Adults. Discontinue diuretic 2-3 days prior to initiating benazepril, then dose as noted above. If unable to discontinue diuretic, begin benazepril at 5 mg/day.
▶ **Dosage in renal impairment**
For adult patients with creatinine clearance less than 30 ml/min, initially, 5 mg/day titrated up to maximum of 40 mg/day.

OFF-LABEL USES
Treatment of CHF

CONTRAINDICATIONS
History of angioedema from previous treatment with ACE inhibitors

INTERACTIONS
Drug
Alcohol, antihypertensives, diuretics: May increase the effects of benazepril.
Lithium: May increase the lithium blood concentration and risk of lithium toxicity.
NSAIDs: May decrease the effects of benazepril.
Potassium-sparing diuretics, potassium supplements: May cause hyperkalemia.
Herbal
None known.
Food
None known.

DIAGNOSTIC TEST EFFECTS
May increase BUN, serum alkaline phosphatase, serum bilirubin, serum potassium, AST (SGOT), and ALT (SGPT) levels. May decrease serum sodium levels. May cause positive antinuclear antibody titer.

SIDE EFFECTS
Frequent (6%-3%)
Cough, headache, dizziness
Occasional (2%)
Fatigue, somnolence or drowsiness, nausea
Rare (less than 1%)
Rash, fever, myalgia, diarrhea, loss of taste

SERIOUS REACTIONS
• Excessive hypotension ('first-dose syncope') may occur in patients with CHF and in those who are severely salt or volume depleted.
• Angioedema (swelling of the face and lips) and hyperkalemia occur rarely.
• Agranulocytosis and neutropenia may be noted in those with collagen vascular disease, including scleroderma and systemic lupus erythematosus, and impaired renal function.
• Nephrotic syndrome may be noted in patients with history of renal disease.

PRECAUTIONS & CONSIDERATIONS
Caution is warranted with cerebrovascular and coronary insufficiency, diabetes mellitus, hypovolemia, renal impairment, and sodium depletion as well as persons on dialysis and in those receiving diuretics. Benazepril crosses the placenta and it is unknown if it is distributed in breast milk. Benazepril may cause fetal or neonatal morbidity or mortality. Safety and efficacy of benazepril have not been established in children. The elderly may be more sensitive to the hypotensive effects of benazepril.
Dizziness and orthostatic hypotension may occur. Rise slowly from lying to sitting position and permit legs to dangle from the bed momentarily before standing to reduce

the hypotensive effect of benazepril. Full therapeutic effect of benazepril may take 2 to 4 weeks. B/P should be obtained immediately before giving each benazepril dose, in addition to regular monitoring. Be alert to fluctuations in B/P. If an excessive reduction in B/P occurs, place the person in the supine position with legs elevated. CBC and blood chemistry should be obtained before beginning benazepril therapy, then every 2 weeks for the next 3 months, and periodically thereafter in patients with autoimmune disease, or renal impairment, and in those who are taking drugs that affect immune response or leukocyte count.

Administration

! Expect the physician to discontinue diuretics 2 to 3 days before beginning benazepril therapy.

May take without regard to food. Do not skip doses.

Bentoquatam
ben'toe-kwa-tam
(IvyBlock)

CATEGORY AND SCHEDULE
Pregnancy Risk Category: NR

CLASSIFICATION
Rhus dermatitis protectant

MECHANISM OF ACTION
An organoclay substance that absorbs and binds to urushiol, the active principle in poison oak, ivy, and sumac. *Therapeutic Effect:* Blocks urushiol skin contact and absorption.

PHARMACOKINETICS
None reported.

AVAILABILITY
Lotion: 5% (IvyBlock).

INDICATIONS AND DOSAGES
▶ **Contact dermatitis prophylaxis caused by poison oak, ivy, or sumac**
TOPICAL
Adults, Elderly, Children 6 yr and older. Apply thin film over skin at least 15 minutes before potential exposure. Re-apply q4hr or sooner if needed.

CONTRAINDICATIONS
Hypersensitivity to bentoquatam or any of its components such as methylparabens

INTERACTIONS
Drug
None known.
Herbal
None known.
Food
None known.

DIAGNOSTIC TEST EFFECTS
None known.

SIDE EFFECTS
Occasional
Erythema

SERIOUS REACTIONS
• None reported.

PRECAUTIONS & CONSIDERATIONS
Caution is necessary with history of allergic-type responses to medications, especially topical formulations, open wounds, psoriatic lesions, or other cutaneous conditions. The use of bentoquatam has not been studied in pregnancy. There are no age-related precautions noted in children or the elderly.

Administration
Bentoquatam is for external use
only. Bentoquatam is a protectant,
not a treatment, for poison oak, ivy,
or sumac. Apply 15 minutes before
exposure. Do not apply after exposure. Re-apply every 4 hours or
sooner if needed.

Benzocaine
ben′zoe-kane
(Americaine Anesthetic
Lubricant, Americaine Otic,
Anbesol, Anbesol Baby Gel,
Anbesol Maximum Strength,
Babee Teething, Benzodent,
Cepacol, Cetacaine, Chiggerex,
Chiggertox, Cylex, Dermoplast,
Detaine, Foille, Foille Medicated
First Aid, Foille Plus, HDA
Toothache, Hurricane, Lanacane,
Mycinettes, Omedia, Orabase-B,
Orajel, Orajel Baby, Orajel Baby
Nighttime, Orajel Maximum
Strength, Orasol, Otricaine,
Otocain, Retre-Gel, Solarcaine,
Topicaine [AUS], Trocaine,
Zilactin, Zilactin Baby)

CATEGORY AND SCHEDULE
Pregnancy Risk Category: C

CLASSIFICATION
Anesthetics, otic, topical, dermatologics

MECHANISM OF ACTION
A local anesthetic that blocks nerve
conduction in the autonomic, sensory,
and motor nerve fibers. Competes
with calcium ions for membrane
binding. Reduces permeability of
resting nerves to potassium and
sodium ions. *Therapeutic Effect:*
Produces local analgesic effect.

PHARMACOKINETICS
Poorly absorbed by topical administration. Well absorbed from mucous
membranes and traumatized skin.
Metabolized in liver and by hydrolysis with cholinesterase. Minimal
excretion in urine.

AVAILABILITY
Cream: 5%, 20% (Lanacane).
Lozenge: 10 mg (Cepacol, Trocaine),
15 mg (Cyclex, Mycinettes).
Oral Aerosol: 14% (Cetacaine), 20%
(Hurricane).
Oral Gel: 6.3% (Anbesol), 6.5%
(HDA Toothache), 7.5% (Anbesol
Baby, Detaine, Orajel Baby), 10%
(Orajel, Orajel Baby Nighttime,
Zilactin-B, Zilactin Baby), 20%
(Anbesol Maximum Strength,
Hurricane).
Oral Liquid: 6.3% (Anbesol), 7.5%
(Orajel Baby), 10% (Orajel), 20%
(Anbesol Maximum Strength,
Hurricane).
Oral Lotion: 2.5% (Babee Teething).
Oral Ointment: 20% (Benzadent).
Otic Solution: 20% (Americane
Otic, Omedia, Oticaine, Otocain).
Paste: 20% (Orabase-B).
Topical Aerosol: 5% (Foille, Foille
Plus), 20% (Dermoplast,
Solarcaine).
Topical Gel: 5% (Retre-Gel),
20% (Americaine Anesthetic
Lubricant).
Topical Liquid: 2% (Chiggertox).
Topical Ointment: 2% (Chiggerex),
5% (Foille Medicated First Aid).

INDICATIONS AND DOSAGES
▸ **Canker sores**
TOPICAL
*Adults, Elderly, Children older than
2 yr.* Apply gel, liquid, or ointment

to affected area. Maximum:
4 times/day.

▸ **Denture irritation**
TOPICAL
Adults, Elderly. Apply thin layer of
gel to affected area up to 4 times/day
or until pain is relieved.

▸ **General lubrication**
TOPICAL
*Adults, Elderly, Children older than
2 yr.* Apply gel to exterior of tube or
instrument prior to use.

▸ **Otitis externa, otitis media**
OTIC
*Adults, Elderly, Children older than
1 yr.* Instill 4-5 drops into external
ear canal of affected ears. Repeat
q1-2hr as needed.

▸ **Pain and itching associated with
sunburn, insect bites, minor cuts,
scrapes, minor burns, minor skin
irritations**
TOPICAL
*Adults, Elderly, Children older
than 2 yr.* Apply to affected area
3-4 times/day.

▸ **Pharyngitis**
PO
Adults, Elderly. 1 lozenge q2hr.
Maximum 8 lozenges/day.

▸ **Toothache/teething pain**
TOPICAL
*Adults, Elderly, Children older than
2 yr.* Apply gel, liquid, or ointment
to affected areas. Maximum:
4 times/day.

▸ **Anesthesia**
TOPICAL
Adults, Elderly. Apply aerosol, gel,
ointment, liquid q4-12hr as needed.

OFF-LABEL USES
Obesity, spasticity

CONTRAINDICATIONS
Hypersensitivity to benzocaine or
ester-type local anesthetics, perforated
tympanic membrane or ear discharge
(otic preparations)

INTERACTIONS
Drug
Hyaluronidase: May increase inci-
dence of systemic reaction to benzo-
caine.
Sulfonamides: May decrease the
antibacterial effect of sulfonamides.
Herbal
St. John's wort: May increase risk
of cardiovascular collapse and delay
effects of benzocaine.
Food
None known.

DIAGNOSTIC TEST EFFECTS
None known.

SIDE EFFECTS
Occasional
Burning, stinging, angioedema,
contact dermatitis, taste disorders

SERIOUS REACTIONS
• Methemoglobinemia occurs rarely
in infants and young children.

PRECAUTIONS & CONSIDERATIONS
Caution should be used with children
younger than 2 years old and infants
and with inflamed skin or open
wounds. It is unknown if benzocaine
crosses the placenta or is distributed
in breast milk. Safety and efficacy
of this drug has not been established
in children younger than 2 years old
for topical preparations and younger
than 1 year old for otic solutions.
There are not age-related precautions
in the elderly. Avoid contact with eyes.
    An allergic reaction with blue
color around mouth, fingers or toes,
fast breathing, redness, pain or
swelling, or unusual tiredness
or weakness should be reported
immediately.
Administration
Do not eat 1 hour prior to topical
oral administration. Rinse mouth
well before reinserting dentures.

Do not use for more than one week.

Do not remove film coating from benzocaine gel.

Clean area before applying topical aerosol benzocaine. Hold can 6-12 inches away from affected area. If applying to face, spray in palm of hand and then apply to affected area.

Benzonatate
ben-zoe'na-tate
(Tessalon Perles)

CATEGORY AND SCHEDULE
Pregnancy Risk Category: C

CLASSIFICATION
Antitussives

MECHANISM OF ACTION
A non-narcotic antitussive that anesthetizes stretch receptors in respiratory passages, lungs, and pleura. *Therapeutic Effect:* Reduces cough production.

AVAILABILITY
Capsules: 100 mg, 200 mg.

INDICATIONS AND DOSAGES
▶ Antitussive
PO
Adults, Elderly, Children older than 10 yr. 100 mg 3 times a day or every 4 hours up to 600 mg/day.

CONTRAINDICATIONS
None known.

INTERACTIONS
Drug
CNS depressants: May increase the effects of benzonatate.

Herbal
None known.
Food
None known.

DIAGNOSTIC TEST EFFECTS
None known.

SIDE EFFECTS
Occasional
Mild somnolence, mild dizziness, constipation, GI upset, skin eruptions, nasal congestion

SERIOUS REACTIONS
• A paradoxical reaction, including restlessness, insomnia, euphoria, nervousness, and tremor, has been noted.

PRECAUTIONS & CONSIDERATIONS
Caution is warranted with a productive cough. Dizziness and drowsiness are common side effects. Avoid tasks that require mental alertness or motor skills until response to the drug has been established. Fluid intake and environmental humidity should be increased to lower the viscosity of secretions.
Administration
Take benzonatate without regard to food. Swallow the capsules whole; chewing them or dissolving them in the mouth may produce temporary local anesthesia or choking.

Metabolized to benzoic acid in skin.
Excreted in urine as benzoate.

B

Benzoyl Peroxide

ben'zoe-ill per-ox'ide
(Acetoxyl [CAN], Benoxyl [CAN],
Benzac, Benzac AC, Benzac AC
Wash, Benzac W, Benzac W
Wash, Benzagel, Benzagel Wash,
Benzashave, Brevoxyl, Brevoxyl
Cleansing, Brevoxyl Wash,
Clearplex, Clinac BPO, Del
Aqua, Desquam-E, Desquam-X,
Exact Acne Medication, Fostex
10% BPO, Loroxide, Neutrogena
Acne Mask, Neutrogena On The
Spot Acne Treatment, Oxy [AUS],
Oxy 10 Balanced Medicated
Face Wash, Oxy 10 Balance Spot
Treatment, Palmer's Skin
Success Acne, Oxyderm [CAN],
PanOxyl, PanOxyl-AQ, PanOxyl
Aqua Gel, PanOxylBar, Seba-
Gel, Solugel [CAN], Triaz, Triaz
Cleanser, Zapzyt)

CATEGORY AND SCHEDULE

Pregnancy Risk Category: C
OTC

CLASSIFICATION

Anti-infectives, topical, dermatologics, keratolytics

MECHANISM OF ACTION

A keratolytic agent that releases
free-radical oxygen which oxidizes
bacterial proteins in the sebaceous
follicles decreasing the number of
anaerobic bacteria and decreasing
irritating-type free fatty acids.
Therapeutic Effect: Bactericidal
action against Propionibacterium
acnes and Staphylococcus
epidermidis.

PHARMACOKINETICS

Minimal absorption through skin.
Gel is more penetrating than cream.

AVAILABILITY

Cream, topical: 2.5 % (Neutrogena
On The Spot Acne Treatment),
5% (Benzashave, Exact Acne
Medication, Neutrogena Acne
Mask), 10% (Benzashave).
Gel, topical: 2.5% (Benzac, Benzac
AC, Benzac W, Desquam-E), 4%
(Brevoxyl), 5% (Benzac, Benzac
AC, Benzac W, Benzagel, Clearplex,
Desquam-E, Desquam-X, Oxy 10
Balance Spot Treatment, PanOxyl,
PanOxyl AQ, Seba-Gel), 6% (Triaz,
Triaz Cleanser), 7% (Clinac BPO),
8% (Brevoxyl), 10% (Benzac, Benzac
AC, Benzac W, Benzagel, Benzagel
Wash, Clearplex, Desquam-E,
Desquam-X, Fostex, Oxy 10 Balance
Spot Treatment, PanOxyl, PanOxyl
AQ, PanOxyl Aqua Gel, Seba-Gel,
Triaz, Triaz Cleanser, Zapzyt).
Liquid, topical: 2.5% (Benzac AC
Wash), 5% (Benzac AC Wash, Benzac
W Wash, Del-Aqua, Desquam-X),
10% Benzac AC Wash, Benzac W
Wash, Del-Aqua, Oxy-10 Balance
Medicated Face Wash).
Lotion, topical: 4% (Brevoxyl
Cleansing, Brevoxyl Wash), 5.5%
(Loroxide), 8% (Brevoxyl Cleansing,
Brevoxyl Wash), 10% (Fostex,
Palmeris Skin Success Acne).
Soap bar, topical: 5% (PanOxyl
Bar), 10% (Desquam-X, Fostex,
PanOxyl Bar).

INDICATIONS AND DOSAGES
▶ **Acne**
TOPICAL
Adults. Apply 2.5%-10% concentra-
tion 1-2 times/day.

OFF-LABEL USES

Dermal ulcers, seborrheic dermatitis,
surgical wounds, tinea pedis, tinea
versicolor

CONTRAINDICATIONS
Hypersensitivity to benzoyl peroxide or any component of the formulation

INTERACTIONS
Drug
Sunscreens containing PABA: May cause skin to change color when both agents are used concomitantly.
Herbal
None known.
Food
None known.

DIAGNOSTIC TEST EFFECTS
None known.

SIDE EFFECTS
Occasional
Irritation, dryness, burning, peeling, stinging, contact dermatitis, bleaching of hair

SERIOUS REACTIONS
• Hypersensitivity reactions have been reported with benzoyl peroxide use.

PRECAUTIONS & CONSIDERATIONS
Caution should be used on skin because benzoyl peroxide may cause contact dermatitis, hair bleaching, and seborrhea. Caution should also be used around the eyes, lips, mucous membranes, and highly inflamed skin. Be aware that cross-sensitization may occur with benzoic acid derivatives such as cinnamon and other topical anesthetics. It is unknown if benzoyl peroxide crosses the placenta or is distributed in breast milk. Safety and efficacy of benzoyl peroxide have not been established in children. There are no age-related precautions noted in the elderly.

Mild stinging and redness may occur. Be aware that benzoyl peroxide may bleach hair and fabric.

Administration
Control frequency or concentration of benzoyl peroxide by the amount of drying or peeling. If excessive dryness or peeling occurs, decrease dose. Use 30 minutes after shaving the area.

Benztropine
benz'troe-peen
(Apo-Benztropine [CAN], Bentrop [AUS], Cogentin)
Do not confuse benztropine with bromocriptine.

CATEGORY AND SCHEDULE
Pregnancy Risk Category: C

CLASSIFICATION
Anticholinergics, antiparkinson agents

MECHANISM OF ACTION
An antiparkinson agent that selectively blocks central cholinergic receptors, helping to balance cholinergic and dopaminergic activity. *Therapeutic Effect:* Reduces the incidence and severity of akinesia, rigidity, and tremor.

AVAILABILITY
Tablets: 0.5 mg, 1 mg, 2 mg.
Injection: 1 mg/ml.

INDICATIONS AND DOSAGES
▸ **Parkinsonism**
PO
Adults. 0.5-6 mg/day as a single dose or in 2 divided doses. Titrate by 0.5 mg at 5-6 day intervals.
Elderly. Initially, 0.5 mg once or twice a day. Titrate by 0.5 mg at 5-6 day intervals. Maximum: 4 mg/day.

▸ **Drug-induced extrapyramidal symptoms**
PO, IM
Adults. 1-4 mg once or twice a day.
Children older than 3 yr. 0.02-0.05 mg/kg/dose once or twice a day.
▸ **Acute dystonic reactions**
IM, IV
Adults. Initially, 1-2 mg; then 1-2 mg PO twice a day to prevent recurrence.

CONTRAINDICATIONS
Angle-closure glaucoma, benign prostatic hyperplasia, children younger than 3 years, GI obstruction, intestinal atony, megacolon, myasthenia gravis, paralytic ileus, severe ulcerative colitis

INTERACTIONS
Drug
Alcohol, other CNS depressants: May increase sedation.
Amantadine, anticholinergics, MAOIs: May increase the effects of benztropine.
Antacids, antidiarrheals: May decrease the absorption and effects of benztropine.
Herbal
None known.
Food
None known.

DIAGNOSTIC TEST EFFECTS
None known.

SIDE EFFECTS
Frequent
Somnolence, dry mouth, blurred vision, constipation, decreased sweating or urination, GI upset, photosensitivity
Occasional
Headache, memory loss, muscle cramps, anxiety, peripheral paresthesia, orthostatic hypotension, abdominal cramps

Rare
Rash, confusion, eye pain

SERIOUS REACTIONS
• Overdose may produce severe anticholinergic effects, such as unsteadiness, somnolence, tachycardia, dyspnea, skin flushing, and severe dryness of the mouth, nose, or throat.
• Severe paradoxical reactions, marked by hallucinations, tremor, seizures, and toxic psychosis, may occur.

PRECAUTIONS & CONSIDERATIONS
Caution is warranted with arrhythmias, heart disease, hypertension, hepatic or renal impairment, obstructive diseases of the GI or GU tracts, urine retention, benign prostatic hyperplasia, tachycardia, and treated open-angle glaucoma. The elderly (older than 60 years) are more likely to develop agitation, disorientation, confusion, and psychotic-like symptoms.
   Dizziness, drowsiness, and dry mouth are expected responses to the drug. Alcohol and tasks that require mental alertness or motor skills should be avoided. Notify the physician of agitation, headache, somnolence, or confusion.
Administration
Take at bedtime or throughout the day to treat tremors. Improvement usually occurs in 1-2 days.

Benzylpenicilloyl; Polylysine

ben'zil-pen-i-sil'oyl
pol-i-lie'seen

(Pre-Pen)

Do not confuse with benzoyl peroxide.

CATEGORY AND SCHEDULE

Pregnancy Risk Category: C

CLASSIFICATION

Diagnostics, nonradioactive

MECHANISM OF ACTION

A diagnostic agent that invokes immunoglobulin E which produce type I accelerated urticarial reactions to penicillins. *Therapeutic Effect:* A positive reaction will suggest penicillin sensitivity.

PHARMACOKINETICS

Not known.

AVAILABILITY

Solution: 0.25 ml (Pre-Pen).

INDICATIONS AND DOSAGES

▸ **Penicillin sensitivity**

INTRADERMAL

Adults, Children. Use a tuberculin syringe with a 26- to 30-gauge, short bevel needle. A dose of 0.01 to 0.02 ml is injected intradermally. A control of 0.9% sodium chloride should be injected about $1\frac{1}{2}$ inches from the test site. Skin response usually occurs within 5 to 15 minutes.

SCRATCH TEST

Adults, Children. Use a 20-gauge needle to make 3 to 5 mm nonbleeding scratch of the epidermis. Apply a small drop of solution to scratch and rub gently with applicator or toothpick. A positive reaction consists of a pale wheal surrounding the scratch site develops within 10 minutes and ranges from 5 to 15 mm in diameter.

CONTRAINDICATIONS

Systemic or marked local reaction to its previous administration or hypersensitivity to penicillin

INTERACTIONS

Drug
None known.
Herbal
None known.
Food
None known.

DIAGNOSTIC TEST EFFECTS

None known.

SIDE EFFECTS

Frequent
Skin rash
Occasional
Nausea

SERIOUS REACTIONS

• None significant.

PRECAUTIONS & CONSIDERATIONS

A scratch test or intradermal injection should be performed before administration. A negative reaction occurs when there is no response. An ambiguous response is indicated by a wheal slightly larger than initial injection bleb, with or without accompanying erythematous flare and larger than the control site. A positive response is indicated by itching and marked increase in size of original bleb. Control site should be reactionless. Epinephrine 1:1000 should be immediately available.

If a positive reaction occurs with a scratch test, intradermal administration should not be used.

Administration
Inspect visually for particulate matter and/or discoloration prior to administration.

Bepridil
beh'prih-dill
(Bepadin, Vascor)

CATEGORY AND SCHEDULE
Pregnancy Risk Category: C

CLASSIFICATION
Calcium channel blockers

MECHANISM OF ACTION
A calcium channel blocker that inhibits calcium ion entry across cell membranes of cardiac and vascular smooth muscle; decreases heart rate, myocardial contractility, slows SA and AV conduction. *Therapeutic Effect:* Dilates coronary arteries, peripheral arteries/arterioles.

PHARMACOKINETICS
Rapidly, completely absorbed from GI tract. Undergoes first-pass metabolism in liver to active metabolite. Primarily excreted in urine. Not removed by hemodialysis. **Half-life:** less than 24 hrs.

AVAILABILITY
Tablets: 200 mg, 300 mg (Vascor).

INDICATIONS AND DOSAGES
▸ **Chronic stable angina**

PO
Adults, Elderly. Initially, 200 mg/day; after 10 days, dosage may be adjusted. Maintenance: 200-400 mg/day.

CONTRAINDICATIONS
Sick sinus syndrome/second- or third-degree AV block (except in presence of pacemaker), severe hypotension (<90 mm Hg, systolic), history of serious ventricular arrhythmias, uncompensated cardiac insufficiency, congenital QT interval prolongation, use with other drugs prolonging QT interval

INTERACTIONS
Drug
Beta blockers: May have additive effect.
Digoxin: May increase digoxin concentration.
Procainamide, quinidine: May increase risk of QT interval prolongation.
Hypokalemia-producing agents: May increase risk of arrhythmias.
Herbal
None known.
Food
None known.

DIAGNOSTIC TEST EFFECTS
QT interval may be increased.

SIDE EFFECTS
Frequent
Dizziness, lightheadedness, nervousness, headache, asthenia (loss of strength), hand tremor, nausea, diarrhea
Occasional
Drowsiness, insomnia, tinnitus, abdominal discomfort, palpitations, dry mouth, shortness of breath, wheezing, anorexia, constipation

Rare
Peripheral edema, anxiety, flatulence, nasal congestion, paresthesia.

SERIOUS REACTIONS
• CHF, second- and third-degree AV block occur rarely.
• Serious arrhythmias can be induced.
• Overdosage produces nausea, drowsiness, confusion, slurred speech, profound bradycardia.

PRECAUTIONS & CONSIDERATIONS
Caution is warranted with CHF or impaired renal or hepatic function. It is unknown if bepridil crosses the placenta or is distributed in breast milk. Safety and efficacy of bepridil has not been established in children. The elderly are more sensitive to bepridil's hypotensive effects and the half-life may be increased.

Drowsiness or dizziness may occur. Rise slowly from lying or sitting position and wait momentarily before standing. Avoid tasks that require alertness and motor skills. Contact physician if irregular heartbeat, shortness of breath, pronounced dizziness, nausea, dyspepsia, ringing/roaring in ears, or constipation occurs. Avoid alcohol, grapefruit, and grapefruit juice.
Storage
Store at room temperature.
Administration
May take without regard to food, however, use with meals or at bedtime may decrease risk of nausea. Do not crush or break film-coated tablets. Do not abruptly discontinue medication.

Beractant
ber-akt'ant
(Survanta)
Do not confuse Survanta with Sufenta.

CATEGORY AND SCHEDULE
Pregnancy Risk Category: This drug is not indicated for use in pregnant women.

CLASSIFICATION
Surfactants, lung

MECHANISM OF ACTION
A natural bovine lung extract that reduces alveolar surface tension, stabilizing alveoli. *Therapeutic Effect:* Improves lung compliance and respiratory gas exchange.

PHARMACOKINETICS
Not absorbed systemically.

AVAILABILITY
Intratracheal Suspension for Inhalation: 25 mg/ml vials.

INDICATIONS AND DOSAGES
▸ **Prevention and rescue treatment of respiratory distress syndrome (RDS) or hyaline membrane disease in premature infants**
INTRATRACHEAL
Infants. 100 mg of phospholipids/kg birth weight (4 ml/kg). Give within 15 min of birth if infant weighs less than 1250 g and has evidence of surfactant deficiency; give within 8 hr when RDS is confirmed by X-ray and requires mechanical ventilation. May repeat 6 hr or longer after preceding dose. Maximum: 4 doses in the first 48 hr of life.

CONTRAINDICATIONS
None known.

INTERACTIONS
Drug
None known.
Herbal
None known.
Food
None known.

DIAGNOSTIC TEST EFFECTS
None known.

SIDE EFFECTS
Frequent
Transient bradycardia, oxygen (O_2) desaturation, increased carbon dioxide (CO_2) retention
Occasional
Endotracheal tube reflux
Rare
Apnea, endotracheal tube blockage, hypotension or hypertension, pallor, vasoconstriction

SERIOUS REACTIONS
• Life-threatening nosocomial sepsis may occur.

PRECAUTIONS & CONSIDERATIONS
Caution should be used in persons at risk for circulatory overload. This drug is for use only in neonates. No age-related precautions have been noted. The infant should be monitored with arterial or transcutaneous measurement of systemic O_2 and CO_2. Visitors should be limited during treatment. Hand washing and other infection control measures should be monitored to minimize the risk of nosocomial infections.
Storage
Refrigerate vials. Unopened, unused vials may be returned to the refrigerator only once and within 8 hours after having been warmed to room temperature.

Administration
Administer beractant in a highly supervised setting. Clinicians caring for the neonate must be experienced with intubation and ventilator management.

Warm the vial by letting it stand at room temperature for 20 minutes or warming in your hand for 8 minutes. Gently swirl the vial, if needed to redisperse contents. Do not shake it. The solution normally appears off-white to light brown. Enter each single-use vial only once; discard unused suspension.

Instill the drug through a catheter inserted into the infant's endotracheal tube. Don't instill it into the main-stem bronchus. Monitor the infant for bradycardia and decreased arterial O_2 saturation during administration. Stop the procedure, as prescribed, if the infant experiences these effects, and take appropriate measures before reinstituting therapy.

Betamethasone
bay-ta-meth'a-sone
(glucocorticoid, synthetic, corticosteroid, systemic, corticosteroid, topical)
(Alphatrex, Betaderm [CAN], Betatrex, Beta-Val, Betnesol [CAN], Celestone, Diprolene, Luxiq, Maxivate)

CATEGORY AND SCHEDULE
Pregnancy Risk Category: C (D if used in first trimester)

CLASSIFICATION
Corticosteroids

MECHANISM OF ACTION
An adrenocortical steroid that controls the rate of protein synthesis,

depresses the migration of polymor-phonuclear leukocytes and fibro-blasts, reduces capillary permeability and prevents or controls inflamma-tion. *Therapeutic Effect:* Decreases tissue response to inflammatory process.

AVAILABILITY
Tablet (Celestone): 0.6 mg.
Cream (Alphatrex, Diprolene, Maxivate): 0.05%.
Cream (Betatrex, Beta-Val): 0.1%.
Foam (Luxiq): 0.12%.
Gel (Diprolene): 0.05%.
Lotion: (Alphatrex, Diprolene, Maxivate): 0.05%.
Lotion (Betatrex, Beta-Val): 0.1%.
Ointment (Alphatrex, Diprolene, Maxivate): 0.05%.
Oinment (Betatrex): 0.1%.
Syrup (Celestone): 0.6 mg/5 ml.
Injection (Celestone, Soluspan): 6 mg/ml.

INDICATIONS AND DOSAGES
▸ **Anti-inflammation, immunosup-pression, corticosteroid replacement therapy**
PO
Adults, Elderly. 0.6-7.2 mg/day.
Children. 0.063-0.25 mg/kg/day in 3-4 divided doses.
▸ **Relief of inflamed and pruritic dermatoses**
TOPICAL
Adults, Elderly. 1-3 times a day.
Foam: Apply twice a day.

CONTRAINDICATIONS
Hypersensitivity to betamethasone, systemic fungal infections

INTERACTIONS
Drug
Amphotericin: May increase hypokalemia.
Digoxin: May increase digoxin toxi-city secondary to hypokalemia.

Diuretics, insulin, oral hypo-glycemics, potassium supplements: May decrease the effects of these drugs.
Hepatic enzyme inducers: May decrease the effect of betamethasone.
Live virus vaccines: May decrease the patient's antibody response to vaccine, increase vaccine side effects, and potentiate virus replication.
Herbal
None known.
Food
None known.

DIAGNOSTIC TEST EFFECTS
May increase blood glucose levels and serum lipids, amylase, and sodium levels. May decrease serum calcium, potassium, and thyroxine levels.

SIDE EFFECTS
Frequent
Systemic: Increased appetite, abdominal distention, nervousness, insomnia, false sense of well-being
Topical: Burning, stinging, pruritus
Occasional
Systemic: Dizziness, facial flushing, diaphoresis, decreased or blurred vision, mood swings
Topical: Allergic contact dermatitis, purpura or blood-containing blisters, thinning of skin with easy bruising, telangiectases or raised dark red spots on skin

SERIOUS REACTIONS
• Overdose may cause systemic hypercorticism and adrenal suppression.

PRECAUTIONS & CONSIDERATIONS
Caution is warranted with persons at increased risk for peptic ulcer disease and in those with cirrhosis, hypothyroidism, or nonspecific ulcerative colitis. Monitor growth

and development of children receiving long-term steroid therapy.

Mood swings, ranging from euphoria to depression, may occur. Initially, tuberculosis skin test, X-rays, and EKG should be evaluated. Blood glucose level, B/P, serum electrolyte levels, height, and weight should be monitored before and during therapy.

Administration

Give oral betamethasone with milk or food to decrease GI upset. Give single doses in the morning before 9 AM; give multiple doses at evenly spaced intervals. Do not abruptly discontinue the drug.

For topical use, gently cleanse area before applying drug. Apply sparingly and rub into area thoroughly. Use occlusive dressings only as ordered. When using aerosol, spray area for 3 seconds from a 15-cm distance; avoid inhalation. Do not use topical form on broken skin or in areas of infection and do not apply to the face or inguinal areas, or to wet skin.

Betaxolol

bay-tax′oh-lol
(Betoptic-S, Betoquin [AUS], Kerlone)
Do not confuse betaxolol with bethanechol.

CATEGORY AND SCHEDULE
Pregnancy Risk Category: C
(D if used in second or third trimester)

CLASSIFICATION
Antiadrenergics, beta blocking, ophthalmics

MECHANISM OF ACTION
An antihypertensive and antiglaucoma agent that blocks beta$_1$-adrenergic receptors in cardiac tissue. Reduces aqueous humor production. *Therapeutic Effect:* Slows sinus heart rate, decreases B/P and reduces intraocular pressure (IOP).

AVAILABILITY
Tablets (Kerlone): 10 mg, 20 mg.
Ophthalmic Solution (Betoptic-S): 0.5%.
Ophthalmic Suspension (Betoptic-S): 0.25%.

INDICATIONS AND DOSAGES
▶ **Hypertension**
PO
Adults. Initially, 5-10 mg/day.
May increase to 20 mg/day after 7-14 days.
Elderly. Initially, 5 mg/day.
▶ **Chronic open-angle glaucoma and ocular hypertension**
EYE DROPS
Adults, Elderly. 1 drop twice a day.
▶ **Dosage in renal impairment**
For adult and elderly patients who are on dialysis, initially give 5 mg/day; increase by 5 mg/day q2wk. Maximum: 20 mg/day.

OFF-LABEL USES
Treatment of angle-closure glaucoma during or after iridectomy, malignant glaucoma, secondary glaucoma; with miotics, to decrease IOP in acute and chronic angle-closure glaucoma

CONTRAINDICATIONS
Cardiogenic shock, overt cardiac failure, second- or third-degree heart block, sinus bradycardia

INTERACTIONS
Drug
Cimetidine: May increase betaxolol blood concentration.

Diuretics, other antihypertensives:
May increase hypotensive effect of
betaxolol.
Insulin, oral hypoglycemics: May
prolong hypoglycemic effect of these
drugs.
NSAIDs: May decrease antihyper-
tensive effect.
Sympathomimetics, xanthines:
May mutually inhibit hypotensive
effects and may mask symptoms of
hypoglycemia.
Herbal
None known.
Food
None known.

DIAGNOSTIC TEST EFFECTS

May increase serum antinuclear
antibody titer and BUN, serum
lipoprotein, creatinine, potassium,
uric acid, and triglyceride
levels.

SIDE EFFECTS

Betaxolol is generally well tolerated,
with mild and transient side
effects.
Frequent
Systemic: Hypotension manifested
as dizziness, nausea, diaphoresis,
headache, fatigue, constipation or
diarrhea, dyspnea
Ophthalmic: Eye irritation, visual
disturbances
Occasional
Systemic: Insomnia, flatulence,
urinary frequency, impotence or
decreased libido, bradycardia,
bronchospasm
Ophthalmic: Increased light sensitivity, watering of eye
Rare
Systemic: Rash, arrhythmias,
arthralgia, myalgia, confusion,
altered taste, increased
urination
Ophthalmic: Dry eye, conjunctivitis,
eye pain

SERIOUS REACTIONS

• Overdose may produce profound
bradycardia, hypotension, and bronchospasm.
• Abrupt withdrawal may result in
diaphoresis, palpitations, headache,
and tremors.
• Betaxolol administration may
precipitate CHF or MI in patients
with cardiac disease; thyroid storm
in those with thyrotoxicosis; and
peripheral ischemia in those with
existing peripheral vascular disease.
• Hypoglycemia may occur in
patients with previously controlled
diabetes.
• Ophthalmic overdose may produce
bradycardia, hypotension, bronchospasm, and acute cardiac failure.

PRECAUTIONS & CONSIDERATIONS

Caution is warranted with diabetes,
hyperthyroidism, impaired hepatic or
renal function, inadequate cardiac
function, and peripheral vascular
disease. Be aware that salt and alcohol intake should be restricted. Nasal
decongestants or OTC cold preparations (stimulants) should not be used
without physician approval.
Orthostatic hypotension may occur,
so rise slowly from a lying to sitting
position and dangle the legs from the
bed momentarily before standing.
Notify the physician of fatigue,
headache, prolonged dizziness, and
shortness of breath. B/P for hypotension, respiratory status for shortness
of breath, pattern of daily bowel
activity and stool consistency, and
pulse for quality, rate, and rhythm
should be monitored during treatment. If pulse rate is 60 beats/minute
or lower or systolic B/P is less than
90 mm Hg, withhold the medication
and contact the physician. Signs and
symptoms of CHF, such as decreased
urine output, distended neck veins,
dyspnea (particularly on exertion or

lying down), night cough, peripheral edema, and weight gain should also be assessed.

Administration

To assess tolerance for betaxolol, obtain a standing systolic B/P 1 hour after giving the drug. Do not abruptly discontinue betaxolol. Compliance is essential to control glaucoma and hypertension.

Bethanechol

be-than'e-kole

(Duvoid [CAN], Myotonachol [CAN], Urecholine, Urocarb [AUS])

Do not confuse bethanechol with betaxolol.

CATEGORY AND SCHEDULE

Pregnancy Risk Category: C

CLASSIFICATION

Cholinergics

MECHANISM OF ACTION

A cholinergic that acts directly at cholinergic receptors in the smooth muscle of the urinary bladder and GI tract. Increases detrusor muscle tone. *Therapeutic Effect:* May initiate micturition and bladder emptying. Improves gastric and intestinal motility.

AVAILABILITY

Tablets (Duvoid): 10 mg, 25 mg, 50 mg.

INDICATIONS AND DOSAGES

▶ **Postoperative and postpartum urine retention, atony of bladder**

PO

Adults, Elderly. 10-50 mg 3-4 times a day. Minimum effective dose

determined by giving 5-10 mg initially, then repeating same amount at 1-hr intervals until desired response is achieved, or maximum of 50 mg is reached.

Children. 0.6 mg/kg/day in 3-4 divided doses.

OFF-LABEL USES

Treatment of congenital megacolon, gastroesophageal reflux, postoperative gastric atony

CONTRAINDICATIONS

Active or latent bronchial asthma, acute inflammatory GI tract conditions, anastomosis, bladder wall instability, cardiac or coronary artery disease, epilepsy, hypertension, hyperthyroidism, hypotension, GI or urinary tract obstruction, parkinsonism, peptic ulcer, pronounced bradycardia, recent GI resection, vasomotor instability

INTERACTIONS

Drug

Cholinesterase inhibitors: May increase the effects and risk of toxicity of bethanechol.

Procainamide, quinidine: May decrease the effects of bethanechol.

Herbal

None known.

Food

None known.

DIAGNOSTIC TEST EFFECTS

May increase serum amylase, lipase, and AST (SGOT) levels.

SIDE EFFECTS

Occasional

Belching, blurred or changed vision, diarrhea, urinary urgency

SERIOUS REACTIONS

• Overdosage produces CNS stimulation (including insomnia, anxiety, and orthostatic hypotension), and cholinergic stimulation (such as headache, increased salivation, diaphoresis, nausea, vomiting, flushed skin, abdominal pain, and seizures).

PRECAUTIONS & CONSIDERATIONS

Notify the physician of difficulty breathing, irregular heartbeat, muscle weakness, nausea and vomiting, diarrhea, severe abdominal pain, and increased salivation or sweating. Intake and output and vital signs should be monitored.

Administration

! Avoid giving IM or IV route because doing so will precipitate a violent cholinergic reaction marked by bloody diarrhea, circulatory collapse, severe hypotension, and shock. The antidote is 0.6-1.2 mg atropine sulfate. Side effects are more noticeable with subcutaneous administration.

Bevacizumab

beh-vah-sif′zoo-mab
(Avastin)

CATEGORY AND SCHEDULE

Pregnancy Risk Category: C

CLASSIFICATION

Antineoplastics, monoclonal antibodies

MECHANISM OF ACTION

An antineoplastic that binds to and inhibits vascular endothelial growth factor, a protein that plays a major role in the formation of new blood vessels to tumors. *Therapeutic Effect:* Inhibits metastatic disease progression.

PHARMACOKINETICS

Clearance varies by body weight, gender, and tumor burden. **Half-life:** 20 days (range, 11-50 days).

AVAILABILITY

Injection: 25 mg/ml vial.

INDICATIONS AND DOSAGES

▸ **First-line treatment of metastatic carcinoma of the colon or rectum in combination with 5-fluorouracil (5-FU)**
IV
Adults, Elderly. 5 mg/kg once every 14 days.

OFF-LABEL USES

Adjunctive therapy in breast cancer, renal cell carcinoma

CONTRAINDICATIONS

GI perforation, hypertensive crisis, nephrotic syndrome, recent hemoptysis, serious bleeding, wound dehiscence requiring medical intervention

INTERACTIONS

Drug
None known.
Herbal
None known.
Food
None known.

DIAGNOSTIC TEST EFFECTS

May decrease serum potassium, sodium, and hemoglobin levels; hematocrit; and WBC and platelet counts.

▥ IV INCOMPATIBILITIES

Do not mix bevacizumab with dextrose solutions.

SIDE EFFECTS

Frequent (73%-25%)
Asthenia, vomiting, anorexia, hypertension, epistaxis, stomatitis, constipation, headache, dyspnea
Occasional (21%-15%)
Altered taste, dry skin, exfoliative dermatitis, dizziness, flatulence, excessive lacrimation, skin discoloration, weight loss, myalgia

Rare (8%-6%)
Nail disorder, skin ulcer, alopecia, confusion, abnormal gait, dry mouth

SERIOUS REACTIONS
• UTIs, manifested as urinary frequency or urgency and protein-uria, occur frequently.
• CHF, deep vein thrombosis, GI perforation, hypertensive crisis, nephrotic syndrome, and severe hemorrhage are the most serious reactions that occur.
• Anemia, neutropenia, and throm-bocytopenia occur occasionally.
• Hypersensitivity reactions occur rarely.

PRECAUTIONS & CONSIDERATIONS
Caution is warranted with CHF, epis-taxis, hypertension, proteinuria, and renal insufficiency. Bevacizumab is teratogenic and has the potential to impair fertility. Its use by pregnant women may decrease maternal and fetal body weight and increase the risk of fetal skeletal abnormalities. Breast-feeding women should not take bevacizumab. The safety and efficacy of bevacizumab have not been established in children. Patients older than 65 years have a higher incidence of serious adverse reac-tions. Avoid receiving immunizations without the physician's approval and avoid contact with crowds, people with known infections, and anyone who has recently received a live-virus vaccine because bevacizumab lowers the body's resistance to infection.
   Notify the physician if asthenia (loss of energy), abdominal pain, chills, fever, or nausea and vomiting occur. B/P, CBC, serum potassium, and sodium levels should be monitored before and regularly during beva-cizumab treatment. Urine should be assessed for proteinuria. Persons with a urine dipstick reading of 2+ or more should have a 24-hour urine collection. Pattern of daily bowel activity and stool consistency should be monitored.

Storage
Refrigerate vials. The diluted solution may be refrigerated for up to 8 hours.

Administration
! Don't give bevacizumab by IV push or IV bolus. Withdraw the amount of bevacizumab needed for a dose of 5 mg/kg, and dilute it in 100 ml 0.9% NaCl. Discard any unused portion. Infuse the initial dose of bevacizumab over 90 minutes after chemotherapy. If the person tolerates the first infu-sion well, the second infusion may be administered over 60 minutes.

Bexarotene
beks-air'oh-teen
(Targretin)

CATEGORY AND SCHEDULE
Pregnancy Risk Category: X

CLASSIFICATION
Antineoplastics, retinoids, dermatologics

MECHANISM OF ACTION
This retinoid antineoplastic agent binds to and activates retinoid X receptor subtypes, which regulate the genes that control cellular differentiation and proliferation. *Therapeutic Effect:* Inhibits growth of tumor cell lines of hematopoietic and squamous cell origin and induces tumor regression.

PHARMACOKINETICS
Moderately absorbed from the GI tract. Protein binding: greater than 99%. Metabolized in the liver. Primarily eliminated through the hepatobiliary system. **Half-life:** 7 hr.

AVAILABILITY
Capsules (Soft Gelatin): 75 mg.

INDICATIONS AND DOSAGES
▸ **Cutaneous T-cell lymphoma refractory to at least one prior systemic therapy**
PO
Adults. 300 mg/m^2/day. If no response and initial dose is well tolerated, may be increased to 400 mg/m^2/day. If not tolerated, may decrease to 200 mg/m^2/day, then to 100 mg/m^2/day.
TOPICAL
Adults. Initially, apply once every other day. May increase at weekly intervals up to 4 times a day.

OFF-LABEL USES
Treatment of diabetes mellitus; head, neck, lung, and renal cell carcinomas; Kaposi's sarcoma

CONTRAINDICATIONS
None known.

INTERACTIONS
Drug
Antidiabetics: May enhance the effects of these drugs.
Erythromycin, itraconazole, ketoconazole: May increase bexarotene blood concentrations.
Phenytoin, rifampin: May decrease bexarotene blood concentrations.
Herbal
None known.
Food
Grapefruit juice: May increase bexarotene blood concentration and risk of toxicity.

DIAGNOSTIC TEST EFFECTS
May increase serum cholesterol, triglyceride, and total and LDL cholesterol levels. May increase CA-125 assay value in patients with ovarian cancer. May decrease serum HDL cholesterol levels. May produce abnormal liver function test results.

SIDE EFFECTS
Frequent
Hyperlipidemia (79%), headache (30%), hypothyroidism (29%), asthenia (20%)
Occasional
Rash (17%); nausea (15%); peripheral edema (13%); dry skin, abdominal pain (11%); chills, exfoliative dermatitis (10%); diarrhea (7%)

SERIOUS REACTIONS
• Pancreatitis, hepatic failure, and pneumonia occur rarely.

PRECAUTIONS & CONSIDERATIONS
Caution is warranted with diabetes mellitus, lipid abnormalities, and hepatic impairment. Bexarotene use should be avoided during pregnancy because the drug may cause fetal harm. Pregnancy should be determined before beginning treatment. Reliable contraceptive methods should be used during therapy and for 1 month afterward. Notify the physician if she plans to become or becomes pregnant. It is unknown if bexarotene is distributed in breast milk; however, breast-feeding is not recommended. The safety and efficacy of bexarotene have not been established in children. No age-related precautions have been noted in the elderly. Abrasive, drying, or medicated soaps should be avoided during therapy.

Baseline lipid profile, liver function, thyroid function, and WBC count should be determined. Serum cholesterol and triglyceride levels, CBC, and liver and thyroid function test results should be monitored during therapy.
Administration
Take oral bexarotene with food.

Bicalutamide
bye-ka-loo'ta-mide
(Casodex, Cosudex [AUS])

CATEGORY AND SCHEDULE
Pregnancy Risk Category: X

CLASSIFICATION
Antineoplastics, antiandrogens, hormones/hormone modifiers

MECHANISM OF ACTION
An antiandrogen antineoplastic agent that competitively inhibits androgen action by binding to androgen receptors in target tissue. *Therapeutic Effect:* Decreases growth of prostatic carcinoma.

PHARMACOKINETICS
Well absorbed from the GI tract. Protein binding: 96%. Metabolized in the liver to inactive metabolite. Excreted in urine and feces. Not removed by hemodialysis. **Half-life:** 5.8 days.

AVAILABILITY
Tablets: 50 mg.

INDICATIONS AND DOSAGES
▸ Prostatic carcinoma
PO
Adults, Elderly. 50-100 mg once a day in morning or evening, given concurrently with a luteinizing hormone-releasing hormone (LHRH) analogue or after surgical castration.

CONTRAINDICATIONS
Pregnancy, use in women, hypersensitivity to any component of the formulation.

INTERACTIONS
Drug

Warfarin: May increase warfarin's effects.
Herbal
None known.
Food
None known.

DIAGNOSTIC TEST EFFECTS
May increase BUN level and serum alkaline phosphatase, bilirubin, AST (SGOT), and ALT (SGPT) levels. May decrease blood Hgb level and WBC count.

SIDE EFFECTS
Frequent
Hot flashes (49%), breast pain (38%), muscle pain (27%), constipation (17%), diarrhea (10%), asthenia (15%), nausea (11%)
Occasional (9%-8%)
Nocturia, abdominal pain, peripheral edema
Rare (7%-3%)
Vomiting, weight loss, dizziness, insomnia, rash, impotence, gynecomastia

SERIOUS REACTIONS
• Sepsis, CHF, hypertension, and iron deficiency anemia may occur.

PRECAUTIONS & CONSIDERATIONS
Caution is warranted with moderate to severe hepatic impairment. Liver function test results should be obtained before beginning therapy. Bicalutamide may inhibit spermatogenesis; this drug is not used in women. The safety and efficacy of bicalutamide have not been established in children. No age-related precautions have been noted in the elderly.
    Potential side effects, such as diarrhea, nausea, and vomiting, may occur. Notify the physician if nausea and vomiting persist.

Administration
Give oral bicalutamide at the same time each day and without regard to food. Avoid abruptly discontinuing the drug. Both bicalutamide and the LHRH analogue must be continued to achieve the desired therapeutic effect.

Biperiden
bye-per′i-den
(Akineton HCl)

CATEGORY AND SCHEDULE
Pregnancy Risk Category: C

CLASSIFICATION
Anticholinergics, antiparkinson agents

MECHANISM OF ACTION
A weak anticholinergic that exhibits competitive antagonism of acetylcholine at cholinergic receptors in the corpus striatum, which restores balance. *Therapeutic Effect:* Antiparkinson activity.

PHARMACOKINETICS
Well absorbed from gastrointestinal (GI) tract. Protein binding: 23%-33%. Widely distributed. **Half-life:** 18-24 hr.

AVAILABILITY
Tablets: 2 mg (Akineton HCl).

INDICATIONS AND DOSAGES
▸ **Extrapyramidal symptoms**
PO
Adults, Elderly. 2 mg 3-4 times/day. Dosage in renal impairment.
▸ **Parkinsonism**
PO
Adults, Elderly. 2 mg 1-3 times/day.

OFF-LABEL USES
Adjunct to methadone maintenance

CONTRAINDICATIONS
None known.

INTERACTIONS
Drug
Anticholinergics, antihistamines, phenothiazine, tricyclic antidepressants: May increase anticholinergic effects of biperiden.
Atenolol: May increase the bioavailability of atenolol.
Cholinergic agents: May decrease the effects of cholinergic agents.
Digoxin: May increase the amount of digoxin by delaying gastric emptying.
Levodopa: May increase the amount of levodopa by delaying gastric emptying.
Herbal
Betel nut: May decrease the anticholinergic effects of biperiden.
Food
Alcohol.

DIAGNOSTIC TEST EFFECTS
None known.

SIDE EFFECTS
Frequent
Orthostatic hypotension, anorexia, headache, blurred vision, urinary retention, dry mouth or nose
Occasional
Insomnia, agitation, euphoria
Rare
Vomiting, depression, irritation or swelling of eyes, rash

SERIOUS REACTIONS
• Overdosage may vary from severe anticholinergic effects, such as unsteadiness, severe drowsiness, dryness of mouth, nose, or throat, tachycardia, shortness of breath, and skin flushing.

• Also produces severe paradoxical reaction, marked by hallucinations, tremor, seizures, and toxic psychosis.

PRECAUTIONS & CONSIDERATIONS

Be alert to elderly patients older than 60 years of age because they tend to develop agitation, disorientation, mental confusion, and psychotic-like symptoms. Caution is also warranted with arrhythmias, heart disease, hypertension, liver or renal impairment, obstructive diseases of the gastrointestinal (GI) or genitourinary (GU) tracts, prostatic hypertrophy, tachycardia, treated open-angle glaucoma, and urinary retention. Biperiden use is not recommended during pregnancy or while breastfeeding. Safety and efficacy of biperiden has not been established in children. Alcoholic beverages should be avoided during biperiden therapy.

Neurologic effects including agitation, headache, lethargy, and mental confusion may be experienced. Dizziness, drowsiness, and dry mouth may be expected responses to the biperiden. Masklike facial expression, muscular rigidity, shuffling gait, and resting tremors of hands and head should be assessed.

Storage

Store at room temperature away from moisture and heat.

Administration

Biperiden should be taken with a full glass of water. It should be taken after a meal if it upsets the stomach.

Bisacodyl

bis-a-koe′dill
(Alophen, Apo-Bisacodyl [CAN], Bisalax [AUS], Dulcolax, Femilax, Gentlax, Modane, Veracolate)
Do not confuse with Accolate, Mudrane.

CATEGORY AND SCHEDULE

Pregnancy Risk Category: C
OTC

CLASSIFICATION

Bowel evacuants, laxatives

MECHANISM OF ACTION

A GI stimulant that has a direct effect on colonic smooth musculature by stimulating the intramural nerve plexi. *Therapeutic Effect:* Promotes fluid and ion accumulation in the colon increasing peristalsis and producing a laxative effect.

PHARMACOKINETICS

Route	Onset	Peak	Duration
PO	6-12 hr	N/A	N/A
Rectal	15-60 min	N/A	N/A

Minimal absorption following oral and rectal administration. Absorbed drug is excreted in urine; remainder is eliminated in feces.

AVAILABILITY

Tablets (Enteric-Coated): 5 mg.
Suppositories: 10 mg.

INDICATIONS AND DOSAGES

▸ **Treatment of constipation**
PO
Adults, Children older than 12 yr.
5-15 mg as needed. Maximum: 30 mg.

Children 3-12 yr. 5-10 mg or 0.3 mg/kg at bedtime or after breakfast.
Elderly. Initially, 5 mg/day.
RECTAL
Adults, Children 12 yr and older. 10 mg to induce bowel movement.
Children 2-11 yr. 5-10 mg as a single dose.
Children younger than 2 yr. 5 mg.
Elderly. 5-10 mg/day.

CONTRAINDICATIONS

Abdominal pain, appendicitis, intestinal obstruction, nausea, undiagnosed rectal bleeding, vomiting

INTERACTIONS

Drug
Antacids, cimetidine, famotidine, ranitidine: May cause rapid dissolution of bisacodyl, producing abdominal cramping, and vomiting.
Oral medications: May decrease transit time of concurrently administered oral medications, decreasing absorption of bisacodyl.
Herbal
None known.
Food
Milk: May cause rapid dissolution of bisacodyl.

DIAGNOSTIC TEST EFFECTS

None known.

SIDE EFFECTS

Frequent
Some degree of abdominal discomfort, nausea, mild cramps, faintness
Occasional
Rectal administration: burning of rectal mucosa, mild proctitis

SERIOUS REACTIONS

• Long-term use may result in laxative dependence, chronic constipation, and loss of normal bowel function.

• Prolonged use or overdose may result in electrolyte or metabolic disturbances (such as hypokalemia, hypocalcemia, and metabolic acidosis or alkalosis), as well as persistent diarrhea, vomiting, muscle weakness, malabsorption, and weight loss.

PRECAUTIONS & CONSIDERATIONS

Excessive use of bisacodyl may lead to fluid and electrolyte imbalance. It is unknown if bisacodyl crosses the placenta or is distributed in breast milk. Avoid bisacodyl use in children younger than 6 years of age because this population is usually unable to describe symptoms or more severe side effects. Repeated use of bisacodyl in the elderly may cause orthostatic hypotension and weakness due to electrolyte loss.

Increasing fluid intake, exercising, and eating a high-fiber diet should be instituted to promote defecation. Notify the physician if unrelieved constipation, dizziness, muscle cramps or pain, rectal bleeding, or weakness occurs. Electrolyte levels, hydration status, daily bowel activity, stool consistency, and record time of evacuation should be assessed.

Administration
Take oral bisacodyl on an empty stomach for faster action. Offer 6 to 8 glasses of water a day to aid in stool softening. Administer tablets whole; do not chew or crush them. Avoid taking within 1 hour of antacids, milk, or other oral medications.

For rectal use, if suppository is too soft, chill for 30 minutes in refrigerator or run cold water wrapper. Moisten suppository with cold water before inserting deep into rectum.

Bismuth Subsalicylate

bis'muth sub-sal-ih'sah-late
(Bismed [CAN], Colo-Fresh, Devrom, Kaopectate, Pepto-Bismol)

CATEGORY AND SCHEDULE
Pregnancy Risk Category: C
OTC

CLASSIFICATION
Antidiarrheals

MECHANISM OF ACTION
An antinauseant and antiulcer agent that absorbs water and toxins in the large intestine and forms a protective coating in the intestinal mucosa. Also possesses antisecretory and antimicrobial effects.
Therapeutic Effect: Prevents diarrhea. Helps treat *Helicobacter-pylori*-associated peptic ulcer disease.

AVAILABILITY
Caplet (Devrom): 200 mg.
Liquid (Kaopectate, Pepto-Bismol): 262 mg/15 ml, 525 mg/15 ml.
Tablet (Colo-Fresh): 324 mg.
Tablets (Chewable [Devrom]): (Devrom): 200 mg.
Tablets (Chewable [Pepto-Bismol]): 262 mg.

INDICATIONS AND DOSAGES
▶ **Diarrhea, gastric distress**
PO
Adults, Elderly. 2 tablets (30 ml) q30-60min. Maximum: 8 doses in 24 hr.
Children 9-12 yr. 1 tablet or 15 ml q30-60min. Maximum: 8 doses in 24 hr.

Children 6-8 yr. Two-thirds of a tablet or 10 ml q30-60min. Maximum: 8 doses in 24 hr.
Children 3-5 yr. One-third of a tablet or 5 ml q30-60min. Maximum: 8 doses in 24 hr.
▶ ***H. pylori*-associated duodenal ulcer, gastritis**
PO
Adults, Elderly. 525 mg 4 times a day, with 500 mg amoxicillin and 500 mg metronidazole, 3 times a day after meals, for 7-14 days.
▶ **Chronic infant diarrhea**
PO
Children 2-24 mo. 2.5 ml q4hr.

OFF-LABEL USES
Prevention of traveler's diarrhea

CONTRAINDICATIONS
Bleeding ulcers, gout, hemophilia, hemorrhagic states, renal impairment

INTERACTIONS
Drug
Anticoagulants, heparin, thrombolytics: May increase the risk of bleeding.
Aspirin, other salicylates: May increase the risk of salicylate toxicity.
Insulin, oral antidiabetics: Large dose may increase the effects of insulin and oral antidiabetics.
Tetracyclines: May decrease the absorption of tetracyclines.
Herbal
None known.
Food
None known.

DIAGNOSTIC TEST EFFECTS
May alter serum alkaline phosphatase, AST (SGOT), ALT (SGPT), and uric acid levels. May decrease serum potassium level. May prolong PT.

SIDE EFFECTS
Frequent
Grayish black stools
Rare
Constipation

SERIOUS REACTIONS
- Debilitated patients and infants may develop impaction.

PRECAUTIONS & CONSIDERATIONS
Caution is warranted with diabetes and in the elderly. Avoid bismuth if taking aspirin or other salicylates because of increased risk of toxicity. Also, inform the physician if taking anticoagulants because this drug combination can dangerously prolong bleeding time. Be aware that stool may appear black or gray. Pattern of daily bowel activity and stool consistency should be monitored.
Administration
Shake the suspension well before administration.

Chew the chewable tablet before swallowing. Alternatively, allow the chewable tablet to dissolve before swallowing.

Bisoprolol
bis-ope′pro-lal
(Zebeta)
Do not confuse Zebeta with DiaBeta.

CATEGORY AND SCHEDULE
Pregnancy Risk Category: C (D if used in second or third trimester)

CLASSIFICATION
Antiadrenergics, beta blocking

MECHANISM OF ACTION
An antihypertensive that blocks beta$_1$-adrenergic receptors in cardiac tissue. *Therapeutic Effect:* Slows sinus heart rate and decreases B/P.

PHARMACOKINETICS
Well absorbed from the GI tract. Protein binding: 26%-33%. Metabolized in the liver. Primarily excreted in urine. Not removed by hemodialysis. **Half-life:** 9-12 hr (increased in impaired renal function).

AVAILABILITY
Tablets: 5 mg, 10 mg.

INDICATIONS AND DOSAGES
▸ **Hypertension**
PO
Adults. Initially, 5 mg/day. May increase up to 20 mg/day.
Elderly. Initially, 2.5-5 mg/day. May increase by 2.5-5 mg/day.
Maximum: 20 mg/day.
▸ **Dosage in hepatic impairment**
For adults and elderly patients with cirrhosis or hepatitis whose creatinine clearance is less than 40 ml/min, initially give 2.5 mg.

OFF-LABEL USES
Angina pectoris, premature ventricular contractions, supraventricular arrhythmias,

CONTRAINDICATIONS
Cardiogenic shock, overt cardiac failure, second- or third-degree heart block

INTERACTIONS
Drug
Cimetidine: May increase bisoprolol blood concentration.
Diuretics, other antihypertensives: May increase the hypotensive effect of bisoprolol.

Insulin, oral hypoglycemics: May mask symptoms of hypoglycemia and prolong the hypoglycemic effect of these drugs.
NSAIDs: May decrease antihypertensive effect.
Sympathomimetics, xanthines: May mutually inhibit effects.
Herbal
None known.
Food
None known.

DIAGNOSTIC TEST EFFECTS
May increase antinuclear antibody titer and BUN, serum lipoprotein, creatinine, potassium, uric acid, and triglyceride levels.

SIDE EFFECTS
Frequent
Hypotension manifested as dizziness, nausea, diaphoresis, headache, cold extremities, fatigue, constipation or diarrhea
Occasional
Insomnia, flatulence, urinary frequency, impotence or decreased libido
Rare
Rash, arthralgia, myalgia, confusion (especially in the elderly), altered taste

SERIOUS REACTIONS
• Overdose may produce profound bradycardia and hypotension.
• Abrupt withdrawal may result in diaphoresis, palpitations, headache, and tremulousness.
• Bisoprolol administration may precipitate CHF and MI in patients with heart disease; thyroid storm in those with thyrotoxicosis; and peripheral ischemia in those with existing peripheral vascular disease.
• Hypoglycemia may occur in patients with previously controlled diabetes.

• Thrombocytopenia, including unusual bruising and bleeding, occurs rarely.

PRECAUTIONS & CONSIDERATIONS
Caution is warranted with bronchospastic disease, diabetes, hyperthyroidism, impaired hepatic or renal function, inadequate cardiac function, and peripheral vascular disease. Bisoprolol readily crosses the placenta and is distributed in breast milk. Bisoprolol use should be avoided in pregnant women after the first trimester because it may result in low-birth-weight infants. The drug may also produce apnea, bradycardia, hypoglycemia, or hypothermia during childbirth. The safety and efficacy of bisoprolol have not been established in children. In the elderly, age-related peripheral vascular disease may increase the risk of decreased peripheral circulation. Be aware that salt and alcohol intake should be restricted. Nasal decongestants or OTC cold preparations (stimulants) should not be used without physician approval.

Orthostatic hypotension may occur, so rise slowly from a lying to sitting position and dangle the legs from the bed momentarily before standing. Tasks that require mental alertness or motor skills should be avoided. B/P for hypotension, respiratory status for shortness of breath, pattern of daily bowel activity and stool consistency, and pulse for quality, rate, and rhythm should be monitored. If pulse rate is 60 beats/minute or lower or systolic B/P is less than 90 mm Hg, withhold the medication and contact the physician. Signs and symptoms of CHF, such as decreased urine output, distended neck veins, dyspnea (particularly on exertion or lying down), night cough, peripheral edema, and weight gain should also be assessed.

Administration
Bisoprolol may be taken without regard to food. If necessary, crush scored tablet. Do not abruptly discontinue bisoprolol. Compliance is essential to control glaucoma and hypertension.

Bitolterol
bye-tole′ter-ol
(Tornalate)

CATEGORY AND SCHEDULE
Pregnancy Risk Category: C

CLASSIFICATION
Adrenergic agonists, bronchodilators

MECHANISM OF ACTION
An antiadrenergic, sympatholytic agent that stimulates beta2-adrenergic receptors in lungs. *Therapeutic Effect:* Relaxes bronchial smooth muscle, relieves bronchospasm, reduces airway resistance.

PHARMACOKINETICS
Onset of action is rapid with duration of 4-8 hr. Rapidly absorbed following aerosol administration. Primarily distributed to lungs. Metabolized in liver. Excreted in urine and feces. **Half-life:** 3 hr.

AVAILABILITY
Aerosol for oral inhalation: 0.8% (Tornalate).
Solution for oral inhalation: 0.2% (Tornalate).

INDICATIONS AND DOSAGES
▸ **Brochospasm**

INHALATION
Adults, Elderly, Children 12 yr and older. Use 2 inhalations, separated by 1-3 minute interval. A third inhalation may be required.
▸ **Prevention of bronchospasm**
INHALATION
Adults, Elderly, Children 12 yr and older. Use 2 inhalations q8hr. Do not exceed 3 inhalations q6hr, or 2 inhalations q4hr.

OFF-LABEL USES
Chronic obstructive pulmonary disease

CONTRAINDICATIONS
History of hypersensitivity to sympathomimetics, bitolterol, or any of its components.

INTERACTIONS
Drug
Beta-blockers: May decrease effects of beta blockers.
Digoxin: May increase risk of arrhythmias.
MAOIs, tricyclic antidepressants, sympathomimetic agents, inhaled anesthetics: May increase the risk of toxicity.
Aminophylline: May increase risk of cardiotoxicity.
Herbal
None known.
Food
None known.

DIAGNOSTIC TEST EFFECTS
May decrease potassium.

▓ IV INCOMPATIBILITIES
Phenytoin, propofol (Diprivan)
▓ **IV Compatibilities**
Amiodarone (Cordarone), atracurium (Tacrium), calcium chloride, calcium gluconate, digoxin, dopamine (Intropin), esmolol (Brevibloc), famotidine (Pepcid),

insulin, isoproterenol, lidocaine, potassium, quinidine, ranitidine (Zantac), sodium bicarbonate, theophylline, verapamil

SIDE EFFECTS
Frequent
Tremor
Occasional
Cough, dry or irritated mouth/throat, headache, nausea, vomiting
Rare
Dizziness, vertigo, palpitations, insomnia

SERIOUS REACTIONS
• Although tolerance to the bronchodilating effect has not been observed, prolonged or too frequent use may lead to tolerance.
• Severe paradoxical bronchoconstriction may occur with excessive use.

PRECAUTIONS & CONSIDERATIONS
Caution is warranted with unstable vasomotor symptoms, cardiovascular disorders, diabetes, hyperthyroidism, prostatic hyperplasia or history of seizures. It is unknown if bitolterol crosses the placenta or is distributed in breast milk. Safety and efficacy of bitolterol has not been established in children. There are no age-related precautions noted in the elderly, but this age group may be more sensitive to drug's effects. Increase fluid intake to decrease lung secretion viscosity.

Bitolterol may cause nervousness, restlessness, and insomnia. If these effects persist, notify the physician.
Storage
Store at room temperature.
Administration
Shake canister well before use. Administer pressurized inhalation during the second half of inspiration, as the airways are open, water and

the aerosol distribution is more extensive. If more than one inhalation per dose is necessary, wait at least 1 full minute between inhalations. Second inhalation is best delivered after 10 minutes. Rinse mouth with water immediately after inhalation to prevent mouth and throat dryness. Administer around-the-clock rather than 3 times/day to promote less variation in peak and trough serum levels. Do not exceed the recommended dosage because excessive use may lead to adverse effects or loss of effectiveness.

Bivalirudin
bye-va-leer'u-din
(Angiomax)

CATEGORY AND SCHEDULE
Pregnancy Risk Category: B

CLASSIFICATION
Anticoagulants, thrombin inhibitors

MECHANISM OF ACTION
An anticoagulant that specifically and reversibly inhibits thrombin by binding to its receptor sites.
Therapeutic Effect: Decreases acute ischemic complications in patients with unstable angina pectoris.

PHARMACOKINETICS

Route	Onset	Peak	Duration
IV	Immediate	N/A	1 hr

Primarily eliminated by kidneys. Twenty-five percent removed by hemodialysis. **Half-life:** 25 min (increased in moderate to severe renal impairment).

AVAILABILITY
Injection (Lyophilized Powder): 250 mg.

INDICATIONS AND DOSAGES
▶ **Anticoagulant in patients with unstable angina who are undergoing percutaneous transluminal coronary angioplasty (PTCA) in conjunction with aspirin**
IV
Adults, Elderly. 1 mg/kg as IV bolus followed by 4-hr IV infusion at rate of 2.5 mg/kg/hr. After initial 4-hr infusion is completed, give additional IV infusion at rate of 0.2 mg/kg/hr for 20 hr or less, if necessary.
▶ **Dosage in renal impairment**

GFR	Dosage Reduced by
30-59 ml/min	20%
10-29 ml/min	60%
Dialysis	90%

CONTRAINDICATIONS
Active major bleeding

INTERACTIONS
Drug
Platelet aggregation inhibitors other than aspirin, thrombolytics, warfarin: May increase the risk of bleeding complications.
Herbal
Ginkgo biloba: May increase the risk of bleeding.
Food
None known.

DIAGNOSTIC TEST EFFECTS
Prolongs aPTT and PT.

▦ IV INCOMPATIBILITIES
Do not mix with other medications.

SIDE EFFECTS
Frequent (42%)
Back pain
Occasional (15%-12%)
Nausea, headache, hypotension, generalized pain
Rare (8%-4%)
Injection site pain, insomnia, hypertension, anxiety, vomiting, pelvic or abdominal pain, bradycardia, nervousness, dyspepsia, fever, urine retention

SERIOUS REACTIONS
• A hemorrhagic event occurs rarely and is characterized by a fall in B/P or Hct.

PRECAUTIONS & CONSIDERATIONS
Caution is warranted with conditions associated with increased risk of bleeding, including bacterial endocarditis, cerebrovascular accident, hemorrhagic diathesis, intracerebral surgery, recent major bleeding, recent major surgery, stroke, severe hypertension, and severe hepatic or renal impairment. It is unknown if bivalirudin is distributed in breast milk or crosses the placenta. Safety and efficacy of bivalirudin have not been established in children. In the elderly, age-related renal impairment may require dosage adjustment. Females should be aware that menstrual flow may be heavier than usual.

Notify the physician of bleeding from femoral vein site, blood in urine or stool, or discomfort or pain (especially chest pain) after treatment. Pulse rate, B/P, aPTT, Hct, BUN and serum creatinine levels, and stool or urine cultures for occult blood should be monitored.
Storage
Store unreconstituted vials at room temperature. Reconstituted solution may be refrigerated for no more than

24 hours. Diluted drug with a concentration of 0.5 to 5 mg/ml is stable at room temperature for 24 hours or less.

Administration

! Bivalirudin is intended for use with aspirin, 300-325 mg daily. Treatment should be initiated immediately before angioplasty.

To each 250-mg vial add 5 ml sterile water for injection. Gently swirl until all material is dissolved. Further dilute each vial in 50 ml D_5W or 0.9% NaCl to yield final concentration of 5 mg/ml: 1 vial in 50 ml, 2 vials in 100 ml, 5 vials in 250 ml. If low-rate infusion is used after the initial infusion, reconstitute the 250-mg vial with an additional 5 ml sterile water for injection. Gently swirl until all material is dissolved. Further dilute each vial in 500 ml D_5W or 0.9% NaCl to yield final concentration of 0.5 mg/ml. Diluting produces a clear, colorless solution; do not use solution if it is cloudy or contains a precipitate. Expect to adjust IV infusion based on aPTT or person's body weight.

Bortezomib

bor-teh'zoe-mib
(Velcade)

CATEGORY AND SCHEDULE

Pregnancy Risk Category: D

CLASSIFICATION

Antineoplastics, proteasome inhibitors

MECHANISM OF ACTION

A proteasome inhibitor, antineoplastic agent that degrades conjugated proteins required for cell-cycle progression and mitosis, disrupting cell proliferation. *Therapeutic Effect:* Produces antitumor and chemosensitizing activity and cell death.

PHARMACOKINETICS

Distributed to tissues and organs, with highest level in the GI tract and liver. Protein binding: 83%. Primarily metabolized by enzymatic action. Rapidly cleared from the circulation. Significant biliary excretion, with lesser amount excreted in the urine. **Half-life:** 9-15 hr.

AVAILABILITY

Powder for Injection: 3.5 mg.

INDICATIONS AND DOSAGES

▶ **Multiple myeloma**

IV

Adults, Elderly. Treatment cycle consists of 1.3 mg/m² twice weekly on days 1, 4, 8, and 11 for 2 wk followed by a 10-day rest period on days 12 to 21. Consecutive doses separated by at least 72 hr.

▶ **Dosage adjustment guidelines**

Therapy is withheld at onset of grade 3 nonhematological or grade 4 hematological toxicities, excluding neuropathy. When symptoms resolve, therapy is restarted at a 25% reduced dosage

▶ **Neuropathic pain, peripheral sensory neuropathy**

IV

Adults, Elderly. For grade 1 with pain or grade 2 (interfering with function but not activities of daily living [ADLs]), 1 mg/m². For grade 2 with pain or grade 3 (interfering with ADLs), withhold drug until toxicity is resolved, then reinitiate with 0.7 mg/m². For grade 4 (permanent sensory loss that interferes with function), discontinue bortezomib.

CONTRAINDICATIONS
Hypersensitivity to boron or mannitol

INTERACTIONS
Drug
Oral antidiabetics: May alter the response of these drugs.
Food
None known.
Herbal
None known.

DIAGNOSTIC TEST EFFECTS
May significantly decrease blood Hgb and Hct levels and neutrophil, platelet, and WBC counts.

SIDE EFFECTS
Expected (65%-36%)
Fatigue, malaise, asthenia, nausea, diarrhea, anorexia, constipation, fever, vomiting
Frequent (28%-21%)
Headache, insomnia, arthralgia, limb pain, edema, paresthesia, dizziness, rash
Occasional (18%-11%)
Dehydration, cough, anxiety, bone pain, muscle cramps, myalgia, back pain, abdominal pain, taste alteration, dyspepsia, pruritus, hypotension (including orthostatic hypotension), rigors, blurred vision

SERIOUS REACTIONS
• Thrombocytopenia occurs in 40% of patients. Platelet count peaks at day 11 and returns to baseline by day 21. GI and intracerebral hemorrhage are associated with drug-induced thrombocytopenia.
• Anemia occurs in 32% of patients.
• New onset or worsening neuropathy occurs in 37% of patients. Symptoms may improve in some patients when bortezomib is discontinued.
• Pneumonia occurs occasionally.

PRECAUTIONS & CONSIDERATIONS
Caution is warranted with history of syncope. Caution should also be used with any medication that increases the risk of dehydration, hypotension, and hepatic or renal function impairment. Bortezomib may induce degenerative effects in the ovaries and testes and may affect male and female fertility. Breast-feeding is not recommended. The safety and efficacy of bortezomib have not been established in children. The elderly are at increased risk for grade 3 and 4 thrombocytopenia.

Notify the physician of orthostatic hypotension, fever, pregnancy, nausea, vomiting, or diarrhea. Tasks that require mental alertness or motor skills should be avoided until response to the drug is established. Signs and symptoms of peripheral neuropathy, including a burning sensation, hyperesthesia, neuropathic pain, and paresthesia of the extremities, should be assessed. CBC, especially platelet count, should be monitored before and throughout bortezomib treatment. Intake and output and B/P should also be monitored. Adequate hydration should be maintained to prevent dehydration. IM injections or rectal medications and performing other procedures that may induce trauma and bleeding should be avoided.
Storage
Store unopened vials at room temperature. The reconstituted solution is stable at room temperature for up to 8 hours.
Administration
Reconstitute the vial with 3.5 ml 0.9% NaCl. Give bortezomib as a bolus IV injection.

Bosentan
bo′sen-tan
(Tracleer)
Do not confuse with Tricor.

CATEGORY AND SCHEDULE
Pregnancy Risk Category: X

CLASSIFICATION
Endothelin receptor antagonist

MECHANISM OF ACTION
An endothelin receptor antagonist
that blocks endothelin-1, the neuro-
hormone that constricts pulmonary
arteries. *Therapeutic Effect:* Improves
exercise ability and slows clinical
worsening of pulmonary arterial
hypertension (PAH).

PHARMACOKINETICS
Highly bound to plasma proteins,
mainly albumin. Metabolized in
the liver. Eliminated by biliary
excretion. **Half-life:** Approximately
5 hr.

AVAILABILITY
Tablets: 62.5 mg, 125 mg.

INDICATIONS AND DOSAGES
▶ **PAH in those with World
Health Organization Class III or
IV symptoms**
PO
Adults, Elderly. 62.5 mg twice a day
for 4 wk; then increase to
maintenance dosage of 125 mg
twice a day.
Children weighing less than 40 kg.
62.5 mg twice a day.

CONTRAINDICATIONS
Administration with cyclosporine or
glyburide, pregnancy

INTERACTIONS
Drug
**Atorvastatin, glyburide, hormonal
contraceptives (including oral,
injectable, and implantable),
lovastatin, simvastatin, warfarin:**
May decrease the plasma concentra-
tions of these drugs.
Cyclosporine, ketoconazole: May
increase plasma concentration of
bosentan.
Herbal
None known.
Food
None known.

DIAGNOSTIC TEST EFFECTS
May increase serum bilirubin, AST
(SGOT), and ALT (SGPT) levels.
May decrease blood Hgb and Hct
levels.

SIDE EFFECTS
Occasional
Headache, nasopharyngitis, flushing
Rare
Dyspepsia (heartburn, epigastric
distress), fatigue, pruritus,
hypotension

SERIOUS REACTIONS
• Abnormal hepatic function, lower
extremity edema, and palpitations
occur rarely.

PRECAUTIONS & CONSIDERATIONS
Caution is warranted with moderate
to severe hepatic function impairment. Bosentan administration may
induce atrophy of seminiferous
tubules of the testes, cause male
infertility, or reduce sperm count.
Bosentan causes fetal harm and has
teratogenic effects on the fetus,
including malformations of the
face, head, large vessels, and mouth.
Breast-feeding is not recommended.
The safety and efficacy of bosentan
have not been established in children.

Use cautiously in the elderly because the higher frequency of decreased cardiac, hepatic, and renal function is more common in this age group.

Because pregnancy must be avoided during bosentan therapy, it should be ruled out before the start of therapy. A negative result from a urine or serum pregnancy test should be performed during the first 5 days of a normal menstrual period and at least 11 days after the last act of sexual intercourse before drug therapy begins. Monthly pregnancy tests should be performed during bosentan therapy. Hepatic enzyme levels [serum aminotransferase, serum alkaline phosphatase, bilirubin, AST (SGOT), and ALT (SGPT)] should be monitored before bosentan therapy begins and monthly thereafter. Changes in monitoring and treatment should be initiated if an elevation in hepatic enzyme levels occurs. Treatment should be stopped if clinical symptoms of hepatic injury, including abdominal pain, fatigue, jaundice, nausea, and vomiting, occur or if bilirubin level increases. Blood Hgb level at 1 and 3 months should also be obtained after treatment begins and every 3 months thereafter; a decrease in blood Hct and Hgb levels signifies anemia.

Administration
Take bosentan in the morning and evening, with or without food. Do not break or crush film-coated tablets. Swallow the film-coated tablets whole and avoid chewing them.

Botulinum Toxin Type A
bot′yoo-lin-num toks′in type A
(Botox, Dysport [AUS])

CATEGORY AND SCHEDULE
Pregnancy Risk Category: C

CLASSIFICATION
Miscellaneous CNS agents

MECHANISM OF ACTION
A neurotoxin that blocks neuromuscular conduction by binding to receptor sites on motor nerve endings, and inhibiting the release of acetylcholine, resulting in muscle denervation. *Therapeutic Effect:* Reduces muscle activity.

AVAILABILITY
Injection: 100 units/vial.

INDICATIONS AND DOSAGES
▸ **Cervical dystonia in patients who have previously tolerated botulinum toxin type A**
IM
Adults, Elderly. Mean dose of 236 units (range: 198-300 units) divided among the affected muscles, based on patient's head and neck position, localization of pain, muscle hypertrophy, patient response, and adverse reaction history.
▸ **Cervical dystonia in patients who have not previously been treated with botulinum toxin type A**
IM
Adults, Elderly. Administer at lower dosage than for patients who have previously tolerated the drug.
▸ **Strabismus**
IM
Adults, Children older then 12 yr. 1.25-2.5 units into any one muscle.

Children 2 mo-12 yr. 1-2.5 units into any one muscle.

▸ **Blepharospasm**
IM
Adults. Initially, 1.25-2.5 units. May increase up to 2.5-5.0 units at repeat treatments. Maximum: 5 units per injection or cumulative dose of 200 units over a 30 day period.

▸ **Cerebral palsy spasticity**
IM
Children older than 18 mo.
1-6 units/kg. Maximum: 50 units per injection site. No more than 400 units per visit or during a 3 month period.

▸ **Improvement of brow furrow**
IM
Adults 65 yr and younger.
Individualized.

OFF-LABEL USES
Treatment of dynamic muscle contracture in children with cerebral palsy, focal task-specific dystonia, head and neck tremor unresponsive to drug therapy, hemifacial spasms, laryngeal dystonia, oromandibular dystonia, spasmoditic torticollis, writer's cramp

CONTRAINDICATIONS
Infection at proposed injection sites, hypersensitivity to albumin, botulinum toxin, or any component of the formulation.

INTERACTIONS
Drug
Aminoglycoside antibiotics, other drugs that interfere with neuromuscular transmission (such as curare-like compounds): May potentiate the effects of botulinum toxin type A.
Herbal
None known.
Food
None known.

DIAGNOSTIC TEST EFFECTS
None known.

SIDE EFFECTS
Frequent (15%-11%)
Localized pain, tenderness, or bruising at injection site; localized weakness in injected muscle; upper respiratory tract infection; neck pain; headache
Occasional (10%-2%)
Increased cough, flu-like symptoms, back pain, rhinitis, dizziness, hypertonia, soreness at injection site, asthenia, dry mouth, nausea, somnolence
Rare
Stiffness, numbness, diplopia, ptosis

SERIOUS REACTIONS
• Mild to moderate dysphagia occurs in approximately 20% of patients.
• Arrhythmias and severe dysphagia (manifested as aspiration, pneumonia, and dyspnea) occur rarely.
• Overdose produces systemic weakness and muscle paralysis.

PRECAUTIONS & CONSIDERATIONS
Caution is warranted with neuromuscular junctional disorders, such as amyotrophic lateral sclerosis, Lambert-Eaton syndrome, motor neuropathy, and myasthenia gravis, because they may experience significant systemic effects, including respiratory compromise, and severe dysphagia. Be aware of signs of dysphagia and aspiration pneumonia, including fever, sputum production, and adventitious breath sounds after treatment.

Clinical improvement should begin within 2 weeks of the injection but the drug's maximum benefit will appear approximately 6 weeks after the injection. Resume normal activity slowly and carefully. Seek medical attention immediately if respiratory, speech, or swallowing difficulties occur.
Storage
Store drug vials in the freezer. The reconstituted solution may be refrigerated for up to 4 hours.

B

Administer the drug within 4 hours after reconstitution. The solution normally appears as clear and colorless; discard the solution if particulate matter is present.

Administration

! Plan to have a physician inject the drug into the affected muscle.

Expect to administer the drug at the lowest effective dosage, and at the longest effective dosing interval to avoid formation of neutralizing antibodies. Dilute drug with 0.9% NaCl. For a resulting dose of units/0.1 ml draw up 1 ml of diluent to provide 10 units, 2 ml to provide 5 units, 4 ml to provide 2.5 units, or 8 ml to provide 1.25 units. Slowly and gently inject the diluent into the vial to avoid producing bubbles. Then, rotate the vial gently to mix the drug. If a vacuum doesn't pull the diluent into the vial, discard it. For IM use, assist the physician, as necessary, while he or she injects the drug into the affected muscles using a 25-, 27-, or 30-gauge needle for superficial muscles, and a 22-gauge needle for deeper muscles.

Botulinum Toxin Type B
bot′yoo-lin-num toks′in type B
(Myobloc)

CATEGORY AND SCHEDULE
Pregnancy Risk Category: C

CLASSIFICATION
Miscellaneous CNS agents

MECHANISM OF ACTION
A neurotoxin that inhibits acetyl-choline release at the neuromuscular

junction. *Therapeutic Effect:* Produces flaccid paralysis.

AVAILABILITY
Injection: 2500 units, 5000 units, 10,000 units.

INDICATIONS AND DOSAGES
▸ **To reduce the severity of symptoms in patients with cervical dystonia who have previously tolerated botulinum toxin type B**
IM
Adults, Elderly. 2500-5000 units divided among the affected muscles.
▸ **To reduce the severity of symptoms in patients with cervical dystonia who have not previously been treated with botulinum toxin type B**
IM
Adults, Elderly. Administer at lower dosage than for patients who have previously tolerated the drug.

CONTRAINDICATIONS
Infection at proposed injection site, hypersensitivity to albumin, botulinum toxin, or any component of the formulation.

INTERACTIONS
Drug
Aminoglycoside antibiotics, other drugs that interfere with neuromuscular transmission (such as curare-like compounds): May potentiate the effects of botulinum toxin type B.
Herbal
None known.
Food
None known.

DIAGNOSTIC TEST EFFECTS
None known.

SIDE EFFECTS
Frequent (19%-12%)
Infection, neck pain, headache, injection site pain, dry mouth

Occasional (10%-4%)
Flu-like symptoms, generalized pain, increased cough, back pain, myasthenia
Rare
Dizziness, nausea, rhinitis, headache, vomiting, edema, allergic reaction

SERIOUS REACTIONS
• Mild to moderate dysphagia occurs in approximately 10% of patients.
• Arrhythmias and severe dysphagia (manifested as aspiration, pneumonia, and dyspnea) occur rarely.
• Overdose produces systemic weakness and muscle paralysis.

PRECAUTIONS & CONSIDERATIONS
Caution is warranted with neuromuscular junctional disorders, such as amyotrophic lateral sclerosis, Lambert-Eaton syndrome, motor neuropathy, and myasthenia gravis, because they may experience significant systemic effects, including respiratory compromise, and severe dysphagia. Be aware of signs of dysphagia and aspiration pneumonia, including fever, sputum production, and adventitious breath sounds after treatment.

Resume normal activity slowly and carefully. Seek medical attention immediately if respiratory, speech, or swallowing difficulties occur.
Storage
Unreconstituted vials may be refrigerated for up to 21 months. Do not freeze them. The reconstituted solution may be stored in the refrigerator for up to 4 hours. Administer the drug within 4 hours after reconstitution. The solution normally appears clear and colorless; discard it if particulate matter is present.
Administration
! Plan to have a physician inject the drug into the affected muscle.

Dilute drug with 0.9% NaCl. Slowly and gently inject the diluent into the vial to avoid producing bubbles. Then rotate the vial gently to mix the drug. If a vacuum doesn't pull the diluent into the vial, discard it. For IM use, assist the physician as necessary, while he or she injects the drug into the affected muscles using a 25-, 27-, or 30-gauge needle for superficial muscles, and a 22-gauge needle for deeper muscles. Know that drug's effect lasts for 12 to 16 weeks at doses of 5000 or 10,000 units.

Bretylium
bre-til′ee-um
(Bretylium Tosylate-Dextrose, Bretylate [CAN])

CATEGORY AND SCHEDULE
Pregnancy Risk Category: C

CLASSIFICATION
Antiarrhythmics, class III

MECHANISM OF ACTION
An antiarrhythmic that directly affects myocardial cell membranes. *Therapeutic Effect:* Contributes to suppression of ventricular tachycardia.

PHARMACOKINETICS
Absorption is not expected to be present in peripheral blood at recommended doses. Protein binding: 1%-6%. Not metabolized. Excreted unchanged in urine. Removed by hemodialysis. **Half-life:** 6-13.5 hr.

AVAILABILITY
Injection: 50 mg/ml (Bretylium Tosylate-Dextrose).

Premix Solutions: 500 mg/250 ml, 1000 mg/250 ml (Bretylium Tosylate-Dextrose).

INDICATIONS AND DOSAGES
▸ **Ventricular arrhythmias, immediate, life threatening**
IV
Adults, Elderly. 5 mg/kg undiluted by rapid IV injection. May increase to 10 mg/kg, repeat as needed. Maintenance: 5-10 mg/kg diluted over 8 minutes or longer, q6hr or IV infusion at 1-2 mg/minute.
Children. 5 mg/kg, then 10 mg/kg at 15-30 minute intervals. Maximum: 30 mg/kg total dose. Maintenance: 5-10 mg/kg q6hr.
▸ **Ventricular arrhythmias, other**
IM
Adults, Elderly. 5-10 mg/kg undiluted, may repeat at 1-2 hour intervals. Maintenance: 5-10 mg/kg q6-8hr
IV
Adults, Elderly. 5-10 mg/kg diluted over 8 minutes or longer, may repeat at 1-2 hour intervals. Maintenance: 5-10 mg/kg q6hr or IV infusion at 1-2 mg/minute.
Children. 5-10 mg/kg/dose diluted q6hr.

OFF-LABEL USES
Treatment of cervical dystonia in patients who have developed resistance to botulinum toxin type A.

CONTRAINDICATIONS
Hypersensitivity to bretylium or any component of the formulation

INTERACTIONS
Drug
Arsenic trioxide, antipsychotics, Class I, IA, and III antiarrhythmics, dolasetron, fluoroquinolones, halofantrine, tricyclic antidepressants: May increase risk of cardiotoxicity (QT prolongation, torsades de pointes, cardiac arrest).
Digoxin: May increase digoxin toxicity (due to initial norepinephrine release).
Herbal
None known.
Food
None known.

DIAGNOSTIC TEST EFFECTS
None known.

SIDE EFFECTS
Frequent
Transitory hypertension followed by postural and supine hypotension in 50% of pts observed as dizziness, lightheadedness, faintness, vertigo
Occasional
Diarrhea, loose stools, nausea, vomiting
Rare
Angina, bradycardia

SERIOUS REACTIONS
• Respiratory depression from possible neuromuscular blockade.

PRECAUTIONS & CONSIDERATIONS
Extreme cautions should be used with digitalis-induced arrhythmias and fixed cardiac output such as severe pulmonary hypertension, and aortic stenosis. Caution is also warranted with impaired renal function, hyperthermia, hypotension, and sinus bradycardia. It is unknown if bretylium crosses the placenta or is distributed in breast milk. There are no age-related precautions noted in children. The elderly are more susceptible to the drug's hypotensive effect. Tolerance to hypotensive effects usually occurs within several days of initial therapy. Rise slowly from lying to sitting position and permit legs to dangle from bed

for at least 5 minutes before standing 1 hour after dose administration.
Storage
Store vials at room temperature.
Administration
Maintain supine position during infusion.

Do not dilute solution for IM injection. Do not give more than 5 ml into one site (over 3 ml may cause pain at injection site). Same-site injection may cause muscular atrophy and necrosis—rotate injection sites.

Reconstitute solution for injection by diluting vials with at least 50 ml D_5W or 0.9% NaCl. Give injection undiluted over 1 minute.

For intermittent IV infusion (piggyback), infuse over at least 8 minutes (too rapid IV produces nausea and vomiting).

For IV infusion, give 1-2 mg/minute of diluted solution.

Bromocriptine
broe-moe-krip'teen
(Apo-Bromocriptine [CAN], Bromohexal [AUS], Kripton [AUS], Parlodel)
Do not confuse bromocriptine with benztropine, or Parlodel with pindolol.

CATEGORY AND SCHEDULE
Pregnancy Risk Category: C

CLASSIFICATION
Antiparkinson agents, dopaminergics, ergot alkaloids and derivatives

MECHANISM OF ACTION
A dopamine agonist that directly stimulates dopamine receptors in the corpus striatum and inhibits prolactin secretion. Also suppresses secretion of growth hormone. *Therapeutic Effect:* Improves symptoms of parkinsonism, suppresses galactorrhea, and reduces serum growth hormone concentrations in acromegaly.

PHARMACOKINETICS

Indication	Onset	Peak	Duration
Prolactin lowering	2 hr	8 hr	24 hr
Antiparkinson	0.5-1.5 hr	2 hr	N/A
Growth hormone suppressant	1-2 hr	4-8 wk	4-8 hr

Minimally absorbed from the GI tract. Protein binding: 90%-96%. Metabolized in the liver. Excreted in feces by biliary secretion. **Half-life:** 15 hr.

AVAILABILITY
Capsules: 5 mg.
Tablets: 2.5 mg.

INDICATIONS AND DOSAGES
▸ **Hyperprolactinemia**
PO
Adults, Elderly. Initially, 1.25-2.5 mg/day. May increase by 2.5 mg/day at 3- to 7-day intervals. Range: 2.5 mg 2-3 times a day.
▸ **Parkinson's disease**
PO
Adults, Elderly. Initially, 1.25 mg twice a day. May increase by 2.5 mg/day every 14-28 days. Range: 30-90 mg/day.
▸ **Acromegaly**
PO
Adults, Elderly. Initially, 1.25-2.5 mg. May increase at

3-7 day intervals. Usual dose 20-30 mg/day.

OFF-LABEL USES
Treatment of cocaine addiction, hyperprolactinemia associated with pituitary adenomas, neuroleptic malignant syndrome

CONTRAINDICATIONS
Hypersensitivity to ergot alkaloids, peripheral vascular disease, pregnancy, severe ischemic heart disease, uncontrolled hypertension

INTERACTIONS
Drug
Alcohol: May produce a disulfiram-like reaction (chest pain, confusion, flushed face, nausea, vomiting).
Erythromycin, ritonavir: May increase bromocriptine blood concentration and risk of toxicity.
Estrogens, progestins: May decrease the effects of bromocriptine.
Haloperidol, MAOIs, pheno-thiazines, risperidone: May decrease bromocriptine's prolactin-lowering effect.
Hypotension-producing medications: May increase hypotension.
Levodopa: May increase the effects of bromocriptine.
Herbal
None known.
Food
None known.

DIAGNOSTIC TEST EFFECTS
May increase plasma growth hormone concentration.

SIDE EFFECTS
Frequent
Nausea (49%), headache (19%), dizziness (17%)
Occasional (7%-3%)
Fatigue, lightheadedness, vomiting, abdominal cramps, diarrhea, constipation, nasal congestion, somnolence, dry mouth
Rare
Muscle cramps, urinary hesitancy

SERIOUS REACTIONS
• Visual or auditory hallucinations have been noted in patients with Parkinson's disease.
• Long-term, high-dose therapy may produce continuing rhinorrhea, syncope, GI hemorrhage, peptic ulcer, and severe abdominal pain.

PRECAUTIONS & CONSIDERATIONS
Caution is warranted with cardiac or hepatic function impairment, hypertension, and psychiatric disorders. Be aware the incidence of side effects is high, especially at the beginning of therapy and with high dosages. Bromocriptine use is not recommended during pregnancy or breast-feeding. Nonhormonal contraceptives are recommended to females during treatment. The safety and efficacy of bromocriptine have not been established in children. The elderly are more prone to CNS adverse effects.

Dizziness, drowsiness, and dry mouth are expected responses to the drug. Alcohol and tasks that require mental alertness or motor skills should be avoided. Also, change positions slowly and dangle the legs momentarily before standing to avoid light-headedness. Notify the physician if watery nasal discharge occurs. Constipation should be assessed during treatment.
Administration
Lie down before taking the first dose to avoid lightheadedness. Take bromocriptine after food to decrease the incidence of nausea.

Brompheniramine
brome-fen-ir'a-meen
(BroveX, BroveX CT, Codimal
A, Colhist, Dimetane, Dimetane
Extentabs, Dimetapp, Lodrane
12 Hour, Nasahist B, ND Stat)

CATEGORY AND SCHEDULE
Pregnancy Risk Category: B
OTC (tablets, elixir)

CLASSIFICATION
Antihistamines, H1

MECHANISM OF ACTION
An alkylamine that competes
with histamine at histaminic
receptor sites. Inhibits central
acetylcholine. *Therapeutic Effect:*
Results in anticholinergic,
antipruritic, antitussive, antiemetic
effects. Produces antidyskinetic,
sedative effect.

PHARMACOKINETICS
Rapidly absorbed after PO
administration. Widely distributed.
Metabolized in liver. Primarily
excreted in urine. **Half-life:** 25 hr.

AVAILABILITY
Tablets: 4 mg (Dimetane).
Tablets, chewable (extended-release):
12 mg (BroveX CT).
Tablets (extended-release): 6 mg
(Lodrane 12 Hour).
Tablets (timed-release): 8 mg, 12 mg
(Dimetane Extentabs).
Elixir: 2 mg/5 ml (Dimetapp).
Oral Suspension: 12 mg/5 ml
(BroveX).

INDICATIONS AND DOSAGES
▸ **Allergic rhinitis, anaphylaxis,
urticarial transfusion reactions,
urticaria**

PO
*Adults, Elderly, Children 12 yr and
older.* 4 mg q4-6hr or 8-12 mg
extended/timed-release q12hr.
Children younger than 12 yr.
1-2 mg q4-6hr.
▸ **Amelioration of allergic reactions
to blood or plasma, anaphylaxis as
an adjunct to epinephrine and other
standard measures after the acute
symptoms have been controlled,
other uncomplicated allergic
conditions of the immediate type
when oral therapy is impossible or
contraindicated**
IM/IV/SC
*Adults, Elderly, Children 12 yr and
older.* 5-20 mg/day in 2 divided
doses. Maximum: 40 mg/day.
Children younger than 12 yr.
0.125 mg/kg/day or 3.75 mg/m^2 in
3-4 divided doses.

CONTRAINDICATIONS
Concurrent MAOI therapy, focal
CNS lesions, newborn or premature
infants, hypersensitivity to
brompheniramine or related
drugs

INTERACTIONS
Drug
Anticholinergics: May increase
anticholinergic effects.
MAOIs: May increase anticholiner-
gic and CNS depressant effects.
Procarbazine: May increase CNS
depressant effects.
Herbal
None known.
Food
None known.

DIAGNOSTIC TEST EFFECTS
May suppress wheal and flare
reactions to antigen skin testing
unless antihistamines are
discontinued 4 days before
testing.

SIDE EFFECTS
Frequent
Drowsiness, dizziness, dry mouth, nose, or throat, urinary retention, thickening of bronchial secretions
Elderly: Sedation, dizziness, hypotension
Occasional
Epigastric distress, flushing, blurred vision, tinnitus, paresthesia, sweating, chills

SERIOUS REACTIONS
• Children may experience dominant paradoxical reactions, including restlessness, insomnia, euphoria, nervousness, and tremors.
• Overdosage in children may result in hallucinations, seizures, and death.
• Hypersensitivity reaction, such as eczema, pruritus, rash, cardiac disturbances, and photosensitivity, may occur.

PRECAUTIONS & CONSIDERATIONS
Caution is warranted with asthma, pyloro-duodenal or bladder neck obstruction, glucose-6-phosphate dehydrogenase (G6PD) deficiency, or prostatic hypertrophy. It is unknown if brompheniramine crosses the placenta or is detected in breast milk. There is an increased risk of seizures in neonates and premature infants if the drug is used during the third trimester of pregnancy. Brompheniramine use is not recommended in newborns or premature infants as these groups are at an increased risk of experiencing paradoxical reaction. The elderly are at an increased risk of developing confusion, dizziness, hyperexcitability, hypotension, and sedation. Dizziness, drowsiness, and dry mouth are expected side effects of brompheniramine. Avoid alcohol during therapy.

Storage
Store at room temperature. Protect from light to prevent discoloration.
Administration
Give oral brompheniramine with meals to minimize GI upset.
  Be aware that IM and subcutaneous brompheniramine injection may be administered without dilution.
  Brompheniramine for IV injection may be administered undiluted or diluted 1-10 ml with sterile saline for injection. Give slowly with patient in recumbent position. May add to 0.9% NaCl, D$_5$W or whole blood for IV administration.

Budesonide
bu-dess'ah-nide
(Entocort EC, Pulmicort Respules, Pulmicort Turbuhaler, Rhinocort Aqua, Rhinocort Aqueous [AUS], Rhinocort Hayfever [AUS])

CATEGORY AND SCHEDULE
Pregnancy Risk Category: B

CLASSIFICATION
Corticosteroids, inhalation

MECHANISM OF ACTION
A glucocorticoid that inhibits the accumulation of inflammatory cells and decreases and prevents tissues from responding to the inflammatory process. *Therapeutic Effect:* Relieves symptoms of allergic rhinitis or Crohn's disease.

PHARMACOKINETICS
Minimally absorbed from nasal tissue; moderately absorbed from inhalation. Protein binding: 88%.

Primarily metabolized in the liver.
Half-life: 2-3 hr.

AVAILABILITY

Capsules (Entocort EC): 3 mg.
*Powder for oral inhalation
(Pulmicort Turbuhaler):* 200 mcg
per inhalation.
*Suspension for oral inhalation
(Pulmicort Respules):* 0.25 mg/2 ml;
0.5 mg/2 mg.
Nasal spray (Rhinocort Aqua):
32 mcg/spray.

INDICATIONS AND DOSAGES
▸ **Rhinitis**
Intranasal (Rhinocort Aqua)
*Adults, Elderly, Children 6 yr and
older.* 1 spray in each nostril once a
day. Maximum: 8 sprays/day for
adults and children 12 yr and older;
4 sprays/day for children younger
than 12 yr.
▸ **Bronchial asthma**
NEBULIZATION
Children 6 mo-8 yr. 0.25-1 mg/day
titrated to lowest effective dosage.
INHALATION
*Adults, Elderly, Children 6 yr and
older.* Initially, 200-400 mcg twice a
day. Maximum: Adults: 800 mcg
twice a day. Children: 400 mcg twice
a day.
▸ **Crohn's disease**
PO
Adults, Elderly. 9 mg once a day for
up to 8 wk.

OFF-LABEL USES
Treatment of vasomotor rhinitis

CONTRAINDICATIONS
Hypersensitivity to any corticosteroid
or its components, persistently positive sputum cultures for *Candida
albicans,* primary treatment of status
asthmaticus, systemic fungal infections, untreated localized infection
involving nasal mucosa

INTERACTIONS
Drug
Cimetidine: May increase the serum
concentrations of budesonide.
CYP 3A4 inhibitors: May increase
the serum level and toxicity of
budesonide.
Herbal
St. John's wort: May increase levels
of budesonide.
Food
None known.

DIAGNOSTIC TEST EFFECTS
None known.

SIDE EFFECTS
Frequent (greater than 3%)
Nasal: Mild nasopharyngeal irritation, burning, stinging, or dryness;
headache; cough
Inhalation: Flu-like symptoms,
headache, pharyngitis
Occasional (3%-1%)
Nasal: Dry mouth, dyspepsia, rebound
congestion, rhinorrhea, loss of taste
Inhalation: Back pain, vomiting,
altered taste, voice changes, abdominal pain, nausea, dyspepsia

SERIOUS REACTIONS
• An acute hypersensitivity reaction
marked by urticaria, angioedema,
and severe bronchospasm, occurs
rarely.

PRECAUTIONS & CONSIDERATIONS
Caution is warranted with adrenal
insufficiency, cirrhosis, glaucoma,
hypothyroidism, osteoporosis,
tuberculosis, and untreated infection.
It is unknown if budesonide crosses
the placenta or is distributed in
breast milk. In children, prolonged
treatment and high doses may
decrease cortisol secretion and short-
term growth rate. No age-related
precautions have been noted in the
elderly.

Symptoms should improve in 24 hours but the drug's full effect may take 3 to 7 days to appear. Those using budesonide intranasally should notify the physician if nasal irritation occurs or if symptoms, such as sneezing, fail to improve.

Administration

For inhalation, first shake the container well. Exhale completely and place the mouthpiece between the lips. Inhale and hold breath for as long as possible before exhaling. Allow at least 1 minute between inhalations. Rinse mouth after each use to decrease dry mouth and hoarseness and prevent fungal infection of the mouth.

For intranasal use, clear nasal passages as much as possible. Tilt the head slightly forward. Insert the spray tip into the nostril, pointing toward the nasal passages, away from the nasal septum. Spray budesonide into the nostril while holding the other nostril closed, and at the same time, inhale through the nose to deliver the medication as high into the nasal passages as possible.

Bumetanide
byoo-met'a-nide
(Bumex, Burinex [CAN])

CATEGORY AND SCHEDULE
Pregnancy Risk Category: C
(D if used in pregnancy-induced hypertension)

CLASSIFICATION
Diuretics, loop

MECHANISM OF ACTION
A loop diuretic that enhances excretion of sodium, chloride, and to lesser degree, potassium, by direct action at the ascending limb of the loop of Henle and in the proximal tubule. *Therapeutic Effect:* Produces diuresis.

PHARMACOKINETICS

Route	Onset	Peak	Duration
PO	30-60 min	60-120 min	4-6 hr
IV	Rapid	15-30 min	2-3 hr
IM	40 min	60-120 min	4-6 hr

Completely absorbed from the GI tract (absorption decreased in CHF and nephrotic syndrome). Protein binding: 94%-96%. Partially metabolized in the liver. Primarily excreted in urine. Not removed by hemodialysis. **Half-life:** 1-1.5 hr.

AVAILABILITY
Tablets: 0.5 mg, 1 mg, 2 mg.
Injection: 0.25 mg/ml.

INDICATIONS AND DOSAGES
▸ **Edema**
PO
Adults, Children older than 18 yr.
0.5-2 mg as a single dose in the morning. May repeat at q4-5hr.
Elderly. 0.5 mg/day, increased as needed.
IV, IM
Adults, Elderly. 0.5-2 mg/dose; may repeat in 2-3 hr. Or 0.5-1 mg/hr by continuous IV infusion.
▸ **Hypertension**
PO
Adults, Elderly. Initially, 0.5 mg/day. Range: 1-4 mg/day. Maximum: 5 mg/day. Larger doses may be given 2-3 doses/day.
▸ **Usual pediatric dosage**
PO, IV, IM
Children. 0.015-0.1 mg/kg/dose q6-24hr.

B

OFF-LABEL USES
Treatment of hypercalcemia, hypertension

CONTRAINDICATIONS
Anuria, hepatic coma, severe electrolyte depletion

INTERACTIONS
Drug
Amphotericin B, nephrotoxic and ototoxic medications: May increase the risk of nephrotoxicity and ototoxicity.
Anticoagulants, heparin: May decrease the effects of these drugs.
Lithium: May increase the risk of lithium toxicity.
Other hypokalemia-causing medications: May increase the risk of hypokalemia.
Herbal
None known.
Food
None known.

DIAGNOSTIC TEST EFFECTS
May increase blood glucose, BUN, serum uric acid, and urinary phosphate levels. May decrease serum calcium, chloride, magnesium, potassium, and sodium levels.

IV INCOMPATIBILITIES
Midazolam (Versed)
IV Compatibilities
Aztreonam (Azactam), cefepime (Maxipime), diltiazem (Cardizem), dobutamine (Dobutrex), furosemide (Lasix), lorazepam (Ativan), milrinone (Primacor), morphine, piperacillin and tazobactam (Zosyn), propofol (Diprivan)

SIDE EFFECTS
Expected
Increased urinary frequency and urine volume
Frequent
Orthostatic hypotension, dizziness
Occasional
Blurred vision, diarrhea, headache, anorexia, premature ejaculation, impotence, dyspepsia
Rare
Rash, urticaria, pruritus, asthenia, muscle cramps, nipple tenderness

SERIOUS REACTIONS
• Vigorous diuresis may lead to profound water and electrolyte depletion, resulting in hypokalemia, hyponatremia, dehydration, coma, and circulatory collapse.
• Ototoxicity—manifested as deafness, vertigo, or tinnitus—may occur, especially in patients with severe renal impairment and those taking other ototoxic drugs.
• Blood dyscrasias and acute hypotensive episodes have been reported.

PRECAUTIONS & CONSIDERATIONS
Caution is warranted with diabetes mellitus, hypersensitivity to sulfonamides, hepatic or renal impairment, and in the elderly and debilitated. It is unknown if bumetanide is distributed in breast milk. The safety and efficacy of bumetanide have not been established in children. The elderly are at increased risk for circulatory collapse or thromboembolic episodes and may be more sensitive to the drug's hypotensive and electrolyte effects. Age-related renal impairment may require reduced dosage or an extended dosage interval in the elderly. Consuming foods high in potassium such as apricots, bananas, legumes, meat, orange juice, raisins, whole grains, including cereals, and white and sweet potatoes, is encouraged.
An increase in the frequency and volume of urination and hearing

abnormalities, such as a sense of fullness or ringing in the ears, may occur. Blood pressure (B/P), vital signs, electrolytes, intake and output, and weight should be monitored before and during treatment. Be aware of signs of electrolyte disturbances such as hypokalemia or hyponatremia. Hypokalemia may cause arrhythmias, altered mental status, muscle cramps, asthenia, and tremor. Hyponatremia may result in cold and clammy skin, confusion, and thirst.

Storage
Store vials at room temperature.

Administration
Take bumetanide with food to avoid GI upset, preferably with breakfast to help prevent nocturia.
Bumetanide is compatible with D_5W, 0.9% NaCl, and lactated Ringer's solution, but it may also be given undiluted. The solution remains stable for 24 hours if diluted. Administer the drug by IV push over 1 to 2 minutes. Bumetanide may also be given as a continuous infusion.

Bupivacaine

byoo-piv'a-caine
(Marcaine, Marcaine Spinal, Sensorcaine, Sensorcaine-MPF)

CATEGORY AND SCHEDULE
Pregnancy Risk Category: C

CLASSIFICATION
Anesthetics, local

MECHANISM OF ACTION
An amide-type anesthetic that stabilizes neuronal membranes and prevents initiation and transmission of nerve impulses thereby effecting local anesthetic actions. *Therapeutic Effect:* Produces local analgesia.

PHARMACOKINETICS
Onset of action occurs within 4-10 minutes depending on route of administration. Duration is 1.5-8.5 hr. Well absorbed. Protein binding: 95%. Metabolized in liver. Excreted in urine. **Half life:** 1.5-5.5 hr (Adults), 8.1 hr (Neonates)

AVAILABILITY
Injection: 0.25% (Marcaine, Sensorcaine-MPF), 0.5% (Marcaine, Sensorcaine-MPF), 0.75% (Marcaine, Marcaine Spinal, Sensorcaine-MPF).

INDICATIONS AND DOSAGES
Dose varies with procedure, depth of anesthesia, vascularity of tissues, duration of anesthesia and condition of patient.
▶ **Analgesic, epidural (partial to moderate motor blockade)**
IV
Adults, Elderly. 10-20 ml (25-50 mg) of a 0.25% solution. Repeat once q3hr as needed.
Children more than 10 kg.
1-2.5 mg/kg single dose as a 0.125% or 0.25% solution or 0.2-0.4 mg/kg/hr continuous infusion as a 0.1%, 0.125%, or 0.25% solution. Maximum: 0.4 mg/kg/hr.
Children less than 10 kg.
1-1.25 mg/kg single dose as a 0.125% or 0.25% solution or 0.1-0.2 mg/kg/hr continuous infusion as a 0.1%, 0.125%, or 0.25% solution. Maximum: 0.2 mg/kg/hr.
▶ **Analgesic, epidural (moderate to complete motor blockade)**
IV
Adults, Elderly. 10-20 ml (50-100 mg) as a 0.5% solution.

Repeat once q3hr as needed.
Children more than 10 kg.
1-2.5 mg/kg single dose as a 0.125%
or 0.25% solution or 0.2-0.4 mg/kg/hr
continuous infusion as a 0.1%,
0.125%, or 0.25% solution.
Maximum: 0.4 mg/kg/hr.
Children less than 10 kg.
1-1.25 mg/kg single dose as a
0.125% or 0.25% solution or
0.1-0.2 mg/kg/hr continuous infusion
as a 0.1%, 0.125%, or 0.25% solution.
Maximum: 0.2 mg/kg/hr.

▸ **Analgesic, epidural (complete motor blockade)**
IV
Adults. 10-20 ml (75-150 mg) as a
0.75% solution. Repeat once q3hr as
needed.
Children more than 10 kg.
1-2.5 mg/kg single dose as a 0.125%
or 0.25% solution or 0.2-0.4 mg/kg/hr
continuous infusion as a 0.1%,
0.125%, or 0.25% solution.
Maximum: 0.4 mg/kg/hr.
Children less than 10 kg.
1-1.25 mg/kg single dose as a
0.125% or 0.25% solution or
0.1-0.2 mg/kg/hr continuous
infusion as a 0.1%, 0.125%, or
0.25% solution. Maximum:
0.2 mg/kg/hr.

▸ **Analgesic, intrapleural**
IV
Adults, Elderly. 10-30 ml bolus of
0.25%, 0.375%, or 0.5% q4-8hr or
0.375% solution with epinephrine
continuous infusion at 6 ml/hr after
20 ml loading dose.

▸ **Analgesic, caudal (moderate to complete blockade)**
IV
Adults, Elderly. 15-30 mL of 0.5%
solution (75-150 mg) OR 0.25%
solution (37.5-75 mg), repeated once
every 3 hr as needed
Children more than 10 kg.
1-2.5 mg/kg single dose as a 0.125%
or 0.25% solution or 0.2-0.4 mg/kg/hr

continuous infusion as a 0.1%,
0.125%, or 0.25% solution.
Maximum: 0.4 mg/kg/hr.
Children less than 10 kg.
1-1.25 mg/kg single dose as a
0.125% or 0.25% solution or
0.1-0.2 mg/kg/hr continuous infusion
as a 0.1%, 0.125%, or 0.25% solution. Maximum: 0.2 mg/kg/hr.

▸ **Analgesic, dental**
IV
Adults, Elderly. 1.8-3.6 ml of 0.5%
solution (9-18 mg) with epinephrine.
A second dose of 9 mg may be
administered. Maximum: 90 mg
total dose.

▸ **Analgesic, peripheral nerve block (moderate to complete motor blockade)**
IV
Adults, Elderly. 5-37.5 ml
(25-175 mg) of 0.5% solution or
5-70 ml (12.5-175 mg) of 0.25%
solution. Repeat q3hr as needed.
Maximum: up to 400 mg/day.
Children 12 yr and older.
0.3-2.5 mg/kg as a 0.25% or 0.5%
solution. Maximum: 1 ml/kg of
0.25% solution or 0.5 ml/kg of 0.5%
solution.

▸ **Analgesic, retrobulbar (complete motor blockade)**
IV
Adults, Elderly. 2-4 ml (15-30 mg)
of 0.75% solution.

▸ **Analgesic, sympathetic blockade**
IV
Adults, Elderly. 20-50 ml (50-
125 mg) of 0.25% (no epinephrine)
solution. Repeat once q3hr as needed.

▸ **Analgesic, hyperbaric spinal (obstetrical, normal vaginal delivery)**
IV
Adults, Elderly. 0.8 ml (6 mg)
bupivacaine in dextrose as 0.75%
solution

▸ **Analgesic, hyperbaric spinal (obstetrical, cesarean section)**

IV
Adults, Elderly. 1-1.4 ml
(7.5-10.5 mg) bupivacaine in
dextrose as 0.75% solution.
▸ **Anesthesia, hyperbaric spinal
(surgical, lower extremity, and
perineal procedures)**
IV
Adults, Elderly. 1 ml (7.5 mg)
bupivacaine in dextrose as 0.75%
solution
Children 12 yr and older.
0.3-0.6 mg/kg bupivacaine in
dextrose as a 0.75% solution
▸ **Anesthesia, spinal (surgical, lower
abdominal procedures)**
IV
Adults, Elderly. 1.6 ml (12 mg)
bupivacaine in dextrose as 0.75%
solution.
Children 12 yr and older.
0.3-0.6 mg/kg bupivacaine in
dextrose as a 0.75% solution
▸ **Anesthesia, spinal (surgical,
hyperbaric, upper abdominal
procedures)**
IV
Adults, Elderly. 2 ml (15 mg)
bupivacaine in dextrose administered
in horizontal position
Children 12 yr and older.
0.3-0.6 mg/kg bupivacaine in
dextrose as a 0.75% solution
▸ **Analgesic, local infiltration**
IV
Adults, Elderly. 0.25% solution.
Maximum: 225 mg with epinephrine
or 175 mg without epinephrine.
Children 12 yr and older.
0.5-2.5 mg/kg as a 0.25% or 0.5%
solution. Maximum: 1 ml/kg of
0.25% solution or 0.5 ml/kg of 0.5%
solution.

CONTRAINDICATIONS
Local infection at the site of
proposed lumbar puncture (spinal
anesthesia), obstetrical paracervical
block anesthesia, septicemia (spinal

anesthesia), severe hemorrhage,
severe hypotension or shock,
arrhythmias such as complete heart
block, which severely restrict cardiac
output (spinal anesthesia), sulfite
allergy (epinephrine containing
solutions only), hypersensitivity to
bupivacaine products or to other
amide-type anesthetics

INTERACTIONS
Drug
**Angiotensin converting enzyme
inhibitors:** May increase risk of
bradycardia and hypotension as well
as loss of consciousness.
**Beta-blockers, ergot-type oxytocics,
MAO inhibitors, TCAs, phenothiazines, vasopressors:** May
increase the risk of bupivacaine
toxicity.
Cisatracurium, rapacuronium:
May increase neuromuscular blocking action.
Hyaluronidase: May increase
incidence of systemic reaction to
bupivacaine.
Propofol: May increase hypnotic
effect of propofol.
Ropivacaine: May prolong effect of
intrathecal bupivacaine.
Verapamil: May increase risk of
heart block.
Herbal
St. John's wort: May increase
risk of cardiovascular collapse
and/or delay emergence from
anesthesia.
Food
None known.

DIAGNOSTIC TEST EFFECTS
None known.

▨ IV INCOMPATIBILITIES
None known.
▯ **IV Compatibilities**
Fentanyl, hydromorphone
(Dilaudid), morphine

SIDE EFFECTS

Occasional

Hypotension, bradycardia, palpitations, respiratory depression, dizziness, headache, vomiting, nausea, restlessness, weakness, blurred vision, tinnitus, apnea

SERIOUS REACTIONS

• Arterial hypotension, bradycardia, ventricular arrhythmias, central nervous system (CNS) depression and excitation, convulsions, respiratory arrest, tinnitus have been reported.

• Solutions with epinephrine contain metabisulfite, a sulfite that may cause allergic-type reactions, including anaphylaxis.

PRECAUTIONS & CONSIDERATIONS

Caution is warranted with pregnancy as well as obstetrical epidural anesthesia. Only concentrations lower than 0.75% should be used. Caution should be used with regional IV anesthesia (Bier block), hyperthyroidism, hepatic disease, impaired cardiovascular function, hypertension, and heart block because there is a higher risk for developing bupivacaine toxicity. Solutions containing vasoconstrictors should be used cautiously in area with limited blood supply, in the presence of disease that may adversely affect the cardiovascular system or with peripheral vascular disease. Caution should also be used cautiously with retrobulbar blocks because bupivacaine has caused respiratory arrest.

Be aware that solutions containing epinephrine or other vasopressors should not be used concomitantly with ergot-type oxytocic drugs. Use in extreme caution in persons receiving MAOIs or tricyclic antidepressants because severe hypertension can occur. Be aware that spinal anesthetics should not be injected during uterine contractions. Be aware that local anesthetic solutions contain antimicrobial preservatives and should not be used for caudal or epidural anesthesia. Be aware that reduced doses should be given to debilitated, elderly, acutely ill, and young people. Be aware that it is unknown if bupivacaine is a triggering agent for malignant hyperthermia. Be aware the bupivacaine may cause severe disturbances of cardiac rhythm, shock, or heart block after spinal anesthesia. Be aware that severe dose-related cardiac arrhythmias may occur if preparations containing a vasoconstrictor such as epinephrine are used during or following the administration of chloroform, cyclopropane, halothane, trichloroethylene, or other related agents.

Bupivicaine is distributed in breast milk. Be aware that fetal bradycardia frequently follows obstetrical paracervical block with some amide-type local anesthetics and may be associated with fetal acidosis. Be aware that bupivacaine spinal with dextrose is not recommended in children younger than 18 years. Be aware that some elderly may require dosage adjustment.

Storage

Store at room temperature. Protect from light. Bupivacaine 1.25 mg/ml in 0.9% NaCl injection is stable for up to 32 days when refrigerated.

Administration

Be aware that solutions containing preservatives should be used for epidural or caudal blocks. Dosage varies with anesthetic procedure, area to be anesthetized, vascularity of the tissues, number of neuronal segments to be blocked, depth of anesthesia and degree of muscle relaxation required, duration of anesthesia desired, individual tolerance, and physical condition of the person. Be aware that 0.75% solutions should not used for obstetrical epidural anesthesia due to reports of cardiac arrest and death occurring with this concentration. Be aware that repeated doses of bupivacaine may cause significant increases in blood levels with each repeated dose due to accumulation of the drug or its metabolites or to slow metabolic degradation. Be aware that concentrated solutions (0.5%-0.75%) should be given in incremental doses of 3-5 ml with sufficient time between doses to detect toxic manifestations of unintentional intravascular or intrathecal injection during epidural administration. Be aware that bupivacaine should be used in dextrose only for spinal analgesia. The lowest bupivacaine dosage that gives effective anesthesia should be used to avoid high plasma levels and serious systemic side effects.

Buprenorphine
byoo-pre-nor′feen
(Buprenex, Subutex, Temgesic [CAN])

CATEGORY AND SCHEDULE
Pregnancy Risk Category: C
Controlled Substance: Schedule V (opioid agonist), III (tablet)

CLASSIFICATION
Analgesics, narcotic

MECHANISM OF ACTION
An opioid agonist-antagonist that binds with opioid receptors in the CNS. *Therapeutic Effect:* Alters the perception of and emotional response to pain; blocks the effects of heroin and produces minimal opioid withdrawal symptoms.

AVAILABILITY
Tablets (Sublingual): 2 mg, 8 mg.
Injection: 0.3 mg/ml.

INDICATIONS AND DOSAGES
▸ **Analgesia**
IV, IM
Adults, Children older than 12 yr.
0.3 mg q6-8hr as needed. May repeat once in 30-60 min. Range: 0.15-0.6 mg q4-8hr as needed.
Children 2-12 yr. 2-6 mcg/kg q4-6hr as needed.
Elderly. 0.15 mg q6hr as needed.
▸ **Opioid dependence**
SUBLINGUAL
Adults, Elderly, Children older than 16 yr. Initially, 12-16 mg/day, beginning at least 4 hr after last use of heroin or short-acting opioid. Maintenance: 16 mg/day. Range: 4-24 mg/day. Patients should be switched to buprenorphine and naloxone combination, is preferred for maintenance treatment.

CONTRAINDICATIONS
Hypersensitivity to buprenorphine; hypersensitivity to naloxone for those receiving the fixed combination product containing naloxone (Suboxone)

INTERACTIONS
Drug
CNS depressants, MAOIs: May increase CNS or respiratory depression and hypotension.
Other opioid analgesics: May decrease the effects of other opioid analgesics.
Herbal
Kava kava, St. John's wort, valerian: May increase CNS depression.

Food
None known.

DIAGNOSTIC TEST EFFECTS
May increase serum amylase and
lipase levels.

SIDE EFFECTS
Frequent
Tablet: Headache, pain, insomnia,
anxiety, depression, nausea, abdominal pain, constipation, back pain,
weakness, rhinitis, withdrawal
syndrome, infection, diaphoresis
Injection (more than 10%): Sedation
Occasional
Injection: Hypotension, respiratory
depression, dizziness, headache,
vomiting, nausea, vertigo

SERIOUS REACTIONS
• Overdose results in cold and
clammy skin, weakness, confusion,
severe respiratory depression,
cyanosis, pinpoint pupils, and
extreme somnolence progressing to
seizures, stupor, and coma.

PRECAUTIONS & CONSIDERATIONS
Caution is warranted with hepatic
impairment and possible neurologic
injury. Dizziness may occur, so
change positions slowly and avoid
tasks that require mental alertness or
motor skills. B/P, pulse rate, respiratory status, and clinical improvement
should be monitored.
Administration
Place the tablet under the tongue
until dissolved. If two or more
tablets are needed, all may be placed
under the tongue at the same time.
For IV use, administer buprenorphine slowly, over at least 2 minutes.

Buspirone
byoo-spir'own
(BuSpar, Buspirex [CAN], Bustab
[CAN])
**Do not confuse buspirone with
bupropion.**

CATEGORY AND SCHEDULE
Pregnancy Risk Category: B

CLASSIFICATION
Anxiolytics

MECHANISM OF ACTION
Although its exact mechanism of
action is unknown, this nonbarbiturate is thought to bind to serotonin
and dopamine receptors in the CNS.
The drug may also increase norepinephrine metabolism in the locus
ceruleus. *Therapeutic Effect:*
Produces anxiolytic effect.

PHARMACOKINETICS
Rapidly and completely absorbed
from the GI tract. Protein binding:
95%. Undergoes extensive first-pass
metabolism. Metabolized in the liver
to active metabolite. Primarily
excreted in urine. Not removed by
hemodialysis. **Half-life**: 2-3 hr.

AVAILABILITY
Tablets: 5 mg, 7.5 mg, 10 mg,
15 mg, 30 mg.

INDICATIONS AND DOSAGES
▶ **Short-term management (up to
4 weeks) of anxiety disorders**
PO
Adults. 5 mg 2-3 times a day or
7.5 mg twice a day. May increase by
5 mg/day every 2-4 days.
Maintenance: 15-30 mg/day in
2-3 divided doses. Maximum:
60 mg/day.

Elderly. Initially, 5 mg twice a day. May increase by 5 mg/day every 2-3 days. Maximum: 60 mg/day. *Children.* Initially, 5 mg/day. May increase by 5 mg/day at weekly intervals. Maximum: 60 mg/day.

OFF-LABEL USES
Management of panic attack, premenstrual syndrome (aches, pain, fatigue, irritability)

CONTRAINDICATIONS
Concurrent use of MAOIs, severe hepatic or renal impairment

INTERACTIONS
Drug
Erythromycin, itraconazole: May increase buspirone blood concentration and risk of toxicity.
MAOIs: May increase B/P.
Other CNS depressants: Potentiates effects of buspirone and may increase sedation.
Herbal
Kava kava: May increase sedation.
Food
Alcohol: Potentiates effects of buspirone and may increase sedation
Grapefruit, grapefruit juice: May increase buspirone blood concentration and risk of toxicity.

DIAGNOSTIC TEST EFFECTS
None known.

SIDE EFFECTS
Frequent (12%-6%)
Dizziness, somnolence, nausea, headache
Occasional (5%-2%)
Nervousness, fatigue, insomnia, dry mouth, lightheadedness, mood swings, blurred vision, poor concentration, diarrhea, paresthesia
Rare
Muscle pain and stiffness, nightmares, chest pain, involuntary movements

SERIOUS REACTIONS
• Buspirone does not appear to cause drug tolerance, psychological or physical dependence, or withdrawal syndrome.
• Overdose may produce severe nausea, vomiting, dizziness, drowsiness, abdominal distention, and excessive pupil contraction.

PRECAUTIONS & CONSIDERATIONS
Caution is warranted with impaired renal or hepatic function. It is unknown if buspirone crosses the placenta or is distributed in breast milk. The safety and efficacy of buspirone have not been established in children. No age-related precautions have been noted in the elderly. Grapefruit juice should be avoided because it may increase the risk of drug toxicity.

Drowsiness may occur but usually disappears with continued therapy. Change positions slowly from recumbent, to sitting, before standing to prevent dizziness. Alcohol and tasks that require mental alertness or motor skills should also be avoided. Autonomic responses, such as cold, clammy hands and diaphoresis, and motor responses, such as agitation, trembling, and tension, should be assessed. Hepatic and renal function should be monitored in long-term therapy.
Administration
Take buspirone without regard to food. Crush tablets as needed. Improvement may be noticed within 7-10 days of starting therapy, but optimum therapeutic effect generally takes 3 to 4 weeks to appear.

Butenafine
byoo-ten'a-feen
(Mentax)

CATEGORY AND SCHEDULE
Pregnancy Risk Category: B

CLASSIFICATION
Antifungals, topical,
dermatologics

MECHANISM OF ACTION
An antifungal agent that locks
biosynthesis of ergosterol, essential
for fungal cell membrane.
Fungicidal. *Therapeutic Effect:*
Relieves athletes foot.

PHARMACOKINETICS
Total amount absorbed into systemic
circulation has not been determined.
Metabolized in liver. Excreted in
urine. **Half-life:** 35 hrs.

AVAILABILITY
Cream: 1% (Mentax).

INDICATIONS AND DOSAGES
▸ **Tinea pedis, tinea
corporis, tinea cruris, tinea
versicolor**
TOPICAL
*Adults, Elderly, Children 12 yr and
older.* Apply to affected area and
immediate surrounding skin daily for
4 wk.

OFF-LABEL USES
Onychomycosis, seborrheic
dermatitis

CONTRAINDICATIONS
Hypersensitivity to butenafine
or any component of the
formulation

INTERACTIONS
Drug
None known.
Herbal
None known.
Food
None known.

DIAGNOSTIC TEST EFFECTS
None known.

SIDE EFFECTS
Occasional
(2%) Contact dermatitis,
burning/stinging, worsening of the
condition
Rare
(Less than 2%) Erythema, irritation,
pruritus

SERIOUS REACTIONS
• None known.

PRECAUTIONS & CONSIDERATIONS
Caution should be used with
sensitivity to naftifine or other
allylamine antifungals. It is unknown
if butenafine is excreted in breast
milk. Safety and efficacy of butenafine has not been established in
children younger than 12 years of
age. There are no age-related precautions noted in the elderly. Avoid
contact with eyes, nose, mouth, or
other mucous membranes.
Administration
Gently cleanse area prior to
application. Use occlusive dressings
only as ordered. Apply sparingly
and rub into area thoroughly. Use
for full course of treatment or until
symptoms improve.

Butoconazole
byoo-toe-ko′na-zole
(Gynazole-1, Femstat One [CAN])
Mycelex-3 2%

CATEGORY AND SCHEDULE
Pregnancy Risk Category: C

CLASSIFICATION
Antifungals, topical,
dermatologics

MECHANISM OF ACTION
An antifungal similar to imidazole
derivatives that inhibits the steroid
synthesis, a vital component of
fungal cell formation, thereby
damaging the fungal cell membrane.
Therapeutic Effect: Fungistatic.

PHARMACOKINETICS
Not known.

AVAILABILITY
Cream: 2% (Mycelex-3, OTC)
Cream: 2% (Gynazole-1, prefilled
applicator)

INDICATIONS AND DOSAGES
▶ Treatment of candidiasis
TOPICAL
Adults, Elderly. Insert one applica-
torful intravaginally at bedtime for
up to 3 or 6 days.

CONTRAINDICATIONS
Hypersensitivity to butoconazole or
any of its components

INTERACTIONS
Drug
Not known.
Herbal
Not known.
Food
Not known.

SIDE EFFECTS
Occasional
Vaginal itching, burning, irritation

SERIOUS REACTIONS
• Soreness, swelling, pelvic pain, or
cramping rarely occurs.

PRECAUTIONS & CONSIDERATIONS
Be aware that butoconazole
contains mineral oil which may
weaken latex or rubber products
such as condoms. Tampons should
not be used while using butoconazole because tampons can absorb
and decrease the efficacy of the
medication. The OTC preparation
should not be used if abdominal
pain, fever, or foul-smelling
discharge is present. It is
unknown if butoconazole crosses
the placenta or is distributed in
breast milk.
Administration
Insert one applicatorful
intravaginally at bedtime as a
single dose.

Butorphanol
byoo-tor′fa-nole
(Stadol, Stadol NS)
**Do not confuse with butabarbi-
tal or Stadol with Haldol.**

CATEGORY AND SCHEDULE
Pregnancy Risk Category: C, D
if used for prolonged time, high
dose at term
Controlled Substance: Schedule
IV

CLASSIFICATION
Analgesics, narcotic agonist-
antagonist

MECHANISM OF ACTION
An opioid that binds to opiate receptor sites in the central nervous system (CNS). Reduces intensity of pain stimuli incoming from sensory nerve endings. *Therapeutic Effect:* Alters pain perception and emotional response to pain.

PHARMACOKINETICS

Route	Onset	Peak	Duration
IM	10-30 min	30-60 min	3-4 hr
IV	Less than 1 min	30 min	2-4 hr
Nasal	15 min	1-2 hr	4-5 hr

Rapidly absorbed after IM injection. Protein binding: 80%. Extensively metabolized in the liver. Primarily excreted in urine. **Half-life:** 2.5-4 hr.

AVAILABILITY
Injection: 1 mg/ml, 2 mg/ml.
Nasal Spray: 10 mg/ml.

INDICATIONS AND DOSAGES
▶ **Analgesia**
IM
Adults. 1-4 mg q3-4hr as needed.
Elderly. 1 mg q4-6hr as needed.
IV
Adults. 0.5-2 mg q3-4hr as needed.
Elderly. 1 mg q4-6hr as needed.
▶ **Migraine**
NASAL
Adults. 1 mg or 1 spray in one nostril. May repeat in 60-90 min. May repeat 2-dose sequence q3-4hr as needed. Alternatively, 2 mg or one spray each nostril if patient remains recumbent, may repeat in 3-4 hr.

CONTRAINDICATIONS
CNS disease that affects respirations, physical dependence on other opioid analgesics, preexisting respiratory depression, pulmonary disease

INTERACTIONS
Drug
Alcohol, CNS depressants: May increase CNS or respiratory depression and hypotension.
Buprenorphine: Effects may be decreased with buprenorphine.
MAOIs: May produce severe, fatal reaction unless dose is reduced by one-fourth.
Herbal
None known.
Food
None known.

DIAGNOSTIC TEST EFFECTS
None known.

▨ IV INCOMPATIBILITIES
Amphotericin B complex (Abelcet, AmBisome, Amphotec)
▨ **IV Compatibilities**
Atropine, diphenhydramine (Benadryl), droperidol (Inapsine), hydroxyzine (Vistaril), morphine, promethazine (Phenergan), propofol (Diprivan)

SIDE EFFECTS
Frequent
Parenteral: Somnolence (43%), dizziness (19%)
Nasal: Nasal congestion (13%), insomnia (11%)
Occasional
Parenteral (3%-9%): Confusion, diaphoresis, clammy skin, lethargy, headache, nausea, vomiting, dry mouth
Nasal (3%-9%): Vasodilation, constipation, unpleasant taste, dyspnea, epistaxis, nasal irritation, upper respiratory tract infection, tinnitus
Rare
Parenteral: Hypotension, pruritus, blurred vision, sensation of heat, CNS stimulation, insomnia
Nasal: Hypertension, tremor, ear pain, paresthesia, depression, sinusitis

B

SERIOUS REACTIONS

• Abrupt withdrawal after prolonged use may produce symptoms of narcotic withdrawal, such as abdominal cramping, rhinorrhea, lacrimation, anxiety, increased temperature, and piloerection or goose bumps.

• Overdose results in severe respiratory depression, skeletal muscle flaccidity, cyanosis, and extreme somnolence progressing to seizures, stupor, and coma.

• Tolerance to analgesic effect and physical dependence may occur with chronic use.

PRECAUTIONS & CONSIDERATIONS

Caution is warranted with head injury, hypertension, impaired liver or renal function, or myocardial infarction, prior to biliary tract surgery (because the drug produces spasm of sphincter of Oddi), and in the elderly or debilitated. During labor, assess fetal heart tones, and uterine contractions. Be aware that the safety and efficacy of butorphanol have not been established in children younger than 18 years of age. Be aware that the elderly may be more sensitive to effects. Adjust drug dose and interval in the elderly.

Dizziness and drowsiness may occur, so change positions slowly and avoid alcohol, CNS depressants, and tasks that require mental alertness or motor skills until response to the drug is established. B/P, pulse rate and quality, respirations, and clinical improvement of pain should be monitored.

Storage

Store at room temperature.

Administration

! May be given by IM or IV push.

For intranasal use, blow nose to clear nasal passages as much as possible. Spray into nostril while holding other nostril closed and concurrently inspire through nose to permit medication as high into nasal passages as possible.

For IV use, butorphanol may be given undiluted. Administer over 3 to 5 minutes.

Cabergoline
cab-err-go-leen
(Dostinex)

CATEGORY AND SCHEDULE
Pregnancy Risk Category: B

CLASSIFICATION
Antiparkinson agents, dopaminergics, ergot alkaloids and derivatives, hormones/hormone modifiers

MECHANISM OF ACTION
Agonist at dopamine D2 receptors suppressing prolactin secretion. *Therapeutic effects:* Shrinks prolactinomas, restores gonadal function.

PHARMACOKINETICS
Cabergoline is administered orally and undergoes significant first-pass metabolism following systemic absorption. Extensively metabolized in the liver. Elimination is primarily in the feces. **Half-life:** 80 hours.

AVAILABILITY
Tablet: 0.5 mg

INDICATIONS AND DOSAGES
▸ **Hyperprolactemia (idiopathic or primary pituitary adenomas)**
PO
Adults, elderly. 0.25 mg 2 times per week, titrate by 0.25 mg/dose no more than every 4 weeks up to 1 mg two times per week
PV
Adults. 0.5 mg two to five times per week
▸ **Parkinson's disease**
PO
Adults. 0.5 mg/day and titrate to response. Mean effective dose is 3 mg/day and ranges from 0.5-6 mg/day.
▸ **Restless leg syndrome (RLS)**
PO
Adults. 0.5 mg once daily at bedtime, slowly titrate up until symptoms resolve or drug-intolerance limits further adjustment. Mean effective dose is 2 mg/day and ranges from 1-4 mg/day.

OFF-LABEL USES
Parkinson's disease, restless leg syndrome (RLS)

CONTRAINDICATIONS
Hypersensitivity to cabergoline, ergot alkaloids or any one of its components.
Uncontrolled hypertension.

INTERACTIONS
Drug
Antihypertensives: May increase hypotensive effect.
Cimetidine, haloperidol, loxapine, MAOIs, methyldopa, metoclopramide, molindone, olanzapine, phenothiazines, pimozide, reserpine, risperidone, thiothixene, tricyclic antidepressants: Antagonizes the prolactin-lowering effect of cabergoline.
Antipsychotics, phenothiazine-type antiemetics: Cabergoline may diminish the effects of these dopamine agonists.
Levodopa: Additive neurologic effects are possible.
Ergot alkaloids: May lead to ergot toxicity.
Anti-retroviral drugs: May lead to ergot toxicity.
Imatinib: May increase the risk of ergot-related side effects.
Herbal
None known.
Food
None known.

DIAGNOSTIC TEST EFFECTS
None known.

SIDE EFFECTS
Frequent
Nausea, orthostatic hypotension, confusion, dyskinesia, hallucinations, peripheral edema
Occasional
Headache, vertigo, dizziness, dyspepsia, postural hypotension, constipation, asthenia, fatigue, abdominal pain, drowsiness
Rare
Vomiting, dry mouth, diarrhea, flatulence, anxiety, depression, dysmenorrheal, dyspepsia, mastalgia, paresthesias, vertigo, visual impairment, pleuropulmonary changes, pleural effusion, pulmonary fibrosis, heart failure, peptic ulcer

SERIOUS REACTIONS
• Overdosage may produce nasal congestion, syncope, or hallucinations.

PRECAUTIONS & CONSIDERATIONS
Caution is warranted with postpartum lactation inhibition or suppression and hepatic impairment. It is unknown if cabergoline crosses the placenta or is distributed into breast milk. In general, dopamine agonists like cabergoline, are not used in pregnant women. Safety and efficacy has not been established in children or the elderly.
    Nausea, headache, constipation, and dizziness may occur during therapy.
Administration
Dosage may be increased by 0.25 mg twice weekly up to a dosage of 1 mg twice weekly according to serum prolactin level. Dosage increases should not occur more rapidly than every 4 weeks.

Caffeine Citrate
kaf'een
(Cafcit)

CATEGORY AND SCHEDULE
Pregnancy Risk Category: C

CLASSIFICATION
Analeptics, stimulants, central nervous system, xanthine derivatives

MECHANISM OF ACTION
A methylxanthine and competitive inhibitor of phosphodiesterase that blocks antagonism of adenosine receptors. *Therapeutic Effect:* Stimulates respiratory center, increases minute ventilation, decreases threshold of or increases response to hypercapnia, increases skeletal muscle tone, decreases diaphragmatic fatigue, increases metabolic rate, and increases oxygen consumption.

PHARMACOKINETICS
Protein binding: 36%. Widely distributed through the tissues and CSF. Metabolized in liver. Excreted in urine. **Half-life:** 4-5 hrs.

AVAILABILITY
Liquid: 20 mg/ml (Cafcit).
Intravenous Solution: 20 mg/ml (Cafcit).
Oral Solution: 20 mg/ml (Cafcit).

INDICATIONS AND DOSAGES
▸ **Neonatal apnea**
IV/PO
Infants between 28-33 wks gestational age. Loading dose: 20 mg/kg over 30 min. Maintenance: 5 mg/kg/day over 10 min. or orally beginning 24 hr. after loading dose.

CONTRAINDICATIONS
Hypersensitivity to caffeine, xanthines, or any other component of the formulation

INTERACTIONS
Drug
Cimetidine: May increase effects of caffeine citrate.
Ketoconazole: May increase effects of caffeine citrate.
Phenobarbital: May decrease effects of caffeine citrate.
Phenytoin: May decrease effects of caffeine citrate.
Theophylline: May increase theophylline concentrations and toxicity.
Herbal
None known.
Food
None known.

DIAGNOSTIC TEST EFFECTS
May report false decreases in phenobarbital levels.

IV INCOMPATIBILITIES
None known.
IV Compatibilities
Amino acid solutions, D_5W, IV fat emulsion, antipyrine, calcium, dopamine, fentanyl, heparin

SIDE EFFECTS
Occasional
Feeding intolerance, irritability, restlessness
Rare
Necrotizing enterocolitis, rash, tachycardia, increased ventricular output, increased stroke volume, GI intolerance, hypo/hyperglycemia, increased creatinine clearance, increased sodium and calcium excretion.

SERIOUS REACTIONS
• Accidental injury, sepsis, hemorrhage, gastritis, GI hemorrhage, disseminated intravascular coagulation, acidosis, abnormal healing, cerebral hemorrhage, dyspnea, lung edema, dry skin, retinopathy, and kidney failure have been reported.
• Overdosage includes symptoms of fever, tachypnea, jitteriness, insomnia, fine tremor of the extremities, hypertonia, opisthotonos, tonic-clonic movements, non-purposeful jaw and lip movements, vomiting, hyperglycemia, elevated blood urea nitrogen, and elevated total leukocyte concentration.

PRECAUTIONS & CONSIDERATIONS
Caution should be used in infants with cardiovascular disorders, hepatic or renal impairment, and seizure disorders. Caffeine readily crosses the placenta and is excreted in breast milk. Safety and efficacy in long-term treatment of infants has not been established. Be aware that necrotizing enterocolitis may occur in infants. There are no age-related precautions noted in the elderly.
Administration
Be aware that 20 mg caffeine citrate = 10 mg caffeine base. May take with or without food. Do not administer if visible particulate matter or discoloration is visible. Discard vial.

Calcipotriene
kal-sip′oh-tri-een
(Dovonex)

CATEGORY AND SCHEDULE
Pregnancy Risk Category: C

CLASSIFICATION
Dermatologics

MECHANISM OF ACTION
A synthetic vitamin D_3 analogue that regulates skin cell (keratinocyte) production and development. *Therapeutic Effect:* preventing abnormal growth and production of psoriasis (abnormal keratinocyte growth).

PHARMACOKINETICS
Minimal absorption through intact skin. Metabolized in liver.

AVAILABILITY
Cream: 0.005% (Dovonex).
Ointment: 0.005% (Dovonex).
Topical Solution: 0.005% (Dovonex).

INDICATIONS AND DOSAGES
▸ **Psoriasis**
TOPICAL
Adults, Elderly, Children 12 yr and older. Apply thin layer to affected skin twice daily (morning and evening); rub in gently and completely.
▸ **Scalp psoriasis**
TOPICAL SOLUTION
Adults, Elderly, Children 12 yr and older. Apply to lesions after combing hair.

CONTRAINDICATIONS
Hypercalcemia or evidence of vitamin D toxicity, use on face, hypersensitivity to calcipotriene or any component of the formulation

INTERACTIONS
Drug
None known.
Herbal
None known.
Food
None known.

DIAGNOSTIC TEST EFFECTS
Excessive use may increase serum calcium level.

SIDE EFFECTS
Frequent
Burning, itching, skin irritation
Occasional
Erythema, dry skin, peeling, rash, worsening of psoriasis, dermatititis
Rare
Skin atrophy, hyperpigmentation, folliculitis

SERIOUS REACTIONS
• Potential for hypercalcemia may occur.

PRECAUTIONS & CONSIDERATIONS
Caution should be used with history of nephrolithiasis. It is unknown if calcipotriene crosses the placenta or is distributed in breast milk. Be aware that children and the elderly are at greater risk for skin reactions. Improvement is usually noted after 2 weeks of therapy and marked improvement after 8 weeks of therapy.
Storage
Store at room temperature.
Administration
Apply cream or ointment by rubbing gently into the affected and surrounding area twice daily (in morning and in the evening). Wash hands after application.

Calcitonin
kal-si-toe'nin
(Calcimar, Caltine [CAN],
Cibacalcin, Miacalcin)
**Do not confuse calcitonin with
calcitriol.**

CATEGORY AND SCHEDULE
Pregnancy Risk Category: C

CLASSIFICATION
Hormones/hormone modifiers

MECHANISM OF ACTION
A synthetic hormone that decreases
osteoclast activity in bones,
decreases tubular reabsorption of
sodium and calcium in the kidneys,
and increases absorption of calcium
in the GI tract. *Therapeutic Effect:*
Regulates serum calcium
concentrations.

PHARMACOKINETICS
Injection form rapidly metabolized
(primarily in kidneys); primarily
excreted in urine. Nasal form rapidly
absorbed. **Half-life:** 70-90 min
(injection); 43 min (nasal).

AVAILABILITY
Injection: 200 international units/ml
(calcitonin-salmon), 500 mg
(calcitonin-human).
Nasal Spray: 200 international
units/activation (calcitonin-salmon).

INDICATIONS AND DOSAGES
▸ **Skin testing before treatment in
patients with suspected sensitivity
to calcitonin-salmon**
Adults, Elderly. Prepare a 10-
international units/ml dilution;
withdraw 0.05 ml from a 200-
international units/ml vial in a tuberculin syringe; fill up to 1 ml with
0.9% NaCl. Take 0.1 ml and inject
intracutaneously on inner aspect of
forearm. Observe after 15 min; a
positive response is the appearance
of more than mild erythema or
wheal.
▸ **Paget's disease**
IM, SUBCUTANEOUS
Adults, Elderly. Initially, 100 international units/day. Maintenance: 50
international units/day or 50-100
international units every 1-3 days.
INTRANASAL
Adults, Elderly. 200-400 international units/day.
▸ **Osteoporosis imperfecta**
IM, SUBCUTANEOUS
Adults. 2 international units/kg
3 times a week.
▸ **Postmenopausal osteoporosis**
IM, SUBCUTANEOUS
Adults, Elderly. 100 international
units/day with adequate calcium and
vitamin D intake.
INTRANASAL
Adults, Elderly. 200 international
units/day as a single spray, alternating nostrils daily.
▸ **Hypercalcemia**
IM, SUBCUTANEOUS
Adults, Elderly. Initially, 4 interna-
tional units/kg q12hr; may increase
to 8 international units/kg q12hr if
no response in 2 days; may further
increase to 8 international units/kg
q6hr if no response in another 2 days.

OFF-LABEL USES
Treatment of secondary osteoporosis
due to drug therapy or hormone
disturbance

CONTRAINDICATIONS
Hypersensitivity to gelatin desserts
or salmon protein

INTERACTIONS
Drug
None known.

Herbal
None known.
Food
None known.

DIAGNOSTIC TEST EFFECTS
None known.

SIDE EFFECTS
Frequent
IM, Subcutaneous (10%): Nausea (may occur 30 min after injection, usually diminishes with continued therapy), inflammation at injection site
Nasal (12%-10%): Rhinitis, nasal irritation, redness, sores
Occasional
IM, Subcutaneous (5%-2%): Flushing of face or hands
Nasal (5%-3%): Back pain, arthralgia, epistaxis, headache
Rare
IM, Subcutaneous: Epigastric discomfort, dry mouth, diarrhea, flatulence
Nasal: Itching of earlobes, edema of feet, rash, diaphoresis

SERIOUS REACTIONS
• Patients with a protein allergy may develop a hypersensitivity reaction.

PRECAUTIONS & CONSIDERATIONS
Caution is warranted with history of allergy and renal dysfunction. Calcitonin does not cross the placenta, and it is unknown if the drug is distributed in breast milk; its safety in breast-feeding women has not been established. The safety and efficacy of this drug have not been established in children. No age-related precautions have been noted in the elderly.
Nausea may occur but usually decreases with continued therapy. Notify the physician if itching, rash, shortness of breath or significant nasal irritation occurs. Electrolyte levels should be checked.
Improvement in biochemical abnormalities and bone pain usually occurs in the first few months of treatment; with neurologic lesions, improvement may take more than a year.
Storage
Refrigerate the nasal spray. It may be stored at room temperature once the pump has been activated.
Administration
Calcitonin may be administered as IM or subcutaneous injection. No more than 2 ml should be given IM at any one site. Bedtime administration may reduce flushing and nausea. For intranasal use, clear nasal passages as much as possible. Tilt head slightly forward and insert the spray tip into the nostril, pointing toward the nasal passages and away from the septum. Spray into the nostril while holding the other nostril closed, and at the same time inhale through the nose to deliver the drug as high into the nasal passage as possible.

Calcitriol
kal-si-trye′ole
(Calcijex, Rocaltrol)

CATEGORY AND SCHEDULE
Pregnancy Risk Category: A (D if used in doses above RDA)

CLASSIFICATION
Vitamins/minerals

MECHANISM OF ACTION
A fat-soluble vitamin that is essential for absorption, utilization of

calcium phosphate, and normal calcification of bone. *Therapeutic Effect:* Stimulates calcium and phosphate absorption from small intestine, promotes secretion of calcium from bone to blood, promotes renal tubule phosphate resorption, acts on bone cells to stimulate skeletal growth and on parathyroid gland to suppress hormone synthesis and secretion.

PHARMACOKINETICS
Rapidly absorbed from small intestine. Extensive metabolism in kidneys. Primarily excreted in feces; minimal excretion in urine. **Half-life:** 5-8 hr.

AVAILABILITY
Capsule: 0.25 mcg, 0.5 mcg (Rocaltrol).
Injection: 1 mcg/ml, 2 mcg/ml (Calcijex).
Oral Solution: 1 mcg/ml (Rocaltrol).

INDICATIONS AND DOSAGES
▸ **Renal failure**
PO
Adults, Elderly. 0.25 mcg/day or every other day.
Children. 0.25-2 mcg/day with hemodialysis; 0.014-0.41 mcg/kg/day without hemodialysis.
IV
Adults, Elderly. 0.5 mcg/day (0.01 mcg/kg) 3 times/week. Dose range: 0.5-3 mcg (0.01-0.05 mcg/kg) 3 times/week.
Children. 0.01-0.05 mcg/kg 3 times/week with hemodialysis.
▸ **Hypoparathyroidism/pseudohypoparathyroidism**
PO
Adults, Elderly. 0.5-2 mcg/day
Children 6 yr and older. 0.5-2 mcg once daily.
Children 5-1 yr. 0.25-0.75 mcg once daily.
Children less than 1 yr. 0.04-0.08 mcg/kg once daily.

▸ **Vitamin D-dependent rickets**
PO
Adults, Elderly, Children. 1 mcg once daily.
▸ **Vitamin D-resistant rickets**
PO
Adults, Elderly, Children. 0.015-0.02 mcg/kg once daily. Maintenance: 0.03-0.06 mcg/kg once daily. Maximum: 2 mcg once daily.

CONTRAINDICATIONS
Hypercalcemia, malabsorption syndrome, vitamin D toxicity, hypersensitivity to other vitamin D products or analogs

INTERACTIONS
Drug
Aluminum-containing antacid (long-term use): May increase aluminum concentration and aluminum bone toxicity.
Calcium-containing preparations, thiazide diuretics: May increase the risk of hypercalcemia.
Magnesium-containing antacids: May increase magnesium concentration.
Herbal
None known.
Food
None known.

DIAGNOSTIC TEST EFFECTS
May increase serum cholesterol, calcium, magnesium, and phosphate levels. May decrease serum alkaline phosphatase.

SIDE EFFECTS
Occasional
Hypercalcemia, headache, irritability, constipation, metallic taste, nausea, polyuria

SERIOUS REACTIONS
• Early signs of overdosage are manifested as weakness, headache,

somnolence, nausea, vomiting, dry mouth, constipation, muscle and bone pain, and metallic taste sensation.

• Later signs of overdosage are evidenced by polyuria, polydipsia, anorexia, weight loss, nocturia, photophobia, rhinorrhea, pruritus, disorientation, hallucinations, hyperthermia, hypertension, and cardiac arrhythmias.

PRECAUTIONS & CONSIDERATIONS

Caution is warranted with coronary artery disease, kidney stones, and renal impairment.

It is unknown if calcitriol crosses the placenta or is distributed in breast milk. Children may be more sensitive to the effects of calcitriol. Serum alkaline phosphatase, BUN, serum calcium, serum creatinine, serum magnesium, serum phosphate, and urinary calcium levels should be monitored. Therapeutic serum calcium level is 9 to 10 mg/dl. Daily dietary calcium intake should be estimated. Maintain adequate fluid intake.

Administration

May be administered undiluted as bolus through catheter at the end of hemodialysis.

Give oral calcitriol without regard to food. Swallow the drug whole and avoid crushing, chewing, or opening the capsules.

Calcium Salts

(PhosLo)(Apo-Cal [CAN], Calsan [CAN], Calsup [AUS], Caltrate, Dicarbosil, OsCal, Titralac, Tums) (Calciject) (Citracal, Calcitrate) (Calcione, Calciquid)

Do not confuse OsCal with Asacol, Citracal with Citrucel, or PhosLo with PhosChol.

CATEGORY AND SCHEDULE

Pregnancy Risk Category: C
OTC (acetate, carbonate, citrate, glubionate, gluconate [tablets only])

CLASSIFICATION

Minerals and electrolytes

MECHANISM OF ACTION

An electrolyte that is essential for the function and integrity of the nervous, muscular, and skeletal systems. Calcium plays an important role in normal cardiac and renal function, respiration, blood coagulation, and cell membrane and capillary permeability. It helps regulate the release and storage of neurotransmitters and hormones, and it neutralizes or reduces gastric acid (increase pH). Calcium acetate combines with dietary phosphate to form insoluble calcium phosphate.
Therapeutic Effects: Replaces calcium in deficiency states; controls hyperphosphatemia in end-stage renal disease.

PHARMACOKINETICS

Moderately absorbed from the small intestine (absorption depends on presence of vitamin D metabolites and patient's pH). Primarily eliminated in feces.

AVAILABILITY
Calcium Acetate
Gelcap (Phoslo): 667 mg (equivalent to 169 mg elemental calcium).
Tablet (Phoslo): 667 mg (equivalent to 169 mg elemental calcium).
Calcium Carbonate
Tablets: (Caltrate 600): equivalent to 600 mg elemental calcium.
Tablets (Os-Cal 500): equivalent to 500 mg elemental calcium.
Tablets (Chewable [Os-Call 500]): equivalent to 500 mg elemental calcium.
Tablets (Chewable [Tums]): equivalent to 200 mg elemental calcium.
Calcium Chloride
Injection: 10% (100 mg/ml) equivalent to 27.2 mg elemental calcium per ml.
Calcium Citrate
Tablets: (Cal-Citrate): 250 mg (equivalent to 53 mg elemental calcium).
Tablets (Citracal): 950 mg (equivalent to 200 mg elemental calcium).
Calcium Glubionate
Syrup. 1.8 g/5 ml (equivalent to 115 mg of elemental calcium per 5 ml).
Calcium Gluconate
Injection: 10% (equivalent to 9 mg elemental calcium per ml).

INDICATIONS AND DOSAGES
▶ **Hyperphosphatemia**
PO (calcium acetate)
Adults, Elderly. 2 tablets 3 times a day with meals.
▶ **Hypocalcemia**
PO (calcium carbonate)
Adults, Elderly. 1-2 g/day in 3-4 divided doses.
Children. 45-65 mg/kg/day in 3-4 divided doses.

PO (calcium glubionate)
Adults, Elderly. 16-18 g/day in 4-6 divided doses.
Children, Infants. 0.6-2 g/kg/day in 4 divided doses.
Neonates. 1.2 g/kg/day in 4-6 divided doses.
IV (calcium chloride)
Adults, Elderly. 0.5-1 g repeated q4-6hr as needed.
Children. 2.5-5 mg/kg/dose q4-6hr.
IV (calcium gluconate)
Adults, Elderly. 2-15 g/24 hr.
Children. 200-500 mg/kg/day.
▶ **Antacid**
PO (calcium carbonate)
Adults, Elderly. 1-2 tabs (5-10 ml) q2hr as needed.
▶ **Osteoporosis**
PO (calcium carbonate)
Adults, Elderly. 1200 mg/day.
▶ **Cardiac arrest**
IV (calcium chloride)
Adults, Elderly. 2-4 mg/kg. May repeat q10min.
Children. 20 mg/kg. May repeat in 10 min.
▶ **Hypocalcemia tetany**
IV (calcium chloride)
Adults, Elderly. 1 g may repeat in 6 hours.
Children. 10 mg/kg over 5-10 min. May repeat in 6-8 hr.
IV (calcium gluconate)
Adults, Elderly. 1-3 g until therapeutic response achieved.
Children. 100-200 mg/kg/dose q6-8hr.

OFF-LABEL USES
Treatment of hyperphosphatemia (calcium carbonate)

CONTRAINDICATIONS
Calcium renal calculi, digoxin toxicity, hypercalcemia, hypercalciuria, sarcoidosis, ventricular fibrillation
Calcium acetate: Decreased renal function, hypoparathyroidism

INTERACTIONS
Drug
Digoxin: May increase the risk of arrhythmias.
Etidronate, gallium: May antagonize the effects of these drugs.
Ketoconazole, phenytoin, tetracyclines: May decrease the absorption of these drugs.
Magnesium (parenteral), methenamine: May decrease the effects of these drugs.
Herbal
None known.
Food
None known.

DIAGNOSTIC TEST EFFECTS
May increase, blood pH, and serum gastrin and calcium levels. May decrease serum phosphate and potassium levels.

🔳 IV INCOMPATIBILITIES
Calcium chloride: amphotericin B complex (Abelcet, AmBisone, Amphotec), propofol (Diprivan), sodium bicarbonate
Calcium gluconate: amphotericin B complex (Abelcet, AmBisome, Amphotec), fluconazole (Diflucan)
🔳 IV Compatibilities
Calcium chloride: Amikacin (Amikin), dobutamine (Dobutrex), lidocaine, milrinone (Primacor), morphine, norepinephrine (Levophed)
Calcium gluconate: Ampicillin, aztreonam (Azactam), cefazolin (Ancef), cefepime (Maxipime), ciprofloxacin (Cipro), dobutamine (Dobutrex), enalapril (Vasotec), famotidine (Pepcid), furosemide (Lasix), heparin, lidocaine, magnesium sulfate, meropenem (Merrem IV), midazolam (Versed), milrinone (Primacor), norepinephrine (Levophed), piperacillin and

tazobactam (Zosyn), potassium chloride, propofol (Diprivan)

SIDE EFFECTS
Frequent
PO: Chalky taste
Parenteral: Hypotension; flushing; feeling of warmth; nausea; vomiting; pain, rash, redness, or burning at injection site; diaphoresis
Occasional
PO: Mild constipation, fecal impaction, peripheral edema, metabolic alkalosis (muscle pain, restlessness, slow breathing, altered taste)
Calcium carbonate: Milk-alkali syndrome (headache, decreased appetite, nausea, vomiting, unusual tiredness)
Rare
Difficult or painful urination

SERIOUS REACTIONS
- Hypercalcemia is a serious adverse effect of calcium acetate use. Early signs include constipation, headache, dry mouth, increased thirst, irritability, decreased appetite, metallic taste, fatigue, weakness, and depression. Later signs include confusion, somnolence, hypertension, photosensitivity, arrhythmias, nausea, vomiting, and increased painful urination.

PRECAUTIONS & CONSIDERATIONS
Caution is warranted with chronic renal impairment, decreased cardiac function, dehydration, history of renal calculi, and ventricular fibrillation during cardiac resuscitation. Calcium acetate is distributed in breast milk; it is unknown whether calcium chloride and gluconate are distributed in breast milk. Restrict IV use in children because their small vasculature increases the risk of developing extreme irritation and

possible tissue necrosis or sloughing. Oral absorption may be decreased in the elderly. Avoid consuming excessive amounts of alcohol, caffeine, and tobacco.

Adequate hydration should be maintained. B/P, EKG, serum magnesium, phosphate and potassium levels, urine calcium concentrations, and renal function test results should be monitored.

Storage
Store vials at room temperature.

Administration
Take tablets with a full glass of water 30 minutes to 1 hour after meals. Dilute the syrup in juice or water and administer it before meals to increase absorption. Chew the chewable tablets well before swallowing them. Do not to take calcium within 2 hours of consuming other oral drugs or fiber-containing foods.

Calcium chloride may be given undiluted or may be diluted with an equal amount 0.9% NaCl or sterile water for injection.

Calcium gluconate may be given undiluted or may be diluted in up to 1000 ml 0.9% NaCl. Give calcium chloride by slow IV push (0.5 to 1 ml/minute). Rapid administration may produce bradycardia, hypotension, peripheral vasodilation, a chalky or metallic taste, and a feeling of warmth. Give calcium gluconate by IV push at a rate of 0.5 to 1 ml/minute. Rapid administration may produce arrhythmias, hypotension, MI, and vasodilation. When administering calcium gluconate by intermittent IV infusion, the maximum rate is 200 mg/minute.

C

Calfactant
cal-fac′tant
(Infasurf)

CATEGORY AND SCHEDULE
Pregnancy Risk Category: This drug is not indicated for use in pregnant women.

CLASSIFICATION
Surfactants, lung

MECHANISM OF ACTION
A natural lung extract that reduces alveolar surface tension, stabilizing the alveoli. *Therapeutic Effect:* Restores surface activity to infant lungs, improves lung compliance and respiratory gas exchange.

PHARMACOKINETICS
No studies have been performed.

AVAILABILITY
Intratracheal Suspension: 35-mg/ml vials.

INDICATIONS AND DOSAGES
▶ **Respiratory distress syndrome (RDS)**
INTRATRACHEAL
Neonates. 3 ml/kg of birth weight administered as soon as possible after birth in 2 doses of 1.5 ml/kg. Repeat 3-ml/kg doses, up to a total of 3 doses given 12 hr apart.

CONTRAINDICATIONS
None known.

INTERACTIONS
Drug
None known.
Herbal
None known.
Food
None known.

DIAGNOSTIC TEST EFFECTS
None known.

SIDE EFFECTS
Frequent
Cyanosis (65%), airway obstruction (39%), bradycardia (34%), reflux of surfactant into endotracheal tube (21%), need for manual ventilation (16%)
Occasional
Need for reintubation (3%)

SERIOUS REACTIONS
• Cyanosis, airway obstruction, bradycardia, and reflux of surfactant into endotracheal tube may occur.

PRECAUTIONS & CONSIDERATIONS
Caution is warranted with a hypersensitivity to calfactant. This drug is for use only in neonates. No age-related precautions have been noted.

The neonate's oxygenation and ventilation should be monitored using arterial or transcutaneous measurement of systemic oxygen (O_2) and carbon dioxide (CO_2). Visitors should be limited during treatment. Hand washing and other infection control measures should be monitored to minimize the risk of nosocomial infections.

Storage
Refrigerate vials. Unopened, unused vials may be returned to refrigerator only once after having been warmed to room temperature.

Administration
Gently swirl the vial, if needed, to redisperse contents. Do not shake it. Enter each single use vial only once; discard unused suspension. Instill the drug intratracheally through a side port adapter into the infant's endotracheal tube. Give each aliquot over 20-30 ventilatory breaths. Administer only during the inspiratory cycle.

Between aliquot dosages, turn the infant so that the opposite lung is in the dependent position.

Candesartan
kan-de-sar'tan
(Atacand)

CATEGORY AND SCHEDULE
Pregnancy Risk Category: C (D if used in second or third trimester)

CLASSIFICATION
Angiotensin II receptor antagonists

MECHANISM OF ACTION
An angiotensin II receptor, type AT_1, antagonist that blocks the vasoconstrictor and aldosterone-secreting effects of angiotensin II, inhibiting the binding of angiotensin II to the AT_1 receptors. *Therapeutic Effect:* Causes vasodilation, decreases peripheral resistance, and decreases B/P.

PHARMACOKINETICS

Route	Onset	Peak	Duration
PO	2-3 hr	6-8 hr	Greater than 24 hr

Rapidly, completely absorbed. Protein binding: greater than 99%. Undergoes minor hepatic metabolism to inactive metabolite. Excreted unchanged in urine and in the feces through the biliary system. Not removed by hemodialysis. **Half-life:** 9 hr.

AVAILABILITY
Tablets: 4 mg, 8 mg, 16 mg, 32 mg.

INDICATIONS AND DOSAGES
▸ **Hypertension alone or in combination with other antihypertensives**
PO
Adults, Elderly, Patient with mildly impaired liver or renal function.
Initially, 16 mg once a day in those who are not volume depleted. Can be given once or twice a day with total daily doses of 8-32 mg. Give lower dosage in those treated with diuretics or with severely impaired renal function.

OFF-LABEL USES
Treatment of heart failure

CONTRAINDICATIONS
Hypersensitivity to candesartan

INTERACTIONS
Drug
None known.
Herbal
None known.
Food
None known.

DIAGNOSTIC TEST EFFECTS
May increase BUN, serum alkaline phosphatase, serum bilirubin, serum creatinine, AST (SGOT), and ALT (SGPT) levels. May decrease blood Hgb and Hct levels.

SIDE EFFECTS
Occasional (6%-3%)
Upper respiratory tract infection, dizziness, back and leg pain
Rare (2%-1%)
Pharyngitis, rhinitis, headache, fatigue, diarrhea, nausea, dry cough, peripheral edema

SERIOUS REACTIONS
• Overdosage may manifest as hypotension and tachycardia. Bradycardia occurs less often. Institute supportive measures.

C

PRECAUTIONS & CONSIDERATIONS
Caution is warranted with hepatic and renal impairment, renal artery stenosis, severe CHF, and dehydration. It is unknown if candesartan is distributed in breast milk. Candesartan may cause fetal or neonatal morbidity or mortality. Safety and efficacy of candesartan have not been established in children. No age-related precautions have been noted in the elderly. Apical pulse and B/P should be assessed immediately before each candesartan dose, and regularly throughout therapy. Be alert to fluctuations in apical pulse and B/P. If an excessive reduction in B/P occurs, place the person in the supine position with feet slightly elevated and notify the physician. Tasks that require mental alertness or motor skills should be avoided. Blood Hgb and Hct and BUN, serum alkaline phosphatase, serum bilirubin, serum creatinine, AST (SGOT), and ALT (SGPT) levels should be obtained before and during therapy. Maintain adequate hydration; exercising outside during hot weather should be avoided in order to decrease the risk of dehydration and hypotension.
Administration
Take candesartan without regard to food.

Capecitabine
ka-pe-site'-a-been
(Xeloda)
Do not confuse Xeloda with Xenical.

CATEGORY AND SCHEDULE
Pregnancy Risk Category: D

CLASSIFICATION
Antineoplastics, antimetabolites

MECHANISM OF ACTION
An antimetabolite that is enzymatically converted to 5-fluorouracil. Inhibits enzymes necessary for synthesis of essential cellular components. *Therapeutic Effect:* Interferes with DNA synthesis, RNA processing, and protein synthesis.

PHARMACOKINETICS
Readily absorbed from the GI tract. Protein binding: less than 60%. Metabolized in the liver. Primarily excreted in urine. **Half-life:** 45 min.

AVAILABILITY
Tablets: 150 mg, 500 mg.

INDICATIONS AND DOSAGES
▸ **Metastatic breast cancer, colon cancer**
PO
Adults, Elderly. Initially, 2500 mg/m^2/day in 2 equally divided doses approximately q12h for 2 wk. Follow with a 1-wk rest period; given in 3-wk cycles.

CONTRAINDICATIONS
Severe renal impairment

INTERACTIONS
Drug
Warfarin: May alter the effects of warfarin.

Herbal
None known.
Food
None known.

DIAGNOSTIC TEST EFFECTS
May increase serum alkaline phosphatase, bilirubin, AST (SGOT), and ALT (SGPT) levels. May decrease blood Hct, Hgb level, and WBC count.

SIDE EFFECTS
Frequent (greater than 5%)
Diarrhea (sometimes severe), nausea, vomiting, stomatitis, hand and foot syndrome (painful palmar-plantar swelling with paresthesia, erythema, and blistering), fatigue, anorexia, dermatitis
Occasional (less than 5%)
Constipation, dyspepsia, nail disorder, headache, dizziness, insomnia, edema, myalgia

SERIOUS REACTIONS
• Serious reactions may include myelosuppression (evidenced by neutropenia, thrombocytopenia, and anemia), cardiovascular toxicity (marked by angina, cardiomyopathy, and deep vein thrombosis), respiratory toxicity (marked by dyspnea, epistaxis, and pneumonia), and lymphedema.

PRECAUTIONS & CONSIDERATIONS
Use cautiously in patients with a history of coronary artery disease, concomitant coumarin-derived anticoagulant therapy, concomitant phenytoin therapy, renal impairment, or liver dysfunction due to liver metastases. Caution is also warranted in the elderly. Avoid use in pregnant women. It is unknown if capecitabine is distributed in breast milk. Safety and efficacy of capecitabine have not been established in children. Monitor for signs of infection.

Monitor for symptoms of hand-and-foot syndrome.
Administration
Take capecitabine within 30 minutes after a meal.

Capreomycin
kap ree-oh-mye'sin
(Capastat Sulfate, Capastat [AUS])
Do not confuse with Captopril, Capsaicin, or Kanamycin.

CATEGORY AND SCHEDULE
Pregnancy Risk Category: C

CLASSIFICATION
Antimycobacterials

MECHANISM OF ACTION
A cyclic polypeptide antimicrobial but the mechanism of action is not well understood. *Therapeutic Effect:* Suppresses mycobacterial multiplication.

PHARMACOKINETICS
Not well absorbed from the gastrointestinal (GI) tract. Undergoes little metabolism. Primarily excreted unchanged in urine. **Half-life:** 4-6 hrs (half-life is increased with impaired renal function).

AVAILABILITY
Injection: 100 mg/ml (Capastat sulfate).

INDICATIONS AND DOSAGES
▸ **Tuberculosis**
IM
Adults, Elderly, Children. 15-20 mg/kg/day for 60-120 days, followed by 1 g 2-3 times/wk. Maximum: 1 g/day.

OFF-LABEL USES
Treatment of atypical mycobacterial infections

CONTRAINDICATIONS
Concurrent use of other ototoxic or nephrotoxic drugs, hypersensitivity to capreomycin

INTERACTIONS
Drug
Aminoglycosides: May increase the risk of aminoglycoside toxicity
Nondepolarizing neuromuscular blocking agents: May increase neuromuscular blockade.
Herbal
None known.
Food
None known.

DIAGNOSTIC TEST EFFECTS
None known.

SIDE EFFECTS
Frequent
Ototoxicity, nephrotoxicity
Occasional
Eosinophilia
Rare
Rash, fever, urticaria, hypokalemia, thrombocytopenia, vertigo

SERIOUS REACTIONS
• Renal failure, ototoxicity, and thrombocytopenia can occur.

PRECAUTIONS & CONSIDERATIONS
Cautiously use with pre-existing hearing impairment and renal dysfunction. It is unknown if capreomycin crosses the placenta and is excreted in breast milk. Age-related renal impairment may require dosage adjustment in the elderly. Complete blood count (CBC) and renal and liver function test results should be obtained before the initiation of therapy. Hearing changes must be reported immediately. Renal function, electrolytes, and acid-base balance should be monitored during therapy.

Administration

Reconstitute by dissolving the vial contents (1 g) in 2 ml of 0.9% sodium chloride injection or sterile water for injection. Allow 2 to 3 minutes for complete dissolution. The solution for injection may acquire a pale straw color and darken with time. This is not associated with a loss of potency or development of toxicity.

Capsaicin

cap-say′sin
(Zostrix)
Do not confuse with Zovirax.

CATEGORY AND SCHEDULE

Pregnancy Risk Category: C
OTC

CLASSIFICATION

Analgesics, topical, dermatologics

MECHANISM OF ACTION

A topical analgesic that depletes and prevents reaccumulation of the chemomediator of pain impulses (substance P) from peripheral sensory neurons to CNS.
Therapeutic Effect: Relieves pain.

PHARMACOKINETICS

None reported.

AVAILABILITY

Cream: 0.025%, 0.075% (Zostrix).

INDICATIONS AND DOSAGES

▸ **Treatment of neuralgia, osteoarthritis, rheumatoid arthritis**
TOPICAL
Adults, Elderly, Children older than 2 yr. Apply directly to affected area 3-4 times/day. Continue for 14 to 28 days for optimal clinical response.

OFF-LABEL USES

Treatment of neurogenic pain

CONTRAINDICATIONS

Hypersensitivity to capsaicin or any component of the formulation

INTERACTIONS

Drug
Anticoagulants, antiplatelet agents, low molecular weight heparins, thrombolytic agents: May increase risk of bleeding.
Herbal
None known.
Food
None known.

DIAGNOSTIC TEST EFFECTS

None known.

SIDE EFFECTS

Frequent
Burning, stinging, erythema at site of application

SERIOUS REACTIONS

• None known.

PRECAUTIONS & CONSIDERATIONS

Caution is warranted with concurrent use of nephrotoxic agents, dehydration, fluid and electrolyte imbalance, neurologic abnormalities and renal or hepatic impairment. It is unknown if capsaicin crosses the placenta or is distributed in breast milk. Safety and efficacy has not been established in children less than 2 years of age. There are no age-related precautions noted in the elderly.

Transient burning may occur on application, and usually disappears after 72 hours.

Storage
Store at room temperature.
Administration
Capsaicin is for external use only.
Avoid eye contact. Wash hands
immediately after application.
If there is no improvement or
condition deteriorates after 28 days,
discontinue use and consult
physician.

Captopril
cap-toe-pril
(Acenorm [AUS], Capoten,
Captohexal [AUS], Novo-Captoril
[CAN], Topace [AUS])
**Do not confuse captopril with
Capitrol.**

CATEGORY AND SCHEDULE
Pregnancy Risk Category: C
(D if used in second or third
trimester)

CLASSIFICATION
Angiotensin converting enzyme
inhibitors

MECHANISM OF ACTION
An ACE inhibitor that suppresses
the renin-angiotensin-aldosterone
system and prevents conversion of
angiotensin I to angiotensin II, a
potent vasoconstrictor; may also
inhibit angiotensin II at local
vascular and renal sites. Decreases
plasma angiotensin II, increases
plasma renin activity, and
decreases aldosterone secretion.
Therapeutic Effect: Reduces
peripheral arterial resistance,
pulmonary capillary wedge
pressure; improves cardiac
output and exercise tolerance.

PHARMACOKINETICS

Route	Onset	Peak	Duration
PO	0.25 hr	0.5-1.5 hr	Dose related

Rapidly, well absorbed from the GI
tract (absorption is decreased in the
presence of food). Protein binding:
25%-30%. Metabolized in the liver.
Primarily excreted in urine.
Removed by hemodialysis. **Half-life:**
less than 3 hr (increased in those
with impaired renal function).

AVAILABILITY
Tablets: 12.5 mg, 25 mg, 50 mg,
100 mg.

INDICATIONS AND DOSAGES
▸ **Hypertension**
PO
Adults, Elderly. Initially,
12.5-25 mg 2-3 times a day. After
1-2 wk, may increase to 50 mg
2-3 times a day. Diuretic may be
added if no response in additional
1-2 wk. If taken in combination with
diuretic, may increase to
100-150 mg 2-3 times a day after
1-2 wk. Maintenance: 25-150 mg
2-3 times a day. Maximum:
450 mg/day.
▸ **CHF**
PO
Adults, Elderly. Initially,
6.25-25 mg 3 times a day. Increase
to 50 mg 3 times a day. After at least
2 wk, may increase to 50-100 mg
3 times a day. Maximum:
450 mg/day.
▸ **Post-myocardial infarction,
impaired liver function**
PO
Adults, Elderly. 6.25 mg a day, then
12.5 mg 3 times a day. Increase to
25 mg 3 times a day over several
days up to 50 mg 3 times a day over
several weeks.

C

▸ **Diabetic nephropathy prevention of kidney failure**
PO
Adults, Elderly. 25 mg 3 times a day.
Children. Initially 0.3-0.5 mg/kg/dose titrated up to a maximum of 6 mg/kg/day in 2-4 divided doses.
Neonates. Initially, 0.05-0.1 mg/kg/dose q8-24hr titrated up to 0.5 mg/kg/dose given q6-24hr.

▸ **Dosage in renal impairment**
Creatinine clearance 10-50 ml/min. 75% of normal dosage.
Creatinine clearance less than 10 ml/min. 50% of normal dosage.

OFF-LABEL USES
Diagnosis of anatomic renal artery stenosis, hypertensive crisis, rheumatoid arthritis

CONTRAINDICATIONS
History of angioedema from previous treatment with ACE inhibitors

INTERACTIONS
Drug
Alcohol, antihypertensives, diuretics: May increase the effects of captopril.
Lithium: May increase lithium blood concentration and risk of lithium toxicity.
NSAIDs: May decrease the effects of captopril.
Potassium-sparing diuretics, potassium supplements: May cause hyperkalemia.
Herbal
None known.
Food
All food. Food significantly reduces drug absorption by 30% to 40%.

DIAGNOSTIC TEST EFFECTS
May increase BUN, serum alkaline phosphatase, serum bilirubin, serum creatinine, serum potassium, AST (SGOT), and ALT (SGPT) levels.

May decrease serum sodium levels. May cause positive antinuclear antibody titer.

SIDE EFFECTS
Frequent (7%-4%)
Rash
Occasional (4%-2%)
Pruritus, dysgeusia (change in sense of taste)
Rare (less than 2%-0.5%)
Headache, cough, insomnia, dizziness, fatigue, paresthesia, malaise, nausea, diarrhea or constipation, dry mouth, tachycardia

SERIOUS REACTIONS
• Excessive hypotension (first-dose syncope) may occur in patients with CHF and in those who are severely salt and volume depleted.
• Angioedema (swelling of face and lips) and hyperkalemia occur rarely.
• Agranulocytosis and neutropenia may be noted in those with collagen vascular disease, including scleroderma and systemic lupus erythematosus, and impaired renal function.
• Nephrotic syndrome may be noted in those with history of renal disease.

PRECAUTIONS & CONSIDERATIONS
Caution is warranted with cerebrovascular or coronary insufficiency, hypovolemia, renal impairment, sodium depletion, those on dialysis and/or receiving diuretics, and in the elderly. Captopril crosses the placenta, is distributed in breast milk, and may cause fetal or neonatal morbidity or mortality. Safety and efficacy of captopril have not been established in children. The elderly may be more sensitive to the hypotensive effects of captopril.
　　Dizziness may occur. B/P should be obtained immediately before

giving each captopril dose, in addition to regular monitoring. Be alert to fluctuations in B/P. If an excessive reduction in B/P occurs, place the person in the supine position with legs elevated. CBC and blood chemistry should be obtained before beginning captopril therapy, then every 2 weeks for the next 3 months, and periodically thereafter in patients with autoimmune disease, or renal impairment, and in those who are taking drugs that affect immune response or leukocyte count. Skin for rash and urinalysis for proteinuria should also be assessed. CBC, BUN, serum creatinine, and serum potassium should be monitored in those who are receiving a diuretic. Full therapeutic effect of captopril may take several weeks.

Administration

! Give captopril 1 hour before meals for maximum absorption because food significantly decreases drug absorption.

Crush tablets if necessary. Do not skip doses.

Carbamazepine

kar-ba-maz′e-peen
(Apo-Carbamazepine [CAN], Carbatrol, Epitol, Tegretol, Tegretol CR [AUS], Tegretol XR, Teril [AUS])
Do not confuse Tegretol with Cartrol, Toradol, or Trental.

CATEGORY AND SCHEDULE
Pregnancy Risk Category: D

CLASSIFICATION
Anticonvulsants, antipsychotics

MECHANISM OF ACTION
An iminostilbene derivative that decreases sodium and calcium ion influx into neuronal membranes, reducing post-tetanic potentiation at synapses. *Therapeutic Effect:* Reduces seizure activity.

PHARMACOKINETICS
Slowly and completely absorbed from the GI tract. Protein binding: 75%. Metabolized in the liver to active metabolite. Primarily excreted in urine. Not removed by hemodialysis. **Half-life:** 25-65 hr (decreased with chronic use).

AVAILABILITY
Capsules (Extended Release [Carbatrol]): 100 mg, 200 mg, 400 mg.
Suspension (Tegretol): 100 mg/5 ml.
Tablets (Epitol, Tegretol): 200 mg.
Tablets (Chewable [Tegretol]): 100 mg.
Tablets (Extended-Release [Tegretol XR]): 100 mg, 200 mg, 400 mg.

INDICATIONS AND DOSAGES
▸ **Seizure control**
PO
Adults, Children older than 12 yr. Initially, 200 mg twice a day. May increase dosage by 200 mg/day at weekly intervals. Range: 400-1200 mg/day in 2-4 divided doses. Maximum: 1.6-2.4 g/day.
Children 6-12 yr. Initially, 100 mg twice a day. May increase by 100 mg/day at weekly intervals. Range: 20-30 mg/kg/day. Maxiumum: 1000 mg/day.
Children younger than 6 yr. Initially 5 mg/kg/day. May increase at weekly intervals to 10 mg/kg/day up to 20 mg/kg/day.
Elderly. Initially 100 mg 1-2 times a day. May increase by 100 mg/day at

weekly intervals. Usual dose
400-1000 mg/day.
▸ **Trigeminal neuralgia, diabetic neuropathy**
PO
Adults. Initially, 100 mg twice a day.
May increase by 100 mg twice a day
up to 400-800 mg/day. Maxiumum:
1200 mg/day.
Elderly. Initially 100 mg 1-2 times a
day. May increase by 100 mg/day at
weekly intervals. Usual dose 400-
1000 mg/day.

OFF-LABEL USES
Treatment of alcohol withdrawal,
bipolar disorder, diabetes insipidus,
neurogenic pain, psychotic disorders

CONTRAINDICATIONS
Concomitant use of MAOIs, history
of myelosuppression, hypersensitivity to tricyclic antidepressants

INTERACTIONS
Drug
**Anticoagulants, clarithromycin,
diltiazem, erythromycin, estrogens,
propoxyphene, quinidine, steroids:**
May decrease the effects of these
drugs.
**Antipsychotics, haloperidol,
tricyclic antidepressants:** May
increase CNS depressant effects.
Cimetidine: May increase carbamazepine blood concentration and
risk of toxicity.
Isoniazid: May increase metabolism of isoniazid; may increase
carbamazepine blood concentration
and risk of toxicity.
MAOIs: May cause seizures and
hypertensive crisis.
**Other anticonvulsants, barbitu-
rates, benzodiazepines, valproic
acid:** May increase the metabolism
of these drugs.
Verapamil: May increase the toxicity of carbamazepine.

Herbal
None known.
Food
Grapefruit: May increase the
absorption and blood concentration
of carbamazepine.

DIAGNOSTIC TEST EFFECTS
May increase BUN and blood
glucose levels and serum alkaline
phosphatase, bilirubin, AST (SGOT),
ALT (SGPT), protein, cholesterol,
HDL, and triglyceride levels. May
decrease serum calcium and thyroid
hormone (T_3, T_4, T_4 index) levels.
Therapeutic serum level is 4-
12 mcg/ml; toxic serum level is
greater than 12 mcg/ml.

SIDE EFFECTS
Frequent
Drowsiness, dizziness, nausea,
vomiting
Occasional
Visual abnormalities (spots before
eyes, difficulty focusing, blurred
vision), dry mouth or pharynx,
tongue irritation, headache, fluid
retention, diaphoresis, constipation
or diarrhea, behavioral changes in
children

SERIOUS REACTIONS
• Toxic reactions may include blood
dyscrasias (such as aplastic anemia,
agranulocytosis, thrombocytopenia,
leukopenia, leukocytosis, and
eosinophilia), cardiovascular disturbances (such as CHF, hypotension or
hypertension, thrombophlebitis and
arrhythmias), and dermatologic
effects (such as rash, urticaria, pruritus, and photosensitivity).
• Abrupt withdrawal may precipitate status epilepticus.

PRECAUTIONS & CONSIDERATIONS
Caution is warranted with impaired
cardiac, hepatic, and renal function.

Be aware that carbamazepine crosses the placenta and accumulates in fetal tissue. It is also distributed in breast milk. Children are more likely than adults to develop behavioral changes. The elderly are more susceptible to agitation, AV block, bradycardia, confusion, and syndrome of inappropriate antidiuretic hormone secretion. Grapefruit juice should be avoided because it may increase the drug's blood concentration.

Drowsiness may occur but disappears with continued therapy, so tasks that require mental alertness or motor skills should be avoided. Notify the physician if visual disturbances, fever, joint pain, mouth ulcerations, sore throat, and unusual bleeding occur. Seizure disorder, including the duration, frequency, and intensity of seizures, should be assessed before and during therapy. BUN level, CBC, serum iron determination, and urinalysis should be obtained before and periodically during carbamazepine therapy.
Storage
Store the tablets, capsules, and oral suspension at room temperature.
Administration
! If the patient must change to another anticonvulsant, plan to decrease the carbamazepine dose gradually as therapy begins with a low dose of the replacement drug. When transferring from tablets to suspension, expect to divide the total daily tablet dose into smaller, more frequent doses of suspension. Also plan to administer extended-release tablets in 2 divided doses. Therapeutic serum level of carbamazepine is 4-12 mcg/ml. Take carbamazepine with meals to reduce the risk of GI distress. Shake the oral suspension well. Don't administer it simultaneously with any other liquid medicine. Don't crush extended-release tablets.

C

Carbamide Peroxide
(Auro Ear Drops, Debrox, ERO Ear, GlyOxide, Mollifene Ear Wax Removing, Murine Ear Drops, Orajel Perioseptic, Proxigel) (gel, solution)

CATEGORY AND SCHEDULE
Pregnancy Risk Category: C

CLASSIFICATION
Cerumenolytic; topical oral anti-inflammatory

MECHANISM OF ACTION
A cerumenolytic that releases oxygen on contact with moist mouth tissues to provide cleansing effects, reduce inflammation, relieve pain, and inhibit odor-forming bacteria. In the ear, oxygen is released and hydrogen peroxide is reduced to water which enables the chemical reaction. *Therapeutic Effect:* Relieves inflammation of gums and lips. Emulsifies and disperses ear wax.

PHARMACOKINETICS
Not known.

AVAILABILITY
Gel, oral: 10% (Proxigel).
Solution, oral: 10% (Gly-Oxide), 15% (Orajel Perioseptic).
Solution, otic: 6.5% (Auro Ear Drops, Debrox, ERO Ear, Mollifene Ear Wax Removing, Murine Ear Drops)

INDICATIONS AND DOSAGES
▶ **Earwax removal**
TOPICAL, SOLUTION
Adults, Elderly, Children 12 yr or older. Tilt head and administer 5-10 drops twice a day for up to 4 days.
Children 12 yr or younger. Tilt head and administer 1-5 drops twice a day for up to 4 days.
▶ **Oral lesions**
TOPICAL, GEL
Adults, Elderly, Children. Apply to affected area 4 times a day.
TOPICAL, SOLUTION
Adults, Elderly, Children. Apply several drops undiluted on affected area 4 times a day after meals and at bedtime.

OFF-LABEL USES
Dental whitener

CONTRAINDICATIONS
Dizziness, ear discharge or drainage, ear injury, ear pain, irritation, or rash, hypersensitivity to carbamide peroxide or any one of its components

INTERACTIONS
Drug
None known.
Herbal
None known.
Food
None known.

DIAGNOSTIC TEST EFFECTS
Not known.

SIDE EFFECTS
Occasional
Oral: Gingival sensitivity

SERIOUS REACTIONS
• Opportunistic infections caused by organisms like Candida albicans is possible with prolonged use.

PRECAUTIONS & CONSIDERATIONS
It is unknown if carbamide peroxide crosses the placenta or is distributed in breast milk. There are no age-related precautions noted in the elderly.
Administration
Use several drops after a meal or at bedtime. Mix with saliva, swish for several minutes, and expectorate. Do not to drink or rinse mouth after use.

Tilt the patient's head sideways to instill in ear. Keep drops in ear for several minutes by keeping head tilted and placing cotton in ear. Tip of the applicator should not enter the ear canal.

Carbenicillin
kar-ben-ih-sill′in
(Geocillin)

CATEGORY AND SCHEDULE
Pregnancy Risk Category: B

CLASSIFICATION
Antibiotics, penicillins

MECHANISM OF ACTION
A penicillin that inhibits cell wall synthesis in susceptible microorganisms. *Therapeutic Effect:* Produces bactericidal effect.

PHARMACOKINETICS
Moderately absorbed from the gastrointestinal (GI) tract. Protein binding: 50%. Widely distributed. Partially metabolized in liver. Primarily excreted in urine. Removed by hemodialysis. **Half-life:** 1-1.5 hrs (half-life increased in impaired renal function).

AVAILABILITY
Tablet: 382 mg (Geocillin).

INDICATIONS AND DOSAGES
▶ **Prostatitis**
PO
Adults, Elderly. 764 mg q6hr.
▶ **Urinary tract infection**
PO
Adults, Elderly. 382-764 mg q6hr.

OFF-LABEL USES
Perioperative prophylaxis

CONTRAINDICATIONS
Hypersensitivity to any penicillin

INTERACTIONS
Drug
Anticoagulants: May increase bleeding effects of anticoagulants.
Oral contraceptives: May decrease effectiveness of oral contraceptives.
Probenecid: May increase carbenicillin blood concentration and risk of toxicity.
Tetracyclines: May decrease the effect of carbenicillin.
Herbal
None known.
Food
None known.

DIAGNOSTIC TEST EFFECTS
May increase SGOT levels. May interfere with urinary glucose tests using cupric sulfate (Benedict's solution, Clinitest). May give false-positives of urine or serum proteins.

▨ IV INCOMPATIBILITIES
Amikacin (Amikin), bleomycin (Blenoxane), gentamicin, pro-methazine (Phenergan)
▨ IV Compatibilities
Cefotetan (Cefotan), dopamine (Inotropin), hydromorphone (Dilaudid), magnesium sulfate, morphine, multivitamins, potassium chloride, ranitidine (Zantac)

SIDE EFFECTS
Frequent
GI disturbances, including mild diarrhea, nausea, or vomiting, oral or vaginal candidiasis
Occasional
Generalized rash, urticaria, phlebitis, headache
Rare
Dizziness, seizures

SERIOUS REACTIONS
• Altered bacterial balance may result in potentially fatal superinfections and antibiotic-associated colitis as evidenced by abdominal cramps, watery or severe diarrhea, and fever.
• Severe hypersensitivity reactions, including seizures, occur rarely.

PRECAUTIONS & CONSIDERATIONS
Caution is warranted with antibiotic-associated colitis or a history of allergies, particularly to cephalosporins. Be aware of a history of allergies, especially to cephalosporins and penicillins, before giving the drug. Carbenicillin readily crosses the placenta, appears in cord blood and amniotic fluid, and is distributed in breast milk in low concentrations. Carbenicillin may lead to allergic sensitization, candidiasis, diarrhea, and skin rash in infants. In the elderly, age-related renal impairment may require dosage adjustment. Intake and output, renal, hepatic and hemato-logic function tests, and urinalysis results should be monitored. Carbenicillin should be withheld and the physician promptly notified if the patient experiences a rash or diarrhea. Although a rash is common with carbenicillin, it also may indicate hypersensitivity. Severe diarrhea

with abdominal pain, blood or mucus in stools, and fever may indicate antibiotic-associated colitis.

Storage
Store capsules at room temperature. Oral suspension, after prepared, is stable for 3 months if refrigerated.

When injection preparation is reconstituted, the solution remains stable for 24 hours at room temperature and 72 hours under refrigeration.

Administration
Give oral preparation 1 hour before or 2 hours after meals for maximum absorption.

Administer IV preparation around the clock to promote less variation in peak and trough levels.

Carbidopa and Levodopa

kar-bee-doe′pa; lee-voe-doe′pa
(Apo-Levocarb [CAN], Kinson [AUS], Sinemet, Sinemet CR)

CATEGORY AND SCHEDULE
Pregnancy Risk Category: C

CLASSIFICATION
Antiparkinson agents, dopaminergics

MECHANISM OF ACTION
Levodopa is converted to dopamine in the basal ganglia thus increasing dopamine concentration in brain and inhibiting hyperactive cholinergic activity. Carbidopa prevents peripheral breakdown of levodopa, allowing more levodopa to be available for transport into the brain. *Therapeutic Effect:* Reduces tremor.

PHARMACOKINETICS
Carbidopa is rapidly and completely absorbed from the GI tract. Widely distributed. Excreted primarily in urine. Levodopa is converted to dopamine. Excreted primarily in urine. **Half-life:** 1-2 hr (carbidopa); 1-3 hr (levodopa).

AVAILABILITY
Tablets: 10 mg carbidopa/ 100 mg levodopa, 25 mg carbidopa/ 100 mg levodopa, 25 mg carbidopa/250 mg levodopa.
Tablets (Extended-Release): 25 mg carbidopa/100 mg levodopa, 50 mg carbidopa/200 mg levodopa.

INDICATIONS AND DOSAGES
▶ **Parkinsonism**
PO
Adults. Initially, 25/100 mg 2-4 times a day. May increase up 200/2000 mg daily.
Elderly. Initially, 25/100 mg twice a day. May increase as necessary.
When converting a patient from Sinemet to Sinemet CR (50 mg/ 200 mg), dosage is based on the total daily dose of levodopa, as follows:

Sinemet	Sinemet CR
300-400 mg	1 tablet twice a day
500-600 mg	1.5 tablet twice a day or 1 tablet 3 times a day
700-800 mg	4 tablets in 3 or more divided doses
900-1000 mg	5 tablets in 3 or more divided doses

Intervals between doses of Sinemet CR should be 4-8 hr while awake.

CONTRAINDICATIONS
Angle-closure glaucoma, use within 14 days of MAOIs

INTERACTIONS
Drug
Anticonvulsants, benzodiazepines, haloperidol, phenothiazines: May decrease the effects of carbidopa and levodopa.
MAOIs: May increase the risk of hypertensive crisis.
Selegiline: May increase levodopa-induced dyskinesias, nausea, orthostatic hypotension, confusion, and hallucinations.
Herbal
None known.
Food
None known.

DIAGNOSTIC TEST EFFECTS
May increase BUN level and serum LDH, alkaline phosphatase, bilirubin, AST (SGOT), and ALT (SGPT) levels.

SIDE EFFECTS
Frequent (90%-10%)
Uncontrolled movements of face, tongue, arms, or upper body; nausea and vomiting (80%); anorexia (50%)
Occasional
Depression, anxiety, confusion, nervousness, urine retention, palpitations, dizziness, lightheadedness, decreased appetite, blurred vision, constipation, dry mouth, flushed skin, headache, insomnia, diarrhea, unusual fatigue, darkening of urine and sweat
Rare
Hypertension, ulcer, hemolytic anemia (marked by fatigue)

SERIOUS REACTIONS
• Patients on long-term therapy have a high incidence of involuntary choreiform, dystonic, and dyskinetic movements.
• Numerous mild to severe CNS and psychiatric disturbances may occur, including reduced attention span, anxiety, nightmares, daytime somnolence, euphoria, fatigue, paranoia, psychotic episodes, depression, and hallucinations.

PRECAUTIONS & CONSIDERATIONS
Caution is warranted with active peptic ulcer, severe cardiac, endocrine, hepatic, pulmonary, or renal impairment, treated open-angle glaucoma, a history of MI, bronchial asthma (because of tartrazine sensitivity), and emphysema. It is unknown if carbidopa and levodopa crosses the placenta or is distributed in breast milk. However, this drug may inhibit lactation. Women should not breast-feed while taking this drug. The safety and efficacy of carbidopa and levodopa have not been established in children younger than 18 years. The elderly are more sensitive to levodopa's effects. The elderly receiving anticholinergics are at increased risk for adverse CNS effects, such as anxiety, confusion, and nervousness.

Dizziness, drowsiness, dry mouth, and darkened urine may occur. Alcohol and tasks that require mental alertness or motor skills should be avoided. Notify the physician if agitation, headache, lethargy, or confusion occurs. Relief of symptoms, such as improvement of mask-like facial expression, muscular rigidity, shuffling gait, and resting tremors of the hands and head, should be assessed.
Administration
! Plan to discontinue levodopa at least 12 hours before giving carbidopa and levodopa. Expect the initial dose to provide at least 25% of the previous levodopa dose. Void before giving carbidopa and levodopa to reduce the risk of urine retention.

Take carbidopa and levodopa without regard to food. If GI upset occurs, take with food. Scored tablets may be crushed as needed. Extended-release tablets may be cut in half but not crushed. Therapeutic effects may be delayed from several weeks to months.

Carboplatin
car-bow′play-tin
(Paraplatin)
Do not confuse carboplatin with Cisplatin or Platinol.

CATEGORY AND SCHEDULE
Pregnancy Risk Category: D

CLASSIFICATION
Antineoplastics, platinum agents

MECHANISM OF ACTION
A platinum coordination complex that inhibits DNA synthesis by cross-linking with DNA strands, preventing cell division. Cell cycle-phase nonspecific. *Therapeutic Effect:* Interferes with DNA function.

PHARMACOKINETICS
Protein binding: Low. Hydrolyzed in solution to active form. Primarily excreted in urine. **Half-life:** 2.6-5.9 hr.

AVAILABILITY
Powder for Injection: 50 mg, 150 mg, 450 mg.
Injection Solution: 10 mg/ml.

INDICATIONS AND DOSAGES
▸ **Ovarian carcinoma (monotherapy)**
IV
Adults. 360 mg/m^2 on day 1, every 4 wk. Don't repeat dose until neutrophil and platelet counts are within acceptable levels. Adjust drug

dosage in previously treated patients based on lowest post-treatment platelet or neutrophil count. Increase dosage only once to no more than 125% of starting dose.
▸ **Ovarian carcinoma (combination therapy)**
IV
Adults. 300 mg/m^2 (with cyclophosphamide) on day 1, every 4 wk. Don't repeat dose until neutrophil and platelet counts are within acceptable levels.
Children. 300-600 mg/m^2 every 4 wk for solid tumor, or 175 mg/m^2 every 4 wk for brain tumor.
▸ **Dosage in renal impairment**
Initial dosage is based on creatinine clearance; subsequent dosages are based on the patient's tolerance and degree of myelosuppression.

Creatinine Clearance	Dosage Day 1
Greater than 60 ml/min	360 mg/m^2
41-59 ml/min	250 mg/m^2
16-40 ml/min	200 mg/m^2

OFF-LABEL USES
Treatment of bony and soft-tissue sarcomas; germ cell tumors; neuroblastoma; pediatric brain tumor; small-cell lung cancer; solid tumors of the bladder, cervix, and testes; squamous cell carcinoma of the esophagus

CONTRAINDICATIONS
History of severe allergic reaction to cisplatin, platinum compounds, or mannitol; severe bleeding, severe myelosuppression

INTERACTIONS
Drug
Bone marrow depressants: May increase myelosuppression.

Live-virus vaccines: May potentiate virus replication, increase vaccine side effects, and decrease the patient's antibody response to the vaccine.
Nephrotoxic, ototoxic medications: May increase the risk of nephrotoxicity.
Herbal
None known.
Food
None known.

DIAGNOSTIC TEST EFFECTS
May decrease serum electrolyte levels, including calcium, magnesium, potassium, and sodium. High dosages (more than 4 times the recommended dosage) may elevate BUN and serum alkaline phosphatase, bilirubin, creatinine, and AST SGOT levels.

▨ IV INCOMPATIBILITIES
Amphotericin B complex (Abelcet, AmBisome, Amphotec)
▨ IV Compatibilities
Etoposide (VePesid), granisetron (Kytril), ondansetron (Zofran), paclitaxel (Taxol)

SIDE EFFECTS
Frequent
Nausea (75%-80%), vomiting (65%)
Occasional
Generalized pain (17%), diarrhea or constipation (6%), peripheral neuropathy (4%)
Rare (3%-2%)
Alopecia, asthenia, hypersensitivity reaction (erythema, pruritus, rash, urticaria)

SERIOUS REACTIONS
• Myelosuppression may be severe, resulting in anemia, infection, (sepsis, pneumonia), and bleeding.
• Prolonged treatment may result in peripheral neurotoxicity.

PRECAUTIONS & CONSIDERATIONS
Caution is warranted in renal impairment. Be aware that prior aminoglycoside therapy may potentiate carboplatin-induced renal toxicity. Use cautiously in elderly previously treated with cisplatin; they are at an increased risk of developing carboplatin-induced peripheral neuropathy. Avoid using carboplatin in pregnant women. The use of a contraceptive is recommended during therapy. It is unknown if carboplatin is distributed in breast milk. Safety and efficacy have not been established in children. Tell the patient of the possibility of hair loss and that normal hair growth should resume after treatment has ended.
Administration
Be aware that aluminum reacts with carboplatin to form an inactive precipitate; intravenous sets and needles containing aluminum that may come in contact with carboplatin should not be used.

Carboprost
kar′boe-prost
(Hemabate)

CATEGORY AND SCHEDULE
Pregnancy Risk Category: X

CLASSIFICATION
Abortifacients, oxytocics, prostaglandins, stimulants, uterine

MECHANISM OF ACTION
A prostaglandin similar to prostaglandin F2 alpha (dinoprost) that directly acts on myometrium and stimulates contraction in gravid uterus. *Therapeutic Effect:* Produces cervical dilation and softening.

PHARMACOKINETICS
None reported.

AVAILABILITY
Injection: 250 mcg carboprost and 83 mcg tromethamine/ml (Hemabate).

INDICATIONS AND DOSAGES
▸ Abortion
IM
Adults. Initially, 100-250 mcg, may repeat at 1.5-3.5 hour intervals. May increase up to 500 mcg if uterine contractility inadequate. Maximum: 12 mg total dose or continuous administration for more than 2 days.
▸ Postpartum hemorrhage
IM
Adults. Initially, 250 mcg, may repeat at 15-90 minute intervals. Maximum: 2 mg total dose.

OFF-LABEL USES
Treatment of incomplete abortion, benign hydatiform mole, induction of labor, ripening of cervix prior to abortion.

CONTRAINDICATIONS
Acute pelvic inflammatory disease, active cardiac disease, pulmonary disease, renal disease, hepatic disease, pregnancy, hypersensitivity to carboprost or other prostaglandins

INTERACTIONS
Drug
Oxytocin, oxytocics: May cause uterine hypertonus leading to uterine rupture or cervical lacerations.
Herbal
None known.
Food
None known.

DIAGNOSTIC TEST EFFECTS
None known.

▨ IV INCOMPATIBILITIES
No information available.
▨ IV Compatibilities
Heparin, potassium

SIDE EFFECTS
Frequent
Nausea
Occasional
Facial flushing
Rare
Vomiting, diarrhea

SERIOUS REACTIONS
• Excessive dosing may cause uterine hypertonicity with spasm and tetanic contraction, leading to cervical laceration/perforation and uterine rupture and hemorrhage.

PRECAUTIONS & CONSIDERATIONS
Caution is warranted with a history of asthma, hypo/hypertension,

anemia, jaundice, diabetes mellitus, epilepsy, compromised (scarred) uterus, cardiovascular, adrenal, or hepatic disease. Be aware that carboprost tromethamine use is contraindicated during pregnancy and that small amounts of the drug are found in breast milk. There is no information available on carboprost tromethamine use in children or the elderly. Avoid smoking because of added effects of vasoconstriction.

Strength, duration, frequency of contractions as well as vital signs should be monitored every 15 min until stable, then hourly until abortion complete. Fever, chills, foul-smelling/increased vaginal discharge, or uterine cramps/pain should be reported immediately.
Storage
Refrigerate ampoules.
Administration
Be aware that carboprost tromethamine should not be injected IV because it may result in bronchospasm, hypertension, vomiting, and anaphylaxis.

Dilute immediately prior to IM administration in 0.9% NaCl for bladder irrigation.

Carisoprodol
kar′i-so-pro′dol
(Soma)

CATEGORY AND SCHEDULE
Pregnancy Risk Category: C

CLASSIFICATION
Musculoskeletal agents, relaxants, skeletal muscle

MECHANISM OF ACTION
A centrally-acting skeletal muscle relaxant whose exact mechanism is unknown. Effects may be due to its CNS depressant actions. *Therapeutic Effect:* Relieves muscle spasms and pain.

AVAILABILITY
Tablets: 350 mg.

INDICATIONS AND DOSAGES
▶ **Adjunct to rest, physical therapy, analgesics, and other measures for relief of discomfort from acute, painful musculoskeletal conditions**
PO
Adults, Elderly. 350 mg 4 times a day.

CONTRAINDICATIONS
Acute intermittent porphyria, sensitivity to meprobamate

INTERACTIONS
Drug
Alcohol, other CNS depressants: May increase CNS depression.
Herbal
None known.
Food
None known.

DIAGNOSTIC TEST EFFECTS
None known.

SIDE EFFECTS
Frequent (greater than 10%)
Somnolence
Occasional (10%-1%)
Tachycardia, facial flushing, dizziness, headache, lightheadedness, dermatitis, nausea, vomiting, abdominal cramps, dyspnea

SERIOUS REACTIONS
• Overdose may cause CNS and respiratory depression, shock, and coma.

PRECAUTIONS & CONSIDERATIONS

Caution is warranted with hepatic and renal impairment. Drowsiness or dizziness may occur. Avoid alcohol, CNS depressants, and tasks that require mental alertness or motor skills. Liver and renal function tests should be obtained at baseline and periodically for those on long-term therapy. Therapeutic response, such as relief muscle spasm and pain, should be assessed.

Administration

Take carisoprodol without regard to food. Take the last dose at bedtime.

Carteolol

kar-tee'oh-lole
(Cartrol, Ocupress)
Do not confuse with carvedilol.

CATEGORY AND SCHEDULE

Pregnancy Risk Category: C/D if after first trimester

CLASSIFICATION

Antiadrenergics, beta blocking, ophthalmics

MECHANISM OF ACTION

An antihypertensive that blocks beta$_1$-adrenergic receptor at normal doses and beta$_2$-adrenergic receptors at large doses. Predominantly blocks beta$_1$-adrenergic receptors in cardiac tissue. Reduces aqueous humor production. *Therapeutic Effect:* Slows sinus heart rate, decreases cardiac output, decreases blood pressure (B/P), increases airway resistance, decreases intraocular pressure.

PHARMACOKINETICS

Well absorbed from the gastrointestinal (GI) tract. Protein binding: unknown. Minimally metabolized in liver. Primarily excreted unchanged in urine. Not removed by hemodialysis. **Half-life:** 6 hrs (increased in decreased renal function).

AVAILABILITY

Ophthalmic solution: 1% (Ocupress).
Tablets: 2.5 mg, 5 mg (Cartrol).

INDICATIONS AND DOSAGES

▶ **Hypertension**
PO
Adults, Elderly. Initially, 2.5 mg/day as single dose either alone or in combination with diuretic. May increase gradually to 5-10 mg/day as a single dose. Maintenance: 2.5-5 mg/day.

▶ **Dosage in renal impairment**

Creatinine Clearance	Dosage Interval
>60 ml/min	24 hr
20-60 ml/min	48 hr
<20 ml/min	72 hr

▶ **Open-angle glaucoma, ocular hypertension**
OPHTHALMIC
Adults, Elderly. 1 drop 2 times/day.

OFF-LABEL USES

Combination with miotics decreases IOP in acute/chronic angle closure glaucoma, treatment of secondary glaucoma, malignant glaucoma, angle closure glaucoma during/after iridectomy

CONTRAINDICATIONS

Bronchial asthma, COPD, bronchospasm, overt cardiac failure, cardiogenic shock, heart block greater than first degree, persistently severe bradycardia

INTERACTIONS
Drug
Cimetidine: May increase carteolol concentrations.
Diuretics, other hypotensives: May increase hypotensive effect.
Insulin, oral hypoglycemics: May mask symptoms of hypoglycemia and prolong hypoglycemic effect of these drugs.
MAOIs: May produce hypertension.
NSAIDs: May decrease antihypertensive effects.
Sympathomimetics, xanthines: May mutually inhibit effects of carteolol.
Herbal
None known.
Food
None known.

DIAGNOSTIC TEST EFFECTS
May increase serum ANA titer, BUN, serum LDH, lipoprotein, alkaline phosphatase, bilirubin, creatinine, potassium, triglyceride, uric acid, SGOT (AST), and SGPT (ALT) levels.

SIDE EFFECTS
Frequent
Oral: Hypotension manifested as dizziness, nausea, diaphoresis, headache, cold extremities, fatigue, constipation/diarrhea
Ophthalmic: Redness of eye or inside of eyelids, decreased night vision
Occasional
Oral: Insomnia, flatulence, urinary frequency, impotence or decreased libido
Ophthalmic: Blepharoconjunctivitis, edema, droopy eyelid, staining of cornea, blurred vision, brow ache, increased light sensitivity, burning, stinging

Rare
Rash, arthralgia, myalgia, confusion (especially elderly), taste disturbances

SERIOUS REACTIONS
* Abrupt withdrawal (particularly in those with coronary artery disease) may produce angina or precipitate MI.
* May precipitate thyroid crisis in those with thyrotoxicosis.
* Beta-blockers may mask signs and symptoms of acute hypoglycemia (tachycardia, B/P changes) in diabetic patients.

PRECAUTIONS & CONSIDERATIONS
Caution is warranted with impaired renal, cardiac or liver function, hypothyroidism, hypothermia during delivery, and small birth weight infants. Be aware that carteolol crosses the placenta and is distributed in small amounts in breast milk. Safety and efficacy of carteolol has not been established in children. Age-related peripheral vascular disease may increase susceptibility to decreased peripheral circulation in the elderly.

Do not abruptly discontinue carteolol. If carteolol is stopped suddenly, it may cause chest pain or heart attack.

Restrict salt and avoid alcohol and tasks that require mental alertness or motor skills. In addition, avoid nasal decongestants and over-the-counter (OTC) cold preparations, especially those containing stimulants, without physician approval.

Stinging or discomfort is common with ophthalmic use.
Storage
Store ophthalmic solution and tablets at room temperature.
Administration
Give oral carteolol without regard to food.

To use ophthalmic preparation, wash hands before instilling. Sit or lie down to instill. Open eye, look at ceiling, and instill prescribed amount. Close eye and apply gentle pressure to inner corner of eye. Do not let tip of applicator touch eye.

Carvedilol
kar-vea′die-lole
(Coreg, Dilatrend [AUS])
Do not confuse carvedilol with carteolol.

CATEGORY AND SCHEDULE
Pregnancy Risk Category: C (D if used in the second or third trimester)

CLASSIFICATION
Antiadrenergics, beta blocking

MECHANISM OF ACTION
An antihypertensive that possesses nonselective beta-blocking and alpha-adrenergic blocking activity. Causes vasodilation. *Therapeutic Effect:* Reduces cardiac output, exercise-induced tachycardia, and reflex orthostatic tachycardia; reduces peripheral vascular resistance.

PHARMACOKINETICS

Route	Onset	Peak	Duration
PO	30 min	1-2 hr	24 hr

Rapidly and extensively absorbed from the GI tract. Protein binding: 98%. Metabolized in the liver. Excreted primarily via bile into feces. Minimally removed by hemodialysis.

Half-life: 7-10 hr. Food delays rate of absorption.

AVAILABILITY
Tablets: 3.125 mg, 6.25 mg, 12.5 mg, 25 mg.

INDICATIONS AND DOSAGES
▶ **Hypertension**
PO
Adults, Elderly. Initially, 6.25 mg twice a day. May double at 7- to 14-day intervals to highest tolerated dosage. Maximum: 50 mg/day.
▶ **CHF**
PO
Adults, Elderly. Initially, 3.125 mg twice a day. May double at 2-wk intervals to highest tolerated dosage. Maximum: For patients weighing more than 85 kg, give 50 mg twice a day, for those weighing 85 kg or less, give 25 mg twice a day.
▶ **Left ventricular dysfunction**
PO
Adults, Elderly. Initially, 3.125-6.25 mg twice a day. May increase at intervals of 3-10 days up to 25 mg twice a day.

OFF-LABEL USES
Treatment of angina pectoris, idiopathic cardiomyopathy

CONTRAINDICATIONS
Bronchial asthma or related bronchospastic conditions, cardiogenic shock, pulmonary edema, second- or third-degree AV block, severe bradycardia

INTERACTIONS
Drug
Calcium blockers: Increase risk of conduction disturbances.
Clonidine: May potentiate B/P effects.
Cimetidine: May increase carvedilol blood concentration.

C

Digoxin: Increases concentrations of this drug.
Diuretics, other antihypertensives: May increase hypotensive effect.
Insulin, oral hypoglycemics: May mask symptoms of hypoglycemia and prolong hypoglycemic effect of these drugs.
Rifampin: Decreases carvedilol blood concentration.
Herbal
None known.
Food
None known.

DIAGNOSTIC TEST EFFECTS
None known.

SIDE EFFECTS
Carvedilol is generally well tolerated, with mild and transient side effects.
Frequent (6%-4%)
Fatigue, dizziness
Occasional (2%)
Diarrhea, bradycardia, rhinitis, back pain
Rare (less than 2%)
Orthostatic hypotension, somnolence, UTI, viral infection

SERIOUS REACTIONS
• Overdose may produce profound bradycardia, hypotension, bronchospasm, cardiac insufficiency, cardiogenic shock, and cardiac arrest.
• Abrupt withdrawal may result in diaphoresis, palpitations, headache, and tremors.
• Carvedilol administration may precipitate CHF and MI in patients with heart disease; thyroid storm in those with thyrotoxicosis; and peripheral ischemia in those with existing peripheral vascular disease.
• Hypoglycemia may occur in patients with previously controlled diabetes.

PRECAUTIONS & CONSIDERATIONS
Caution should be used in those undergoing anesthesia and in those with CHF controlled with ACE inhibitor, digoxin or diuretics, diabetes mellitus; hypoglycemia, impaired hepatic function, peripheral vascular disease, and thyrotoxicosis. It is unknown if carvedilol crosses the placenta or is distributed in breast milk. Carvedilol use should be avoided in pregnant women after the first trimester because it may result in low-birth-weight infants. The drug may also produce apnea, bradycardia, hypoglycemia, or hypothermia during childbirth. The safety and efficacy of carvedilol have not been established in children. In the elderly, the incidence of dizziness may be increased. Be aware that salt and alcohol intake should be restricted. Nasal decongestants or OTC cold preparations (stimulants) should not be used without physician approval.

Orthostatic hypotension may occur, so rise slowly from a lying to sitting position and dangle the legs from the bed momentarily before standing. Tasks that require mental alertness or motor skills should be avoided. Apical pulse and B/P should be assessed immediately before giving carvedilol. B/P for hypotension, respiratory status for shortness of breath, pattern of daily bowel activity and stool consistency, EKG for arrhythmias, and pulse for quality, rate, and rhythm should be monitored during treatment. If pulse rate is 60 beats/minute or lower or systolic B/P is less than 90 mm Hg, withhold the medication and contact the physician. Signs and symptoms of CHF, such as decreased urine output, distended neck veins, dyspnea (particularly on exertion or lying down), night cough, peripheral edema, and weight gain should also be assessed.

Administration
Take carvedilol with food to slow the rate of absorption and reduce the risk of orthostatic hypotension. To assess tolerance for carvedilol, assess a standing systolic B/P 1 hour after giving the drug.

Cascara Sagrada
cass-care'ah sah-graud'ah
(Cascara Sagrada)

CATEGORY AND SCHEDULE
Pregnancy Risk Category: C

CLASSIFICATION
Laxatives

MECHANISM OF ACTION
A GI stimulant that has a direct effect on colonic smooth musculature, by stimulating intramural nerve plexi. *Therapeutic Effect:* Promotes fluid and ion accumulation in the colon, increasing peristalsis and promoting a laxative effect.

AVAILABILITY
Liquid: (18% alcohol) 1 g/ml.

INDICATIONS AND DOSAGES
▶ **Treatment of constipation**
PO
Adults, Elderly. 5 ml at bedtime.
Children 2-11 yr. 2.5 ml, 1-3 ml as a single dose.
Infant. 1.25 ml, 0.5-2 ml as a single dose.

CONTRAINDICATIONS
Abdominal pain, appendicitis, intestinal obstruction, nausea, vomiting

INTERACTIONS
Drug
Oral medications: May decrease transit time of concurrently administered oral medications, decreasing the absorption of cascara sagrada.
Herbal
None known.
Food
None known.

DIAGNOSTIC TEST EFFECTS
May increase blood glucose level. May decrease serum calcium and potassium levels.

SIDE EFFECTS
Frequent
Pink-red, red-violet, red-brown, or yellow-brown discoloration of urine
Occasional
Some degree of abdominal discomfort, nausea, mild cramps, faintness

SERIOUS REACTIONS
• Long-term use may result in laxative dependence, chronic constipation, and loss of normal bowel function.
• Prolonged use or overdose may result in electrolyte or metabolic disturbances (such as hypokalemia, hypocalcemia, and metabolic acidosis or alkalosis), as well as persistent diarrhea, vomiting, muscle weakness, malabsorption, and weight loss.

PRECAUTIONS & CONSIDERATIONS
Be aware excessive use of cascara sagrada may lead to fluid and electrolyte imbalance. Be aware the liquid form contains alcohol. Because cascara sagrada is a strong stimulant, use cautiously in pregnant women.
Urine may temporarily turn pink-red, red-violet, red-brown, or yellow-brown. Maintain adequate fluid intake.

Pattern of daily bowel activity and stool consistency and serum electrolyte levels should be monitored.
Administration
Take cascara sagrada on an empty stomach for faster action. Avoid taking within 1 hour of antacids, milk, or other oral medications. Do not use cascara sagrada if abdominal pain, nausea, or vomiting lasting longer than 1 week occurs. To promote defecation increase fluid intake, exercise, and eat a high-fiber diet.

Caspofungin Acetate
kas-poe-fun'jin
(Cancidas)

CATEGORY AND SCHEDULE
Pregnancy Risk Category: C

CLASSIFICATION
Antifungals

MECHANISM OF ACTION
An antifungal that inhibits the synthesis of glucan, a vital component of fungal cell formation, thereby damaging the fungal cell membrane. *Therapeutic Effect:* Fungistatic.

PHARMACOKINETICS
Distributed in tissue. Extensively bound to albumin. Protein binding: 97%. Slowly metabolized in liver to active metabolite. Excreted primarily in urine and to a lesser extent in feces. Not removed by hemodialysis. **Half-life:** 40-50 hr.

AVAILABILITY
Powder for Injection: 50-mg, 70-mg vials.

INDICATIONS AND DOSAGES
▶ **Aspergillosis**
IV
Adults, Elderly, Children older than 12 yr. Give single 70-mg loading dose on day 1, followed by 50 mg/day thereafter. For patients with moderate hepatic insufficiency, daily dose reduced to 35 mg.
▶ **Invasive candidiasis**
IV
Adults, Elderly. Initially, 70 mg followed by 50 mg daily.
▶ **Esophageal candidiasis**
IV
Adult, Elderly. 50 mg a day.

CONTRAINDICATIONS
None known.

INTERACTIONS
Drug
Carbamazepine, cyclosporine, dexamethasone, efavirenz, nelfinavir, nevirapine, phenytoin, rifampin: May increase blood concentration of caspofungin.
Tacrolimus: May decrease the effect of tacrolimus.
Herbal
None known.
Food
None known.

DIAGNOSTIC TEST EFFECTS
May increase PT as well as serum alkaline phosphatase, serum bilirubin, serum creatinine, LDH, SGOT (AST), SGPT (ALT), serum uric acid, urine pH, urine protein, urine RBC, and urine WBC levels. May decrease Hgb, Hct, platelet count, and serum albumin, serum bicarbonate, serum protein, and serum potassium levels.

▨ IV INCOMPATIBILITIES
Don't mix caspofungin with any other medication or use dextrose as a diluent.

SIDE EFFECTS
Frequent (26%)
Fever
Occasional (11%-4%)
Headache, nausea, phlebitis
Rare (3% or less)
Paresthesia, vomiting, diarrhea,
abdominal pain, myalgia, chills,
tremor, insomnia

SERIOUS REACTIONS
• Hypersensitivity reactions (characterized by rash, facial swelling,
pruritus, and a sensation of warmth)
may occur.

PRECAUTIONS & CONSIDERATIONS
Caution is warranted with liver function impairment. Be aware that
caspofungin crosses the placental
barrier, may be embryotoxic, and is
distributed in breast milk. Be aware
that the safety and efficacy of caspofungin have not been established in
children. In the elderly, age-related
moderate renal impairment may
require dosage adjustment.
   Baseline temperature, liver
function test results, and history of
allergies should be obtained before
giving the drug. Signs and symptoms of liver function should be
assessed. If increased shortness of
breath, itching, facial swelling, or a
rash occurs, notify the physician.
Report pain, burning, or swelling at
the IV infusion site.
Storage
Refrigerate but warm it to room
temperature before preparing it with
the diluent. The reconstituted solution, before prepared as the patient
infusion solution, may be stored at
room temperature for 1 hour before
infusion. The final infusion solution
can be stored at room temperature
for 24 hours. Discard the solution
if it contains particulate or is
discolored.

Administration
For a 50- to 70-mg loading dose, add
10.5 ml 0.9% NaCl to the vial.
Transfer 10 ml of the reconstituted
solution to 250 ml 0.9% NaCl. For
35-mg dose in persons with moderate liver insufficiency, add 10.5 ml
0.9% NaCl to the vial. Transfer 10 ml
of reconstituted solution to 100 or
250 ml 0.9% NaCl for 50- to 70-mg
a day dose. For moderate liver
insufficiency, transfer 7 ml to 100
or 250 ml 0.9% NaCl. Infuse over
60 minutes.

Castor Oil
(Emulsoil, Purge)

CATEGORY AND SCHEDULE
Pregnancy Risk Category: X
OTC

CLASSIFICATION
Laxative, stimulant

MECHANISM OF ACTION
A laxative prepared from the bean of
the castor plant but the exact mechanism of action is unknown. Acts
primarily in the small intestine. May
be hydrolyzed to ricinoleic acid
which reduces net absorption of fluid
and electrolytes and stimulates peristalsis. *Therapeutic Effect:* Increases
peristalsis, promotes laxative effect.

PHARMACOKINETICS
Minimal absorption by the gastrointestinal (GI) tract. May be metabolized like other fatty acids.

AVAILABILITY
Emulsion: 36.4%/ml.
Oral liquid: 95% (Emulsoil, Purge).

INDICATIONS AND DOSAGES
▶ **Constipation**
PO
*Adults, Elderly, Children 12 yr
and older.* 15-60 ml as a single
dose.
Children 2-12 yr. 5-15 ml as a
single dose.
Children less than 2 yr. 1-2 ml as a
single dose. Maximum: 5 ml as a
single dose.

CONTRAINDICATIONS
Abdominal pain, appendicitis,
intestinal obstruction, nausea,
vomiting, pregnancy

INTERACTIONS
Drug
Droperidol: May increase risk of
cardiotoxicity.
Levomethadyl: May increase risk
of QT prolongation.
Herbal
Licorice: May increase risk of
hypokalemia.
Food
None known.

DIAGNOSTIC TEST EFFECTS
None known.

SIDE EFFECTS
Occasional
Some degree of abdominal discomfort, nausea, mild cramps, griping,
faintness

SERIOUS REACTIONS
• Long-term use may result in
laxative dependence, chronic
constipation, and loss of normal
bowel function.
• Chronic use or overdosage may
result in electrolyte disturbances,
such as hypokalemia, hypocalcemia,
and metabolic acidosis or alkalosis,
persistent diarrhea, malabsorption, and
weight loss. Electrolyte disturbance

may produce vomiting and muscle
weakness.

PRECAUTIONS & CONSIDERATIONS
Caution should be used for extended
periods (greater than 1 week) of
castor oil use. Be aware castor oil is
contraindicated in pregnancy. It is
unknown if castor oil is distributed
in breast milk. Safety and efficacy of
castor oil has not been established in
children younger than 2 years of age.
There are no age-related precautions
noted in the elderly, but monitor for
signs of dehydration and electrolyte
loss. Avoid taking within 1 hour of
other oral medication because it
decreases drug absorption.
Storage
Store at room temperature.
Administration
Take castor oil on an empty stomach
for faster results. Drink at least 6 to
8 glasses of water a day to aid in
stool softening.

Cefaclor
sef′a-klor
(Apo-Cefaclor [CAN], Ceclor,
Ceclor CD, Cefkor [AUS], Cefkor
CD [AUS], Keflor [AUS])

CATEGORY AND SCHEDULE
Pregnancy Risk Category: B

CLASSIFICATION
Antibiotics, cephalosporins

MECHANISM OF ACTION
A second-generation cephalosporin
that binds to bacterial cell
membranes and inhibits cell wall
synthesis. *Therapeutic Effect:*
Bactericidal.

PHARMACOKINETICS

Well absorbed from the GI tract. Protein binding: 25%. Widely distributed. Primarily excreted unchanged in urine. Moderately removed by hemodialysis. **Half-life:** 0.6-0.9 hr (increased in impaired renal function).

AVAILABILITY

Capsules (Ceclor): 250 mg, 500 mg.
Oral Suspension (Ceclor):
125 mg/5 ml, 187 mg/5 ml,
250 mg/5 ml, 375 mg/5 ml.
Tablets, extended-release (Ceclor CD): 375 mg, 500 mg.
Tablets, chewable (Raniclor):
125 mg, 187 mg, 250 mg, 375 mg.

INDICATIONS AND DOSAGES

▸ **Bronchitis**
PO
Adults, Elderly (extended-release).
500 mg q12hr for 7 days.
▸ **Lower respiratory tract infections**
PO
Adults, Elderly. 250-500 mg q8hr.
▸ **Otitis media**
PO
Children. 20-40 mg/kg/day in 2-3 divided doses. Maximum: 1 g/day.
▸ **Pharyngitis, skin/skin structure infections, tonsillitis**
PO
Adults, Elderly (extended-release).
375 mg q12hr.
Adults, Elderly (regular-release).
250-500 mg q8hr.
Children. 20-40 mg/kg/day in 2-3 divided doses. Maximum: 1 g/day.
▸ **Urinary tract infections**
PO
Adults, Elderly. 250-500 mg q8hr.
Children. 20-40 mg/kg/day in 2-3 divided doses q8hr. Maximum: 1 g/day.
PO (Extended-Release Tablets)
Adults, Children older than 16 yr.
375-500 mg q12hr.

▸ **Otitis media**
PO
Children older than 1 mo.
40 mg/kg/day in divided doses q8hr. Maximum: 1 g/day.
▸ **Dosage in renal impairment**
Decreased dosage may be necessary in patients with creatinine clearance less than 40 ml/min.

CONTRAINDICATIONS

History of anaphylactic reaction to penicillins or hypersensitivity to cephalosporins

INTERACTIONS

Drug
Probenecid: May increase cefaclor blood concentration.
Herbal
None known.
Food
None known.

DIAGNOSTIC TEST EFFECTS

May increase BUN level and serum alkaline phosphatase, bilirubin, creatinine, LDH, AST (SGOT), and ALT (SGPT) levels. May cause a positive direct or indirect Coombs' test.

SIDE EFFECTS

Frequent
Oral candidiasis, mild diarrhea, mild abdominal cramping, vaginal candidiasis
Occasional
Nausea, serum sickness-like reaction (marked by fever and joint pain; usually occurs after the second course of therapy and resolves after the drug is discontinued)
Rare
Allergic reaction (pruritus, rash, and urticaria)

SERIOUS REACTIONS

• Antibiotic-associated colitis and other superinfections may result

from altered bacterial balance.
• Nephrotoxicity may occur, especially in patients with pre-existing renal disease.
• Patients with a history of allergies, especially to penicillin, are at increased risk for developing a severe hypersensitivity reaction, marked by severe pruritus, angioedema, bronchospasm, and anaphylaxis.

PRECAUTIONS & CONSIDERATIONS
Caution is warranted with a history of GI disease (especially antibiotic-associated colitis or ulcerative colitis), renal impairment, and concurrent use of nephrotoxic medications. Be aware that cefaclor readily crosses the placenta and is distributed in breast milk. There are no age-related precautions noted in children older than 1 month. In the elderly, age-related renal impairment may require dosage adjustment.

Although mild GI effects may be tolerable, an increase in their severity may indicate the onset of antibiotic-associated colitis. The mouth for white patches on the mucous membranes and tongue, pattern of daily bowel activity and stool consistency, signs and symptoms of superinfection including abdominal pain, moderate to severe diarrhea, severe anal or genital pruritus, and severe mouth soreness should be assessed. Renal function should be assessed.

Storage
After reconstitution, oral solution is stable for 14 days if refrigerated.

Administration
Take without regard to meals; if GI upset occurs, give with food or milk. Do not cut, crush, or chew extended-release tablets.

Shake oral suspension well before using.

Cefadroxil
sef-a-drox'ill
(Duricef)

C

CATEGORY AND SCHEDULE
Pregnancy Risk Category: B

CLASSIFICATION
Antibiotics, cephalosporins

MECHANISM OF ACTION
A first-generation cephalosporin that binds to bacterial cell membranes and inhibits cell wall synthesis. *Therapeutic Effect:* Bactericidal.

PHARMACOKINETICS
Well absorbed from the GI tract. Protein binding: 15%-20%. Widely distributed. Primarily excreted unchanged in urine. Removed by hemodialysis. **Half-life:** 1.2-1.5 hr (increased in impaired renal function).

AVAILABILITY
Capsules: 500 mg.
Oral Suspension: 250 mg/5 ml, 500 mg/5 ml.
Tablets: 1000 mg.

INDICATIONS AND DOSAGES
▶ **UTIs**
PO
Adults, Elderly. 1-2 g/day as a single dose or in 2 divided doses.
Children. 30 mg/kg/day in 2 divided doses. Maximum: 2 g/day.
▶ **Skin and skin-structure infections, group A beta-hemolytic streptococcal pharyngitis, tonsillitis**
PO
Adults, Elderly. 1-2 g in 2 divided doses.
Children. 30 mg/kg/day in 2 divided doses. Maximum: 2 g/day.

▸ **Impetigo**
PO
Children. 30 mg/kg/day as a single or in 2 divided doses. Maximum: 2 g/day.
▸ **Dosage in renal impairment**
After an initial 1-g dose, dosage and frequency are modified based on creatinine clearance and the severity of the infection.

Creatinine Clearance	Dosage Interval
25-50 ml/min	500 mg q12hr
10-25 ml/min	500 mg q24hr
0-10 ml/min	500 mg q36hr

CONTRAINDICATIONS
History of anaphylactic reaction to penicillins or hypersensitivity to cephalosporins

INTERACTIONS
Drug
Probenecid: Increases cefadroxil blood concentration.
Herbal
None known.
Food
None known.

DIAGNOSTIC TEST EFFECTS
May increase BUN level and serum alkaline phosphatase, bilirubin, creatinine, LDH, AST (SGOT), and ALT (SGPT) levels. May cause a positive direct or indirect Coombs' test.

SIDE EFFECTS
Frequent
Oral candidiasis, mild diarrhea, mild abdominal cramping, vaginal candidiasis
Occasional
Nausea, unusual bruising or bleeding, serum sickness-like reaction (marked by fever and joint pain; usually occurs after the second course of therapy and resolves after the drug is discontinued)
Rare
Allergic reaction (rash, pruritus, urticaria), thrombophlebitis (pain, redness, swelling at injection site)

SERIOUS REACTIONS
• Antibiotic-associated colitis and other superinfections may result from altered bacterial balance.
• Nephrotoxicity may occur, especially in patients with pre-existing renal disease.
• Patients with a history of allergies, especially to penicillin, are at increased risk for developing a severe hypersensitivity reaction, marked by severe pruritus, angioedema, bronchospasm, and anaphylaxis.

PRECAUTIONS & CONSIDERATIONS
Caution is warranted with a history of GI disease (especially antibiotic-associated colitis or ulcerative colitis), renal impairment and concurrent use of nephrotoxic medications. Be aware that cefadroxil readily crosses the placenta and is distributed in breast milk. There are no age-related precautions noted in children. In the elderly, age-related renal impairment may require dosage adjustment.

Although mild GI effects may be tolerable, an increase in their severity may indicate the onset of antibiotic-associated colitis. The mouth for white patches on the mucous membranes and tongue, pattern of daily bowel activity and stool consistency, signs and symptoms of superinfection including abdominal pain, moderate to severe diarrhea, severe anal or genital pruritus, and severe mouth soreness should be assessed. Renal function should be assessed.

Storage
After reconstitution, oral solution is
stable for 14 days if refrigerated.
Administration
Take without regard to meals; if GI
upset occurs, give with food or milk.
Shake oral suspension well before
using.

Cefamandole
sef-a-man'dole
(Mandol)

CATEGORY AND SCHEDULE
Pregnancy Risk Category: B

CLASSIFICATION
Antibiotics, cephalosporins

MECHANISM OF ACTION
A second-generation cephalosporin
that binds to bacterial cell
membranes. *Therapeutic Effect:*
Inhibits synthesis of bacterial cell
wall. Bactericidal.

PHARMACOKINETICS
Well absorbed from the gastrointestinal (GI) tract. Protein binding: 56%-
78%. Widely distributed. Primarily
excreted unchanged in urine and high
concentrations in feces. Moderately
removed by hemodialysis. **Half-life:**
0.5-1 hr (half-life is increased with
impaired renal function).

AVAILABILITY
Injection: 1 g, 2 g, 10 g (Mandol).

INDICATIONS AND DOSAGES
▶ **Severe infections**
IV/IM
Adults, Elderly. 500-1000 mg q4-8hr.
Maximum: 2 g q4hr.

Children older than 1 mo.
50-150 mg/kg/day in divided doses
q4-8hr.

Creatinine Clearance	Dose
25-50 ml/min	1-2 g q8hr
10-25 ml/min	1 g q8hr
10 ml/min or less	1 g q12hr

OFF-LABEL USES
None known.

CONTRAINDICATIONS
Hypersensitivity to
cephalosporins, any component of
the formulation, or other
cephalosporins

INTERACTIONS
Drug
Aminoglycosides, furosemide:
May increase nephrotoxicity.
Probenecid: may increase cefaman-
dole blood concentration.
Herbal
None known.
Food
Ethanol: May cause disulfiram-like
reactions.

DIAGNOSTIC TEST EFFECTS
Positive direct or indirect Coombs'
test. May give false-positive urinary
glucose test using cupric sulfate.
May give false-positive serum or
urine creatinine with Jaffe
reaction.

IV INCOMPATIBILITIES
Amikacin (Amikin), amiodarone
(Cordarone, Pacerone),
cimetidine (Tagamet),
metronidazole (Flagyl), vancomycin
(Vancocin)
IV Compatibilities
Dopamine (Inotropin), heparin,
hydromorphone (Dilaudid),
morphine, ranitidine (Zantac)

SIDE EFFECTS
Frequent
Diarrhea, thrombophlebitis (pain, redness, swelling at injection site)
Occasional
Nausea, fever, vomiting
Rare
Allergic reaction as evidenced by pruritus, rash, and urticaria

SERIOUS REACTIONS
• Antibiotic-associated colitis manifested as severe abdominal pain and tenderness, fever, and watery and severe diarrhea, and other superinfections, may result from altered bacterial balance.
• Nephrotoxicity may occur, especially in patients with preexisting renal disease.
• Severe hypersensitivity reaction including severe pruritus, angioedema, bronchospasm, and anaphylaxis, particularly in patients with a history of allergies, especially to penicillin, may occur.

PRECAUTIONS & CONSIDERATIONS
Caution should be used with history of GI disease (especially antibiotic-associated colitis or ulcerative colitis), renal impairment as well as those using nephrotoxic medications. History of allergies, particularly cephalosporins and penicillins, should be determined before beginning drug therapy. Be alert for signs and symptoms of superinfection including abdominal pain, moderate to severe diarrhea, severe anal or genital pruritus, and severe mouth soreness. Cefamandole readily crosses the placenta and is distributed in breast milk. There are no age-related precautions noted in children older than 1 month. In the elderly, age-related renal impairment may require dosage adjustment. White patches on the mucous membranes or tongue should be reported.

Induration and tenderness should be monitored at the site of IM injection. Daily bowel activity and stool consistency should also be monitored. Mild GI effects may be tolerable, but increasing severity may indicate the onset of antibiotic-associated colitis.

Administration
Reconstitute IM preparation 1-g vial with 3 ml sterile or bacteriostatic water for injection, 0.9% Sodium Chloride. Administer deep into large muscle mass.

Reconstitute IV preparation with 10 ml sterile water for injection, 5% Dextrose or 0.9% Sodium Chloride injection, then further dilute in 100 ml piggyback set and infuse over 30 minutes. Discard the solution if precipitate forms.

Cefazolin
sef-a′zoe-lin
(Ancef, Kefzol)
Do not confuse cefazolin with cefprozil or Cefzil.

CATEGORY AND SCHEDULE
Pregnancy Risk Category: B

CLASSIFICATION
Antibiotics, cephalosporins

MECHANISM OF ACTION
A first-generation cephalosporin that binds to bacterial cell membranes and inhibits cell wall synthesis. *Therapeutic Effect:* Bactericidal.

PHARMACOKINETICS
Widely distributed. Protein binding: 85%. Primarily excreted unchanged

in urine. Moderately removed by hemodialysis. **Half-life:** 1.4-1.8 hr (increased in impaired renal function).

AVAILABILITY
Injection: 500 mg, 1 g.
Ready-to-Hang Infusion: 1 g/50 ml, 2 g/100 ml.

INDICATIONS AND DOSAGES
▶ **Uncomplicated UTIs**
IV, IM
Adults, Elderly. 1 g q12hr.
▶ **Mild to moderate infections**
IV, IM
Adults, Elderly. 250-500 mg q8-12hr.
▶ **Severe infections**
IV, IM
Adults, Elderly. 0.5-1 g q6-8hr.
▶ **Life-threatening infections**
IV, IM
Adults, Elderly. 1-1.5 g q6hr. Maximum: 12 g/day.
▶ **Perioperative prophylaxis**
IV, IM
Adults, Elderly. 1 g 30-60 min before surgery, 0.5-1 g during surgery, and q6-8hr for up to 24 hr postoperatively.
▶ **Usual pediatric dosage**
Children. 50-100 mg/kg/day in divided doses q8hr. Maximum: 6 g/day.
Neonates older than 7 days. 40-60 mg/kg/day in divided doses q8-12hr.
Neonates 7 days and younger. 40 mg/kg/day in divided doses q12hr.
▶ **Dosage in renal impairment**
Dosing frequency is modified based on creatinine clearance.

Creatinine Clearance	Dosage Interval
10-30 ml/min	Usual dose q12hr
Less than 10 ml/min	Usual dose q24hr

CONTRAINDICATIONS
History of anaphylactic reaction to penicillins or hypersensitivity to cephalosporins

INTERACTIONS
Drug
Probenecid: Increases cefazolin blood concentration.
Herbal
None known.
Food
None known.

DIAGNOSTIC TEST EFFECTS
May increase BUN level and serum alkaline phosphatase, bilirubin, creatinine, LDH, AST (SGOT), and ALT (SGPT) levels. May cause a positive direct or indirect Coombs' test

▓ IV INCOMPATIBILITIES
Amikacin (Amikin), amiodarone (Cordarone), hydromorphone (Dilaudid)
▓ IV Compatibilities
Calcium gluconate, diltiazem (Cardizem), famotidine (Pepcid), heparin, insulin (regular), lidocaine, magnesium sulfate, midazolam (Versed), morphine, multivitamins, potassium chloride, propofol (Diprivan), vecuronium (Norcuron)

SIDE EFFECTS
Frequent
Discomfort with IM administration, oral candidiasis, mild diarrhea, mild abdominal cramping, vaginal candidiasis
Occasional
Nausea, serum sickness-like reaction (marked by fever and joint pain; usually occurs after the second course of therapy and resolves after the drug is discontinued)

Rare
Allergic reaction (rash, pruritus, urticaria), thrombophlebitis (pain, redness, swelling at injection site)

SERIOUS REACTIONS

• Antibiotic-associated colitis and other superinfections may result from altered bacterial balance.
• Nephrotoxicity may occur, especially in patients with pre-existing renal disease.
• Patients with a history of allergies, especially to penicillin, are at increased risk for developing a severe hypersensitivity reaction, marked by severe pruritus, angioedema, bronchospasm, and anaphylaxis.

PRECAUTIONS & CONSIDERATIONS

Caution is warranted with a history of GI disease (especially antibiotic-associated colitis or ulcerative colitis), renal impairment, and concurrent use of nephrotoxic medications. Be aware that cefazolin readily crosses the placenta and is distributed in breast milk. There are no age-related precautions noted in children older than 1 month. In the elderly, age-related renal impairment may require dosage adjustment.

Although mild GI effects may be tolerable, an increase in their severity may indicate the onset of antibiotic-associated colitis. The mouth for white patches on the mucous membranes and tongue, pattern of daily bowel activity and stool consistency, signs and symptoms of superinfection including abdominal pain, moderate to severe diarrhea, severe anal or genital pruritus, and severe mouth soreness should be assessed. Renal function should be assessed.

Storage

Solution normally appears light yellow to yellow. IV infusion (piggyback) is stable for 24 hours at room temperature and 96 hours if refrigerated. Discard solution if precipitate forms.

Administration

To minimize discomfort, give IM injection deep and slowly. To minimize injection site discomfort, give the IM injection in the gluteus maximus rather than lateral aspect of thigh. Take cefazolin for the full length of treatment and evenly space doses around the clock.

For IV use, reconstitute each 1 g with at least 10 ml sterile water for injection. May further dilute in 50 to 100 ml D_5W or 0.9% NaCl to decrease the incidence of thrombophlebitis. For IV push, administer over 3 to 5 minutes. For intermittent IV infusion (piggyback), infuse over 20 to 30 minutes.

Cefdinir
sef′di-neer
(Omnicef)

CATEGORY AND SCHEDULE
Pregnancy Risk Category: B

CLASSIFICATION
Antibiotics, cephalosporins

MECHANISM OF ACTION
A third-generation cephalosporin that binds to bacterial cell membranes and inhibits cell wall synthesis. *Therapeutic Effect:* Bactericidal.

PHARMACOKINETICS
Moderately absorbed from the GI tract. Protein binding: 60%-70%. Widely distributed. Not appreciably metabolized. Primarily excreted unchanged in urine.

Minimally removed by hemodialysis.
Half-life: 1-2 hr (increased in impaired renal function).

AVAILABILITY

Capsules: 300 mg.
Oral Suspension: 125 mg/5 ml.

INDICATIONS AND DOSAGES
▶ **Community-acquired pneumonia**
PO
Adults, Elderly, Children 13 yr and older. 300 mg q12hr for 10 days.
▶ **Acute exacerbation of chronic bronchitis**
PO
Adults, Elderly. 300 mg q12hr for 5-10 days.
▶ **Acute maxillary sinusitis**
PO
Adults, Elderly, Children 13 yr and older. 300 mg q12hr or 600 mg q24hr for 10 days.
Children 6 mo-12 yr. 7 mg/kg q12hr or 14 mg/kg q24hr for 10 days.
▶ **Pharyngitis or tonsillitis**
PO
Adults, Elderly, Children 13 yr and older. 300 mg q12hr for 5-10 days or 600 mg q24hr for 10 days.
Children 6 mos-12 yrs. 7 mg/kg q12hr for 5-10 days or 14 mg/kg q24hr for 10 days.
▶ **Uncomplicated skin or skin-structure infections**
PO
Adults, Elderly, Children 13 yr and older. 300 mg q12hr for 10 days.
Children 6 mo-12 yr. 7 mg/kg q12hr for 10 days.
▶ **Acute bacterial otitis media**
PO (Capsules)
Children 6 mo-12 yr. 7 mg/kg q12hr or 14 mg/kg q24hr for 10 days.
▶ **Usual pediatric dosage for oral suspension**
Children weighing 81-95 lb (37-43 kg). 12.5 ml (2.5 tsp) q12hr or 25 ml (5 tsp) q24hr.

Children weighing 61-80 lb (28-36 kg). 10 ml (2 tsp) q12hr or 20 ml (4 tsp) q24hr.
Children weighing 41-60 lb (19-27 kg). 7.5 ml (1 tsp) q12hr or 15 ml (3 tsp) q24hr.
Children weighing 20-40 lb (9-18 kg). 5 ml (1 tsp) q12hr or 10 ml (2 tsp) q24hr.
Infants weighing less than 20 lb (9 kg). 2.5 ml ($\frac{1}{2}$ tsp) q12hr or 5 ml (1 tsp) q24hr.
▶ **Dosage in renal impairment**
For patients with creatinine clearance less than 30 ml/min, dosage is 300 mg/day as single daily dose. For hemodialysis patients, dosage is 300 mg or 7 mg/kg/dose every other day.

CONTRAINDICATIONS

History of anaphylactic reaction to penicillins or hypersensitivity to cephalosporins

INTERACTIONS
Drug
Antacids: Decrease cefdinir blood concentration.
Probenecid: Increases cefdinir blood concentration.
Herbal
None known.
Food
None known.

DIAGNOSTIC TEST EFFECTS

May increase serum alkaline phosphatase, bilirubin, LDH, AST (SGPT), and ALT (SGOT) levels. May produce a false-positive reaction for ketones in urine.

SIDE EFFECTS
Frequent
Oral candidiasis, mild diarrhea, mild abdominal cramping, vaginal candidiasis

Occasional
Nausea, serum sickness-like reaction
(marked by fever and joint pain;
usually occurs after the second
course of therapy and resolves after
the drug is discontinued)
Rare
Allergic reaction (rash, pruritus,
urticaria)

SERIOUS REACTIONS

• Antibiotic-associated colitis and
other superinfections may result
from altered bacterial balance.
• Nephrotoxicity may occur,
especially in patients with pre-
existing renal disease.
• Patients with a history of allergies, especially to penicillin, are at
increased risk for developing a
severe hypersensitivity reaction,
marked by severe pruritus,
angioedema, bronchospasm, and
anaphylaxis.

PRECAUTIONS & CONSIDERATIONS

Caution is warranted with hypersensitivity to penicillins or other drugs,
a history of GI disease (especially
antibiotic-associated colitis or ulcerative colitis), and liver or renal
impairment. Be aware that cefdinir
readily crosses the placenta and is
not detected in breast milk. Be aware
that infants and newborns may have
lower renal clearance of cefdinir. In
the elderly, age-related decreases in
renal function may require decreased
cefdinir dosage or increased dosing
interval.

Although mild GI effects may be
tolerable, an increase in their severity
may indicate the onset of antibiotic-
associated colitis. The mouth for
white patches on the mucous
membranes and tongue, pattern of
daily bowel activity and stool consistency, signs and symptoms of superinfection including abdominal pain,

moderate to severe diarrhea, severe
anal or genital pruritus, and severe
mouth soreness should be assessed.
Renal function should be assessed.
Storage
Store mixed suspension at room
temperature. Discard unused portion
after 10 days.
Administration
Take without regard to meals; if GI
upset occurs, give with food or milk.
To reconstitute oral suspension, for
the 60-ml bottle, add 39 ml water; for
the 120-ml bottle, add 65 ml water.
Shake oral suspension well before
administering. Continue therapy for
the full length of treatment and
evenly space doses around the clock.

Cefditoren
seff-di-tore'en
(Spectracef)

CATEGORY AND SCHEDULE
Pregnancy Risk Category: B

CLASSIFICATION
Antibiotics, cephalosporins

MECHANISM OF ACTION
A third-generation cephalosporin
that binds to bacterial cell
membranes and inhibits cell wall
synthesis. *Therapeutic effect:*
Bactericidal.

PHARMACOKINETICS
Moderately absorbed from the
gastrointestinal (GI) tract. Protein
binding: 88%. Not metabolized.
Excreted in the urine. Minimally
removed by hemodialysis. **Half-life:**
1.6 hrs (half-life increased with
impaired renal function).

AVAILABILITY
Tablets: 200 mg.

INDICATIONS AND DOSAGES
▶ **Pharyngitis, tonsillitis, skin infections**
PO
Adults, Elderly, Children older than 12 yr. 200 mg twice a day for 10 days.
▶ **Acute exacerbation of chronic bronchitis**
PO
Adults, Elderly, Children older than 12 yr. 400 mg twice a day for 10 days.
▶ **Community-acquired pneumonia**
PO
Adults, Elderly, Children older than 12 yr. 400 mg twice a day for 14 days.
▶ **Dosage in renal impairment**
Dosage and frequency are modified based on creatinine clearance.

Creatinine Clearance	Dosage
50-80 ml/min	No adjustment necessary.
30-49 ml/min	200 mg twice a day
Less than 30 ml/min	200 mg once a day

CONTRAINDICATIONS
Carnitive deficiency, inborn errors of metabolism, known allergy to cephalosporins, hypersensitivity to milk protein

INTERACTIONS
Drug
Antacids containing magnesium or aluminum, H_2 receptor antagonists: May decrease the absorption of cefditoren.
Probenecid: May increase the absorption of cefditoren.
Herbal
None known.

Food
High fat meals. Increase the cefditoren plasma concentration.

DIAGNOSTIC TEST EFFECTS
May cause a positive direct or indirect Coombs' test and a false-positive reaction to glycosuria.

SIDE EFFECTS
Occasional (11%)
Diarrhea
Rare (4%-1%)
Nausea, headache, abdominal pain, vaginal candidiasis, dyspepsia, vomiting

SERIOUS REACTIONS
• Antibiotic-associated colitis and other superinfections may occur.
• Patients with a history of allergies, especially to penicillin, are at increased risk for developing a severe hypersensitivity reaction, marked by severe pruritus, angioedema, bronchospasm, and anaphylaxis.

PRECAUTIONS & CONSIDERATIONS
Caution is warranted with allergies, renal impairment, a history of GI disease, and hypersensitivity to penicillins or other drugs. It is unknown if cefditoren is distributed in breast milk. The safety and efficacy of cefditoren have not been established in children younger than 12 years. Age-related renal impairment may require a dosage adjustment in the elderly.

Although mild GI effects may be tolerable, an increase in their severity may indicate the onset of antibiotic-associated colitis. The mouth for white patches on the mucous membranes and tongue, pattern of daily bowel activity and stool consistency, signs and symptoms of super-infection including abdominal pain, moderate to severe diarrhea, severe anal or genital pruritus, and severe mouth soreness should be assessed. Renal function should be assessed.

Administration

Take with meals to enhance drug absorption. Take for the full length of treatment. Do not skip doses.

Cefepime

sef′e-peem
(Maxipime)
Do not confuse with ceftidine.

CATEGORY AND SCHEDULE
Pregnancy Risk Category: B

CLASSIFICATION
Antibiotics, cephalosporins

MECHANISM OF ACTION
A fourth-generation cephalosporin that binds to bacterial cell membranes and inhibits cell wall synthesis. *Therapeutic Effect:* Bactericidal.

PHARMACOKINETICS
Well absorbed after IM administration. Protein binding: 20%. Widely distributed. Primarily excreted unchanged in urine. Removed by hemodialysis. **Half-life:** 2-2.3 hr (increased in impaired renal function, and in the elderly).

AVAILABILITY
Powder for Injection: 500 mg, 1 g, 2 g.

INDICATIONS AND DOSAGES
▶ **Pneumonia**
IV
Adults, Elderly. 1-2 g q12hr for 7-10 days.

Children 2 mo and older. 50 mg/kg q12hr. Maximum: 2 g/dose.
▶ **Intra-abdominal infections**
IV
Adults, Elderly. 2 g q12hr for 10 days.
▶ **Skin and skin structure infections**
IV
Adults, Elderly. 2 g q12hr for 10 days.
Children 2 mo and older. 50 mg/kg q12hr. Maximum: 2 g/dose.
▶ **UTIs**
IV
Adults, Elderly. 0.5-2 g q12hr for 7-10 days.
Children 2 mo and older. 50 mg/kg q12hr. Maximum: 2 g/dose.
▶ **Febrile neutropenia**
IV
Adults, Elderly. 2 g q8hr.
Children 2 mo and older. 50 mg/kg q8hr. Maximum: 2 g/dose.
▶ **Dosage in renal impairment**
Dosage and frequency are modified based on creatinine clearance and the severity of the infection.

Creatinine Clearance	Dose
30-60 ml/min	0.5-2 g q24hr
11-29 ml/min	0.5-1 g q24hr
10 ml/min or less	0.25-0.5 g q24hr

CONTRAINDICATIONS
History of anaphylactic reaction to penicillins or hypersensitivity to cephalosporins

INTERACTIONS
Drug
Probenecid: May increase cefepime blood concentration.
Herbal
None known.
Food
None known.

DIAGNOSTIC TEST EFFECTS
May increase serum alkaline phosphatase, bilirubin, LDH, AST (SGOT), and ALT (SGPT) levels. May cause a positive direct or indirect Coombs' test.

▒ IV INCOMPATIBILITIES
Acyclovir (Zovirax), amphotericin (Fungizone), cimetidine (Tagamet), ciprofloxacin (Cipro), cisplatin (Platinol), dacarbazine (DTIC), daunorubicin (Cerubidine), diazepam (Valium), diphenhydramine (Benadryl), dobutamine (Dobutrex), dopamine (Intropin), doxorubicin (Adriamycin), droperidol (Inapsine), famotidine (Pepcid), ganciclovir (Cytovene), haloperidol (Haldol), magnesium, magnesium sulfate, mannitol, meperidine (Demerol), metoclopramide (Reglan), morphine, ofloxacin (Floxin), ondansetron (Zofran), vancomycin (Vancocin)

▒ IV Compatibilities
Bumetanide (Bumex), calcium gluconate, furosemide (Lasix), hydromorphone (Dilaudid), lorazepam (Ativan), propofol (Diprivan)

SIDE EFFECTS
Frequent
Discomfort with IM administration, oral candidiasis, mild diarrhea, mild abdominal cramping, vaginal candidiasis
Occasional
Nausea, serum sickness-like reaction (marked by fever and joint pain; usually occurs after the second course of therapy and resolves after the drug is discontinued)
Rare
Allergic reaction (rash, pruritus, urticaria), thrombophlebitis (pain, redness, swelling at injection site)

SERIOUS REACTIONS
• Antibiotic-associated colitis manifested and other superinfections may result from altered bacterial balance.
• Nephrotoxicity may occur, especially in patients with pre-existing renal disease.
• Patients with a history of allergies, especially to penicillin, are at increased risk for developing a severe hypersensitivity reaction, marked by severe pruritus, angioedema, bronchospasm, and anaphylaxis.

PRECAUTIONS & CONSIDERATIONS
Caution is warranted with renal impairment. It is unknown if cefepime is distributed in breast milk. There are no age-related precautions noted in children older than 2 months. Age-related renal impairment may require dosage adjustment in the elderly.

Although mild GI effects may be tolerable, an increase in their severity may indicate the onset of antibiotic-associated colitis. The pattern of daily bowel activity and stool consistency, the mouth for white patches on the mucous membranes and tongue, signs and symptoms of superinfection including abdominal pain, moderate to severe diarrhea, severe anal or genital pruritus, and severe mouth soreness should be assessed. Renal function should be assessed.

Storage
Solution is stable for 24 hours at room temperature or 7 days if refrigerated.

Administration
For IM use, add 1.3 ml sterile water for injection, 0.9% NaCl, or D_5W to 500-mg vial (2.4 ml for 1-g and 2-g vials). To minimize the pain experienced by the patient, give IM

injection slowly and deeply into a large muscle mass (e.g., upper gluteus maximus) instead of the lateral aspect of the thigh.

For IV use, add 5 ml to 500-mg vial (10 ml for 1-g and 2-g vials). Further dilute with 50 to 100 ml 0.9% NaCl, or D$_5$W. For IV push, administer over 3 to 5 minutes. For intermittent IV infusion (piggyback), infuse over 30 minutes.

Cefixime
sef-ix'ime
(Suprax)
Do not confuse Suprax with Sporanox, Surbex, or Surfak.

CATEGORY AND SCHEDULE
Pregnancy Risk Category: B

CLASSIFICATION
Antibiotics, cephalosporins

MECHANISM OF ACTION
A third-generation cephalosporin that binds to bacterial cell membranes and inhibits cell wall synthesis. *Therapeutic Effect:* Bactericidal.

PHARMACOKINETICS
Moderately absorbed from the GI tract. Protein binding: 65%-70%. Widely distributed. Primarily excreted unchanged in urine. Minimally removed by hemodialysis. **Half-life:** 3-4 hr (increased in renal impairment).

AVAILABILITY
Oral Suspension: 100 mg/5 ml.
Tablets: 200 mg, 400 mg.

INDICATIONS AND DOSAGES
▸ **Otitis media, acute bronchitis, acute exacerbations of chronic bronchitis, pharyngitis, tonsillitis, and uncomplicated UTIs**
PO
Adults, Elderly, Children weighing more than 50 kg. 400 mg/day as a single dose or in 2 divided doses.
Children 6 mo-12 yr weighing less than 50 kg. 8 mg/kg/day as a single dose or in 2 divided doses.
Maximum: 400 mg.
▸ **Uncomplicated gonorrhea**
PO
Adults. 400 mg as a single dose.
▸ **Dosage in renal impairment**
Dosage is modified based on creatinine clearance.

Creatinine Clearance	% of Usual Dose
21-60 ml/min	75%
Less than 20 ml/min	50%

CONTRAINDICATIONS
History of anaphylactic reaction to penicillins, hypersensitivity to cephalosporins

INTERACTIONS
Drug
Probenecid: Increases serum concentration of cefixime.
Herbal
None known.
Food
None known.

DIAGNOSTIC TEST EFFECTS
May increase BUN and serum alkaline phosphatase, bilirubin, creatinine, AST (SGOT), and ALT (SGPT) levels. May increase LDH level. May cause a positive direct or indirect Coombs' test.

SIDE EFFECTS
Frequent
Oral candidiasis, mild diarrhea, mild abdominal cramping, vaginal candidiasis
Occasional
Nausea, serum sickness-like reaction (marked by arthralgia and fever; usually occurs after second course of therapy and resolves after drug is discontinued)
Rare
Allergic reaction (rash, pruritus, urticaria)

SERIOUS REACTIONS
• Antibiotic-associated colitis and other superinfections may result from altered bacterial balance.
• Nephrotoxicity may occur, especially in patients with pre-existing renal disease.
• Patients with a history of allergies, especially to penicillin, are at increased risk for developing a severe hypersensitivity reaction, marked by severe pruritus, angioedema, bronchospasm, and anaphylaxis.

PRECAUTIONS & CONSIDERATIONS
Caution is warranted with hypersensitivity to penicillin, history of gastrointestinal disease (particularly colitis), and renal impairment. Cefixime crosses the placenta. It is not known if it is distributed in the breast milk. There are no age-related precautions noted in children. Age-related renal impairment may require dose adjustment.

Stool changes, abdominal cramps, diarrhea, nausea, vomiting, headache, sore mouth or tongue may occur. If fever, skin itching, rash, or swelling occurs, notify the physician immediately.
Storage
Suspension is stable at room temperature or under refrigeration for 14 days.

Store tablets at room temperature.
Administration
For otitis media, give suspension only. Shake well before using. Take tablets or suspension with food if GI irritation occurs. Continue for the full length of treatment.

Cefoperazone
sef-oh-per'a-zone
(Aerosporin)

CATEGORY AND SCHEDULE
Pregnancy Risk Category: NR

CLASSIFICATION
Antibiotics, cephalosporins

MECHANISM OF ACTION
An antibiotic that alters cell membrane permeability in susceptible microorganisms. *Therapeutic Effect:* Bactericidal activity.

PHARMACOKINETICS
Negligible absorption. Protein binding: low. Excreted in urine. Poor removal in hemodialysis. **Half-life:** 6 hr.

AVAILABILITY
Powder: 500,000 (Aerosporin).

INDICATIONS AND DOSAGES
▸ **Mild to moderate infections**
IV
Adults, Elderly, Children 2 yr and older. 15,000-25,000 units/kg/day in divided doses q12hr.
Infants. Up to 40,000 units/kg/day.

IM
Adults, Elderly, Children 2 yr and older. 25,000-30,000 units/kg/day in divided doses q4-6hr.
Infants. Up to 40,000 units/kg/day.
Usual irrigation dosage
Continuous Bladder Irrigation
Adults, Elderly. 1 ml urogenital concentrate (contains 200,000 units polymyxin B, 57 mg neomycin) added to 1000 ml 0.9% NaCl. Give each 1000 ml >24 hrs for up to 10 days (may increase to 2000 ml/day when urine output >2 L/day).
Usual ophthalmic dosage
OPHTHALMIC
Adults, Elderly, Children. 1 drop q3-4hr.

CONTRAINDICATIONS
Hypersensitivity to polymyxin B or any component of the formulation

INTERACTIONS
Drug
Neuromuscular blocking agents or anesthetics: May produce muscle paralysis and prolonged or increased skeletal muscle relaxation.
Aminoglycosides, other nephrotoxic drugs: may increase nephrotoxicity.
Herbal
None known.
Food
None known.

DIAGNOSTIC TEST EFFECTS
None known.

🏵 IV INCOMPATIBILITIES
Acid solutions, alkali solutions, amphotericin B, calcium, cefazolin (Ancef), cephalothin (Keflin), cephapirin (Cefadyl), chloramphenicol (Chloromycetin), chlorothiazide (Diuril), cobalt, heparin, iron, magnesium, manganese, nitrofurantoin, prednisolone, tetracycline

🏵 IV Compatibilities
Acetylcysteine (Mucomyst), amikacin (Amikin), ascorbic acid, carbenicillin (Geocillin), cimetidine (Tagamet), diphenhydramine (Benadryl), erythromycin, hydrocortisone, kanamycin (Kantrex), lincomycin (Lincocin), penicillin G (Pfizerpen), phenobarbital (Luminal), procaine (Novocain), ranitidine (Zantac)

SIDE EFFECTS
Frequent
Severe pain, irritation at IM injection sites, phlebitis, thrombophlebitis with IV administration
Occasional
Fever, urticaria

SERIOUS REACTIONS
• Nephrotoxicity, especially with concurrent/sequential use of other nephrotoxic drugs, renal impairment, concurrent/sequential use of muscle relaxants.
• Superinfection, especially with fungi, may occur.

PRECAUTIONS & CONSIDERATIONS
Caution is warranted with a history of gastrointestinal (GI) disease especially antibiotic-associated colitis, ulcerative colitis, and renal or hepatic impairment. Cefoperazone readily crosses the placenta and is distributed in breast milk. There are no age-related precautions noted in children. Age-related renal impairment may require dosage adjustment in the elderly. History of allergies, particularly to cephalosporins and penicillins should be determined before beginning drug therapy. Alcohol and alcohol-containing preparations should be avoided during and for 72 hours after last dose of cefoperazone.

Be aware of signs of superinfection including abdominal pain, moderate to severe diarrhea, severe anal or genital pruritus, and severe mouth soreness.

Storage

Reconstituted solution with 0.9% NaCl or D$_5$W is stable for 24 hours at room temperature, 5 days when refrigerated, or 3 weeks when frozen. After freezing, thawed solution is stable for 48 hours at room temperature or 10 days when refrigerated.

Administration

Space drug doses evenly around the clock.

For IM injection, reconstitute by adding sterile water or bacteriostatic water for injection. Depending on dose, divide dose and give in separate IM sites. May administer smaller doses to avoid discomfort. Administer IM injections deeply into large muscle.

For IV injection, reconstitute with sterile water for injection, and further dilute in 50-100 ml 0.9% NaCl or D$_5$W and infuse over 15-30 minutes at maximum concentration of 50 mg/ml.

Cefotaxime

sef-oh-taks′eem

(Claforan)

Do not confuse cefotaxime with cefoxitin, ceftizoxime, cefuroxime, or Claritin.

CATEGORY AND SCHEDULE

Pregnancy Risk Category: B

CLASSIFICATION

Antibiotics, cephalosporins

MECHANISM OF ACTION

A third-generation cephalosporin that binds to bacterial cell membranes and inhibits cell wall synthesis. *Therapeutic Effect:* Bactericidal.

PHARMACOKINETICS

Widely distributed, including to CSF. Protein binding: 30%-50%. Partially metabolized in the liver to active metabolite. Primarily excreted in urine. Moderately removed by hemodialysis. **Half-life:** 1 hr (increased in impaired renal function).

AVAILABILITY

Powder for Injection: 500 mg, 1 g, 2 g.

INDICATIONS AND DOSAGES

▸ **Uncomplicated infections**

IV, IM

Adults, Elderly. 1 g q12hr.

▸ **Mild to moderate infections**

IV, IM

Adults, Elderly. 1-2 g q8hr.

▸ **Severe infections**

IV, IM

Adults, Elderly. 2 g q6-8hr.

▸ **Life-threatening infections**

IV, IM

Adults, Elderly. 2 g q4hr.

Children: 2 g q4hr. Maximum: 12 g/day.

▸ **Gonorrhea**

IM

Adults. (Male): 1 g as a single dose. (Female): 0.5 g as a single dose.

▸ **Perioperative prophylaxis**

IV, IM

Adults, Elderly. 1 g 30-90 min before surgery.

▸ **Cesarean section**

IV

Adults. 1 g as soon as umbilical cord is clamped, then 1 g 6 and 12 hr after first dose.

▸ **Usual pediatric dosage**
Children weighing 50 kg or more.
1-2 g q6-8hr.
Children 1 mo-12 yr weighing less than 50 kg. 100-200 mg/kg/day in divided doses q6-8hr.
▸ **Dosage in renal impairment**
For patients with creatinine clearance less than 20 ml/min give half of dose at usual dosing intervals.

OFF-LABEL USES
Treatment of Lyme disease

CONTRAINDICATIONS
History of anaphylactic reaction to penicillins or hypersensitivity to cephalosporins

INTERACTIONS
Drug
Probenecid: May increase cefotaxime blood concentration.
Herbal
None known.
Food
None known.

DIAGNOSTIC TEST EFFECTS
May increase liver function test results and produce a positive direct or indirect Coombs' test

🔲 IV INCOMPATIBILITIES
Allopurinol (Aloprim), filgrastim (Neupogen), fluconazole (Diflucan), hetastarch (Hespan), pentamidine (Pentam IV), vancomycin (Vancocin)
🔲 **IV Compatibilities**
Diltiazem (Cardizem), famotidine (Pepcid), hydromorphone (Dilaudid), lorazepam (Ativan), magnesium sulfate, midazolam (Versed), morphine, propofol (Diprivan)

SIDE EFFECTS
Frequent
Discomfort with IM administration, oral candidiasis, mild diarrhea, mild abdominal cramping, vaginal candidiasis
Occasional
Nausea, serum sickness-like reaction (marked by fever and joint pain; usually occurs after the second course of therapy and resolves after the drug is discontinued)
Rare
Allergic reaction (rash, pruritus, urticaria), thrombophlebitis (pain, redness, swelling at injection site)

SERIOUS REACTIONS
• Antibiotic-associated colitis and other superinfections may result from altered bacterial balance.
• Nephrotoxicity may occur, especially in patients with pre-existing renal disease.
• Patients with a history of allergies, especially to penicillin, are at increased risk for developing a severe hypersensitivity reaction, marked by severe pruritus, angioedema, bronchospasm, and anaphylaxis.

PRECAUTIONS & CONSIDERATIONS
Caution is warranted with history of GI disease (especially antibiotic-associated or ulcerative colitis) and renal impairment. Cefotaxime readily crosses the placenta and is distributed in the breast milk. There are no age-related precautions noted in children. Age-related renal impairment may require dosage adjustment in the elderly.
Although mild GI effects may be tolerable, an increase in their severity may indicate the onset of antibiotic-associated colitis. The pattern of daily bowel activity and stool consistency, the mouth for white patches on the mucous membranes and tongue, signs and symptoms of superinfection including abdominal pain, moderate to severe diarrhea,

severe anal or genital pruritus, and severe mouth soreness should be assessed. Renal function should be assessed.

Storage

The solution for IV use normally appears light yellow to amber. The IV infusion (piggyback) may become darker, but this doesn't affect potency. The IV infusion (piggyback) is stable for 24 hours at room temperature, and 5 days if refrigerated. Discard the solution if a precipitate forms.

Administration

For IV use, add 10 ml of sterile water for injection to each 500-mg, 1-g, or 2-g vial to provide a concentration of 50, 95, or 180 mg/ml, respectively. The resulting solution may be further diluted with 50 to 100 ml of 0.9% NaCl or D_5W. Administer the IV push over 3 to 5 minutes. Administer the intermittent IV infusion (piggyback) over 20 to 30 minutes.

For IM use, reconstitute the drug with sterile water for injection or bacteriostatic water for injection. Add 2, 3, or 5 ml to each 500-mg, 1-g, or 2-g vial, respectively, to yield a concentration of 230, 300, or 330 mg/ml, respectively. To minimize patient discomfort, slowly inject the drug deep into the gluteus maximus rather than the lateral aspect of the thigh. Administer a 2-g IM dose at two separate sites.

Cefotetan

sef'oh-tee-tan
(Cefotan)
Do not confuse cefotetan with cefoxitin or Ceftin.

CATEGORY AND SCHEDULE

Pregnancy Risk Category: B

CLASSIFICATION

Antibiotics, cephalosporins

MECHANISM OF ACTION

A second-generation cephalosporin that binds to bacterial cell membranes and inhibits cell wall synthesis. *Therapeutic Effect:* Bactericidal.

PHARMACOKINETICS

Protein binding: 78%-91%. Primarily excreted unchanged in urine. Minimally removed by hemodialysis. **Half-life:** 3-4.6 hr (increased in impaired renal function).

AVAILABILITY

Powder for Injection: 1 g, 2 g.

INDICATIONS AND DOSAGES

▸ **UTIs**
IV, IM
Adults, Elderly. 1-2 g in divided doses q12-24hr.
▸ **Mild to moderate infections**
IV, IM
Adults, Elderly. 1-2 g q12hr.
▸ **Severe infections**
IV, IM
Adults, Elderly. 2 g q12hr.
▸ **Life-threatening infections**
IV, IM
Adults, Elderly. 3 g q12hr.
▸ **Perioperative prophylaxis**
IV
Adults, Elderly. 1-2 g 30-60 min before surgery.

▶ **Cesarean section**
IV
Adults. 1-2 g as soon as umbilical cord is clamped.
▶ **Usual pediatric dosage**
Children. 40-80 mg/kg/day in divided doses q12hr. Maximum: 6 g/day.
▶ **Dosage in renal impairment**
Dosing frequency is modified based on creatinine clearance and the severity of the infection.

Creatinine Clearance	Dosage Interval
10-30 ml/min	Usual dose q24hr
Less than 10 ml/min	Usual dose q48hr

CONTRAINDICATIONS
History of anaphylactic reaction to penicillins or hypersensitivity to cephalosporins

INTERACTIONS
Drug
Alcohol: May produce a disulfiram-like reaction (facial flushing, headache, nausea, pruritus, tachycardia).
Heparin, other anticoagulants: May increase the risk of bleeding.
Herbal
None known.
Food
None known.

DIAGNOSTIC TEST EFFECTS
May increase BUN level and serum alkaline phosphatase, creatinine, AST (SGOT), and ALT (SGPT) levels. May prolong prothrombin time and produce a positive direct or indirect Coombs' test. Interferes with crossmatching procedures and hematologic tests.

IV INCOMPATIBILITIES
Vancomycin (Vancocin)

IV Compatibilities
Diltiazem (Cardizem), famotidine (Pepcid), heparin, insulin (regular), morphine, propofol (Diprivan)

SIDE EFFECTS
Frequent
Discomfort with IM administration, oral candidiasis, mild diarrhea, mild abdominal cramping, vaginal candidiasis
Occasional
Nausea, unusual bleeding or bruising, serum sickness-like reaction (marked by fever and joint pain; usually occurs after the second course of therapy and resolves after the drug is discontinued)
Rare
Allergic reaction (rash, pruritus, urticaria), thrombophlebitis (pain, redness, swelling at injection site)

SERIOUS REACTIONS
• Antibiotic-associated colitis and other superinfections may result from altered bacterial balance.
• Nephrotoxicity may occur, especially in patients with pre-existing renal disease.
• Patients with a history of allergies, especially to penicillin, are at increased risk for developing a severe hypersensitivity reaction, marked by severe pruritus, angioedema, bronchospasm, and anaphylaxis.

PRECAUTIONS & CONSIDERATIONS
Caution is warranted with history of GI disease (especially antibiotic-associated or ulcerative colitis), renal impairment, and concurrent use of nephrotoxic drugs. Cefotetan readily crosses the placenta and is distributed in the breast milk. The safety and efficacy have not been established in children. Age-related renal

impairment may require dosage adjustment in the elderly.

Although mild GI effects may be tolerable, an increase in their severity may indicate the onset of antibiotic-associated colitis. The pattern of daily bowel activity and stool consistency, the mouth for white patches on the mucous membranes and tongue, signs and symptoms of superinfection including abdominal pain, moderate to severe diarrhea, severe anal or genital pruritus, and severe mouth soreness should be assessed. Renal function should be assessed.

Storage

The solution normally appears colorless to light yellow. A deeper yellow does not indicate loss of potency. The IV infusion (piggyback) is stable for 24 hours at room temperature and 96 hours if refrigerated. Discard the solution if a precipitate forms.

Administration

! Give by IM injection, IV push, or intermittent IV infusion (piggyback) only.

For IV use, reconstitute each 1-g vial with 10 ml of sterile water for injection to provide a concentration of 95 mg/ml. The resulting solution may be further diluted with 50 to 100 ml of 0.9% NaCl or D$_5$W. Administer IV push over 3 to 5 minutes. Administer intermittent IV infusion (piggyback) over 20 to 30 minutes.

For IM use, add 2 ml of sterile water for injection or other appropriate diluent to each 1-g vial, or 3 ml to each 2-g vial, to provide a concentration of 400 mg/ml or 500 mg/ml, respectively. To minimize discomfort, slowly inject the drug deep into the gluteus maximus rather than the lateral aspect of thigh.

Cefoxitin
se-fox′i-tin
(Mefoxin)
Do not confuse cefoxitin with cefotaxime, cefotetan, or Cytoxan.

CATEGORY AND SCHEDULE
Pregnancy Risk Category: B

CLASSIFICATION
Antibiotics, cephalosporins

MECHANISM OF ACTION
A second-generation cephalosporin that binds to bacterial cell membranes and inhibits cell wall synthesis. *Therapeutic Effect:* Bactericidal.

AVAILABILITY
Powder for Injection: 1 g, 2 g.

INDICATIONS AND DOSAGES
▸ **Mild to moderate infections**
IV, IM
Adults, Elderly. 1-2 g q6-8hr.
▸ **Severe infections**
IV, IM
Adults, Elderly. 1 g q4hr or 2 g q6-8hr up to 2 g q4hr.
▸ **Uncomplicated gonorrhea**
IM
Adults. 2 g one time with 1 g probenecid.
▸ **Perioperative prophylaxis**
IV, IM
Adults, Elderly. 2 g 30-60 min before surgery, then q6hr for up to 24 hr after surgery.
Children older than 3 mo. 30-40 mg/kg 30-60 min before surgery, then q6hr for up to 24 hr after surgery.
▸ **Cesarean section**
IV
Adults. 2 g as soon as umbilical cord is clamped, then 2 g 4 and 8 hr

after first dose, then q6hr for up to 24 hr.

▶ **Usual pediatric dosage**
Children older than 3 mo.
80-160 mg/kg/day in 4-6 divided doses. Maximum: 12 g/day.
Neonates. 90-100 mg/kg/day in divided doses q6-8hr.

▶ **Dosage in renal impairment**
After a loading dose of 1-2 g, dosage and frequency are modified based on creatinine clearance and the severity of the infection.

Creatinine Clearance	Dosage
30-50 ml/min	1-2 g q8-12hr
10-29 ml/min	1-2 g q12-24hr
5-9 ml/min	500 mg-1 g q12-24hr
Less than 5 ml/min	500 mg-1 g q24-48hr

CONTRAINDICATIONS
History of anaphylactic reaction to penicillins or hypersensitivity to cephalosporins

INTERACTIONS
Drug
Probenecid: Increases serum concentration of cefoxitin.
Herbal
None known.
Food
None known.

DIAGNOSTIC TEST EFFECTS
May increase BUN level and serum alkaline phosphatase, creatinine, AST (SGOT), and ALT (SGPT) levels. May produce a positive direct or indirect Coombs' test. Interferes with crossmatching procedures and hematologic tests.

🖳 IV INCOMPATIBILITIES
Filgrastim (Neupogen), pentamidine (Pentam IV), vancomycin (Vancocin)

🖳 IV Compatibilities
Diltiazem (Cardizem), famotidine (Pepcid), heparin, hydromorphone (Dilaudid), magnesium sulfate, morphine, multivitamins, propofol (Diprivan)

SIDE EFFECTS
Frequent
Discomfort with IM administration, oral candidiasis, mild diarrhea, mild abdominal cramping, vaginal candidiasis
Occasional
Nausea, serum sickness-like reaction (marked by fever and joint pain; usually occurs after the second course of therapy and resolves after the drug is discontinued).
Rare
Allergic reaction (pruritus, rash, urticaria), thrombophlebitis (pain, redness, swelling at injection site)

SERIOUS REACTIONS
• Antibiotic-associated colitis and other superinfections may result from altered bacterial balance.
• Nephrotoxicity may occur, especially in patients with pre-existing renal disease.
• Patients with a history of allergies, especially to penicillin, are at increased risk for developing a severe hypersensitivity reaction, marked by severe pruritus, angioedema, bronchospasm, and anaphylaxis.

PRECAUTIONS & CONSIDERATIONS
Caution is warranted with history of GI disease (especially antibiotic-associated or ulcerative colitis), renal impairment, and concurrent use of nephrotoxic drugs.

Although mild GI effects may be tolerable, an increase in their severity may indicate the onset of antibiotic-associated colitis. The pattern of daily bowel activity and stool consistency, the mouth for white patches on the mucous membranes and tongue, signs and symptoms of superinfection including abdominal pain, moderate to severe diarrhea, severe anal or genital pruritus, and severe mouth soreness should be assessed. Renal function should be assessed.

Storage
The solution normally appears colorless to light amber; a darker color does not indicate loss of potency. The IV infusion (piggyback) is stable for 24 hours at room temperature and 48 hours if refrigerated. Discard the solution if a precipitate forms.

Administration
! Give by IM injection, intermittent IV infusion (piggyback), or IV push. Space doses evenly around the clock.

For IM use, reconstitute each 1-g vial with 2 ml of sterile water for injection or lidocaine to provide a concentration of 400 mg/ml. To minimize patient discomfort, slowly inject the drug deep into the gluteus maximus rather than the lateral aspect of the thigh.

For IV use, reconstitute each 1-g vial with 10 ml of sterile water for injection to provide a concentration of 95 mg/ml. The resulting solution may be further diluted with 50 to 100 ml of sterile water for injection, 0.9% NaCl, or D_5W. Administer IV push, administer over 3 to 5 minutes. Administer intermittent IV infusion (piggyback) over 15 to 30 minutes.

Cefpodoxime
sef-pod′ox-ime
(Vantin)
Do not confuse Vantin with Ventolin.

C

CATEGORY AND SCHEDULE
Pregnancy Risk Category: B

CLASSIFICATION
Antibiotics, cephalosporins

MECHANISM OF ACTION
A third-generation cephalosporin that binds to bacterial cell membranes and inhibits cell wall synthesis. *Therapeutic Effect:* Bactericidal.

PHARMACOKINETICS
Well absorbed from the GI tract (food increases absorption). Protein binding: 21%-40%. Widely distributed. Primarily excreted unchanged in urine. Partially removed by hemodialysis. **Half-life:** 2.3 hr (increased in impaired renal function and elderly patients).

AVAILABILITY
Oral Suspension: 50 mg/5 ml, 100 mg/5 ml.
Tablets: 100 mg, 200 mg.

INDICATIONS AND DOSAGES
▶ **Chronic bronchitis, pneumonia**
PO
Adults, Elderly, Children older than 13 yr. 200 mg q12hr for 10-14 days.
▶ **Gonorrhea, rectal gonococcal infection (female patients only)**
PO
Adults, Children older than 13 yr. 200 mg as a single dose.

▶ **Skin and skin-structure infections**
PO
Adults, Elderly, Children older than 13 yr. 400 mg q12hr for 7-14 days.
▶ **Pharyngitis, tonsillitis**
PO
Adults, Elderly, Children older than 13 yr. 100 mg q12hr for 5-10 days.
Children 6 mo-13 yr. 5 mg/kg q12hr for 5-10 days. Maximum: 100 mg/dose.
▶ **Acute maxillary sinusitis**
PO
Adults, Children older than 13 yr. 200 mg twice a day for 10 days.
Children 2 mo-13 yr. 5 mg/kg q12hr for 10 days. Maximum: 400 mg/day.
▶ **UTIs**
PO
Adults, Elderly, Children older than 13 yr. 100 mg q12hr for 7 days.
▶ **Acute otitis media**
PO
Children 6 mo-13 yr. 5 mg/kg q12hr for 5 days. Maximum: 400 mg/dose.
▶ **Dosage in renal impairment**
For patients with creatinine clearance less than 30 ml/min, usual dose is given q24hr. For patients on hemodialysis, usual dose is given 3 times/wk after dialysis.

CONTRAINDICATIONS
History of anaphylactic reaction to penicillins or hypersensitivity to cephalosporins

INTERACTIONS
Drug
Antacids, H$_2$ antagonists: May decrease cefpodoxime absorption.
Probenecid: May increase cefpodoxime blood concentration.
Herbal
None known.
Food
None known.

DIAGNOSTIC TEST EFFECTS
May increase BUN level and serum alkaline phosphatase, bilirubin, creatinine, LDH, AST (SGOT), and ALT (SGPT) levels. May produce a positive direct or indirect Coombs' test.

SIDE EFFECTS
Frequent
Oral candidiasis, mild diarrhea, mild abdominal cramping, vaginal candidiasis
Occasional
Nausea, serum sickness-like reaction (marked by fever and joint pain; usually occurs after the second course of therapy and resolves after the drug is discontinued)
Rare
Allergic reaction (pruritus, rash, urticaria)

SERIOUS REACTIONS
• Antibiotic-associated colitis and other superinfections may result from altered bacterial balance.
• Nephrotoxicity may occur, especially in patients with pre-existing renal disease.
• Patients with a history of allergies, especially to penicillin, are at increased risk for developing a severe hypersensitivity reaction, marked by severe pruritus, angioedema, bronchospasm, and anaphylaxis.

PRECAUTIONS & CONSIDERATIONS
Caution is warranted with history of GI disease (especially antibiotic-associated or ulcerative colitis), renal impairment, and concurrent use of nephrotoxic drugs. Cefpodoxime readily crosses the placenta and is distributed in breast milk. The safety and efficacy of cefpodoxime have not been established in children younger than 6 months. Age-related renal impairment may require a dosage adjustment in the elderly.

Although mild GI effects may be tolerable, an increase in their severity may indicate the onset of antibiotic-associated colitis. The pattern of daily bowel activity and stool consistency, the mouth for white patches on the mucous membranes and tongue, signs and symptoms of superinfection including abdominal pain, moderate to severe diarrhea, severe anal or genital pruritus, and severe mouth soreness should be assessed. Renal function should be assessed.

Storage

After reconstitution, the oral suspension is stable for 14 days if refrigerated.

Administration

Administer cefpodoxime with food to enhance drug absorption.

Cefprozil
sef-pro′zil
(Cefzil)
Do not confuse cefprozil with Cefazolin, Cefol, Ceftin, or Kefzol.

CATEGORY AND SCHEDULE
Pregnancy Risk Category: B

CLASSIFICATION
Antibiotics, cephalosporins

MECHANISM OF ACTION
A second-generation cephalosporin that binds to bacterial cell membranes and inhibits cell wall synthesis. *Therapeutic Effect:* Bactericidal.

PHARMACOKINETICS
Well absorbed from the GI tract. Protein binding: 36%-45%.

Widely distributed. Primarily excreted unchanged in urine. Moderately removed by hemodialysis. **Half-life:** 1.3 hr (increased in impaired renal function).

AVAILABILITY
Oral Suspension: 125 mg/5 ml, 250 mg/5 ml.
Tablets: 250 mg, 500 mg.

INDICATIONS AND DOSAGES
▸ **Pharyngitis, tonsillitis**
PO
Adults, Elderly. 500 mg q24hr for 10 days.
Children 2-12 yr. 7.5 mg/kg q12hr for 10 days.
▸ **Acute bacterial exacerbation of chronic bronchitis, secondary bacterial infection of acute bronchitis**
PO
Adults, Elderly. 500 mg q12hr for 10 days.
▸ **Skin and skin-structure infections**
PO
Adults, Elderly. 250-500 mg q12hr for 10 days.
Children. 20 mg/kg q24hr for 10 days.
▸ **Acute sinusitis**
PO
Adults, Elderly. 250-500 mg q12hr for 10 days.
Children 6 mo-12 yr. 7.5-15 mg/kg q12hr for 10 days.
▸ **Otitis media**
PO
Children 6 mo-12 yr. 15 mg/kg q12hr for 10 days. Maximum: 1 g/day.
▸ **Dosage in renal impairment**
Patients with creatinine clearance less than 30 ml/min receive 50% of usual dose at usual interval.

CONTRAINDICATIONS
History of anaphylactic reaction to penicillins or hypersensitivity to cephalosporins

INTERACTIONS
Drug
Probenecid: Increases serum concentration of cefprozil.
Herbal
None known.
Food
None known.

DIAGNOSTIC TEST EFFECTS
May increase liver function test results. May produce a positive direct or indirect Coombs' test. Interferes with crossmatching procedures and hematologic tests.

SIDE EFFECTS
Frequent
Oral candidiasis, mild diarrhea, mild abdominal cramping, vaginal candidiasis
Occasional
Nausea, serum sickness reaction (marked by fever and joint pain; usually occurs after the second course of therapy and resolves after the drug is discontinued)
Rare
Allergic reaction (pruritus, rash, urticaria)

SERIOUS REACTIONS
• Antibiotic-associated colitis and other superinfections may result from altered bacterial balance.
• Nephrotoxicity may occur, especially in patients with pre-existing renal disease.
• Patients with a history of allergies, especially to penicillin, are at increased risk for developing a severe hypersensitivity reaction, marked by severe pruritus, angioedema, bronchospasm, and anaphylaxis.

PRECAUTIONS & CONSIDERATIONS
Caution is warranted with history of GI disease (especially antibiotic-associated or ulcerative colitis), renal impairment, and concurrent use of nephrotoxic drugs. Cefprozil readily crosses the placenta and is distributed in breast milk. The safety and efficacy of cefprozil have not been established in children younger than 6 months. Age-related renal impairment may require a dosage adjustment in the elderly.

Although mild GI effects may be tolerable, an increase in their severity may indicate the onset of antibiotic-associated colitis. The pattern of daily bowel activity and stool consistency, the mouth for white patches on the mucous membranes and tongue, signs and symptoms of superinfection including abdominal pain, moderate to severe diarrhea, severe anal or genital pruritus, and severe mouth soreness should be assessed. Renal function should be assessed.

Storage
After reconstitution, the oral suspension is stable for 14 days if refrigerated.

Administration
Shake the oral suspension well before using. Take cefprozil without regard to meals; however, if GI upset occurs, give it with food or milk.

Ceftazidime
sef-taz'i-deem
(Ceptaz, Fortaz, Fortum [AUS], Tazicef, Tazidime)
Do not confuse ceftazidime with ceftizoxime.

CATEGORY AND SCHEDULE
Pregnancy Risk Category: B

CLASSIFICATION
Antibiotics, cephalosporins

MECHANISM OF ACTION
A third-generation cephalosporin that binds to bacterial cell membranes and inhibits cell wall synthesis. *Therapeutic Effect:* Bactericidal.

PHARMACOKINETICS
Widely distributed (including to CSF). Protein binding: 5%-17%. Primarily excreted unchanged in urine. Removed by hemodialysis. **Half-life:** 2 hr (increased in impaired renal function).

AVAILABILITY
Powder for Injection (Fortaz, Tazicef, Tazidime): 500 mg, 1 g, 2 g.

INDICATIONS AND DOSAGES
▸ **UTIs**
IV, IM
Adults. 250-500 mg q8-12hr.
▸ **Mild to moderate infections**
IV, IM
Adults. 1 g q8-12hr.
▸ **Uncomplicated pneumonia, skin and skin-structure infections**
IV, IM
Adults. 0.5-1 g q8hr.
▸ **Bone and joint infections**
IV, IM
Adults. 2 g q12hr.

▸ **Meningitis, serious gynecologic and intra-abdominal infections**
IV, IM
Adults. 2 g q8hr.
▸ **Pseudomonal pulmonary infections in patients with cystic fibrosis**
IV
Adults. 30-50 mg/kg q8hr. Maximum: 6 g/day.
▸ **Usual elderly dosage**
Elderly (normal renal function). 500 mg-1 g q12hr.
▸ **Usual pediatric dosage**
Children 1 mo-12 yr. 100-150 mg/kg/day in divided doses q8hr. Maximum: 6 g/day.
Neonates 0-4 wk. 100-150 mg/kg/day in divided doses q8-12hr.
▸ **Dosage in renal impairment**
After an initial 1-g dose, dosage and frequency are modified based on creatinine clearance and the severity of the infection.

Creatinine Clearance	Dosage
30-50 ml/min	1 g q12hr
16-30 ml/min	1 g q24hr
6-15 ml/min	500 mg q24hr
Less than 5 ml/min	500 mg q48hr

CONTRAINDICATIONS
History of anaphylactic reaction to penicillins or hypersensitivity to cephalosporins

INTERACTIONS
Drug
None known.
Herbal
None known.
Food
None known.

DIAGNOSTIC TEST EFFECTS
May increase BUN level and serum alkaline phosphatase, creatinine, LDH, AST (SGOT), and ALT (SGPT) levels. May produce a

positive direct or indirect Coombs' test. Interferes with crossmatching procedures and hematologic tests.

▓ IV INCOMPATIBILITIES

Amphotericin B complex (AmBisome, Amphotec, Abelcet), doxorubicin liposomal (Doxil), fluconazole (Diflucan), idarubicin (Idamycin), midazolam (Versed), pentamidine (Pentam IV), vancomycin (Vancocin)

▓ IV Compatibilities

Diltiazem (Cardizem), famotidine (Pepcid), heparin, hydromorphone (Dilaudid), morphine, propofol (Diprivan)

SIDE EFFECTS

Frequent
Discomfort with IM administration, oral candidiasis, mild diarrhea, mild abdominal cramping, vaginal candidiasis
Occasional
Nausea, serum sickness-like reaction (marked by fever and joint pain; usually occurs after the second course of therapy and resolves after the drug is discontinued)
Rare
Allergic reaction (pruritus, rash, urticaria), thrombophlebitis (pain, redness, swelling at injection site)

SERIOUS REACTIONS

• Antibiotic-associated colitis and other superinfections may result from altered bacterial balance.
• Nephrotoxicity may occur, especially in patients with pre-existing renal disease.
• Patients with a history of allergies, especially to penicillin, are at increased risk for developing a severe hypersensitivity reaction, marked by severe pruritus, angioedema, bronchospasm, and anaphylaxis.

PRECAUTIONS & CONSIDERATIONS

Caution is warranted with history of GI disease (especially antibiotic-associated or ulcerative colitis), renal impairment, and concurrent use of nephrotoxic drugs. Ceftazidime readily crosses the placenta and is distributed in breast milk. No age-related precautions have been noted in children. Age-related renal impairment may require a dosage adjustment in the elderly.

Although mild GI effects may be tolerable, an increase in their severity may indicate the onset of antibiotic-associated colitis. The pattern of daily bowel activity and stool consistency, the mouth for white patches on the mucous membranes and tongue, signs and symptoms of superinfection including abdominal pain, moderate to severe diarrhea, severe anal or genital pruritus, and severe mouth soreness should be assessed. Renal function should be assessed.

Storage
The solution normally appears light yellow to amber, but tends to darken; color change does not indicate loss of potency. The IV infusion (piggyback) is stable for 18 hours at room temperature and 7 days if refrigerated. Discard the solution if a precipitate forms.

Administration
! Give ceftazidime by IM injection, direct IV injection, or intermittent IV infusion (piggyback).

For IV use, add 10 ml of sterile water for injection to each 1-g vial to provide a concentration of 90 mg/ml. The resulting solution may be further diluted with 50 to 100 ml of 0.9% NaCl, D_5W, or another compatible diluent. Administer IV push over 3 to 5 minutes. Administer intermittent IV infusion (piggyback) over 15 to 30 minutes.

For IM use, to reconstitute, add 1.5 ml of sterile water for injection or lidocaine 1% to 500-mg vial, if prescribed, or 3 ml to 1-g vial to provide a concentration of 280 mg/ml. To minimize patient discomfort, slowly inject the drug deep into the gluteus maximus rather than the lateral aspect of the thigh.

Ceftibuten
cef'te-bute-in
(Cedax)

CATEGORY AND SCHEDULE
Pregnancy Risk Category: B

CLASSIFICATION
Antibiotics, cephalosporins

MECHANISM OF ACTION
A third-generation cephalosporin that binds to bacterial cell membranes and inhibits cell wall synthesis. *Therapeutic Effect:* Bactericidal.

PHARMACOKINETICS
Rapidly absorbed from the gastrointestinal tract. Excreted primarily in urine. **Half-Life:** 2-3hr.

AVAILABILITY
Capsules: 400 mg.
Oral Suspension: 90 mg/5 ml.

INDICATIONS AND DOSAGES
▶ **Chronic bronchitis**
PO
Adults, Elderly. 400 mg/day once a day for 10 days.
▶ **Pharyngitis, tonsillitis**
PO
Adults, Elderly. 400 mg once a day for 10 days.

Children older than 6 mo. 9 mg/kg once a day for 10 days. Maximum: 400 mg/day.
▶ **Otitis media**
PO
Children older than 6 mo. 9 mg/kg once a day for 10 days. Maximum: 400 mg/day.
▶ **Dosage in renal impairment**
Dosage is modified based on creatinine clearance.

Creatinine Clearance	Dosage
50 ml/min and higher	400 mg or 9 mg/kg q24hr
30-49 ml/min	200 mg or 4.5 mg/kg q24hr
Less than 30 ml/min	100 mg or 2.25 mg/kg q24hr

CONTRAINDICATIONS
History of anaphylactic reaction to penicillins or hypersensitivity to cephalosporins

INTERACTIONS
Drug
Aminoglycosides: Increased risk of nephrotoxicity.
Probenecid: Increases serum ceftibuten level.
Herbal
None known.
Food
None known.

DIAGNOSTIC TEST EFFECTS
May increase BUN level and serum alkaline phosphatase, bilirubin, creatinine, LDH, AST (SGOT), and ALT (SGPT) levels. May produce a positive direct or indirect Coombs' test.

SIDE EFFECTS
Frequent
Oral candidiasis, mild diarrhea (discharge, itching)

Occasional
Nausea, serum sickness-like reaction (marked by fever and joint pain; usually occurs after the second course of therapy and resolves after the drug is discontinued)
Rare
Allergic reaction (rash, pruritus, urticaria)

SERIOUS REACTIONS

• Antibiotic-associated colitis and other superinfections may result from altered bacterial balance.
• Nephrotoxicity may occur, especially in patients with pre-existing renal disease.
• Patients with a history of allergies, especially to penicillin, are at increased risk for developing a severe hypersensitivity reaction, marked by severe pruritus, angioedema, bronchospasm, and anaphylaxis.

PRECAUTIONS & CONSIDERATIONS

Caution is warranted with history of GI disease (especially antibiotic-associated or ulcerative colitis), renal impairment, and allergies to peni-cillins or other drugs.

Although mild GI effects may be tolerable, an increase in their severity may indicate the onset of antibiotic-associated colitis. The pattern of daily bowel activity and stool consis-tency, the mouth for white patches on the mucous membranes and tongue, signs and symptoms of superinfection including abdominal pain, moderate to severe diarrhea, severe anal or genital pruritus, and severe mouth soreness should be assessed. Renal function should be assessed.

Administration
! Use oral suspension when treating otitis media to achieve higher peak blood levels.

Take with food or milk if GI upset occurs. Take full course of treatment and space drug doses evenly around the clock.

Ceftizoxime
sef-ti-zox'eem
(Cefizox)
Do not confuse ceftizoxime with cefotaxime or ceftazidime.

CATEGORY AND SCHEDULE
Pregnancy Risk Category: B

CLASSIFICATION
Antibiotics, cephalosporins

MECHANISM OF ACTION
A third-generation cephalosporin that binds to bacterial cell membranes and inhibits cell wall synthesis. *Therapeutic Effect:* Bactericidal.

PHARMACOKINETICS
Widely distributed (including to CSF). Protein binding: 30%. Primarily excreted unchanged in urine. Moderately removed by hemodialysis. **Half-life:** 1.7 hr (increased in impaired renal function).

AVAILABILITY
Powder for Injection: 500 mg, 1 g, 2 g.

INDICATIONS AND DOSAGES
▶ **Uncomplicated UTIs**
IV, IM
Adults, Elderly. 500 mg q12hr.
▶ **Mild, moderate, or severe infec-tions of the biliary, respiratory, and GU tracts; skin, bone, and**

intra-abdominal infections; meningitis; and septicemia
IV, IM
Adults, Elderly. 1-2 g q8-12hr.
▶ **Life-threatening infections of the biliary, respiratory, and GU tracts; skin, bone and intra-abdominal infections; meningitis; and septicemia**
IV
Adults, Elderly. 3-4 g q8hr, up to 2 g q4hr.
▶ **Pelvic inflammatory disease (PID)**
IV
Adults. 2 g q4-8hr.
▶ **Uncomplicated gonorrhea**
IM
Adults. 1 g one time.
▶ **Usual pediatric dosage**
Children older than 6 mo: 50 mg/kg q6-8hr. Maximum: 12 g/day.
▶ **Dosage in renal impairment**
After a loading dose of 0.5-1 g, dosage and frequency are modified based creatinine clearance and the severity of the infection.

Creatinine Clearance	Dosage
50-79 ml/min	0.5 g-1.5 g q8hr
5-49 ml/min	0.25 g-1 g q12hr
Less than 5 ml/min	0.25-0.5 g q24hr or 0.5 g-1 g q48hr

CONTRAINDICATIONS
History of anaphylactic reaction to penicillins or hypersensitivity to cephalosporins

INTERACTIONS
Drug
Probenecid: Increases serum concentration of ceftizoxime.
Herbal
None known.
Food
None known.

DIAGNOSTIC TEST EFFECTS
May increase BUN level and serum alkaline serum phosphatase, creatinine, AST (SGOT), and ALT (SGPT) levels. May produce a positive direct or indirect Coombs' test.

▨ IV INCOMPATIBILITIES
Filgrastim (Neupogen)
▨ IV Compatibilities
Hydromorphone (Dilaudid), morphine, propofol (Diprivan)

SIDE EFFECTS
Frequent
Discomfort with IM administration, oral candidiasis, mild diarrhea, mild abdominal cramping, vaginal candidiasis
Occasional
Nausea, serum sickness-like reaction (fever, joint pain; usually occurs after the second course of therapy and resolves after the drug is discontinued)
Rare
Allergic reaction (rash, pruritus, urticaria), thrombophlebitis (pain, redness, swelling at injection site)

SERIOUS REACTIONS
• Antibiotic-associated colitis manifested and other superinfections may result from altered bacterial balance.
• Nephrotoxicity may occur, especially in patients with pre-existing renal disease.
• Patients with a history of allergies, especially to penicillin, are at increased risk for developing a severe hypersensitivity reaction, marked by severe pruritus, angioedema, bronchospasm, and anaphylaxis.

PRECAUTIONS & CONSIDERATIONS
Caution is warranted with history of GI disease (especially antibiotic-associated or ulcerative colitis) and

hepatic or renal impairment. Ceftizoxime readily crosses the placenta and is distributed in breast milk. Ceftizoxime use in children is associated with transient elevations of blood eosinophil count and serum CK, AST (SGOT), and ALT (SGPT) levels. Age-related renal impairment may require a dosage adjustment in the elderly.

Although mild GI effects may be tolerable, an increase in their severity may indicate the onset of antibiotic-associated colitis. The pattern of daily bowel activity and stool consistency, the mouth for white patches on the mucous membranes and tongue, signs and symptoms of superinfection including abdominal pain, moderate to severe diarrhea, severe anal or genital pruritus, and severe mouth soreness should be assessed. Renal function should be assessed.

Storage

The solution normally appears clear to pale yellow. A change from yellow to amber does not indicate loss of potency. The IV infusion (piggyback) is stable for 24 hours at room temperature and 96 hours if refrigerated. Discard the solution if a precipitate forms.

Administration

For IV use, to reconstitute, add 5 ml of sterile water for injection to each 0.5-g vial to provide a concentration of 95 mg/ml. The resulting solution may be further diluted with 50 to 100 ml of 0.9% NaCl, D_5W, or another compatible fluid. Administer IV push over 3 to 5 minutes. Infuse intermittent IV infusion (piggyback) over 15 to 30 minutes.

For IM use, add 1.5 ml of sterile water for injection to each 0.5-g vial to provide a concentration of 270 mg/ml. Give deep IM injections slowly to minimize patient discomfort.

When giving a 2-g dose, divide the dose and give in different large muscle masses.

Ceftriaxone
sef-try-ax'one
(Rocephin)

CATEGORY AND SCHEDULE
Pregnancy Risk Category: B

CLASSIFICATION
Antibiotics, cephalosporins

MECHANISM OF ACTION
A third-generation cephalosporin that binds to bacterial cell membranes and inhibits cell wall synthesis. *Therapeutic Effect:* Bactericidal.

PHARMACOKINETICS
Widely distributed (including to CSF). Protein binding: 83%-96%. Primarily excreted unchanged in urine. Not removed by hemodialysis. **Half-life:** 4.3-4.6 hr IV; 5.8-8.7 hr IM (increased in impaired renal function).

AVAILABILITY
Powder for Injection: 250 mg, 500 mg, 1 g, 2 g.

INDICATIONS AND DOSAGES
▸ **Mild to moderate infections**
IV, IM
Adults, Elderly. 1-2 g as a single dose or in 2 divided doses.
▸ **Serious infections**
IV, IM
Adults, Elderly. Up to 4 g/day in 2 divided doses.

Children. 50-75 mg/kg/day in divided doses q12hr. Maximum: 2 g/day.
▸ **Skin and skin-structure infections**
IV, IM
Children. 50-75 mg/kg/day as a single dose or in 2 divided doses. Maximum: 2 g/day.
▸ **Meningitis**
IV
Children. Initially, 75 mg/kg, then 100 mg/kg/day as a single dose or in divided doses q12hr. Maximum: 4 g/day.
▸ **Lyme disease**
IV
Adults, Elderly. 2-4 g a day for 10-14 days.
▸ **Acute bacterial otitis media**
IM
Children. 50 mg/kg once a day for 3 days. Maximum: 1 g/day.
▸ **Perioperative prophylaxis**
IV, IM
Adults, Elderly. 1 g 0.5-2 hrs before surgery.
▸ **Uncomplicated gonorrhea**
IM
Adults. 250 mg plus doxycycline one time.
▸ **Dosage in renal impairment**
Dosage modification is usually unnecessary but liver and renal function test results should be monitored in those with both renal and liver impairment or severe renal impairment.

CONTRAINDICATIONS
History of anaphylactic reaction to penicillins or hypersensitivity to cephalosporins

INTERACTIONS
Drug
None known.
Herbal
None known.
Food
None known.

DIAGNOSTIC TEST EFFECTS
May increase BUN level and serum alkaline phosphatase, bilirubin, creatinine, AST (SGOT), and ALT (SGPT) levels. May produce a positive direct or indirect Coombs' test. Interferes with crossmatching procedures and hematologic tests.

▨ IV INCOMPATIBILITIES
Aminophylline, amphotericin B complex (AmBisome, Amphotec, Abelcet), filgrastim (Neupogen), fluconazole (Diflucan), labetalol (Normodyne), pentamidine (Pentam IV), vancomycin (Vancocin)
▨ IV Compatibilities
Diltiazem (Cardizem), heparin, lidocaine, morphine, propofol (Diprivan)

SIDE EFFECTS
Frequent
Discomfort with IM administration, oral candidiasis, mild diarrhea, mild abdominal cramping, vaginal candidiasis
Occasional
Nausea, serum sickness-like reaction (marked by fever and joint pain; usually occurs after the second course of therapy and resolves after the drug is discontinued)
Rare
Allergic reaction (rash, pruritus, urticaria), thrombophlebitis (pain, redness, swelling at injection site)

SERIOUS REACTIONS
• Antibiotic-associated colitis and other superinfections may result from altered bacterial balance.
• Nephrotoxicity may occur, especially in patients with pre-existing renal disease.
• Patients with a history of allergies, especially to penicillin, are at increased risk for developing a severe hypersensitivity reaction, marked by severe pruritus,

angioedema, bronchospasm, and
anaphylaxis.

Caution is warranted with history of
GI disease (especially antibiotic-
associated or ulcerative colitis),
hepatic or renal impairment, and
concurrent use of nephrotoxic drugs.
Ceftriaxone readily crosses the
placenta and is distributed in breast
milk. Ceftriaxone use in children
may displace serum bilirubin from
serum albumin. Use ceftriaxone
cautiously in neonates, who may
become hyperbilirubinemic. Age-
related renal impairment may require
a dosage adjustment in the elderly.

Although mild GI effects may be
tolerable, an increase in their severity
may indicate the onset of antibiotic-
associated colitis. The pattern of
daily bowel activity and stool consistency, the mouth for white patches on
the mucous membranes and tongue,
signs and symptoms of superinfection including abdominal pain,
moderate to severe diarrhea, severe
anal or genital pruritus, and severe
mouth soreness should be assessed.
Renal function should be assessed.

Storage
The solution normally appears light
yellow to amber. The IV infusion
(piggyback) is stable for 3 days at
room temperature and 10 days if
refrigerated. Discard the solution if a
precipitate forms.

Administration
For IV use, add 2.4 ml of sterile
water for injection to each 250-mg
vial, 4.8 ml to each 500-mg vial,
9.6 ml to each 1-g vial, and 19.2 ml
to each 2-g vial to provide a concentration of 100 mg/ml. The resulting
solution may be further diluted with
50 to 100 ml of 0.9% NaCl or D_5W.
Infuse the intermittent IV infusion
(piggyback) over 15 to 30 minutes

for adults and over 10 to 30 minutes
for children or neonates. Alternate
IV sites and use large veins to
reduce the risk of phlebitis.

For IM use, add 0.9 ml of sterile
water for injection, 0.9% NaCl,
D_5W, bacteriostatic water and 0.9%
benzyl alcohol, or lidocaine to each
250-mg vial, 1.8 ml to each 500-mg
vial, 3.6 ml to each 1-g vial, and
7.2 ml to each 2-g vial to provide a
concentration of 250 mg/ml. To
minimize patient discomfort, slowly
inject the drug deep into the gluteus
maximus rather than the lateral
aspect of the thigh.

Cefuroxime
sef-yoor-ox′eem
(Ceftin, Zinnat [AUS]) (Kefurox,
Zinacef)
**Do not confuse cefuroxime
with cefotaxime, Cefzil, or
deferoxamine.**

CATEGORY AND SCHEDULE
Pregnancy Risk Category: B

CLASSIFICATION
Antibiotics, cephalosporins

MECHANISM OF ACTION
A second-generation cephalosporin
that binds to bacterial cell membranes
and inhibits cell wall synthesis.
Therapeutic Effect: Bactericidal.

PHARMACOKINETICS
Rapidly absorbed from the GI tract.
Protein binding: 33%-50%. Widely
distributed (including to CSF).
Primarily excreted unchanged in
urine. Moderately removed by
hemodialysis. **Half-life:** 1.3 hr

(increased in impaired renal function).

AVAILABILITY
Oral Suspension: 125 mg/5 ml, 250 mg/5 ml.
Tablets: 250 mg, 500 mg.
Powder for Injection: 750 mg, 1.5 g.

INDICATIONS AND DOSAGES
▸ **Ampicillin-resistant influenza; bacterial meningitis; early Lyme disease; GU tract, gynecologic, skin, and bone infections; septicemia; gonorrhea, and other gonococcal infections**
IV, IM
Adults, Elderly. 750 mg-1.5 g q8hr.
Children. 75-100 mg/kg/day divided q8hr. Maximum: 8 g/day.
Neonates. 50-100 mg/kg/day divided q12hr.
PO
Adults, Elderly. 125-500 mg twice a day, depending on the infection.
▸ **Pharyngitis, tonsillitis**
PO
Children 3 mo-12 yr. 125 mg (tablets) q12hr or 20 mg/kg/day (suspension) in 2 divided doses.
▸ **Acute otitis media, acute bacterial maxillary sinusitis, impetigo**
PO
Children 3 mo-12 yr. 250 mg (tablets) q12hr or 30 mg/kg/day (suspension) in 2 divided doses.
▸ **Bacterial meningitis**
IV
Children 3 mo-12 yr. 200-240 mg/kg/day in divided doses q6-8hr.
▸ **Perioperative prophylaxis**
IV
Adults, Elderly. 1.5 g 30-60 min before surgery and 750 mg q8hr after surgery.
▸ **Usual neonatal dosage**
IV, IM
Neonates. 20-100 mg/kg/day in divided doses q12hr.

▸ **Dosage in renal impairment**
Adult dosage and frequency are modified based on creatinine clearance and the severity of the infection.

Creatinine Clearance	Dosage
Greater than 20 ml/min	750 mg-1 g q8hr
10-20 ml/min	750 mg q12hr
Less than 10 ml/min	750 mg q24hr

CONTRAINDICATIONS
History of anaphylactic reaction to penicillins or hypersensitivity to cephalosporins

INTERACTIONS
Drug
Probenecid: Increases serum concentration of cefuroxime.
Herbal
None known.
Food
None known.

DIAGNOSTIC TEST EFFECTS
May increase serum alkaline phosphatase, bilirubin, LDH, AST (SGOT), and ALT (SGPT) levels. May produce a positive direct or indirect Coombs' test. Interferes with crossmatching procedures, hematologic tests.

▦ IV INCOMPATIBILITIES
Filgrastim (Neupogen), fluconazole (Diflucan), midazolam (Versed), vancomycin (Vancocin)
▦ IV Compatibilities
Diltiazem (Cardizem), hydromorphone (Dilaudid), morphine, propofol (Diprivan)

SIDE EFFECTS
Frequent
Discomfort with IM administration, oral candidiasis, mild diarrhea, mild

abdominal cramping, vaginal candidiasis

Occasional

Nausea, serum sickness-like reaction (marked by fever and joint pain; usually occurs after the second course of therapy and resolves after the drug is discontinued)

Rare

Allergic reaction (rash, pruritus, urticaria), thrombophlebitis (pain, redness, swelling at injection site)

SERIOUS REACTIONS

• Antibiotic-associated colitis and other superinfections may result from altered bacterial balance.

• Nephrotoxicity may occur, especially in patients with pre-existing renal disease.

• Patients with a history of allergies, especially to penicillin, are at increased risk for developing a severe hypersensitivity reaction, marked by severe pruritus, angioedema, bronchospasm, and anaphylaxis.

PRECAUTIONS & CONSIDERATIONS

Caution is warranted with history of GI disease (especially antibiotic-associated or ulcerative colitis), renal impairment, and concurrent use of nephrotoxic drugs. Cefuroxime readily crosses the placenta and is distributed in breast milk. No age-related precautions have been noted in children. Age-related renal impairment may require a dosage adjustment in the elderly.

Although mild GI effects may be tolerable, an increase in their severity may indicate the onset of antibiotic-associated colitis. The pattern of daily bowel activity and stool consistency, the mouth for white patches on the mucous membranes and tongue, signs and symptoms of superinfection including

abdominal pain, moderate to severe diarrhea, severe anal or genital pruritus, and severe mouth soreness should be assessed. Renal function should be assessed.

Storage

The solution normally appears light yellow to amber; a darker color does not indicate loss of potency. The IV infusion (piggyback) is stable for 24 hours at room temperature and 7 days if refrigerated. Discard the solution if a precipitate forms.

Administration

Take cefuroxime tablets without regard to food. However, if GI upset occurs, give with food or milk. Avoid crushing tablets because they have a bitter taste. Give the oral suspension with food.

For IV use, to reconstitute, add 8 ml of sterile water for injection to each 750-mg vial, or 14 ml to each 1.5-g vial to provide a concentration of 100 mg/ml. For intermittent IV infusion (piggyback), further dilute with 50 to 100 ml of 0.9% NaCl or D_5W. Administer the IV push over 3 to 5 minutes. Infuse the intermittent IV infusion (piggyback) over 15 to 60 minutes.

For IM use, to minimize patient discomfort, slowly inject the drug deep into the gluteus maximus rather than the lateral aspect of the thigh.

Celecoxib

sel-eh-cox′ib

(Celebrex, DisperDose, Panixine)

Do not confuse with Celebrex, Cerebyx, or Celexa.

CATEGORY AND SCHEDULE

Pregnancy Risk Category: C (D if used in third trimester or near delivery)

CLASSIFICATION

Analgesics, non-narcotic, COX-2 inhibitors, nonsteroidal anti-inflammatory drugs

MECHANISM OF ACTION

An NSAID that inhibits cyclo-oxygenase-2, the enzyme responsible for prostaglandin synthesis. Mechanism of action in treating familial adenomatous polyposis is unknown. *Therapeutic Effect:* Reduces inflammation and relieves pain.

PHARMACOKINETICS

Widely distributed. Protein binding: 97%. Metabolized in the liver. Primarily eliminated in feces. **Half-life:** 11.2 hr.

AVAILABILITY

Capsules: 100 mg, 200 mg, 400 mg.

INDICATIONS AND DOSAGES

▸ **Osteoarthritis**

PO

Adults, Elderly. 200 mg/day as a single dose or 100 mg twice a day.

▸ **Rheumatoid arthritis**

PO

Adults, Elderly. 100-200 mg twice a day.

▸ **Acute pain**

PO

Adults, Elderly. Initially, 400 mg with additional 200 mg on day 1, if needed. Maintenance: 200 mg twice a day as needed.

▸ **Familial adenomatous polyposis**

PO

Adults, Elderly. 400 mg twice daily (with food).

CONTRAINDICATIONS

Hypersensitivity to aspirin, NSAIDs, or sulfonamides

INTERACTIONS

Drug

Fluconazole: May increase celecoxib blood level.

Lithium: May increase lithium blood levels.

Warfarin: May increase the risk of bleeding.

Herbal

None known.

Food

None known.

DIAGNOSTIC TEST EFFECTS

May increase AST (SGOT) and ALT (SGPT) levels.

SIDE EFFECTS

Frequent (greater than 5%)

Diarrhea, dyspepsia, headache, upper respiratory tract infection

Occasional (5%-1%)

Abdominal pain, flatulence, nausea, back pain, peripheral edema, dizziness, rash

SERIOUS REACTIONS

• None known.

PRECAUTIONS & CONSIDERATIONS

Be aware of the potential for increased risk of cardiovascular events and gastrointestinal bleeding associated with celecoxib use. Caution is warranted with smokers, active alcoholism, history of peptic ulcer disease, and receiving anticoagulant or steroid therapy, and in the elderly. It is unknown if celecoxib crosses the placenta or is distributed in breast milk. Celecoxib should not be used during the third trimester of pregnancy because it may cause adverse effects in the fetus, such as premature closure of the ductus arteriosus. The safety and efficacy of celecoxib have not been established in children younger than 18 years. No age-related precautions have been noted in the elderly. Alcohol and aspirin should be avoided during celecoxib therapy because these substances increase the risk of GI bleeding.

Therapeutic response, such as decreased pain, stiffness, swelling, and tenderness, improved grip strength, and increased joint mobility, should be evaluated.

Administration
Take celecoxib without regard to food. If GI upset occurs, take celecoxib with food. Don't crush or break capsules.

Cellulose Sodium Phosphate
(Calcibind)
Do not confuse with cellulite.

CATEGORY AND SCHEDULE
Pregnancy Risk Category: C

CLASSIFICATION
Metabolics

MECHANISM OF ACTION
A nonabsorbable compound that alters urinary composition of calcium, magnesium, phosphate, and oxalate. Calcium binds to cellulose sodium phosphate therefore preventing intestinal absorption of it. *Therapeutic Effect:* Prevents the formation of kidney stones.

PHARMACOKINETICS
Not absorbed from gastrointestinal (GI) tract. Eliminated in the feces.

AVAILABILITY
Powder for reconstitution: 300 g (Calcibind).

INDICATIONS AND DOSAGES
▸ **Absorptive hypercalciuria Type I**
Acute bleeding
PO
Adults, Elderly. Initially, 15 g/day (5 g with each meal). Decrease dosage to 10 g/day when urinary calcium is less than 150 mg/day.

OFF-LABEL USES
Absorptive hypercalciuria Type II

CONTRAINDICATIONS
Primary or secondary hyperparathyroidism, including renal hypercalciuria (renal calcium leak), hypomagnesemic states (serum magnesium <1.5 mg/dl), bone disease (osteoporosis, osteomalacia, osteitis), hypocalcemic states (e.g., hypoparathyroidism, intestinal malabsorption), normal or low intestinal absorption and renal excretion of calcium, enteric hyperoxaluria, and patients with high fasting urinary calcium or hypophosphatemia.

INTERACTIONS
Drug
Calcium-containing medications: May decrease effectiveness of cellulose sodium phosphate.
Magnesium: May decrease effectiveness of magnesium.

Herbal
None known.
Food
Milk, dairy products: May
decrease effectiveness of cellulose
sodium phosphate.
**Foods high in oxalate (spinach,
rhubarb, chocolate, brewed tea):**
May increase risk of hyperoxaluria
which decreases the effect of cellulose sodium phosphate.

DIAGNOSTIC TEST EFFECTS
None known.

SIDE EFFECTS
Occasional
GI disturbance, manifested by poor
taste of the drug, loose bowel movements, diarrhea, dyspepsia.

SERIOUS REACTIONS
• Hyperoxaluria and hypomagne-
siuria, which negate the beneficial
effect of hypocalciuria on new stone
formation, magnesium depletion,
and depletion of trace metals
(copper, zinc, iron) may occur.

PRECAUTIONS & CONSIDERATIONS
Caution should be used with congestive heart failure or ascites. Cellulose
sodium phosphate is not recommended in pregnant women. It is
unknown if cellulose sodium phosphate is distributed in breast milk.
Safety and efficacy of cellulose
sodium phosphate has not been
established in children less than
16 years of age.
  Reduction in urinary calcium
(less than 200 mg/day) should be
assessed every 3-6 months. Magnesium, copper, zinc, iron, parathyroid hormone, and complete blood
count (CBC) should be checked
every 3-6 months. Serum PTH
should also be monitored at least
once between the first 2 weeks

to 3 months of treatment and
adjusted or stopped if there is a rise
in serum PTH above normal.
Reduction in renal stone formation
during therapy should be assessed.
Administration
Take with meals or within
30 minutes of meals. Cellulose
sodium phosphate is usually taken
with magnesium to replace dietary
magnesium. Mix cellulose sodium
phosphate with a large glass of
water, fruit juice, or soft drink. Do
not mix with milk or products that
have electrolytes such as Gatorade or
Powerade.

Cephalexin
sef-a-lex'in
(Apo-Cephalex [CAN],
Biocef, Ceporex [AUS],
Ibilex [AUS], Keflex, Keftab,
Novolexin [CAN])

CATEGORY AND SCHEDULE
Pregnancy Risk Category: B

CLASSIFICATION
Antibiotics, cephalosporins

MECHANISM OF ACTION
A first-generation cephalosporin
that binds to bacterial cell
membranes and inhibits cell wall
synthesis. *Therapeutic Effect:*
Bactericidal.

PHARMACOKINETICS
Rapidly absorbed from the GI tract.
Protein binding: 10%-15%. Widely
distributed. Primarily excreted
unchanged in urine. Moderately
removed by hemodialysis. **Half-life:**
0.9-1.2 hr (increased in impaired
renal function).

AVAILABILITY

Capsules (Biocef): 500 mg.
Capsules (Keflex): 250 mg, 500 mg.
Powder for Oral Suspension:
125 mg/5 ml, 250 mg/5 ml.
Tablets: 250 mg, 500 mg.
Tablets (Keftab): 500 mg.

INDICATIONS AND DOSAGES

▶ **Bone infections, prophylaxis of rheumatic fever, follow-up to parenteral therapy**
PO
Adults, Elderly. 250-500 mg q6hr up to 4 g/day.
▶ **Streptococcal pharyngitis, skin and skin-structure infections, uncomplicated cystitis**
PO
Adults, Elderly. 500 mg q12hr.
▶ **Usual pediatric dosage**
Children. 25-100 mg/kg/day in 2-4 divided doses.
▶ **Otitis media**
PO
Children. 75-100 mg/kg/day in 4 divided doses.
▶ **Dosage in renal impairment**
After usual initial dose, dosing frequency is modified based on creatinine clearance and the severity of the infection.

Creatinine Clearance	Dosage Interval
10-40 ml/min	Usual dose q8-12hr
Less than 10 ml/min	Usual dose q12-24hr

CONTRAINDICATIONS

History of anaphylactic reaction to penicillins or hypersensitivity to cephalosporins

INTERACTIONS

Drug
Probenecid: Increases serum concentration of cephalexin.

Herbal
None known.
Food
None known.

DIAGNOSTIC TEST EFFECTS

May increase serum alkaline phosphatase, AST (SGOT), and ALT (SGPT) levels. May produce a positive direct or indirect Coombs' test. Interferes with crossmatching procedures and hematologic tests.

SIDE EFFECTS

Frequent
Oral candidiasis, mild diarrhea, mild abdominal cramping, vaginal candidiasis
Occasional
Nausea, serum sickness-like reaction (marked by fever and joint pain; ususally occurs after the second course of therapy and resolves after the drug is discontinued)
Rare
Allergic reaction (rash, pruritus, urticaria)

SERIOUS REACTIONS

• Antibiotic-associated colitis and other superinfections may result from altered bacterial balance.
• Nephrotoxicity may occur, especially in patients with pre-existing renal disease.
• Patients with a history of allergies, especially to penicillin, are at increased risk for developing a severe hypersensitivity reaction, marked by severe pruritus, angioedema, bronchospasm, and anaphylaxis.

PRECAUTIONS & CONSIDERATIONS

Caution is warranted with history of GI disease (especially antibiotic-associated or ulcerative colitis), renal impairment, and concurrent use of nephrotoxic drugs. Cephalexin readily crosses the placenta and is distributed in breast milk. No age-related precautions have been noted in children. Age-related renal impairment may require a dosage adjustment in the elderly.

Although mild GI effects may be tolerable, an increase in their severity may indicate the onset of antibiotic-associated colitis. The pattern of daily bowel activity and stool consistency, the mouth for white patches on the mucous membranes and tongue, signs and symptoms of superinfection including abdominal pain, moderate to severe diarrhea, severe anal or genital pruritus, and severe mouth soreness should be assessed. Renal function should be assessed.

Storage
After reconstitution, the oral suspension is stable for 14 days if refrigerated.

Administration
! Space drug doses evenly around the clock.

Shake the oral suspension well before using. Take oral cephalexin without regard to meals. However, if GI upset occurs, give with food or milk.

Cephradine
sef′ra-deen
(Velosef)

CATEGORY AND SCHEDULE
Pregnancy Risk Category: B

CLASSIFICATION
Antibiotics, cephalosporins

MECHANISM OF ACTION
A first-generation cephalosporin that binds to bacterial cell membranes. Inhibits synthesis of bacterial cell wall. *Therapeutic Effect:* Bactericidal.

PHARMACOKINETICS
Well absorbed from the gastrointestinal (GI) tract. Protein binding: 18%-20%. Widely distributed. Primarily excreted unchanged in urine. Removed by hemodialysis. **Half-life:** 1-2 hrs (half-life is increased with impaired renal function).

AVAILABILITY
Capsules: 250 mg, 500 mg (Velosef).
Oral Suspension: 125 mg/5 ml, 250 mg/5 ml (Velosef).

INDICATIONS AND DOSAGES
▸ **Mild, moderate, or severe infections of the respiratory, and genitourinary (GU) tracts; bone, joint, and skin infections; prostatitis; otitis media**
PO
Adults, Elderly. 250-500 mg q6hr. Maximum: 8 g/day.
Children older than 9 mo. 25-50 mg/kg/day in divided doses q6-12hr. Maximum: 4 g/day.
Dosage in renal impairment
Dosage and frequency are based on the degree of renal impairment and the severity of infection. After initial 1-g dose:

Creatinine Clearance	Dosage Interval
10-50 ml/min	250 mg q6hr
0-10 ml/min	125 mg q6hr

CONTRAINDICATIONS
History of hypersensitivity to penicillins and cephalosporins

INTERACTIONS
Drug
Diuretics: Increases risk of nephrotoxicity.

Probenecid: Increases cephradine blood concentration.
Herbal
None known.
Food
Delays absorption and reduces peak levels when administered immediately before oral cephradine.

DIAGNOSTIC TEST EFFECTS

Positive direct or indirect Coombs' test. False-positive serum or urine creatinine with Jaffe reaction, urinary proteins and steroids, and glucose test using cupric sulfate (Benedict's solution, Clinitest, Fehling's solution).

SIDE EFFECTS

Frequent
Diarrhea, mild abdominal cramping, vaginal candidiasis (discharge, itching)
Occasional
Nausea, headache, unusual bruising or bleeding, serum sickness reaction (fever, joint pain)
Rare
Allergic reaction (rash, pruritus, urticaria)

SERIOUS REACTIONS

• Antibiotic-associated colitis as evidenced by severe abdominal pain and tenderness, fever, and watery and severe diarrhea, and other superinfections may result from altered bacterial balance.
• Nephrotoxicity may occur, especially in patients with preexisting renal disease.
• Severe hypersensitivity reaction including severe pruritus, angioedema, bronchospasm, and anaphylaxis, particularly in patients with history of allergies, especially penicillin, may occur.

PRECAUTIONS & CONSIDERATIONS

History of allergies, particularly cephalosporins and penicillins, should be determined before initiating drug therapy. Be alert for signs and symptoms of superinfection including anal or genital pruritus, changes or ulceration of the oral mucosa, moderate to severe diarrhea and new or increased fever. Caution should be used with history of GI disease (especially antibiotic-associated colitis or ulcerative colitis), renal impairment, and concurrent use of nephrotoxic medications. Cephradine readily crosses the placenta and is distributed in breast milk. There are no age-related precautions noted in children. Age-related renal impairment may require dosage adjustment.
Storage
Store mixed suspension at room temperature. Discard unused portion after 10-14 days.
Administration
Give without regard to meals. Shake oral suspension well before administering. Continue therapy for full length of treatment and space doses evenly around the clock. Antacids should be taken 2 hours prior to or 2 hours after taking this medication.

Cetirizine
si-tear'a-zeen
(Reactine [CAN], Zyrtec)
**Do not confuse Zyrtec
with Zantac or
Zyprexa.**

CATEGORY AND SCHEDULE
Pregnancy Risk Category: B

CLASSIFICATION
Antihistamines, H1

MECHANISM OF ACTION
A second-generation piperazine that
competes with histamine for
H_1-receptor sites on effector cells in
the GI tract, blood vessels, and
respiratory tract. *Therapeutic Effect:*
Prevents allergic response, produces
mild bronchodilation, blocks
histamine-induced bronchitis.

PHARMACOKINETICS

Route	Onset	Peak	Duration
PO	Less than 1 hr	4-8 hr	Less than 24 hr

Rapidly and almost completely
absorbed from the GI tract (absorption not affected by food). Protein
binding: 93%. Undergoes low first-
pass metabolism; not extensively
metabolized. Primarily excreted in
urine (more than 80% as unchanged
drug). **Half-life:** 6.5-10 hr.

AVAILABILITY
Syrup: 5 mg/5 ml.
Tablets: 5 mg, 10 mg.
Tablets (Chewable): 5 mg, 10 mg.

INDICATIONS AND DOSAGES
▸ **Allergic rhinitis, urticaria**
PO

*Adults, Elderly, Children older than
5 yr.* Initially, 5-10 mg/day as a
single or in 2 divided doses.
Children 2-5 yr. 2.5 mg/day. May
increase up to 5 mg/day as a single
or in 2 divided doses.
Children 12-23 mo. Initially,
2.5 mg/day. May increase up to
5 mg/day in 2 divided doses.
Children 6-11 mo. 2.5 mg once
a day.
▸ **Dosage in renal or hepatic
impairment**
For adult and elderly patients with
renal impairment (creatinine
clearance of 11-31 ml/min), those
receiving hemodialysis (creatinine
clearance of less than 7 ml/min), and
those with hepatic impairment,
dosage is decreased to 5 mg once
a day.

OFF-LABEL USES
Treatment of bronchial asthma

CONTRAINDICATIONS
Hypersensitivity to cetirizine or
hydroxyzine

INTERACTIONS
Drug
Alcohol, other CNS depressants:
May increase CNS depression.
Herbal
None known.
Food
None known.

DIAGNOSTIC TEST EFFECTS
May suppress wheal and flare reactions to antigen skin testing, unless
drug is discontinued 4 days before
testing.

SIDE EFFECTS
Occasional (10%-2%)
Pharyngitis; dry mucous membranes,
nose, or throat; nausea and vomiting;
abdominal pain; headache; dizziness;

fatigue; thickening of mucus; somnolence; photosensitivity; urine retention

SERIOUS REACTIONS
• Children may experience paradoxical reactions, including restlessness, insomnia, euphoria, nervousness, and tremor.
• Dizziness, sedation, and confusion are more likely to occur in elderly patients.

PRECAUTIONS & CONSIDERATIONS
Caution is warranted with renal or hepatic impairment. Cetirizine use is not recommended during the early months of pregnancy. It is unknown if cetirizine is excreted in breast milk. Breast-feeding is not recommended. Cetirizine is less likely to cause anticholinergic effects in children. The elderly are more likely to experience anticholinergic effects, such as dry mouth and urine retention, as well as dizziness, sedation, and confusion. Avoid drinking alcoholic beverages, prolonged exposure to sunlight, and tasks that require alertness or motor skills until response to the drug is established.

Drowsiness may occur at dosages greater than 10 mg/day. Baseline liver function test results should be performed to assess hepatic function. Therapeutic response should also be monitored.

Administration
Take cetirizine without regard to food.

Cetuximab
ceh-tux′ih-mab
(Erbitux)

CATEGORY AND SCHEDULE
Pregnancy Risk Category: C

CLASSIFICATION
Antineoplastics, monoclonal antibodies

MECHANISM OF ACTION
A monoclonal antibody that binds to the epidermal growth factor receptor (EGFR), a glycoprotein on normal and tumor cells, thus inhibiting cell growth and inducing apoptosis. *Therapeutic Effect:* Inhibits the growth and survival of tumor cells that overexpress EGFR.

PHARMACOKINETICS
Reaches steady state levels by the third weekly infusion. Clearance decreases as dose increases. **Half-life:** 114 hr (range, 75-188 hr).

AVAILABILITY
Injection: 2 mg/ml.

INDICATIONS AND DOSAGES
▶ Metastatic colorectal carcinoma
IV
Adults, Elderly. Initially, 400 mg/m^2 as a loading dose. Maintenance: 250 mg/m^2 infused over 60 minutes weekly.

CONTRAINDICATIONS
None known.

INTERACTIONS
Drug
None known.
Herbal
None known.

Food
None known.

DIAGNOSTIC TEST EFFECTS
May decrease WBC count, hematocrit, and hemoglobin level.
⚕ IV Compatibilities
Irinotecan (Camptosar)

SIDE EFFECTS
Frequent (90%-25%)
Acneiform rash, malaise, fever, nausea, diarrhea, constipation, headache, abdominal pain, anorexia, vomiting
Occasional (16%-10%)
Nail disorder, back pain, stomatitis, peripheral edema, pruritus, cough, insomnia
Rare (9%-5%)
Weight loss, depression, dyspepsia, conjunctivitis, alopecia

SERIOUS REACTIONS
• Anemia occurs in 10% of patients.
• A severe infusion reaction, characterized by rapid onset of airway obstruction, a precipitous drop in blood pressure, and severe urticaria, occurs rarely.
• Dermatologic toxicity, pulmonary embolus, leukopenia, and renal failure occur rarely.

PRECAUTIONS & CONSIDERATIONS
Caution is warranted with hypersensitivity to murine proteins. Cetuximab crosses the placental barrier and may cause fetal harm or spontaneous abortion. Females should not breast-feed while taking cetuximab. The safety and efficacy of cetuximab have not been established in children. No age-related precautions have been noted in the elderly. Vaccinations and contact with crowds, persons with a known infection, and anyone who has recently received a live-virus vaccine should be avoided. Sun exposure should be limited and sunscreen should be worn outdoors during cetuximab therapy because sunlight can exacerbate skin reactions.

Signs and symptoms of an infusion reaction, such as rapid onset of bronchospasm, hoarseness, hypotension, stridor, and urticaria, should be monitored. The first severe infusion reaction may occur during subsequent infusions. Skin should be assessed for evidence of dermatologic toxicity, such as dry skin, exfoliative dermatitis or rash, and inflammatory sequelae. Hemoglobin and hematocrit should be monitored.
Storage
Refrigerate vials. Preparations in infusion containers are stable for up to 8 hours at room temperature or 12 hours if refrigerated. Discard any unused portion. The solution should appear clear and colorless; it may contain a small amount of visible white particulates.
Administration
! Premedicate the patient with 50 mg diphenhydramine IV. Cetuximab may be used as monotherapy or in combination with irinotecan. Do not give cetuximab by IV push or bolus. Don't shake or dilute the vials. Infuse the drug using a low-protein-binding 0.22-micron in-line filter. Give the first dose as a 120-minute IV infusion. Administer maintenance infusions over 60 minutes. The maximum infusion rate is 5 ml/minute.

Cevimeline
sev-im'el-ine
(Evoxac)
Do not confuse Evoxac with Eurax.

CATEGORY AND SCHEDULE
Pregnancy Risk Category: C

CLASSIFICATION
Cholinergics

MECHANISM OF ACTION
A cholinergic agonist that binds to muscarinic receptors of effector cells, thereby increasing secretion of exocrine glands, such as salivary glands. *Therapeutic Effect:* Relieves dry mouth.

AVAILABILITY
Capsules: 30 mg.

INDICATIONS AND DOSAGES
▶ **Dry mouth**
PO
Adults. 30 mg 3 times a day.

CONTRAINDICATIONS
Acute iritis, angle-closure glaucoma, uncontrolled asthma

INTERACTIONS
Drug
Amiodarone, diltiazem, erythromycin, fluoxetine, itraconazole, ketoconazole, paroxetine, quinidine, ritonavir, verapamil: May increase the effects of cevimeline.
Atropine, phenothiazines, tricyclic antidepressants: May decrease the effects of cevimeline.
Beta blockers: May increase the risk of conduction disturbances.

Herbal
None known.
Food
All foods: Decreases the absorption rate of cevimeline.

DIAGNOSTIC TEST EFFECTS
None known.

SIDE EFFECTS
Frequent (19%-11%)
Diaphoresis, headache, nausea, sinusitis, rhinitis, upper respiratory tract infection, diarrhea
Occasional (10%-3%)
Dyspepsia, abdominal pain, cough, UTI, vomiting, back pain, rash, dizziness, fatigue
Rare (2%-1%)
Skeletal pain, insomnia, hot flashes, excessive salivation, rigors, anxiety

SERIOUS REACTIONS
• Cevimeline use may result in decreased visual acuity, especially at night, and impaired depth perception.

PRECAUTIONS & CONSIDERATIONS
Caution is warranted with cardiovascular disease, CHF, chronic bronchitis, COPD, cholelithiasis, and history of nephrolithiasis. Avoid driving at night or performing hazardous duties in reduced lighting because cevimeline use may decrease visual acuity or impair depth perception.
Adequate hydration should be maintained to prevent dehydration.
Vital signs should be monitored.
Administration
Take cevimeline without regard to food.

Charcoal, Activated
(Actidose-Aqua, Actidose with
Sorbitol, Aqueous Charcodote
[CAN], CharcoAid, Charcoal
Plus DS, Charcocaps,
EZ-Char, Kerr Insta-Char,
Liqui-Char)

CATEGORY AND SCHEDULE
Pregnancy Risk Category: C

CLASSIFICATION
Antidiarrheal, antidote,
antiflatulent

MECHANISM OF ACTION
An antidote that adsorbs (detoxifies)
ingested toxic substances, irritants,
intestinal gas. *Therapeutic Effect:*
Inhibits gastrointestinal (GI) absorption and absorbs intestinal gas.

PHARMACOKINETICS
Not orally absorbed from the GI
tract. Not metabolized. Excreted in
feces as charcoal. **Half-life:**
Unknown.

AVAILABILITY
Capsules, activated: 260 mg
(Charcocaps).
Granules, activated: 15 g
(CharcoAid-G).
Liquid, activated: 15 g (Actidose-
Aqua, Liqui-Char), 25 g (Actidose-
Aqua, Kerr Insta-Char, Liqui-Char),
50 g (Actidose-Aqua, Kerr Insta-
Char).
Liquid, activated: 25 g (Actidose
with Sorbitol, Liqui-Char, Kerr Insta-
Char), 50 g (Actidose with Sorbitol,
Liqui-Char, Kerr Insta-Char).
Pellets, activated: 25 g (EZ-Char).
Powder for suspension, activated:
30 g, 240 g.
Tablets, activated: 250 mg (Charcol
Plus DS).

INDICATIONS AND DOSAGES
▸ **Acute poisoning**
PO
*Adults, Elderly, Children 12 yr and
older.* Give 30-100 g as slurry (30 g
in at least 8 oz H$_2$O) or 12.5-50 g in
aqueous or sorbitol suspension.
Usually given as single dose.
*Children more than 1 yr and less
than 12 yr.* 25-50 g as a single dose.
Smaller doses (10-25 g) may be used
in children 1-5 yr due to smaller gut
lumen capacity.

CONTRAINDICATIONS
Intestinal obstruction, GI tract not
anatomically intact; patients at risk of
hemorrhage or GI perforation, if use
would increase risk and severity of
aspiration, not effective for cyanide,
mineral acids, caustic alkalis, organic
solvents, iron, ethanol, methanol
poisoning, lithium, do not use charcoal
with sorbitol in patients with fructose
intolerance, charcoal with sorbitol not
recommended in children <1 year of
age, hypersensitivity to charcoal or
any component of the formation

INTERACTIONS
Drug
Orally administered medications:
May decrease absorption of orally
administered medications.
Ipecac: May decrease the effect of
ipecac.
Herbal
None known.
Food
**Ice cream, sherbet, marmalade,
milk:** May reduce the effects of
charcoal.

DIAGNOSTIC TEST EFFECTS
None known.

SIDE EFFECTS
Occasional
Diarrhea, GI discomfort, intestinal gas

SERIOUS REACTIONS
• Hypernatremia, hypokalemia, and hypermagnesemia may occur with coadministration of cathartics.

PRECAUTIONS & CONSIDERATIONS
Caution should be used with decreased peristalsis. It is unknown if charcoal crosses the placenta or is distributed in breast milk. Safety and efficacy of charcoal have not been established in children less than 1 year old. There are no age-related precautions noted in the elderly. Be aware that charcoal causes the stools to turn black.

Be aware that charcoal may cause vomiting which is hazardous in petroleum distillate and caustic ingestions. Be aware that vomiting should be induced with ipecac before administering activated charcoal since charcoal absorbs ipecac syrup. Be aware that if charcoal and sorbitol is administered, doses should be limited to prevent excessive fluid and electrolyte loss.

Storage
Store in closed container because it absorbs gases from air.

Administration
Charcoal is most effective when administered within 1 hour of ingestion for most ingestions. Flavoring agents, such as chocolate, can enhance charcoal's palatability.

Be aware about 10 g of activated charcoal for each 1 g of toxin is considered adequate but may require multiple doses. If sorbitol is also used, sorbitol dose should not exceed 1.5 g/kg. When using multiple doses of charcoal, sorbitol should be given with every other dose (not to exceed 2 doses/day).

Be aware that if treatment includes ipecac syrup, induce vomiting prior to administration of charcoal.

Chloral Hydrate
klor-al hye′drate
(Aquachloral Supprettes, PMS-Chloral Hydrate [CAN], Somnote)

CATEGORY AND SCHEDULE
Pregnancy Risk Category: C

CLASSIFICATION
Sedatives/hypnotics

MECHANISM OF ACTION
A nonbarbiturate chloral derivative that produces CNS depression. *Therapeutic Effect:* Induces quiet, deep sleep, with only a slight decrease in respiratory rate and B/P.

AVAILABILITY
Capsules (Somnote): 500 mg.
Syrup: 500 mg/5 ml.
Suppositories (Aquachloral Supprettes): 324 mg, 648 mg.

INDICATIONS AND DOSAGES
▸ **Premedication for dental or medical procedures**
PO, Rectal
Adults. 0.5-1 g.
Children. 75 mg/kg up to 1 g total.
▸ **Premedication for EEG**
PO, Rectal
Adults. 0.5-1.5 g.
Children. 25-50 mg/kg/dose 30-60 min prior to EEG. May repeat in 30 min. Maximum: 1 g for infants, 2 g for children.

CONTRAINDICATIONS
Gastritis, marked hepatic or renal impairment, severe cardiac disease

INTERACTIONS
Drug
Alcohol, other CNS depressants:
May increase the effects of chloral
hydrate.
Furosemide (IV): May alter B/P
and cause diaphoresis if given within
24 hours after chloral hydrate.
Warfarin: May increase the effect
of warfarin.
Herbal
None known.
Food
None known.

DIAGNOSTIC TEST EFFECTS
None known.

SIDE EFFECTS
Occasional
Gastric irritation (nausea, vomiting,
flatulence, diarrhea), rash, sleep-
walking
Rare
Headache, paradoxical CNS hyperactivity or nervousness in children,
excitement or restlessness in the elderly
(particularly in patients with pain).

SERIOUS REACTIONS
• Overdose may produce somnolence, confusion, slurred speech,
severe incoordination, respiratory
depression, and coma.

PRECAUTIONS & CONSIDERATIONS
Caution is warranted with clinical
depression and history of drug
abuse. Do not drive if taking chloral
hydrate before a procedure. B/P,
pulse rate, and respiratory rate,
rhythm, and depth should be assessed
immediately before and during chloral hydrate use. The elderly should be
monitored for paradoxical reactions,
such as excitability.
Storage
Store suppositories at room temperature; don't refrigerate them.

Administration
Take chloral hydrate capsules with a
full glass of water or fruit juice.
Swallow the capsules whole and do
not chew them. Dilute the dose of
syrup in water to minimize gastric
irritation.
For rectal use, if the suppository is
too soft to insert, chill in the refrigerator for 30 minutes or run cold
water over it before removing the
foil wrapper. First remove the foil
wrapper and moisten the suppository
with cold water. Lie down on
side and use finger to push the
suppository well up into the rectum.

Chloramphenicol
klor-am-fen'i-kole
(Chloromycetin, Chloroptic,
Chlorsig [AUS])
**Do not confuse chlorampheni-
col with chlorambucil.**

CATEGORY AND SCHEDULE
Pregnancy Risk Category: C

CLASSIFICATION
Anti-infectives, ophthalmics,
otics, antibiotics, chloramicheni-
col and derivatives

MECHANISM OF ACTION
A dichloroacetic acid derivative that
inhibits bacterial protein synthesis
by binding to bacterial ribosomal
receptor sites. *Therapeutic Effect:*
Bacteriostatic (may be bactericidal
in high concentrations).

AVAILABILITY
Powder for Injection: 100 mg/ml.
Ophthalmic Ointment: 10 mg/g.
Ophthalmic Solution: 5 mg/ml.

INDICATIONS AND DOSAGES

▸ **Mild to moderate infections caused by organisms resistant to other less toxic antibiotics**

IV
Adults, Elderly. 50-100 mg/kg/day in divided doses q6hr. Maximum: 4 g/day.
Children older than 1 mo. 50-75 mg/kg/day in divided doses q6hr. Maximum: 4 g/day

▸ **Meningitis**

IV
Children older than 1 mo.
50-100 mg/kg/day in divided doses q6hr.

▸ **Usual ophthalmic dosage**
Adults, Elderly, Children. 1-2 drops 4-6 times/day.

CONTRAINDICATIONS

Hypersensitivity to chloramphenicol

INTERACTIONS

Drug
Anticonvulsants, bone marrow depressants: May increase myelosuppression.
Clindamycin, erythromycin: May antagonize the effects of these drugs.
Oral antidiabetics: May increase the effects of these drugs.
Phenobarbital, phenytoin, warfarin: May increase blood concentrations of these drugs.
Vitamin B$_{12}$: May decrease the effects of vitamin B$_{12}$ in patients with pernicious anemia.
Herbal
None known.
Food
None known.

DIAGNOSTIC TEST EFFECTS

Therapeutic blood level: 10-20 mcg/ml; toxic blood level: greater than 25 mcg/ml. When administered with iron salts, may increase serum iron levels.

SIDE EFFECTS

Occasional
Systemic: Nausea, vomiting, diarrhea
Ophthalmic: Blurred vision, burning, stinging, hypersensitivity reaction
Otic: Hypersensitivity reaction
Rare
"Gray baby" syndrome in neonates (abdominal distention, blue-gray skin color, cardiovascular collapse, unresponsiveness), rash, shortness of breath, confusion, headache, optic neuritis (blurred vision, eye pain), peripheral neuritis (numbness and weakness in feet and hands)

SERIOUS REACTIONS

• Superinfection due to bacterial or fungal overgrowth may occur.
• There is a narrow margin between effective therapy and toxic levels producing blood dyscrasias.
• Myelosuppression, with resulting aplastic anemia, hypoplastic anemia, and pancytopenia, may occur weeks or months later.

PRECAUTIONS & CONSIDERATIONS

Caution is warranted with myelosuppression, or renal or hepatic impairment, and in those who have previously undergone cytotoxic drug therapy or radiation therapy. Caution should be used in children younger than 2 years.

Concurrent use of other drugs that cause myelosuppression should be determined before therapy because chloramphenicol should not be given concurrently with these drugs, if possible. Baseline blood studies should also be determined before beginning chloramphenicol therapy.

Nausea, vomiting, visual disturbances should be reported. Pattern of daily bowel activity and stool consistency, mental status, and skin for rash should be assessed. Be alert for signs and symptoms of superinfection, such as anal or genital pruritus, a change in the oral mucosa, diarrhea, and increased fever. Know and monitor the drug's therapeutic blood level which is 10 to 20 mcg/ml and toxic blood level is greater than 25 mcg/ml.

Administration
Space drug doses evenly around the clock and continue taking chloramphenicol for the full course of treatment. Continue treatment of the ophthalmic form for at least 48 hours after the eye returns to normal appearance.

Chlordiazepoxide
klor-dye-az-e-pox′ide
(Apo-Chlordiazepoxide [CAN], Librium, Novopoxide [CAN])
Do not confuse with Librax.

CATEGORY AND SCHEDULE
Pregnancy Risk Category: D

CLASSIFICATION
Anxiolytics, benzodiazepines

MECHANISM OF ACTION
A benzodiazepine that enhances the action of the inhibitory neurotransmitter gamma-aminobutyric acid in the CNS. *Therapeutic Effect:* Produces anxiolytic effect.

AVAILABILITY
Capsules: 5 mg, 10 mg, 25 mg.
Injection Powder for Reconstitution. 100 mg.

INDICATIONS AND DOSAGES
▸ **Alcohol withdrawal symptoms**
PO
Adults, Elderly. 50-100 mg. May repeat q2-4hr. Maximum: 300 mg/24 hr.
▸ **Anxiety**
PO
Adults. 15-100 mg/day in 3-4 divided doses.
Elderly. 5 mg 2-4 times a day.

OFF-LABEL USES
Treatment of panic disorder, tension headache, tremors

CONTRAINDICATIONS
Acute alcohol intoxication, acute angle-closure glaucoma

INTERACTIONS
Drug
Other CNS depressants: May increase CNS depression.
Herbal
Kava kava, valerian: May increase CNS depression.
Food
Alcohol: May increase CNS depression.

DIAGNOSTIC TEST EFFECTS
None known. Therapeutic serum drug level is 1-3 mcg/ml; toxic serum drug level is greater than 5 mcg/ml.

SIDE EFFECTS
Frequent
Pain at IM injection site; somnolence, ataxia, dizziness, confusion with oral dose (particularly in elderly or debilitated patients)
Occasional
Rash, peripheral edema, GI disturbances
Rare
Paradoxical CNS reactions, such as hyperactivity or nervousness in children and excitement or restlessness in the elderly (generally noted during first 2 weeks of therapy, particularly in presence of uncontrolled pain)

SERIOUS REACTIONS
• IV administration may produce pain, swelling, thrombophlebitis, and carpal tunnel syndrome.
• Abrupt or too rapid withdrawal may result in pronounced restlessness, irritability, insomnia, hand tremors, abdominal or muscle cramps, diaphoresis, vomiting, and seizures.
• Overdose results in somnolence, confusion, diminished reflexes, and coma.

PRECAUTIONS & CONSIDERATIONS
Caution is warranted with impaired renal or hepatic function.
Drowsiness may occur. Change positions slowly from recumbent, to sitting, before standing to prevent dizziness. Alcohol and tasks that require mental alertness or motor skills should also be avoided. Autonomic responses, such as cold, clammy hands and diaphoresis, and motor responses, such as agitation, trembling, and tension, should be assessed. B/P, pulse rate, and respiratory rate, rhythm, and depth should be monitored immediately before giving the drug.

Administration
! Expect to use the smallest effective chlordiazepoxide dose in the elderly or debilitated and those with hepatic disease or a low serum albumin level. Be aware that therapeutic serum level for chlordiazepoxide is 1-3 mcg/ml, and the toxic serum level is greater than 5 mcg/ml. Stay recumbent for up to 3 hours after parenteral administration to reduce the drug's hypotensive effect. IM injection may produce discomfort. Do not discontinue the drug abruptly after long-term therapy.

Chloroquine/ Chloroquine Phosphate
klor'oh-kwin
(Aralen hydrochloride, Aralen [CAN]) (Aralen phosphate)

CATEGORY AND SCHEDULE
Pregnancy Risk Category: C

CLASSIFICATION
Antiprotozoals

MECHANISM OF ACTION
An amebecide that concentrates in parasite acid vesicles and may interfere with parasite protein synthesis. *Therapeutic Effect:* Increases pH and inhibits parasite growth.

PHARMACOKINETICS
Rate of absorption is variable. Chloroquine is almost completely absorbed from the gastrointestinal (GI) tract. Protein binding: 50%-65%. Widely distributed into body tissues such as eyes, heart, kidneys, liver, and lungs. Partially metabolized to active de-ethylated metabolites (principal metabolite is desethylchloroquine). Excreted in urine. Removed by hemodialysis. **Half-life:** 1-2 mo.

AVAILABILITY
Tablets: 250 mg, 500 mg (Aralen).

INDICATIONS AND DOSAGES
▸ **Chloroquine Phosphate**
Treatment of malaria (acute attack): Dose (mg base)

Dose	Time	Adults	Children
Initial	Day 1	600 mg	10 mg/kg
Second	6 hrs later	300 mg	5 mg/kg
Third	Day 2	300 mg	5 mg/kg
Fourth	Day 3	300 mg	5 mg/kg

▸ **Suppression of malaria**
PO
Adults. 300 mg (base)/wk on same day each week beginning 2 wk before exposure; continue for 6-8 wks after leaving endemic area.
Children. 5 mg (base)/kg/wk.
▸ **Malaria prophylaxis**
PO
Adults. 600 mg base initially given in 2 divided doses 6 hr apart.
Children. 10 mg base/kg.
▸ **Amebiasis**
PO
Adults. 1 g (600 mg base) daily for 2 days; then, 500 mg (300 mg base)/day for at least 2-3 wk.
▸ **Chloroquine HCl**
Treatment of malaria
IM
Adults. Initially, 160-200 mg base (4-5 ml), repeat in 6 hr. Maximum: 800 mg base in first 24 hr. Begin oral therapy as soon as possible and continue for 3 days until approximately 1.5 g base given.
Children. Initially, 5 mg base/kg, repeat in 6 hr. Do not exceed 10 mg base/kg/24 hr.
▸ **Amebiasis**
IM
Adults. 160-200 mg base (4-5 ml) daily for 10-12 days. Change to oral therapy as soon as possible.

OFF-LABEL USES

Treatment of sarcoid-associated hypercalcemia, juvenile arthritis, rheumatoid arthritis, systemic lupus erythematosus, solar urticaria, chronic cutaneous vasculitis

CONTRAINDICATIONS

Hypersensitivity to 4-aminoquinoline compounds, retinal or visual field changes

INTERACTIONS

Drug
Alcohol: May increase GI irritation.
Penicillamine: May increase concentration of penicillamine and increase risk of hematologic, renal or severe skin reaction.
Ampicillin: May reduce the absorption of ampicillin. Separate administration by 2 hours.
Antacids and kaolin: May be decreased due to GI binding with kaolin or magnesium trisilicate.
Cimetidine: May increase levels of chloroquine.
Cyclosporine: May increase cyclosporine concentrations.
CYP2D6 inhibitors (chlorpromazine, delavirdine, fluoxetine, miconazole, paroxetine, pergolide, quinidine, quinine, ritonavir, ropinirole): May increase the levels and effects of chloroquine.
CYP2D6 substrates (amphetamines, selected beta-blockers, dextromethorphan, fluoxetine, lidocaine, mirtazapine, nefazodone, paroxetine, risperidone, ritonavir, thioridazine, tricyclic antidepressants, venlafaxine): May increase the levels and effects of CYP2D6 substrates.
CYP2D6 prodrug substrates: Chloroquine may decrease the levels and effects of CYP2D6 prodrug substrates.
CYP3A4 inducers (aminoglutethimide, carbamazepine, nafcillin, nevirapine, phenobarbital, phenytoin, and rifamycins): CYP3A4 inducers may decrease the levels and effects of chloroquine.

CYP3A4 inhibitors (azole antifungals, ciprofloxacin, clarithromycin, diclofenac, doxycycline, erythromycin, imatinib, isoniazid, nefazodone, nicardipine, propofol, protease inhibitors, quinidine, and verapamil): May increase the levels and effects of chloroquine.

Praziquantel: May decrease praziquantel concentrations.

Herbal
None known.

Food
None known.

DIAGNOSTIC TEST EFFECTS

Acute decrease in Hct, Hgb, RBC count may occur.

SIDE EFFECTS

Frequent
Discomfort with IM administration, mild transient headache, anorexia, nausea, vomiting

Occasional
Visual disturbances (blurring, difficulty focusing); nervousness, fatigue, pruritus esp. of palms, soles, scalp; bleaching of hair, irritability, personality changes, diarrhea, skin eruptions

Rare
Phlebitis or thrombophlebitis at IV injection site, abdominal cramps, headache, hypotension

SERIOUS REACTIONS

• Ocular toxicity and ototoxicity have been reported.
• Prolonged therapy: peripheral neuritis and neuromyopathy, hypotension, ECG changes, agranulocytosis, aplastic anemia, thrombocytopenia, convulsions, psychosis.
• Overdosage includes symptoms of headache, vomiting, visual disturbance, drowsiness, convulsions, hypokalemia followed by cardiovascular collapse, and death.

PRECAUTIONS & CONSIDERATIONS

Caution is warranted with alcoholism, severe blood disorders, liver disease, neurologic disorders, and G6PD deficiency. It is unknown if chloroquine crosses the placenta or is distributed in breast milk. Be aware that children are especially susceptible to chloroquine fatalities. There are no age-related precautions noted in the elderly.

History of allergies, especially to antibiotics, should be determined before giving chloroquine.

Visual disturbances should be reported immediately.

Storage
Store tablets and solution for injection at room temperature.

Administration
Chloroquine PO_4 500 mg = 300 mg base; chloroquine HCl 50 mg = 40 mg base.

Give oral chloroquine with food or milk to minimize GI irritation. May mix with chocolate syrup or enclosed in gelatin capsules to mask the bitter taste.

For IM injection, inject deeply into a large muscle mass. Administer very slowly.

Chlorothiazide
klor-oh-thye′a-zide
(Diuril, Diuril Sodium)

CATEGORY AND SCHEDULE
Pregnancy Risk Category: C

CLASSIFICATION
Diuretics, thiazide and derivatives

MECHANISM OF ACTION
A sulfonamide derivative that acts as a thiazide diuretic and antihypertensive. As a diuretic blocks reabsorption of water, the electrolytes sodium and potassium at cortical diluting segment of distal tubule. As an antihypertensive reduces plasma, extracellular fluid volume decreases peripheral vascular resistance (PVR) by direct effect on blood vessels. *Therapeutic Effect:* Promotes diuresis, reduces blood pressure (B/P).

PHARMACOKINETICS
Poorly absorbed from the gastrointestinal (GI) tract. Not metabolized. Primarily excreted unchanged in urine. Not removed by hemodialysis. **Half-life:** 45-120 min.

AVAILABILITY
Powder for injection, lyophilized: 0.5 g.
Oral suspension: 250 mg/5 ml (Diuril).
Tablets: 250 mg, 500 mg (Diuril).

INDICATIONS AND DOSAGES
▶ **Edema, hypertension**
PO
Adults. 0.5-1 g 1-2 times/day. May give every other day or 3-5 days/wk.
Children 12 yr and older. 10-20 mg/kg/dose in divided doses q8-12hr. Maximum: 2 g/day.
Children 2-12 yr. 1 g/day.
Children 6 mo-2 yr. 10-20 mg/kg/day in divided doses q12-24hr. Maximum: 375 mg/day.
Children younger than 6 mo. 20-30 mg/kg/day in divided doses q12hr. Maximum: 375 mg/day.
▶ **Hypertension**
IV
Adults. 0.5-1 g in divided doses q12-24hr.

OFF-LABEL USES
Treatment of diabetes insipidus, prevention of calcium-containing renal stones

CONTRAINDICATIONS
Anuria, history of hypersensitivity to sulfonamides or thiazide diuretics, renal decompensation

INTERACTIONS
Drug
Cholestyramine, colestipol: May decrease the absorption and effects of chlorothiazide.
Digoxin: May increase the risk of toxicity of digoxin caused by hypokalemia.
Lithium: May increase the risk of toxicity of lithium.
NSAIDs: May decrease the absorption and effects of chlorothiazide.
Probenecid: May increase concentrations of chlorothiazide.
Herbal
Ginkgo biloba: May increase blood pressure.
Licorice: May increase risk of hypokalemia and decrease effectiveness of chlorothiazide.
Ma Huang: May decrease hypotensive effect of chlorothiazide.
Yohimbe: May decrease effects of chlorothiazide.
Food
None known.

DIAGNOSTIC TEST EFFECTS
None known.

SIDE EFFECTS
Expected
Increase in urine frequency and volume
Frequent
Potassium depletion
Occasional
Postural hypotension, headache, gastrointestinal (GI) disturbances,

photosensitivity reaction, muscle spasms, alopecia, rash, urticaria

SERIOUS REACTIONS

• Vigorous diuresis may lead to profound water loss and electrolyte depletion, resulting in hypokalemia, hyponatremia, and dehydration.
• Acute hypotensive episodes may occur.
• Hyperglycemia may be noted during prolonged therapy.
• GI upset, pancreatitis, dizziness, paresthesias, headache, blood dyscrasias, pulmonary edema, allergic pneumonitis, and dermatologic reactions occur rarely.
• Overdosage can lead to lethargy and coma without changes in electrolytes or hydration.

PRECAUTIONS & CONSIDERATIONS

Caution should be used with diabetes mellitus, electrolyte imbalance, hyperuricemia or gout, hypotension, systemic lupus erythematosus, impaired liver function and severe renal disease. Chlorothiazide crosses the placenta and a small amount is distributed in breast milk. Breast-feeding is not recommended in this patient population. Safety and efficacy of IV chlorothiazide have not been established in children and infants. Be aware that the elderly may be more sensitive to the drug's electrolyte and hypotensive effects. Age-related renal impairment may require caution in the elderly.

Frequency and volume of urination is expected to increase. Be aware that chlorothiazide may aggravate digitalis toxicity. Be aware that sensitivity reactions may occur with or without history of allergy or asthma. Skin should be protected from sunlight.

Hypokalemia may result in change in mental status, muscle cramps, nausea, tachycardia, tremor, vomiting, and weakness.

Hyponatremia may result in clammy and cold skin, confusion, and thirst. Be especially alert for potassium depletion in persons taking digoxin, such as cardiac arrhythmias. Foods high in potassium such as apricots, bananas, legumes, meat, orange juice, white and sweet potatoes, raisins, and whole grains, such as cereals should be eaten during treatment.

Administration

May take oral chlorothiazide on alternate days or 3-5 days weekly. May take with food or milk if GI upset occurs, preferably with breakfast to help prevent nocturia.

A fresh solution for injection should be prepared before each administration because chlorothiazide does not contain preservatives. Discard unused portion. Do not administer subcutaneously or intramuscularly. May be given slowly by direct IV injection or infusion. Reconstitute with 18 ml sterile water for injection for a final concentration of 28 mg/ml.

Chloroxine
klor-ox′ine
(Capitrol)
Do not confuse with chloroquine.

CATEGORY AND SCHEDULE
Pregnancy Risk Category: C

CLASSIFICATION
Anti-infectives, topical, dermatologics

MECHANISM OF ACTION
An antifungal that reduces scaling of the epidermis by slowing down

mitotic activity. *Therapeutic Effect:* Reduces the excess scaling in patients with dandruff or seborrheic dermatitis.

PHARMACOKINETICS
No studies have investigated the absorption/pharmacokinetics of chloroxine.

AVAILABILITY
Shampoo: 2% (Capitrol).

INDICATIONS AND DOSAGES
▸ **Dandruff, seborrheic dermatitis**
Adults. Shampoo affected area twice weekly.

OFF-LABEL USES
Not known.

CONTRAINDICATIONS
Acutely inflamed lesions, hypersensitivity to chloroxine or any one of its components.

INTERACTIONS
Drug
None known.
Herbal
None known.
Food
None known.

DIAGNOSTIC TEST EFFECTS
None known.

SIDE EFFECTS
Discoloration of light hair, skin irritation, burning

SERIOUS REACTIONS
• None known.

PRECAUTIONS & CONSIDERATIONS
Discoloration of light colored hair may occur. Irritation and hair discoloration should be reported. It is unknown if chloroxine is distributed

in breast milk. There are no age-related precautions noted in children or the elderly.
Administration
Shake well before administration. Massage shampoo thoroughly onto the wet scalp, avoiding contact with the eyes. Lather should remain on the scalp for approximately 3 minutes, then rinse. The application should be repeated and the scalp rinsed thoroughly. Shampoo should be used twice weekly.

Chlorpheniramine
klor-fen-ir'a-meen
(Aller-Chlor, Chlor-Trimeton, Chlor-Trimeton Allergy, Chlor-Trimeton Allergy 12 Hour, Chlor-Trimeton Allergy 8 Hour, Chlor-Tripolon [CAN], Chlorate, Chlorphen, Diabetic Tussin Allergy Relief)
Do not confuse with chlorpromazine or chlorpropamide.

CATEGORY AND SCHEDULE
Pregnancy Risk Category: C
OTC (tablets, syrup)

CLASSIFICATION
Antihistamines, H1

MECHANISM OF ACTION
A propylamine derivative antihistamine that competes with histamine for histamine receptor sites on cells in the blood vessels, gastrointestinal (GI) tract, and respiratory tract. *Therapeutic Effect:* Inhibits symptoms associated with seasonal allergic rhinitis such as increased mucus production and sneezing.

PHARMACOKINETICS
Well absorbed after PO and parenteral administration. Food delays absorption. Widely distributed. Metabolized in liver. Primarily excreted in urine. Not removed by dialysis. **Half-life:** 20 hr.

AVAILABILITY
Injection: 10 mg/ml, 100 mg/ml.
Syrup: 2 mg/5 ml (Aller-Chlor, Diabetic Tussin Allergy Relief [sugar free]).
Tablets: 4 mg (Aller-Chlor, Chlor-Trimeton, Chlorate, Chlorphen).
Tablets (sustained-release): 8 mg (Chlor-Trimeton Allergy 8 Hour), 12 mg (Chlor-Trimeton Allergy 12 Hour).

INDICATIONS AND DOSAGES
▶ **Allergic rhinitis, common cold**
PO
Adults, Elderly. 4 mg q6-8hr or 8-12 mg (sustained-release) q8-12hr. Maximum: 24 mg/day.
Children 12 yr and older. 4 mg q6-8hr or 8 mg (sustained-release) q12hr. Maximum: 24 mg/day.
Children 6-11 yr. 2 mg q4-6hr. Maximum: 12 mg/day.
IM/IV/SC
Adults, Elderly. 5-40 mg as a single dose. Maximum: 40 mg/day.
SC
Children 6 yr and older.
87.5 mcg/kg or 2.5 mg/m^2 4 times/day.

CONTRAINDICATIONS
Hypersensitivity to chlorpheniramine or its components

INTERACTIONS
Drug
Alcohol, central nervous system (CNS) depressants: May increase CNS depressant effects.
Anticholinergics: May increase anticholinergic effects.

MAOIs: May increase anticholinergic and CNS depressant effects.
Phenytoin, fosphenytoin: May increase the risk of phenytoin toxicity.
Procarbazine: May increase CNS depressant effects.
Herbal
None known.
Food
None known.

DIAGNOSTIC TEST EFFECTS
None known.

▨ IV INCOMPATIBILITIES
Calcium, iodipamide, kanamycin (Kantrex), norepinephrine (Levophed), pentobarbital (Nembutal)
▨ IV Compatibilities
Amikacin (Amikin), corticotropin, cortisone, hyaluronidase (Wydase), penicillin G

SIDE EFFECTS
Frequent
Drowsiness, dizziness, muscular weakness, hypotension, dry mouth, nose, throat, and lips, urinary retention, thickening of bronchial secretions
Elderly: Sedation, dizziness, hypotension
Occasional
Epigastric distress, flushing, visual or hearing disturbances, paresthesia, diaphoresis, chills

SERIOUS REACTIONS
• Children may experience dominant paradoxical reactions, including restlessness, insomnia, euphoria, nervousness, and tremors.
• Overdosage in children may result in hallucinations, seizures, and death.
• Hypersensitivity reaction, such as eczema, pruritus, rash, cardiac disturbances, and photosensitivity, may occur.

- Overdosage may vary from CNS depression, including sedation, apnea, hypotension, cardiovascular collapse, or death to severe paradoxical reaction, such as hallucinations, tremor, and seizures.

PRECAUTIONS & CONSIDERATIONS

Caution is warranted with asthma, cardiovascular disease, chronic obstructive pulmonary disease (COPD), hypertension, hyperthyroidism, narrow-angle glaucoma, increased intraocular pressure (IOP), peptic ulcer disease, prostatic hypertrophy, pyloro-duodenal or bladder neck obstruction, and seizure disorders. It is unknown if chlorpheniramine crosses the placenta or is detected in breast milk. Be aware that chlorpheniramine use is not recommended in newborns or premature infants as these groups are at an increased risk of experiencing paradoxical reaction. Be aware that the elderly are at an increased risk of developing confusion, dizziness, hyperexcitability, hypotension, and sedation.

Dizziness, drowsiness, and dry mouth are expected side effects. Mental alertness or motor skills should be avoided. Tolerance to the drug's sedative effects can occur.

Administration

Give oral chlorpheniramine without regard to meals. Do not crush, break, or chew sustained-release tablets.

Give deep IM injection into large muscle mass.

Chlorpromazine
klor-proe′ma-zeen
(Chlorpromanyl [CAN], Largactil [CAN], Thorazine)
Do not confuse chlorpromazine with chlorpropamide, clomipramine, or prochlorperazine, or Thorazine with thiamide or thioridazine.

CATEGORY AND SCHEDULE
Pregnancy Risk Category: C

CLASSIFICATION
Antiemetics/antivertigo, antipsychotics, phenothiazines

MECHANISM OF ACTION
A phenothiazine that blocks dopamine neurotransmission at postsynaptic dopamine receptor sites. Possesses strong anticholinergic, sedative, and antiemetic effects; moderate extrapyramidal effects; and slight antihistamine action.
Therapeutic Effect: Relieves nausea and vomiting; improves psychotic conditions; controls intractable hiccups and porphyria.

PHARMACOKINETICS
Rapidly absorbed after oral or IM administration. Protein binding: 92%-97%. Metabolized in the liver. Excreted in urine.
Half-life: 6 hr.

AVAILABILITY
Oral concentrate: 30 mg/ml, 100 mg/ml.
Syrup: 10 mg/5 ml.
Tablets: 10 mg, 25 mg, 50 mg, 100 mg, 200 mg.
Capsules (Sustained-Release): 30 mg, 75 mg, 150 mg.

Injection (Thorazine): 25 mg/ml.
Suppositories: 25 mg, 100 mg.

INDICATIONS AND DOSAGES
▸ **Severe nausea or vomiting**
PO
Adults, Elderly. 10-25 mg q4-6hr.
Children. 0.5-1 mg/kg q4-6hr.
IM, IV
Adults, Elderly. 25-50 mg q4-6hr.
Children. 0.5-1 mg/kg q6-8hr.
RECTAL
Adults, Elderly. 50-100 mg q6-8hr.
Children. 1 mg/kg q6-8hr.
▸ **Psychotic disorders**
PO
Adults, Elderly. 30-800 mg/day in
1-4 divided doses.
Children older than 6 mo.
0.5-1 mg/kg q4-6hr.
IM, IV
Adults, Elderly. Initially, 25 mg;
may repeat in 1-4 hr. May gradually
increase to 400 mg q4-6hr.
Maximum: 300-800 mg/day.
Children older than 6 mo.
0.5-1 mg/kg q6-8hr. Maximum:
75 mg/day for children 5-12 yr;
40 mg/day for children younger than
5 yr.
▸ **Intractable hiccups**
PO, IV, IM
Adults. 25-50 mg 3 times a day.
▸ **Porphyria**
PO
Adults. 25-50 mg 3-4 times a day.
IM
Adults, Elderly. 25 mg 3-4 times
a day.

OFF-LABEL USES
Treatment of choreiform movement
of Huntington's disease

CONTRAINDICATIONS
Comatose states, myelosuppression,
severe cardiovascular disease, severe
CNS depression, subcortical brain
damage

INTERACTIONS
Drug
Alcohol, other CNS depressants:
May increase respiratory depression
and the hypotensive effects of chlor-
promazine.
Antithyroid agents: May increase
the risk of agranulocytosis.
**Extrapyramidal symptom-
producing medications:** Increased
risk of extrapyramidal symptoms.
Hypotensives: May increase
hypotension.
Levodopa: May decrease the effects
of levodopa.
Lithium: May decrease the absorp-
tion of chlorpromazine and produce
adverse neurologic effects.
MAOIs, tricyclic antidepressants:
May increase the anticholinergic and
sedative effects of chlorpromazine.
Herbal
None known.
Food
None known.

DIAGNOSTIC TEST EFFECTS
May produce false-positive pregnancy and phenylketonuria (PKU)
test results. May cause EKG
changes, including Q- and T-wave
disturbances. Therapeutic serum
drug level is 50-300 mcg/ml; toxic
serum drug level is greater than
750 mcg/ml.

SIDE EFFECTS
Frequent
Somnolence, blurred vision,
hypotension, color vision or night
vision disturbances, dizziness,
decreased sweating, constipation,
dry mouth, nasal congestion
Occasional
Urinary retention, photosensitivity,
rash, decreased sexual function,
swelling or pain in breasts, weight
gain, nausea, vomiting, abdominal
pain, tremors

SERIOUS REACTIONS

• Extrapyramidal symptoms appear to be dose related and are divided into three categories: akathisia (including inability to sit still, tapping of feet), parkinsonian symptoms (such as masklike face, tremors, shuffling gait, hypersalivation), and acute dystonias (including torticollis, opisthotonos, and oculogyric crisis). A dystonic reaction may also produce diaphoresis and pallor.

• Tardive dyskinesia, including tongue protrusion, puffing of the cheeks, and puckering of the mouth is a rare reaction that may be irreversible.

• Abrupt discontinuation after long-term therapy may precipitate nausea, vomiting, gastritis, dizziness, and tremors.

• Blood dyscrasias, particularly agranulocytosis and mild leukopenia, may occur.

• Chlorpromazine may lower the seizure threshold.

PRECAUTIONS & CONSIDERATIONS

Caution is warranted with alcoholism, glaucoma, history of seizures, hypocalcemia (increases susceptibility to dystonias), impaired cardiac, hepatic, renal or respiratory function, benign prostatic hyperplasia, and urine retention. Alcohol, tasks that require mental alertness or motor skills, and excessive exposure to sunlight should be avoided. Skin should not come in contact with the oral concentrate and syrup because it can cause contact dermatitis.

Drowsiness may occur and urine may darken. Notify the physician of visual disturbances. CBC, calcium, hydration status, and skin should be assessed.

Administration

A slight yellow color in the oral concentrate or syrup won't affect the drug's potency. However, discard the drug if it is markedly discolored or contains precipitate.

Dilute each dose of oral concentrate immediately before administration with 60 ml or more of water, coffee, tea, milk, carbonated beverage, tomato or fruit juice, simple syrup, orange syrup, soup, or pudding. Use immediately and discard any remaining mixture.

! Do not give chlorpromazine by the subcutaneous route because severe tissue necrosis may occur. Be aware the therapeutic serum level for chlorpromazine is 50 to 300 mcg/ml, and the toxic serum level is greater than 750 mcg/ml.

For IM use, to prevent irritation at the injection site, dilute the injection solution with sodium chloride for injection or add 2% procaine, as prescribed.

Chlorpropamide
klor-pro′pa-mide
(Apo-Chlorpropamide [CAN], Diabinese)
Do not confuse with chlorpromazine.

CATEGORY AND SCHEDULE
Pregnancy Risk Category: C

CLASSIFICATION
Antidiabetic agents, sulfonylureas, first generation

MECHANISM OF ACTION
A first-generation sulfonylurea that promotes release of insulin from beta cells of pancreas. *Therapeutic Effect:* Lowers blood glucose concentration.

PHARMACOKINETICS
Rapidly absorbed from the gastrointestinal (GI) tract. Protein binding: 60%-90%. Extensively metabolized in liver. Excreted primarily in urine. Removed by hemodialysis. **Half-life:** 30-42 hr.

AVAILABILITY
Tablets: 100 mg, 250 mg (Diabenese).

INDICATIONS AND DOSAGES
▶ **Diabetes mellitus, combination therapy**
PO
Adults. Initially, 250 mg once a day. Maintenance: 250-500 mg once a day. Maximum: 750 mg/day.
Elderly. Initially, 100-125 mg once a day. Maintenance: 100-250 mg once a day. Increase or decrease by 50-125 mg a day for 3-5 day intervals.
▶ **Renal function impairment**
Not recommended.

OFF-LABEL USES
Neurogenic diabetes insipidus

CONTRAINDICATIONS
Diabetic complications, such as ketosis, acidosis, and diabetic coma, severe liver or renal impairment, sole therapy for type 1 diabetes mellitus, or hypersensitivity to sulfonylureas

INTERACTIONS
Drug
Alcohol: Disulfiram-like reactions may occur. Symptoms of low blood sugar including sweating, shaking, weakness, drowsiness, and trouble concentrating will occur.
Beta-blockers, MAOIs, NSAIDs, salicylates: May increase hypoglycemic effect.
Fluoroquinolone antibiotics: May increase the risk of hypoglycemia.

Glucocorticoids, thiazide diuretics: May increase blood glucose.
Oral contraceptives: May increase blood glucose.
Herbal
Bitter melon: May increase the risk of hypoglycemia.
St. John's wort: May increase the risk of hypoglycemia.
Food
None known.

DIAGNOSTIC TEST EFFECTS
None known.

SIDE EFFECTS
Frequent
Headache, upper respiratory tract infection
Occasional
Sinusitis, myalgia (muscle aches), pharyngitis, aggravated diabetes mellitus

SERIOUS REACTIONS
• Possible increased risk of cardiovascular mortality with this class of drugs.
• Overdosage can cause severe hypoglycemia prolonged by extended half-life.

PRECAUTIONS & CONSIDERATIONS
Caution is necessary with the elderly and liver function impairment. Chlorpropamide should be avoided in the elderly because of the high risk for hypoglycemia. Blood glucose should be checked before giving chlorpropamide. Chlorpropamide crosses the placenta and is distributed in breast milk and is not recommended in pregnant or breast-feeding women. Abdominal or chest pain, dark urine or light stool, hypoglycemic reactions, fever, nausea, palpitations, rash, vomiting, or yellowing of the eyes or skin should be reported immediately.

Be alert to conditions that alter blood glucose requirements, such as fever, increased activity, stress, or a surgical procedure. Hypoglycemia, such as anxiety, cool, wet skin, diplopia, dizziness, headache, hunger, numbness in mouth, tachycardia, and tremors, or hyperglycemia, including deep, rapid breathing, dim vision, fatigue, nausea, polydipsia, polyphagia, polyuria, and vomiting can occur. Blood glucose levels, Hgb, and liver function tests should be monitored during therapy. Candy, sugar packets, or other sugar supplements for immediate response to hypoglycemia should be carried.

Administration

Give chlorpropamide with or without regard to meals.

Chlorthalidone
klor-thal′i-doan
(Apo-Chlorthalidone [CAN], Hygroton [AUS], Thalitone)

CATEGORY AND SCHEDULE
Pregnancy Risk Category: B
(D if used in pregnancy-induced hypertension)

CLASSIFICATION
Diuretics, thiazide and derivatives

MECHANISM OF ACTION
A thiazide diuretic that blocks reabsorption of sodium, potassium, and water at the distal convoluted tubule; also decreases plasma and extracellular fluid volume and peripheral vascular resistance. *Therapeutic Effect:* Produces diuresis; lowers B/P.

PHARMACOKINETICS

Route	Onset	Peak	Duration
PO (diuretic)	2 hr	2-6 hr	Up to 36 hr

Rapidly absorbed from the GI tract. Excreted unchanged in urine.
Half-life: 35-50 hr. Onset of antihypertensive effect: 3-4 days; optimal therapeutic effect: 3-4 wk.

AVAILABILITY
Tablets: 15 mg, 25 mg, 50 mg, 100 mg.

INDICATIONS AND DOSAGES
▶ **Hypertension, edema**
PO
Adults. 25-100 mg/day or 100 mg 3 times a week.
Elderly. Initially, 12.5-25 mg/day or every other day.

CONTRAINDICATIONS
Anuria, history of hypersensitivity to sulfonamides or thiazide diuretics, renal decompensation

INTERACTIONS
Drug
Cholestyramine, colestipol: May decrease the absorption and effects of chlorthalidone.
Digoxin: May increase the risk of digoxin toxicity associated with chlorthalidone-induced hyperkalemia.
Lithium: May increase the risk of lithium toxicity.
Herbal
None known.
Food
None known.

DIAGNOSTIC TEST EFFECTS
May increase blood glucose and serum cholesterol, LDL, bilirubin, calcium, creatinine, uric acid, and triglyceride levels. May decrease

urinary calcium and serum magnesium, potassium, and sodium levels.

SIDE EFFECTS

Expected
Increase in urinary frequency and urine volume
Frequent
Potassium depletion (rarely produces symptoms)
Occasional
Anorexia, impotence, diarrhea, orthostatic hypotension, GI disturbances, photosensitivity
Rare
Rash

SERIOUS REACTIONS

• Vigorous diuresis may lead to profound water and electrolyte depletion, resulting in hypokalemia, hyponatremia, and dehydration.
• Acute hypotensive episodes may occur.
• Hyperglycemia may occur during prolonged therapy.
• Overdose can lead to lethargy and coma without changes in electrolytes or hydration.

PRECAUTIONS & CONSIDERATIONS

Caution is warranted with diabetes mellitus, gout, hypercholesterolemia, hepatic impairment, severe renal disease, and in the elderly and debilitated. It is unknown if chlorthalidone is distributed in breast milk. Chlorthalidone crosses the placenta and a small amount is distributed in breast milk. Breast-feeding is not recommended for patients taking this drug. No age-related precautions have been noted in children. The elderly may be more sensitive to the drug's hypotensive and electrolyte effects. Consuming foods high in potassium such as apricots, bananas, legumes, meat, orange juice, raisins, whole grains, including cereals,

and white and sweet potatoes, is encouraged. Avoid prolonged exposure to sunlight.

Dizziness or lightheadedness may occur, so change positions slowly to reduce the drug's hypotensive effect. An increase in the frequency and volume of urination may also occur. Blood pressure (B/P), vital signs, electrolytes, intake and output, and weight should be monitored before and during treatment. Blood glucose levels should be checked after prolonged therapy because hyperglycemia may occur. Be aware of signs of electrolyte disturbances such as hypokalemia. Hypokalemia may cause arrhythmias, altered mental status, muscle cramps, asthenia, and tremor.

Administration
Take chlorthalidone with food or milk if GI upset occurs, preferably with breakfast to help prevent nocturia. Crush scored tablets if needed.

Chlorzoxazone
klor-zox′a-zone
(Parafon Forte DSC, Remular, Remular-S)
Do not confuse with chlorthalidone.

CATEGORY AND SCHEDULE
Pregnancy Risk Category: C

CLASSIFICATION
Musculoskeletal agents, relaxants, skeletal muscle

MECHANISM OF ACTION
A skeletal muscle relaxant that inhibits transmission of reflexes at

the spinal cord level. *Therapeutic Effect:* Relieves muscle spasticity.

PHARMACOKINETICS
Readily absorbed from the gastrointestinal (GI) tract. Metabolized in liver. Primarily excreted in urine. **Half-life:** 1.1 hr.

AVAILABILITY
Caplets: 500 mg (Parafon Forte DSC).
Tablets: 250 mg.

INDICATIONS AND DOSAGES
▶ **Musculoskeletal pain**
PO
Adults, Elderly. 250-500 mg 3-4 times/day. Maximum: 750 mg 3-4 day.
Children. 20 mg/kg/day in 3-4 divided doses.

CONTRAINDICATIONS
Hypersensitivity to chlorzoxazone or any one of its components.

INTERACTIONS
Drug
Alcohol, central nervous system (CNS) depressants: May increase CNS depression.
Herbal
Garlic: May decrease the effectiveness of chlorzoxazone.
Kava: May increase CNS depression.
St. John's wort: May decrease the effectiveness of chlorzoxazone.
Food
None known.

DIAGNOSTIC TEST EFFECTS
False-positive for serum aprobarbital when using Toxi-Lab Screen.

SIDE EFFECTS
Frequent
Drowsiness, fever, headache

Occasional
Nausea, vomiting, stomach cramps, rash

SERIOUS REACTIONS
• Overdosage results in nausea, vomiting, diarrhea, and hypotension.

PRECAUTIONS & CONSIDERATIONS
Caution is necessary with liver impairment. Blood counts and liver and renal function tests should be performed periodically for those on long-term therapy. There is an increased risk of central nervous system (CNS) toxicity, manifested as confusion, hallucinations, mental depression, and sedation in the elderly. Age-related renal impairment may require a decreased dosage.
  Drowsiness may occur during treatment but usually diminishes with continued therapy. Tasks that require mental alertness or motor skills should be avoided until response to baclofen is established. Alcohol and CNS depressants should be avoided.
Administration
Take without regard to meals.

C

Cholestyramine
koe-less-tir′a-meen
(Novo-Cholamine [CAN], Prevalite, Questran [CAN], Questran Lite [AUS])
Do not confuse Questran with Quarzan.

CATEGORY AND SCHEDULE
Pregnancy Risk Category: B

CLASSIFICATION
Antihyperlipidemics, bile acid sequestrants

MECHANISM OF ACTION

An antihyperlipoproteinemic that binds with bile acids in the intestine, forming an insoluble complex. Binding results in partial removal of bile acid from enterohepatic circulation. *Therapeutic Effect:* Removes LDL cholesterol from plasma.

PHARMACOKINETICS

Not absorbed from the GI tract. Decreases in serum LDL apparent in 5 to 7 days and in serum cholesterol in 1 mo. Serum cholesterol returns to baseline levels about 1 mo after drug is discontinued.

AVAILABILITY

Powder for Oral Suspension: 4 g.

INDICATIONS AND DOSAGES

▶ **Primary hypercholesterolemia**
PO
Adults, Elderly. 3-4 g 3-4 times a day. Maximum: 16-32 g/day in 2-4 divided doses.
Children older than 10 yr. 2 g/day. Maximum: 8 g/day in 2 or more divided doses.
Children 10 yr and younger. Initially, 2 g/day. Range: 1-4 g/day.
▶ **Pruritis**
PO
Adults, Elderly. 4 g 1-2 times a day. Maintenance: Up to 24 g/day in divided doses.

OFF-LABEL USES

Treatment of diarrhea (due to bile acids), hyperoxaluria

CONTRAINDICATIONS

Complete biliary obstruction, hypersensitivity to cholestyramine or tartrazine (frequently seen in aspirin hypersensitivity)

INTERACTIONS

Drug

Anticoagulants: May increase effects of these drugs by decreasing level of vitamin K.
Digoxin, folic acid, penicillins, propranolol, tetracyclines, thiazides, thyroid hormones, other medications: May bind and decrease absorption of these drugs.
Oral vancomycin: Binds and decreases the effects of oral vancomycin.
Warfarin: May decrease warfarin absorption.

Herbal

None known.

Food

None known.

DIAGNOSTIC TEST EFFECTS

May increase serum alkaline phosphatase, serum magnesium, AST (SGOT), and ALT (SGPT) levels. May decrease serum calcium, potassium, and sodium levels. May prolong prothrombin time.

SIDE EFFECTS

Frequent

Constipation (may lead to fecal impaction), nausea, vomiting, abdominal pain, indigestion

Occasional

Diarrhea, belching, bloating, headache, dizziness

Rare

Gallstones, peptic ulcer disease, malabsorption syndrome

SERIOUS REACTIONS

• GI tract obstruction, hyperchloremic acidosis, and osteoporosis secondary to calcium excretion may occur.
• High dosage may interfere with fat absorption, resulting in steatorrhea.

PRECAUTIONS & CONSIDERATIONS

Caution is warranted with bleeding disorders, GI dysfunction (especially constipation), hemorrhoids, and osteoporosis. Cholestyramine is not systemically absorbed and may interfere with maternal absorption of fat-soluble vitamins. No age-related precautions have been noted in children. Cholestyramine use is limited in children younger than 10 years of age. The elderly are at increased risk for experiencing adverse nutritional effects and GI side effects.

Notify the physician of abdominal discomfort, flatulence, and food intolerance. Pattern of daily bowel activity and stool consistency should be assessed. High-fiber foods, such as fruits, whole grain cereals, and vegetables will reduce the risk of constipation. History of hypersensitivity to aspirin, cholestyramine, and tartrazine should be determined before beginning cholestyramine therapy. Serum cholesterol and triglyceride levels should be checked at baseline and periodically thereafter.

Administration

Take other drugs at least 1 hour before or 4 to 6 hours after cholestyramine because this drug is capable of binding drugs in the GI tract. Don't take cholestyramine in its dry form because it is highly irritating. Mix with 3 to 6 ounces fruit juice, milk, soup, or water. Allow the powder to sit on the surface of the liquid for 1 to 2 minutes to prevent lumping; then mix thoroughly. When mixing the powder with carbonated beverages, use an extra large glass and stir the liquid slowly to avoid excessive foaming. Take before meals.

Choline Magnesium Trisalicylate

koe'leen mag-nees'ee-um tri-sal'eh-cye'late
(Tricosal, Trilisate)

CATEGORY AND SCHEDULE

Pregnancy Risk Category: C
(D if full dose used in third trimester of pregnancy)

CLASSIFICATION

Analgesics, non-narcotic, salicylates

MECHANISM OF ACTION

A nonsteroidal salicylate that inhibits prostaglandin synthesis and acts on the hypothalamus heat-regulating center. *Therapeutic Effect:* Reduces inflammatory response and intensity of pain stimulus reaching sensory nerve endings.

PHARMACOKINETICS

Rapidly absorbed from gastrointestinal (GI) tract. Oral route onset 1 hour, peak 2 hours and duration 9-17 hours. Protein binding: High. Widely distributed. Excreted in the urine. **Half-life:** 2-3 hr.

AVAILABILITY

Tablets: 500 mg, 750 mg, 1000 mg (Tricosal, Trilisate).
Liquid: 500 mg/5 ml (Trilisate).

INDICATIONS AND DOSAGES

▸ **Analgesic, acute painful shoulder, anti-inflammatory, antipyretic**
PO
Adults, Elderly. Initially, 500 mg-1500 mg q8-12hr, then 1-4.5 g/day.
Children less than 37 kg.
50 mg/kg/day in divided doses.

CONTRAINDICATIONS

Allergy to tartrazine dye, bleeding disorders, GI bleeding or ulceration, history of hypersensitivity to choline magnesium trisalicylate, aspirin, or NSAIDs.

INTERACTIONS

Drug

Alcohol, NSAIDs: May increase the risk of adverse GI effects, including ulceration.

Antacids, urinary alkalinizers: Increase the excretion of choline magnesium trisalicylate.

Anticoagulants, heparin, thrombolytics: Increase the risk of bleeding.

Platelet aggregation inhibitors, valproic acid: May increase the risk of bleeding.

Probenecid: May decrease the effect of these drugs.

Herbal

Cat's claw, dong quai, evening primrose, feverfew, garlic, ginger, ginkgo, red clover, horse chestnut, green tea, ginseng: May increase the risk of bleeding.

Food

Curry powder, paprika, licorice, Benedictine liqueur, prunes, raisins, tea, gherkins: May increase the risk of salicylate accumulation.

DIAGNOSTIC TEST EFFECTS

May yield false-negative results for glucose oxidase urinary glucose tests (Clinitest); false-positive results using the cupric sulfate method (Clinitest). May interfere with Gerhardt test (urinary ketone analysis). May prolong bleeding time, and prothrombin time (PT). May decrease T3 and T4 levels.

SIDE EFFECTS

Side effects appear less frequently with short-term treatment.

Occasional

Nausea, dyspepsia (heartburn, indigestion, epigastric pain), tinnitus

Rare

Anorexia, headache, vomiting, flatulence, dizziness, somnolence, insomnia, fatigue, hearing impairment

SERIOUS REACTIONS

• High doses may produce GI bleeding.

• Overdosage may be characterized by ringing in ears, generalized pruritus (may be severe), headache, dizziness, flushing, tachycardia, hyperventilation, sweating, and thirst.

PRECAUTIONS & CONSIDERATIONS

Caution should be used with dehydration, erosive gastritis, peptic ulcer disease, and chronic renal insufficiency. Caution is also warranted in children with acute febrile illness because choline magnesium trisalicylate increases the risk of developing Reye's syndrome. Choline magnesium trisalicylate crosses the placenta and is distributed in breast milk. It should be avoided during the last trimester of pregnancy because the drug may adversely affect the fetal cardiovascular system causing premature closure of ductus arteriosus. Lower choline magnesium trisalicylate dosages are recommended in the elderly because this age group may be more susceptible to toxicity.

Administration

Take choline magnesium trisalicylate with meals to avoid GI upset. Mix with fruit juice just before drinking.

Ciclopirox
sye-kloe-peer'ox
(Loprox, Penlac)
**Do not confuse with
ciprofloxacin.**

CATEGORY AND SCHEDULE
Pregnancy Risk Category: B

CLASSIFICATION
Antifungals, topical,
dermatologics

MECHANISM OF ACTION
An antifungal that inhibits
the transport of essential elements
in the fungal cell, thereby
interfering with biosynthesis
in fungi. *Therapeutic Effect:*
Results in fungal cell
death.

PHARMACOKINETICS
Absorbed through intact skin.
Distributed to epidermis, dermis,
including hair, hair follicles, and
sebaceous glands. Protein binding:
98%. Primarily excreted in urine
and to a lesser extent in feces.
Half-life: 1.7 hr.

AVAILABILITY
Cream: 0.77% (Loprox).
Gel: 0.77% (Loprox).
Lotion: 0.77% (Loprox TS).
Shampoo: 0.77% (Loprox).
Topical Solution, nail lacquer: 8%
(Penlac).

INDICATIONS AND DOSAGES
▶ **Tinea pedis**
TOPICAL
*Adults, Elderly, Children 10 yr and
older.* Apply 2 times a day until
signs and symptoms significantly
improve.

▶ **Tinea cruris, Tinea corporis**
TOPICAL
*Adults, Elderly, Children 10 yr and
older.* Apply 2 times a day until
signs and symptoms significantly
improve.
▶ **Onychomycosis**
Topical (solution)
*Adults, Elderly, Children 10 yr and
older.* Apply to the affected area
(nails) daily. Remove with alcohol
every 7 days.
▶ **Seborrheic dermatitis**
SHAMPOO
*Adults, Elderly, Children 10 yr and
older.* Apply to affected scalp areas
2 times a day, in the morning and
evening for 4 weeks.

CONTRAINDICATIONS
Hypersensitivity to ciclopirox or any
one of its components

INTERACTIONS
Drug
Not known.
Herbal
Not known.
Food
Not known.

DIAGNOSTIC TEST EFFECTS
None known.

SIDE EFFECTS
Rare
Topical: Irritation, burning, redness,
pain at the site of application

SERIOUS REACTIONS
• None known.

PRECAUTIONS & CONSIDERATIONS
Avoid use of occlusive wrappings or
dressings. Avoid contact with eyes.
If local irritation occurs, ciclopirox
should be discontinued. It is unknown
if ciclopirox crosses the placenta or
is distributed in breast milk.

Safety and efficacy has not been established in children younger than 12 years old. There are no age-related precautions in the elderly.

Administration

Apply topical formulation by rubbing gently into the affected and surrounding area 2 times daily until signs and symptoms improve.

Apply nail lacquer once daily, preferably at bedtime or 8 hours before washing, to the affected nails with the applicator brush provided. Cover evenly over the entire nail plate. Ciclopirox should be removed on a daily basis. Daily applications should be made over the previous coat. Remove with alcohol every 7 days. Repeat cycle throughout the duration of therapy. File away with emery board loose nail material and trim nails every 7 days after ciclopirox is removed with alcohol.

Apply to shampoo to affected scalp areas 2 times a day, in the morning and evening for 4 weeks. Clinical improvement usually occurs within the first week with continuing resolution of signs and symptoms through the fourth week of treatment.

Cidofovir
ci-dah′fo-veer
(Vistide)

CATEGORY AND SCHEDULE
Pregnancy Risk Category: C

CLASSIFICATION
Antivirals

MECHANISM OF ACTION
An anti-infective that inhibits viral DNA synthesis by incorporating itself into the growing viral DNA chain. *Therapeutic Effect:* Suppresses replication of cytomegalovirus (CMV).

PHARMACOKINETICS
Protein binding: less than 6%. Excreted primarily unchanged in urine. Effect of hemodialysis unknown. Elimination **half-life:** 1.4-3.8 hr.

AVAILABILITY
Injection: 75 mg/ml (5-ml ampule).

INDICATIONS AND DOSAGES
▸ **CMV retinitis in patients with AIDS (in combination with probenecid)**
IV INFUSION
Adults. Induction: Usual dosage, 5 mg/kg at constant rate over 1 hr once weekly for 2 consecutive wk. Give 2 g of PO probenecid 3 hr before cidofovir dose, and then give 1 g 2 hr and 8 hr after completion of the 1-hr cidofovir infusion (total of 4 g). In addition, give 1 L of 0.9% NaCl over 1-2 hr immediately before the cidofovir infusion. If tolerated, a second liter may be infused over 1-3 hr at the start of the infusion or immediately afterward. Maintenance: 5 mg/kg cidofovir at constant rate over 1 hr once every 2 wk.
▸ **Dosage in renal impairment**
Dosages are modified based on creatinine clearance.

Creatinine Clearance	Induction Dose	Maintenance Dose
41-55 ml/min	2 mg/kg	2 mg/kg
30-40 ml/min	1.5 mg/kg	1.5 mg/kg
20-29 ml/min	1 mg/kg	1 mg/kg
19 ml/min or less	0.5 mg/kg	0.5 mg/kg

OFF-LABEL USES
Treatment of ganciclovir-resistant CMV, foscarnet-resistant CMV, adenovirus, and acyclovir-resistant herpes simplex virus or varicella-zoster virus

CONTRAINDICATIONS
Direct intraocular injection, history of clinically severe hypersensitivity to probenecid or other sulfa-containing drugs, hypersensitivity to cidofovir, renal function impairment (serum creatinine level greater than 1.5 mg/dl, creatinine clearance of 55 ml/min or less, or urine protein level greater than 100 mg/dl)

INTERACTIONS
Drug
Nephrotoxic medications (such as aminoglycosides, amphotericin B, foscarnet, IV pentamidine): Increase the risk of nephrotoxicity.
Herbal
None known.
Food
None known.

DIAGNOSTIC TEST EFFECTS
May decrease neutrophil count and serum bicarbonate, phosphate, and uric acid levels. May elevate serum creatinine levels.

▒ IV INCOMPATIBILITIES
No information available for Y-site administration.

SIDE EFFECTS
Frequent
Nausea, vomiting (65%), fever (57%), asthenia (46%), rash (30%), diarrhea (27%), headache (27%), alopecia (25%), chills (24%), anorexia (22%), dyspnea (22%), abdominal pain (17%)

SERIOUS REACTIONS
• Serious adverse reactions may include proteinuria (80%), nephrotoxicity (53%), neutropenia (31%), elevated serum creatinine levels (29%), infection (24%), anemia (20%), ocular hypotony (a decrease in intraocular pressure, 12%), and pneumonia (9%).
• Concurrent use of probenecid may produce a hypersensitivity reaction characterized by a rash, fever, chills, and anaphylaxis.
• Acute renal failure occurs rarely.

PRECAUTIONS & CONSIDERATIONS
Caution is warranted with preexisting diabetes. Be aware that cidofovir is embryotoxic and results in reduced fetal body weight in animals. Females of childbearing age should use effective contraception during and for 1 month after cidofovir treatment; male patients should practice barrier contraceptive methods during and for 3 months after treatment. Be aware that it is unknown if cidofovir is excreted in breast milk. Do not administer to breast-feeding women. Breast-feeding is not recommended in this population because of the possibility of HIV transmission. Be aware that the safety and efficacy of cidofovir have not been established in children. In the elderly, age-related renal impairment may require dosage adjustment.

For persons also taking zidovudine (AZT), expect to temporarily discontinue zidovudine administration or decrease zidovudine dose by 50% on days of cidofovir infusion. Be aware that concurrent probenecid use reduces the metabolic clearance of zidovudine. Renal function should be closely monitored through serum creatinine levels and urinalysis during therapy. Urine protein and white blood cell (WBC) count should also be monitored. Visual acuity and ocular symptoms should be evaluated.

Storage
Store cidofovir at controlled room temperature (68° to 77° F). Refrigerate admixtures for no more than 24 hours. Allow refrigerated admixtures to warm to room temperature before use.

Administration
! Do not exceed the recommended dosage, frequency, or infusion rate. Dilute in 100 ml 0.9% NaCl and infuse over 1 hour. Prepare to administer IV hydration with 0.9% NaCl and probenecid with each cidofovir infusion to minimize the risk of nephrotoxicity. Eat food before each dose of probenecid to help reduce nausea and vomiting. As prescribed, administer an antiemetic to reduce the risk of nausea.

Cilostazol
sil-os'tah-zol
(Pletal)
Do not confuse Pletal with Plendil.

CATEGORY AND SCHEDULE
Pregnancy Risk Category: C

CLASSIFICATION
Platelet inhibitors

MECHANISM OF ACTION
A phosphodiesterase III inhibitor that inhibits platelet aggregation. Dilates vascular beds with greatest dilation in femoral beds. *Therapeutic Effect:* Improves walking distance in patients with intermittent claudication.

PHARMACOKINETICS
Moderately absorbed from the GI tract. Protein binding: 95%-98%. Extensively metabolized in the liver. Excreted primarily in the urine and, to a lesser extent, in the feces. Not removed by hemodialysis. **Half-life:** 11-13 hr. Therapeutic effect is usually noted in 2-4 wk but may take as long as 12 wk.

AVAILABILITY
Tablets: 50 mg, 100 mg.

INDICATIONS AND DOSAGES
▸ **Intermittent claudication**
PO
Adults, Elderly. 100 mg twice a day at least 30 min before or 2 hr after meals.

CONTRAINDICATIONS
CHF of any severity

INTERACTIONS
Drug
Clarithromycin, diltiazem, erythromycin, fluconazole, fluoxetine, omeprazole, sertraline: May incease concentration of cilostazol.
Aspirin: May potentiate inhibition of platelet aggregation.
Herbal
None known.
Food
Grapefruit juice: May increase blood concentration and risk of toxicity of cilostazol.

DIAGNOSTIC TEST EFFECTS
May increase BUN and serum creatinine levels. May decrease Hgb and Hct.

SIDE EFFECTS
Frequent (34%-10%)
Headache, diarrhea, palpitations, dizziness, pharyngitis

Occasional (7%-3%)
Nausea, rhinitis, back pain, peripheral edema, dyspepsia, abdominal pain, tachycardia, cough, flatulence, myalgia
Rare (2%-1%)
Leg cramps, paresthesia, rash, vomiting

SERIOUS REACTIONS
• Signs and symptoms of overdose are noted by severe headache, diarrhea, hypotension, and cardiac arrhythmias.

PRECAUTIONS & CONSIDERATIONS
It is unknown if cilostazol crosses the placenta or is distributed in breast milk. Safety and efficacy of cilostazol have not been established in children. No age-related precautions have been noted in the elderly. Hgb, Hct, and platelet counts should be obtained before and periodically during treatment.
Administration
Take cilostazol at least 30 minutes before or 2 hours after meals. Do not give with grapefruit juice because grapefruit juice may increase the drug's blood concentration and risk of toxicity.

Cimetidine
sye-met′i-deen
(Apo-Cimetidine [CAN], Cimehexal [AUS], Magicul [AUS], Novocimetine [CAN], Peptol [CAN], Sigmetadine [AUS], Tagamet, Tagamet HB)
Do not confuse cimetidine with simethicone.

CATEGORY AND SCHEDULE
Pregnancy Risk Category: B
OTC Tablets: 100 mg

CLASSIFICATION
Antihistamines, H2, gastrointestinals

MECHANISM OF ACTION
An antiulcer agent and gastric acid secretion inhibitor that inhibits histamine action at histamine 2 receptor sites of parietal cells. *Therapeutic Effect*: Inhibits gastric acid secretion during fasting, at night, or when stimulated by food, caffeine, or insulin.

PHARMACOKINETICS
Well absorbed from the GI tract. Protein binding: 15%-20%. Widely distributed. Metabolized in the liver. Primarily excreted in urine. Not removed by hemodialysis. **Half-life:** 2 hr; increased with impaired renal function.

AVAILABILITY
Tablets (Tagamet HB): 200 mg.
Tablets (Tagamet): 300 mg, 400 mg.
Liquid: 300 mg/5 ml.
Liquid (Tagamet HB): 200 mg/20 ml.
Injection: 150 mg/ml.

INDICATIONS AND DOSAGES
▶ **Active ulcer**
PO
Adults, Elderly. 300 mg 4 times a day or 400 mg twice a day or 800 mg at bedtime.
IM, IV
Adults, Elderly. 300 mg q6hr or 150 mg as single dose followed by 37.5 mg/hr continuous infusion.
▶ **Prevention of duodenal ulcer**
PO
Adults, Elderly. 400-800 mg at bedtime.
▶ **Gastric hypersecretory secretions**
PO, IV, IM
Adults, Elderly. 300-600 mg q6hr. Maximum: 2400 mg/day.
Children. 20-40 mg/kg/day in divided doses q6hr.
Infants. 10-20 mg/kg/day in divided doses q6-12hr.
Neonates. 5-10 mg/kg/day in divided doses q8-12hr.
▶ **Gastrointestinal reflux disease**
PO
Adults, Elderly. 800 mg twice a day or 400 mg 4 times a day for 12 wks.
▶ **OTC use**
PO
Adults, Elderly. 100 mg up to 30 min before meals. Maximum: 2 doses/day.
▶ **Prevention of upper GI bleeding**
IV infusion
Adults, Elderly. 50 mg/hr.
▶ **Dosage in renal impairment**
Dosage is based on a 300-mg dose in adults. Dosage interval is modified based on creatinine clearance.

Creatinine Clearance	Dosage Interval
Greater than 40 ml/min	q6hr
20-40 ml/min	q8hr or decrease dose by 25%
Less than 20 ml/min	q12hr or decrease dose by 50%

Give after hemodialysis and q12hr between dialysis sessions.

OFF-LABEL USES
Prevention of aspiration pneumonia; treatment of acute urticaria, chronic warts, upper GI bleeding

CONTRAINDICATIONS
Hypersensitivity to cimetidine or other H2-antagonists.

INTERACTIONS
Drug
Antacids: May decrease the absorption of cimetidine.
Calcium channel blockers, cyclosporine, lidocaine, metoprolol, metronidazole, oral anticoagulants, oral antidiabetics, phenytoin, propranolol, theophylline, tricyclic antidepressants: May decrease the metabolism and increase the blood concentrations of these drugs.
Ketoconazole: May decrease the absorption of ketoconazole.
Herbal
None known.
Food
None known.

DIAGNOSTIC TEST EFFECTS
Interferes with skin tests using allergen extracts. May increase prolactin, serum creatinine, and transaminase levels. May decrease parathyroid hormone concentration.

▓ IV INCOMPATIBILITIES
Allopurinol (Aloprim), amphotericin B complex (AmBisome, Amphotec, Abelcet), cefepime (Maxipime)
▓ IV Compatibilities
Aminophylline, diltiazem (Cardizem), furosemide (Lasix), heparin, hydromorphone (Dilaudid), insulin (regular), lidocaine, lorazepam (Ativan), midazolam (Versed), morphine, potassium chloride, propofol (Diprivan)

C

SIDE EFFECTS
Occasional (4%-2%)
Headache
Elderly and severely ill patients, patients with impaired renal function: Confusion, agitation, psychosis, depression, anxiety, disorientation, hallucinations. Effects reverse 3 to 4 days after discontinuance.
Rare (less than 2%)
Diarrhea, dizziness, somnolence, nausea, vomiting, gynecomastia, rash, impotence

SERIOUS REACTIONS
- Rapid IV administration may produce cardiac arrhythmias and hypotension.

PRECAUTIONS & CONSIDERATIONS
Caution is warranted with impaired hepatic or renal function and in the elderly. Cimetidine crosses the placenta and is distributed in breast milk. Cimetidine use in infants may suppress gastric acidity, inhibit drug metabolism, and produce CNS stimulation. Long-term use in children may induce cerebral toxicity and affect the hormonal system. The elderly are more likely to experience confusion, especially those with impaired renal function. Do not take antacids within 1 hour of oral cimetidine administration. Avoid smoking. Tasks that require mental alertness or motor skills should also be avoided until response to the drug has been established. Alcohol and aspirin, both of which may cause GI distress, should also be avoided during cimetidine therapy.

Notify the physician if blood in emesis or stool, or dark, tarry stool occurs. Pattern of daily bowel activity and stool consistency, electrolytes, and hydration status should be monitored.

Storage
Store parenteral form at room temperature. Reconstituted IV solution is stable for 48 hours at room temperature.

Administration
Dilute each 300 mg (2 ml) with 18 ml 0.9% NaCl, 0.45% NaCl, 0.2% NaCl, D_5W, $D_{10}W$, Ringer's solution, or lactated Ringer's solution to a total volume of 20 ml. For IV push, administer over not less than 2 minutes to prevent arrhythmias and hypotension. For intermittent IV (piggyback) administration, infuse over 15 to 20 minutes. For IV infusion, dilute with 100 to 1000 ml 0.9% NaCl, D_5W, or other compatible solution, and infuse over 24 hours.

For IM use, administer undiluted. Inject deep into large muscle mass, such as the gluteus maximus muscle. IM administration may produce transient discomfort at the injection site.

Cinacalcet
sin-a-cal′set
(Sensipar)

CATEGORY AND SCHEDULE
Pregnancy Risk Category: C

CLASSIFICATION
Calcimimetic agent

MECHANISM OF ACTION
A calcium receptor agonist that increases the sensitivity of the calcium-sensing receptor on the parathyroid gland to extracellular calcium, thus lowering the parathyroid hormone (PTH) level.
Therapeutic Effect: Decreases serum calcium and PTH levels.

PHARMACOKINETICS
Extensively distributed after PO administration. Protein binding: 93%-97%. Rapidly and extensively metabolized by multiple enzymes. Primarily eliminated in urine with a lesser amount excreted in feces. **Half-life:** 30-40 hr.

AVAILABILITY
Tablets: 30 mg, 60 mg, 90 mg.

INDICATIONS AND DOSAGES
▸ **Hypercalcemia in parathyroid carcinoma**
PO
Adults, Elderly. Initially, 30 mg twice a day. Titrate dosage sequentially (60 mg twice a day, 90 mg twice a day, and 90 mg 3-4 times a day) every 2-4 wk as needed to normalize serum calcium levels.
▸ **Secondary hyperparathyroidism in patients on dialysis**
PO
Adults, Elderly. Initially, 30 mg once a day. Titrate dosage sequentially (60, 90, 120, and 180 mg once a day) every 2-4 wk.

CONTRAINDICATIONS
None known.

INTERACTIONS
Drug
Amitriptyline: Increases amitriptyline plasma concentration.
Flecainide, thioridazine, tricyclic antidepressants, vinblastine: May require dosage adjustment of these drugs
Erythromycin, itraconazole, ketoconazole: Increase cinacalcet plasma concentration.
Herbal
None known.
Food
High-fat meals: Increase cinacalcet plasma concentration.

DIAGNOSTIC TEST EFFECTS
Reduces serum calcium level.

SIDE EFFECTS
Frequent (31%-21%)
Nausea, vomiting, diarrhea
Occasional (15%-10%)
Myalgia, dizziness
Rare (7%-5%)
Asthenia, hypertension, anorexia, non-cardiac chest pain

SERIOUS REACTIONS
• Overdose may lead to hypocalcemia.

PRECAUTIONS & CONSIDERATIONS
Caution is warranted with hepatic impairment. Cinacalcet may cross the placental barrier. Cinacalcet's safe use during breast-feeding has not been established; the drug may cause adverse reactions in breast-fed infants. The safety and efficacy of cinacalcet have not been established in children. No age-related precautions have been noted in the elderly. Notify the physician if diarrhea or vomiting occurs. Serum electrolyte levels and pattern of daily bowel activity and stool consistency should be monitored.
Storage
Store tablets at room temperature.
Administration
Don't break or crush film-coated tablets. Take the drug with food or shortly after a meal.

Ciprofloxacin
sip-ro-floks'a-sin
(C-Flox [AUS], Ciloquin
[AUS], Ciloxan, Cipro,
Ciproxin [AUS])
**Do not confuse ciprofloxacin or
Ciproxin with Ciloxan,
cinoxacin, or Cytoxan.**

CATEGORY AND SCHEDULE
Pregnancy Risk Category: C

CLASSIFICATION
Anti-infectives, ophthalmics,
antibiotics, quinolones

MECHANISM OF ACTION
A fluoroquinolone that inhibits the
enzyme DNA gyrase in susceptible
bacteria, interfering with bacterial
cell replication. *Therapeutic Effect:*
Bactericidal.

PHARMACOKINETICS
Well absorbed from the GI tract
(food delays absorption). Protein
binding: 20%-40%. Widely distributed (including to CSF). Metabolized
in the liver to active metabolite.
Primarily excreted in urine.
Minimal removal by hemodialysis.
Half-life: 4-6 hr (increased in
impaired renal function and the
elderly).

AVAILABILITY
Tablets (Cipro): 100 mg, 250 mg,
500 mg, 750 mg.
*Tablets, extended-release (Cipro
XR):* 500 mg, 1000 mg.
Infusion: 200 mg/100 ml,
400 mg/200 ml.
Ophthalmic Ointment (Ciloxan):
0.3%.
Ophthalmic Suspension (Ciloxan):
0.3%.

INDICATIONS AND DOSAGES
▶ **Mild to moderate UTIs**
PO
Adults, Elderly. 250 mg q12hr.
IV
Adults, Elderly. 200 mg q12hr.
▶ **Complicated UTIs, mild to moderate
respiratory tract, bone, joint, skin
and skin-structure infections;
infectious diarrhea**
PO
Adults, Elderly. 500 mg q12hr.
IV
Adults, Elderly. 400 mg q12hr.
▶ **Severe, complicated infections**
PO
Adults, Elderly. 750 mg q12hr.
IV
Adults, Elderly. 400 mg q12hr.
▶ **Prostatitis**
PO
Adults, Elderly. 500 mg q12hr for
28 days.
▶ **Uncomplicated bladder
infection**
PO
Adults. 100 mg twice a day for
3 days.
▶ **Acute sinusitis**
PO
Adults. 500 mg q12hr.
▶ **Uncomplicated gonorrhea**
PO
Adults. 250 mg as a single dose.
▶ **Cystic fibrosis**
IV
Children. 30 mg/kg/day in 2-3
divided doses. Maximum:
1.2 g/day.
PO
Children. 40 mg/kg/day. Maximum:
2 g/day.
▶ **Corneal ulcer**
OPHTHALMIC
Adults, Elderly. 2 drops q15min for
6 hr, then 2 drops q30min for the
remainder of first day, 2 drops q1hr
on second day, and 2 drops q4hr on
days 3-14.

C

▸ **Conjunctivitis**
OPHTHALMIC
Adults, Elderly. 1-2 drops q2hr for 2 days, then 2 drops q4hr for next 5 days.
▸ **Dosage in renal impairment**
Dosage and frequency are modified based on creatinine clearance and the severity of the infection.

Creatinine Clearance	Dosage Interval
Less than 30 ml/min	Usual dose q18-24hr

▸ **Hemodialysis**
250-500 mg q24hr (after dialysis).
▸ **Peritoneal Dialysis**
250-500 mg q24hr (after dialysis).

OFF-LABEL USES
Treatment of chancroid

CONTRAINDICATIONS
Hypersensitivity to ciprofloxacin or other quinolones; for ophthalmic administration: vaccinia, varicella, epithelial herpes simplex, keratitis, mycobacterial infection, fungal disease of ocular structure, use after uncomplicated removal of a foreign body.

INTERACTIONS
Drug
Antacids, iron preparations, sucralfate: May decrease ciprofloxacin absorption.
Caffeine, oral anticoagulants: May increase the effects of these drugs.
Theophylline: Decreases clearance and may increase blood concentration and risk of toxicity of theophylline.
Herbal
None known.

Food
None known.

DIAGNOSTIC TEST EFFECTS
May increase BUN and serum alkaline phosphatase, bilirubin, creatinine, LDH, AST (SGOT), and ALT (SGPT) levels.

▨ IV INCOMPATIBILITIES
Aminophylline, ampicillin and sulbactam (Unasyn), cefepime (Maxipime), dexamethasone (Decadron), furosemide (Lasix), heparin, hydrocortisone (Solu-Cortef), methylprednisolone (Solu-Medrol), phenytoin (Dilantin), sodium bicarbonate
▨ IV Compatibilities
Calcium gluconate, diltiazem (Cardizem), dobutamine (Dobutrex), dopamine (Intropin), lidocaine, lorazepam (Ativan), magnesium, midazolam (Versed), potassium chloride

SIDE EFFECTS
Frequent (5%-2%)
Nausea, diarrhea, dyspepsia, vomiting, constipation, flatulence, confusion, crystalluria
Ophthalmic: Burning, crusting in corner of eye
Occasional (less than 2%)
Abdominal pain or discomfort, headache, rash
Ophthalmic: Bad taste, sensation of something in eye, eyelid redness or itching
Rare (less than 1%)
Dizziness, confusion, tremors, hallucinations, hypersensitivity reaction, insomnia, dry mouth, paresthesia

SERIOUS REACTIONS
• Superinfection (especially enterococcal or fungal), nephropathy, cardiopulmonary arrest, chest pain, and cerebral thrombosis may occur.

- Hypersensitivity reactions, including photosensitivity (as evidenced by rash, pruritus, blisters, edema, and burning skin), have occurred in patients receiving fluoroquinolones.
- Arthropathy may occur if the drug is given to children younger than 18 years.
- Sensitization to the ophthalmic form of the drug may contraindicate later systemic use of ciprofloxacin.

PRECAUTIONS & CONSIDERATIONS

Caution is warranted with CNS disorders, renal impairment, seizures, and those taking caffeine or theophylline. Be aware that the oral suspension should not be administered by NG tube. It is unknown if ciprofloxacin is distributed in breast milk. If possible, pregnant or breast-feeding women should avoid taking the drug because of the risk of arthropathy in the fetus or infant. The safety and efficacy of ciprofloxacin have not been established in children younger than 18 years. Age-related renal impairment may require a dosage adjustment in the elderly.

Dizziness, headache, tremors, visual problems, chest and joint pain should be reported. Food tolerance and pattern of daily bowel activity and stool consistency should be assessed. A crystal precipitate may form when using the ophthalmic preparation but resolves in 1 to 7 days. History of hypersensitivity to ciprofloxacin and other quinolones should be determined before therapy.

Storage

The oral suspension may be stored for 14 days at room temperature. Store the injection form at room temperature. The solution normally appears clear and colorless or slightly yellow.

Administration

Oral ciprofloxacin may be taken without regard to food, but the preferred administration time is 2 hours after a meal. Shake the oral suspension well before taking it and do not chew the microcapsules in the suspension. Do not administer antacids containing aluminum or magnesium within 2 hours of ciprofloxacin. Consume sufficient amounts of citrus fruits and cranberry juice to acidify urine and drink several glasses of water between meals. Take full course of therapy and do not skip doses.

For IV use, after withdrawing the drug from a 200-mg or 400-mg vial, further dilute it with D_5W or 0.9% NaCl for injection to a final concentration of 1 to 2 mg/ml. Infuse the drug over 60 minutes. IV ciprofloxacin is also available prediluted in ready-to-use infusion containers.

For ophthalmic use, tilt the head back, and place the solution in the conjunctival sac of the affected eye. Close the eye and then press gently on the lacrimal sac for 1 minute. Don't use ophthalmic solutions for injection. Unless the infection is very superficial, systemic administration generally accompanies ophthalmic use.

C

Citalopram
sy-tal'oh-pram
(Celexa, Cipramil [AUS])
**Do not confuse Celexa
with Celebrex, Zyprexa, or
Cerebyx.**

CATEGORY AND SCHEDULE
Pregnancy Risk Category: C

CLASSIFICATION
Antidepressants, serotonin
specific reuptake inhibitors

MECHANISM OF ACTION
A selective serotonin reuptake
inhibitor that blocks the uptake of
the neurotransmitter serotonin at
CNS presynaptic neuronal
membranes, increasing its availability at postsynaptic receptor sites.
Therapeutic Effect: Relieves
depression.

PHARMACOKINETICS
Well absorbed after PO administration. Protein binding: 80%. Primarily
metabolized in the liver. Primarily
excreted in feces with a lesser
amount eliminated in urine.
Half-life: 35 hr.

AVAILABILITY
Oral Solution: 10 mg/5 ml.
Tablets: 10 mg, 20 mg, 40 mg.

INDICATIONS AND DOSAGES
▸ **Depression**
PO
Adults. Initially, 20 mg once a day
in the morning or evening. May
increase in 20-mg increments at
intervals of no less than 1 wk.
Maximum: 60 mg/day.
*Elderly, Patients with hepatic
impairment.* 20 mg/day. May titrate
to 40 mg/day only for nonresponding
patients.

OFF-LABEL USES
Treatment of alcohol abuse,
dementia, diabetic neuropathy,
obsessive-compulsive disorder,
smoking cessation

CONTRAINDICATIONS
Sensitivity to citalopram, use within
14 days of MAOIs

INTERACTIONS
Drug
**Antifungals, cimetidine,
macrolide antibiotics:** May
increase the citalopram plasma
level.
Carbamazepine: May decrease the
citalopram plasma level.
MAOIs: May cause serotonin
syndrome, marked by autonomic
hyperactivity, coma, diaphoresis,
excitement, hyperthermia, and
rigidity, and neuroleptic malignant
syndrome.
Metoprolol: Increases the metoprolol plasma level.
Herbal
None known.
Food
None known.

DIAGNOSTIC TEST EFFECTS
May reduce serum sodium level.

SIDE EFFECTS
Frequent (21%-11%)
Nausea, dry mouth, somnolence,
insomnia, diaphoresis
Occasional (8%-4%)
Tremor, diarrhea, abnormal ejacula-
tion, dyspepsia, fatigue, anxiety,
vomiting, anorexia
Rare (3%-2%)
Sinusitis, sexual dysfunction,
menstrual disorder, abdominal pain,
agitation, decreased libido

SERIOUS REACTIONS
• Overdose is manifested as dizziness, drowsiness, tachycardia, somnolence, confusion, and seizures.

PRECAUTIONS & CONSIDERATIONS
Caution is warranted with hepatic and renal impairment and in those with a history of hypomania, mania, and seizures. Citalopram is distributed in breast milk. Citalopram use in children may increase anticholinergic effects and hyperexcitability. The elderly are more sensitive to the drug's anticholinergic effects, such as dry mouth, and are more likely to experience confusion, dizziness, hyperexcitability, and sedation.

Alcohol and tasks that require mental alertness or motor skills should be avoided. CBC and blood chemistry tests should be performed before and periodically during therapy, especially with long-term use.

Administration
! Make sure at least 14 days elapse between the use of MAOIs and citalopram.

Take citalopram without regard to food. Crush scored tablets if necessary. Do not abruptly discontinue citalopram or increase the dosage.

Clarithromycin
clare-i-thro-mye′sin
(Biaxin, Biaxin XL, Klacid [AUS])

CATEGORY AND SCHEDULE
Pregnancy Risk Category: C

CLASSIFICATION
Antibiotics, macrolides

MECHANISM OF ACTION
A macrolide that binds to ribosomal receptor sites of susceptible organisma, inhibiting protein synthesis of the bacterial cell wall. *Therapeutic Effect:* Bacteriostatic; may be bactericidal with high dosages or very susceptible microorganisms.

PHARMACOKINETICS
Well absorbed from the GI tract. Protein binding: 65%-75%. Widely distributed. Metabolized in the liver to active metabolite. Primarily excreted in urine. Not removed by hemodialysis. **Half-life:** 3-7 hr; metabolite 5-7 hr (increased in impaired renal function).

AVAILABILITY
Oral Suspension: 125 mg/5 ml, 250 mg/5 ml.
Tablets: 250 mg, 500 mg.
Tablets (Extended-Release): 500 mg.

INDICATIONS AND DOSAGES
▶ **Bronchitis**
PO
Adults, Elderly. 500 mg q12hr for 7-14 days.
▶ **Skin, soft tissue infections**
PO
Adults, Elderly. 250 mg q12hr for 7-14 days.
Children. 7.5 mg/kg q12hr for 10 days.
▶ **MAC prophylaxis**
PO
Adults, Elderly. 500 mg 2 times/day.
Children. 7.5 mg/kg q12hr.
Maximum: 500 mg 2 times/day.
▶ **MAC treatment**
PO
Adults, Elderly. 500 mg 2 times/day in combination.
Children. 7.5 mg/kg q12hr in combination. Maximum: 500 mg 2 times/day.

▶ **Pharyngitis, tonsillitis**
PO
Adults, Elderly. 250 mg q12hr for
10 days.
Children. 7.5 mg/kg q12hr for
10 days.
▶ **Pneumonia**
PO
Adults, Elderly. 250 mg q12hr for
7-14 days.
Children. 7.5 mg/kg q12hr.
▶ **Maxillary sinusitis**
PO
Adults, Elderly. 500 mg q12hr for
14 days.
Children. 7.5 mg/kg q12hr.
Maximum: 500 mg 2 times/day.
▶ ***H. pylori***
PO
Adults, Elderly. 500 mg q12hr for
10-14 days in combination.
▶ **Acute otitis media**
PO
Children. 7.5 mg/kg q12hr for
10 days.
▶ **Dosage in renal impairment**
For patients with creatinine clearance
less than 30 ml/min, reduce dose by
50% and administer once or twice
a day.

CONTRAINDICATIONS
Hypersensitivity to clarithromycin or
other macrolide antibiotics

INTERACTIONS
Drug
**Carbamazepine, digoxin, theo-
phylline:** May increase blood
concentration and toxicity of these
drugs.
Rifampin: May decrease clar-
ithromycin blood concentration.
Warfarin: May increase warfarin
effects.
Zidovudine: May decrease blood
concentration of zidovudine.
Herbal
None known.

Food
None known.

DIAGNOSTIC TEST EFFECTS
May (rarely) increase BUN, AST
(SGOT), and ALT (SGPT) levels.

SIDE EFFECTS
Occasional (6%-3%)
Diarrhea, nausea, altered taste,
abdominal pain
Rare (2%-1%)
Headache, dyspepsia

SERIOUS REACTIONS
• Antibiotic-associated colitis and
other superinfections may result
from altered bacterial balance.
• Hepatotoxicity and thrombocytopenia occur rarely.

PRECAUTIONS & CONSIDERATIONS
Caution is warranted with hepatic or
renal dysfunction and in the elderly
with severe renal impairment.
Determine if there is a history of
hepatitis or allergies to clarithromycin
or other macrolides before beginning therapy. It is unknown if clarithromycin is distributed in breast
milk. The safety and efficacy of clarithromycin have not been established
in children younger than 6 months.
Age-related renal impairment may
require a dosage adjustment in the
elderly.
    Daily bowel activity and stool
consistency should be assessed. Mild
GI effects may be tolerable, but
severe symptoms may indicate the
onset of antibiotic-associated colitis.
Be alert for signs and symptoms of
superinfection, including abdominal
pain, anal or genital pruritus, moderate to severe diarrhea, and mouth
soreness.
Administration
Take tablets and oral suspension
with or without food.

Take clarithromycin tablets with 8 oz of water. Don't crush or break tablets. Space doses evenly around the clock and continue taking clarithromycin for the full course of therapy.

Clemastine
klem′as-teen
(Dayhistol Allergy, Tavist Allergy)

CATEGORY AND SCHEDULE
Pregnancy Risk Category: B

CLASSIFICATION
Antihistamines, H1

MECHANISM OF ACTION
An ethanolamine that competes with histamine on effector cells in the gastrointestinal (GI) tract, blood vessels, and respiratory tract. *Therapeutic Effect:* Relieves allergy symptoms, including urticaria, rhinitis, and pruritus.

PHARMACOKINETICS

Route	Onset	Peak	Duration
PO	15-60 min	5-7 hr	10-12 hr

Well absorbed from the GI tract. Metabolized in the liver. Excreted primarily in urine.

AVAILABILITY
Syrup (Dayhist, Tavist):
0.67 mg/5 ml.
Tablets (Dayhist, Tavist): 1.34 mg, 2.68 mg.

INDICATIONS AND DOSAGES
▶ **Allergic rhinitis, urticaria**
PO
Adults, Children older than 11 yr.
1.34 mg twice a day up to 2.68 mg 3 times a day. Maximum: 8.04 mg/day.
Children 6-11 yr. 0.67-1.34 mg twice a day. Maximum: 4.02 mg/day.
Children younger than 6 yr. 0.05 mg/kg/day divided into 2-3 doses per day. Maximum: 1.34 mg/day.
Elderly. 1.34 mg 1-2 times a day.

CONTRAINDICATIONS
Angle-closure glaucoma, hypersensitivity to clemastine, use within 14 days of MAOIs

INTERACTIONS
Drug
Alcohol, other CNS depressants: May increase CNS depression.
MAOIs: May increase the anticholinergic and CNS depressant effects of clemastine.
Herbal
None known.
Food
None known.

DIAGNOSTIC TEST EFFECTS
May suppress wheal and flare reactions to antigen skin testing unless drug is discontinued 4 days before testing.

SIDE EFFECTS
Frequent
Somnolence, dizziness, urine retention, thickening of bronchial secretions, dry mouth, nose, or throat; in elderly, sedation, dizziness, hypotension
Occasional
Epigastric distress, flushing, blurred vision, tinnitus, paresthesia, diaphoresis, chills

SERIOUS REACTIONS

• A hypersensitivity reaction, marked by eczema, pruritus, rash, cardiac disturbances, angioedema, and photosensitivity, may occur.
• Overdose symptoms may vary from CNS depression, including sedation, apnea, cardiovascular collapse, and death to severe paradoxical reaction, such as hallucinations, tremor, and seizures.
• Children may experience paradoxical reactions, such as restlessness, insomnia, euphoria, nervousness, and tremors.
• Overdose in children may result in hallucinations, seizures, and death.

PRECAUTIONS & CONSIDERATIONS

Caution is warranted with asthma, GI or GU obstruction, peptic ulcer disease, and benign prostatic hyperplasia. Clemastine is excreted in breast milk and should not be used in breast-feeding women. The safety and efficacy of clemastine have not been established in children younger than 6 years. Age-related renal impairment may require a dosage adjustment in the elderly. Avoid drinking alcoholic beverages and tasks that require alertness or motor skills until response to the drug is established.

Drowsiness, dizziness, and dry mouth may occur; tolerance may develop to the sedative effects. Blood pressure (B/P) and therapeutic response should be monitored.

Administration

! Be aware that the fixed-combination form Tavist-D may produce mild CNS stimulation. Take clemastine without regard to food. Crush scored tablets as needed.

Clindamycin

klin-da-mye′sin
(Cleocin, Dalacin [CAN])

CATEGORY AND SCHEDULE

Pregnancy Risk Category: B

CLASSIFICATION

Anti-infectives, topical, antibiotics, lincosamides, dermatologics

MECHANISM OF ACTION

A lincosamide antibiotic that inhibits protein synthesis of the bacterial cell wall by binding to bacterial ribosomal receptor sites. Topically, it decreases fatty acid concentration on the skin. *Therapeutic Effect:* Bacteriostatic. Prevents outbreaks of acne vulgaris.

PHARMACOKINETICS

Rapidly absorbed from the GI tract. Protein binding: 92%-94%. Widely distributed. Metabolized in the liver to some active metabolites. Primarily excreted in urine. Not removed by hemodialysis. **Half-life:** 2.4-3 hr (increased in impaired renal function and premature infants).

AVAILABILITY

Capsules: 75 mg, 150 mg, 300 mg.
Oral Solution: 75 mg/5 ml.
Injection: 150 mg/ml.
Topical Gel: 1%.
Topical Solution: 1%.
Vaginal Cream: 2%.
Vaginal Suppository: 100 mg.

INDICATIONS AND DOSAGES

▸ **Chronic bone and joint, respiratory tract, skin and soft-tissue, intra-abdominal, and female GU infections; endocarditis; septicemia**

PO
Adults, Elderly. 150-450 mg/dose
q6-8hr.
Children. 10-30 mg/kg/day in 3-4
divided doses. Maximum: 1.8 g/day.
IV, IM
Adults, Elderly. 1.2-1.8 g/day in
2-4 divided doses.
Children. 25-40 mg/kg/day in 3-4
divided doses. Maximum: 4.8 g/day.
▶ **Bacterial vaginosis**
PO
Adults, Elderly. 300 mg twice a day
for 7 days.
INTRAVAGINAL
Adults. One applicatorful at bedtime
for 3-7 days or 1 suppository at
bedtime for 3 days.
▶ **Acne vulgaris**
TOPICAL
Adults. Apply thin layer to affected
area twice a day.

OFF-LABEL USES
Treatment of malaria, otitis media,
Pneumocystis carinii pneumonia,
toxoplasmosis

CONTRAINDICATIONS
History of antibiotic-associated
colitis, regional enteritis, or ulcerative colitis; hypersensitivity to
clindamycin or lincomycin; known
allergy to tartrazine dye

INTERACTIONS
Drug
Adsorbent antidiarrheals: May
delay absorption of clindamycin.
Chloramphenicol, erythromycin:
May antagonize the effects of clin-
damycin.
Neuromuscular blockers:
May increase the effects of these
drugs.
Herbal
None known.
Food
None known.

DIAGNOSTIC TEST EFFECTS
May increase serum alkaline phos-
phatase, AST (SGOT), and ALT
(SGPT) levels.

▧ IV INCOMPATIBILITIES
Allopurinol (Aloprim), filgrastim
(Neupogen), fluconazole (Diflucan),
idarubicin (Idamycin)
⬚ IV Compatibilities
Amiodarone (Cordarone),
diltiazem (Cardizem), heparin,
hydromorphone (Dilaudid), magnesium sulfate, midazolam (Versed),
morphine, multivitamins, propofol
(Diprivan)

SIDE EFFECTS
Frequent
Systemic: Abdominal pain, nausea,
vomiting, diarrhea
Topical: Dry scaly skin
Vaginal: Vaginitis, pruritus
Occasional
Systemic: Phlebitis or thrombophlebitis with IV administration,
pain and induration at IM injection
site, allergic reaction, urticaria,
pruritus
Topical: Contact dermatitis, abdominal pain, mild diarrhea, burning or
stinging
Vaginal: Headache, dizziness,
nausea, vomiting, abdominal
pain
Rare
Vaginal: Hypersensitivity
reaction

SERIOUS REACTIONS
• Antibiotic-associated colitis and
other superinfections may occur
during and several weeks after clindamycin therapy (including the topical form).
• Blood dyscrasias (leukopenia,
thrombocytopenia) and nephrotoxicity (proteinuria, azotemia, oliguria)
occur rarely.

PRECAUTIONS & CONSIDERATIONS

Caution is warranted with severe renal or hepatic dysfunction and in patients using neuromuscular blockers concurrently. Don't apply topical preparations to abraded areas or near the eyes. Systemic clindamycin readily crosses the placenta and is distributed in breast milk. It is unknown if the topical and vaginal forms of clindamycin are distributed in breast milk. Use clindamycin cautiously in children less than 1 month old. No age-related precautions have been noted in the elderly. Use caution when applying topical clindamycin concurrently with abrasive, peeling acne agents, soaps, or alcohol-containing cosmetics to avoid a cumulative effect. Sexual intercourse during treatment with the vaginal form of clindamycin should be avoided.

Diarrhea should be reported promptly to the physician because of the potential for developing serious colitis (even with topical or vaginal clindamycin). Pattern of daily bowel activity and stool consistency should be assessed. Skin should be assessed for dryness, irritation, and rash. Be alert for signs and symptoms of superinfection, such as anal or genital pruritus, a change in oral mucosa, increased fever, and severe diarrhea. History of allergies, particularly to aspirin, clindamycin, or lincomycin, should be determined before beginning drug therapy. Use of neuromuscular blockers should also be determined because their concurrent use should be avoided, if possible.

Storage
Store capsules at room temperature. After reconstitution, the oral solution is stable for 2 weeks at room temperature. Don't refrigerate the oral solution to avoid thickening it. The IV infusion (piggyback) is stable at room temperature for up to 16 days.

Administration
Take capsules with 8 oz of water and without regard to food.

The IV infusion (piggyback) is stable at room temperature for up to 16 days. Dilute 300 to 600 mg with 50 ml D_5W or 0.9% NaCl (900 to 1200 mg with 100 ml). Never exceed a concentration of 18 mg/ml. Infuse 50-ml (300- to 600-mg) piggyback solution over 10 to 20 minutes; infuse 100-ml (900-mg to 1.2-g) piggyback solution over 30 to 40 minutes. Be aware that severe hypotension or cardiac arrest can occur with too-rapid administration. Don't administer more than 1.2 g in a single infusion.

For IM use, don't exceed 600 mg/ dose. Give by deep IM injection.

Do not apply topical preparations near the eyes or on abraded areas. Rinse eyes with copious amounts of cool tap water if the vaginal form of clindamycin accidentally comes in contact with eyes.

Clioquinol

klee-oh-kwee′nole
(Ala-Quin, Dek-Quin, Vioform-Hydrocortisone Cream, Vioform-Hydrocortisone Mild Cream, Vioform-Hydrocortisone Mild Ointment, Vioform-Hydrocortisone Ointment)

CATEGORY AND SCHEDULE
Pregnancy Risk Category: C

CLASSIFICATION
Anti-infectives, topical, antifungals, topical, corticosteroids, topical, dermatologics

MECHANISM OF ACTION

Clioquinol is a broad-spectrum antibacterial agent but the mechanism of action is unknown. Hydrocortisone is a corticosteroid that diffuses across cell membranes, forms complexes with specific receptors and further binds to DNA and stimulates transcription of mRNA (messenger RNA) and subsequent protein synthesis of various enzymes thought to be ultimately responsible for the anti-inflammatory effects of corticosteroids applied topically to the skin. *Therapeutic Effect:* Alters membrane function and produces antibacterial activity.

PHARMACOKINETICS

Clioquinol may be absorbed through the skin in sufficient amounts.

AVAILABILITY

Cream: 3% clioquinol and 0.5% hydrocortisone (Ala-QuinVioform-Hydrocortisone Mild Cream, 3% clioquinol and 1% hydrocortisone (Vioform-Hydrocortisone Cream, Dek-Quin).
Ointment: 3% clioquinol and 1% hydrocortisone (Vioform-Hydrocortisone Mild Ointment).

INDICATIONS AND DOSAGES
▸ **Antibacterial, antifungal skin conditions**
TOPICAL
Adults, Elderly, Children 12 yr and older. Apply to skin 3-4 times/day.

CONTRAINDICATIONS

Lesions of the eye, tuberculosis of skin, diaper rash, hypersensitivity to clioquinol or hydrocortisone or any other component of the formulation.

INTERACTIONS
Drug
None known.
Herbal
None known.
Food
None known.

DIAGNOSTIC TEST EFFECTS

May alter thyroid function tests. Clioquinol may produce false-positivity ferric chloride test results for phenylketonuria (PKU).

SIDE EFFECTS
Occasional
Blistering, burning, itching, peeling, skin rash, redness, swelling

SERIOUS REACTIONS

• Thinning of skin with easy bruising may occur with prolonged use.

PRECAUTIONS & CONSIDERATIONS

Caution is warranted with herpes simplex, eczema vaccinatum, varicella, or other viral infections of the skin as well as intolerance to chloroxine, iodine, or iodine-containing preparations. It is unknown if clioquinol and hydrocortisone crosses the placenta or is distributed in breast milk. There are no age-related precautions noted in children or the elderly.
This medication may stain fabrics, skin, hair, and nails yellow. The affected area should be kept clean and dry. Light clothing should be worn to promote ventilation.
Storage
Store at room temperature.
Administration
Before applying, wash affected area with soap and water, and dry thoroughly. Apply a thin layer to affected area. Wash hands after application.

Clobetasol
klo-bet′a-sol
(Alti-Clobetasol [CAN], Cormax, Dermovate [CAN], Gen-Clobetasol [CAN], Olux, Novo-Clobetasol [CAN], Temovate)

CATEGORY AND SCHEDULE
Pregnancy Risk Category: C

CLASSIFICATION
Corticosteroids, topical, dermatologics

MECHANISM OF ACTION
A corticosteroid that inhibits accumulation of inflammatory cells at inflammation sites, phagocytosis, lysosomal enzyme release and synthesis or release of mediators of inflammation. *Therapeutic Effect:* Decreases or prevents tissue response to inflammatory process.

PHARMACOKINETICS
May be absorbed from intact skin. Metabolized in liver. Excreted in the urine.

AVAILABILITY
Cream: 0.05% (Cormax, Temovate).
Cream, in emollient base: 0.05% (Temovate).
Foam: 0.05% (Olux).
Gel: 0.05% (Temovate).
Ointment: 0.05% (Cormax, Temovate).
Topical Solution: 0.05% (Cormax, Temovate).

INDICATIONS AND DOSAGES
▶ Anti-inflammatory, corticosteroid replacement therapy

TOPICAL
Adults, Elderly, Children more than 12 yr and older. Apply 2 times/day for 2 weeks.
FOAM
Adults, Elderly, Children more than 12 yr and older. Apply 2 times/day for 2 wk.

CONTRAINDICATIONS
Hypersensitivity to clobetasol or other corticosteroids.

INTERACTIONS
Drug
None known.
Herbal
None known.
Food
None known.

DIAGNOSTIC TEST EFFECTS
None known.

SIDE EFFECTS
Frequent
Local irritation, dry skin, itching, redness
Occasional
Allergic contact dermatitis
Rare
Cushing's syndrome, numbness of fingers, skin atrophy

SERIOUS REACTIONS
• Overdosage can occur from topically applied clobetasol propionate absorbed in sufficient amounts to produce systemic effects producing reversible adrenal suppression, manifestations of Cushing's syndrome, hyperglycemia, and glucosuria in some patients.

PRECAUTIONS & CONSIDERATIONS
Avoid use of occlusive dressings on affected area. Skin irritation should be reported. HPA axis suppression should be evaluated by ACTH

stimulation test, AM plasma cortisol test, or urinary free cortisol test. It is unknown if clobetasol propionate crosses the placenta or is distributed in the breast milk. Safety and efficacy of clobetasol propionate has not been established in children. There are no age-related precautions noted in the elderly.

Administration
Apply sparingly to skin or scalp and rub into area thoroughly. Use for two weeks. If using for the scalp, part the hair and apply to the area.

Clocortolone
klo-kort′o-lone
(Cloderm, Cloderm [CAN])

CATEGORY AND SCHEDULE
Pregnancy Risk Category: C

CLASSIFICATION
Corticosteroids, topical, dermatologics

MECHANISM OF ACTION
A topical corticosteroid that inhibits accumulation of inflammatory cells at inflammation sites, suppresses mitotic activity, and cause vasocon-striction. *Therapeutic Effect:* Decreases or prevents tissue response to inflammatory process.

PHARMACOKINETICS
Absorption is variable and dependent upon many factors including integrity of skin, dose, vehicle used, and use of occlusive dressings. Small amounts may be absorbed from the skin. Metabolized in liver. Excreted in the urine and feces.

AVAILABILITY
Cream: 0.1%.

INDICATIONS AND DOSAGES
▸ **Dermatoses**
TOPICAL
Adults, Elderly, Children 12 yr and older. Apply 1-4 times/day.

CONTRAINDICATIONS
Hypersensitivity to clocortolone pivalate or other corticosteroids; viral, fungal, or tubercular skin lesions

INTERACTIONS
Drug
None known.
Herbal
None known.
Food
None known.

DIAGNOSTIC TEST EFFECTS
None known.

SIDE EFFECTS
Occasional
Local irritation, burning, itching, redness, allergic contact dermatitis
Rare
Hypertrichosis, hypopigmentation, maceration of skin, miliaria, perioral dermatitis, skin atrophy, striae

SERIOUS REACTIONS
• Overdosage can occur from topi-cally applied clocortolone pivalate absorbed in sufficient amounts to produce systemic effects in some patients.

PRECAUTIONS & CONSIDERATIONS
Avoid use of occlusive dressings on affected area. Skin irritation should be reported. HPA axis suppression should be evaluated by ACTH stimu-lation test, AM plasma cortisol test, or urinary free cortisol test. It is unknown if clocortolone crosses the

placenta or is distributed in the breast milk. Safety and efficacy of clocortolone has not been established in children. There are no age-related precautions noted in the elderly.

Administration
Apply topical preparation sparingly. Do not use on broken skin. Avoid use of occlusive dressings only as ordered.

Clofazimine
kloe-faz′i-meen
(Lamprene)

CATEGORY AND SCHEDULE
Pregnancy Risk Category: C

CLASSIFICATION
Antimycobacterials

MECHANISM OF ACTION
An antibiotic that binds to mycobacterial DNA. *Therapeutic Effect:* Inhibits mycobacterial growth and produces anti-inflammatory action.

AVAILABILITY
Capsules: 50 mg.

INDICATIONS AND DOSAGES
▶ **Leprosy**
PO
Adults, Elderly. 100 mg/day in combination with dapsone and rifampin for 3 yr then 100 mg/day as monotherapy.
Children. 1 mg/kg/day in combination with dapsone and rifampin.
▶ **Erythema nodosum**
PO
Adults, Elderly. 100-200 mg/day for up to 3 mo, then 100 mg/day.

CONTRAINDICATIONS
None significant.

INTERACTIONS
Drug
Dapsone: May decrease the effects of clofazimine.
Herbal
None significant.
Food
All foods: May increase the absorption of clofazimine.

DIAGNOSTIC TEST EFFECTS
May increase blood glucose levels.

SIDE EFFECTS
Frequent (greater than 10%)
Dry skin, abdominal pain, nausea, vomiting, diarrhea, skin discoloration (pink to brownish-black)
Occasional (10%-1%)
Rash; pruritus; eye irritation; discoloration of sputum; sweat and urine

SERIOUS REACTIONS
• None significant.

PRECAUTIONS & CONSIDERATIONS
Caution is warranted with GI problems, including abdominal pain and diarrhea. Sensitivity to clofazimine should be assessed before beginning therapy. Notify the physician if crampy or colicky abdominal pain occurs. Be aware that clofazimine may cause skin discoloration.
Administration
Take clofazimine with food.

Clomiphene

kloe′mi-feen

(Clomhexal [AUS], Clomid,
Clomid [CAN], Milophene,
Milophene [CAN], Serophene,
Serophene [CAN])

**Do not confuse with
chlomipramine.**

CATEGORY AND SCHEDULE

Pregnancy Risk Category: X

CLASSIFICATION

Hormones/hormone
modifiers, stimulants,
ovarian

MECHANISM OF ACTION

An ovulation stimulator that
promotes release of pituitary
gonadotropins. *Therapeutic Effect:*
Stimulates ovulation.

PHARMACOKINETICS

Readily absorbed. Time to peak
occurs within 6.5 hr. Undergoes
enterohepatic recirculation.
Primarily excreted in feces.
Half-life: 5-7 days.

AVAILABILITY

Tablets: 50 mg (Clomid, Milophene,
Serophene).

INDICATIONS AND DOSAGES

▶ **Ovulatory failure, females**
PO
Adults. 50 mg/day for 5 days (first
course); start the regimen on the
fifth day of cycle. Increase dose
only if unresponsive to cyclic
50 mg. Maximum: 100 mg/day
for 5 days.

OFF-LABEL USES

Infertility in males

CONTRAINDICATIONS

Liver dysfunction, abnormal uterine
bleeding, enlargement or development of ovarian cyst, uncontrolled
thyroid or adrenal dysfunction in the
presence of an organic intracranial
lesion such as pituitary tumor,
pregnancy, hypersensitivity to
clomiphene

INTERACTIONS

Drug
Danazol: May decrease the
response of clomiphene.
Estradiol: May decrease estradiol.
Herbal
None known.
Food
None known.

DIAGNOSTIC TEST EFFECTS

Altered levels of thyroid function tests.

SIDE EFFECTS

Frequent (13%-10%)
Hot flashes, ovarian enlargement
Occasional (5%-2%)
Abdominal/pelvic discomfort,
bloating, nausea, vomiting, breast
discomfort (females)
Rare (less than 1%)
Vision disturbances, abnormal
menstrual flow, breast enlargement
(males), headache, mental depression,
ovarian cyst formation, thromboembolism, uterine fibroid enlargement

SERIOUS REACTIONS

• Thrombophlebitis, alopecia, and
polyuria occurs rarely.

PRECAUTIONS & CONSIDERATIONS

Caution should be used with liver
dysfunction, polycystic ovary
disease, and multiple pregnancies.
Clomiphene use should be avoided
during pregnancy, and it is distributed in breast milk. Safety and
efficacy have not been established

in children or the elderly. Pregnancy should be immediately reported. Visual disturbances, dizziness, lightheadedness may occur.

Administration
Take clomiphene without meals.

Clomipramine
klom-ip′ra-meen
(Anafranil, Apo-Clomipramine [CAN], Clopram [AUS], Novo-Clopamine [CAN], Placil [AUS])
Do not confuse clomipramine with chlorpromazine or clomiphene, or Anafranil with alfentanil, enalapril, or nafarelin.

CATEGORY AND SCHEDULE
Pregnancy Risk Category: C

CLASSIFICATION
Antidepressants, tricyclic

MECHANISM OF ACTION
A tricyclic antidepressant that blocks the reuptake of neurotransmitters, such as norepinephrine and serotonin, at CNS presynaptic membranes, increasing their availability at postsynaptic receptor sites. *Therapeutic Effect:* Reduces obsessive-compulsive behavior.

AVAILABILITY
Capsules: 25 mg, 50 mg, 75 mg.

INDICATIONS AND DOSAGES
▸ **Obsessive-compulsive disorder**
PO
Adults, Elderly. Initially, 25 mg/day. May gradually increase to 100 mg/day in the first 2 wk. Maximum: 250 mg/day.
Children 10 yr and older. Initially, 25 mg/day. May gradually increase up to maximum of 200 mg/day.

OFF-LABEL USES
Treatment of bulimia nervosa, cataplexy associated with narcolepsy, mental depression, neurogenic pain, panic disorder

CONTRAINDICATIONS
Acute recovery period after MI, use within 14 days of MAOIs

INTERACTIONS
Drug
Antithyroid agents: May increase the risk of agranulocytosis.
Cimetidine: May increase clomipramine blood concentration and risk of toxicity.
Clonidine, guanadrel: May decrease the effects of these drugs.
MAOIs: May increase the risk of neuroleptic malignant syndrome, seizures, hyperpyresis, and hypertensive crisis.
Other CNS depressants: May increase CNS and respiratory depression and the hypotensive effects of clomipramine.
Phenothiazines: May increase the anticholinergic and sedative effects of clomipramine.
Sympathomimetics: May increase the risk of cardiac effects.
Herbal
None known.
Food
Alcohol. May increase CNS and respiratory depression and the hypotensive effects of clomipramine.

DIAGNOSTIC TEST EFFECTS
May alter the blood glucose level and EKG readings.

SIDE EFFECTS
Frequent
Somnolence, fatigue, dry mouth, blurred vision, constipation, sexual dysfunction (42%), ejaculatory failure (20%), impotence, weight gain (18%), delayed micturition, orthostatic hypotension, diaphoresis, impaired concentration, increased appetite, urine retention
Occasional
GI disturbances (such as nausea, GI distress, and metallic taste), asthenia, aggressiveness, muscle weakness
Rare
Paradoxical reactions (agitation, restlessness, nightmares, insomnia), extrapyramidal symptoms, (particularly fine hand tremor), laryngitis, seizures

SERIOUS REACTIONS
• Overdose may produce seizures; cardiovascular effects, such as severe orthostatic hypotension, dizziness, tachycardia, palpitations, and arrhythmias; and altered temperature regulation, including hyperpyrexia or hypothermia.
• Abrupt discontinuation after prolonged therapy may produce headache, malaise, nausea, vomiting, and vivid dreams.
• Anemia and agranulocytosis have been noted.

PRECAUTIONS & CONSIDERATIONS
Caution is warranted with cardiac disease, diabetes mellitus, glaucoma, hiatal hernia, history of seizures, history of urinary obstruction or urine retention, hyperthyroidism, increased IOP, benign prostatic hyperplasia, renal or hepatic disease, and schizophrenia. Clomipramine is minimally distributed in breast milk. Clomipramine use is not recommended for children younger than 10 years. A lower dosage should be given to the elderly because they're at increased risk for drug toxicity.

Dizziness may occur, so change positions slowly and avoid alcohol and tasks that require mental alertness or motor skills. CBC to detect signs of anemia and agranulocytosis and EKG to detect arrhythmias should be performed before and periodically during therapy.
Administration
! Make sure at least 14 days elapse between the use of MAOIs and clomipramine.

Take clomipramine with food or milk if GI distress occurs. Full therapeutic effect may be noted in 2 to 4 weeks. Do not abruptly discontinue clomipramine.

Clonazepam
kloe-na′zi-pam
(Apo-Clonazepam [CAN], Clonapam [CAN], Klonopin, Paxam [AUS], Rivotril [CAN])
Do not confuse clonazepam with clonidine or lorazepam.

CATEGORY AND SCHEDULE
Pregnancy Risk Category: D

CLASSIFICATION
Anxiolytics, benzodiazepines

MECHANISM OF ACTION
A benzodiazepine that depresses all levels of the CNS; inhibits nerve impulse transmission in the motor cortex and suppresses abnormal discharge in petit mal seizures. *Therapeutic Effect:* Produces anxiolytic and anticonvulsant effects.

PHARMACOKINETICS

Well absorbed from the GI tract. Protein binding: 85%. Metabolized in the liver. Excreted in urine. Not removed by hemodialysis. **Half-life:** 18-50 hr.

AVAILABILITY

Tablets: 0.5 mg, 1 mg, 2 mg.
Tablets (Disintegrating): 0.125 mg, 0.25 mg, 0.5 mg, 1 mg, 2 mg.

INDICATIONS AND DOSAGES

▸ **Adjunctive treatment of Lennox-Gastaut syndrome (petit mal variant) and akinetic, myoclonic, and absence (petit mal) seizures**
PO
Adults, Elderly, Children 10 yr and older. 1.5 mg/day; may be increased in 0.5- to 1-mg increments every 3 days until seizures are controlled. Do not exceed maintenance dosage of 20 mg/day.
Infants, Children younger than 10 yr or weighing less than 30 kg. 0.01-0.03 mg/kg/day in 2-3 divided doses; may be increased by up to 0.5 mg every 3 days until seizures are controlled. Don't exceed maintenance dosage of 0.2 mg/kg/day.
▸ **Panic disorder**
PO
Adults, Elderly. Initially, 0.25 mg twice a day; increased in increments of 0.125-0.25 mg twice a day every 3 days. Maximum: 4 mg/day.

OFF-LABEL USES

Adjunctive treatment of seizures; treatment of simple, complex partial, and tonic-clonic seizures

CONTRAINDICATIONS

Narrow-angle glaucoma, significant hepatic disease

INTERACTIONS

Drug
Alcohol, other CNS depressants: May increase CNS depressant effect.
Herbal
Kava kava: May increase sedation.
Food
None known.

DIAGNOSTIC TEST EFFECTS

None known.

SIDE EFFECTS

Frequent
Mild, transient drowsiness; ataxia; behavioral disturbances (aggression, irritability, agitation), especially in children
Occasional
Rash, ankle or facial edema, nocturia, dysuria, change in appetite or weight, dry mouth, sore gums, nausea, blurred vision
Rare
Paradoxical CNS reactions, including hyperactivity or nervousness in children and excitement or restlessness in the elderly (particularly in the presence of uncontrolled pain).

SERIOUS REACTIONS

• Abrupt withdrawal may result in pronounced restlessness, irritability, insomnia, hand tremors, abdominal or muscle cramps, diaphoresis, vomiting, and status epilepticus.
• Overdose results in somnolence, confusion, diminished reflexes, and coma.

PRECAUTIONS & CONSIDERATIONS

Caution is warranted with chronic respiratory disease and impaired renal and hepatic function. Clonazepam crosses the placenta and may be distributed in breast milk. Chronic clonazepam use during pregnancy may produce withdrawal symptoms and CNS depression in neonates. Long-term clonazepam use may adversely affect the mental and physical development of children. The elderly are usually more sensitive to clonazepam's CNS effects, such as ataxia, dizziness, and oversedation. Expect to give them a lower dosage and increase it gradually. Alcohol, smoking, and tasks that require mental alertness or motor skills should be avoided.

Drowsiness and dizziness may occur. History of the seizure disorder, including the duration, frequency, and intensity of seizures should be assessed. Autonomic responses, such as cold or clammy hands and diaphoresis, and motor responses, such as agitation, trembling, and tension, in those with panic disorder should also be assessed. CBC and blood chemistry tests and hepatic and renal function should be periodically monitored.

Administration
! If the patient must switch to another anticonvulsant, expect to decrease the clonazepam dose gradually as therapy begins with a low dose of the replacement drug.

Take clonazepam without regard to meals. Crush tablets as needed. Do not abruptly discontinue the drug after long-term therapy. Strict maintenance of drug therapy is essential for seizure control.

Clonidine
klon'ih-deen
(Catapres, Catapres TTS, Dixarit [CAN], Duraclon)
Do not confuse clonidine with clomiphene, Klonopin, or quinidine, or Catapres with Cetapred.

CATEGORY AND SCHEDULE
Pregnancy Risk Category: C

CLASSIFICATION
Antiadrenergics, central

MECHANISM OF ACTION
An antiadrenergic, sympatholytic agent that prevents pain signal transmission to the brain and produces analgesia at pre- and post-alpha-adrenergic receptors in the spinal cord. *Therapeutic Effect:* Reduces peripheral resistance; decreases BP and heart rate.

PHARMACOKINETICS

Route	Onset	Peak	Duration
PO	0.5-1 hr	2-4 hr	Up to 8 hr

Well absorbed from the GI tract. Transdermal best absorbed from the chest and upper arm; least absorbed from the thigh. Protein binding: 20%-40%. Metabolized in the liver. Primarily excreted in urine. Minimally removed by hemodialysis. **Half-life:** 12-16 hr (increased with impaired renal function).

AVAILABILITY
Tablets (Catapres): 0.1 mg, 0.2 mg, 0.3 mg.

Transdermal Patch (Catapres TTS):
2.5 mg (release at 0.1 mg/24 hr),
5 mg (release at 0.2 mg/24 hr),
7.5 mg (release at 0.3 mg/24 hr).
Injection (Duraclon): 100 mcg/ml,
500 mcg/ml.

INDICATIONS AND DOSAGES
▸ **Hypertension**
PO
Adults. Initially, 0.1 mg twice a day.
Increase by 0.1-0.2 mg q2-4 days.
Maintenance: 0.2-1.2 mg/day in
2-4 divided doses up to maximum of
2.4 mg/day.
Elderly. Initially, 0.1 mg at bedtime.
May increase gradually.
Children. 5-25 mcg/kg/day in
divided doses q6hr. Increase at 5- to
7-day intervals. Maximum:
0.9 mg/day.
TRANSDERMAL
Adults, Elderly. System delivering
0.1 mg/24 hr up to 0.6 mg/24 hr
q7 days.
▸ **Attention deficit hyperactivity
disorder (ADHD)**
PO
Children. Initially 0.05 mg/day. May
increase by 0.05 mg/day q3-7 days.
Maximum: 0.3-0.4 mg/day.
▸ **Severe pain**
EPIDURAL
Adults, Elderly. 30-40 mcg/hr.
Children. Initially, 0.5 mcg/kg/hr,
not to exceed adult dose.

OFF-LABEL USES
ADHD, diagnosis of pheochromocytoma, opioid withdrawal, prevention
of migraine headaches, treatment of
dysmenorrhea or menopausal flushing

CONTRAINDICATIONS
Epidural contraindicated in those
patients with bleeding diathesis or
infection at the injection site, and
in those receiving anticoagulation
therapy

INTERACTIONS
Drug
Beta blockers: Discontinuing these
drugs may increase risk of clonidine-
withdrawal hypertensive crisis.
Tricyclic antidepressants: May
decrease effect of clonidine.
Herbal
None known.
Food
None known.

DIAGNOSTIC TEST EFFECTS
None known.

▦ IV INCOMPATIBILITIES
None known.
 IV Compatibilities
Bupivacaine (Marcaine, Sensorcaine),
fentanyl (Sublimaze), heparin, keta-
mine (Ketalar), lidocaine, lorazepam
(Ativan)

SIDE EFFECTS
Frequent
Dry mouth (40%), somnolence
(33%), dizziness (16%), sedation,
constipation (10%)
Occasional (5%-1%)
Tablets, injection: Depression,
swelling of feet, loss of appetite,
decreased sexual ability, itching
eyes, dizziness, nausea, vomiting,
nervousness
Transdermal: Itching, reddening or
darkening of skin
Rare (less than 1%)
Nightmares, vivid dreams, cold feeling in fingers and toes

SERIOUS REACTIONS
• Overdose produces profound
hypotension, irritability, bradycardia,
respiratory depression, hypothermia,
miosis (pupillary constriction),
arrhythmias, and apnea.
• Abrupt withdrawal may result in
rebound hypertension associated
with nervousness, agitation, anxiety,

insomnia, hand tingling, tremor, flushing, and diaphoresis.

PRECAUTIONS & CONSIDERATIONS

Caution is warranted with cerebrovascular disease, chronic renal failure, Raynaud's disease, recent MI, severe coronary insufficiency, and thromboangiitis obliterans. Clonidine crosses the placenta and is distributed in breast milk. Children are more sensitive to clonidine's effects. Use clonidine with caution in children. The elderly may be more sensitive to the hypotensive effect of clonidine. Age-related renal impairment may require dosage adjustment in the elderly.

Dizziness and lightheadedness may occur. Rise slowly from a lying to a sitting position and permit legs to dangle momentarily before standing to avoid clonidine's hypotensive effect. B/P should be obtained immediately before giving each dose, in addition to regular monitoring. Be alert for B/P fluctuations. Daily bowel activity and stool consistency should also be assessed. Expect concurrent beta-blocker therapy to be discontinued several days before discontinuing clonidine therapy to prevent clonidine withdrawal hypertensive crisis; and clonidine dosage should be reduced over 2 to 4 days.

Administration

Take oral clonidine without regard to food. Tablets may be crushed. Take last oral dose just before bedtime. Avoid skipping doses or voluntarily discontinuing clonidine because it can produce severe, rebound hypertension.

For transdermal use, apply the system to dry, hairless area of intact skin on upper arm or chest. Rotate sites to prevent skin irritation. Do not trim patch to adjust dose.

Clopidogrel
clo-pid′o-grill
(Iscover [AUS], Plavix)
Do not confuse Plavix with Paxil.

CATEGORY AND SCHEDULE
Pregnancy Risk Category: B

CLASSIFICATION
Platelet inhibitors

MECHANISM OF ACTION
A thienopyridine derivative that inhibits binding of the enzyme adenosine phosphate (ADP) to its platelet receptor and subsequent ADP-mediated activation of a glycoprotein complex. *Therapeutic Effect:* Inhibits platelet aggregation.

PHARMACOKINETICS

Route	Onset	Peak	Duration
PO	1 hr	2 hr	N/A

Rapidly absorbed. Protein binding: 98%. Extensively metabolized by the liver. Eliminated equally in the urine and feces. **Half-life:** 8 hr.

AVAILABILITY
Tablets: 75 mg.

INDICATIONS AND DOSAGES
▸ **Myocardial infarction (MI), stroke reduction**
PO
Adults, Elderly. 75 mg once a day.
▸ **Acute coronary syndrome**
PO
Adults, Elderly. Initially, 300 mg loading dose, then 75 mg once a day (in combination with aspirin).

CONTRAINDICATIONS

Active bleeding, coagulation disorders, severe hepatic disease

INTERACTIONS

Drug
Fluvastatin, other NSAIDs, phenytoin, tamoxifen, tolbutamide, torsemide, warfarin: May interfere with metabolism of these drugs.
Herbal
Ginger, ginkgo biloba: May increase the risk of bleeding.
Food
None known.

DIAGNOSTIC TEST EFFECTS

Prolongs bleeding time.

SIDE EFFECTS

Frequent (15%)
Skin disorders
Occasional (8%-6%)
Upper respiratory tract infection, chest pain, flu-like symptoms, headache, dizziness, arthralgia
Rare (5%-3%)
Fatigue, edema, hypertension, abdominal pain, dyspepsia, diarrhea, nausea, epistaxis, dyspnea, rhinitis

SERIOUS REACTIONS

• None known.

PRECAUTIONS & CONSIDERATIONS

Caution is warranted with hematologic disorders, history of bleeding, hypertension, hepatic or renal impairment, and in preoperative persons. Be aware it may take longer to stop bleeding during drug therapy.

Notify the physician of unusual bleeding. Also, notify dentists and other physicians before surgery is scheduled or when new drugs are prescribed. Platelet count for thrombocytopenia, Hgb, WBC count, and BUN, serum bilirubin, creatinine, AST (SGOT) and ALT (SGPT) levels should be monitored. Platelet count should be obtained before clopidogrel therapy, every 2 days during the first week of treatment and weekly thereafter until therapeutic maintenance dose is reached. Be aware abrupt discontinuation of clopidogrel produces an elevated platelet count within 5 days.

Administration
Take clopidogrel without regard to food. Do not crush coated tablets.

Clorazepate

klor-az′e-pate
(Novoclopate [CAN], Tranxene, Tranxene SD, Tranxene SD Half-Strength, T-Tab)
Do not confuse clorazepate with clofibrate.

CATEGORY AND SCHEDULE

Pregnancy Risk Category: D

CLASSIFICATION

Anxiolytics, benzodiazepines

MECHANISM OF ACTION

A benzodiazepine that depresses all levels of the CNS, including limbic and reticular formation, by binding to benzodiazepine receptor sites on the gamma-aminobutyric acid (GABA) receptor complex. Modulates GABA, a major inhibitory neurotransmitter in the brain. *Therapeutic Effect:* Produces anxiolytic effect, suppresses seizure activity.

AVAILABILITY

Tablets (Tranxene, T-Tab): 3.75 mg, 7.5 mg, 15 mg.
Tablets (Extended Release [Tranxene SD]): 22.5 mg.

Tablets (Extended-Release [Tranxene SD Half-Strength]): 11.25 mg.

INDICATIONS AND DOSAGES
▸ **Anxiety**
PO
Adults, Elderly. (Regular release): 7.5-15 mg 2-4 times a day. (Sustained release): 11.25 mg or 22.5 mg once a day at bedtime.
▸ **Anticonvulsant**
PO
Adults, Elderly, Children older than 12 yr. Initially, 7.5 mg 2-3 times a day. May increase by 7.5 mg at weekly intervals. Maximum: 90 mg/day.
Children 9-12 yr. Initially, 3.75-7.5 mg twice a day. May increase by 2.75 mg at weekly intervals. Maximum: 60 mg/day.
▸ **Alcohol withdrawal**
PO
Adults, Elderly. Initially, 30 mg, then 15 mg 2-4 times a day on first day. Gradually decrease dosage over subsequent days. Maximum: 90 mg/day.

CONTRAINDICATIONS
Acute narrow-angle glaucoma

INTERACTIONS
Drug
Other CNS depressants: May increase CNS depressant effects.
Herbal
Kava kava, valerian: May increase CNS depression.
Food
Alcohol: May increase CNS depressant effects.

DIAGNOSTIC TEST EFFECTS
None known. Therapeutic serum drug level is 0.12-1.5 mcg/ml; toxic serum drug level is greater than 5 mcg/ml.

SIDE EFFECTS
Frequent
Somnolence
Occasional
Dizziness, GI disturbances, nervousness, blurred vision, dry mouth, headache, confusion, ataxia, rash, irritability, slurred speech
Rare
Paradoxical CNS reactions, such as hyperactivity or nervousness in children and excitement or restlessness in the elderly or debilitated (generally noted during first 2 weeks of therapy, particularly in presence of uncontrolled pain)

SERIOUS REACTIONS
• Abrupt or too-rapid withdrawal may result in pronounced restlessness, irritability, insomnia, hand tremors, abdominal or muscle cramps, diaphoresis, vomiting, and seizures.
• Overdose results in somnolence, confusion, diminished reflexes, and coma.

PRECAUTIONS & CONSIDERATIONS
Caution is warranted with acute alcohol intoxication and renal and hepatic impairment. Females should use effective contraception during therapy and notify their physician immediately if they become or may be pregnant.

Drowsiness and dizziness may occur. Change positions slowly from recumbent to sitting, before standing, to prevent dizziness. Alcohol, smoking, and tasks that require mental alertness or motor skills should also be avoided. Autonomic responses, such as cold, clammy hands and diaphoresis, and motor responses, such as agitation, trembling, and tension, should be assessed. Seizure frequency and intensity should be assessed.

Administration
! If the person must change to another anticonvulsant, plan to decrease clorazepate dosage gradually as low-dose therapy begins with the replacement drug. Be aware the therapeutic peak serum level is 0.12-1.5 mcg/ml; the toxic serum level is greater than 5 mcg/ml.

Do not abruptly discontinue the medication after long-term use because this may precipitate seizures. Strict compliance with the drug regimen is essential for seizure control.

Clotrimazole
kloe-try-mah-zole
(Canesten [CAN], Clotrimaderm [CAN], Mycelex, Mycelex OTC, Lotrimin, Gyne-Lotrimin, Trivagizole 3)

CATEGORY AND SCHEDULE
Pregnancy Risk Category: B (topical), C (troches)

CLASSIFICATION
Antifungals, topical, dermatologics

MECHANISM OF ACTION
An antifungal that binds with phospholipids in fungal cell membrane. The altered cell membrane permeability. *Therapeutic Effect:* Inhibits yeast growth.

PHARMACOKINETICS
Poorly, erratically absorbed from GI tract. Bound to oral mucosa. Absorbed portion metabolized in liver. Eliminated in feces. Topical: Minimal systemic absorption (highest concentration in stratum corneum).

Intravaginal: Small amount systemically absorbed. **Half-life:** 3.5-5 hr.

AVAILABILITY
Combination pack: Vaginal tablet 100 mg and vaginal cream 1% (Mycelex-7).
Lotion: 1% (Lotrimin).
Topical Cream: 1% (Lotrimin, Lotrimin AF, Mycelex, Mycelex OTC).
Topical Solution: 1% (Lotrimin, Lotrimin AF, Mycelex, Mycelex OTC).
Troches: 10 mg (Mycelex).
Vaginal Cream: 1% (Gyne-Lotrimin, Mycelex-7), 2% (Gyne-Lotrimin 3, Mycelex-3, Trivagizole 3).
Vaginal Tablets: 100 mg, 500 mg (Gyne-Lotrimin, Mycelex-7).

INDICATIONS AND DOSAGES
▸ **Oropharyngeal candidiasis treatment**
PO
Adults, Elderly. 10 mg 5 times/day for 14 days.
▸ **Oropharyngeal candidiasis prophylaxis**
PO
Adults, Elderly. 10 mg 3 times/day.
▸ **Dermatophytosis, cutaneous candidiasis**
TOPICAL
Adults, Elderly. 2 times/day. Therapeutic effect may take up to 8 wk.
▸ **Vulvovaginal candidiasis**
VAGINAL (TABLETS)
Adults, Elderly. 1 tablet (100 mg) at bedtime for 7 days; 2 tablets (200 mg) at bedtime for 3 days; or 500-mg tablet one time.
VAGINAL (CREAM)
Adults, Elderly. 1 applicatorful at bedtime for 7-14 days.

OFF-LABEL USES
Topical: Treatment of paronychia, tinea barbae, tinea capitias.

CONTRAINDICATIONS

Hypersensitivity to clotrimazole or any component of the formulation, children <3 yr

INTERACTIONS
Drug

Benzodiazepines: May increase benzodiazepine serum concentrations and increase risk of toxicity.
Ergot derivatives: May increase risk of ergotism (nausea, vomiting, vasospastic ischemia).
Fentanyl: May increase or prolong opioid effects (CNS depression).
Tacrolimus: May increase risk of tacrolimus toxicity.
Trimetrexate: May increase risk of trimetrexate toxicity.
Herbal
None known.
Food
None known.

DIAGNOSTIC TEST EFFECTS
May increase SGOT (AST).

SIDE EFFECTS
Frequent
Oral: Nausea, vomiting, diarrhea, abdominal pain
Occasional
Topical: Itching, burning, stinging, erythema, urticaria
Vaginal: Mild burning (tablets/cream); irritation, cystitis (cream)
Rare
Vaginal: Itching, rash, lower abdominal cramping, headache

SERIOUS REACTIONS
• None reported.

PRECAUTIONS & CONSIDERATIONS

Caution is warranted with hepatic disorder with oral therapy. It is unknown if clotrimazole crosses the placenta or is distributed in breast milk. Be aware that clotrimazole use is contraindicated in children less than 3 years. There are no age-related precautions noted in children more than 5 years or in the elderly. Refrain from sexual intercourse or advise partner to use condom during clotrimazole therapy. Separate personal items and linens.

Itching, burning, and stinging may occur with topical preparations. Vulvovaginal irritation, abdominal cramping, urinary frequency, and discomfort may occur with vaginal therapy.

Administration

Lozenges must be dissolved in mouth more than 15-30 minutes for oropharyngeal therapy. Swallow saliva.

When using topical preparation, rub well into affected, surrounding areas. Do not apply occlusive covering or other preparations. Keep area clean and dry. Wear light clothing to promote ventilation.

To use vaginally, use vaginal applicator and insert high in vagina. Continue to use during menses.

Clozapine

klo′za-peen
(Clopine [AUS], Clozaril, FazaClo)
Do not confuse clozapine with Cloxapen or clofazimine, or Clozaril with Clinoril, or Colazal.

CATEGORY AND SCHEDULE
Pregnancy Risk Category: B

CLASSIFICATION
Antipsychotics

MECHANISM OF ACTION
A dibenzodiazepine derivative that interferes with the binding of dopamine at dopamine receptor sites; binds primarily at nondopamine receptor sites. *Therapeutic Effect:* Diminishes schizophrenic behavior.

AVAILABILITY
Tablets (Clozaril): 12.5 mg, 25 mg, 100 mg.
Oral disintegrating tablets (FazaClo): 25 mg, 100 mg.

INDICATIONS AND DOSAGES
▸ **Schizophrenic disorders, reduce suicidal behavior**
PO
Adults. Initially, 25 mg once or twice a day. May increase by 25-50 mg/day over 2 wk until dosage of 300-450 mg/day is achieved. May further increase by 50-100 mg/day no more than once or twice a week, Range: 200-600 mg/day. Maximum: 900 mg/day.
Elderly. Initially, 25 mg/day. May increase by 25 mg/day. Maximum: 450 mg/day.

CONTRAINDICATIONS
Coma, concurrent use of other drugs that may suppress bone marrow function, history of clozapine-induced agranulocytosis or severe granulocytopenia, myeloproliferative disorders, severe CNS depression

INTERACTIONS
Drug
Alcohol, other CNS depressants: May increase CNS depressant effects.
Bone marrow depressants: May increase myelosuppression.
Lithium: May increase the risk of confusion, dyskinesia, and seizures.
Phenobarbital: Decreases clozapine blood concentration.

Herbal
None known.
Food
None known.

DIAGNOSTIC TEST EFFECTS
May increase serum glucose levels.

SIDE EFFECTS
Frequent
Somnolence (39%), salivation (31%), tachycardia (25%), dizziness (19%), constipation (14%)
Occasional
Hypotension (9%); headache (7%); tremor, syncope, diaphoresis, dry mouth (6%); nausea, visual disturbances (5%); nightmares, restlessness, akinesia, agitation, hypertension, abdominal discomfort or heartburn, weight gain (4%)
Rare
Rigidity, confusion, fatigue, insomnia, diarrhea, rash

SERIOUS REACTIONS
• Seizures occur in about 3% of patients.
• Overdose produces CNS depression (including sedation, coma, and delirium), respiratory depression, and hypersalivation.
• Blood dyscrasias, particularly agranulocytosis; and mild leukopenia, may occur.

PRECAUTIONS & CONSIDERATIONS
Caution is warranted with alcohol withdrawal and in those with cardiovascular disease, glaucoma, history of seizures, benign prostatic hyperplasia, myocarditis, urine retention, and impaired hepatic, renal, or respiratory function.

Drowsiness may occur but generally subsides with continued therapy. Alcohol and tasks that require mental alertness or motor skills should be avoided. B/P for hypertension or hypotension, heart rate for tachycardia, and CBC for blood dyscrasias (particularly agranulocytosis and mild leukopenia) should be assessed. WBC count should be monitored every week for the first 6 months of continuous therapy, then biweekly when WBC counts are acceptable.

Administration

Take clozapine without regard to food. Do not abruptly discontinue clozapine. It is required to monitor blood work before prescription can be filled.

Co-Trimoxazole (Sulfamethoxazole and Trimethoprim)

koe-trye-mox′a-zole
(Apo-Sulfatrim [CAN], Bactrim, Bactrim DS, Cosig Forte [AUS], Novotrimel [CAN], Resprim [AUS], Resprim Forte [AUS], Septra, Septra DS, Septrin [AUS], Septrin Forte [AUS], Sulfatrim Pediatric)
Do not confuse Bactrim with bacitracin, co-trimoxazole with clotrimazole, or Septra with Sectral or Septa.

CATEGORY AND SCHEDULE

Pregnancy Risk Category: C

CLASSIFICATION

Antibiotics, folate antagonists, sulfonamides

MECHANISM OF ACTION

A sulfonamide and folate antagonist that blocks bacterial synthesis of essential nucleic acids. *Therapeutic Effect:* Bactericidal in susceptible microorganisms.

PHARMACOKINETICS

Rapidly and well absorbed from the GI tract. Protein binding: 45%-60%. Widely distributed. Metabolized in the liver. Excreted in urine. Minimally removed by hemodialysis. **Half-life:** sulfamethoxazole 6-12 hr, trimethoprim 8-10 hr (increased in impaired renal function).

AVAILABILITY

! All dosage forms have same 5:1 ratio of sulfamethoxazole (SMX) to trimethoprim (TMP).
Oral Suspension (Septra, Sulfatrim Pediatric): SMX 200 mg and TMP 40 mg per 5 ml.
Tablets (Bactrim, Septra): SMX 400 mg and TMP 80 mg.
Tablets, double strength (Bactrim DS, Septra DS): SMX 800 mg and TMP 160 mg.
Injection (Septra): SMX 80 mg and TMP 16 mg per ml.

INDICATIONS AND DOSAGES

▸ **Mild to moderate infections**
PO, IV
Adults, Elderly, Children older than 2 mo. 6-12 mg/kg/day in divided doses q12hr.
▸ **Serious infections, *Pneumocystis Carinii* pneumonia (PCP)**
PO, IV
Adults, Elderly, Children older than 2 mo. 15-20 mg/kg/day in divided doses q6-8hr.
▸ **Prevention of PCP**
PO
Adults. One double-strength tablet each day.
Children. 150 mg/m^2/day on 3 consecutive days/wk.
▸ **Traveler's diarrhea**
PO
Adults, Elderly. One double-strength tablet q12hr for 5 days.
▸ **Acute exacerbation of chronic bronchitis**

PO

Adults, Elderly. One double-strength tablet q12hr for 14 days.

▶ **Prevention of UTIs**

PO

Adults, Elderly, Children older than 2 mo. 2 mg/kg/dose once a day.

▶ **Dosage in renal impairment**

Dosage and frequency are modified based on creatinine clearance, the severity of the infection and the serum concentration of the drug. For those with creatinine clearance of 15-30 ml/min, a 50% dosage reduction is recommended.

OFF-LABEL USES

Treatment of bacterial endocarditis; gonorrhea; meningitis; septicemia; sinusitis; and biliary tract, bone, joint, chancroid, chlamydial, intra-abdominal, skin and soft-tissue infections

CONTRAINDICATIONS

Hypersensitivity to trimethoprim or any sulfonamides, infants younger than 2 months old, megaloblastic anemia due to folate deficiency.

INTERACTIONS

Drug

Hemolytics: May increase the risk of toxicity.

Hepatotoxic medications: May increase the risk of hepatotoxicity.

Hydantoin anticonvulsants, oral antidiabetics, warfarin: May increase or prolong the effects of these drugs and increase their risk of toxicity.

Methenamine: May form a precipitate.

Methotrexate: May increase the effects of methotrexate.

Herbal

None known.

Food

None known.

DIAGNOSTIC TEST EFFECTS

May increase BUN and serum alkaline phosphatase, creatinine, potassium, AST (SGOT), and ALT (SGPT) levels.

▧ IV INCOMPATIBILITIES

Fluconazole (Diflucan), foscarnet (Foscavir), midazolam (Versed), vinorelbine (Navelbine)

▧ IV Compatibilities

Diltiazem (Cardizem), heparin, hydromorphone (Dilaudid), lorazepam (Ativan), magnesium sulfate, morphine

SIDE EFFECTS

Frequent

Anorexia, nausea, vomiting, rash (generally 7-14 days after therapy begins), urticaria

Occasional

Diarrhea, abdominal pain, pain or irritation at the IV infusion site

Rare

Headache, vertigo, insomnia, seizures, hallucinations, depression

SERIOUS REACTIONS

• Rash, fever, sore throat, pallor, purpura, cough, and shortness of breath may be early signs of serious adverse reactions.

• Fatalities have occasionally occurred after Stevens-Johnson syndrome, toxic epidermal necrolysis, fulminant hepatic necrosis, agranulocytosis, aplastic anemia, and other blood dyscrasias in patients taking sulfonamides.

• Myelosuppression, decreased platelet count and severe dermatologic reactions may occur, especially in the elderly.

PRECAUTIONS & CONSIDERATIONS

Caution is warranted with impaired renal or hepatic function or glucose-6-phosphate dehydrogenase deficiency.

Co-trimoxazole use is contraindicated during pregnancy at term and during breastfeeding. Co-trimoxazole readily crosses the placenta and is distributed in breast milk. Co-trimoxazole use is contraindicated in children younger than 2 months old; if given to newborns, it may produce kernicterus. Elderly patients have an increased risk of developing myelosuppression, decreased platelet count, and severe skin reactions.

History of bronchial asthma, hypersensitivity to trimethoprim or any sulfonamide, or sulfite sensitivity, should be determined before beginning drug therapy. Report any new symptoms, especially bleeding, bruising, fever, sore throat, and a rash or other skin changes. Intake and output, pattern of daily bowel activity and stool consistency, skin for rash, renal and liver function, CNS symptoms such as hallucinations, headache, insomnia, and vertigo, should be assessed. Vital signs should be monitored at least twice a day.

Storage
Store tablets and oral suspension at room temperature. Be aware that the piggyback IV infusion solution is stable for 2 to 6 hours. Use the solution immediately. Discard the solution if it is cloudy or contains a precipitate.

Administration
! Be aware that drug potency is expressed in terms of trimethoprim content.

Take the oral form with 8 oz water on an empty stomach. Have the patient drink several additional glasses of water each day.

For piggyback IV infusion, dilute each 5-ml vial with 75 to 125 ml D₅W. Don't mix co-trimoxazole with other drugs or solutions. Infuse the solution over 60 to 90 minutes.

Avoid bolus or rapid infusion and IM injection. Ensure that the patient is adequately hydrated.

Codeine
koe′deen
(Actacode [AUS], Codeine Phosphate Injection, Codeine Linctus [AUS])
(Contin [CAN])
Do not confuse codeine with Cardene or Lodine.

CATEGORY AND SCHEDULE
Pregnancy Risk Category: C (D if used for prolonged periods or at high dosages at term)
Controlled Substance: Schedule II (analgesic), III (fixed-combination form)

CLASSIFICATION
Analgesics, narcotic, antitussives

MECHANISM OF ACTION
An opioid agonist that binds to opioid receptors at many cites in the CNS, particularly in the medulla. This action inhibits the ascending pain pathways. *Therapeutic Effect:* Alters the perception of and emotional response to pain, suppresses cough reflex.

AVAILABILITY
Tablets: 15 mg, 30 mg, 60 mg.
Oral Solution: 15 mg/5 ml.
Injection: 15 mg/ml, 30 mg/ml.

INDICATIONS AND DOSAGES
▸ **Analgesia**
PO, IM, SUBCUTANEOUS
Adults, Elderly. 30 mg q4-6hr.
Range: 15-60 mg.

Children. 0.5-1 mg/kg q4-6hr.
Maximum: 60 mg/dose.
▸ **Cough**
PO
Adults, Elderly, Children 12 yr and older. 10-20 mg q4-6hr.
Children 6-11 yr. 5-10 mg q4-6hr.
Children 2-5 yr. 2.5-5 mg q4-6hr.
▸ **Dosage in renal impairment**
Dosage is modified based on creatinine clearance.

Creatinine Clearance	Dosage
10-50 ml/min	75% of usual dose
Less than 10 ml/min	50% of usual dose

OFF-LABEL USES
Treatment of diarrhea

CONTRAINDICATIONS
None known.

INTERACTIONS
Drug
Alcohol, other CNS depressants: May increase CNS or respiratory depression, and hypotension.
MAOIs: May produce a severe, sometimes fatal reaction; plan to administer a test dose, which is one-quarter of usual codeine dose.
Herbal
None known.
Food
None known.

DIAGNOSTIC TEST EFFECTS
May increase serum amylase and lipase levels.

SIDE EFFECTS
Frequent
Constipation, somnolence, nausea, vomiting
Occasional
Paradoxical excitement, confusion, palpitations, facial flushing, decreased urination, blurred vision, dizziness, dry mouth, headache, hypotension (including orthostatic hypotension), decreased appetite, injection site redness, burning, or pain
Rare
Hallucinations, depression, abdominal pain, insomnia

SERIOUS REACTIONS
• Too-frequent use may result in paralytic ileus.
• Overdose may produce cold and clammy skin, confusion, seizures, decreased B/P, restlessness, pinpoint pupils, bradycardia, respiratory depression, decreased LOC, and severe weakness.
• The patient who uses codeine repeatedly may develop a tolerance to the drug's analgesic effect as well as physical dependence.

PRECAUTIONS & CONSIDERATIONS
Extreme caution should be used with acute alcoholism, anoxia, CNS depression, hypercapnia, respiratory depression or dysfunction, seizures, shock, and untreated myxedema. Caution is also warranted with acute abdominal conditions, Addison's disease, COPD, hypothyroidism, hepatic impairment, increased intracranial pressure, benign prostatic hyperplasia, and urethral stricture. Codeine crosses the placenta and is distributed in breast milk. Regular use of opioids during pregnancy may produce withdrawal symptoms in the neonate, such as diarrhea, excessive crying, fever, hyperactive reflexes, irritability, seizures, sneezing, tremors, vomiting, and yawning. Codeine may prolong labor if administered in the latent phase of the first stage of labor or before the cervix is dilated 4 to 5 cm. The neonate may develop respiratory depression if the mother

receives codeine during labor. Children and the elderly are more prone to experience paradoxical excitement. Children younger than 2 years and the elderly are more susceptible to the drug's respiratory depressant effects. In the elderly, age-related renal impairment may increase the risk of codeine-induced urine retention.

Dizziness and drowsiness may occur, so change positions slowly and avoid alcohol, CNS depressants, and tasks that require mental alertness or motor skills until response to the drug is established. Vital signs, pattern of daily bowel activity and stool consistency, and clinical improvement of pain should be monitored.

Administration

! Be aware that ambulatory patients and patients not in severe pain may be more prone to dizziness, hypotension, nausea, and vomiting than patients in the supine position and those in severe pain. Expect to reduce the initial dosage in elderly and debilitated patients; those with hypothyroidism, Addison's disease, or renal insufficiency; and those using other CNS depressants concurrently.

For oral use, take codeine with food or milk to minimize adverse GI effects.

For IM and subcutaneous use, inspect drug for cloudiness or precipitate. If present, discard drug.

Colchicine
kol′chi-seen
(Colchicine, Colgout [AUS])

CATEGORY AND SCHEDULE
Pregnancy Risk Category: D

CLASSIFICATION
Antigout agents

MECHANISM OF ACTION
An alkaloid that decreases leukocyte motility, phagocytosis, and lactic acid production. *Therapeutic Effect:* Decreases urate crystal deposits and reduces inflammatory process.

PHARMACOKINETICS
Rapidly absorbed from the GI tract. Highest concentration is in the liver, spleen, and kidney. Protein binding: 30%-50%. Reenters the intestinal tract by biliary secretion and is reabsorbed from the intestines. Partially metabolized in the liver. Eliminated primarily in feces.

AVAILABILITY
Tablets: 0.6 mg.
Injection: 1 mg.

INDICATIONS AND DOSAGES
▸ **Acute gouty arthritis**
PO
Adults, Elderly. 0.6-1.2 mg; then 0.6 mg q1-2hr or 1-1.2 mg q2hr, until pain is relieved or nausea, vomiting, or diarrhea occurs. Total dose: 4-8 mg.
IV
Adults, Elderly. Initially, 2 mg; then 0.5 mg q6hr until satisfactory response. Maximum: 4 mg/wk or 4 mg/one course of treatment. If pain recurs, may give 1-2 mg/day for

several days but no sooner than
7 days after a full course of IV therapy (total of 4 mg).
▶ Chronic gouty arthritis
PO
Adults, Elderly. 0.5-0.6 mg once
weekly up to once a day, depending
on number of attacks per year.

OFF-LABEL USES
To reduce frequency of recurrence of
familial Mediterranean fever; treatment of acute calcium pyrophos-
phate deposition, amyloidosis, biliary
cirrhosis, recurrent pericarditis,
sarcoid arthritis

CONTRAINDICATIONS
Blood dyscrasias; severe cardiac, GI,
hepatic, or renal disorders

INTERACTIONS
Drug
Bone marrow depressants:
May increase the risk of blood
dyscrasias.
NSAIDs: May increase the risk of
bone marrow depression, neutropenia,
and thrombocytopenia.
Herbal
None known.
Food
None known.

DIAGNOSTIC TEST EFFECTS
May increase serum alkaline phos-
phatase and AST (SGOT) levels.
May decrease platelet count.

▓ IV INCOMPATIBILITIES
No information available via Y-site
administration.

SIDE EFFECTS
Frequent
PO: Nausea, vomiting, abdominal
discomfort
Occasional
PO: Anorexia

Rare
Hypersensitivity reaction, including
angioedema
Parenteral: Nausea, vomiting, diarrhea, abdominal discomfort, pain or
redness at injection site, neuritis in
injected arm

SERIOUS REACTIONS
• Bone marrow depression, including
aplastic anemia, agranulocytosis, and
thrombocytopenia, may occur with
long-term therapy.
• Overdose initially causes a burning feeling in the skin or throat,
severe diarrhea, and abdominal pain.
The patient then experiences fever,
seizures, delirium, and renal impairment, marked by hematuria and oliguria. The third stage of overdose
causes hair loss, leukocytosis, and
stomatitis.

PRECAUTIONS & CONSIDERATIONS
Caution is warranted with impaired
hepatic function and in the elderly or
debilitated. It is unknown if colchicine
crosses the placenta or is distributed
in breast milk. Safety and efficacy of
colchicine have not been established
in children. The elderly may be more
susceptible to cumulative toxicity
and age-related renal impairment
may increase risk of myopathy. The
drug should be discontinued immediately if GI symptoms occur. Limit
intake of high purine foods, such as
fish and organ meats, and drink 8 to
10 eight-ounce glasses of fluid daily
while taking colchicine.
   Notify the physician if fever,
numbness, skin rash, sore throat,
fatigue, unusual bleeding or bruising,
or weakness occurs. The drug should
be discontinued as soon as gout pain
is relieved, or at the first appearance
of diarrhea, nausea, or vomiting.
High fluid intake (3000 ml/day)
should be encouraged; intake and

output should be monitored; output should be at least 2000 ml/day. Signs and symptoms of a therapeutic response, including improved joint range of motion and reduced joint tenderness, redness, and swelling, should be evaluated.

Storage
Store at room temperature.

Administration
Take colchicine without regard to meals.

For IV use, may dilute with 0.9% NaCl or sterile water for injection; do not dilute with D₅W. Administer over 2 to 5 minutes.

Colesevelam
koh-le-sev′e-lam
(Welchol)

CATEGORY AND SCHEDULE
Pregnancy Risk Category: B

CLASSIFICATION
Antihyperlipidemics, bile acid sequestrants

MECHANISM OF ACTION
A bile acid sequestrant and nonsystemic polymer that binds with bile acids in the intestines, preventing their reabsorption and removing them from the body. *Therapeutic Effect:* Decreases LDL cholesterol.

AVAILABILITY
Tablets: 625 mg.

INDICATIONS AND DOSAGES
▸ **To decrease LDL cholesterol level in primary hypercholesterolemia (Fredrickson type IIa)**

PO
Adults, Elderly. 3 tablets with meals twice a day or 6 tablets once a day with a meal. May increase daily dose to 7 tablets a day.

CONTRAINDICATIONS
Complete biliary obstruction, hypersensitivity to colesevelam

INTERACTIONS
Drug
Aspirin, clindamycin, digoxin, furosemide, glipizide, hydrocortisone, imipramine, NSAIDs, phenytoin, propranolol, tetracyclines, thiazide diuretics, vitamins A, D, E, K: May decrease the absorption of these drugs.
Herbal
None known.
Food
None known.

DIAGNOSTIC TEST EFFECTS
None known.

SIDE EFFECTS
Frequent (12%-8%)
Flatulence, constipation, infection, dyspepsia (heartburn, epigastric distress)

SERIOUS REACTIONS
• GI tract obstruction may occur.

PRECAUTIONS & CONSIDERATIONS
Caution is warranted with dysphagia, severe GI motility disorders, those who have had major GI tract surgery and in those susceptible to fat-soluble vitamin deficiency. Colesevelam is not absorbed systemically. It may decrease proper maternal vitamin absorption and may affect breast-feeding infants. Safety and efficacy of colesevelam have not been established in children. No age-related

precautions have been noted in the elderly.

Pattern of daily bowel activity and stool consistency should be assessed. Serum cholesterol and triglyceride levels should be checked at baseline and periodically thereafter.

Administration
Take with meals and with a liquid.

Colestipol
koe-les'ti-pole
(Colestid, Colestid [CAN])

CATEGORY AND SCHEDULE
Pregnancy Risk Category: C

CLASSIFICATION
Antihyperlipidemics, bile acid sequestrants

MECHANISM OF ACTION
An antihyperlipoproteinemic that binds with bile acids in the intestine, forming an insoluble complex. Binding results in partial removal of bile acid from enterohepatic circulation.
Therapeutic Effect: Removes low-density lipoproteins (LDL) and cholesterol from plasma.

PHARMACOKINETICS
Not absorbed from the gastrointestinal (GI) tract. Excreted in the feces.

AVAILABILITY
Granules: 5 g packet (Colestid).
Tablet: 1 g (Colestid).

INDICATIONS AND DOSAGES
▸ **Primary hypercholesterolemia**

PO, GRANULES
Adults, Elderly. Initially, 5 g 1-2 times/day. Range: 5-30 g/day once or in divided doses.
PO, TABLETS
Adults, Elderly. Initially, 2 g 1-2 times/day. Range: 2-16 g/day.

OFF-LABEL USES
Treatment of diarrhea (due to bile acids); hyperoxaluria

CONTRAINDICATIONS
Complete biliary obstruction, hypersensitivity to bile acid sequestering resins

INTERACTIONS
Drug
Anticoagulants: May increase effects of these drugs by decreasing vitamin K.
Digoxin, folic acid, penicillins, propranolol, tetracyclines, thiazides, thyroid hormones, and other medications: May bind and decrease absorption of these drugs.
Oral vancomycin: Binds and decreases the effects of oral vancomycin.
Warfarin: May decrease warfarin absorption.
Herbal
Vitamin A, vitamin E: May decrease vitamin A and E absorption.
Food
None known.

DIAGNOSTIC TEST EFFECTS
May decrease serum calcium, potassium, and sodium levels. May prolong prothrombin time.

SIDE EFFECTS
Frequent
Constipation (may lead to fecal impaction), nausea, vomiting, stomach pain, indigestion

Occasional
Diarrhea, belching, bloating, headache, dizziness
Rare
Gallstones, peptic ulcer, malabsorption syndrome

SERIOUS REACTIONS
• GI tract obstruction, hyperchloremic acidosis, and osteoporosis secondary to calcium excretion may occur.
• High dosage may interfere with fat absorption, resulting in steatorrhea.

PRECAUTIONS & CONSIDERATIONS
Caution is warranted with bleeding disorders, GI dysfunction (especially constipation), hemorrhoids, and osteoporosis. Abdominal discomfort, flatulence, and food tolerance may occur during therapy. Colestipol may interfere with maternal absorption of fat-soluble vitamins. There are no age-related precautions noted in children. The elderly are at an increased risk of experiencing adverse nutritional effects and GI side effects. Electrolytes and serum cholesterol and triglyceride levels should be monitored during therapy.
Administration
Take other drugs at least 1 hour before or 4 to 6 hours after colestipol because this drug is capable of binding drugs in the GI tract. Do not take colestipol in its dry form because it is highly irritating. Mix with 3 to 6 oz fruit juice, milk, soup, or water. Place powder on the surface of the liquid for 1 to 2 minutes to prevent lumping, then mix thoroughly. When mixing the powder with carbonated beverages, use an extra large glass and stir the liquid slowly to avoid excessive foaming. Take before meals. Drink water between meals. High-fiber foods such as fruits, whole grain cereals, and vegetables are encouraged to reduce the risk of constipation.

Cortisone
kor′ti-sone
(Cortate [AUS], Cortone [CAN])
Do not confuse cortisone with Cort-Dome.

CATEGORY AND SCHEDULE
Pregnancy Risk Category: C (D if used in the first trimester)

CLASSIFICATION
Corticosteroids

MECHANISM OF ACTION
An adrenocortical steroid that inhibits the accumulation of inflammatory cells at inflammation sites, phagocytosis, lysosomal enzyme release and synthesis, and release of mediators of inflammation. *Therapeutic Effect:* Prevents or suppresses cell-mediated immune reactions. Decreases or prevents tissue response to inflammatory process.

AVAILABILITY
Tablets: 25 mg.

INDICATIONS AND DOSAGES
Dosage is dependent on the condition being treated and patient response.
▸ **Anti-inflammation, immunosuppression**
PO
Adults, Elderly. 25-300 mg/day in divided doses q12-24hr.
Children. 2.5-10 mg/kg/day in divided doses q6-8hr.

▸ **Physiologic replacement**
PO
Adults, Elderly. 25-35 mg/day.
Children. 0.5-0.75 mg/kg/day in
divided doses q8hr.

CONTRAINDICATIONS
Hypersensitivity to corticosteroids,
administration of live virus
vaccine, peptic ulcers (except in
life-threatening situations), systemic
fungal infection

INTERACTIONS
Drug
Amphotericin: May increase
hypokalemia.
Digoxin: May increase digoxin
toxicity caused by hypokalemia.
**Diuretics, insulin, oral hypo-
glycemics, potassium supplements:**
May decrease the effects of these
drugs.
Hepatic enzyme inducers: May
decrease the effects of cortisone.
Live virus vaccines: May decrease
the patient's antibody response to
vaccine, increase vaccine side effects,
and potentiate virus replication.
Herbal
None known.
Food
None known.

DIAGNOSTIC TEST EFFECTS
May increase blood glucose and
serum lipid, amylase, and sodium
levels. May decrease serum calcium,
potassium, and thyroxine levels.

SIDE EFFECTS
Frequent
Insomnia, heartburn, anxiety,
abdominal distention, increased
diaphoresis, acne, mood swings,
increased appetite, facial flushing,
delayed wound healing, increased
susceptibility to infection, diarrhea
or constipation

Occasional
Headache, edema, change in skin
color, frequent urination
Rare
Tachycardia, allergic reaction (such
as rash and hives), psychological
changes, hallucinations, depression

SERIOUS REACTIONS
• Long-term therapy may cause
hypocalcemia, hypokalemia, muscle
wasting in arms and legs, osteoporosis, spontaneous fractures, amenorrhea, cataracts, glaucoma, peptic
ulcer disease, and CHF.
• Abrupt withdrawal following
long-term therapy may cause
anorexia, nausea, fever, headache,
joint pain, rebound inflammation,
fatigue, weakness, lethargy, dizziness,
and orthostatic hypotension.

PRECAUTIONS & CONSIDERATIONS
Caution is warranted with cirrhosis,
CHF, history of tuberculosis (it may
reactivate disease), hypertension,
hypothyroidism, nonspecific ulcerative colitis, psychosis, seizure disorders, and thromboembolic disorders.
Monitor growth and development of
children receiving long-term corticosteroid therapy. Dentist or other
physicians should be informed of
cortisone therapy if taken within the
past 12 months.
   Mood swings, ranging from
euphoria to depression, may occur.
Notify the physician of fever, muscle
aches, sore throat, and sudden weight
gain or swelling. Blood glucose level,
B/P, serum electrolyte levels, height,
and weight should be monitored
before and during therapy. Be alert
to signs and symptoms of infection
caused by reduced immune response,
including fever, sore throat, and
vague symptoms. In long-term therapy, signs and symptoms of hypocalcemia (such as muscle twitching,

cramps, and positive Chvostek's or Trousseau's signs) or hypokalemia (such as EKG changes, nausea and vomiting, irritability, weakness and muscle cramps, and numbness or tingling, especially in the lower extremities) should be assessed.

Administration
Do not change the dosage of or schedule for cortisone. Do not abruptly discontinue the drug; the drug must be withdrawn gradually under medical supervision.

Cosyntropin
kos-syn-troe′pin
(Cortrosyn)

CATEGORY AND SCHEDULE
Pregnancy Risk Category: C

CLASSIFICATION
Hormones/hormone modifiers

MECHANISM OF ACTION
A glucocorticoid that stimulates initial reaction in synthesis of adrenal steroids from cholesterol. *Therapeutic Effect:* Increases endogenous corticoid synthesis.

PHARMACOKINETICS
None reported.

AVAILABILITY
Powder for reconstitution: 0.25 mg (Cortrosyn).

INDICATIONS AND DOSAGES
▸ **Screening test for adrenal function**
IM
Adults, Elderly, Children 2 yr and older. 0.25-0.75 mg one time.

Children less than 2 yr. 0.125 mg one time.
Neonates. 0.015 mg/kg/dose.
IV, INFUSION
Adults. 0.25 mg in D_5W or 0.9% NaCl infused at rate of 0.04 mg/hr.

CONTRAINDICATIONS
Hypersensitivity to cosyntropin or corticotropin

INTERACTIONS
Drug
Fluoroquinolones: May increase risk for tendon rupture.
Itraconazole: May increase cosyntropin plasma concentrations and side effects.
Rotavirus vaccine: May increase risk of infection by live vaccine.
Bupropion: May lower seizure threshold.
Herbal
Echinacea, ma huang: May decrease effectiveness of cosyntropin.
Licorice: May increase risk of corticosteroid side effects.
Saiboku-to: May increase and prolong effect of cosyntropin.
Food
None known.

DIAGNOSTIC TEST EFFECTS
None known.

SIDE EFFECTS
Occasional
Nausea, vomiting
Rare
Hypersensitivity reaction (fever, pruritus)

SERIOUS REACTIONS
• None reported.

PRECAUTIONS & CONSIDERATIONS
Be aware that short duration for diagnostic use does not produce effects of long-term cosyntropin therapy. It is

unknown if cosyntropin crosses the placenta or is distributed in breast milk. There are no age-related precautions noted in children or the elderly.

If an allergic reaction with itching, hives, swelling in face or hands, swelling or tingling in mouth or throat, tightness in chest, and trouble breathing occurs, notify the physician.

The following criteria may be used as guidelines to determine whether there has been a normal response to cosyntropin:
— Morning control plasma cortisol concentration exceeds 5 mcg (0.005 mg) per 100 ml.
— 30-minute cortisol concentration shows an increase of at least 7 mcg (0.007 mg) per 100 ml above the control level.
— 30-minute cortisol concentration exceeds 18 mcg (0.018 mg) per 100 ml.
— If a 60-minute test interval is used, a normal response to cosyntropin is shown by a plasma cortisol concentration that is approximately 2 times the baseline concentration.

Storage
Be aware when constituted with 0.9% NaCl, cosyntropin is stable for 24 hours at room temperature. It is stable for up to 21 days when refrigerated under a nitrogen atmosphere.

Administration
Be aware that each 0.25 mg of cosyntropin is equivalent to 25 units of corticotrophin. Be aware that peak plasma cortisol concentrations usually occur 45-60 minutes after cosyntropin administration.

For IM injection, 1 ml of diluent provided (0.9% NaCl injection) should be added to the vial containing 250 mcg (0.25 mg) of cosyntropin. The resultant solution contains 250 mcg (0.25 mg) of cosyntropin per ml.

For intravenous infusion, cosyntropin may be further diluted with D_5W or 0.9% NaCl injection. Administer 0.25 mg in D_5W or 0.9% NaCl infused at rate of 0.04 mg per hour.

Cromolyn
kroe′moe-lin
(Apo-Cromolyn [CAN], Crolom, Gastrocom, Intal, Nasalcrom, Opticrom, Rynacrom [AUS])

CATEGORY AND SCHEDULE
Pregnancy Risk Category: B

CLASSIFICATION
Mast cell stabilizers, ophthalmics

MECHANISM OF ACTION
An antiasthmatic and antiallergic agent that prevents mast cell release of histamine, leukotrienes, and slow-reacting substances of anaphylaxis by inhibiting degranulation after contact with antigens. *Therapeutic Effect:* Helps prevent symptoms of asthma, allergic rhinitis, mastocytosis, and exercise-induced bronchospasm.

PHARMACOKINETICS
Minimal absorption after PO, inhalation, or nasal administration. Absorbed portion excreted in urine or by biliary system. **Half-life:** 80-90 min.

AVAILABILITY
Oral Concentrate (Gastrocrom): 100 mg/5 ml.
Nasal Spray (Nasalcrom): 40 mg/ml.
Solution for Nebulization (Intal): 10 mg/ml.

Solution for Oral Inhalation (Intal):
800 mcg/inhalation.
Ophthalmic Solution (Crolom,
Opticrom): 4%.

INDICATIONS AND DOSAGES
▸ **Asthma**
INHALATION (NEBULIZATION)
Adults, Elderly, Children older than
2 yr. 20 mg 3-4 times a day.
AEROSOL SPRAY
Adults, Elderly, Children 12 yr and
older. Initially, 2 sprays 4 times a
day. Maintenance: 2-4 sprays
3-4 times a day.
Children 5-11 yr. Initially, 2 sprays
4 times a day, then 1-2 sprays 3-
4 times a day.
▸ **Prevention of bronchospasm**
INHALATION (NEBULIZATION)
Adults, Elderly, Children older than
2 yr. 20 mg within 1 hr before
exercise or exposure to allergens.
AEROSOL SPRAY
Adults, Elderly, Children older than
5 yr. 2 sprays within 1 hr before
exercise or exposure to allergens.
▸ **Food allergy, inflammatory bowel**
disease
PO
Adults, Elderly, Children older than
12 yr. 200-400 mg 4 times a day.
Children 2-12 yr. 100-200 mg
4 times a day. Maximum:
40 mg/kg/day.
▸ **Allergic rhinitis**
INTRANASAL
Adults, Elderly, Children older than
6 yr. 1 spray each nostril 3-4 times a
day. May increase up to 6 times a day.
▸ **Systemic mastocytosis**
PO
Adults, Elderly, Children older than
12 yr. 200 mg 4 times a day.
Children 2-12 yr. 100 mg 4 times a
day. Maximum: 40 mg/kg/day.
Children younger than 2 yr. 20 mg/
kg/day in 4 divided doses. Maximum:
30 mg/kg/day (children 6 mo-2 yr).

▸ **Conjunctivitis**
OPHTHALMIC
Adults, Elderly, Children older than
4 yr. 1-2 drops in both eyes 4-
6 times a day.

CONTRAINDICATIONS
Status asthmaticus

INTERACTIONS
Drug
None known.
Herbal
None known.
Food
None known.

DIAGNOSTIC TEST EFFECTS
None known.

SIDE EFFECTS
Frequent
PO: Headache, diarrhea
Inhalation: Cough, dry mouth and
throat, stuffy nose, throat irritation,
unpleasant taste
Nasal: Nasal burning, stinging, or
irritation; increased sneezing
Ophthalmic: Eye burning or stinging
Occasional
PO: Rash, abdominal pain, arthralgia,
nausea, insomnia
Inhalation: Bronchospasm, hoarse-
ness, lacrimation
Nasal: Cough, headache, unpleasant
taste, postnasal drip
Ophthalmic: Lacrimation and itching
of eye
Rare
Inhalation: Dizziness, painful
urination, arthralgia, myalgia, rash
Nasal: Epistaxis, rash
Ophthalmic: Chemosis or edema of
conjunctiva, eye irritation

SERIOUS REACTIONS
• Anaphylaxis occurs rarely when
cromolyn is given by the inhalation,
nasal, or oral route.

PRECAUTIONS & CONSIDERATIONS

Caution is warranted with arrhythmias and coronary artery disease. When discontinuing the drug, taper the dosage cautiously because symptoms may recur. It is unknown if cromolyn crosses the placenta or is distributed in breast milk. No age-related precautions have been noted in children. Age-related hepatic and renal impairment may require a dosage adjustment in the elderly. Drink plenty of fluids to decrease the thickness of lung secretions.

Baseline exercise and activity tolerance should be established. Pulse rate and quality and respiratory rate, depth, rhythm, and type should be monitored. Observe for cyanosis manifested as lips and fingernails with a blue or dusky color in light-skinned patients; a gray color in dark-skinned patients.

Administration

Take oral cromolyn at least 30 minutes before meals. Pour contents of capsule into hot water and stir until completely dissolved; add an equal amount of cold water while stirring. Don't mix the drug with food, fruit juice, or milk.

For inhalation, first shake the container well. Exhale completely and place the mouthpiece between the lips. Inhale and hold breath for as long as possible before exhaling. Allow 1 to 10 before inhaling a second dose to promote deeper bronchial penetration. Rinse mouth after each use to decrease dry mouth and hoarseness and prevent fungal infection of the mouth.

For intranasal use, clear nasal passages as much as possible; a nasal decongestant may be required. Tilt the head slightly forward. Insert the spray tip into the nostril, pointing toward the nasal passages, away from the nasal septum. Spray into the nostril while holding the other nostril closed, and at the same time, inhale through the nose to deliver the medication as high into the nasal passages as possible

For ophthalmic use, place a finger on the lower eyelid and pull it down until a pocket is formed between the eye and lower lid. Hold the dropper above the pocket and instill the prescribed number of drops into the pocket. Close the eyes gently so that the drug isn't squeezed out of the lacrimal sac. Apply gentle finger pressure to the lacrimal sac at the inner canthus for 1 minute after installation to lessen the risk of systemic absorption.

Crotamiton

kroe-tam'i-ton
(Eurax)
Do not confuse with Euflex, Eulexin, or Evoxac.

CATEGORY AND SCHEDULE

Pregnancy Risk Category: C

CLASSIFICATION

Anti-infectives, topical, dermatologics, scabicides/pediculicides

MECHANISM OF ACTION

A scabicidal agent whose exact mechanism is unknown. *Therapeutic Effect:* Scabicidal activity against Sarcoptes scabiei.

PHARMACOKINETICS

Not known.

AVAILABILITY

Cream: 10% (Eurax).
Lotion: 10% (Eurax).

C

INDICATIONS AND DOSAGES
▸ **Treatment of scabies**
TOPICAL
Adults, Elderly, Children. Wash and scrub away loose scales and towel dry. Apply a thin layer and massage into skin over the entire body with special attention to skin folds, creases, and interdigital spaces. Repeat application in 24 hours. Take a cleansing bath 48 hours after the final application. Treatment may be repeated after 7-10 days if live mites are still present.
▸ **Pruritus**
TOPICAL
Adults, Elderly, Children. Massage into affected areas until medication is completely absorbed. Repeat as needed.

OFF-LABEL USES
Folliculitis, pediculosis

CONTRAINDICATIONS
Hypersensitivity to crotamiton or any one of its components

INTERACTIONS
Drug
None known.
Herbal
None known.
Food
None known.

DIAGNOSTIC TEST EFFECTS
None known.

SIDE EFFECTS
Occasional
Itching, burning, irritation, warm sensation, contact dermatitis

SERIOUS REACTIONS
• None known.

PRECAUTIONS & CONSIDERATIONS
All contaminated clothing and bed linens should be cleaned to avoid reinfestation. It is unknown if crotamiton crosses the placenta or is distributed in the breast milk. Safety and efficacy of crotamiton has not been established in children. There are no age-related precautions noted in the elderly.
Administration
Avoid contact with eyes. Shake lotion well before using. Apply a thin layer and massage onto the entire body from the neck to the toes especially to skin folds, digits, and creases.

Cyanocobalamin (Vitamin B12)
sye-an-oh-koe-bal'a-min
(Bedoz [CAN], Cytamen [AUS])

CATEGORY AND SCHEDULE
Pregnancy Risk Category: A (C if used in doses above recommended daily allowance)

CLASSIFICATION
Hematinics, vitamins/minerals

MECHANISM OF ACTION
Acts as a coenzyme for various metabolic functions, including fat and carbohydrate metabolism and protein synthesis. *Therapeutic Effect:* Necessary for cell growth and replication, hematopoiesis, and myelin synthesis.

PHARMACOKINETICS
In the presence of calcium, absorbed systemically in lower half of ileum. Initially, bound to intrinsic factor; this complex passes down intestine, binding to receptor sites on ileal mucosa.

Protein binding: High. Metabolized in the liver. Primarily eliminated unchanged in urine.
Half-life: 6 days.

AVAILABILITY
Tablets: 50 mcg, 100 mcg, 250 mcg, 500 mcg, 1000 mcg, 5000 mcg.
Tablet (Extended-Release): 1500 mcg.
Injection: 1000 mcg/ml.

INDICATIONS AND DOSAGES
▸ **Pernicious anemia**
IM, SUBCUTANEOUS
Adults, Elderly. 100 mcg/day for 7 days, then every other day for 7 days, then every 3-4 days for 2-3 wk. Maintenance: 100 mcg/mo (oral 1000-2000 mcg/day).
Children. 30-50 mcg/day for 2 or more wk. Maintenance: 100 mcg/mo.
Neonates. 1000 mcg/day for 2 or more wk. Maintenance: 50 mcg/mo.
▸ **Uncomplicated vitamin B_{12} deficiency**
PO
Adults, Elderly. 1000-2000 mcg/day
IM, SUBCUTANEOUS
Adults, Elderly. 100 mcg/day for 5-10 days, followed by 100-200 mcg/mo.
▸ **Complicated vitamin B_{12} deficiency**
IM, SUBCUTANEOUS
Adults, Elderly. 1000 mcg (with IM or IV folic acid 15 mg) as a single dose, then 1000 mcg/day plus oral folic acid 5 mg/day for 7 days.

CONTRAINDICATIONS
Folic acid deficiency anemia, hereditary optic nerve atrophy, history of allergy to cobalamins

INTERACTIONS
Drug
Alcohol, colchicines: May decrease the absorption of cyanocobalamin.

Ascorbic acid: May destroy cyanocobalamin.
Folic acid (large doses): May decrease cyanocobalamin blood concentration.
Herbal
None known.
Food
None known.

DIAGNOSTIC TEST EFFECTS
None known.

SIDE EFFECTS
Occasional
Diarrhea, pruritus

SERIOUS REACTIONS
• Impurities in preparation may cause a rare allergic reaction.
• Peripheral vascular thrombosis, pulmonary edema, hypokalemia, and CHF may occur.

PRECAUTIONS & CONSIDERATIONS
Cyanocobalamin crosses the placenta and is excreted in breast milk. No age-related precautions have been noted in children or the elderly. Eating foods rich in vitamin B_{12}, including clams, dairy products, egg yolks, fermented cheese, herring, muscle and organ meats, oysters, and red snapper, is encouraged.

Notify the physician of symptoms of infection. Serum potassium level, which normally ranges from 3.5 to 5 mEq/L, and serum cyanocobalamin level, which normally ranges from 200 to 800 mcg/ml, should be monitored. Also, watch for a rise in the blood reticulocyte count, which peaks in 5 to 8 days. Reversal of deficiency symptoms (anorexia, ataxia, fatigue, hyporeflexia, insomnia, irritability, loss of positional sense, pallor, and palpitations on exertion) should also be assessed. A therapeutic response to treatment usually occurs within 48 hours.

Administration
Take cyanocobalamin with meals to increase absorption.

Cyclobenzaprine
sye-kloe-ben′za-preen
(Flexeril, Flexitec [CAN], Novo-Cycloprine [CAN])
Do not confuse cyclobenzaprine with cycloserine or cyproheptadine, or Flexeril with Floxin.

CATEGORY AND SCHEDULE
Pregnancy Risk Category: B

CLASSIFICATION
Musculoskeletal agents, relaxants, skeletal muscle

MECHANISM OF ACTION
A centrally acting skeletal muscle relaxant that reduces tonic somatic muscle activity at the level of the brainstem. *Therapeutic Effect:* Relieves local skeletal muscle spasm.

PHARMACOKINETICS

Route	Onset	Peak	Duration
PO	1 hr	3-4 hr	12-24 hr

Well but slowly absorbed from the GI tract. Protein binding: 93%. Metabolized in the GI tract and the liver. Primarily excreted in urine.
Half-life: 1-3 days.

AVAILABILITY
Tablets: 5 mg, 10 mg.

INDICATIONS AND DOSAGES
▶ **Acute, painful musculoskeletal conditions**
PO
Adults. Initially, 5 mg 3 times a day. May increase to 10 mg 3 times a day.
Elderly. 5 mg 3 times a day.
▶ **Dosage in hepatic impairment**
Mild: 5 mg 3 times a day.
Moderate and severe: Not recommended.

OFF-LABEL USES
Treatment of fibromyalgia

CONTRAINDICATIONS
Acute recovery phase of MI, arrhythmias, CHF, heart block, conduction disturbances, hyperthyroidism, use within 14 days of MAOIs

INTERACTIONS
Drug
Alcohol, other CNS depression-producing medications (such as tricyclic antidepressants): May increase CNS depression.
MAOIs: May increase the risk of hypertensive crisis and severe seizures.
Herbal
None known.
Food
None known.

DIAGNOSTIC TEST EFFECTS
None known.

SIDE EFFECTS
Frequent
Somnolence (39%), dry mouth (27%), dizziness (11%)
Rare (3%-1%)
Fatigue, asthenia, blurred vision, headache, nervousness, confusion, nausea, constipation, dyspepsia, unpleasant taste

SERIOUS REACTIONS
• Overdose may result in visual hallucinations, hyperactive reflexes, muscle rigidity, vomiting, and hyperpyrexia.

PRECAUTIONS & CONSIDERATIONS
Caution is warranted with angle-closure glaucoma, impaired hepatic or renal function, increased intraocular pressure, and history of urine retention. It is unknown if cyclobenzaprine crosses the placenta or is distributed in breast milk. The safety and efficacy of cyclobenzaprine have not been established in children. The elderly have an increased sensitivity to the drug's anticholinergic effects, such as confusion and urine retention.

Drowsiness may occur but usually diminishes with continued therapy. Avoid alcohol, CNS depressants, and tasks that require mental alertness or motor skills. Change positions slowly to help avoid the drug's hypotensive effects. Therapeutic response, such as decreased skeletal muscle pain, stiffness, and tenderness and improved mobility, should be assessed.

Administration
! Do not administer cyclobenzaprine for longer than 2 to 3 weeks.
Take cyclobenzaprine without regard to food.

Cycloserine
sye-kloe-ser′een
(Closina [AUS],
Seromycin)

CATEGORY AND SCHEDULE
Pregnancy Risk Category: C

CLASSIFICATION
Antimycobacterials

MECHANISM OF ACTION
An antitubercular that inhibits cell wall synthesis by competing with the amino acid, D-alanine, for incorporation into the bacterial cell wall. *Therapeutic Effect:* Causes disruption of bacterial cell wall. Bactericidal or bacteriostatic.

PHARMACOKINETICS
Readily absorbed from the gastrointestinal (GI) tract. No protein binding. Widely distributed (including cerebrospinal fluid [CSF]). Metabolized in liver. Primarily excreted in urine. Removed by hemodialysis.
Half-life: 10 hr.

AVAILABILITY
Capsules: 250 mg (Seromycin).

INDICATIONS AND DOSAGES
▸ **Tuberculosis**
Adults, Elderly. 250 mg q12hr for 14 days, then 500 mg to 1g/day in 2 divided doses for 18-24 months. Maximum: 1 g as a single daily dose.
Children. 10-20 mg/kg/day in 2 divided doses. Maximum: 1000 mg/day for 18-24 months.
Dosage in renal impairment

Creatinine Clearance	Dosage Interval
10-50 ml/min	q24hr
Less than 10 ml/min	q36-48hr

OFF-LABEL USES
Gaucher's disease, acute urinary tract infections

CONTRAINDICATIONS
Epilepsy, depression, severe anxiety, psychosis, severe renal insufficiency, excessive concurrent use of alcohol, history of hypersensitivity reactions with previous cycloserine therapy

INTERACTIONS
Drug
Alcohol: May increase central nervous system (CNS) effects.
Isoniazid, ethionamide: May increase cycloserine toxicity.
Phenytoin: May increase the risk of epileptic seizures.
Herbal
Vitamin B12: May decrease vitamin B12.
Folic acid: May decrease folic acid.
Food
None known.

DIAGNOSTIC TEST EFFECTS
None known.

SIDE EFFECTS
Occasional
Drowsiness, headache, dizziness, vertigo, seizures, confusion, psychosis, paresis, tremor, vitamin B12 deficiency, folate deficiency, cardiac arrhythmias, increased liver enzymes

SERIOUS REACTIONS
• Neurotoxicity, as evidenced by confusion, agitation, CNS depression, psychosis, coma, and seizures, occur rarely.

• Neurotoxic effects of cycloserine may be treated and prevented with the administration of 200 to 300 mg of pyridoxine daily.

PRECAUTIONS & CONSIDERATIONS
Caution is warranted with epilepsy, depression, severe anxiety, psychosis, severe renal disease, and chronic alcoholism. Hypersensitivity reactions to cycloserine should be determined before starting treatment. Cycloserine crosses the placenta and is excreted in breast milk. There are no age-related precautions noted in children or elderly. Cycloserine concentrations should be monitored. Toxicity is greatly increased at levels more than 30 mcg/ml.

Drowsiness, mental confusion, dizziness, or tremors may occur during treatment. Excessive amounts of alcoholic beverages should be avoided.
Administration
May be taken with food. Vitamin B12 and folic acid dietary requirements may need to be increased during therapy.

Cyclosporine
sye-kloe-spor'in
(Cysporin [AUS], Gengraf, Neoral, Restasis, Sandimmune, Sandimmune Neoral [AUS])
Do not confuse cyclosporine with cycloserine, cyclophosphamide, or Cyklokapron.

CATEGORY AND SCHEDULE
Pregnancy Risk Category: C

CLASSIFICATION
Immunologic agents

MECHANISM OF ACTION
A cyclic polypeptide that inhibits both cellular and humoral immune responses by inhibiting interleukin-2, a proliferative factor needed for T-cell activity. *Therapeutic Effect:* Prevents organ rejection and relieves symptoms of psoriasis and arthritis.

PHARMACOKINETICS
Variably absorbed from the GI tract. Protein binding: 90%. Widely distributed. Metabolized in the liver. Eliminated primarily by biliary or fecal excretion. Not removed by hemodialysis. **Half-life:** Adults, 10-27 hr; children, 7-19 hr.

AVAILABILITY
Capsules, softgel (Gengraf, Neoral, Sandimmune): 25 mg, 100 mg.
Oral Solution (Sandimmune): 50-ml bottle with calibrated liquid measuring device.
Injection (Sandimmune): 50 mg/ml.
Ophthalmic Emulsion (Restasis): 0.05%.

INDICATIONS AND DOSAGES
▶ **Transplantation, prevention of organ rejection**
PO
Adults, Elderly, Children. 10-18 mg/kg/dose given 4-12 hr before organ transplantation. Maintenance: 5-15 mg/kg/day in divided doses then tapered to 3-10 mg/kg/day.
IV
Adults, Elderly, Children. Initially, 5-6 mg/kg/dose given 4-12 hr before to organ transplantation.
Maintenance: 2-10 mg/kg/day in divided doses.
▶ **Rheumatoid arthritis**
PO
Adults, Elderly. Initially, 2.5 mg/kg a day in 2 divided doses. May increase by 0.5-0.75 mg/kg/day. Maximum: 4 mg/kg/day.

▶ **Psoriasis**
PO
Adults, Elderly. Initially, 2.5 mg/kg/day in 2 divided doses. May increase by 0.5 mg/kg/day. Maximum: 4 mg/kg/day.
▶ **Dry eye**
OPHTHALMIC
Adults, Elderly. Instill 1 drop in each affected eye q12hr.

OFF-LABEL USES
Treatment of alopecia areata, aplastic anemia, atopic dermatitis, Behçet's disease, biliary cirrhosis, prevention of corneal transplant rejection

CONTRAINDICATIONS
History of hypersensitivity to cyclosporine or polyoxyethylated castor oil

INTERACTIONS
Drug
ACE inhibitors, potassium-sparing diuretics, potassium supplements: May cause hyperkalemia.
Cimetidine, danazol, diltiazem, erythromycin, ketoconazole: May increase cyclosporine concentration and risk of hepatotoxicity and nephrotoxicity.
Immunosuppressants: May increase risk of infection and lymphoproliferative disorders.
Live-virus vaccines: May increase vaccine side effects, potentiate virus replication, and decrease the patient's antibody response to the vaccine.
Lovastatin: May increase the risk of acute renal failure and rhabdomyolysis.
Herbal
St. John's wort: May alter cyclosporine absorption.
Food
Grapefruit, grapefruit juice: May increase the absorption and risk of toxicity of cyclosporine.

DIAGNOSTIC TEST EFFECTS

May increase BUN and serum alkaline phosphatase, amylase, bilirubin, creatinine, potassium, uric acid, AST (SGOT), and ALT (SGPT) levels. May decrease serum magnesium level. Therapeutic peak serum level is 50-300 ng/ml; toxic serum level is greater than 400 ng/ml.

▓ IV INCOMPATIBILITIES

Amphotericin B complex (Abelcet, AmBisome, Amphotec), magnesium

💧 IV Compatibilities

Propofol (Diprivan)

SIDE EFFECTS

Frequent
Mild to moderate hypertension (26%), hirsutism (21%), tremor (12%)
Occasional (4%-2%)
Acne, leg cramps, gingival hyperplasia (marked by red, bleeding, and tender gums), paresthesia, diarrhea, nausea, vomiting, headache
Rare (less than 1%)
Hypersensitivity reaction, abdominal discomfort, gynecomastia, sinusitis

SERIOUS REACTIONS

• Mild nephrotoxicity occurs in 25% of renal transplant patients, 38% of cardiac transplant patients, and 37% of liver transplant patients, generally 2 to 3 months after transplantation (more severe toxicity generally occurs soon after transplantation). Hepatotoxicity occurs in 4% of renal transplant patients, 7% of cardiac transplant patients, and 4% of liver transplant patients, generally within the first month after transplantation. Both toxicities usually respond to dosage reduction.
• Severe hyperkalemia and hyperuricemia occur occasionally.

PRECAUTIONS & CONSIDERATIONS

Caution is warranted with cardiac impairment, chickenpox, herpes zoster infection, hypokalemia, malabsorption syndrome, renal or hepatic impairment, and pregnant women. Use ophthalmic form cautiously with an active eye infection. Cyclosporine readily crosses the placenta and is distributed in breast milk. Women taking this drug should not breast-feed. No age-related precautions have been noted in transplant children. The elderly are at increased risk for hypertension and an increased serum creatinine level. Avoid consuming grapefruit and grapefruit juice because they increase the drug's blood concentration and risk of side effects.

Headache, excessive hair growth, gum disease, and tremor may occur. Good oral hygiene should be maintained to prevent gingivitis. Blood test results, including renal function studies, liver function tests, and drug blood levels, should be monitored before beginning cyclosporine therapy and regularly during treatment. Mild toxicity is characterized by a slow rise in serum levels; more overt toxicity, by a rapid rise in serum levels. Hematuria is also noted in nephrotoxicity. Know that the therapeutic peak serum level of cyclosporine is 50 to 300 ng/ml and the toxic serum level is over 400 ng/ml; the dose should be taken after a trough serum level has been drawn. Serum potassium level for hyperkalemia and B/P for hypertension should also be assessed.

Storage

The capsules should be kept in original foil wrapping and stored in a dry, cool environment, away from direct light. Don't refrigerate the oral solution because it may separate. The liquid form should be kept in the amber-colored glass container. Discard the oral solution 2 months after the bottle has been opened. Store the parenteral form at room temperature and protect it from light. After diluted, solution is stable for 24 hours.

Administration
! The oral solution is available in 50-ml bottles and comes with a calibrated liquid measuring device. Expect to begin therapy with the oral form as soon as possible. Expect to give cyclosporine with adrenal corticosteroids. Know that administering other immunosuppressive agents with cyclosporine increases the patient's susceptibility to infection and lymphoma.

In a glass container, mix oral solution with room-temperature milk, chocolate milk, or orange juice. Stir the mixture well and have the patient drink it immediately. Avoid using Styrofoam containers because the liquid form of the drug may adhere to the wall of the container. Add more diluent to the glass container and mix it with the remaining solution to ensure that the total amount of cyclosporine is swallowed. Dry the outside of the measuring device before replacing it in its cover. Don't rinse it with water. Take the drug at the same time each day.

For IV use, dilute each milliliter of concentrate with 20 to 100 ml 0.9% NaCl or D₅W. Infuse the solution over 2 to 6 hours. Monitor continuously for the first 30 minutes of the infusion, and frequently thereafter for a hypersensitivity reaction, marked by facial flushing and dyspnea.

For ophthalmic use, invert vial several times to obtain a uniform suspension. Remove any contact lenses prior to administration. May re-insert lenses 15 minutes after drug administration. May use with artificial tears.

Cyproheptadine
si-proe-hep'ta-deen
(Periactin)

CATEGORY AND SCHEDULE
Pregnancy Risk Category: B

CLASSIFICATION
Antihistamines, H1

MECHANISM OF ACTION
An antihistamine that competes with histamine at histaminic receptor sites. Anticholinergic effects cause drying of nasal mucosa. *Therapeutic Effect:* Relieves allergic conditions (urticaria, pruritus).

PHARMACOKINETICS
Well absorbed from GI tract. Metabolized in liver. Primarily eliminated in feces.
Half-life: 16 hr.

AVAILABILITY
Syrup: 2 mg/5 ml (Periactin).
Tablets: 4 mg (Periactin).

INDICATIONS AND DOSAGES
▸ **Allergic condition**
PO
Adults, Children older than 15 yr. 4 mg 3 times/day. May increase dose but do not exceed 0.5 mg/kg/day.
Children 7-14 yr. 4 mg 2-3 times/day, or 0.25 mg/kg daily in divided doses.
Children 2-6 yr. 2 mg 2-3 times/day, or 0.25 mg/kg daily in divided doses.
Usual elderly dosage
PO
Initially, 4 mg 2 times/day.

CONTRAINDICATIONS
Acute asthmatic attack, patients receiving MAO inhibitors, history of hypersensitivity to antihistamines

INTERACTIONS
Drug
Alcohol, central nervous system (CNS) depressants: May increase CNS depression.
Fluoxetine, paroxetine: May decrease fluoxetine efficacy.
MAOIs: May increase anticholinergic and CNS depressant effects.
Protirelin: May decrease TSH response.
Herbal
None known.
Food
None known.

DIAGNOSTIC TEST EFFECTS
May suppress flare and wheal reaction to antigen skin testing unless drug is discontinued 4 days before testing. May increase SGPT (AST) levels.

SIDE EFFECTS
Frequent
Drowsiness, dizziness, muscular weakness, dry mouth/nose/throat/lips, urinary retention, thickening of bronchial secretions
Elderly
Frequent
Sedation, dizziness, hypotension
Occasional
Epigastric distress, flushing, visual disturbances, hearing disturbances, paresthesia, sweating, chills

SERIOUS REACTIONS
• Children may experience dominant paradoxical reaction (restlessness, insomnia, euphoria, nervousness, tremors).
• Overdosage in children may result in hallucinations, convulsions, death.

• Hypersensitivity reaction (eczema, pruritus, rash, cardiac disturbances, angioedema, photosensitivity) may occur.
• Overdosage may vary from CNS depression (sedation, apnea, cardiovascular collapse, death) to severe paradoxical reaction (hallucinations, tremor, seizures).

C

PRECAUTIONS & CONSIDERATIONS
Caution is warranted with narrow-angle glaucoma, peptic ulcer, prostatic hypertrophy, pyloroduodenal or bladder neck obstruction, asthma, COPD, increased intraocular pressure, cardiovascular disease, hyperthyroidism, hypertension, and seizure disorders. It is unknown if cyproheptadine crosses the placenta or is distributed in breast milk. Safety and efficacy of cyproheptadine have not been established in newborns. Be aware that elderly patients are more likely to experience dizziness, sedation, confusion, and hypotension.
Dry mouth, drowsiness, and dizziness are expected side effects. Tolerance to sedative effects may occur. Avoid alcohol and tasks that require alertness and motor skills.
Administration
Give without regard to meals. Scored tablets may be crushed.

Cytarabine
sye-tare′a-been
(Ara-C, Cytosar [CAN], Cytosar-U)
Do not confuse cytarabine with Cytadren, Cytovene, or vidarabine.

CATEGORY AND SCHEDULE
Pregnancy Risk Category: D

CLASSIFICATION
Antineoplastics, antimetabolites

MECHANISM OF ACTION
An antimetabolite that is converted intracellularly to a nucleotide. Cell cycle-specific for S phase of cell division. *Therapeutic Effect:* May inhibit DNA synthesis. Potent immunosuppressive activity.

PHARMACOKINETICS
Widely distributed; moderate amount crosses the blood-brain barrier. Protein binding: 15%. Primarily excreted in urine. **Half-life:** 1-3 hr.

AVAILABILITY
Injection Powder: 100 mg, 500 mg, 1 g, 2 g.
Injection Solution: 20 mg/ml, 100 mg/ml.

INDICATIONS AND DOSAGES
▸ **To induce remission in acute lymphocytic leukemia, acute and chronic myelocytic leukemia, meningeal leukemia, or non-Hodgkin's lymphoma in children**
IV
Adults, Elderly, Children.
200 mg/m^2/day for 5 days q2wk as monotherapy or 100-200 mg/m^2/day for 5- to 10-day course of therapy every q2-4wk in combination therapy.

INTRATHECAL
Adults, Elderly, Children.
5-7.5 mg/m^2 every 2-7 days.
▸ **To maintain remission in acute lymphocytic leukemia, acute and chronic myelocytic leukemia, meningeal leukemia, or non-Hodgkin's lymphoma in children**
IV
Adults, Elderly, Children.
70-200 mg/m^2/day for 2-5 days every month.
IM, SUBCUTANEOUS
Adults, Elderly, Children.
1-1.5 mg/m^2 as single dose q1-4wk.
INTRATHECAL
Adults, Elderly, Children.
5-7.5 mg/m^2 every 2-7 days.

OFF-LABEL USES
Treatment of Hodgkin's disease, myelodysplastic syndrome

CONTRAINDICATIONS
None known.

INTERACTIONS
Drug
Antigout medications: May decrease the effects of these drugs.
Bone marrow depressants: May increase myelosuppression.
Cyclophosphamide: May increase the risk of cardiomyopathy.
Live-virus vaccines: May potentiate virus replication, increase vaccine side effects, and decrease the patient's antibody response to the vaccine.
Herbal
None known.
Food
None known.

DIAGNOSTIC TEST EFFECTS
May increase serum alkaline phosphatase, bilirubin, uric acid, and AST (SGOT) levels.

IV INCOMPATIBILITIES

Amphotericin B complex (Abelcet, AmBisome, Amphotec), ganciclovir (Cytovene), insulin (regular)

IV Compatibilities

Dexamethasone (Decadron), diphenhydramine (Benadryl), filgrastim (Neupogen), granisetron (Kytril), hydromorphone (Dilaudid), lorazepam (Ativan), morphine, ondansetron (Zofran), potassium chloride, propofol (Diprivan)

SIDE EFFECTS

Frequent

IV, SUBCUTANEOUS (33%-16%): Asthenia, fever, pain, altered taste and smell, nausea, vomiting (risk greater with IV push than with continuous IV infusion)

INTRATHECAL (28%-11%): Headache, asthenia, altered taste and smell, confusion, somnolence, nausea, vomiting

Occasional

IV, SUBCUTANEOUS (11%-7%): Abnormal gait, somnolence, constipation, back pain, urinary incontinence, peripheral edema, headache, confusion

INTRATHECAL (7%-3%): Peripheral edema, back pain, constipation, abnormal gait, urinary incontinence

SERIOUS REACTIONS

• Myelosuppression may result in blood dyscrasias, such as leukopenia, anemia, thrombocytopenia, megaloblastosis, and reticulocytopenia, after a single IV dose.

• Leukopenia, anemia, and thrombocytopenia should be expected with daily or continuous IV therapy.

• Cytarabine syndrome, (as evidenced by fever, myalgia, rash, conjunctivitis, malaise, and chest pain) and hyperuricemia may occur.

• High-dose cytarabine therapy may produce severe CNS, GI, and pulmonary toxicity.

PRECAUTIONS & CONSIDERATIONS

Caution is warranted in cardiomyopathy, hepatic impairment, and pre-existing drug-induced bone marrow suppression. Caution should also be used in women of child-bearing age. The use of contraception should be advised. It is unknown if cytarabine is distributed in breast milk. Monitor leukocyte and platelet counts daily during the induction phase. Perform bone marrow examinations and liver and kidney function tests periodically. Monitor uric acid serum concentrations.

Storage

Unopened vials may be stored at room temperature. Reconstituted solutions are stable at room temperature for 48 hours.

Administration

Avoid using diluents containing benzyl alcohol; preservative-free normal saline is usually used.

Dacarbazine

da-kar'ba-zeen
(DTIC [CAN], DTIC-Dome)
**Do not confuse dacarbazine
with Dicarbosil or procarbazine.**

CATEGORY AND SCHEDULE
Pregnancy Risk Category: C

CLASSIFICATION
Antineoplastics, alkylating agents

MECHANISM OF ACTION
An alkylating antineoplastic agent
that forms methyldiazonium ions,
which attack nucleophilic groups in
DNA. Cross-links DNA strands.
Therapeutic Effect: Inhibits DNA,
RNA, and protein synthesis.

PHARMACOKINETICS
Minimally crosses the blood-brain
barrier. Protein binding: 5%.
Metabolized in the liver. Excreted in
urine. **Half-life:** 5 hr (increased in
impaired renal function).

AVAILABILITY
Powder for Injection: 100-mg vials,
200-mg vials, 500-mg vials.

INDICATIONS AND DOSAGES
▸ **Malignant melanoma**
IV
Adults, Elderly. 2-4.5 mg/kg/day
for 10 days, repeated q4wk; or
250 mg/m^2 a day for 5 days,
repeated q3wk.
▸ **Hodgkin's disease**
IV
Adults, Elderly. 150 mg/m^2/day for
5 days, repeated q4wk; or
375 mg/m^2 once, repeated every
15 days (as combination therapy).
Children. 375 mg/m^2 on days 1
and 15; repeated every 28 days
(as combination therapy).

▸ **Solid tumors**
IV
Children. 200-470 mg/m^2/day over
5 days every 21-28 days.
▸ **Neuroblastoma**
IV
Children. 800-900 mg/m^2 as
single dose on day 1 of therapy,
repeated q3-4wk (as combination
therapy).

OFF-LABEL USES
Treatment of islet cell carcinoma,
neuroblastoma, soft-tissue
sarcoma

CONTRAINDICATIONS
Demonstrated hypersensitivity to
dacarbazine

INTERACTIONS
Drug
Bone marrow depressants: May
enhance myelosuppression.
Live-virus vaccines: May potentiate
virus replication, increase vaccine
side effects, and decrease the
patient's antibody response to the
vaccine.
Herbal
None known.
Food
None known.

DIAGNOSTIC TEST EFFECTS
May increase BUN, serum
alkaline phosphatase, AST
(SGOT), and ALT (SGPT)
levels.

▓ IV INCOMPATIBILITIES
Allopurinol (Aloprim),
cefepime (Maxipime), heparin,
piperacillin, and tazobactam
(Zosyn)
▓ IV Compatibilities
Etoposide (VePesid), granisetron
(Kytril), ondansetron (Zofran),
paclitaxel (Taxol)

SIDE EFFECTS
Frequent (90%)
Nausea, vomiting, anorexia (occurs within 1 hr of initial dose, may last up to 12 hr)
Occasional
Facial flushing, paresthesia, alopecia, flu-like symptoms (fever, myalgia, malaise), dermatologic reactions, confusion, blurred vision, headache, lethargy
Rare
Diarrhea, stomatitis, photosensitivity

SERIOUS REACTIONS
• Myelosuppression may result in blood dyscrasias, such as leukopenia and thrombocytopenia, generally 2-4 weeks after the last dacarbazine dose.
• Hepatotoxicity occurs rarely.

PRECAUTIONS & CONSIDERATIONS
Caution is warranted with hepatic impairment. Because of the risk of fetal harm, pregnant women should not take dacarbazine, especially during the first trimester. Breast-feeding women also should not take this drug. The safety and efficacy of dacarbazine have not been established in children. In the elderly, age-related renal impairment may require a dosage adjustment. Immunizations and coming in contact with those who have recently received a live-virus vaccine should be avoided during treatment.

Notify the physician if easy nausea and vomiting, bruising, fever, signs of local infection, sore throat, or unusual bleeding from any site occurs. Adequate hydration should be maintained to avoid dehydration from vomiting. Erythrocyte, leukocyte, and platelet counts for evidence of myelosuppression should be monitored.

Storage
Refrigerate unopened vials and protect them from light. The reconstituted solution containing 10 mg/ml is stable for up to 8 hours at room temperature or up to 72 hours if refrigerated. Solutions further diluted with D_5W or 0.9% NaCl are stable for up to 8 hours at room temperature or up to 24 hours if refrigerated.

Administration
! Dacarbazine dosage is individualized based on clinical response and tolerance of the drug's adverse effects. When administering this drug in combination therapy, consult specific protocols for optimum dosage and sequence of drug administration.

! Give dacarbazine by IV push or IV infusion, as prescribed. Because dacarbazine may be carcinogenic, mutagenic, or teratogenic, handle the drug with extreme care during preparation and administration.

For IV use, reconstitute the 100-mg vial with 9.9 ml (or the 200-mg vial with 19.7 ml) sterile water for injection to provide a concentration of 10 mg/ml. Give by IV push over 2 to 3 minutes. For IV infusion, further dilute with up to 250 ml D_5W or 0.9% NaCl. Infuse the drug over 15 to 30 minutes. Discard it if the color changes from ivory to pink because this indicates decomposition. Apply hot packs if the patient develops a burning sensation, irritation, or local pain at the injection site. Monitor the injection site for signs and symptoms of extravasation, including coolness, stinging, swelling, and slight or no blood return.

Daclizumab
da-kliz'yoo-mab
(Zenapax)

CATEGORY AND SCHEDULE
Pregnancy Risk Category: C

CLASSIFICATION
Immunosuppressives,
monoclonal antibodies

MECHANISM OF ACTION
A monoclonal antibody that binds
to the interleukin-2 (IL-2) receptor
complex, inhibiting the IL-2-
mediated activation of T lymphocytes, a critical pathway in the
cellular immune response involved
in allograft rejection. *Therapeutic
Effect:* Prevents organ rejection.

PHARMACOKINETICS
Half-life: Adults, 20 days.

AVAILABILITY
Injection: 25 mg/5 ml.

INDICATIONS AND DOSAGES
▶ **Prevention of acute renal
transplant rejection (in combination
with an immunosuppressive)**
IV
Adults, Children. 1 mg/kg over
15 min q14 days for 5 doses,
beginning no more than 24 hr
before transplantation. Maximum:
100 mg.

OFF-LABEL USES
Treatment of graft vs. host disease

CONTRAINDICATIONS
None known.

INTERACTIONS
Drug
None known.

Herbal
None known.
Food
None known.

DIAGNOSTIC TEST EFFECTS
None known.

▨ IV INCOMPATIBILITIES
Don't mix daclizumab with any
other drugs.

SIDE EFFECTS
Occasional (greater than 2%)
Constipation, nausea, diarrhea,
vomiting, abdominal pain, edema,
headache, dizziness, fever, pain,
fatigue, insomnia, weakness,
arthralgia, myalgia, diaphoresis

SERIOUS REACTIONS
• Hypersensitivity reaction, which
occurs rarely, is characterized by
dyspnea, tachycardia, dysphagia,
peripheral edema, rash, and pruritus.

PRECAUTIONS & CONSIDERATIONS
Caution is warranted with an
infection and history of malignancy.
Pregnancy should be avoided. It is
unknown if daclizumab crosses the
placenta or is distributed in breast
milk. No age-related precautions
have been noted in children or the
elderly. Avoid crowded areas and
other circumstances that increase
risk for infection.
   Notify the physician of GI disturbances, urinary changes, difficulty
breathing or swallowing, itching or
swelling of the lower extremities,
rash, rapid heartbeat, or weakness.
Laboratory values, including a CBC,
and vital signs, particularly B/P and
pulse rate, should be monitored.
Storage
Refrigerate vials and protect them
from light. Once reconstituted, the
solution is stable for 4 hours at

room temperature, 24 hours if refrigerated.
Administration
! Daclizumab is given in combination with an immunosuppresive regimen (cyclosporine, corticosteriods) for prevention of organ rejection.

For IV use, dilute the drug in 50 ml 0.9% NaCl. Invert the vial gently. Avoid shaking it. Infuse the drug over 15 minutes.

Dalteparin
doll'teh-pare-in
(Fragmin)

CATEGORY AND SCHEDULE
Pregnancy Risk Category: B

CLASSIFICATION
Anticoagulants

MECHANISM OF ACTION
An antithrombin that inhibits factor Xa and thrombin in the presence of low-molecular-weight heparin. Only slightly influences platelet aggregation, PT, and aPTT. *Therapeutic Effect:* Produces anticoagulation.

PHARMACOKINETICS

Route	Onset	Peak	Duration
Subcutaneous	N/A	4 hr	N/A

Protein binding: less than 10%.
Half-life: 3-5 hr.

AVAILABILITY
Syringe: 2500 international units/ 0.2 ml, 5000 international units/ 0.2 ml, 7500 international units/ 0.3 ml, 10,000 international units/ml.

Vial: 10,000 international units/ml, 25,000 international units/ml.

INDICATIONS AND DOSAGES
▶ **Low- to moderate-risk abdominal surgery**
SUBCUTANEOUS
Adults, Elderly. 2500 international units 1-2 hr before surgery, then daily for 5-10 days.
▶ **High-risk abdominal surgery**
SUBCUTANEOUS
Adults, Elderly. 5000 international units 1-2 hr before surgery, then daily for 5-10 days.
▶ **Total hip surgery**
SUBCUTANEOUS
Adults, Elderly. 2500 international units 1-2 hr before surgery, then 2500 units 6 hr after surgery, then 5000 units/day for 7-10 days.
▶ **Unstable angina, non-Q-wave MI**
SUBCUTANEOUS
Adults, Elderly. 120 international units/kg q12hr (maximum: 10,000 international units/dose) given with aspirin until clinically stable.
▶ **Prevention of DVT or PE in the acutely ill patient**
SUBCUTANEOUS
Adults, Elderly. 5000 international units once a day.

CONTRAINDICATIONS
Active major bleeding; concurrent heparin therapy; hypersensitivity to dalteparin, heparin, or pork products; thrombocytopenia associated with positive in vitro test for antiplatelet antibody

INTERACTIONS
Drug
Anticoagulants, platelet inhibitors: May increase risk of bleeding.
Herbal
None known.

Food
None known.

DIAGNOSTIC TEST EFFECTS
Increases (reversible) LDH, serum alkaline phosphatase, AST (SGOT), and ALT (SGPT) levels.

SIDE EFFECTS
Occasional (7%-3%)
Hematoma at injection site
Rare (less than 1%)
Hypersensitivity reaction (chills, fever, pruritus, urticaria, asthma, rhinitis, lacrimation, headache); mild, local skin irritation

SERIOUS REACTIONS
• Overdose may lead to bleeding complications ranging from local ecchymoses to major hemorrhage.
• Thrombocytopenia occurs rarely.

PRECAUTIONS & CONSIDERATIONS

Caution is warranted with bacterial endocarditis, conditions with increased risk of hemorrhage, history of heparin-induced thrombocytopenia, recent GI ulceration and hemorrhage, hypertensive or diabetic retinopathy, impaired hepatic or renal function, and uncontrolled arterial hypertension. Dalteparin should be used with caution in pregnant women, particularly during the last trimester and immediately postpartum because it increases the risk of maternal hemorrhage. It is unknown if dalteparin is distributed in breast milk. Safety and efficacy of dalteparin have not been established in children. No age-related precautions have been noted in the elderly. Other medications, including OTC drugs, should be avoided.

Notify the physician of signs of bleeding, breathing difficulty, bruising, dizziness, fever, itching, lightheadedness, rash, or swelling.

Baseline CBC and B/P should be established. CBC and stool for occult blood should be monitored throughout therapy.
Storage
Store drug at room temperature.
Administration
The patient should sit or lie down before administering by deep subcutaneous injection. Inject into U-shaped area around the navel, upper outer side of thigh, or upper outer quadrangle of buttock. Use a fine needle (25- to 26-gauge) to minimize tissue trauma. Introduce the entire length of the needle (one-half inch) into skin-fold held between the thumb and forefinger, holding the needle during injection at a 45°- to 90°-angle. Do not rub injection site after administration to avoid bruising. Alternate administration site with each injection. The usual length of dalteparin therapy is 5 to 10 days. Perform an ice massage at the injection site shortly before injection to prevent excessive bruising.

Danazol
da′na-zole
(Cyclomen [CAN], Danocrine)

CATEGORY AND SCHEDULE
Pregnancy Risk Category: X

CLASSIFICATION
Hormones/hormone modifiers

MECHANISM OF ACTION
A testosterone derivative that suppresses the pituitary-ovarian axis by inhibiting the output of pituitary gonadotropins. Causes atrophy of both normal and ectopic endometrial

tissue in endometriosis. Follicle-stimulating hormone (FSH) and luteinizing hormone (LH) are depressed in fibrocystic breast disease. Inhibits steroid synthesis and binding of steroids to their receptors in breast tissues. Increases serum levels of esterase inhibitor. *Therapeutic Effect:* Produces anovulation and amenorrhea, reduces the production of estrogen, corrects biochemical deficiency as seen in hereditary angioedema.

PHARMACOKINETICS
Well absorbed from gastrointestinal (GI) tract. Metabolized in liver, primarily to 2-hydroxymethylethisterone. Excreted in urine. **Half-life:** 4.5 hr.

AVAILABILITY
Capsules: 50 mg, 100 mg, 200 mg (Danocrine).

INDICATIONS AND DOSAGES
▸ **Endometriosis**
PO
Adults. 200-800 mg/day in 2 divided doses for 3-9 mo.
▸ **Fibrocystic breast disease**
PO
Adults. 100-400 mg/day in 2 divided doses.
▸ **Hereditary angioedema**
PO
Adults. Initially, 200 mg 2-3 times/day. Decrease dose by 50% or less at 1-3 mo intervals. If attack occurs, increase dose by up to 200 mg/day.

OFF-LABEL USES
Treatment of gynecomastia, menorrhagia, precocious puberty

CONTRAINDICATIONS
Cardiac impairment, hypercalcemia, pregnancy, prostatic or breast cancer in males, severe liver or renal disease

INTERACTIONS
Drug
Carbamazepine, cyclosporine, tacrolimus, and warfarin: May increase serum levels and increase risk of toxicity of these drugs.
HMG-CoA reductase inhibitors: May increase chance of developing myopathy or rhabdomyolysis.
Hormonal contraceptives: May decrease effectiveness of contraceptives.
Hypoglycemic agents: May increase the risk of hypoglycemia.
Herbal
None known.
Food
Food may delay time to peak. High fat meal increases plasma concentration.

DIAGNOSTIC TEST EFFECTS
May increase blood Hgb and Hct, LDL concentrations, serum alkaline phosphatase, bilirubin, calcium, potassium, SGOT (AST) levels, and sodium levels. May decrease HDL concentrations. May alter levels of testosterone, androstenedione, dehydroepiandrosterone.

SIDE EFFECTS
Frequent
Females: Amenorrhea, breakthrough bleeding/spotting, decreased breast size, increased weight, irregular menstrual period.
Occasional
Males/females: Edema, rhabdomyolysis (muscle cramps, unusual fatigue), virilism (acne, oily skin), flushed skin, altered moods
Rare
Males/females: Hematuria, gingivitis, carpal tunnel syndrome, cataracts,

severe headache, vomiting, rash, photosensitivity
Females: Enlarged clitoris, hoarseness, deepening voice, hair growth, monilial vaginitis
Males: Decreased testicle size.

SERIOUS REACTIONS
• Jaundice may occur in those receiving 400 mg/day or more. Liver dysfunction, eosinophilia, thrombocytopenia, pancreatitis occur rarely.

PRECAUTIONS & CONSIDERATIONS
Caution should be used with seizure disorder, migraine, or conditions influenced by edema. Be aware that danazol use is contraindicated during lactation. If pregnancy is suspected, notify the physician. Safety and efficacy of danazol have not been established in children. Be aware that danazol should be used with caution in the elderly.
If masculinizing effects, weight gain, muscle cramps, or fatigue occur, notify the physician. Spotting or bleeding may occur in the first months of therapy. Nonhormonal contraceptive should be used during therapy.
Storage
Store at room temperature.
Administration
Take full course of treatment as prescribed by the physician. Be aware that therapy should be initiated during menstruation or when patient is not pregnant.

Dantrolene
dan′troe-leen
(Dantrium)
Do not confuse Dantrium with Daraprim.

CATEGORY AND SCHEDULE
Pregnancy Risk Category: C

CLASSIFICATION
Musculoskeletal agents, relaxants, skeletal muscle

MECHANISM OF ACTION
A skeletal muscle relaxant that reduces muscle contraction by interfering with release of calcium ion. Reduces calcium ion concentration. *Therapeutic Effect:* Dissociates excitation-contraction coupling. Interferes with catabolic process associated with malignant hyperthermic crisis.

PHARMACOKINETICS
Poorly absorbed from the gastrointestinal (GI) tract. Protein binding: High. Metabolized in the liver. Primarily excreted in urine.
Half-life: IV: 4-8 hr; PO: 8.7 hr.

AVAILABILITY
Capsules: 25 mg, 50 mg, 100 mg.
Powder for Injection: 20-mg vial.

INDICATIONS AND DOSAGES
▸ Spasticity
PO
Adults, Elderly. Initially, 25 mg/day. Increase to 25 mg 2-4 times a day, then by 25-mg increments up to 100 mg 2-4 times a day.
Children. Initially, 0.5 mg/kg twice a day. Increase to 0.5 mg/kg 3-4 times a day, then in increments

of 0.5 mg/kg/day up to 3 mg/kg
2-4 times a day. Maximum:
400 mg/day.
▶ **Prevention of malignant
hyperthermic crisis**
PO
Adults, Elderly, Children. 4-8 mg/
kg/day in 3-4 divided doses 1-2 days
before surgery; give last dose 3-4 hr
before surgery.
IV
Adults, Elderly, Children. 2.5 mg/kg
about 1.25 hr before surgery.
▶ **Management of malignant
hyperthermic crisis**
IV
Adults, Elderly, Children. Initially a
minimum of 1 mg/kg rapid IV; may
repeat up to total cumulative dose of
10 mg/kg. May follow with 4-8 mg/
kg/day PO in 4 divided doses up to
3 days after crisis.

OFF-LABEL USES
Relief of exercise-induced pain
in patients with muscular
dystrophy, treatment of flexor
spasms and neuroleptic malignant
syndrome

CONTRAINDICATIONS
Active hepatic disease

INTERACTIONS
Drug
**Central nervous system
(CNS) depressants:** May
increase CNS depression with
short-term use.
Liver toxic medications: May
increase the risk of liver toxicity
with chronic use.
Herbal
None known.
Food
None known.

DIAGNOSTIC TEST EFFECTS
May alter liver function test results.

▦ IV INCOMPATIBILITIES
None known.

SIDE EFFECTS
Frequent
Drowsiness, dizziness, weakness,
general malaise, diarrhea (mild)
Occasional
Confusion, diarrhea (may be severe),
headache, insomnia, constipation,
urinary frequency
Rare
Paradoxical CNS excitement or
restlessness, paresthesia, tinnitus,
slurred speech, tremor, blurred
vision, dry mouth, nocturia,
impotence, rash, pruritus

SERIOUS REACTIONS
• There is a risk of liver toxicity,
most notably in females, those
35 years of age and older, and those
taking other medications concurrently.
• Overt hepatitis noted most
frequently between 3rd and 12th
month of therapy.
• Overdosage results in vomiting,
muscular hypotonia, muscle twitching, respiratory depression, and
seizures.

PRECAUTIONS & CONSIDERATIONS
Caution is warranted with a history
of previous liver disease and
impaired cardiac or pulmonary function. Be aware that dantrolene readily crosses the placenta and should
not be used in breastfeeding mothers.
There are no age-related precautions
noted in children 5 years and older.
There is no information available on
dantrolene use in the elderly.
Drowsiness may occur but usually
diminishes with continued therapy.
Avoid alcohol, CNS depressants, and
tasks that require mental alertness or
motor skills. Notify the physician if
bloody or tarry stools, continued
weakness, diarrhea, fatigue, itching,

nausea, or skin rash occurs. Blood tests, such as liver and renal function tests, should be performed before and during therapy. Therapeutic response, such as decreased intensity of skeletal muscle pain or spasm, should be assessed.

Storage
Store at room temperature. Use within 6 hours after reconstitution. Solution normally appears clear, colorless; discard if cloudy or precipitate is present

Administration
! Begin with low-dose therapy, as prescribed, then increase gradually at 4- to 7-day intervals to reduce incidence of side effects.

Take oral dantrolene without regard to meals.

For IV use, reconstitute 20-mg vial with 60 ml sterile water for injection to provide a concentration of 0.33 mg/ml. For IV infusion, administer over 1 hour. Diligently monitor for extravasation because of high pH of IV preparation. May produce severe complications.

Dapsone
dap'sone
(Dapsone)

CATEGORY AND SCHEDULE
Pregnancy Risk Category: C

CLASSIFICATION
Antimycobacterials

MECHANISM OF ACTION
An antibiotic that is a competitive antagonist of para-aminobenzoic acid (PABA); it prevents normal bacterial utilization of PABA for synthesis of folic acid. *Therapeutic Effect:* Inhibits bacterial growth.

AVAILABILITY
Tablets: 25 mg, 100 mg.

INDICATIONS AND DOSAGES
▸ **Leprosy**
PO
Adults, Elderly. 50-100 mg/day for 3-10 yr.
Children. 1-2 mg/kg/24 hr. Maximum: 100 mg/day.
▸ **Dermatitis herpetiformis**
PO
Adults, Elderly. Initially, 50 mg/day. May increase up to 300 mg/day.
▸ ***Pneumocystis carinii*** **pneumonia (PCP)**
PO
Adults, Elderly. 100 mg/day in combination with trimethoprim for 21 days.
▸ **Prevention of PCP**
PO
Adults, Elderly. 100 mg/day.
Children older than 1 mo. 2 mg/kg/day. Maximum: 100 mg/day.

OFF-LABEL USES
Treatment of inflammatory bowel disorders, malaria

CONTRAINDICATIONS
None significant.

INTERACTIONS
Drug
Methotrexate: May increase hematologic reactions.
Probenecid: May decrease the excretion of dapsone.
Protease inhibitors (including ritonavir): May increase dapsone blood concentration.
Rifampin: May decrease rifampin blood concentration.
Trimethoprim: May increase the risk of toxic effects.

Herbal
St. John's wort: May decrease dapsone blood concentration.
Food
None significant.

DIAGNOSTIC TEST EFFECTS
None significant.

SIDE EFFECTS
Frequent (greater than 10%)
Hemolytic anemia, methemoglobine-mia, rash
Occasional (10%-1%)
Hemolysis, photosensitivity reaction

SERIOUS REACTIONS
• Agranulocytosis and blood dyscrasias may occur.

PRECAUTIONS & CONSIDERATIONS
Caution is warranted with agranulo-cytosis, severe anemia, aplastic anemia, glucose-6 phosphate dehydrogenase deficiency, or a hypersensitivity to dapsone or its derivatives (such as sulfoxone sodium). Overexposure to sun or ultraviolet light should be avoided.
Baseline CBC should be obtained. Hypersensitivity to dapsone or its derivatives should be determined before therapy. Skin should be assessed for a dermatologic reaction. Signs and symptoms of hemolysis, such as jaundice, should be moni-tored. Persistent fatigue, fever, or sore throat should be reported.
Administration
Take dapsone without regard to food.

Daptomycin
dap'toe-my-sin
(Cubicin)

CATEGORY AND SCHEDULE
Pregnancy Risk Category: B

D

CLASSIFICATION
Antibiotics, lipopeptides

MECHANISM OF ACTION
A lipopeptide antibacterial agent that binds to bacterial membranes and causes a rapid depolarization of the membrane potential. The loss of membrane potential leads to inhibition of protein, DNA, and RNA synthesis. *Therapeutic Effect:* Bactericidal.

PHARMACOKINETICS
Widely distributed. Protein binding: 90%. Primarily excreted unchanged in urine. Moderately removed by hemodialysis. **Half-life:** 7-8 hr (increased in impaired renal function).

AVAILABILITY
Powder for Injection: 250 mg/vial, 500 mg/vial.

INDICATIONS AND DOSAGES
▸ **Complicated skin and skin-structure infections**
IV
Adults, Elderly. 4 mg/kg every 24 hr for 7-14 days.
▸ **Dosage in renal impairment**
For patients with creatinine clear-ance of less than 30 ml/min, dosage is 4 mg/kg q48hr for 7-14 days.

CONTRAINDICATIONS
None known.

INTERACTIONS
Drug
HMG-CoA reductase inhibitors:
May cause myopathy.
Tobramycin: Increases the serum concentration of daptomycin.
Herbal
None known.
Food
None known.

DIAGNOSTIC TEST EFFECTS
May increase serum CPK levels.
May alter liver function test results.

▓ IV INCOMPATIBILITIES
Diluents containing dextrose. If the same IV line is used to administer different drugs, the line should be flushed with 0.9% NaCl.

SIDE EFFECTS
Frequent (6%-5%)
Constipation, nausea, peripheral injection site reactions, headache, diarrhea
Occasional (4%-3%)
Insomnia, rash, vomiting
Rare (less than 3%)
Pruritus, dizziness, hypotension

SERIOUS REACTIONS
• Skeletal muscle myopathy, characterized by muscle pain and weakness, particularly of the distal extremities, occurs rarely.
• Antibiotic-associated colitis and other superinfections may result from altered bacterial balance.

PRECAUTIONS & CONSIDERATIONS
Caution is warranted with pregnancy, musculoskeletal disorders, and renal impairment. Avoid concurrent use of HMG-CoA reductase inhibitors because they may cause myopathy. It is unknown if daptomycin is distributed in breast milk. The safety and efficacy of this drug have not been established in children younger than 18 years of age. No age-related precautions have been noted in the elderly.

Report headache, dizziness, nausea, rash, severe diarrhea, new muscle weakness, or any other new symptoms. Mild GI effects may be tolerable, but severe symptoms may indicate the onset of antibiotic-associated colitis. Pattern of daily bowel activity and stool consistency should be monitored. Culture and sensitivity tests should be obtained before giving the first dose of daptomycin; therapy may begin before the test results are known. Check for white patches on the mucous membranes and tongue. Be alert for signs and symptoms of superinfection, including abdominal pain, moderate to severe diarrhea, severe anal or genital pruritus, and severe mouth soreness.

Storage
Store the drug in the refrigerator. The reconstituted solution is stable for 12 hours at room temperature and up to 48 hours if refrigerated.

Administration
The drug normally appears as a pale yellow to light brown lyophilized cake. Discard the solution if it contains particulate matter. Reconstitute the 250-mg vial with 5 ml 0.9% NaCl and the 500-mg vial with 10 ml 0.9% NaCl. Further dilute in 50 ml 0.9% NaCl. Infuse the intermittent IV (piggyback) infusion over 30 minutes.

Darbepoetin Alfa
dar-beh-poe′ee-tin
(Aranesp)
Do not confuse Aranesp with Aricept.

CATEGORY AND SCHEDULE
Pregnancy Risk Category: C

CLASSIFICATION
Hematopoietic agents, hormones/hormone modifiers

MECHANISM OF ACTION
A glycoprotein that stimulates formation of RBCs in bone marrow; increases serum half-life of epoetin. *Therapeutic Effect:* Induces erythropoiesis and release of reticulocytes from bone marrow.

PHARMACOKINETICS
Well absorbed after subcutaneous administration. **Half-life:** 48.5 hr.

AVAILABILITY
Injection: 25 mcg/ml, 40 mcg/ml, 60 mcg/ml, 100 mcg/ml, 150 mcg/ml, 200 mcg/ml, 300 mcg/ml.

INDICATIONS AND DOSAGES
▸ **Anemia in chronic renal failure**
IV BOLUS, SUBCUTANEOUS
Adults, Elderly. Initially, 0.45 mcg/kg once weekly. Adjust dosage to achieve and maintain a target Hgb not to exceed 12 g/dl. Do not increase dosage more frequently than once monthly. Limit increases in Hgb by less than 1 g/dl over any 2-week period.
▸ **Anemia associated with chemotherapy**
IV, SUBCUTANEOUS
Adults, Elderly. 2.25 mcg/kg/dose once a week.

CONTRAINDICATIONS
History of sensitivity to mammalian cell-derived products or human albumin, uncontrolled hypertension

INTERACTIONS
Drug
None known.
Herbal
None known.
Food
None known.

DIAGNOSTIC TEST EFFECTS
May increase BUN, serum phosphorus, potassium, serum creatinine, serum uric acid, and sodium levels. May decrease bleeding time, serum iron concentration, and serum ferritin.

▨ IV INCOMPATIBILITIES
Do not mix with other medications.

SIDE EFFECTS
Frequent
Myalgia, hypertension or hypotension, headache, diarrhea
Occasional
Fatigue, edema, vomiting, reaction at administration site, asthenia, dizziness

SERIOUS REACTIONS
• Vascular access thrombosis, CHF, sepsis, arrhythmias, and anaphylactic reaction occur rarely.

PRECAUTIONS & CONSIDERATIONS
Caution is warranted with hemolytic anemia, history of seizures, known porphyria (impairment of erythrocyte formation in bone marrow), sickle cell anemia, and thalassemia. It is unknown if darbepoetin alfa crosses the placenta or is distributed in breast milk. Safety and efficacy of darbepoetin alfa have not been established in children. In the elderly, age-related renal impairment may

require dosage adjustment. Avoid tasks that require mental alertness or motor skills until response to the drug is established.

Notify the physician of severe headache. Hct level should be monitored diligently. The dosage should be reduced if Hct level increases more than 4 points in 2 weeks. CBC with differential, Hgb, reticulocyte count, BUN, phosphorus, potassium, serum creatinine, and serum ferritin levels should also be monitored before and during therapy. In addition, B/P must be monitored aggressively for an increase because 25% of persons taking darbepoetin alfa require antihypertensive therapy and dietary restrictions. Keep in mind most patients will eventually need supplemental iron therapy.

Storage
Refrigerate vials. Do not shake vials vigorously because doing so may denature medication, rendering it inactive.

Administration
! Avoid excessive agitation of vial; do not shake because it will cause foaming.

For IV use, reconstitution is not necessary. May be given as an IV bolus.

For subcutaneous administration, use one dose per vial; do not reenter vial. Discard unused portion. May be mixed in a syringe with bacteriostatic 0.9% NaCl with benzyl alcohol 0.9% or bacteriostatic saline at a 1:1 ratio. Benzyl alcohol acts as a local anesthetic and may reduce injection site discomfort.

Darifenacin Hydrobromide
dare-ih-fen′ah-sin
(Enablex)

CATEGORY AND SCHEDULE
Pregnancy Risk Category: C

CLASSIFICATION
Anticholinergics

MECHANISM OF ACTION
A urinary antispasmodic agent that acts as a direct antagonist at muscarinic receptor sites in cholinergically innervated organs. Blockade of the receptors limits bladder contractions. *Therapeutic Effect:* Reduces symptoms of bladder irritability and overactivity; improves bladder capacity.

AVAILABILITY
Tablets (Extended-Release): 7.5 mg, 15 mg.

INDICATIONS AND DOSAGES
▸ **Overactive bladder**
PO
Adults, Elderly. Initially, 7.5 mg once daily. If response is not adequate after at least 2 wk, dosage may be increased to 15 mg once daily.
▸ **Dosage in hepatic impairment**
For patients with moderate hepatic impairment, maximum dosage is 7.5 mg once daily.

CONTRAINDICATIONS
GI or GU obstruction, paralytic ileus, severe hepatic impairment, uncontrolled angle-closure glaucoma, urine retention

INTERACTIONS
Drug
Aminoglutethimide, carbamazepine, nafcillin, nevirapine,

phenobarbital, phenytoin, rifamycins: May decrease the effects and blood level of darifenacin.
Amphetamines, beta-blockers (selected), dextromethorphan, fluoxetine, lidocaine, mirtazapine, nefazodone, paroxetine, risperidone, ritonavir, thioridazine, tricyclic antidepressants, venlafaxine: May increase the effects and blood levels of these drugs.
Azole antifungals, ciprofloxacin, clarithromycin, diclofenac, doxycycline, erythromycin, imatinib, isoniazid, nefazodone, nicardipine, propofol, protease inhibitors, quinidine, verapamil: May increase the effects and blood level of darifenacin.
Codeine, hydrocodone, oxycodone, tramadol: May decrease the effects and blood levels of these drugs.
Herbal
None known.
Food
None known.

DIAGNOSTIC TEST EFFECTS
None known.

SIDE EFFECTS
Frequent (35%-21%)
Dry mouth, constipation
Occasional (8%-4%)
Dyspepsia, headache, nausea, abdominal pain
Rare (3%-2%)
Asthenia, diarrhea, dizziness, dry eyes

SERIOUS REACTIONS
• UTI occurs occasionally.

PRECAUTIONS & CONSIDERATIONS
Caution is warranted with bladder outflow obstruction, constipation, controlled angle-closure glaucoma, decreased GI motility, GI obstructive disorders, hiatal hernia, myasthenia gravis, nonobstructive prostatic hyperplasia, reflux esophagitis, ulcerative colitis, and urine retention.
Administration
Take darifenacin without regard to food. Swallow extended-release tablets whole; don't crush them.

D

Daunorubicin
daw-noe-roo′bi-sin
(Cerubidine, DaunoXome)
Do not confuse daunorubicin with dactinomycin or doxorubicin

CATEGORY AND SCHEDULE
Pregnancy Risk Category: D

CLASSIFICATION
Antineoplastics, antibiotics

MECHANISM OF ACTION
An anthracycline antibiotic that inhibits DNA and DNA-dependent RNA synthesis by binding with DNA strands. Liposomal encapsulation increases uptake by tumors, prolongs drug action, and may decrease toxicity. *Therapeutic Effect:* Prevents cell division.

PHARMACOKINETICS
Widely distributed. Protein binding: High. Does not cross the blood-brain barrier. Metabolized in the liver to active metabolite. Excreted in urine; eliminated by biliary excretion.
Half-life: 18.5 hr; metabolite: 26.7 hr.

AVAILABILITY
Cerubidine
Powder for Injection: 20 mg.
Solution for Injection: 5 mg/ml.
DaunoXome
Injection: 2 mg/ml.

INDICATIONS AND DOSAGES
▸ **Acute lymphocytic leukemia**
IV
Adults. 45 mg/m² on days 1-3 of induction course.
Children. 25-45 mg/m² on days 1 and 8 of cycle.
▸ **Acute lymphocytic leukemia (ALL)**
IV
Adults, Elderly. 45 mg/m² on days 1-3 of induction course.
Children. 25-45 mg/m² on days 1 and 8 of cycle.
▸ **Acute myeloid leukemia (AML), Acute non-lympocytic leukemia (ANLL)**
IV
Adults, Elderly. 45 mg/m² on days 1-3 of first cycle and on days 1 and 2 of subsequent courses.
Children. 30-60 mg/m² on days 1-3 of cycle.
▸ **Kaposi's sarcoma**
IV
Adults. 20-40 mg/m² (DaunoXome) over 1 hr repeated q2wk; or 100 mg/m² q3wk.
▸ **Dosage in renal impairment**
ALL, AML, ANLL
Creatinine clearance less than 10 ml/min. 75% of normal dose.
Serum creatinine greater than 3 mg/dl. 50% of normal dose.
Kaposi's sarcoma
Serum creatinine greater than 3 mg/dl. 50% of normal dose.
▸ **Dosage in hepatic impairment**
ALL, AML, ANLL
Bilirubin 1.2-3 mg/dl. 75% of normal dose.
Bilirubin 3.1-5 mg/dl. 50% of normal dose.
Bilirubin greater than 5 mg/dl. Daunorubicin is not recommended for use in this patient population.
Kaposi's sarcoma
Bilirubin 1.2-3 mg/dl. 75% of normal dose.

Bilirubin greater than 3 mg/dl. 50% of normal dose.

OFF-LABEL USES
Treatment of chronic myelocytic leukemia, Ewing's sarcoma, neuroblastoma, non-Hodgkin's lymphoma, Wilms' tumor

CONTRAINDICATIONS
Arrhythmias, CHF, left ventricular ejection fraction less than 40%, pre-existing myelosuppression

INTERACTIONS
Drug
Antigout medications: May decrease the effects of these drugs.
Bone marrow depressants: May enhance myelosuppression.
Live-virus vaccines: May potentiate virus replication, increase vaccine side effects, and decrease the patient's antibody response to the vaccine.
Herbal
None known.
Food
None known.

DIAGNOSTIC TEST EFFECTS
May increase serum alkaline phosphatase, bilirubin, uric acid, and AST (SGOT) levels.

▓ IV INCOMPATIBILITIES
Allopurinol (Aloprim), aztreonam (Azactam), cefepime (Maxipime), fludarabine (Fludara), piperacillin and tazobactam (Zosyn)
DaunoXome: Don't mix with any other solution, especially NaCl or bacteriostatic agents (such as benzyl alcohol).
⬙ IV Compatibilities
Cytarabine (Cytosar), etoposide (VePesid), filgrastim (Neupogen), granisetron (Kytril), ondansetron (Zofran)

SIDE EFFECTS
Frequent
Complete alopecia (scalp, axillary, pubic), nausea, vomiting (beginning a few hours after administration and lasting 24-48 hours)
DaunoXome: Mild to moderate nausea, fatigue, fever
Occasional
Diarrhea, abdominal pain, esophagitis, stomatitis, transverse pigmentation of fingernails and toenails
Rare
Transient fever, chills

SERIOUS REACTIONS
• Myelosuppression may cause hematologic toxicity, manifested as severe leukopenia, anemia, and thrombocytopenia. Platelet and WBC counts typically decrease in 10-14 days and return to normal levels by the third week of daunorubicin treatment.
• The risk of cardiotoxicity (either acute, manifested as transient EKG abnormalities, or chronic, manifested as CHF) increases when the total cumulative dose exceeds 550 mg/m^2 in adults, 300 mg/m^2 in children older than 2 years, or 10 mg/kg in children younger than 2 years.

PRECAUTIONS & CONSIDERATIONS
Caution is warranted in elderly patients, pre-existing cardiac disease, congestive heart failure (CHF), hepatic or renal function impairment, myelosuppression, hyperuricemia, and secondary leukemias. Avoid using daunorubicin in pregnant women. It is unknown if daunorubicin is distributed in breast milk. Safety and efficacy of daunorubicin have not been established in children. Cardiac, hepatic, and renal function should be monitored prior to each cycle.
Storage
Reconstituted solutions are stable for 24 hours at room temperature. Protect from light.

Administration
Do not administer IM or SC. Avoid extravasation. Reconstitute by adding 4 ml of sterile water for injection to the vial and shaking gently to dissolve to produce 5 mg of daunorubicin per ml.

Deferoxamine
de-fer-ox′a-meen
(Desferal [CAN], Desferal Mesylate)

CATEGORY AND SCHEDULE
Pregnancy Risk Category: C

CLASSIFICATION
Antidotes, chelators

MECHANISM OF ACTION
An antidote that binds with iron to form complex. *Therapeutic Effect:* Promotes urine excretion of acute iron poisoning.

PHARMACOKINETICS
Well absorbed after IM, SC administration. Widely distributed. Rapidly metabolized in tissues, plasma. Excreted in urine, eliminated in feces via biliary excretion. Removed by hemodialysis. **Half-life:** 6 hr.

AVAILABILITY
Injection: 500 mg (Desferal Mesylate).

INDICATIONS AND DOSAGES
▶ **Acute iron intoxication**
IM
Adults: Initially, 90 mg/kg, then 45 mg/kg up to 1 g q4-12hr. Maximum: 6 g/day.
IV
Adults: 15 mg/kg/hr up to 90 mg/kg q8hr. Maximum: 6 g/day.
Children: 15 mg/kg/hr.

▸ **Chronic iron overload**
SUBCUTANEOUS
Adults. 1-2 g/day (20-40 mg/kg)
over 8-24 hr.
Children: 10 mg/kg/day.
IM
Adults. 0.5-1 g/day. In addition to
IM, 2 g infused at rate not to exceed
15 mg/kg/hr.

CONTRAINDICATIONS
Severe renal disease, anuria, primary
hemochromatosis, hypersensitivity to
deferoxamine mesylate or any
component of the formulation

INTERACTIONS
Drug
Vitamin C: May increase effect of
deferoxamine.
Herbal
None known.
Food
None known.

DIAGNOSTIC TEST EFFECTS
May cause a falsely high total
iron-binding capacity (TIBC).

▓ IV INCOMPATIBILITIES
Do not mix with any other
intravenous medications.

SIDE EFFECTS
Frequent
Pain, induration at injection site,
urine color change (to orange-rose)
Occasional
Abdominal discomfort, diarrhea, leg
cramps, impaired vision

SERIOUS REACTIONS
• Neurotoxicity, including high-
frequency hearing loss, has been
reported.

PRECAUTIONS & CONSIDERATIONS
Caution should be used with
aluminum overload or

aluminum-related encephalopathy.
  It is unknown if drug crosses
placenta or is distributed in breast
milk. Use only when absolutely
necessary. Be aware that skeletal
anomalies may present in neonate.
There are no age-related precautions
noted in children less than 3 years of
age. Be aware that age-related renal
impairment may require caution.
Reddish color urine may occur.
Administration
In general, IM route is preferred
unless in shock. Reconstitute each
500-mg vial with 2 ml sterile water
for injection to provide a concentration of 250 mg/ml.
  For IM administration, inject
deeply into upper outer quadrant of
buttock. May give undiluted.
  For subcutaneous injection,
administer very slowly. May give
undiluted.
  For IV administration, further
dilute with 0.9% NaCl, D_5W or
lactated ringers and administer at
maximum rate of 15 mg/kg/hr. A
too-rapid IV administration may
produce skin flushing, urticaria,
hypotension, or shock.

Delavirdine
deh-la′ver-deen
(Rescriptor)

CATEGORY AND SCHEDULE
Pregnancy Risk Category: C
**Do not confuse with Retrovin,
Ritonavir.**

CLASSIFICATION
Antivirals, non-nucleoside
reverse transcriptase inhibitors

MECHANISM OF ACTION
A nonnucleoside reverse transcriptase inhibitor that binds directly to HIV-1 reverse transcriptase and blocks RNA- and DNA-dependent DNA polymerase activities. *Therapeutic Effect:* Interrupts HIV replication, slowing the progression of HIV infection.

PHARMACOKINETICS
Rapidly absorbed after PO administration. Protein binding: 98%. Primarily distributed in plasma. Metabolized in the liver. Eliminated in feces and urine. **Half-life:** 2-11 hr.

AVAILABILITY
Tablets: 100 mg, 200 mg.

INDICATIONS AND DOSAGES
▸ **HIV infection (in combination with other antiretrovirals)**
PO
Adults. 400 mg 3 times a day.

CONTRAINDICATIONS
None known.

INTERACTIONS
Drug
Benzodiazepines, calcium channel blockers: May cause life-threatening adverse reactions.
Carbamazepine, phenobarbital, phenytoin: May decrease delavirdine blood concentration.
H$_2$ blockers: May decrease delavirdine absorption.
Rifampin: May decrease delavirdine blood concentrations.
Herbal
None known.
Food
None known.

DIAGNOSTIC TEST EFFECTS
May increase AST (SGOT) and ALT (SGPT) levels. May decrease neutrophil count.

SIDE EFFECTS
Frequent (18%)
Rash, pruritus
Occasional (greater than 2%)
Headache, nausea, diarrhea, fatigue, anorexia

SERIOUS REACTIONS
• Severe skin rashes, including Stevens-Johnson syndrome, have been reported.

PRECAUTIONS & CONSIDERATIONS
Caution should be used with impaired liver function. It is unknown whether delavirdine crosses the placenta or is distributed in breast milk. Be aware that the safety and efficacy of delavirdine have not been established in children younger than 16 years and in the elderly. Delavirdine is not a cure for HIV infection, nor does it reduce the risk of transmission to others.

Expect to obtain baseline laboratory testing, especially liver function tests, before beginning therapy and at periodic intervals during therapy. Assess for any nausea or vomiting or for skin rash. Determine pattern of bowel activity and stool consistency. Monitor eating pattern and weight loss. Consume small, frequent meals to help offset anorexia and nausea. Medications, including over-the-counter (OTC) drugs, should not be taken without consulting the physician.
Administration
May take without regard to food. May disperse in water before consumption. Persons with achlorhydria should take delavirdine with orange juice or cranberry juice.

Demeclocycline
dem-e-kloe-sye'kleen
(Declomycin, Ledermycin [AUS])

CATEGORY AND SCHEDULE
Pregnancy Risk Category: D

CLASSIFICATION
Antibiotics, tetracyclines

MECHANISM OF ACTION
A tetracycline antibiotic that inhibits bacterial protein synthesis by binding to ribosomal receptor sites; also inhibits ADH-induced water reabsorption. *Therapeutic Effect:* Bacteriostatic; also produces water diuresis.

AVAILABILITY
Tablets: 150 mg, 300 mg.

INDICATIONS AND DOSAGES
▶ **Mild to moderate infections, including acne, pertussis, chronic bronchitis, and UTIs**
PO
Adults, Elderly. 150 mg 4 times a day or 300 mg 2 times a day.
Children older than 8 yr. 8-12 mg/kg/day in 2-4 divided doses.
▶ **Uncomplicated gonorrhea**
PO
Adults. Initially, 600 mg, then 300 mg q12hr for 4 days for total of 3 g.
▶ **Syndrome of inappropriate ADH secretion (SIADH)**
PO
Adults, Elderly. Initially, 900-1200 mg/day in 3-4 divided doses, then decrease dose to 600-900 mg/day in divided doses.

CONTRAINDICATIONS
Children 8 years and younger, last half of pregnancy

INTERACTIONS
Drug
Antacids containing aluminum, calcium, or magnesium; laxatives containing magnesium; oral iron preparations: Impair the absorption of demeclocycline.
Cholestyramine, colestipol: May decrease demeclocycline absorption.
Oral contraceptives: May decrease the effects of oral contraceptives.
Herbal
None known.
Food
Dairy products: May decrease demeclocycline absorption.

DIAGNOSTIC TEST EFFECTS
May increase BUN and serum alkaline phosphatase, amylase, bilirubin, AST (SGOT), and ALT (SGPT) levels.

SIDE EFFECTS
Frequent
Anorexia, nausea, vomiting, diarrhea, dysphagia, possibly severe photosensitivity, (with moderate to high demeclocycline dosage).
Occasional
Urticaria, rash; diabetes insipidus syndrome, marked by polydipsia, polyuria, and weakness (with long-term therapy).

SERIOUS REACTIONS
• Superinfection (especially fungal), anaphylaxis, and benign intracranial hypertension occur rarely.
• Bulging fontanelles occur rarely in infants.

PRECAUTIONS & CONSIDERATIONS
Caution is warranted with renal impairment, and in those who can't avoid sun or ultraviolet exposure, because such exposure may produce a severe photosensitivity reaction.

History of allergies, especially to tetracyclines, should be determined before drug therapy. Pattern of daily bowel activity, stool consistency, food intake and tolerance, renal function, and skin for rash should be assessed. Be alert for signs and symptoms of superinfection, such as anal or genital pruritus, diarrhea, and ulceration or changes of the oral mucosa or tongue. B/P and LOC should be monitored because of the potential for increased intracranial pressure.

Administration

Take demeclocycline doses on an empty stomach with a full glass of water. Space drug doses evenly around the clock and continue taking demeclocycline for the full course of treatment. Take antacids containing aluminum, calcium, or magnesium; laxatives containing magnesium; or oral iron preparations 1 to 2 hours before or after demeclocycline because they may impair the drug's absorption.

Desipramine

dess-ip'ra-meen
(Apo-Desipramine [CAN],
Norpramin,
Novo-Desipramine [CAN],
Pertofran [AUS])
Do not confuse desipramine with disopyramide or imipramine.

CATEGORY AND SCHEDULE

Pregnancy Risk Category: C

CLASSIFICATION

Antidepressants, tricyclic

MECHANISM OF ACTION

A tricyclic antidepressant that blocks the reuptake of neurotransmitters, such as norepinephrine and serotonin, at presynaptic membranes, increasing their availability at postsynaptic receptor sites. Also has strong anticholinergic activity. *Therapeutic Effect:* Relieves depression.

PHARMACOKINETICS

Rapidly, and well absorbed from the GI tract. Protein binding: 90%. Metabolized in the liver. Primarily excreted in urine. Minimally removed by hemodialysis.
Half-life: 12-27 hr.

AVAILABILITY

Tablets: 10 mg, 25 mg, 50 mg, 75 mg, 100 mg, 150 mg.

INDICATIONS AND DOSAGES

▸ **Depression**
PO
Adults. 75 mg/day. May gradually increase to 150-200 mg/day. Maximum: 300 mg/day.
Elderly. Initially, 10-25 mg/day. May gradually increase to 75-100 mg/day. Maximum: 300 mg/day.
Children older than 12 yr. Initially, 25-50 mg/day. May gradually increase to 100 mg/day. Maximum: 150 mg/day.
Children 6-12 yr. 1-3 mg/kg/day. Maximum: 5 mg/kg/day.

OFF-LABEL USES

Treatment of attention deficit hyperactivity disorder, bulimia nervosa, cataplexy associated with narcolepsy, cocaine withdrawal, neurogenic pain, panic disorder

CONTRAINDICATIONS

Angle-closure glaucoma, use within 14 days of MAOIs

INTERACTIONS
Drug
Alcohol, other CNS depressants:
May increase CNS and respiratory depression and the hypotensive effects of desipramine.
Antithyroid agents: May increase the risk of agranulocytosis.
Cimetidine: May increase desipramine blood concentration and risk of toxicity.
Clonidine, guanadrel: May decrease the effects of these drugs.
MAOIs: May increase the risk of neuroleptic malignant syndrome, hyperpyrexia, hypertensive crisis, and seizures.
Phenothiazines: May increase the anticholinergic and sedative effects of desipramine.
Phenytoin: May decrease the desipramine blood concentration.
Sympathomimetics: May increase the risk of cardiac effects.
Herbal
St. John's wort: May increase desipramine's pharmacologic effects and risk of toxicity.
Food
None known.

DIAGNOSTIC TEST EFFECTS
May alter blood glucose level and EKG readings. Therapeutic serum drug level is 115-300 ng/ml; toxic serum drug level is greater than 400 ng/ml.

SIDE EFFECTS
Frequent
Somnolence, fatigue, dry mouth, blurred vision, constipation, delayed micturition, orthostatic hypotension, diaphoresis, impaired concentration, increased appetite, urine retention
Occasional
GI disturbances (such as nausea, GI distress, metallic taste)

Rare
Paradoxical reactions (agitation, restlessness, nightmares, insomnia), extrapyramidal symptoms (particularly fine hand tremor)

SERIOUS REACTIONS
• Overdose may produce confusion, seizures, somnolence, arrhythmias, fever, hallucinations, dyspnea, vomiting, and unusual fatigue or weakness.
• Abrupt discontinuation after prolonged therapy may produce severe headache, malaise, nausea, vomiting, and vivid dreams.

PRECAUTIONS & CONSIDERATIONS
Caution is warranted with cardiac conduction disturbances, cardiovascular disease, hyperthyroidism, seizure disorders, urine retention, and in those taking thyroid replacement therapy. Desipramine crosses the placenta and is minimally distributed in breast milk. Desipramine use is not recommended for children younger than 6 years. Expect to administer lower dosages to elderly patients because they're at increased risk for drug toxicity.

Anticholinergic, sedative, and hypotensive effects may occur during early therapy, but tolerance to these effects usually develop. Since dizziness may occur, change positions slowly and avoid alcohol and avoid tasks that require mental alertness or motor skills. CBC and blood chemistry tests to assess hepatic and renal function and EKG to detect arrhythmias should be performed before and periodically during therapy.
Administration
! Make sure at least 14 days elapse between the use of MAOIs and desipramine. Be aware that the therapeutic serum level for desipramine is

115 to 300 ng/ml, and the toxic serum level is greater than 400 ng/ml.

Take desipramine with food or milk if GI distress occurs. Full therapeutic effect may be noted in 2 to 4 weeks. Do not abruptly discontinue desipramine.

Desirudin
(Iprivask)

CATEGORY AND SCHEDULE
Pregnancy Risk Category: C

CLASSIFICATION
Anticoagulants, thrombin inhibitors

MECHANISM OF ACTION
An anticoagulant that binds specifically and directly to thrombin, inhibiting free circulating and clot-bound thrombin. *Therapeutic Effect:* Prolongs the clotting time of human plasma.

PHARMACOKINETICS
Completely absorbed. Distributed in extracellular space. Metabolized and eliminated by the kidney. **Half-life:** 2-3 hr.

AVAILABILITY
Powder for Injection: 15-mg vial with diluent (diluent includes 0.6 ml mannitol [3%] in water for injection).

INDICATIONS AND DOSAGES
▸ **Prevention of deep vein thrombosis in patients undergoing hip replacement surgery**
SUBCUTANEOUS
Adults, Elderly. Initially, 15 mg q12hr given 5-15 min before surgery

but following induction of regional block anesthesia, if used. May administer up to 12 days post surgery.
▸ **Moderate renal impairment (creatinine clearance 31-60 ml/min or higher)**
SUBCUTANEOUS
Adults, Elderly. 5 mg q12hr.
▸ **Severe renal impairment (creatinine clearance less than 31 ml/min)**
SUBCUTANEOUS
Adults, Elderly. 1.7 mg q12hr.

CONTRAINDICATIONS
Hypersensitivity to natural or recombinant hirudins (anticoagulation factors), active bleeding, irreversible coagulation disorders

INTERACTIONS
Drug
Anticoagulants, dextran 40, systemic glucocorticoids, thrombolytics: Increase the risk of bleeding and should be discontinued before start of desirudin therapy.
Herbal
None known.
Food
None known.

DIAGNOSTIC TEST EFFECTS
May increase aPTT. May decrease Hgb, and Hct concentrations.

SIDE EFFECTS
Frequent (6%)
Hematoma
Occasional (4%-2%)
Injection site mass, wound secretion, nausea, hypersensitivity reaction

SERIOUS REACTIONS
• Serious or major hemorrhage and anaphylactic reaction occur rarely.

PRECAUTIONS & CONSIDERATIONS

Caution is warranted with epidural or spinal anesthesia, renal impairment, increased risk of hemorrhage, including bacterial endocarditis, hemophilia, history of GI or pulmonary bleeding within the past 3 months, history of hemorrhagic stroke, intracranial or intraocular bleeding, organ biopsy, puncture of a non-compressible vessel within the last month, recent major surgery, and severe uncontrolled hypertension. Desirudin may be teratogenic and it is unknown if the drug is distributed in breast milk. Safety and efficacy of desirudin have not been established in children. In the elderly, age-related renal impairment may require dosage adjustment. Females may experience heavier menstrual flow. Other medications, including OTC drugs, should be avoided. An electric razor and soft toothbrush should be used to prevent bleeding during therapy.

Notify the physician of abdominal or back pain, severe headache, black or red stool, coffee-ground vomitus, dark or red urine, or red-speckled mucus from cough. B/P, Hct, pulse rate, aPTT, and serum creatinine levels should be monitored.
Storage
Store vials at room temperature. Reconstitute each vial with 0.5 ml provided diluent. Gently agitate or rotate. Use reconstituted solution immediately; however, it is stable for up to 24 hours if stored at room temperature. Discard unused portion.
Administration
Using a 26- or 27-gauge needle about one-half inch long, withdraw reconstituted solution and administer by deep subcutaneous injection, alternating sites between left and right anterolateral and left and right posterolateral abdominal wall. Introduce entire length of needle into skin fold held between thumb and forefinger, holding skin fold during injection. Dosage should be reduced if peak aPTT exceeds 2 times control.

Desloratidine
des-loer-at′ah-deen
(Aerius, Clarinex, Clarinex Redi-Tabs)
Do not confuse with Claritin.

CATEGORY AND SCHEDULE
Pregnancy Risk Category: C

CLASSIFICATION
Antihistamines

MECHANISM OF ACTION
A nonsedating antihistamine that exhibits selective peripheral histamine H_1 receptor blocking action. Competes with histamine at receptor sites. *Therapeutic Effect:* Prevents allergic responses mediated by histamine, such as rhinitis and urticaria.

PHARMACOKINETICS
Rapidly and almost completely absorbed from the GI tract. Distributed mainly in liver, lungs, GI tract, and bile. Metabolized in the liver to active metabolite and undergoes extensive first-pass metabolism. Eliminated in urine and feces.
Half-life: 27 hr (increased in the elderly and in renal or hepatic impairment).

AVAILABILITY
Tablets: 5 mg.
Tablets (Orally Disintegrating [Reditabs]): 5 mg.

INDICATIONS AND DOSAGES
▶ **Allergic rhinitis, urticaria**
PO
Adults, Elderly, Children older than 12 yr. 5 mg once a day.
▶ **Dosage in hepatic or renal impairment**
Dosage is decreased to 5 mg every other day.

CONTRAINDICATIONS
None known.

INTERACTIONS
Drug
Erythromycin, ketoconazole: May increase desloratadine blood concentration.
Herbal
None known.
Food
None known.

DIAGNOSTIC TEST EFFECTS
May suppress wheal and flare reactions to antigen skin testing unless the drug is discontinued 4 days before testing.

SIDE EFFECTS
Frequent (12%)
Headache
Occasional (3%)
Dry mouth, somnolence
Rare (less than 3%)
Fatigue, dizziness, diarrhea, nausea

SERIOUS REACTIONS
• None known.

PRECAUTIONS & CONSIDERATIONS
Caution is warranted with hepatic impairment. Desloratidine is excreted in breast milk and should not be used by breast-feeding women. The safety and efficacy of desloratidine have not been established in children younger than 6 years. Children and the elderly are more sensitive to the drug's anticholinergic effects, such as dry mouth, nose, and throat. Avoid drinking alcoholic beverages and performing tasks that require alertness or motor skills until response to the drug is established.

Drowsiness may occur. Increase fluid intake with upper respiratory allergies to decrease the viscosity of secretions, offset thirst, and replace fluids lost from diaphoresis. Therapeutic response should be monitored.
Administration
Don't crush or break film-coated tablets.
❗ Desloratidine is 2.5-4 times more potent than its parent compound, loratadine.

D

Desmopressin
des-moe-press′in
(DDAVP, Minirin [AUS], Octostim [CAN], Stimate)

CATEGORY AND SCHEDULE
Pregnancy Risk Category: B

CLASSIFICATION
Antidiuretics, hormones/ hormone modifiers

MECHANISM OF ACTION
A synthetic pituitary hormone that increases reabsorption of water by increasing permeability of collecting ducts of the kidneys. Also serves as a plasminogen activator. *Therapeutic Effect:* Increases plasma factor VIII (antihemophilic factor). Decreases urinary output.

PHARMACOKINETICS

Route	Onset	Peak	Duration
PO	1 hr	2-7 hr	6-8 hr
IV	15-30 min	1.5-3 hr	N/A
Intranasal	15 min-1 hr	1-5 hr	5-21 hr

Poorly absorbed after oral or nasal administration. Metabolism: Unknown. **Half-life:** Oral: 1.5- 2.5 hr. Intranasal: 3.3-3.5 hr. IV: 0.4-4 hr.

AVAILABILITY

Tablets (DDAVP): 0.1 mg, 0.2 mg.
Injection (DDAVP): 4 mcg/ml.
Nasal Solution (DDAVP): 100 mcg/ml.
Nasal Spray (Stimate): 1.5 mg/ml (150 mcg/spray).
Nasal Spray (DDAVP): 100 mcg/ml (10 mcg/spray).

INDICATIONS AND DOSAGES
▶ **Primary nocturnal enuresis**
PO
Children 12 yr and older. 0.2-0.6 mg once before bedtime.
INTRANASAL
Children 6 yr and older. Initially, 20 mcg (0.2 ml) at bedtime; use one-half dose in each nostril. Adjust to maximum of 40 mcg/day.
▶ **Central cranial diabetes insipidus**
PO
Adults, Elderly, Children 12 yr and older. Initially, 0.05 mg twice a day. Range: 0.1-1.2 mg/day in 2-3 divided doses.
Children younger than 12 yr. Initially, 0.05 mg; then twice a day. Range: 0.1-0.8 mg daily.
INTRANASAL
Adults, Elderly, Children older than 12 yr. 5-40 mcg (0.05-0.4 ml) in 1-3 doses/day.
Children 3 mo-12 yr. Initially, 5 mcg (0.05 ml)/day. Range: 5-30 mcg (0.05-0.3 ml)/day.

IV, SUBCUTANEOUS
Adults, Elderly, Children older than 12 yr. 2-4 mcg/day in 2 divided doses or 1/10 of maintenance intranasal dose.
▶ **Hemophilia A, von Willebrand's Disease (Type I)**
IV INFUSION
Adults, Elderly, Children weighing 10 kg or more. 0.3 mcg/kg diluted in 50 ml 0.9% NaCl.
Children weighing less than 10 kg. 0.3 mcg/kg diluted in 10 ml 0.9% NaCl.
INTRANASAL
Adults, Elderly, Children 12 yr and older weighing 50 kg or more. 300 mcg; use 1 spray in each nostril.
Adults, Elderly, Children 12 yr and older weighing less than 50 kg. 150 mcg as a single spray.

CONTRAINDICATIONS
Hemophilia A with factor VIII levels less than 5%; hemophilia B; severe type I, type IIB, or platelet-type von Willebrand's disease

INTERACTIONS
Drug
Carbamazepine, chlorpropamide, clofibrate: May increase the effects of desmopressin.
Demeclocycline, lithium, norepinephrine: May decrease effects of desmopressin.
Herbal
None known.
Food
None known.

DIAGNOSTIC TEST EFFECTS
None known.

SIDE EFFECTS
Occasional
IV: Pain, redness, or swelling at injection site; headache; abdominal cramps; vulval pain; flushed skin;

mild B/P elevation; nausea with high dosages
Nasal: Rhinorrhea, nasal congestion, slight B/P elevation

SERIOUS REACTIONS

• Water intoxication or hyponatremia, marked by headache, somnolence, confusion, decreased urination, rapid weight gain, seizures, and coma, may occur in overhydration. Children, elderly patients, and infants are especially at risk.

PRECAUTIONS & CONSIDERATIONS

Caution is warranted with fluid or electrolyte imbalances, coronary artery disease, hypertensive cardiovascular disease, and predisposition to thrombus formation. Use cautiously in neonates younger than 3 months old because this age-group is at increased risk for fluid balance problems. Careful fluid restrictions are recommended in infants. The elderly are at increased risk for hyponatremia and water intoxication. Avoid overhydration.

Notify the physician of abdominal cramps, headache, heartburn, nausea, or shortness of breath. Signs and symptoms of diabetes insipidus should be monitored. Also, serum electrolyte levels, fluid intake, serum osmolality, urine volume, urine specific gravity, and weight should be assessed. Factor VIII antigen level, aPTT, and factor VIII activity level should be assessed for hemophilia.

Storage

Store oral desmopressin away from light and excessive heat. Refrigerate desmopressin for injection; it is stable for 2 weeks at room temperature. Refrigerate DDAVP nasal solution and Stimate nasal spray. Nasal solution and Stimate nasal spray are stable for 3 weeks at room temperature if unopened; DDAVP nasal spray is stable at room temperature.

Administration

For IV infusion, dilute in 10 to 50 ml 0.9% NaCl and prepare to infuse over 15 to 30 minutes. For preoperative use, administer 30 minutes before procedure, as prescribed. Monitor B/P and pulse during infusion. Remember that the IV dose is one tenth the intranasal dose.

To administer nasal preparation, draw up a measured quantity of desmopressin with a calibrated catheter (rhinyle). Insert one end in nose and blow on the other end to deposit the solution deep in the nasal cavity. For infants, young children, and obtunded patients, an air-filled syringe may be attached to the catheter to deposit the solution.

For subcutaneous use, estimate therapeutic response by adequacy of sleep duration. Expect to adjust morning and evening dosages separately.

Desonide
dess'oh-nide
(Delonide, Desocrot [CAN], DesOwen, Scheinpharm Desonide [CAN], Tridesilon)

CATEGORY AND SCHEDULE
Pregnancy Risk Category: C

CLASSIFICATION
Corticosteroids, topical, dermatologics

MECHANISM OF ACTION
A topical corticosteroid that has anti-inflammatory, antipruritic, and vasoconstrictive properties. The exact mechanism of the anti-inflammatory

process is unclear. *Therapeutic Effect:*
Reduces or prevents tissue response
to the inflammatory process.

PHARMACOKINETICS
Large variation in absorption
determined by many factors.
Metabolized in the liver. Primarily
excreted by the kidneys and small
amounts in the bile.

AVAILABILITY
Lotion: 0.05% (DesOwen).
Cream: 0.05% (DesOwen).
Ointment: 0.05% (DesOwen,
Tridesilon).

INDICATIONS AND DOSAGES
▸ **Dermatoses**
TOPICAL
Adults, Elderly. Apply sparingly
2-3 times/day.
▸ **Otitis externa**
AURAL
Adults, Elderly, Children. Instill 3 to
4 drops into the ear 3-4 times/day.

CONTRAINDICATIONS
Perforated eardrum, history of
hypersensitivity to desonide or other
corticosteroids

INTERACTIONS
Drug
Bupropion: May lower the seizure
threshold.
Herbal
None known.
Food
None known.

DIAGNOSTIC TEST EFFECTS
None known.

SIDE EFFECTS
Occasional
Burning and stinging at site of application, dryness, skin peeling, contact
dermatitis

SERIOUS REACTIONS
• The serious reactions of long-term
therapy and the addition of occlusive
dressings are reversible hypothalamic-
pituitary-adrenal (HPA) axis suppression, manifestations of Cushing's
syndrome, hyperglycemia, and
glucosuria.

PRECAUTIONS & CONSIDERATIONS
Caution should be used over large
surface areas, with prolonged use,
and in addition to occlusive dressings as well as uncontrolled or
untreated infections. Avoid use
of occlusive dressings on affected
area. Skin irritation should be
reported. It is unknown if desonide
crosses the placenta or is distributed
in the breast milk. Children may
absorb larger amounts of the
topical form and may be more
susceptible to toxicity. There are
no age-related precautions noted in
the elderly.
Administration
Gently cleanse area before topical
application. Use occlusive dressings
only as directed. Apply sparingly
and rub into area gently and
thoroughly.
  For the otic preparation, remove
all ceruminous material and debris
prior to instillation. May use a gauze
or cotton wick saturated with solution, insert in the ear canal, and
allow to remain. Keep moist by
further addition of the solution.

Desoximetasone

des-ox-i-met′a-sone
(Taro-Desoximetason [CAN],
Topicort, Topicort-LP)
**Do not confuse with
dexamethasone.**

CATEGORY AND SCHEDULE
Pregnancy Risk Category: C

CLASSIFICATION
Corticosteroids, topical,
dermatologics

MECHANISM OF ACTION
A high potency, fluorinated
topical corticosteroid that has
anti-inflammatory, antipruritic,
and vasoconstrictive properties.
The exact mechanism of the anti-
inflammatory process is unclear.
Therapeutic Effect: Reduces tissue
response to the inflammatory
process.

PHARMACOKINETICS
Large variation in absorption
among sites. Protein binding in
varying degrees. Metabolized
in liver. Primarily excreted in
urine.

AVAILABILITY
Cream: 0.25% (Topicort), 0.05%
(Topicort-LP).
Gel: 0.05% (Topicort).
Ointment: 0.25% (Topicort).

INDICATIONS AND DOSAGES
▶ **Dermatoses**
TOPICAL
Adults, Elderly. Apply sparingly
2 times/day.
Children. Apply sparingly
1-2 times/day.

OFF-LABEL USES
Eczema, psoriasis vulgaris

CONTRAINDICATIONS
History of hypersensitivity to
desoximetasone or other corticosteroids

D

INTERACTIONS
Drug
None known.
Herbal
None known.
Food
None known.

DIAGNOSTIC TEST EFFECTS
None known.

SIDE EFFECTS
Frequent
Itching, redness, irritation, burning
at site of application
Occasional
Dryness, folliculitis, hypertrichosis,
acneiform eruptions, hypopigmenta-
tion, perioral dermatitis
Rare
Allergic contact dermatitis, adrenal
suppression, atrophy, striae, miliaria,
photosensitivity

SERIOUS REACTIONS
• Serious reactions of long-term
therapy and addition of occlusive
dressings are reversible hypothalamic-
pituitary-adrenal (HPA) axis
suppression, manifestations of
Cushing's syndrome, hyperglycemia,
and glucosuria.
• Abruptly withdrawing the drug
after long-term therapy may require
supplemental systemic corticosteroids.

PRECAUTIONS & CONSIDERATIONS
Urinary free cortisol test and ACTH
stimulation test should be evaluated
before therapy. It is unknown if

desoximetasone is excreted in breast milk. There are no age-related precautions in the elderly. Pediatric patients may absorb larger amounts and may be more susceptible to toxicity.

Caution should be used over large surface areas, with prolonged use, and in addition of occlusive dressings.

Administration

Gently cleanse area before application. Use occlusive dressings only as directed. Apply sparingly. Rub into area gently and thoroughly.

Dexamethasone

dex-a-meth′a-sone
(Decadron, Dexasone [CAN], Dexmethsone [AUS], Diodex [CAN], Hexadrol [CAN], Maxidex)
Do not confuse dexamethasone with desoximetasone or dextromethorphan, or Maxidex with Maxzide.

CATEGORY AND SCHEDULE

Pregnancy Risk Category: C (D if used in the first trimester)

CLASSIFICATION

Corticosteroids, ophthalmic, topical, dermatologics, ophthalmics

---

MECHANISM OF ACTION

A long-acting glucocorticoid that inhibits accumulation of inflammatory cells at inflammation sites, phagocytosis, lysosomal enzyme release and synthesis, and release of mediators of inflammation.
Therapeutic Effect: Prevents and suppresses cell and tissue immune reactions and inflammatory process.

PHARMACOKINETICS

Rapidly, completely absorbed from the GI tract after oral administration. Widely distributed. Protein binding: High. Metabolized in the liver. Primarily excreted in urine. Minimally removed by hemodialysis. **Half-life:** 3-4.5 hr.

AVAILABILITY

Elixir: 0.5 mg/5 ml, 1 mg/ml.
Inhalant, Intranasal, Ophthalmic: Solution, suspension, ointment.
Oral Solution: 0.5 mg/5 ml, 0.5 mg/0.5 ml.
Tablets: 0.25 mg, 0.5 mg, 0.75 mg, 1 mg, 1.5 mg, 2 mg, 4 mg, 6 mg.
Topical: Aerosol, cream. Injection: 4 mg/ml.

INDICATIONS AND DOSAGES

▸ **Anti-inflammatory**
PO/IV/IM
Adults, Elderly. 0.75-9 mg/day in divided doses q6-12hr.
Children. 0.08-0.3 mg/kg/day in divided doses q6-12hr.
▸ **Cerebral edema**
IV
Adults, Elderly. Initially, 10 mg, then 4 mg (IM/IV) q6hr.
PO/IV/IM
Children. Loading dose of 1-2 mg/kg, then 1-1.5 mg/kg/day in divided doses q4-6hr.
▸ **Nausea and vomiting in chemotherapy patients**
IV
Adults, Elderly. 8-20 mg once, then 4 mg (PO) q4-6hr or 8 mg q8hr.
Children. 10 mg/m^2/dose (Maximum: 20 mg), then 5 mg/m^2/dose q6hr.
▸ **Physiologic replacement**
PO/IV/IM
Children. 0.03-0.15 mg/kg/day in divided doses q6-12hr.
▸ **Usual ophthalmic dosage, ocular inflammatory conditions**

OINTMENT
Adults, Elderly, Children. Thin coating 3-4 times/day.
SUSPENSION
Adults, Elderly, Children. Initially, 2 drops q1hr while awake and q2hr at night for 1 day, then reduce to 3-4 times/day.

CONTRAINDICATIONS
Active untreated infections, fungal, tuberculosis, or viral diseases of the eye

INTERACTIONS
Drug
Amphotericin: May increase hypokalemia.
Digoxin: May increase digoxin toxicity caused by hypokalemia.
Diuretics, insulin, oral hypoglycemics, potassium supplements: May decrease the effects of these drugs.
Hepatic enzyme inducers: May decrease the effects of dexamethasone.
Live virus vaccines: May decrease the patient's antibody response to vaccine, increase vaccine side effects, and potentiate virus replication.
Herbal
None known.
Food
None known.

DIAGNOSTIC TEST EFFECTS
May increase blood glucose and serum lipid, amylase, and sodium levels. May decrease serum calcium, potassium, and thyroxine levels.

▓ IV INCOMPATIBILITIES
Ciprofloxacin (Cipro), daunorubicin (Cerubidine), idarubicin (Idamycin), midazolam (Versed)
⬚ IV Compatibilities
Aminophylline, cimetidine (Tagamet), cisplatin (Platinol),

cyclophosphamide (Cytoxan), cytarabine (Cytosar), docetaxel (Taxotere), doxorubicin (Adriamycin), etoposide (VePesid), granisetron (Kytril), heparin, hydromorphone (Dilaudid), lorazepam (Ativan), morphine, ondansetron (Zofran), paclitaxel (Taxol), potassium chloride, propofol (Diprivan)

SIDE EFFECTS
Frequent
Inhalation: Cough, dry mouth, hoarseness, throat irritation
Intranasal: Burning, mucosal dryness
Ophthalmic: Blurred vision
Systemic: Insomnia, facial swelling or cushingoid appearance, moderate abdominal distention, indigestion, increased appetite, nervousness, facial flushing, diaphoresis
Occasional
Inhalation: Localized fungal infection, such as thrush
Intranasal: Crusting inside nose, nosebleed, sore throat, ulceration of nasal mucosa.
Ophthalmic: Decreased vision, watering of eyes, eye pain, burning, stinging, redness of eyes, nausea, vomiting
Systemic: Dizziness, decreased or blurred vision
Topical: Allergic contact dermatitis, purpura or blood-containing blisters, thinning of skin with easy bruising, telangiectasis or raised dark red spots on skin
Rare
Inhalation: Increased bronchospasm, esophageal candidiasis
Intranasal: Nasal and pharyngeal candidiasis, eye pain
Systemic: General allergic reaction (such as rash and hives); pain, redness, or swelling at injection site; psychological changes; false sense of well-being; hallucinations; depression

SERIOUS REACTIONS

• Long-term therapy may cause muscle wasting (especially in the arms and legs), osteoporosis, spontaneous fractures, amenorrhea, cataracts, glaucoma, peptic ulcer disease, and CHF.

• The ophthalmic form may cause glaucoma, ocular hypertension, and cataracts.

• Abrupt withdrawal following long-term therapy may cause severe joint pain, severe headache, anorexia, nausea, fever, rebound inflammation, fatigue, weakness, lethargy, dizziness, and orthostatic hypotension.

PRECAUTIONS & CONSIDERATIONS

Caution is warranted with cirrhosis, CHF, diabetes mellitus, high thromboembolic risk, hypertension, hyperthyroidism, ocular herpes simplex, osteoporosis, peptic ulcer disease, respiratory tuberculosis, seizure disorders, ulcerative colitis, and untreated systemic infections. The ophthalmic form should be used cautiously in long-term therapy because prolonged use may result in cataracts or glaucoma. Dexamethasone crosses the placenta and is distributed in breast milk. Prolonged treatment with high dosages may decrease the short-term growth rate and cortisol secretion in children. The elderly are at higher risk for developing hypertension or osteoporosis. Severe stress, including serious infection, surgery, or trauma, may require an increase in dexamethasone dosage. Dentists or other physicians should be informed of dexamethasone therapy of if taken within the past 12 months.

Mood swings, ranging from euphoria to depression, may occur. Notify the physician of fever, muscle aches, sore throat, and sudden weight gain or swelling. Blood glucose level, intake and output, B/P, serum electrolyte levels, height, and weight should be monitored before and during therapy. Be alert to signs and symptoms of infection caused by reduced immune response, including fever, sore throat, and vague symptoms. In long-term therapy, signs and symptoms of hypocalcemia (such as muscle twitching, cramps, and positive Chvostek's or Trousseau's signs) or hypokalemia (such as EKG changes, nausea and vomiting, irritability, weakness and muscle cramps, and numbness or tingling, especially in the lower extremities) should be assessed.

Administration

Take oral dexamethasone with milk or food. Do not abruptly discontinue the drug or change the dosage or schedule.

! Dexamethasone sodium phosphate may be given by IV push or IV infusion.

For IV push, give over 1 to 4 minutes. For IV infusion, mix with 0.9% NaCl or D_5W and infuse over 15 to 30 minutes. If administering to a neonate, solution must be preservative free. IV solution must be used within 24 hours.

May give deep IM, preferably in the gluteus maximus.

For ophthalmic use, to administer the solution or ointment, place a gloved finger on the lower eyelid and pull it out until a pocket is formed between the eye and lower lid. Hold the dropper above the pocket and place the correct number of drops (or one-quarter to half-inch ointment) into the pocket. Close the eye gently. For the ophthalmic solution, apply digital pressure to the lacrimal sac for 1 to 2 minutes to minimize the drainage to the nose and throat, thereby reducing the risk of systemic effects. For the ophthalmic ointment, close the eye for 1 to 2 minutes.

Roll the eyeball to increase the contact area of drug to eye. Remove excess solution or ointment around the eye with a tissue. Use ointment at night to reduce the frequency of solution administration. Expect to taper the dosage slowly when discontinuing the drug.

For topical use, gently cleanse the area before applying the drug. Apply sparingly and rub into area thoroughly after bath or shower for best absorption. Use occlusive dressings only as ordered.

Dexchlorpheniramine
dex′klor-fen-eer′a-meen
(Polaramine, Polaramine Repetabs)

CATEGORY AND SCHEDULE
Pregnancy Risk Category: B

CLASSIFICATION
Antihistamines, H1

MECHANISM OF ACTION
A propylamine derivative that competes with histamine for H1-receptor sites on effector cells in the gastrointestinal (GI) tract, blood vessels, and respiratory tract. Dexchlorpheniramine is the dextro-isomer of chlorpheniramine and is approximately two times more active. *Therapeutic Effect:* Prevents allergic response, produces mild bronchodilation, blocks histamine-induced bronchitis.

PHARMACOKINETICS

Route	Onset	Peak	Duration
PO	0.5 hr	1-2 hr	3-6 hr

Well absorbed from the gastrointestinal (GI) tract. Protein binding: 70%. Widely distributed. Metabolized in liver to active metabolite, undergoes extensive first-pass metabolism. Excreted primarily in urine. Not removed by hemodialysis. **Half-life:** 20 hr.

AVAILABILITY
Tablets: 2 mg (Polaramine [DSC]).
Extended-Release Tablets: 4 mg, 6 mg (Polaramine Repetabs).
Syrup: 2 mg/5 ml (Polaramine).

INDICATIONS AND DOSAGES
▶ **Allergic rhinitis, common cold**
PO
Adults, Elderly, Children 12 yr or older. 2 mg q4-6hr or 4-6 mg timed release at bedtime or q8-10hr.
Children 6-11 yr. 4 mg timed release at bedtime or 1 mg q4-6hr.
Children 2-5 yr. 0.5 mg q4-6hr. Do not use timed release.

OFF-LABEL USES
Asthma, chemotherapy-induced stomatitis, dermographia, familial immunodeficiency disease, malaria, mastocytosis, Meniere's disease, nausea, neurocysticercosis, otitis media, psoriasis, radiocontrast media reactions, urticaria

CONTRAINDICATIONS
History of hypersensitivity to anti-histamines, newborn or premature infants, nursing mothers, third trimester of pregnancy

INTERACTIONS
Drug
Alcohol, central nervous system (CNS) depressants: May increase CNS depression.
Methacholine: May interfere with interpretation of pulmonary function

404   Dexmedetomidine Hydrochloride

tests after a methacholine bronchial challenge.
Procarbazine: May increase CNS depression.
Herbal
None known.
Food
None known.

DIAGNOSTIC TEST EFFECTS
May interfere with the interpretation of the pulmonary function tests after a methacholine bronchial challenge test.

SIDE EFFECTS
Frequent
Drowsiness; dizziness; headache; dry mouth, nose, or throat; urinary retention; thickening of bronchial secretions; sedation; hypotension
Occasional
Epigastric distress, flushing, blurred vision, tinnitus, paresthesia, sweating, chills

SERIOUS REACTIONS
• Children may experience dominant paradoxical reactions, including restlessness, insomnia, euphoria, nervousness, and tremors.
• Hypersensitivity reaction, such as eczema, pruritus, rash, cardiac disturbances, and photosensitivity, may occur.
• Overdosage may vary from CNS depression, including sedation, apnea, hypotension, cardiovascular collapse, or death to severe paradoxical reaction, such as hallucinations, tremor, and seizures.

PRECAUTIONS & CONSIDERATIONS
Caution is warranted with asthma, chronic obstructive pulmonary disease (COPD), narrow-angle glaucoma, peptic ulcer disease, prostatic hypertrophy, pyloro-duodenal or bladder

neck obstruction, and severe CNS depression or coma. Be aware that timed release tablets should be avoided in children 5 years and younger. It is unknown if dexchlorpheniramine crosses the placenta or is distributed in breast milk. Dexchlorpheniramine should not be used in patients during the third trimester of pregnancy. There are no age-related precautions noted in the elderly.

Dizziness, drowsiness, and dry mouth are expected side effects of dexchlorpheniramine. Tasks that require mental alertness or motor skills should be avoided until the effects are established. Alcohol should be avoided during therapy.
Administration
Take without regard to meals.

Dexmedetomidine Hydrochloride
decks-meh-deh-tome'-ih-deen
(Precedex)
Do not confuse Precedex with Peridex or Percocet.

CATEGORY AND SCHEDULE
Pregnancy Risk Category: C

CLASSIFICATION
Adrenergic agonists, sedatives/hypnotics

MECHANISM OF ACTION
A selective alpha$_2$-adrenergic agonist. *Therapeutic Effect:* Produces analgesic, hypnotic, and sedative effects.

AVAILABILITY
Injection: 100 mcg/ml.

INDICATIONS AND DOSAGES
▶ **Sedation before, during, and after intubation and mechanical ventilation while in ICU**
IV
Adults. Loading dose of 1 mcg/kg over 10 min followed by maintenance infusion of 0.2-0.7 mcg/kg/hr.
Elderly. May require decreased dosage. No guidelines available.

CONTRAINDICATIONS
None known.

INTERACTIONS
Drug
Anesthetics, opioids, other sedative-hypnotics: May enhance the effects of dexmedetomidine.
Herbal
None known.
Food
None known.

DIAGNOSTIC TEST EFFECTS
May increase serum potassium, alkaline phosphatase, AST (SGOT), and ALT (SGPT) levels.

▓IV INCOMPATIBILITIES
Do not mix dexmedetomidine with any other medications.

SIDE EFFECTS
Frequent
Hypotension (30%), nausea (11%)
Occasional (3%-2%)
Pain, fever, oliguria, thirst

SERIOUS REACTIONS
• Bradycardia, atrial fibrillation, hypoxia, anemia, pain, and pleural effusion may occur with too-rapid IV infusion.

PRECAUTIONS & CONSIDERATIONS
Caution is warranted with CHF, advanced heart block, hypovolemia,

hepatic or renal impairment, and those on a continuous cardiac monitor and pulse oximeter. Be aware that dexmedetomidine will provide relaxation and sedation before, during, and after insertion of the endotracheal tube, and during mechanical ventilation. Comfort measures, such as mouth care and repositioning, should be provided.

Before dexmedetomidine use, baseline vital signs, EKG, and liver function tests should be obtained. EKG for atrial fibrillation, B/P for hypotension and level of sedation, pulse rate for bradycardia, and respiratory rate and rhythm should be monitored during therapy.
Storage
Store vials at room temperature.
Administration
! Dilute dexmedetomidine with 48 ml 0.9% NaCl before use. Don't infuse the drug for longer than 24 hours.

For IV use, dilute 2 ml of dexmedetomidine with 48 ml of 0.9% NaCl. Administer the drug as a maintenance infusion, as prescribed.

Dexmethylphenidate
dex-meth-ill-fen'i-date
(Focalin)

CATEGORY AND SCHEDULE
Pregnancy Risk Category: C
Controlled Substance Schedule: II

CLASSIFICATION
Stimulants, central nervous system

MECHANISM OF ACTION

A CNS stimulant that blocks the reuptake of norepinephrine and dopamine into presynaptic neurons, increasing the release of these neurotransmitters into the synaptic cleft. *Therapeutic Effect:* Decreases motor restlessness and fatigue; increases motor activity, mental alertness, and attention span; elevates mood.

PHARMACOKINETICS

Route	Onset	Peak	Duration
PO	N/A	N/A	4-5 hr

Readily absorbed from the GI tract. Plasma concentrations increase rapidly. Metabolized in the liver. Excreted unchanged in urine.
Half-life: 2.2 hr.

AVAILABILITY

Tablets: 2.5 mg, 5 mg, 10 mg.

INDICATIONS AND DOSAGES

▶ **Attention deficit hyperactivity disorder (ADHD)**
PO
Patients new to dexmethylphenidate or methylphenidate. 2.5 mg twice a day (5 mg/day). May adjust dosage in 2.5- to 5-mg increments. Maximum: 20 mg/day.
Patients currently taking methylphenidate. Half the methylphenidate dosage. Maximum: 20 mg/day.

CONTRAINDICATIONS

Diagnosis or family history of Tourette syndrome; glaucoma; history of marked agitation, anxiety, or tension; motor tics; use within 14 days of MAOIs

INTERACTIONS

Drug
Amitriptyline, phenobarbital, phenytoin, primidone: Dosage of these drugs may need to be decreased.
MAOIs: May increase the effects of dexmethylphenidate.
Other CNS stimulants: May have an additive effect.
Warfarin: May inhibit the metabolism of warfarin.
Herbal
None known.
Food
None known.

DIAGNOSTIC TEST EFFECTS

None known.

SIDE EFFECTS

Frequent
Abdominal pain, nausea, anorexia, fever
Occasional
Tachycardia, arrhythmias, palpitations, insomnia, twitching
Rare
Blurred vision, rash, arthralgia, insomnia

SERIOUS REACTIONS

• Withdrawal after prolonged therapy may unmask symptoms of the underlying disorder.
• Dexmethylphenidate may lower the seizure threshold in those with a history of seizures.
• Overdose produces excessive sympathomimetic effects, including vomiting, tremor, hyperreflexia, seizures, confusion, hallucinations, and diaphoresis.
• Prolonged administration to children may delay growth.

PRECAUTIONS & CONSIDERATIONS

Caution is warranted with cardiovascular disease, psychosis, seizure disorders, and history of substance abuse. It is unknown if dexmethylphenidate is excreted in breast milk. Children are more prone to develop abdominal pain, insomnia, anorexia, and weight loss. Long-term dexmethylphenidate use may inhibit growth in children. In psychotic children, dexmethylphenidate use may exacerbate behavior disturbances and abnormal thoughts. No age-related precautions have been noted in the elderly.

Tasks that require mental alertness and motor skills should be avoided until response to the drug is established. CBC, WBC count with differential, and platelet should be monitored. Baseline height and weight should be obtained at the beginning and periodically throughout therapy.

Administration
Take dexmethylphenidate without regard to food. Crush tablets as needed. Take the last dose of the day several hours before bedtime to prevent insomnia.

Dextran; Dextrose
dex′tran
(Gentran, Rheomacrodex [CAN])
Do not confuse with Genprine.

CATEGORY AND SCHEDULE
Pregnancy Risk Category: C

CLASSIFICATION
Plasma expanders

MECHANISM OF ACTION
A branched polysaccharide that produces plasma volume expansion due to high colloidal osmotic effect. Draws interstitial fluid into the intravascular space. May also increase blood flow in microcirculation. *Therapeutic Effect:* Increases central venous pressure, cardiac output, stroke volume, B/P, urine output, capillary perfusion, and pulse pressure. Decreases heart rate, peripheral resistance, and blood viscosity. Corrects hypovolemia.

AVAILABILITY
Injection (High Molecular Weight [Gentran]): 6% dextran 70 in 500 ml 0.9% NaCl.
Injection (Low Molecular Weight [Gentran LMD]): 10% dextran 40 in 500 ml D_5W, 10% dextran 40 in 500 ml 0.9% NaCl.

INDICATIONS AND DOSAGES
▶ **Volume expansion, shock**
IV
Adults, Elderly. 500-1000 ml at a rate of 20-40 ml/min. Maximum: 20 ml/kg for first 24 hr, and 10 ml/kg thereafter.
Children. Total dose not to exceed 20 ml/kg on day 1 and 10 ml/kg/day thereafter.

CONTRAINDICATIONS
Hypervolemia, renal failure, severe bleeding disorders, severe CHF, severe thrombocytopenia

INTERACTIONS
Drug
None known.
Herbal
None known.
Food
None known.

DIAGNOSTIC TEST EFFECTS
Prolongs bleeding time and depresses platelet count. Decreases clotting factors V, VIII, and IX.

🔲 IV INCOMPATIBILITIES
Do not add medications to dextran solution.

SIDE EFFECTS
Occasional
Mild hypersensitivity reaction, including urticaria, nasal congestion, wheezing

SERIOUS REACTIONS
- Severe or fatal anaphylaxis, manifested by marked hypotension and cardiac or respiratory arrest, may occur early during IV infusion, generally in those not previously exposed to IV dextran.

PRECAUTIONS & CONSIDERATIONS
Caution is warranted with chronic hepatic disease and extreme dehydration. Females may experience a heavier menstrual flow than usual. An electric razor and soft toothbrush should be used to prevent bleeding during dextran therapy. Do not take any medications, including OTC drugs (especially aspirin), without physician approval.

Notify the physician of bleeding from the surgical site, chest pain, dyspnea, black or red stool, coffee-ground emesis, dark or red urine, or red-speckled mucus from cough. Urine output, vital signs, and laboratory values, such as bleeding time, platelet count, and clotting factors, should be monitored. CVP should also be assessed to detect blood volume overexpansion. Be aware of signs and symptoms of fluid overload, such as peripheral or pulmonary edema, and impending CHF.

Storage
Store at room temperature. Use only clear solutions, and discard partially used containers.

Administration
! Therapy should not continue longer than 5 days.

Give by IV infusion only. Monitor closely during first 15 minutes of infusion for anaphylactic reaction.

Monitor vital signs every 5 minutes. Monitor urine flow rate during administration. Discontinue dextran 40 and give an osmotic diuretic, as prescribed, if oliguria or anuria occurs to minimize vascular overloading. If dextran is given by rapid injection, monitor central venous pressure (CVP). Immediately discontinue the drug and notify the physician if CVP rises precipitously. Monitor B/P diligently during infusion. Stop the infusion immediately if marked hypotension occurs, a sign of imminent anaphylactic reaction. If evidence of blood volume overexpansion occurs, discontinue the drug until blood volume is adjusted by diuresis.

Dextroamphetamine
dex-troe-am-fet´a-meen
(Dexamphetamine [AUS], Dexedrine, Dexedrine Spansule, Dextrostat)
Do not confuse dextroamphetamine with dextromethorphan, or Dexedrine with Dextran or Excedrin.

CATEGORY AND SCHEDULE
Pregnancy Risk Category: C
Controlled Substance Schedule: II

CLASSIFICATION
Adrenergic agonists, amphetamines, stimulants, central nervous system

MECHANISM OF ACTION
An amphetamine that enhances the action of dopamine and norepinephrine by blocking their

reuptake from synapses; also inhibits monoamine oxidase and facilitates the release of catecholamines.
Therapeutic Effect: Increases motor activity and mental alertness; decreases motor restlessness, drowsiness, and fatigue; suppresses appetite.

AVAILABILITY

Capsules, sustained-release (Dexedrine, Spansule): 5 mg, 10 mg, 15 mg.
Tablets (Dexedrine): 5 mg.
Tablets (Dextrostat): 5 mg, 10 mg.

INDICATIONS AND DOSAGES
▸ **Narcolepsy**
PO
Adults, Children older than 12 yr. Initially, 10 mg/day. Increase by 10 mg/day at weekly intervals until therapeutic response is achieved.
Children 6-12 yr. Initially, 5 mg/day. Increase by 5 mg/day at weekly intervals until therapeutic response is achieved. Maximum: 60 mg/day.
▸ **Attention deficit hyperactivity disorder (ADHD)**
PO
Children 6 yr and older. Initially, 5 mg once or twice a day. Increase by 5 mg/day at weekly intervals until therapeutic response is achieved.
Children 3-5 yr. Initially, 2.5 mg/day. Increase by 2.5 mg/day at weekly intervals until therapeutic response is achieved. Maximum: 40 mg/day.
▸ **Appetite suppressant**
PO
Adults. 5-30 mg daily in divided doses of 5-10 mg each, given 30-60 min before meals; or 1 extended-release capsule in the morning.

CONTRAINDICATIONS
Advanced arteriosclerosis, agitated states, glaucoma, history of drug abuse, hypersensitivity to sympathomimetic amines, hyperthyroidism, moderate to severe hypertension, symptomatic cardiovascular disease, use within 14 days of MAOIs

INTERACTIONS
Drug
Beta-blockers: May increase the risk of bradycardia, heart block, and hypertension.
Digoxin: May increase the risk of arrhythmias.
MAOIs: May prolong and intensify the effects of dextroamphetamine.
Meperidine: May increase the risk of hypotension, respiratory depression, seizures, and vascular collapse.
Other CNS stimulants: May increase the effects of dextroamphetamine.
Thyroid hormones: May increase the effects of either drug.
Tricyclic antidepressants: May increase cardiovascular effects.
Herbal
None known.
Food
None known.

DIAGNOSTIC TEST EFFECTS
May increase plasma corticosteroid concentrations.

SIDE EFFECTS
Frequent
Irregular pulse, increased motor activity, talkativeness, nervousness, mild euphoria, insomnia
Occasional
Headache, chills, dry mouth, GI distress, worsening depression in patients who are clinically depressed, tachycardia, palpitations, chest pain, dizziness, decreased appetite

SERIOUS REACTIONS
• Overdose may produce skin pallor or flushing, arrhythmias, and psychosis.

• Abrupt withdrawal after prolonged use of high doses may produce lethargy lasting for weeks.
• Prolonged administration to children with ADHD may inhibit growth.

PRECAUTIONS & CONSIDERATIONS

Caution is warranted in debilitated, elderly, and those who are tartrazine-sensitive. Mental status, B/P, and weight should be assessed. Tasks that require mental alertness or motor skills should be avoided until response to the drug has been established. Notify the physician if decreased appetite, dizziness, dry mouth, or pronounced nervousness occurs.

Administration

Take the last dose of the day several hours before bedtime to prevent insomnia. Tolerance to the drug's appetite suppressant and mood-elevating effects usually occurs within a few weeks.

Dextromethorphan

dex-troe-meth-or'fan
(Babee Cof Syrup, Benylin Adult, Benylin Pediatric, Creomulsion Cough, Creomulsion for Children, Creo-Terpin, Delsym, Dexalone, ElixSure Cough, Hold DM, PediaCare Infants' Long-Acting Cough, Robitussion [AUS], Robitussin CoughGels, Robitussin Honey Cough, Robitussin Maximum Strength Cough, Robitussin Pediatric Cough, Scot-Tussin DM Cough Chasers, Silphen DM, Simply Cough, Vicks 44 Cough Relief)

CATEGORY AND SCHEDULE

Pregnancy Risk Category: C
OTC

CLASSIFICATION

Antitussive

MECHANISM OF ACTION

A chemical relative of morphine without the narcotic properties that acts on the cough center in the medulla oblongata by elevating the threshold for coughing. *Therapeutic Effect:* Suppresses cough.

PHARMACOKINETICS

Rapidly absorbed from the gastrointestinal (GI) tract. Distributed into cerebrospinal fluid (CSF). Extensively and poorly metabolized in liver to dextrorphan (active metabolite). Excreted unchanged in urine. **Half-life:** 1.4-3.9 hr (parent compound), 3.4-5.6 hr (dextrorphan).

AVAILABILITY
Gelcap: 15 mg (Robitussin
CoughGels), 30 mg (Dexalone).
Liquid: 5 mg/5 ml (Simply Cough),
10 mg/5 ml (Vicks Cough Relief),
10 mg/15 ml (Creo-Terpin).
Liquid drops: 7.5 mg/0.8 ml
(PediaCare Infants' Long-Acting
Cough).
Lozenges: 5 mg (Hold DM, Scot-
Tussin DM Cough Chasers).
Suspension (extended-release):
30 mg/5 ml (Delsym).
Syrup: 7.5 mg/5 ml (Babee Cof
Syrup, Benylin Pediatric, ElixSure,
Robitussin Pediatric Cough),
10 mg/5 ml (Robitussin Honey
Cough, Silphen DM), 15 mg/5 ml
(Benylin Adult, Robitussin
Maximum Strength Cough),
20 mg/15 ml (Creomulsion Cough,
Creomulsion for Children)

INDICATIONS AND DOSAGES
▸ **Cough**
PO
*Adults, Elderly, Children 12 yr
and older.* 10-20 mg q4hr.
Maximum: 120 mg/day.
Children 6- 12 yr. 5-10 mg q4hr.
Maximum: 60 mg/day.
Children 2-5 yr. 2.5-5 mg q4hr.
Maximum: 30 mg/day.

OFF-LABEL USES
N-methyl-D-aspartate (NMDA)
antagonist in cerebral injury

CONTRAINDICATIONS
Coadministration with monoamine
oxidase inhibitors (MAOIs), hypersensitivity to dextromethorphan or
its components

INTERACTIONS
Drug
**MAOIs, phenelzine, SSRIs,
sibutramine:** May increase the risk
of serotonin syndrome.

Haloperidol, quinidine: May
increase adverse effects associated
with dextromethorphan.
Herbal
None known.
Food
None known.

DIAGNOSTIC TEST EFFECTS
None known.

SIDE EFFECTS
Rare
Abdominal discomfort, constipation,
dizziness, drowsiness, GI upset,
nausea

SERIOUS REACTIONS
• Overdosage may result in muscle
spasticity, increase or decrease in
blood pressure (B/P), blurred vision,
blue fingernails and lips, nausea,
vomiting, hallucinations, and respiratory depression.

PRECAUTIONS & CONSIDERATIONS
Be aware that dextromethorphan
should not be used for chronic and
persistent cough accompanying a
disease state or cough associated
with excessive secretions. It is
unknown if dextromethorphan
crosses the placenta or is distributed
in breast milk. Be aware that
dextromethorphan is not recommended in children younger than
2 years of age. There are no age-
related precautions noted in the
elderly. If fever, rash, headache,
or sore throat persists, notify the
physician.
Storage
Store syrup, suspension, liquid,
lozenges, or gelcaps at room
temperature.
Administration
Give dextromethorphan without
regard to meals.

Diazepam

dye-az′e-pam
(Antenex [AUS],
Apo-Diazepam [CAN],
Diastat, Diazemuls [CAN],
Dizac, Ducene [AUS],
Valium, Valpam [AUS],
Vivol [CAN])

**Do not confuse diazepam
with diazoxide or
Ditropan, or Valium with
Valcyte.**

CATEGORY AND SCHEDULE

Pregnancy Risk Category: D
Controlled Substance:
Schedule IV

CLASSIFICATION

Anxiolytics, benzodiazepines,
relaxants, skeletal muscle

MECHANISM OF ACTION

A benzodiazepine that depresses
all levels of the CNS by enhancing
the action of gamma-aminobutyric
acid, a major inhibitory neurotransmitter in the brain. *Therapeutic
Effect:* Produces anxiolytic
effect, elevates the seizure
threshold, produces skeletal muscle
relaxation.

PHARMACOKINETICS

Route	Onset	Peak	Duration
PO	30 min	1-2 hr	2-3 hr
IV	1-5 min	15 min	15-60 min
IM	15 min	30-90 min	30-90 min

Well absorbed from the GI tract.
Widely distributed. Protein binding:
98%. Metabolized in the liver to
active metabolite. Excreted in urine.
Minimally removed by hemodialysis.

Half-life: 20-70 hr (increased in
hepatic dysfunction and the elderly).

AVAILABILITY

*Oral Concentrate (Diazepam
Intensol):* 5 mg/ml.
Oral Solution: 5 mg/5 ml.
Tablets (Valium): 2 mg, 5 mg, 10 mg.
Injection: 5 mg/ml.
Rectal Gel (Diastat): 5 mg/ml.

INDICATIONS AND DOSAGES
▸ **Anxiety, skeletal muscle
relaxation**
PO
Adults. 2-10 mg 2-4 times a day.
Elderly. 2.5 mg twice a day.
Children. 0.12-0.8 mg/kg/day in
divided doses q6-8hr.
IV, IM
Adults. 2-10 mg repeated in
3-4 hr.
Children. 0.04-0.3 mg/kg/dose
q2-4hr. Maximum: 0.5 mg/kg in an
8-hr period.
▸ **Preanesthesia**
IV
Adults, Elderly. 5-15 mg 5-10 min
before procedure.
Children. 0.2-0.3 mg/kg. Maximum:
10 mg.
▸ **Alcohol withdrawal**
PO
Adults, Elderly. 10 mg 3-4 times
during first 24 hr, then reduced to
5-10 mg 3-4 times a day as needed.
IV, IM
Adults, Elderly. Initially, 10 mg,
followed by 5-10 mg q3-4hr.
▸ **Status epilepticus**
IV
Adults, Elderly. 5-10 mg q10-15 min
up to 30 mg/8 hr.
Children 5 yr and older. 0.05-0.3 mg/
kg/dose q15-30 min. Maximum:
10 mg/dose.
Children 1 mo to younger than 5 yr.
0.05-0.3 mg/kg/dose q15-30 min.
Maximum: 5 mg/dose.

▸ **Control of increased seizure activity in patients with refractory epilepsy who are on stable regimens of anticonvulsants**
RECTAL GEL
Adults, Children 12 yr and older.
0.2 mg/kg; may be repeated in 4-12 hr.
Children 6-11 yr. 0.3 mg/kg; may be repeated in 4-12 hr.
Children 2-5 yr. 0.5 mg/kg; may be repeated in 4-12 hr.

OFF-LABEL USES
Treatment of panic disorder, tension headache, tremors

CONTRAINDICATIONS
Angle-closure glaucoma, coma, pre-existing CNS depression, respiratory depression, severe, uncontrolled pain

INTERACTIONS
Drug
Alcohol, other CNS depressants: May increase CNS depression.
Herbal
Kava kava, valerian: May increase CNS depression.
Food
None known.

DIAGNOSTIC TEST EFFECTS
May elevate serum LDH, alkaline phosphatase, bilirubin, AST (SGOT), and ALT (SGPT) levels. May produce abnormal renal function test results. Therapeutic serum drug level is 0.5-2 mcg/ml; toxic serum drug level is greater than 3 mcg/ml.

▧ IV INCOMPATIBILITIES
Amphotericin B complex (Abelcet, AmBisome, Amphotec), cefepime (Maxipime), diltiazem (Cardizem), fluconazole (Diflucan), foscarnet (Foscavir), heparin, hydrocortisone (Solu-Cortef), hydromorphone (Dilaudid), meropenem

(Merrem IV), potassium chloride, propofol (Diprivan), vitamins
▧ IV Compatibilities
Dobutamine (Dobutrex), fentanyl, morphine

SIDE EFFECTS
Frequent
Pain with IM injection, somnolence, fatigue, ataxia
Occasional
Slurred speech, orthostatic hypotension, headache, hypoactivity, constipation, nausea, blurred vision
Rare
Paradoxical CNS reactions, such as hyperactivity or nervousness in children and excitement or restlessness in the elderly or debilitated (generally noted during first 2 weeks of therapy, particularly in presence of uncontrolled pain)

SERIOUS REACTIONS
• IV administration may produce pain, swelling, thrombophlebitis, and carpal tunnel syndrome.
• Abrupt or too-rapid withdrawal may result in pronounced restlessness, irritability, insomnia, hand tremor, abdominal or muscle cramps, diaphoresis, vomiting, and seizures.
• Abrupt withdrawal in patients with epilepsy may produce an increase in the frequency or severity of seizures.
• Overdose results in somnolence, confusion, diminished reflexes, and coma.

PRECAUTIONS & CONSIDERATIONS
Caution is warranted with hypoalbuminemia, hepatic and renal impairment, and in those who are taking other CNS depressants. Diazepam crosses the placenta and is distributed in breast milk. Diazepam may increase the risk of fetal abnormalities if administered during the first

trimester of pregnancy. Chronic diazepam use during pregnancy may produce withdrawal symptoms in the patient and CNS depression in the neonate. For children and the elderly, expect to administer a reduced dose initially and to increase dosage gradually to prevent ataxia and excessive sedation. Females should use effective contraception during therapy and notify the physician immediately if they become or suspect they are pregnant.

Drowsiness and dizziness may occur. Change positions slowly from recumbent to sitting, before standing to prevent dizziness. Alcohol, caffeine, and tasks that require mental alertness or motor skills should also be avoided. Autonomic responses, such as cold, clammy hands and diaphoresis, and motor responses, such as agitation, trembling, and tension, should be assessed. Seizure frequency and intensity should be assessed. B/P, pulse rate, and respiratory rate, rhythm, and depth should be obtained immediately before giving diazepam. The duration, location, onset, and type of pain should be recorded and immobility, stiffness, and swelling should be assessed in those being treated for musculoskeletal spasm.

Storage
Store unopened vials at room temperature.

Administration
Take oral diazepam without regard to food. Crush tablets as needed, but don't crush or break capsules. Dilute the oral concentrate with juice, water, or a carbonated beverage or mix it with a semisolid food, such as applesauce or pudding.

For IV use, administer IV push into the tubing of a free-flowing IV solution as close to the vein insertion point as possible. Administer directly into a large vein to reduce the risk of phlebitis and thrombosis. Don't use small veins, such as those of the wrist or dorsum of hand. Administer IV at a rate not exceeding 5 mg/minute. For children, give over a 3-minute period because a too-rapid IV may result in hypotension and respiratory depression. Monitor respirations every 5-15 minutes for 2 hours. Stay recumbent for up to 3 hours after parenteral administration to reduce the drug's hypotensive effect.

For IM use, inject the IM dose deep into the deltoid muscle. IM injection may be painful.

! For rectal use, don't administer the rectal gel more often than once every 5 days or 5 times a month.

Diclofenac
dye-kloe′fen-ak
(Cataflam, Diclohexal [AUS], Diclotek [CAN], Fenac [AUS], Novo-Difenac [CAN], Solaraze, Voltaren, Voltaren Emulgel [AUS], Voltaren Ophthalmic, Voltaren Rapid [AUS], Voltaren XR)
Do not confuse diclofenac with Diflucan or Duphalac, or Voltaren with Verelan.

CATEGORY AND SCHEDULE
Pregnancy Risk Category: B (D if used in third trimester or near delivery; C for ophthalmic solution)

CLASSIFICATION
Analgesics, non-narcotic, nonsteroidal anti-inflammatory drugs, ophthalmics

MECHANISM OF ACTION

An NSAID that inhibits prostaglandin synthesis, reducing the intensity of pain. Also constricts the iris sphincter. May inhibit angiogenesis (the formation of blood vessels) by inhibiting substance P or blocking the angiogenic effects of prostaglandin E. *Therapeutic Effect:* Produces analgesic and anti-inflammatory effects. Prevents miosis during cataract surgery. May reduce angiogenesis in inflamed tissue.

PHARMACOKINETICS

Route	Onset	Peak	Duration
PO	30 min	2-3 hr	Up to 8 hr

Completely absorbed from the GI tract; penetrates cornea after ophthalmic administration (may be systemically absorbed). Protein binding: greater than 99%. Widely distributed. Metabolized in the liver. Primarily excreted in urine. Minimally removed by hemodialysis. **Half-life:** 1.2-2 hr.

AVAILABILITY

Topical Gel (Solaraze): 3%.
Tablets (Cataflam): 50 mg.
Tablets (Enteric-Coated [Voltaren]): 25 mg, 50 mg, 75 mg.
Tablets (Extended-Release [Voltaren XR]): 100 mg.
Ophthalmic Solution (Voltaren Ophthalmic): 0.1%.

INDICATIONS AND DOSAGES

▶ **Osteoarthritis**
PO (Cataflam, Voltaren)
Adults, Elderly. 50 mg 2-3 times a day.
PO (Voltaren XR)
Adults, Elderly. 100 mg/day as a single dose.
▶ **Rheumatoid arthritis**
PO (Cataflam, Voltaren)

Adults, Elderly. 50 mg 2-4 times a day. Maximum: 225 mg/day.
PO (Voltaren XR)
Adults, Elderly. 100 mg once a day. Maximum: 100 mg twice a day.
▶ **Ankylosing spondylitis**
PO (Voltaren)
Adults, Elderly. 100-125 mg/day in 4-5 divided doses.
▶ **Analgesia, primary dysmenorrhea**
PO (Cataflam)
Adults, Elderly. 30 mg 3 times a day.
▶ **Usual pediatric dosage**
Children. 2-3 mg/kg/day in 2-4 divided doses.
▶ **Actinic keratoses**
TOPICAL
Adults, Adolescents. Apply twice a day to lesion for 60-90 days.
▶ **Cataract surgery**
OPHTHALMIC
Adults, Elderly. Apply 1 drop to eye 4 times a day commencing 24 hr after cataract surgery. Continue for 2 wk afterward.
▶ **Pain, relief of photophobia in patients undergoing corneal refractive surgery**
OPHTHALMIC
Adults, Elderly. Apply 1 drop to affected eye 1 hr before surgery, within 15 min after surgery, then 4 times a day for 3 days.

OFF-LABEL USES

Treatment of vascular headaches (oral); to reduce the occurrence and severity of cystoid macular edema after cataract surgery (ophthalmic form)

CONTRAINDICATIONS

Hypersensitivity to aspirin, diclofenac, and other NSAIDs; porphyria

INTERACTIONS
Drug

Acetylcholine, carbachol: May decrease the effects of these drugs (with ophthalmic diclofenac).

Antihypertensives, diuretics: May decrease the effects of these drugs.

Aspirin, other salicylates: May increase the risk of GI side effects such as bleeding.

Bone marrow depressants: May increase the risk of hematologic reactions.

Epinephrine, other antiglaucoma medications: May decrease the antiglaucoma effect of these drugs.

Heparin, oral anticoagulants, thrombolytics: May increase the effects of these drugs.

Lithium: May increase the blood concentration and risk of toxicity of lithium.

Methotrexate: May increase the risk of methotrexate toxicity.

Probenecid: May increase diclofenac blood concentration.
Herbal

Ginkgo biloba: May increase the risk of bleeding.
Food

None known.

DIAGNOSTIC TEST EFFECTS

May increase BUN level; urine protein level; and serum LDH, potassium, alkaline phosphatase, creatinine, AST (SGOT), and ALT (SGPT) levels. May decrease serum uric acid level.

SIDE EFFECTS
Frequent (9%-4%)

PO: Headache, abdominal cramps, constipation, diarrhea, nausea, dyspepsia
Ophthalmic: Burning or stinging on instillation, ocular discomfort

Occasional (3%-1%)

PO: Flatulence, dizziness, epigastric pain
Ophthalmic: Ocular itching or tearing
Rare (less than 1%)

PO: Rash, peripheral edema or fluid retention, visual disturbances, vomiting, drowsiness

SERIOUS REACTIONS

- Overdose may result in acute renal failure.
- Rare reactions with long-term use include peptic ulcer disease, GI bleeding, gastritis, a severe hepatic reaction (jaundice), nephrotoxicity (hematuria, dysuria, proteinuria), and a severe hypersensitivity reaction (bronchospasm or angioedema).

PRECAUTIONS & CONSIDERATIONS

Caution is warranted with CHF, hypertension, hepatic or renal impairment, and history of GI disease. Don't use diclofenac topical gel on children, infants, or neonates. Avoid applying the gel around eyes or on open skin wounds, infected areas, or areas affected by exfoliative dermatitis. Diclofenac crosses the placenta; it is unknown if the drug is distributed in breast milk. Notify the physician of pregnancy. Diclofenac should not be used during the last trimester of pregnancy because it may cause adverse effects in the fetus, such as premature closure of the ductus arteriosus. The safety and efficacy of diclofenac have not been established in children. In the elderly, GI bleeding or ulceration is more likely to cause serious complications and age-related renal impairment may increase the risk of hepatotoxicity or renal toxicity; a decreased drug dosage is recommended. Avoid alcohol and aspirin during therapy because these

substances increase the risk of GI
bleeding.

Notify the physician of persistent
headache, black stools, changes in
vision, pruritus, rash, or weight gain.
Pattern of daily bowel activity and
stool consistency should be assessed.
Therapeutic response, such as
decreased pain, stiffness, swelling,
and tenderness, improved grip
strength, and increased joint
mobility, should be evaluated.

Administration
Don't crush or break enteric-coated
tablets. Take diclofenac with food,
milk, or antacids if GI distress
occurs.

For ophthalmic use, place a finger
on the lower eyelid, and pull it out
until a pocket is formed between the
eye and lower lid. Hold the dropper
above the pocket, and place the
prescribed number of drops in the
pocket. Gently close the eye, and
apply digital pressure to the lacrimal
sac for 1 to 2 minutes to minimize
drainage into the nose and throat,
reducing the risk of systemic effects.
Remove excess solution with a
tissue. Do not use hydrogel soft
contact lenses during ophthalmic
therapy.

Dicloxacillin
dye-klox´a-sill-in
(Dycil, Pathocil)
**Do not confuse with
dicyclomine.**

CATEGORY AND SCHEDULE
Pregnancy Risk Category: B

CLASSIFICATION
Antibiotics, penicillins

MECHANISM OF ACTION
A penicillin that acts as a bactericidal
in susceptible microorganisms.
Therapeutic Effect: Inhibits bacterial
cell wall synthesis.

PHARMACOKINETICS
Well absorbed from gastrointestinal
(GI) tract. Rate and extent reduced
by food. Distributed throughout
body including CSF. Protein binding:
96%. Partially metabolized in liver.
Primarily excreted in feces and
urine. Not removed by hemodialysis.
Half-life: 0.7 hr.

AVAILABILITY
Capsules: 250 mg, 500 mg (Dycil,
Pathocil).

INDICATIONS AND DOSAGES
▸ **Respiratory tract infection,
staphylococcal and streptococcal
infections**
PO
*Adults, Elderly, Children weighing
more than 40 kg.* 125-250 mg q6hr.
Children weighing less than 40 kg.
12.5-25 mg/kg/day q6hr.

CONTRAINDICATIONS
Hypersensitivity to any penicillin

INTERACTIONS
Drug
Allopurinol: May increase
incidence of rash.
Aminoglycosides: May decrease
aminoglycoside efficacy.
Oral contraceptives: May decrease
effects of oral contraceptives.
Probenecid: May increase amoxicillin blood concentration and risk
for dicloxacillin toxicity.
Warfarin: May decrease effects of
warfarin.

DIAGNOSTIC TEST EFFECTS
May cause positive Coombs' test.

SIDE EFFECTS

Frequent
Gastrointestinal (GI) disturbances (mild diarrhea, nausea, or vomiting), headache

Occasional
Generalized rash, urticaria

SERIOUS REACTIONS

• Altered bacterial balance may result in potentially fatal superinfections and antibiotic-associated colitis as evidenced by abdominal cramps, watery or severe diarrhea, and fever.
• Severe hypersensitivity reactions, including anaphylaxis and acute interstitial nephritis occur rarely.

PRECAUTIONS & CONSIDERATIONS

Be aware that dicloxacillin crosses the placenta and is distributed in breast milk in low concentrations. Be aware that dicloxacillin use should be avoided in neonates. There are no age-related precautions noted in the elderly. History of allergies, especially to cephalosporins or penicillins, should be determined before giving the drug. If diarrhea, rash, or symptoms occur during treatment, notify the physician.

Storage
Store at room temperature.

Administration
Take without regard to meals. Continue dicloxacillin for the full length of treatment.

Dicyclomine
dye-sye'kloe-meen
(Bentyl, Bentylol [CAN], Formulex [CAN], Lomine [CAN], Merbentyl [AUS])
Do not confuse dicyclomine with doxycycline or dyclomine, or Bentyl with Aventyl or Benadryl.

CATEGORY AND SCHEDULE
Pregnancy Risk Category: B

CLASSIFICATION
Anticholinergics, gastrointestinals

MECHANISM OF ACTION
A GI antispasmodic and anticholinergic agent that directly acts as a relaxant on smooth muscle. *Therapeutic Effect:* Reduces tone and motility of GI tract.

PHARMACOKINETICS

Route	Onset	Peak	Duration
PO	1-2 hr	N/A	4 hr

Readily absorbed from the GI tract. Widely distributed. Metabolized in the liver. **Half-life:** 9-10 hr.

AVAILABILITY
Capsules: 10 mg.
Tablets: 20 mg.
Syrup: 10 mg/5 ml.
Injection: 10 mg/ml.

INDICATIONS AND DOSAGES
▸ **Functional disturbances of GI motility**
PO
Adults. 10-20 mg 3-4 times a day up to 40 mg 4 times/day.

Children older than 2 yr. 10 mg
3-4 times a day.
Children 6 mo-2 yr. 5 mg 3-4 times
a day.
Elderly. 10-20 mg 4 times a day.
May increase up to 160 mg/day.
IM
Adults. 20 mg q4-6hr.

CONTRAINDICATIONS

Bladder neck obstruction due to
prostatic hyperplasia, coronary
vasospasm, intestinal atony,
myasthenia gravis in patients not
treated with neostigmine, narrow-
angle glaucoma, obstructive disease
of the GI tract, paralytic ileus, severe
ulcerative colitis, tachycardia
secondary to cardiac insufficiency or
thyrotoxicosis, toxic megacolon,
unstable cardiovascular status in
acute hemorrhage

INTERACTIONS
Drug
Antacids, antidiarrheals: May
decrease the absorption of dicyclomine.
Ketoconazole: May decrease the
absorption of ketoconazole.
Other anticholinergics:
May increase the effects of
dicyclomine.
Potassium chloride: May increase
the severity of GI lesions with the
wax matrix formulation of potassium
chloride.
Herbal
None known.
Food
None known.

DIAGNOSTIC TEST EFFECTS
None known.

SIDE EFFECTS
Frequent
Dry mouth (sometimes severe), constipation, diminished sweating ability

Occasional
Blurred vision; photophobia; urinary
hesitancy; somnolence (with high
dosage); agitation, excitement,
confusion, or somnolence noted in
elderly (even with low dosages);
transient light-headedness (with IM
route), irritation at injection site
(with IM route)
Rare
Confusion, hypersensitivity reaction,
increased IOP, nausea, vomiting,
unusual fatigue

SERIOUS REACTIONS
• Overdose may produce temporary
paralysis of ciliary muscle; pupillary
dilation; tachycardia; palpitations;
hot, dry, or flushed skin; absence of
bowel sounds; hyperthermia;
increased respiratory rate; EKG
abnormalities; nausea; vomiting;
rash over face or upper trunk; CNS
stimulation; and psychosis (marked
by agitation, restlessness, rambling
speech, visual hallucinations,
paranoid behavior, and delusions,
followed by depression).

PRECAUTIONS & CONSIDERATIONS
Extreme caution should be used with
autonomic neuropathy, diarrhea,
known or suspected GI infections,
and mild to moderate ulcerative
colitis. Caution is also warranted
with CHF, COPD, coronary artery
disease, esophageal reflux or hiatal
hernia associated with reflux
esophagitis, gastric ulcer, hyperthyroidism, hypertension, hepatic or
renal disease, tachyarrhythmias, and
in the elderly. It is unknown if
dicyclomine crosses the placenta or
is distributed in breast milk. Infants
and young children are more susceptible to the drug's toxic effects.
Dicyclomine use in the elderly may
cause agitation, confusion, somnolence, or excitement. Avoid hot

baths, saunas, and becoming over-heated while exercising in hot weather because this may cause heat stroke. Tasks that require mental alertness or motor skills should also be avoided until response to the drug has been established. Antacids or antidiarrheals should not be taken within 1 hour of taking dicyclomine because they will decrease dicyclomine's effectiveness.

B/P, body temperature, pattern of daily bowel activity and stool consistency, and hydration status should be monitored. The person should void before giving the drug to reduce the risk of urine retention.

Storage
Store capsules, tablets, syrup, and parenteral form at room temperature.

Administration
For oral use, dilute syrup with an equal volume of water just before administration. May give dicyclomine without regard to meals because food may slightly decrease absorption.

The injection normally appears colorless. Do not administer IV or subcutaneously. Inject IM deep in large muscle mass. Do not give for longer than 2 days, as prescribed.

Didanosine (ddl)
dye-dan′o-seen
(Videx, Videx-EC)

CATEGORY AND SCHEDULE
Pregnancy Risk Category: B

CLASSIFICATION
Antivirals, nucleoside reverse transcriptase inhibitors

MECHANISM OF ACTION
A purine nucleoside analogue that is intracellularly converted into a triphosphate, which interferes with RNA-directed DNA polymerase (reverse transcriptase). *Therapeutic Effect:* Inhibits replication of retroviruses, including HIV.

PHARMACOKINETICS
Variably absorbed from the GI tract. Protein binding: less than 5%. Rapidly metabolized intracellularly to active form. Primarily excreted in urine. Partially (20%) removed by hemodialysis. **Half-life:** 1.5 hr; metabolite: 8-24 hr.

AVAILABILITY
Capsules (Delayed-Release): 125 mg, 200 mg, 250 mg, 400 mg.
Pediatric Powder for Oral Solution: 10 mg/ml.
Powder for Oral Solution (Single-Dose Packet): 100 mg.
Tablets (Chewable): 25 mg, 50 mg, 100 mg, 150 mg, 200 mg.

INDICATIONS AND DOSAGES
▸ **HIV infection (in combination with other antiretrovirals)**
TABLETS (CHEWABLE)
Adults, children 13 yr and older weighing 60 kg or more. 200 mg q12hr or 400 mg once a day.
Adults, Children 13 yr and older weighing 60 kg or less. 125 mg q12hr or 250 mg once a day.
Children 3 mo to less than 13 yr. 180-300 mg/m^2/day in divided doses q12hr.
Children younger than 3 mo. 50 mg/m^2/day in divided doses q12hr.
DELAYED-RELEASE CAPSULES
Adults, Children 13 yr and older, weighing 60 kg or more. 400 mg once a day.

Adults, Children 13 yr and older,
weighing 60 kg or less. 250 mg
once a day.
ORAL SOLUTION
Adults, Children 13 yr and older
weighing 60 kg or more. 250 mg
q12hr.
Adults, Children 13 yr and older
weighing 60 kg or less. 167 mg
q12hr.
PEDIATRIC POWDER FOR ORAL
SOLUTION
Children 3 mo to younger than 13 yr.
180-300 mg/m^2/day in divided doses
q12hr.
Children younger than 3 mo.
50 mg/m^2/day in divided doses q12hr.
▸ **Dosage in renal impairment**
Patients weighing less than 60 kg:

CrCl	Tablets	Oral Solution	Delayed-Release Capsules
30-59 ml/min	75 mg twice a day	100 mg twice a day	125 mg once a day
10-29 ml/min	100 mg once a day	100 mg once a day	125 mg once a day
less than 10 ml/min	75 mg once a day	100 mg once a day	N/A

CrCl = creatinine clearance

Patients weighing 60 kg or more:

CrCl	Tablets	Oral Solution	Delayed-Release Capsules
30-59 ml/min	100 mg twice a day	100 mg twice a day	200 mg once a day
10-29 ml/min	150 mg once a day	167 mg once a day	125 mg once a day
Less than 10 ml/min	100 mg once a day	100 mg once a day	125 mg once a day

CrCl = creatinine clearance

CONTRAINDICATIONS
Hypersensitivity to didanosine or
any of its components

INTERACTIONS
Drug
Dapsone, fluoroquinolones,
itraconazole, ketoconazole,
tetracyclines: May decrease
absorption of these drugs.
Medications producing pancreati-
tis or peripheral neuropathy: May
increase the risk of pancreatitis or
peripheral neuropathy.
Stavudine: May increase the
risk of fatal lactic acidosis in
pregnancy.
Herbal
None known.
Food
All foods: Decreases absorption of
didanosine.

DIAGNOSTIC TEST EFFECTS
May increase serum alkaline phosphatase, amylase, bilirubin, lipase,
triglyceride, AST (SGOT), ALT
(SGPT), and uric acid levels. May
decrease serum potassium levels.

SIDE EFFECTS
Frequent
Adults (greater than 10%)
Diarrhea, neuropathy, chills and fever
Children (greater than 25%)
Chills, fever, decreased appetite,
pain, malaise, nausea, vomiting,
diarrhea, abdominal pain, headache,
nervousness, cough, rhinitis, dyspnea,
asthenia, rash, pruritus
Occasional
Adults (9%-2%)
Rash, pruritus, headache, abdominal
pain, nausea, vomiting, pneumonia,
myopathy, decreased appetite, dry
mouth, dyspnea
Children (25%-10%)
Failure to thrive, weight loss,
stomatitis, oral thrush, ecchymosis, ·

arthritis, myalgia, insomnia, epistaxis, pharyngitis

SERIOUS REACTIONS

• Pneumonia and opportunistic infections occur occasionally.
• Peripheral neuropathy, potentially fatal pancreatitis, retinal changes, and optic neuritis are the major toxic effects.

PRECAUTIONS & CONSIDERATIONS

Extreme caution should be used with history of pancreatitis. Caution is warranted with alcoholism, elevated triglycerides, renal or liver dysfunction, T-cell counts less than 100 cells/mm^3, and phenylketonuria and sodium-restricted diets because didanosine contains phenylalanine and sodium. Be aware that didanosine should be used during pregnancy only if clearly needed and that breastfeeding should be discontinued during didanosine therapy. Be aware that didanosine is well tolerated in children older than 3 months. In the elderly, age-related renal impairment may require dosage adjustment. Didanosine is not a cure for HIV infection, nor does it reduce risk of transmission to others. Avoid alcohol.

! Contact the physician if abdominal pain, elevated serum amylase or triglycerides, nausea, and vomiting before administering the medication occur because these symptoms may indicate pancreatitis. Assess for signs and symptoms of peripheral neuropathy, including burning feet, "restless leg syndrome" (unable to find comfortable position for legs and feet), and lack of coordination and for signs and symptoms of opportunistic infections, including cough or other respiratory symptoms, fever, or oral mucosa changes. Assess for nausea, abdominal pain, vomiting, and weight loss as well as visual or hearing difficulty. Expect to obtain baseline values for complete blood count (CBC), renal and liver function tests, vital signs, and weight.

Storage

Store at room temperature. Tablets dispersed in water are stable for 1 hour at room temperature; after reconstitution of buffered powder, oral solution is stable for 4 hours at room temperature. Pediatric powder for oral solution following reconstitution, as directed, is stable for 30 days refrigerated.

Administration

Take oral didanosine 1 hour before or 2 hours after meals because food decreases the rate and extent of didanosine absorption.

Thoroughly crush and disperse chewable tablets in at least 30 ml water before swallowing. Stir the mixture well (up to 2 to 3 minutes) and immediately swallow it. Reconstitute buffered powder for oral solution before giving it by pouring the contents of the packet into 4 oz of water; stir until completely dissolved (up to 2 to 3 minutes). Do not mix with fruit juice or other acidic liquid because didanosine is unstable with an acidic pH.

Add 100 to 200 ml water to 2 or 4 g of the unbuffered pediatric powder, respectively, to provide a concentration of 20 mg/ml. Immediately mix with an equal amount of an antacid to provide a concentration of 10 mg/ml. Shake thoroughly before removing each dose.

Swallow enteric-coated capsules whole; take them on an empty stomach.

Diethylpropion
die-ethyl-prop'ion
Tenuate, Tenuate Dospan

CATEGORY AND SCHEDULE
Pregnancy Risk Category: B
Controlled Substance:
Schedule IV

CLASSIFICATION
Anorexiants, stimulants, central
nervous system

MECHANISM OF ACTION
A sympathomimetic amine that stimulates the release of norepinephrine
and dopamine. *Therapeutic Effect:*
Decreases appetite.

PHARMACOKINETICS
Rapidly absorbed from the
gastrointestinal (GI) tract. Widely
distributed. Metabolized in liver to
active metabolite and undergoes
extensive first-pass metabolism.
Excreted in urine. Unknown if
removed by hemodialysis.
Half-life: 4-6 hr.

AVAILABILITY
Tablets: 25 mg (Tenuate).
Tablets (Extended-Release): 75 mg
(Tenuate Dospan).

INDICATIONS AND DOSAGES
▸ **Obesity**
PO
Adults. 25 mg 3 times/day before
meals. (Extended-Release) 75 mg at
midmorning.

OFF-LABEL USES
Migraines

CONTRAINDICATIONS
Agitated states, use of MAOIs
within 14 days, glaucoma, history
of drug abuse, hyperthyroidism,
advanced arteriosclerosis or severe
cardiovascular disease, severe
hypertension, and hypersensitivity
to sympathomimetic amines

INTERACTIONS
Drug
Anorectic agents: May increase
the risk of cardiac effects of diethyl-
propion.
Anesthetics: May increase the risk
of arrhythmias.
Antidiabetic agents, insulin: May
alter blood glucose concentrations.
Guanethidine: May decrease the
effects of guanethidine.
MAOIs: May increase the risk of
hypertensive crisis.
Phenothiazines: May decrease the
effects of diethylpropion.
Tricyclic antidepressants: May
increase the cardiac and CNS effects
of diethylpropion.
Herbal
None known.
Food
None known.

DIAGNOSTIC TEST EFFECTS
Urine screen for amphetamines.

SIDE EFFECTS
Frequent
Elevated blood pressure, nervous-
ness, insomnia
Occasional
Dizziness, drowsiness, tremor,
headache, nausea, stomach pain,
fever, rash
Rare
Agranulocytosis, leukopenia, blurred
vision, psychosis, CVA, seizure

SERIOUS REACTIONS
• Overdose may produce agitation,
tachycardia, palpitations, cardiac
irregularities, chest pain, psychotic
episode, seizures, and coma.

• Hypersensitivity reactions and blood dyscrasias occur rarely.

PRECAUTIONS & CONSIDERATIONS
Caution is required with diabetes, epilepsy, hypertension, and cardiovascular disease. Diethylpropion crosses the placenta and is distributed in breast milk. There are no age-related precautions noted in the elderly. Alcohol should be avoided during therapy.

Administration
Do not take in afternoon or evening because the drug can cause insomnia. Do not crush or break sustained-release capsules. Take 30 to 45 minutes before meals.

Diflorasone
die-floor'a-sone
(Florone [CAN], Maxiflor, Psorcon, Psorcon-e)

CATEGORY AND SCHEDULE
Pregnancy Risk Category: C

CLASSIFICATION
Corticosteroids, topical, dermatologics

MECHANISM OF ACTION
A high potency, fluorinated corticosteroid that decreases inflammation by suppression of migration of polymorphonuclear leukocytes and reversal of increased capillary permeability. The exact mechanism of the anti-inflammatory process is unclear. *Therapeutic Effect:* Decreases or prevents tissue response to the inflammatory process.

PHARMACOKINETICS
Poor absorption; occlusive dressings increase absorption. Metabolized in liver. Primarily excreted in urine.

AVAILABILITY
Cream: 0.05% (Maxiflor, Psorcon).
Ointment: 0.05% (Maxiflor, Psorcon).
Ointment, emollient: 0.05% (Psorcon-e).

INDICATIONS AND DOSAGES
▸ **Dermatoses**
TOPICAL
Adults, Elderly. (Cream) Apply sparingly 2-4 times/day. (Ointment) Apply sparingly 1-3 times/day.

OFF-LABEL USES
Psoriasis

CONTRAINDICATIONS
History of hypersensitivity to diflorasone or other corticosteroids

INTERACTIONS
Drug
None known.
Herbal
None known.
Food
None known.

DIAGNOSTIC TEST EFFECTS
None known.

SIDE EFFECTS
Rare
Itching, redness, dryness, irritation, burning at site of application, arthralgia, folliculitis, maceration, muscle atrophy, secondary infection

SERIOUS REACTIONS
• Overdosage symptoms include moon face, central obesity, hypertension, diabetes, hyperlipidemia, peptic ulcer, increased susceptibility to

infection, electrolyte and fluid imbalance, psychosis, and hallucinations.

• The serious reactions of long-term therapy and the addition of occlusive dressings are reversible hypothalamic-pituitary-adrenal (HPA) axis suppression, manifestations of Cushing's syndrome, hyperglycemia, and glucosuria.

PRECAUTIONS & CONSIDERATIONS

Caution should be used over large surface areas, with prolonged use, addition of occlusive dressings, and uncontrolled infections. Skin irritation should be reported. HPA axis suppression should be evaluated by ACTH stimulation test, AM plasma cortisol test, or urinary free cortisol test. It is unknown if diflorasone diacetate crosses the placenta or is distributed in the breast milk. Children may absorb larger amounts and may be more susceptible to toxicity. Safety and efficacy of diflorasone diacetate have not been established in children or the elderly.

Administration

Diflorasone diacetate ointments are recommended for dry, scaly lesions; creams are recommended for moist lesions. Gently cleanse area before application. Use occlusive dressings only as directed. Apply a thin film over affected area and rub into area gently and thoroughly.

Diflunisal
dye-floo′ni-sal
(Apo-Diflunisal [CAN], Dolobid, Novo-Diflunisal [CAN])
Do not confuse with Dicarbosil or Slo-bid.

CATEGORY AND SCHEDULE
Pregnancy Risk Category: C (D if used in third trimester or near delivery)

CLASSIFICATION
Analgesics, non-narcotic, salicylates

MECHANISM OF ACTION
A nonsteroidal anti-inflammatory that inhibits prostaglandin synthesis, reducing inflammatory response and intensity of pain stimulus reaching sensory nerve endings. *Therapeutic Effect:* Produces analgesic and anti-inflammatory effect.

PHARMACOKINETICS

Route	Onset	Peak	Duration
PO	1 hr	2-3 hr	8-12 hr

Completely absorbed from the gastrointestinal (GI) tract. Widely distributed. Protein binding: greater than 99%. Metabolized in liver. Primarily excreted in urine. Not removed by hemodialysis.
Half-life: 8-12 hr.

AVAILABILITY
Tablets: 250 mg, 500 mg.

INDICATIONS AND DOSAGES
▸ **Mild to moderate pain**

PO
Adults, Elderly. Initially, 0.5-1 g,
then 250-500 mg q8-12hr.
Maximum: 1.5 g/day.
▸ **Rheumatoid arthritis, osteoarthritis**
PO
Adults, Elderly. 0.5-1 g/day in 2
divided doses. Maximum: 1.5 g/day.

OFF-LABEL USES
Treatment of psoriatic arthritis,
vascular headache

CONTRAINDICATIONS
Active GI bleeding, factor VII or
factor IX deficiencies, hypersensitivity to aspirin or NSAIDs

INTERACTIONS
Drug
Antihypertensives, diuretics: May
decrease the effects of these drugs.
Aspirin, salicylates: May increase
the risk of GI bleeding and side
effects.
Bone marrow depressants: May
increase the risk of hematologic
reactions.
**Heparin, oral anticoagulants,
thrombolytics:** May increase the
effects of these drugs.
Lithium: May increase the blood
concentration and risk of toxicity of
lithium.
Methotrexate: May increase the
risk of toxicity of methotrexate.
Probenecid: May increase diflunisal
blood concentration.
Herbal
Ginkgo biloba: May increase the
risk of bleeding.
Food
None known.

DIAGNOSTIC TEST EFFECTS
May increase serum AST (SGOT)
and ALT (SGPT) levels. May
decrease serum uric acid levels.

SIDE EFFECTS
Side effects are less common with
short-term treatment.
Occasional (9%-3%)
Nausea, dyspepsia (heartburn,
indigestion, epigastric pain),
diarrhea, headache, rash
Rare (3%-1%)
Vomiting, constipation, flatulence,
dizziness, somnolence, insomnia,
fatigue, tinnitus

SERIOUS REACTIONS
• Overdosage may produce drowsiness, vomiting, nausea, diarrhea,
hyperventilation, tachycardia,
diaphoresis, stupor, and coma.
• Peptic ulcer, GI bleeding, gastritis, and severe hepatic reaction,
including cholestasis, jaundice occur
rarely.
• Nephrotoxicity, including dysuria,
hematuria, proteinuria, and nephrotic
syndrome, and severe hypersensitivity
reaction, marked by bronchospasm
and angioedema, occur rarely.

PRECAUTIONS & CONSIDERATIONS
Caution is warranted with edema,
elevated liver function tests, erosive
gastritis, impaired renal or liver
function, peptic ulcer disease,
platelet and bleeding disorders, and
vitamin K deficiency. Be aware that
diflunisal crosses the placenta and is
distributed in breast milk. Avoid
diflunisal use during the last
trimester of pregnancy as the drug
may adversely affect the fetal cardiovascular system, causing premature
closure of ductus arteriosus. Be
aware that the safety and efficacy of
this drug have not been established
in children. In the elderly, GI bleeding or ulceration is more likely to
cause serious adverse effects. In the
elderly, age-related renal impairment
may increase risk of liver or renal

toxicity; a decreased drug dosage is recommended.

Notify the physician if GI distress, headache, or rash occurs. Baseline laboratory tests, including PT, aPTT, renal and liver function studies, and CBC, should be obtained. Skin for rash, pattern of daily bowel activity and stool consistency, and therapeutic response should be assessed.

Administration

Take diflunisal with meals, milk, or water. Don't crush or break film-coated tablets.

Digoxin
di-jox′in
(Digitek, Lanoxicaps, Lanoxin, Sigmaxin [AUS])
Do not confuse digoxin with Desoxyn or doxepin, or Lanoxin with Levsinex or Lonox.

CATEGORY AND SCHEDULE
Pregnancy Risk Category: C

CLASSIFICATION
Antiarrhythmics, cardiac glycosides, inotropes

MECHANISM OF ACTION
A cardiac glycoside that increases the influx of calcium from extracellular to intracellular cytoplasm. *Therapeutic Effect:* Potentiates the activity of the contractile cardiac muscle fibers and increases the force of myocardial contraction. Slows the heart rate by decreasing conduction through the SA and AV nodes.

PHARMACOKINETICS

Route	Onset	Peak	Duration
PO	0.5-2 hr	28 hr	3-4 days
IV	5-30 min	1-4 hr	3-4 days

Readily absorbed from the GI tract. Widely distributed. Protein binding: 30%. Partially metabolized in the liver. Primarily excreted in urine. Minimally removed by hemodialysis. **Half-life:** 36-48 hr (increased with impaired renal function and in the elderly).

AVAILABILITY
Capsules (Lanoxicaps): 50 mcg, 100 mcg, 200 mcg.
Elixir (Lanoxin): 50 mcg/ml.
Tablets (Digitek, Lanoxin): 125 mcg, 250 mcg.
Injection (Lanoxin): 250 mcg/ml, 100 mcg/ml.

INDICATIONS AND DOSAGES
▶ **Rapid loading dose for the management and treatment of CHF; control of ventricular rate in patients with atrial fibrillation; treatment and prevention of recurrent paroxysmal atrial tachycardia**
PO
Adults, Elderly. Initially, 0.5-0.75 mg, additional doses of 0.125-0.375 mg at 6- to 8-hr intervals. Range: 0.75-1.25 mg.
Children 10 yr and older. 10-15 mcg/kg.
Children 5-9 yr. 20-35 mcg/kg.
Children 2-4 yr. 30-40 mcg/kg.
Children 1-23 mo. 35-60 mcg/kg.
Neonate, full-term. 25-35 mcg/kg.
Neonate, premature. 20-30 mcg/kg.
IV
Adults, Elderly. 0.6-1 mg.
Children 10 yr and older. 8-12 mcg/kg.

Children 5-9 yr. 15-30 mcg/kg.
Children 2-4 yr. 25-35 mcg/kg.
Children 1-23 mo. 30-50 mcg/kg.
Neonates, full-term. 20-30 mcg/kg.
Neonates, premature. 15-25 mcg/kg.
▶ **Maintenance dosage for CHF;
control of ventricular rate in patients
with atrial fibrillation; treatment and
prevention of recurrent paroxysmal
atrial tachycardia**
PO, IV
Adults, Elderly. 0.125-0.375 mg/day.
Children. 25%-35% loading
dose (20%-30% for premature
neonates)
▶ **Dosage in renal impairment**
Dosage adjustment is based on crea-
tinine clearance. Total digitalizing
dose: decrease by 50% in end-stage
renal disease.

Creatinine Clearance	Dosage
10-50 ml/min	25%-75% usual
Less than 10 ml/min	10%-25% usual

CONTRAINDICATIONS
Ventricular fibrillation, ventricular
tachycardia unrelated to CHF

INTERACTIONS
Drug
Amiodarone: May increase digoxin
blood concentration and risk of toxicity; may have an additive effect on
the SA and AV nodes.
**Amphotericin, glucocorticoids,
potassium-depleting diuretics:**
May increase risk of toxicity due to
hypokalemia.
**Antiarrhythmics, parenteral
calcium, sympathomimetics:** May
increase risk of arrhythmias.
**Antidiarrheals, cholestyramine,
colestipol, sucralfate:** May
decrease absorption of digoxin.
**Diltiazem, fluoxetine, quinidine,
verapamil:** May increase digoxin
blood concentration.

Parenteral magnesium: May cause
cardiac conduction changes and
heart block.
Herbal
Siberian ginseng: May increase
serum digoxin levels.
Food
None known.

DIAGNOSTIC TEST EFFECTS
None known.

▓ IV INCOMPATIBILITIES
Amphotericin B complex (Abelcet,
Amphotec, AmBisome), fluconazole
(Diflucan), foscarnet (Foscavir),
propofol (Diprivan)
▓ IV Compatibilities
Cimetidine (Tagamet), diltiazem
(Cardizem), furosemide (Lasix),
heparin, insulin (regular),
lidocaine, midazolam (Versed),
milrinone (Primacor), morphine,
potassium chloride, propofol
(Diprivan)

SIDE EFFECTS
None known. However, there is a
very narrow margin of safety
between a therapeutic and toxic
result. Long-term therapy may
produce mammary gland
enlargement in women but is
reversible when drug is
withdrawn.

SERIOUS REACTIONS
• The most common early manifestations of digoxin toxicity are GI
disturbances (anorexia, nausea,
vomiting) and neurologic abnormalities (fatigue, headache, depression,
weakness, drowsiness, confusion,
nightmares).
• Facial pain, personality change,
and ocular disturbances (photophobia, light flashes, halos around bright
objects, yellow or green color
perception) may be noted.

PRECAUTIONS & CONSIDERATIONS

Caution is warranted with acute MI, advanced cardiac disease, cor pulmonale, hypokalemia, hypothyroidism, impaired hepatic or renal function, incomplete AV block, and pulmonary disease. Digoxin crosses the placenta and is distributed in breast milk. Premature infants are more susceptible to toxicity. Keep in mind that infants and children experience signs of overdose differently than adults. The first sign of overdose in children is usually an arrhythmia, such as bradycardia, followed by nausea, vomiting, diarrhea, anorexia, and CNS disturbances. In the elderly, age-related hepatic or renal function impairment may require dosage adjustment. Also, there is an increased risk of loss of appetite in this age group.

Notify the physician if decreased appetite, diarrhea, nausea, visual changes, or vomiting occurs. Apical pulse should be assessed for 60 seconds, or 30 seconds if the person is receiving maintenance therapy. If the pulse rate is 60 beats/minute or lower in adults or 70 beats/minute or less in children, withhold the drug and contact the physician. Blood samples for digoxin level should be obtained 6 to 8 hours after digoxin administration or just before administration of next digoxin dose. Be aware that signs and symptoms of digoxin toxicity are GI disturbances and neurologic abnormalities.

Administration

! Avoid giving digoxin by the IM route because the drug may cause severe local irritation and is erratically absorbed. If no other route is possible, give deep into the muscle followed by massage. Give no more than 2 ml at any one site. Expect to adjust the digoxin dosage in elderly patients and those with renal

dysfunction. Know that larger digoxin doses are often required for adequate control of ventricular rate with atrial fibrillation or flutter. Administer digoxin loading dosage in several doses at 4- to 8-hour intervals, as prescribed.

May take oral digoxin without regard to meals. Crush tablets if necessary. Do not increase or skip digoxin doses.

For IV use, give undiluted or dilute with at least a four-fold volume of sterile water for injection, or D_5W because using less than this amount may cause a precipitate to form. Use immediately. Give IV slowly over at least 5 minutes.

Digoxin Immune Fab

di-jox'in
(Digibind, DigiFab)
Do not confuse with Desoxyn, doxepin.

CATEGORY AND SCHEDULE
Pregnancy Risk Category: C

CLASSIFICATION
Antidotes

MECHANISM OF ACTION
An antidote that binds molecularly to digoxin in the extracellular space. *Therapeutic Effect:* Makes digoxin unavailable for binding at its site of action on cells in the body.

PHARMACOKINETICS

Route	Onset	Peak	Duration
IV	30 min	N/A	3-4 days

Widely distributed into extracellular space. Excreted in urine. **Half-life:** 15-20 hr.

AVAILABILITY

Powder for Injection (Digibind):
38-mg vial.
Powder for Injection (DigiFab):
40-mg vial.

INDICATIONS AND DOSAGES

▸ **Potentially life-threatening digoxin overdose**
IV
Adults, Elderly, Children. Dosage varies according to amount of digoxin to be neutralized. Refer to manufacturer's dosing guidelines.

CONTRAINDICATIONS

None known.

INTERACTIONS

Drug
None known.
Herbal
None known.
Food
None known.

DIAGNOSTIC TEST EFFECTS

May alter serum potassium level. Serum digoxin concentration may increase precipitously and persist for up to 1 week until FAB/digoxin complex is eliminated from the body.

🖼 IV INCOMPATIBILITIES

None known.

SIDE EFFECTS

None known.

SERIOUS REACTIONS

• Hyperkalemia may occur as a result of digitalis toxicity. Signs and symptoms of hyperkalemia include diarrhea, paresthesia of extremities,

heaviness of legs, decreased BP, cold skin, grayish pallor, hypotension, mental confusion, irritability, flaccid paralysis, tented T waves, widening QRS interval, and ST depression.
• Hypokalemia may develop rapidly when the effect of digitalis is reversed. Signs and symptoms of hypokalemia include muscle cramping, nausea, vomiting, hypoactive bowel sounds, abdominal distention, difficulty breathing, and orthostatic hypotension.
• Low cardiac output and CHF may occur rarely.

PRECAUTIONS & CONSIDERATIONS

Caution is warranted with impaired cardiac and renal function. Be aware of signs and symptoms of digoxin toxicity, including anorexia, nausea, and vomiting, as well as visual changes. It is unknown if digoxin immune FAB crosses the placenta or is distributed in breast milk. No age-related precautions have been noted in children. In the elderly, age-related renal impairment may require cautious use.

B/P, EKG, serum potassium level, and temperature should be monitored during and after drug administration. Changes from the initial assessment should be assessed. Hypokalemia may result in cardiac arrhythmias, changes in mental status, muscle cramps, muscle strength changes, or tremor. Hyperkalemia may result in cold and clammy skin, confusion, and diarrhea. Signs and symptoms of an arrhythmia (such as palpitations) or heart failure (such as dyspnea and edema) should also be assessed if the digoxin level falls below the therapeutic level.

Storage
Refrigerate vials. After reconstitution, use the solution immediately. If it's not used immediately, store the

solution in the refrigerator for up to 4 hours.

Administration
Serum digoxin level should be obtained before administering the drug. If the serum digoxin level was drawn less than 6 hours before the last digoxin dose, the serum digoxin level may be unreliable. Impaired renal function may require more than 1 week before serum digoxin assay is reliable.

Reconstitute each 38-mg vial with 4 ml sterile water for injection to provide a concentration of 9.5 mg/ml. Reconstitute each 40-mg vial with 4 ml of sterile water for injection to provide a concentration of 10 mg/ml. Further dilute with 50 ml 0.9% NaCl. Infuse over 30 minutes. It is recommended that the solution be infused through a 0.22- micron filter. If cardiac arrest is imminent, may give drug by IV push.

Dihydroergotamine
dye-hye-droe-er-got'-a-meen
(D.H.E.45, Dihydergot [AUS], Ergomar [CAN], Migranal)

CATEGORY AND SCHEDULE
Pregnancy Risk Category: X

CLASSIFICATION
Ergot alkaloids and derivatives

MECHANISM OF ACTION
An ergotamine derivative, alpha-adrenergic blocker that directly stimulates vascular smooth muscle. May also have antagonist effects on serotonin. *Therapeutic Effect:* Peripheral and cerebral vasoconstriction.

PHARMACOKINETICS
Slow, incomplete absorption from the gastrointestinal (GI) tract; rate of absorption of intranasal varies. Protein binding: greater than 90%. Undergoes extensive first-pass metabolism in liver. Metabolized to active metabolite. Eliminated in feces via biliary system. **Half-life:** 7-9 hr.

AVAILABILITY
Injection: 1 mg/ml (D.H.E.45).
Nasal spray: 4 mg/ml (0.5 mg/spray) (Migranal).

INDICATIONS AND DOSAGES
▶ **Migraine headaches, cluster headaches**
IM/SUBCUTANEOUS
Adults, Elderly. 1 mg at onset of headache; repeat hourly. Maximum: 3 mg/day; 6 mg/wk.
IV
Adults, Elderly. 1 mg at onset of headache; repeat hourly. Maximum: 2 mg/day; 6 mg/wk.
INTRANASAL
Adults, Elderly. 1 spray (0.5 mg) into each nostril; repeat in 15 min. Maximum: 4 sprays/day; 8 sprays/wk.

CONTRAINDICATIONS
Coronary artery disease, hypertension, impaired liver or renal function, malnutrition, peripheral vascular diseases, such as thromboangiitis obliterans, syphilitic arteritis, severe arteriosclerosis, thrombophlebitis, Raynaud's disease, sepsis, severe pruritus

INTERACTIONS
Drug
Beta-blockers, erythromycin: May increase the risk of vasospasm.
Ergot alkaloids, systemic vasoconstrictors: May increase pressor effect.

Fluoxetine: May increase risk of ergotism.
Nitroglycerin: May decrease the effect of nitroglycerin.
Protease inhibitors: May increase the risk of toxicity of dihydroergotamine.
Herbal
None known.
Food
None known.

DIAGNOSTIC TEST EFFECTS
None known.

SIDE EFFECTS
Occasional
Cough, dizziness, rhinitis, altered taste, throat and nose irritation
Rare
Muscle pain, fatigue, diarrhea, upper respiratory infection, dyspepsia

SERIOUS REACTIONS
• Prolonged administration or excessive dosage may produce ergotamine poisoning manifested as nausea, vomiting, weakness of legs, pain in limb muscles, numbness and tingling of fingers or toes, precordial pain, tachycardia or bradycardia, and hypertension or hypotension.
• Localized edema and itching due to vasoconstriction of peripheral arteries and arterioles may occur.
• Feet or hands will become cold, pale, and numb.
• Muscle pain will occur when walking and later, even at rest.
• Gangrene may occur.
• Occasionally confusion, depression, drowsiness, and seizures appear.

PRECAUTIONS & CONSIDERATIONS
Dihydroergotamine use is contraindicated in pregnancy as it produces uterine stimulant action resulting in possible fetal death or retarded fetal growth and increases vasoconstriction of placental vascular bed. It is distributed in breast milk and may prohibit lactation.

Dihydroergotamine use may produce diarrhea or vomiting in the neonate. It may be used safely in children older than 6 years, but only use when the patient is unresponsive to other medication. In the elderly, age-related occlusive peripheral vascular disease increases risk of peripheral vasoconstriction. In the elderly, age-related renal impairment may require caution.

Irregular heartbeat, nausea, numbness or tingling of the fingers and toes, pain or weakness of the extremities, and vomiting should be reported.

Storage
Do not refrigerate or freeze injection formulation.

Administration
Take injection at the first signs of acute migraine or cluster headache.

Prior to intranasal administration, nasal spray must be primed (pumped 4 times). Inhale deeply through the nose while spraying or immediately after spraying in order to let the drug be absorbed through the skin in the nose. Do not tilt head back or inhale through the nose. Initiate treatment at the first sign of symptom of an attack. Nasal spray may be administered at any time during a migraine attack. Once spray is prepared, use within 8 hours. Discard unused solution.

Dihydrotachysterol
dye-hye-droe-tak-iss′ter-ole
(DHT, DHT Intensol,
Hytakerol)

CATEGORY AND SCHEDULE
Pregnancy Risk Category: A
(D if used in doses above RDA)

CLASSIFICATION
Vitamins/minerals

MECHANISM OF ACTION
A fat-soluble vitamin that is
essential for absorption, utilization
of calcium phosphate, and normal
calcification of bone. *Therapeutic
Effect:* Stimulates calcium and
phosphate absorption from small
intestine, promotes secretion of
calcium from bone to blood,
promotes renal tubule phosphate
resorption, acts on bone cells
to stimulate skeletal growth
and on parathyroid gland to suppress
hormone synthesis and secretion.

PHARMACOKINETICS
Well absorbed from small intestine.
Metabolized in liver. Eliminated via
biliary system; excreted in urine.
Half-life: Unknown.

AVAILABILITY
Oral Solution: 0.2 mg/ml (DHT
Intensol).
Capsule: 0.125 mg (Hytakerol).
Tablets: 0.125 mg, 0.2 mg, 0.4 mg
(DHT).

INDICATIONS AND DOSAGES
▶ **Hypoparathyroidism**
PO
Adults, Elderly, Older Children.
Initially, 0.8-2.4 mg/day for
several days. Maintenance:
0.2-1 mg/day.

Infants, Young Children. Initially,
1-5 mg/day for 4 days, then
0.1-0.5 mg/day.
▶ **Nutritional rickets**
PO
Adults, Elderly, Children. 0.5 mg as
a single dose or 13-50 mcg/day until
healing occurs.
▶ **Renal osteodystrophy**
PO
Adults, Elderly. 0.25-0.6 mg/
24 hrs adjusted as necessary
to achieve normal serum
calcium levels and promote
bone healing.

CONTRAINDICATIONS
Hypercalcemia, malabsorption
syndrome, vitamin D toxicity, hypersensitivity to vitamin D products or
analogs

INTERACTIONS
Drug
**Aluminum-containing antacid
(long-term use):** May increase
aluminum concentration and
aluminum bone toxicity.
**Calcium-containing
preparations, thiazide
diuretics:** May increase the
risk of hypercalcemia.
Magnesium-containing antacids:
May increase magnesium
concentration.
Herbal
None known.
Food
None known.

DIAGNOSTIC TEST EFFECTS
May increase serum cholesterol,
calcium, magnesium, and phosphate
levels. May decrease serum alkaline
phosphatase.

SIDE EFFECTS
Occasional
Nausea, vomiting

SERIOUS REACTIONS
• Early signs of overdosage are manifested as weakness, headache, somnolence, nausea, vomiting, dry mouth, constipation, muscle and bone pain, and metallic taste sensation.
• Later signs of overdosage are evidenced by polyuria, polydipsia, anorexia, weight loss, nocturia, photophobia, rhinorrhea, pruritus, disorientation, hallucinations, hyperthermia, hypertension, and cardiac arrhythmias.

PRECAUTIONS & CONSIDERATIONS

Caution is necessary with coronary artery disease, kidney stones, and renal impairment. Mineral oil should be avoided during dihydrotachysterol use. It is unknown if dihydrotachysterol crosses the placenta or is distributed in breast milk. Safety and efficacy have not been established in children. There are no age-related precautions noted in the elderly. Consume foods rich in vitamin D including eggs, leafy vegetables, margarine, meats, milk, vegetable oils, and vegetable shortening.

Serum alkaline phosphatase, BUN, serum calcium, serum creatinine, serum magnesium, serum phosphate, and urinary calcium levels should be monitored. The therapeutic serum calcium level is 9 to 10 mg/dl.

Administration
Take without regard to food. Swallow the vitamin whole and avoid crushing, chewing, or opening the capsules.

Diltiazem
dil-tye'a-zem
(Apo-Diltiaz [CAN], Auscard [AUS], Cardcal [AUS], Cardizem, Cardizem CD, Cardizem LA, Cardizem SR, Cartia, Coras [AUS], Dilacor XR, Diltahexal [AUS], Diltia XT, Diltiamax [AUS], Dilzem [AUS], Novo-Diltiazem [CAN], Taztia XT, Tiazac, Vasocardal CD [AUS])
Do not confuse Cardizem with Cardene or Cardene SR, or Tiazac with Ziac.

CATEGORY AND SCHEDULE
Pregnancy Risk Category: C

CLASSIFICATION
Antiarrhythmics, class IV, calcium channel blockers

MECHANISM OF ACTION
An antianginal, antihypertensive, and antiarrhythmic agent that inhibits calcium movement across cardiac and vascular smooth-muscle cell membranes. This action causes the dilation of coronary arteries, peripheral arteries, and arterioles. *Therapeutic Effect:* Decreases heart rate and myocardial contractility, slows SA and AV conduction and decreases total peripheral vascular resistance by vasodilation.

PHARMACOKINETICS

Route	Onset	Peak	Duration
PO	0.5-1 hr	N/A	N/A
PO (extended-release)	2-3 hr	N/A	N/A
IV	3 min	N/A	N/A

Well absorbed from the GI tract.
Protein binding: 70%-80%.
Undergoes first-pass metabolism in
the liver to active metabolite.
Primarily excreted in urine. Not
removed by hemodialysis. **Half-life:**
3-8 hr.

AVAILABILITY

*Capsules (Sustained-Release
[Cardizem SR]):* 60 mg, 90 mg,
120 mg.
*Capsules (Extended-Release
[Cardizem CD]):* 120 mg, 180 mg,
240 mg, 300 mg, 360 mg.
*Capsules (Extended-Release [Cartia
XT]):* 120 mg, 180 mg, 240 mg,
300 mg.
*Capsules (Extended-Release
[Dilacor XR])* 120 mg, 180 mg,
240 mg.
*Capsules (Extended-Release [Diltia
XT]):* 120 mg, 180 mg, 240 mg.
*Capsules (Extended-Release [Taztia
XT]):* 120 mg, 180 mg, 240 mg,
300 mg, 360 mg.
*Capsules (Extended-Release
[Tiazac]):* 120 mg, 180 mg, 240 mg,
300 mg, 360 mg, 420 mg.
Tablets (Cardizem): 30 mg, 60 mg,
90 mg, 120 mg.
*Tablets (Extended-Release
[Cardizem LA]):* 120 mg, 180 mg,
240 mg, 300 mg, 360 mg, 420 mg.
Injection (Ready-to-Hang Infusion):
1 mg/ml.

INDICATIONS AND DOSAGES
▸ **Angina related to coronary
artery spasm (Prinzmetal's variant),
chronic stable angina (effort-
associated)**
PO
Adults, Elderly. Initially, 30 mg
4 times a day. Increase up to 180-
360 mg/day in 3-4 divided doses at
1- to 2-day intervals.
Adults, Elderly (Cardizem LA).
Initially, 180 mg/day. May increase

at intervals of 7-14 days up to
360 mg/day.
Adults, Elderly (Cardizem CD).
Initially, 120-180 mg/day; titrate
over 7-14 days. Range: Up to
480 mg/day.
▸ **Essential hypertension**
PO
Adults, Elderly. (Cardizem CD,
Cartia XT): Initially, 180-240 mg
once a day. May increase at
2-week intervals. Maintenance
240-360 mg/day. Maximum: 480 mg
once a day. (Cardizem SR): Initially,
60-120 mg twice a day. May increase
at 2-week intervals. Maintenance:
240-360 mg/day. (Cardizem LA):
Initially, 180-240 mg once a day.
May increase at 2-week intervals.
Maintenance: 120-540 mg/day.
(Dilacor XR): 180-240 mg once
a day. (Dilacor XT): Initially,
180-240 mg a day. May increase
at 2-week intervals. Maximum:
540 mg once a day. (Taztia XT):
Initially, 120-240 mg once a
day. May increase at 2-week
intervals. Maximum: 540 mg
once a day.
▸ **Temporary control of rapid
ventricular rate in atrial fibrillation
or flutter, rapid conversion of
paroxysmal supraventricular
tachycardia to normal sinus
rhythm.**
IV PUSH
Adults, Elderly. Initially,
0.25 mg/kg actual body weight
over 2 min. May repeat in 15 min
at dose of 0.35 mg/kg actual body
weight. Subsequent doses
individualized.
IV INFUSION
Adults, Elderly. After initial bolus
injection, may begin infusion at
5-10 mg/hr; may increase by
5 mg/hr up to a maximum of
15 mg/hr. Infusion duration should
not exceed 24 hr.

CONTRAINDICATIONS

Acute MI, pulmonary congestion, severe hypotension (less than 90 mm Hg, systolic), sick sinus syndrome, second- or third-degree AV block (except in the presence of a pacemaker)

INTERACTIONS
Drug
Beta blockers: May have additive effect.
Carbamazepine, quinidine, theophylline: May increase diltiazem blood concentration and risk of toxicity.
Digoxin: May increase serum digoxin concentration.
Procainamide, quinidine: May increase risk of QT-interval prolongation.
Herbal
None known.
Food
None known.

DIAGNOSTIC TEST EFFECTS

PR interval may be increased.

▧ IV INCOMPATIBILITIES

Acetazolamide (Diamox), acyclovir (Zovirax), aminophylline, ampicillin, ampicillin/sulbactam (Unasyn), cefoperazone (Cefobid), diazepam (Valium), furosemide (Lasix), heparin, insulin, nafcillin, phenytoin (Dilantin), rifampin (Rifadin), sodium bicarbonate

▧ IV Compatibilities

Albumin, aztreonam (Azactam), bumetanide (Bumex), cefazolin (Ancef), cefotaxime (Claforan), ceftazidime (Fortaz), ceftriaxone (Rocephin), cefuroxime (Zinacef), cimetidine (Tagamet), ciprofloxacin (Cipro), clindamycin (Cleocin), digoxin (Lanoxin), dobutamine (Dobutrex), dopamine (Intropin), gentamicin (Garamycin), hydromorphone (Dilaudid), lidocaine, lorazepam (Ativan), metoclopramide (Reglan), metronidazole (Flagyl), midazolam (Versed), morphine, multivitamins, nitroglycerin, norepinephrine (Levophed), potassium chloride, potassium phosphate, tobramycin (Nebcin), vancomycin (Vancocin)

SIDE EFFECTS
Frequent (10%-5%)
Peripheral edema, dizziness, light-headedness, headache, bradycardia, asthenia (loss of strength, weakness)
Occasional (5%-2%)
Nausea, constipation, flushing, EKG changes
Rare (less than 2%)
Rash, micturition disorder (polyuria, nocturia, dysuria, frequency of urination), abdominal discomfort, somnolence

SERIOUS REACTIONS
• Abrupt withdrawal may increase frequency or duration of angina.
• CHF and second- and third-degree AV block occur rarely.
• Overdose produces nausea, somnolence, confusion, slurred speech, and profound bradycardia.

PRECAUTIONS & CONSIDERATIONS

Caution is warranted with CHF and impaired hepatic function. It is unclear if diltiazem crosses the placenta. It should be used during pregnancy only if the benefit to the mother outweighs the risk to the fetus. Diltiazem is distributed in breast milk. No age-related precautions have been noted in children. In the elderly, age-related renal impairment may require cautious use. Tasks that require alertness and motor skills should also be avoided.

Dizziness or lightheadedness may occur. Rise slowly from a lying to a sitting position and wait momentarily before standing to avoid diltiazem's hypotensive effect. Notify the physician of constipation, irregular heartbeat, nausea, pronounced dizziness, or shortness of breath. The onset, type (sharp, dull, or squeezing), radiation, location, intensity, and duration of anginal pain and its precipitating factors, such as exertion and emotional stress, should be documented before therapy. Pulse, B/P, and renal and hepatic function test results should be monitored before and during therapy. Skin should be assessed for flushing and peripheral edema, especially behind the medial malleolus.

Storage
Refrigerate vials. After dilution, solution is stable for 24 hours.

Administration
Take oral diltiazem before meals and at bedtime. Crush tablets as needed. Do not crush or open sustained-release capsules.

! Refer to manufacturer's information for dose concentration and infusion rates.

Add 125 mg to 100 ml D_5W or 0.9% NaCl to provide a concentration of 1 mg/ml. Add 250 mg to 250 or 500 ml diluent to provide a concentration of 0.83 mg/ml or 0.45 mg/ml, respectively. The maximum concentration is 1.25 g/250 ml or 5 mg/ml. Infuse per dilution or rate chart provided by manufacturer.

Dimenhydrinate
dye-men-hye′dri-nate
(Dramamine)

CATEGORY AND SCHEDULE
Pregnancy Risk Category: B

D

CLASSIFICATION
Anticholinergics, antiemetics/antivertigo

MECHANISM OF ACTION
An antihistamine and anticholinergic that competes for H1 receptor sites on effector cells of the GI tract, blood vessels, and respiratory tract. The anticholinergic action diminishes vestibular stimulation and depresses labyrinthine function. *Therapeutic Effect:* Prevents symptoms of motion sickness.

AVAILABILITY
Chewable Tablets: 50 mg.
Tablets: 50 mg.

INDICATIONS AND DOSAGES
▶ **Motion sickness**
PO
Adults, Elderly, Children older than 12 yr. 50-100 mg q4-6hr. Maximum: 400 mg/day.
Children 6-12 yr. 25-50 mg q6-8hr. Maximum: 150 mg/day.
Children 2-5 yr. 12.5-25 mg q6-8hr. Maximum: 75 mg/day.

CONTRAINDICATIONS
Hypersensitivity to dimenhydrinate or diphenhydramine.

INTERACTIONS
Drug
Alcohol, other CNS depressants: May increase CNS depression.

Aminoglycosides: Masks signs and symptoms of ototoxicity associated with aminoglycosides.
Other anticholinergics: Increases anticholinergic effect.
Herbal
None known.
Food
None known.

DIAGNOSTIC TEST EFFECTS
None known.

SIDE EFFECTS
Frequent
Dry mouth
Occasional
Hypotension, palpitations, tachycardia, headache, somnolence, dizziness, paradoxical stimulation (especially in children), anorexia, constipation, dysuria, blurred vision, tinnitus, wheezing, chest tightness
Rare
Photosensitivity, rash, urticaria

SERIOUS REACTIONS
• None significant.

PRECAUTIONS & CONSIDERATIONS
Caution is warranted with asthma, bladder neck obstruction, history of seizures, angle-closure glaucoma, and benign prostatic hyperplasia. Alcohol, tasks that require mental alertness or motor skills, and excessive exposure to sunlight should be avoided. Skin should not come in contact with the oral concentrate and syrup because it can cause contact dermatitis.

Drowsiness, dizziness, and dry mouth may occur. B/P should be monitored. Be alert for paradoxical reactions, especially in children, and signs and symptoms of motion sickness.
Administration
Tablets may be swallowed whole, chewed, or allowed to dissolve.

For motion sickness, take dimenhydrinate 1 to 2 hours before the activity that may cause motion sickness.

Dimercaprol
dye-mer-kap´role
(BAL in Oil)

CATEGORY AND SCHEDULE
Pregnancy Risk Category: C

CLASSIFICATION
Antidotes, chelators

MECHANISM OF ACTION
A chelating agent that contains two sulfhydryl groups that form a stable, nontoxic chelate 5-membered heterocyclic ring with heavy metals. *Therapeutic Effect:* Prevents the metal from combining with sulfhydryl groups on physiologic proteins and keeps them inactive until they can be excreted.

PHARMACOKINETICS
Time to peak after IM administration occurs in 30 to 60 minutes. Widely distributed to all tissues including the brain and, mainly, intracellular space. Rapidly metabolized by the liver to inactive metabolites. Excreted in the urine and bile. Removed by hemodialysis. **Half-life:** 4 hr.

AVAILABILITY
Injection, oil: 100 mg/ml
(BAL in Oil).

INDICATIONS AND DOSAGES
▸ **Poisoning, arsenic (mild)**
IM
Adults, Elderly, Children. 2.5 mg/kg 4 times/day for 2 days, 2 times on

day 3, then once daily for 10 days or recovery.
▶ **Poisoning, arsenic (severe)**
IM
Adults, Elderly, Children. 3 mg/kg q4hr for 2 days, 4 times on day 3, then twice daily for 10 days or recovery.
▶ **Poisoning, gold (mild)**
IM
Adults, Elderly, Children. 2.5 mg/kg 4 times/day for 2 days, 2 times on day 3, then once daily for 10 days or recovery.
IM
Adults, Elderly, Children. 3 mg/kg q4hr for 2 days, 4 times on day 3, then twice daily for 10 days or until recovery.
▶ **Poisoning, lead (mild)**
IM
Adults, Elderly, Children. Initially, 4 mg/kg, then 3 mg/kg q4hr for 2-7 days in combination with edetate calcium disodium injection at different injection sites
▶ **Poisoning, lead (severe)**
IM
Adults, Elderly, Children. 4 mg/kg q4hr for 2-7 days in combination with edetate calcium disodium injection at different injection sites
▶ **Poisoning, mercury**
IM
Adults, Elderly, Children. 5 mg/kg for 1 day, followed by 2.5 mg/kg 1 or 2 times/day for 10 days
▶ **Dosage in renal impairment**
Adults, Elderly. 2 mg/kg q12hr during dialysis.

OFF-LABEL USES
Antimony poisoning, bismuth poisoning, selenium poisoning, silver poisoning, vanadium poisoning

CONTRAINDICATIONS
Acute renal impairment, alkyl mercuring poisoning, G6PD

deficiency (unless a life-threatening situation exists), hepatic insufficiency (unless due to arsenic poisoning), use of iron, cadmium or selenium poisoning, hypersensitivity to dimercaprol or any component of the formulations

INTERACTIONS
Drug
Iron, cadmium, selenium, uranium: May increase risk of toxicity.
Herbal
None known.
Food
None known.

DIAGNOSTIC TEST EFFECTS
Iodine (^{131}I) thyroidal uptake values may be decreased. May result in false-positive reaction with nitroprusside test. May increase ALT and AST values.

▓ IV INCOMPATIBILITIES
Edentate calcium disodium

SIDE EFFECTS
Frequent
Hypertension, dose-related tachycardia, headache
Occasional
Nausea, vomiting
Rare
Burning eyes, lips, mouth, throat and penis, nervousness, pain at injection site, salivation, fever, dysuria

SERIOUS REACTIONS
• Abscess formation at injection site, blepharospasm, convulsions, thrombocytopenia, and transient neutropenia occur rarely.

PRECAUTIONS & CONSIDERATIONS
Caution is warranted with hypotension due to dose-related increase in blood pressure and heart rate and renal impairment including oliguria

and glucose 6-phosphate dehydrogenase (G6PD) deficiency. Ensure alkalinization of urine to protect the kidney. Caution is also necessary with people receiving iron supplementation. Avoid use until 24 hours after last dose of dimercaprol.
Be aware that dimercaprol is effective for acute poisoning by mercury salts if therapy is initiated within 1-2 hours after ingestion.
Dimercaprol is not effective for chronic mercury poisoning. Serum alkaline phosphatase concentration, blood urea nitrogen (BUN) concentration, serum calcium, creatinine, electrolyte concentrations, hemoglobin (especially in mercury toxicity), and phosphorus concentrations should be monitored.

Storage
Store ampoules at room temperature.

Administration
Be aware not to mix in the same syringe with edentate calcium disodium. Administer at different sites.
Administer deep IM injection only. Adjust dose if receiving dialysis.

Dinoprostone (PGE2)

dye-noe-prost'one
(Cervidil, Prepidil Gel, Prostin E₂)
Do not confuse Cervidil or Prepidil with bepridil or Prostin with Prostigmin.

CATEGORY AND SCHEDULE
Pregnancy Risk Category: C

CLASSIFICATION
Oxytocics, prostaglandins, stimulants, uterine

MECHANISM OF ACTION
A prostaglandin that directly acts on the myometrium, causing softening and dilation effect of the cervix. *Therapeutic Effect:* Stimulates myometrial contractions in gravid uterus.

PHARMACOKINETICS
Undergoes rapid enzymatic deactivation primarily in maternal lungs. Protein binding: 73%. Primarily excreted in urine. **Half-life:** Less than 5 min.

AVAILABILITY
Vaginal Gel (Prepidil): 0.5 mg .
Vaginal Inserts (Cervidil):
10 mg .
Vaginal Suppositories: 20 mg.

INDICATIONS AND DOSAGES
▶ **Abortifacient**
INTRAVAGINAL
Adults. 20 mg or one suppository high into vagina. May repeat at 3- to 5-hr intervals until abortion occurs. Do not administer for longer than 2 days.
▶ **Ripening of unfavorable cervix**
INTRACERVICAL
Adults. Initially, 0.5 mg (2.5 ml) (Prepidil); if no cervical or uterine response, may repeat 0.5-mg dose in 6 hr. Maximum: 1.5 mg (7.5 ml) for a 24-hr period. Or 10 mg (Cervidil) over 12-hr period; remove upon onset of active labor or 12 hr after insertion.

CONTRAINDICATIONS
Active cardiac, hepatic, pulmonary or renal disease; acute pelvic inflammatory disease; fetal malpresentation; hypersensitivity to dinoprostone or other prostaglandins; significant cephalopelvic disproportion

INTERACTIONS
Drug
Oxytocics: May cause uterine hypertonus, possibly resulting in uterine rupture or cervical laceration.
Herbal
None known.
Food
None known.

DIAGNOSTIC TEST EFFECTS
None known.

SIDE EFFECTS
Frequent
Vomiting (66%), diarrhea (40%), nausea (33%)
Occasional
Headache (10%), chills or shivering (10%), hives, bradycardia, increased uterine pain accompanying abortion, peripheral vasoconstriction
Rare
Flushing, vulvae edema

SERIOUS REACTIONS
• Overdose may cause uterine hypertonicity with spasm and tetanic contraction, leading to cervical laceration or perforation, and uterine rupture or hemorrhage.

PRECAUTIONS & CONSIDERATIONS
Caution is warranted with anemia, cardiovascular disease, cervicitis, compromised or scarred uterus, diabetes mellitus, epilepsy, hepatic disease, history of asthma, hypertension or hypotension, infected endocervical lesions or acute vaginitis, jaundice, renal disease, and uterine fibroids. Notify the physician if chills, fever, foul-smelling or increased vaginal discharge, or uterine cramps or pain occurs.

The character of the cervix, including dilation and effacement, fetal status, including heart rate, as well as uterine activity, including the onset of uterine contractions, should be monitored in those receiving the vaginal gel. Bishop score should be monitored before and after therapy. Uterine tone and duration, frequency, and strength of contractions should be checked if receiving the suppository form. Vital signs should be monitored every 15 minutes until stable, and then hourly until abortion is complete. Expect to give medications to relieve GI adverse effects, if indicated, or abdominal cramps in those receiving the suppository form.

Storage
Refrigerate gel; bring to room temperature just before use to avoid forcing warming process. Keep suppository frozen (less than 4° F [15.6° C]); bring to room temperature just before use. Remove foil wrapper after suppository reaches room temperature.

Administration
Use gel with caution when handling to prevent skin contact. Wash hands thoroughly with soap and water following administration. Assemble dosing apparatus as described in manufacturer's insert. Place the person in the dorsal position and use a speculum to visualize the cervix. Introduce gel into cervical canal just below level of internal os. After administration, remain in the supine position for at least 15 to 30 minutes to minimize leakage of the drug from the cervical canal.

Administer suppository only in a hospital setting, with emergency equipment available. Avoid skin contact because of risk of absorption. Insert high in the vagina. Remain supine for 10 minutes after administration.

Diphenhydramine
dye-fen-hye′dra-meen
(Allerdryl [CAN], Banophen,
Benadryl, Diphen, Diphenhist,
Genahist, Nytol [CAN], Unisom
Sleepgels [AUS])
**Do not confuse diphenhy-
dramine with dimenhydrinate,
or Benadryl with benazepril,
Bentyl, or Benylin, or
Banophen with Baclophen.**

CATEGORY AND SCHEDULE
Pregnancy Risk Category: B
OTC (capsules, tablets, chewable
tablets, syrup, elixir, cream,
spray)

CLASSIFICATION
Antihistamines, anti-Parkinson's
agent, antianaphylactic (adjunct),
antipruritic, antivertigo agent,
hypnotic

MECHANISM OF ACTION
An ethanolamine that competitively
blocks the effects of histamine at
peripheral H_1 receptor sites.
Therapeutic Effect: Produces anticholinergic, antipruritic, antitussive,
antiemetic, antidyskinetic, and sedative effects.

PHARMACOKINETICS

Route	Onset	Peak	Duration
PO	15-30 min	1-4 hr	4-6 hr
IV, IM	Less than 15 min	1-4 hr	4-6 hr

Well absorbed after PO or parenteral
administration. Protein binding:
98%-99%. Widely distributed.
Metabolized in the liver. Primarily
excreted in urine. **Half-life:**
1-4 hr.

AVAILABILITY
*Capsules (Banophen, Diphen,
Genahist):* 25 mg.
Capsules (Nytol): 50 mg.
Syrup (Diphen, Diphenhist):
12.5 mg/5 ml.
*Tablets (Banophen, Benadryl,
Genahist, Nytol)* : 25 mg,
50 mg.
Injection (Benadryl):
50 mg/ml.
Cream (Benadryl): 1%, 2%.
Spray: 1%, 2%.

INDICATIONS AND DOSAGES
▸ **Moderate to severe
allergic reaction, dystonic
reaction**
PO, IV, IM
Adults, Elderly. 25-50 mg q4hr.
Maximum: 400 mg/day.
Children. 5 mg/kg/day in divided
doses q6-8hr. Maximum:
300 mg/day.
▸ **Motion sickness, minor allergic
rhinitis**
PO, IV, IM
*Adults, Elderly, Children 12 yr and
older.* 25-50 mg q4-6hr. Maximum:
300 mg/day.
Children 6-11 yr. 12.5-25 mg
q4-6hr. Maximum: 150 mg/day.
Children 2-5 yr. 6.25 mg q4-6hr.
Maximum: 37.5 mg/day.
▸ **Antitussive**
PO
*Adults, Elderly, Children 12 yr and
older.* 25 mg q4hr. Maximum:
150 mg/day.
Children 6-11 yr. 12.5 mg q4hr.
Maximum: 75 mg/day.
Children 2-5 yr. 6.25 mg q4hr.
Maximum: 37.5 mg/day.
▸ **Nighttime sleep aid**
PO
*Adults, Elderly, Children 12 yr and
older.* 50 mg at bedtime.
Children 2-11 yr. 1 mg/kg/dose.
Maximum: 50 mg.

‣ **Pruritus**
TOPICAL
Adults, Elderly, Children 12 yr and older. Apply 1% or 2% cream or spray 3-4 times a day.
Children 2-11 yr. Apply 1% cream or spray 3-4 times a day.

CONTRAINDICATIONS
Acute exacerbation of asthma, use within 14 days of MAOIs

INTERACTIONS
Drug
Alcohol, other CNS depressants: May increase CNS depressant effects.
Anticholinergics: May increase anticholinergic effects.
MAOIs: May increase the anticholinergic and CNS depressant effects of diphenhydramine.
Herbal
None known.
Food
None known.

DIAGNOSTIC TEST EFFECTS
May suppress wheal and flare reactions to antigen skin testing unless the drug is discontinued 4 days before testing.

▩ IV INCOMPATIBILITIES
Allopurinol (Aloprim), amphotericin B complex (Abelcet, AmBisome, Amphotec), cefepime (Maxipime), dexamethasone (Decadron), foscarnet (Foscavir)

▨ IV Compatibilities
Atropine, cisplatin (Platinol), cyclophosphamide (Cytoxan), cytarabine (Ara-C), droperidol (Inapsine), fentanyl, glycopyrrolate (Robinul), heparin, hydrocortisone (Solu-Cortef), hydromorphone (Dilaudid), hydroxyzine (Vistaril), lidocaine, metoclopramide (Reglan), ondansetron (Zofran), promethazine (Phenergan), potassium chloride, propofol (Diprivan)

SIDE EFFECTS
Frequent
Somnolence, dizziness, muscle weakness, hypotension, urine retention, thickening of bronchial secretions, dry mouth, nose, throat, or lips; in elderly, sedation, dizziness, hypotension
Occasional
Epigastric distress, flushing, visual or hearing disturbances, paresthesia, diaphoresis, chills

SERIOUS REACTIONS
• Hypersensitivity reactions, such as eczema, pruritus, rash, cardiac disturbances, and photosensitivity, may occur.
• Overdose symptoms may vary from CNS depression, including sedation, apnea, hypotension, cardiovascular collapse, and death, to severe paradoxical reactions, such as hallucinations, tremor, and seizures.
• Children and neonates may experience paradoxical reactions, including restlessness, insomnia, euphoria, nervousness, and tremors.
• Overdosage in children may result in hallucinations, seizures, and death.

PRECAUTIONS & CONSIDERATIONS
Caution is warranted with asthma, cardiovascular disease, COPD, hypertension, hyperthyroidism, angle-closure glaucoma, increased IOP, peptic ulcer disease, benign prostatic hyperplasia, pyloroduodenal or bladder neck obstruction, and seizure disorders. Diphenhydramine crosses the placenta and appears in breast milk. Its use by breast-feeding women may inhibit lactation and produce irritability in breast-feeding infants. Use of the drug during the third trimester of pregnancy increases the risk of

seizures in neonates and premature infants. Diphenhydramine is not recommended for children, neonates, or premature infants because they're at an increased risk for paradoxical reactions. The elderly are at increased risk for developing confusion, dizziness, hyperexcitability, hypotension, and sedation. Avoid drinking alcoholic beverages and performing tasks that require alertness or motor skills until response to the drug is established.

Drowsiness, dizziness, and dry mouth may occur; tolerance usually develops to sedative effects. Respiratory rate, depth, and rhythm; pulse rate, and quality; B/P; and therapeutic response should be monitored.

Administration

Take diphenhydramine without regard to food. Crush scored tablets as needed. Don't crush, break, or open capsules or film-coated tablets.

For IM use, inject diphenhydramine deep into a large muscle mass.

For IV use, diphenhydramine may be given undiluted. Administer IV injection over at least 1 minute.

Diphenoxylate and Atropine

dye-fen-ox′i-late
(Lofenoxal [AUS], Lomotil, Lonox)

Do not confuse Lomotil with Lamictal, or Lofenoxal or Lonox with Lanoxin, Loprox, or Lovenox.

CATEGORY AND SCHEDULE

Pregnancy Risk Category: C

CLASSIFICATION

Anticholinergics, antidiarrheals

MECHANISM OF ACTION

A meperidine derivative that acts locally and centrally on gastric mucosa. *Therapeutic Effect:* Reduces intestinal motility.

PHARMACOKINETICS

Well absorbed from the GI tract. Metabolized in the liver to active metabolite. Primarily eliminated in feces. **Half-life:** 2.5 hr; metabolite, 12-24 hr.

AVAILABILITY

Tablets (Lomotil, Lonox): 2.5 mg.
Liquid (Lomotil): 2.5 mg/5 ml.

INDICATIONS AND DOSAGES
▶ **Diarrhea**
PO
Adults, Elderly. Initially, 15-20 mg/day in 3-4 divided doses; then 5-15 mg/day in 2-3 divided doses.
Children 9-12 yr. 2 mg 5 times a day.
Children 6-8 yr. 2 mg 4 times a day.
Children 2-5 yr. 2 mg 3 times a day.

CONTRAINDICATIONS

Children younger than 2 years, dehydration, jaundice, narrow-angle glaucoma, severe hepatic disease

INTERACTIONS
Drug
Alcohol, other CNS depressants: May increase CNS depressant effects.
Anticholinergics: May increase the effects of atropine.
MAOIs: May precipitate hypertensive crisis.
Herbal
None known.
Food
None known.

DIAGNOSTIC TEST EFFECTS
May increase serum amylase level.

SIDE EFFECTS
Frequent
Somnolence, light-headedness, dizziness, nausea
Occasional
Headache, dry mouth
Rare
Flushing, tachycardia, urine retention, constipation, paradoxical reaction (marked by restlessness and agitation), blurred vision

SERIOUS REACTIONS
• Dehydration may predispose to diphenoxylate toxicity.
• Paralytic ileus and toxic megacolon (marked by constipation, decreased appetite, and stomach pain with nausea or vomiting) occur rarely.
• Severe anticholinergic reaction, manifested by severe lethargy, hypotonic reflexes, and hyperthermia, may result in severe respiratory depression and coma.

PRECAUTIONS & CONSIDERATIONS
Caution is warranted with acute ulcerative colitis, cirrhosis, hepatic or renal disease, and renal impairment. It is unknown if diphenoxylate crosses the placenta or is distributed in breast milk. Diphenoxylate is not recommended for use in children because of the increased risk of toxicity, which can lead to respiratory depression. The elderly are more susceptible to the anticholinergic effects of diphenoxylate, and they may experience confusion and respiratory depression. Tasks that require mental alertness or motor skills should be avoided until response to the drug has been established. Alcohol and barbiturates should also be avoided during drug therapy.

Notify the physician if abdominal distention, fever, palpitations, or persistent diarrhea occurs. Pattern of daily bowel activity and stool consistency and hydration status should be monitored.
Administration
Take without regard to meals. If GI irritation occurs, give with food. Administer the liquid form to children 2 to 12 years of age, using a graduated dropper for accurate measurement.

Dipyridamole
dye-peer-id'a-mole
(Apo-Dipyridamole [CAN], Novodipiradol [CAN], Persantin [AUS], Persantin 100 [AUS], Persantin SR [AUS], Persantine)
Do not confuse Aggrenox with Aggrastat or dipyridamole with disopyramide, or Persantin with Periactin.

CATEGORY AND SCHEDULE
Pregnancy Risk Category: C

CLASSIFICATION
Platelet inhibitors

MECHANISM OF ACTION
A blood modifier and platelet aggregation inhibitor that inhibits the activity of adenosine deaminase and phosphodiesterase, enzymes causing accumulation of adenosine and cyclic adenosine monophosphate. *Therapeutic Effect:* Inhibits platelet aggregation; may cause coronary vasodilation.

PHARMACOKINETICS
Slowly, variably absorbed from the GI tract. Widely distributed. Protein binding: 91%-99%. Metabolized in the liver. Primarily eliminated via biliary excretion. **Half-life:** 10-15 hr.

AVAILABILITY
Tablets: 25 mg, 50 mg, 75 mg.
Injection: 5 mg/ml.

INDICATIONS AND DOSAGES
▶ **Prevention of thromboembolic disorders**
PO
Adults, Elderly. 75-400 mg/day in combination with other medications.
Children. 3-6 mg/kg/day in 3 divided doses.
▶ **Diagnostic aid**
IV
Adults, Elderly (based on weight). 0.142 mg/kg/min infused over 4 min; although a maximum hasn't been determined, doses greater than 60 mg have been determined to be unnecessary for any patient.

OFF-LABEL USES
Prevention of myocardial reinfarction, treatment of transient ischemic attacks

CONTRAINDICATIONS
None known.

INTERACTIONS
Drug
Anticoagulants, aspirin, heparin, salicylates, thrombolytics: May increase the risk of bleeding with these drugs.
Herbal
None known.
Food
None known.

DIAGNOSTIC TEST EFFECTS
None known.

IV INCOMPATIBILITIES
No information available via Y-site administration.

SIDE EFFECTS
Frequent (14%)
Dizziness
Occasional (6%-2%)
Abdominal distress, headache, rash
Rare (less than 2%)
Diarrhea, vomiting, flushing, pruritus

SERIOUS REACTIONS
• Overdose produces peripheral vasodilation, resulting in hypotension.

PRECAUTIONS & CONSIDERATIONS
Caution is warranted with hypotension. Dipyridamole is distributed in breast milk. Safety and efficacy of dipyridamole have not been established in children. No age-related precautions have been noted in the elderly. Avoid alcohol because it increases the risk of stomach bleeding and dizziness, possibly resulting in a fall.

Dizziness may occur. Do not rise suddenly from a lying or sitting position. Notify the physician of unusual bleeding or chest pain. B/P for hypotension and skin for erythema and rash should be monitored.
Administration
Take oral dipyridamole on an empty stomach with full glass of water. Therapeutic response may not be achieved before 2 to 3 months of continuous therapy.

For IV use, dilute to at least 1:2 ratio with 0.9% NaCl or D_5W for total volume of 20 to 50 ml because undiluted solution may cause irritation. Infuse over 4 minutes. Inject thallium within 5 minutes after dipyridamole infusion has ended, as prescribed.

Dirithromycin
die-rith-ro-my'sin
(Dynabac)
Do not confuse Dynabac with Dynacin or DynaCirc.

CATEGORY AND SCHEDULE
Pregnancy Risk Category: C

CLASSIFICATION
Antibiotics, macrolides

MECHANISM OF ACTION
A macrolide that binds to ribosomal receptor sites of susceptible organisms, inhibiting bacterial protein synthesis. *Therapeutic Effect:* Bactericidal or bacteriostatic, depending on drug dosage.

PHARMACOKINETICS
Rapidly absorbed from the GI tract. Protein binding: 15%-30%. Widely distributed into tissues and within cells. Eliminated primarily unchanged by biliary excretion. Not removed by hemodialysis. **Half-life:** 30-44 hr.

AVAILABILITY
Tablets (Enteric-Coated): 250 mg.

INDICATIONS AND DOSAGES
▸ **Pharyngitis, tonsillitis**
PO
Adults, Elderly, Children 12 yr and older. 500 mg once a day for 10 days.
▸ **Acute or chronic bronchitis, skin and skin-structure infections**
PO
Adults, Elderly, Children 12 yr and older. 500 mg once a day for 7 days.
▸ **Community-acquired pneumonia**
PO
Adults, Elderly, Children 12 yr and older. 500 mg once a day for 14 days.

CONTRAINDICATIONS
Hypersensitivity to dirithromycin or other macrolide antibiotics

INTERACTIONS
Drug
Aluminum- and magnesium-containing antacids: May decrease dirithromycin blood concentration.
H$_2$ antagonists: Increase dirithromycin absorption.
Herbal
None known.
Food
None known.

DIAGNOSTIC TEST EFFECTS
May increase serum CK and potassium levels as well as blood eosinophil, neutrophil, and platelet counts.

SIDE EFFECTS
Frequent (10%-8%)
Abdominal pain, headache, nausea, diarrhea
Occasional (3%-2%)
Vomiting, dyspepsia, dizziness, nonspecific pain, asthenia
Rare (less than 2%)
Increased cough, flatulence, rash, dyspnea, pruritus and urticaria, insomnia

SERIOUS REACTIONS
• Antibiotic-associated colitis and other superinfections may result from altered bacterial balance.

PRECAUTIONS & CONSIDERATIONS
Caution is warranted with hepatic or renal dysfunction. Determine if there is a history of hepatitis or allergies to dirithromycin or other macrolides before beginning therapy. It is unknown if dirithromycin is distributed in breast milk. The safety and efficacy of dirithromycin have not been established in children younger

than 12 years. No age-related precautions have been noted in elderly patients with normal renal function. WBC should be monitored to determine if the infection is improving. Diarrhea, GI discomfort, headache, nausea, pattern of daily bowel activity and stool consistency, as well as signs and symptoms of superinfection, including anal or genital pruritus, moderate to severe diarrhea, abdominal cramps, fever, and sore mouth or tongue, should be assessed.

Administration

Administer dirithromycin with food or within 1 hour after a meal because food increases absorption. Swallow the tablets whole, do not chew them. Don't crush or cut the tablets. Take the full course of treatment. Take dirithromycin at least 1 hour before or 2 hours after antacids with aluminum or magnesium.

Disopyramide

dye-soe-peer′a-mide
(Norpace, Norpace CR, Rythmodan [CAN])
Do not confuse with desipramine, dipyridamole, or Rythmol.

CATEGORY AND SCHEDULE

Pregnancy Risk Category: C

CLASSIFICATION

Antiarrhythmics, class IA

MECHANISM OF ACTION

An antiarrhythmic that prolongs the refractory period of the cardiac cell by direct effect, decreasing myocardial excitability and conduction velocity. *Therapeutic*

Effect: Depresses myocardial contractility. Has anticholinergic and negative inotropic effects.

AVAILABILITY

Capsules (Norpace): 100 mg, 150 mg.
Capsules (Extended-Release [Norpace CR]): 100 mg, 150 mg.

INDICATIONS AND DOSAGES

▸ **Suppression and prevention of ventricular ectopy, unifocal or multifocal premature ventricular contractions, paired ventricular contractions (couplets), and episodes of ventricular tachycardia**
PO
! Do not use extended release capsules for rapid control
Adults, Elderly weighing 50 kg and more. 150 mg q6hr (300 mg q12hr with extended-release).
Adults, Elderly weighing less than 50 kg. 100 mg q6hr (200 mg q12hr with extended-release).
▸ **Rapid control of arrhythmias**
PO
Adults, elderly weighing 50 kg and more. Initially, 300 mg, then 150 mg q6hr or 300 mg (controlled release) q12hr.
Adults, elderly weighing less than 50 kg. Initially, 200 mg, then 100 mg q6hr or 200 mg (controlled release) q12hr.
▸ **Severe refractory arrhythmias**
PO
Adults, Elderly. Up to 400 mg q6hr.
Children 12-18 yr. 6-15 mg/kg/day in divided doses q6hr.
Children 4-12 yr. 10-15 mg/kg/day in divided doses q6hr.
Children 1-4 yr. 10-20 mg/kg/day in divided doses q6hr.
Children younger than 1 yr. 10-30 mg/kg/day in divided doses q6hr.

▶ **Dosage in renal impairment**
With or without loading dose of
150 mg:

Creatinine Clearance	Dosage
40 ml/min and higher	100 mg q6hr (extended-release 200 mg q12hr)
30-39 ml/min	100 mg q8hr
15-29 ml/min	100 mg q12hr
Less than 15 ml/min	100 mg q24hr

▶ **Dosage in liver impairment**
*Adults, Elderly weighing 50 kg and
more.* 100 mg q6hr (200 mg q12hr
with extended-release).
▶ **Dosage in cardiomyopathy, cardiac
decompensation**
*Adults, Elderly weighing 50 kg
and more.* No loading dose; 100 mg
q6-8hr with gradual dosage
adjustments.

OFF-LABEL USES
Prophylaxis and treatment of
supraventricular tachycardia

CONTRAINDICATIONS
Cardiogenic shock, narrow-angle
glaucoma (unless patient is undergoing cholinergic therapy), preexisting
second- or third-degree atrioventricular (AV) block, preexisting urinary
retention

INTERACTIONS
Drug
**Other antiarrhythmics,
including diltiazem, propranolol,
verapamil:** May prolong
cardiac conduction, decrease
cardiac output.
Pimozide: May increase cardiac
arrhythmias.
Herbal
None known.
Food
None known.

DIAGNOSTIC TEST EFFECTS
May decrease blood glucose levels.
May cause EKG changes. May
increase serum cholesterol and
triglyceride levels. Therapeutic
serum level is 2 to 8 mcg/ml and the
toxic serum level is greater than
8 mcg/ml.

SIDE EFFECTS
Frequent (greater than 9%)
Dry mouth (32%), urinary hesitancy,
constipation
Occasional (9%-3%)
Blurred vision, dry eyes, nose, or
throat, urinary retention, headache,
dizziness, fatigue, nausea
Rare (less than 1%)
Impotence, hypotension, edema,
weight gain, shortness of breath,
syncope, chest pain, nervousness,
diarrhea, vomiting, decreased
appetite, rash, itching

SERIOUS REACTIONS
• May produce or aggravate
congestive heart failure (CHF).
• May produce severe hypotension,
shortness of breath, chest pain,
syncope (especially in patients with
primary cardiomyopathy or CHF).
• Hepatotoxicity occurs rarely.

PRECAUTIONS & CONSIDERATIONS
Caution is warranted with bundle-
branch block, CHF, impaired liver or
renal function, myasthenia gravis,
prostatic hypertrophy, sick sinus
syndrome (sinus bradycardia alternating with tachycardia), and Wolff-
Parkinson-White syndrome. Nasal
decongestants or over-the-counter
(OTC) cold preparations, especially
those containing stimulants should
be avoided without the physician's
approval. Alcohol and salt consumption should also be avoided.
Dizziness and lightheadedness may
occur. Notify the physician if cough

or shortness of breath occurs. The patient should urinate before taking this drug to reduce the risk of urine retention. B/P, EKG for cardiac changes, blood glucose, liver enzyme, and serum alkaline phosphatase, bilirubin, and potassium, AST (SGOT), and ALT (SGPT) levels should be assessed. Disopyramide's therapeutic serum level is 2-8 mcg/ml and toxic serum level is greater than 8 mcg/ml.

Administration

Dosage must be individualized.

Dobutamine

doe-byoo′ta-meen
(Dobutrex)
Do not confuse dobutamine with Dopamine.

CATEGORY AND SCHEDULE

Pregnancy Risk Category: B

CLASSIFICATION

Adrenergic agonists, inotropes

MECHANISM OF ACTION

A direct-acting inotropic agent acting primarily on beta$_1$-adrenergic receptors. *Therapeutic Effect:* Decreases preload and afterload, and enhances myocardial contractility, stroke volume, and cardiac output. Improves renal blood flow and urine output.

PHARMACOKINETICS

Route	Onset	Peak	Duration
IV	1-2 min	10 min	Length of infusion

Metabolized in the liver. Primarily excreted in urine. Not removed by hemodialysis. **Half-life:** 2 min.

AVAILABILITY

Infusion (ready-to-use): 1 mg/ml, 2 mg/ml, 4 mg/ml.
Injection: 12.5-mg/ml vial.

INDICATIONS AND DOSAGES

▶ **Short-term management of cardiac decompensation**

IV INFUSION
Adults, Elderly, Children. 2.5-15 mcg/kg/min. Rarely, drug can be infused at a rate of up to 40 mcg/kg/min to increase cardiac output.
Neonates. 2-15 mcg/kg/min.

CONTRAINDICATIONS

Hypovolemia patients, idiopathic hypertrophic subaortic stenosis, sulfite sensitivity

INTERACTIONS

Drug
Beta blockers: May antagonize the effects of dobutamine.
Digoxin: May increase the risk of arrhythmias and enhance the inotropic effect of both drugs.
MAOIs, oxytocics, tricyclic antidepressants: May increase the adverse effects of dobutamine, such as arrhythmias and hypertension.
Herbal
None known.
Food
None known.

DIAGNOSTIC TEST EFFECTS

Decreases serum potassium level

🔲 IV INCOMPATIBILITIES

Acyclovir (Zovirax), alteplase (Activase), amphotericin B complex (Abelcet, AmBisome, Amphotec), bumetanide (Bumex), cefepime

(Maxipime), foscarnet (Foscavir), furosemide (Lasix), heparin, piperacillin/tazobactam (Zosyn)

IV Compatibilities

Amiodarone (Cordarone), calcium chloride, calcium gluconate, diltiazem (Cardizem), dopamine (Intropin), enalapril (Vasotec), famotidine (Pepcid), hydromorphone (Dilaudid), insulin (regular), lidocaine, lorazepam (Ativan), magnesium sulfate, midazolam (Versed), milrinone (Primacor), morphine, nitroglycerin, norepinephrine (Levophed), potassium chloride, propofol (Diprivan)

SIDE EFFECTS

Frequent (greater than 5%)
Increased heart rate, increased B/P
Occasional (5%-3%)
Pain at injection site
Rare (3%-1%)
Nausea, headache, anginal pain, shortness of breath, fever

SERIOUS REACTIONS

• Overdose may produce a marked increase in heart rate (by 30 beats/minute or higher) marked increase in B/P (by 50 mm Hg or higher), anginal pain, and premature ventricular contractions (PVCs).

PRECAUTIONS & CONSIDERATIONS

Caution is warranted with atrial fibrillation and hypertension. It is unknown if dobutamine crosses the placenta or is distributed in breast milk; therefore, it is not administered to pregnant women. No age-related precautions have been noted in children or the elderly.

Notify the physician of chest pain or palpitations during infusion or pain or burning at the IV site. Cardiac monitoring should be performed continuously to check for arrhythmias. B/P, heart rate, urine output and respiration should be checked before and during treatment. Serum potassium and dobutamine plasma levels should be monitored; keep in mind dobutamine's therapeutic range is 40 to 190 ng/ml.

Storage

Store at room temperature because freezing produces crystallization. Pink discoloration of the solution, caused by oxidation, does not indicate loss of potency if the solution is used within the recommended time period. Further diluted solution for infusion must be used within 24 hours.

Administration

! Dobutamine dosage is determined by the patient's response to the drug. Plan to correct hypovolemia with volume expanders before dobutamine infusion. Expect to administer digoxin to patients with atrial fibrillation before infusion. Administer by IV infusion only.

For IV use, dilute 250-mg ampoule with 10 ml sterile water for injection or D_5W for injection; the resulting solution is 25 mg/ml. Add additional 10 ml of diluent if contents of ampoule are not completely dissolved; the resulting solution is 12.5 mg/ml. Further dilute 250-mg vial with D_5W or 0.9% NaCl. Maximum concentration is 3.125 g/250 ml, or 12.5 mg/ml. Use infusion pump to control flow rate. Titrate dosage to individual response, as prescribed.

Docusate
dok'yoo-sate
(Coloxyl [AUS], Pro-Cal-Sof,
Surfak)(Apo-Docusate [CAN],
Colace, Colax-C [CAN], Diocto,
Docusoft-S, Novo-Ducosate
[CAN], PMS-Docusate [CAN],
Regulex [CAN], Selax [CAN],
Soflax [CAN], Surfak)

CATEGORY AND SCHEDULE
Pregnancy Risk Category: C
OTC

CLASSIFICATION
Laxatives

MECHANISM OF ACTION
A bulk-producing laxative that
decreases surface film tension by
mixing liquid and bowel contents.
Therapeutic Effect: Increases
infiltration of liquid to form a softer
stool.

PHARMACOKINETICS
Minimal absorption from the
GI tract. Acts in small and large
intestines. Results usually occur
1-2 days after first dose, but may
take 3-5 days.

AVAILABILITY
Capsules (Colace): 50 mg, 100 mg.
Capsules (Docusoft-S): 100 mg.
Capsules (Surfak): 240 mg.
Liquid (Colace): 50 mg/5 ml
(sodium).
Syrup (Colace, Diocto):
60 mg/15 ml.

INDICATIONS AND DOSAGES
▸ Stool softener
PO
*Adults, Elderly, Children 12 yr and
older.* 50-500 mg/day in 1-4 divided
doses.
Children 6-11 yr. 40-150 mg/day in
1-4 divided doses.
Children 3-5 yr. 20-60 mg/day in 1-
4 divided doses.
Children younger than 3 yr. 10-
40 mg in 1-4 divided doses.

CONTRAINDICATIONS
Acute abdominal pain, concomitant
use of mineral oil, intestinal obstruction, nausea, vomiting

INTERACTIONS
Drug
Danthron, mineral oil: May
increase the absorption of danthron
or mineral oil.
Herbal
None known.
Food
None known.

DIAGNOSTIC TEST EFFECTS
None known.

SIDE EFFECTS
Occasional
Mild GI cramping, throat irritation
(with liquid preparation)
Rare
Rash

SERIOUS REACTIONS
• None known.

PRECAUTIONS & CONSIDERATIONS
It is unknown if docusate is distributed in breast milk. Docusate use is
not recommended in children
younger than 6 years of age. No age-
related precautions have been noted
in the elderly.
  Notify the physician if unrelieved
constipation, dizziness, muscle
cramps or pain, rectal bleeding, or
weakness occurs. Maintain adequate
fluid intake. Pattern of daily bowel
activity and stool consistency should
be monitored.

Administration
Drink 6 to 8 glasses of water a day to aid in stool softening. Take each dose with full glass of water or fruit juice. Administer docusate liquid with infant formula, fruit juice, or milk to mask the bitter taste. To promote defecation, increase fluid intake, exercise, and eat a high-fiber diet.

Dofetilide
doe-fet′ill-ide
(Tikosyn)

CATEGORY AND SCHEDULE
Pregnancy Risk Category: C

CLASSIFICATION
Antiarrhythmics, class III

MECHANISM OF ACTION
A selective potassium channel blocker that prolongs repolarization without affecting conduction velocity by blocking one or more time-dependent potassium currents. Dofetilide has no effect on sodium channels or adrenergic alpha or beta receptors. *Therapeutic Effect:* Terminates reentrant tachyarrhythmias, preventing reinduction.

AVAILABILITY
Capsules: 125 mcg, 250 mcg, 500 mcg.

INDICATIONS AND DOSAGES
▸ **Maintain normal sinus rhythm after conversion from atrial fibrillation or flutter**
PO
Adults, Elderly. Individualized using a seven-step dosing algorithm

dependent upon calculated creatinine clearance and QT interval measurements.

CONTRAINDICATIONS
Concurrent use of drugs that prolong the QT interval; concurrent use of amiodarone, megestrol, prochlorperazine, or verapamil; congenital or acquired prolonged QT syndrome; paroxysmal atrial fibrillation; severe renal impairment

INTERACTIONS
Drug
Amiloride, megestrol, metformin, prochlorperazine, triamterene: May increase plasma levels of dofetilide.
Bepridil, phenothiazines, tricyclic antidepressants: May prolong the QT interval.
Cimetidine, verapamil: Increases levels of dofetilide.
Ketoconazole, trimethoprim: Increases plasma concentration of dofetilide.
Herbal
None known.
Food
Grapefruit juice: Can increase dofetilide plasma levels.

DIAGNOSTIC TEST EFFECTS
None known.

SIDE EFFECTS
Occasional (less than 5%)
Headache, chest pain, dizziness, dyspnea, nausea, insomnia, back and abdominal pain, diarrhea, rash

SERIOUS REACTIONS
• Angioedema, bradycardia, cerebral ischemia, facial paralysis, and serious ventricular arrhythmias or various forms of heart block may be noted.

PRECAUTIONS & CONSIDERATIONS

Continuous cardiac and B/P monitoring should be instituted. EKG for ventricular arrhythmias and for prolongation of the QT interval and serum creatinine level for changes should be monitored. Notify the physician if dizziness, severe diarrhea, or other adverse effects occurs.

Administration

Administer dofetilide at the same time each day without regard to food. Follow dosing instructions diligently.

Dolasetron

doe-lass'eh-tron
(Anzemet)
Do not confuse Anzemet with Aldomet.

CATEGORY AND SCHEDULE

Pregnancy Risk Category: B

CLASSIFICATION

Antiemetics/antivertigo, serotonin receptor antagonists

MECHANISM OF ACTION

A 5-HT$_3$ receptor antagonist that acts centrally in the chemoreceptor trigger zone and peripherally at the vagal nerve terminals. *Therapeutic Effect:* Prevents nausea and vomiting.

PHARMACOKINETICS

Readily absorbed from the GI tract after PO administration. Protein binding: 69%-77%. Metabolized in the liver. Primarily excreted in urine. Unknown if removed by hemodialysis. **Half-life:** 5-10 hr.

AVAILABILITY

Tablets: 50 mg, 100 mg.

Injection: 20 mg/ml in single use 0.625 ml amps, 0.625 ml fill in 2 ml Carpuject and 5-ml vials.

INDICATIONS AND DOSAGES

▸ **Prevention of chemotherapy-induced nausea and vomiting**
PO
Adults. 100 mg within 1 hr of chemotherapy.
Children 2-16 yr. 1.8 mg/kg within 1 hr of chemotherapy. Maximum: 100 mg.
IV
Adults, Children 1-16 yr. 1.8 mg/kg as a single dose 30 min before chemotherapy. Maximum: 100 mg.
▸ **Treatment or prevention of postoperative nausea or vomiting**
PO
Adults. 100 mg within 2 hr of surgery.
Children 2-16 yr. 1.2 mg/kg within 2 hr of surgery. Maximum: 100 mg.
IV
Adults. 12.5 mg 15 min before cessation of anesthesia or as soon as nausea occurs.
Children 2-16 yr. 0.35 mg/kg 15 min before cessation of anesthesia or as soon as nausea occurs. Maximum: 12.5 mg.

OFF-LABEL USES

Radiation therapy-induced nausea and vomiting

CONTRAINDICATIONS

None known.

INTERACTIONS

Drug

Agents that cause QTc prolongation: Caution should be used with these agents.
Herbal
None known.
Food
None known.

DIAGNOSTIC TEST EFFECTS

May transiently increase AST (SGOT) and ALT (SGPT) levels.

▓ IV INCOMPATIBILITIES

No information available for Y-site administration.

SIDE EFFECTS

Frequent (10%-5%)

Headache, diarrhea, fatigue

Occasional (5%-1%)

Fever, dizziness, tachycardia, dyspepsia

SERIOUS REACTIONS

* Overdose may produce a combination of CNS stimulant and depressant effects.

PRECAUTIONS & CONSIDERATIONS

Caution is warranted with congenital prolonged QT interval syndrome, hypokalemia, hypomagnesemia, and prolonged cardiac conduction intervals. Caution should also be used with concurrent use of diuretics because it can cause electrolyte disturbances, antiarrhythmics that may lead to prolonged QT interval, and high doses of anthracyclines. It is unknown if dolasetron is distributed in breast milk. The safety and efficacy of this drug have not been established in children younger than 2 years. No age-related precautions have been noted in the elderly.

Storage

Store vials at room temperature. After dilution, store solution for up to 24 hours at room temperature or up to 48 hours if refrigerated.

Administration

Do not cut, break, or chew film-coated tablets. For children 2-16 years, injection form may be mixed in apple or apple-grape juice and given orally, if needed, at a dosage of 1.8 mg/kg up to a maximum of 100 mg.

For IV use, dilute the injection in 0.9% NaCl, D_5W, dextrose 5% in 0.45% NaCl, lactated Ringer's (LR) solution, D_5LR, or 10% mannitol injection to 50 ml. Administer by IV push as rapidly as 100 mg/30 seconds or by intermittent or piggyback IV infusion over 15 minutes.

Donepezil

dah-nep'eh-zil

(Aricept)

Do not confuse Aricept with Aciphex or Ascriptin.

CATEGORY AND SCHEDULE

Pregnancy Risk Category: C

CLASSIFICATION

Cholinesterase inhibitors

MECHANISM OF ACTION

A cholinesterase inhibitor that inhibits the enzyme acetyl-cholinesterase, thus increasing the concentration of acetylcholine at cholinergic synapses and enhancing cholinergic function in the CNS. *Therapeutic Effect:* Slows the progression of Alzheimer's disease.

PHARMACOKINETICS

Well absorbed after PO administration. Protein binding: 96%. Extensively metabolized. Eliminated in urine and feces. **Half-life:** 70 hr.

AVAILABILITY

Tablets: 5 mg, 10 mg.

INDICATIONS AND DOSAGES

▶ **Alzheimer's disease**

PO
Adults, Elderly. 5-10 mg/day as a single dose. If initial dose is 5 mg, do not increase to 10 mg for 4-6 wk.

OFF-LABEL USES
Treatment of autism

CONTRAINDICATIONS
History of hypersensitivity to donepezil or piperidine derivatives

INTERACTIONS
Drug
Anticholinergics: May decrease the effect of anticholinergics.
Cholinergic agonists, neuromuscular blockers, succinylcholine: May increase the synergistic effects of these drugs.
Ketoconazole, quinidine: May inhibit the metabolism of donepezil.
NSAIDs: May increase gastric acid secretion of NSAIDs.
Paroxetine: May decrease the metabolism and increase the blood concentration of donepezil.
Herbal
None known.
Food
None known.

DIAGNOSTIC TEST EFFECTS
May increase blood glucose and serum creatine kinase and LDH concentrations. May decrease the serum potassium level.

SIDE EFFECTS
Frequent (11%-8%)
Nausea, diarrhea, headache, insomnia, nonspecific pain, dizziness
Occasional (6%-3%)
Mild muscle cramps, fatigue, vomiting, anorexia, ecchymosis
Rare (3%-2%)
Depression, abnormal dreams, weight loss, arthritis, somnolence, syncope, frequent urination

SERIOUS REACTIONS
• Overdose may result in cholinergic crisis, characterized by severe nausea, increased salivation, diaphoresis, bradycardia, hypotension, flushed skin, abdominal pain, respiratory depression, seizures, and cardiorespiratory collapse. Increasing muscle weakness may result in death if respiratory muscles are involved. The antidote is 1-2 mg IV atropine sulfate with subsequent doses based on therapeutic response.

PRECAUTIONS & CONSIDERATIONS
Caution is warranted with asthma, bladder outflow obstruction, COPD, peptic ulcer disease, history of seizures, sick sinus syndrome or other supraventricular conduction disturbances, and concurrent use of NSAIDs. It is unknown if donepezil is distributed in breast milk. Donepezil is not prescribed for children. No age-related precautions have been noted in the elderly. Be aware donepezil is not a cure for Alzheimer's disease but may slow the progression of its symptoms. Notify the physician if abdominal pain, diarrhea, excessive sweating or salivation, dizziness, or nausea and vomiting occur. Baseline vital signs should be assessed. Cholinergic reactions, such as diaphoresis, dizziness, excessive salivation, facial warmth, abdominal cramps or discomfort, lacrimation, pallor, and urinary urgency should be monitored.
Administration
Take donepezil without regard to food. The drug may be given in the morning or evening; however, best results may be achieved if it's given at bedtime.

Dopamine
doe′pa-meen
(Dopamine Injection [AUS],
Intropin)
**Do not confuse dopamine with
dobutamine or Dopram, or
Inotropin with Isoptin.**

CATEGORY AND SCHEDULE
Pregnancy Risk Category: C

CLASSIFICATION
Adrenergic agonists, inotropes

MECHANISM OF ACTION
A sympathomimetic (adrenergic
agonist) that stimulates adrenergic
receptors. Effects are dose dependent. Low dosages (1-5 mcg/kg/min)
stimulate dopaminergic receptors,
causing renal vasodilation. Low to
moderate dosages (5-15 mcg/
kg/min) have a positive inotropic
effect by direct action and release
of norepinephrine. High dosages
(greater than 15 mcg/kg/min)
stimulate alpha-receptors.
Therapeutic Effect: With low
dosages, increases renal blood
flow, urine flow, and sodium
excretion. With low to moderate
dosages, increases myocardial
contractility, stroke volume, and
cardiac output. With high dosages,
increases peripheral resistance, renal
vasoconstriction, and systolic and
diastolic BP.

PHARMACOKINETICS

Route	Onset	Peak	Duration
IV	1-2 min	N/A	Less than 10 min

Widely distributed. Does not cross
blood-brain barrier. Metabolized in
the liver, kidney, and plasma.
Primarily excreted in urine. Not
removed by hemodialysis.
Half-life: 2 min.

AVAILABILITY
Injection: 40 mg/ml, 80 mg/ml,
160 mg/ml.
Injection (premix with dextrose):
80 mg/100 ml, 160 mg/100 ml,
320 mg/100 ml.

INDICATIONS AND DOSAGES
▶ **Treatment and prevention of acute
hypotension; shock (associated with
cardiac decompensation, MI, open
heart surgery, renal failure, or
trauma), treatment of low cardiac
output, treatment of CHF**
IV
Adults, Elderly. 1 mcg/kg/min up to
50 mcg/kg/min titrated to desired
response.
Children. 1-20 mcg/kg/min.
Maximum: 50 mcg/kg/min.
Neonates. 1-20 mcg/kg/min.

CONTRAINDICATIONS
Pheochromocytoma, sulfite sensitivity, uncorrected tachyarrhythmias,
ventricular fibrillation

INTERACTIONS
Drug
Beta blockers: May decrease the
effects of dopamine.
Digoxin: May increase the risk of
arrhythmias.
Ergot alkaloids: May increase
vasoconstriction.
MAOIs: May increase cardiac
stimulation and vasopressor
effects.
Tricyclic antidepressants: May
increase cardiovascular effects.
Herbal
None known.
Food
None known.

D

DIAGNOSTIC TEST EFFECTS
None known.

🔲 IV INCOMPATIBILITIES
Acyclovir (Zovirax), amphotericin B complex (Abelcet, AmBisome, Amphotec), cefepime (Maxipime), furosemide (Lasix), insulin, sodium bicarbonate

🔲 IV Compatibilities
Amiodarone (Cordarone), calcium chloride, diltiazem (Cardizem), dobutamine (Dobutrex), enalapril (Vasotec), heparin, hydromorphone (Dilaudid), labetalol (Trandate), levofloxacin (Levaquin), lidocaine, lorazepam (Ativan), methylpred-nisolone (Solu-Medrol), midazolam (Versed), milrinone (Primacor), morphine, nicardipine (Cardene), nitroglycerin, norepinephrine (Levophed), piperacillin tazobactam (Zosyn), potassium chloride, propofol (Diprivan)

SIDE EFFECTS
Frequent
Headache, ectopic beats, tachycardia, anginal pain, palpitations, vasoconstriction, hypotension, nausea, vomiting, dyspnea

Occasional
Piloerection or goose bumps, bradycardia, widening of QRS complex.

SERIOUS REACTIONS
• High doses may produce ventricular arrhythmias.
• Patients with occlusive vascular disease are at high-risk for further compromise of circulation to the extremities, which may result in gangrene.
• Tissue necrosis with sloughing may occur with extravasation of IV solution.

PRECAUTIONS & CONSIDERATIONS
Caution is warranted with ischemic heart disease and occlusive vascular disease. Be aware that dopamine dosage may have to be reduced if MAOIs were taken within the last 2 to 3 weeks. It is unknown if dopamine crosses the placenta or is distributed in breast milk. Closely monitor children because gangrene due to extravasation has been reported. No age-related precautions have been noted in the elderly.

Cardiac monitoring should be performed continuously to check for arrhythmias. B/P, heart rate, urine output, and respiration should be checked before and during treatment. Notify the physician of chest pain, palpitation, arrhythmias, decreased peripheral circulation (marked by cold, pale, or mottled extremities), decreased urine output, or significant changes in B/P or heart rate, or burning at the IV site.

Storage
Dopamine is stable for 24 hours after dilution. Do not use solutions darker than slightly yellow or solutions that have discolored to brown or pink to purple because these discolorations indicate decomposition of drug.

Administration
❗ Expect to correct blood volume depletion before administering dopamine. Blood volume replacement may occur simultaneously with dopamine infusion.

For IV use, dilute 200-400 mg ampoule in 250-500 ml 0.9% NaCl, $D_5W/0.45\%$ NaCl, D_5W/lactated Ringer's or lactated Ringer's. Keep in mind the concentration is dependent on the dosage and the patient's fluid requirements. Remember that a 200 mg/250 ml solution yields 800 mcg/ml, and a

200 mg/500 ml solution yields 400 mcg/ml. The maximum concentration is 3.2 g/ 250 ml or 12.8 mg/ml. The drug is available prediluted in 250 or 500 ml of D_5W. Administer into large vein, such as the antecubital or subclavian vein, to prevent drug extravasation. Use an infusion pump to control rate of flow. Titrate dosage to the desired hemodynamic values or optimum urine flow, as prescribed. If extravasation occurs, immediately infiltrate the affected tissue with 10 to 15 ml 0.9% NaCl solution containing 5 to 10 mg phentolamine mesylate, as ordered.

Dornase Alfa
door'nace al'fa
(Pulmozyme)

CATEGORY AND SCHEDULE
Pregnancy Risk Category: B

CLASSIFICATION
Enzymes, respiratory, mucolytics, recombinant DNA origin

MECHANISM OF ACTION
An enzyme that selectively splits and hydrolyzes DNA in sputum. *Therapeutic Effect*: Reduces sputum viscosity and elasticity.

AVAILABILITY
Inhalation: 2.5-mg ampoules for nebulization.

INDICATIONS AND DOSAGES
▸ **To improve management of pulmonary function in patients with cystic fibrosis**

NEBULIZATION
Adults, Children older than 5 yr.
2.5 mg (1 ampoule) once daily by recommended nebulizer. May increase to 2.5 mg twice daily.

CONTRAINDICATIONS
Sensitivity to dornase alfa or epoetin alfa

INTERACTIONS
Drug
None known.
Herbal
None known.
Food
None known.

DIAGNOSTIC TEST EFFECTS
None known.

SIDE EFFECTS
Frequent (greater than 10%)
Pharyngitis, chest pain or discomfort, voice changes
Occasional (10%-3%)
Conjunctivitis, hoarseness, rash

SERIOUS REACTIONS
• None significant.

PRECAUTIONS & CONSIDERATIONS
Hoarseness, chest pain, and sore throat may occur during dornase alfa therapy. Viscosity of pulmonary secretions should be checked. Drink plenty of fluids.
Storage
Refrigerate unopened ampoules and protect them from light. Don't expose them to room temperature longer than 24 hours.
Administration
For nebulization, don't mix any other medications in the nebulizer with dornase alfa.

Doxapram
dox′a-pram
(Dopram)
Do not confuse with doxepin or ultram.

CATEGORY AND SCHEDULE
Pregnancy Risk Category: C

CLASSIFICATION
Analeptics, stimulants, central nervous system

MECHANISM OF ACTION
A central nervous system stimulant that directly stimulates the respiratory center in the medulla or indirectly by effects on the carotid. *Therapeutic Effect:* Increases pulmonary ventilation by increasing resting minute ventilation, tidal volume, respiratory frequency, and inspiratory neuromuscular drive, and enhances the ventilatory response to carbon dioxide.

PHARMACOKINETICS
IV onset 20-40 sec, peak 1-2 min, duration 5-12 min. Metabolized in the liver to metabolites, ketodoxapram (active) and desethyldoxapram (inactive). Partially excreted in the urine. Not removed by hemodialysis. **Half-life:** 2.4-9.9 hr.

AVAILABILITY
Injection: 20 mg/ml (Dopram).

INDICATIONS AND DOSAGES
▸ **Chronic obstructive pulmonary disease (COPD)**
IV INFUSION
Adults, Elderly, Children older than 12 yr. Initially, 1-2 mg/min. Maximum: 3 g/day for no more than 2 hours.

▸ **Drug-induced CNS depression**
IV INJECTION
Adults, Elderly, Children older than 12 yr. Initially, 1-2 mg/kg, repeat after 5 min. May repeat at 1-2 hour intervals, until sustained consciousness. Maximum: 3 g/day.
IV INFUSION
Adults, Elderly, Children older than 12 yr. Initially, bolus dose of 2 mg/kg, repeat after 5 min. If no response, wait 1-2 hours and repeat. If stimulation is noted, initiate infusion at 1-3 mg/min. Infusion should not be continued for more than 2 hours. Maximum: 3 g/day.

▸ **Respiratory depression**
IV INJECTION
Adults, Elderly, Children older than 12 yr. Initially, 0.5-1 mg/kg. May repeat at 5 minute intervals in patients who demonstrate initial response. Maximum: 2 mg/kg.
IV INFUSION
Adults, Elderly, Children older than 12 yr. Initially, 5 mg/min until adequate response or adverse effects are seen. Decrease to 1-3 mg/min. Maximum: 4 mg/kg.

OFF-LABEL USES
Apnea of prematurity, sleep apnea, congenital central hypoventilation syndrome, obesity-hypoventilation syndrome, post-anesthetic respiratory depression, shivering

CONTRAINDICATIONS
Convulsive disorders, cardiovascular impairment, head injury or cerebral vascular accident, severe hypertension, mechanical ventilation disorders, newborns, hypersensitivity to doxapram.

INTERACTIONS
Drug
Cyclopropane, enflurane, halothane: May increase

catecholamine release. Delay the initiation of doxapram therapy for at least 10 minutes following discontinuation of these anesthetics known to sensitize the myocardium.

CNS stimulant medications: May increase risk of stimulation to excessive levels, causing nervousness, insomnia, irritability, or possibly cardiac arrhythmias or seizures.

Monoamine oxidase (MAO) inhibitors, sympathomimetic agents: May increase the pressor effects of these medications or doxapram

Herbal
None known.

Food
None known.

DIAGNOSTIC TEST EFFECTS

May decrease hemoglobin, hematocrit, or red blood cell counts. May further decrease WBC in the presence of pre-existing leukopenia. May increase BUN and albuminuria.

IV INCOMPATIBILITIES

Alkaline solutions, aminophylline (Theophylline), ascorbic acid, carbenicillin (Geocillin), cefoperazone (Cefobid), cefotaxime (Claforan), cefotetan (Cefotan), cefuroxime (Kefurox, Zinacef), dexamethasone (Dexasone LA, Solurex LA), diazepam (Valium), digoxin, dobutamine (Dobutrex), folic acid, furosemide (Lasix), hydrocortisone, ketamine (Ketalar), methylprednisolone, minocycline (Minocin), sodium bicarbonate, thiopental (Pentothal), ticarcillin (Ticar)

IV Compatibilities

Amikacin (Amikin), bumetanide (Bumex), chlorpromazine (Thorazine), cimetidine (Tagamet), cisplatin (Platinol), cyclophosphamide (Neosar), deslanoside, dopamine (Intropin), doxycycline (Doxy-100), epinephrine (Adrenalin), hydroxyzine (Vistaril), imipramine (Tofranil), isoniazid (Nydrazid), lincomycin, methotrexate, netilmicin, phytonadione (Aquamephyton), pyridoxine, terbutaline (Brethine), thiamine, tobramycin (Nebcin), vincristine (Oncovin)

SIDE EFFECTS

Occasional

Flushing, sweating, pruritus, disorientation, headache, dizziness, hyperactivity, convulsions, dyspnea, cough, tachypnea, hiccough, rebound hypoventilation, phlebitis, variations in heart rate, arrhythmias, chest pain, nausea, vomiting, diarrhea, stimulation of urinary bladder with spontaneous voiding.

SERIOUS REACTIONS

• Overdosage may produce extensions of the pharmacologic effects of the drug. Excessive pressor effect, skeletal muscle hyperactivity, tachycardia, and enhanced deep tendon reflexes may be early signs of overdosage.

PRECAUTIONS & CONSIDERATIONS

Caution is warranted with hypermetabolic states, such as hyperthyroidism and pheochromocytoma as well as arrhythmias, diabetes mellitus, glaucoma, hypertension, impaired cardiac, impaired renal or liver function, peptic ulcer disease, and seizure disorder. It is unknown if doxapram crosses the placenta or is excreted in breast milk, so it is not administered to pregnant women. Be aware that doxapram is contraindicated in neonates. There are no age-related precautions noted for the elderly.

Administration

Doxapram dosage is determined by response to the drug. Discontinue if sudden hypotension or dyspnea develops. The rate of infusion should not be increased in severely ill patients with chronic obstructive pulmonary disease. Monitor closely during administration and for some time afterwards until the patient is fully alert for 30 to 60 minutes, to ensure reflexes have been restored and to prevent rebound hypoventilation. Prior to doxapram administration, ensure adequate airway and oxygenation in postanesthetic or drug-induced respiratory depression. Avoid extravasation or use a single injection site over an extended period. Local irritation or thrombophlebitis may result. Doxapram is stable and compatible with D_5W, $D_{10}W$, or 0.9% NaCl.

Doxepin

dox'eh-pin

(Deptran [AUS], Novo-Doxepin [CAN], Prudoxin, Sinequan, Zonalon)
Do not confuse doxepin with doxapram, doxazosin, or Doxidan, or Sinequan with saquinavir.

CATEGORY AND SCHEDULE

Pregnancy Risk Category: C (B for topical form)

CLASSIFICATION

Antidepressants, tricyclic, dermatologics

MECHANISM OF ACTION

A tricyclic antidepressant, antianxiety agent, antineuralgic agent, antipruritic, and antiulcer agent that increases synaptic concentrations of norepinephrine and serotonin. *Therapeutic Effect:* Produces antidepressant and anxiolytic effects.

PHARMACOKINETICS

Rapidly and well absorbed from the GI tract. Protein binding: 80%-85%. Metabolized in the liver to active metabolite. Primarily excreted in urine. Not removed by hemodialysis. **Half-life:** 6-8 hr. Topical: Absorbed through the skin. Distributed to body tissues. Metabolized to active metabolite. Excreted in urine.

AVAILABILITY

Capsules (Sinequan): 10 mg, 25 mg, 50 mg, 75 mg, 100 mg, 150 mg.
Oral Concentrate (Sinequan): 10 mg/ml.
Cream (Prudoxin, Zonalon): 5%.

INDICATIONS AND DOSAGES
▶ **Depression, anxiety**
PO
Adults. 30-150 mg/day at bedtime or in 2-3 divided doses. May increase to 300 mg/day.
Elderly. Initially, 10-25 mg at bedtime. May increase by 10-25 mg/day every 3-7 days. Maximum: 75 mg/day.
Adolescents. Initially, 25-50 mg/day as a single dose or in divided doses. May increase to 100 mg/day.
Children 12 yr and younger. 1-3 mg/kg/day.
▶ **Pruritus associated with eczema**
TOPICAL
Adults, Elderly. Apply thin film 4 times a day.

OFF-LABEL USES
Treatment of neurogenic pain, panic disorder; prevention of vascular headache, pruritus in idiopathic urticaria

CONTRAINDICATIONS
Angle-closure glaucoma, hypersensitivity to other tricyclic antidepressants, urine retention

INTERACTIONS
Drug
Alcohol, other CNS depressants: May increase CNS and respiratory depression and the hypotensive effects of doxepin.
Antithyroid agents: May increase the risk of agranulocytosis.
Cimetidine: May increase doxepin blood concentration and risk of toxicity.
Clonidine, guanadrel: May decrease the effects of these drugs.
MAOIs: May increase the risk of seizures, hyperpyrexia, and hypertensive crisis.
Phenothiazines: May increase the anticholinergic and sedative effects of doxepin.
Sympathomimetics: May increase cardiac effects.
Herbal
None known.
Food
None known.

DIAGNOSTIC TEST EFFECTS
May alter blood glucose levels and EKG readings. Therapeutic serum drug level is 110-250 ng/ml; toxic serum drug level is greater than 300 ng/ml.

SIDE EFFECTS
Frequent
Oral: Orthostatic hypotension, somnolence, dry mouth, headache, increased appetite, weight gain, nausea, unusual fatigue, unpleasant taste
Topical: Edema, increased itching, eczema, burning, or stinging at application site; altered taste, dizziness, somnolence, dry skin, dry mouth, fatigue, headache, thirst
Occasional
Oral: Blurred vision, confusion, constipation, hallucinations, difficult urination, eye pain, irregular heartbeat, fine muscle tremors, nervousness, impaired sexual function, diarrhea, diaphoresis, heartburn, insomnia
Topical: Anxiety, skin irritation or cracking, nausea
Rare
Oral: Allergic reaction, alopecia, tinnitus, breast enlargement
Topical: Fever, photosensitivity

SERIOUS REACTIONS
• Overdose may produce confusion; seizures; severe somnolence; fast, slow, or irregular heartbeat; fever; hallucinations; agitation; dyspnea; vomiting; and unusual fatigue or weakness.
• Abrupt withdrawal after prolonged therapy may produce headache, malaise, nausea, vomiting, and vivid dreams.

PRECAUTIONS & CONSIDERATIONS
Caution is warranted with cardiac disease, diabetes mellitus, glaucoma, hiatal hernia, history of seizures, history of urinary obstruction or urine retention, hyperthyroidism, increased intraocular pressure, renal or hepatic disease, benign prostatic hyperplasia and schizophrenia. Doxepin crosses the placenta and is distributed in breast milk. The safety and efficacy of this drug have not been established in children. Lower doxepin dosages are recommended for the elderly because they're at increased risk for toxicity. Exposure

to sunlight or artificial light sources should be avoided.

Drowsiness and dizziness may occur. Change positions slowly from recumbent to sitting, before standing, to prevent dizziness. Alcohol, caffeine, and tasks that require mental alertness or motor skills should also be avoided. B/P, pulse rate, weight, and EKG should also be monitored. Appearance, behavior, level of interest, mood, and speech pattern should be assessed.

Administration

Take doxepin with food or milk if GI distress occurs. Dilute the oral concentrate in 8 oz fruit juice (such as grapefruit, orange, pineapple, or prune), milk, or water. Avoid diluting in carbonated drinks because they are incompatible with the doxepin. An improvement should occur within 2 to 5 days of starting therapy but the maximum therapeutic effect usually takes 2 to 3 weeks to appear. The therapeutic serum level for doxepin is 110-250 ng/ml; the toxic serum level is greater than 300 ng/ml.

Doxercalciferol
dox-er-cal-sif′-er-ol
(Hectorol)

CATEGORY AND SCHEDULE
Pregnancy Risk Category: B

CLASSIFICATION
Vitamins/minerals

MECHANISM OF ACTION
A fat-soluble vitamin that is essential for absorption, utilization of calcium phosphate, and normal calcification of bone. *Therapeutic*

Effect: Stimulates calcium and phosphate absorption from small intestine, promotes secretion of calcium from bone to blood, promotes renal tubule phosphate resorption, acts on bone cells to stimulate skeletal growth and on parathyroid gland to suppress hormone synthesis and secretion.

PHARMACOKINETICS
Readily absorbed from small intestine. Metabolized in liver. Partially eliminated in urine. Not removed by hemodialysis. **Half-life:** up to 96 hr.

AVAILABILITY
Capsule: 2.5 mcg (Hectorol).
Injection: 2 mcg/ml (Hectorol).

INDICATIONS AND DOSAGES
▸ **Secondary hyperparathyroidism, dialysis patients**
IV
Adults, Elderly. Titrate dose to lower iPTH to 150-300 pg/ml. Adjust dose at 8-week intervals to a maximum dose of 18 mcg/week. Initially, if iPTH level is more than 400 pg/ml, give 4 mcg 3 times/week after dialysis, administered as a bolus dose.
Dose titration:
iPTH level decreased by 50% and more than 300 pg/ml: Dose may be increased by 1-2 mcg at 8-week intervals as needed.
iPTH level 150-300 pg/ml: Maintain the current dose.
iPTH level <100 pg/ml: suspend drug for 1 week and resume at a reduced dose of at least 1 mcg lower.
PO
Adults, Elderly. Dialysis patients: Titrate dose to lower iPTH to 150-300 pg/ml. Adjust dose at 8-week intervals to a maximum dose of 20 mcg 3 times/week. Initially, if iPTH is more than 400 pg/ml, give 10 mcg 3 times/week at dialysis

Dose titration:
iPTH level decreased by 50% and more than 300 pg/ml: Increase dose to 12.5 mcg 3 times/week for 8 more weeks. This titration process may continue at 8-week intervals. Each increase should be by 2.5 mcg/dose.
iPTH level 150-300 pg/ml: Maintain current dose.
iPTH level less than 100 pg/ml: Suspend drug for 1 week and resume at a reduced dose. Decrease each dose by at least 2.5 mcg.

▸ **Secondary hyperparathyroidism, predialysis patients**
PO
Adults, Elderly. Titrate dose to lower iPTH to 35-70 pg/ml with stage 3 disease or to 70-110 pg/ml with stage 4 disease. Dose may be adjusted at 2-week intervals with a maximum dose of 3.5 mcg/day. Begin with 1 mcg/day.
Dose titration:
iPTH level more than 70 pg/ml with stage 3 disease or more than 110 pg/ml with stage 4 disease: Increase dose by 0.5 mcg every 2 weeks as needed.
iPTH level 35-70 pg/ml with stage 3 disease or 70-110 pg/ml with stage 4 disease: Maintain current dose.
iPTH level is less than 35 pg/ml with stage 3 disease or less than 70 pg/ml with stage 4 disease: Suspend drug for 1 week, then resume at a reduced dose of at least 0.5 mcg lower.

CONTRAINDICATIONS
Hypercalcemia, malabsorption syndrome, vitamin D toxicity, hypersensitivity to doxercalciferol or other vitamin D analogs

INTERACTIONS
Drug
Aluminum-containing antacid (long-term use): May increase aluminum concentration and aluminum bone toxicity.

Calcium-containing preparations, thiazide diuretics: May increase the risk of hypercalcemia.
Magnesium-containing antacids: May increase magnesium concentration.
Herbal
None known.
Food
None known.

DIAGNOSTIC TEST EFFECTS
May increase serum cholesterol, calcium, magnesium, and phosphate levels. May decrease serum alkaline phosphatase.

SIDE EFFECTS
Occasional
Edema, headache, malaise, dizziness, nausea, vomiting, dyspnea
Rare
Bradycardia, sleep disorder, pruritus, anorexia, constipation

SERIOUS REACTIONS
• Early signs of overdosage are manifested as weakness, headache, somnolence, nausea, vomiting, dry mouth, constipation, muscle and bone pain, and metallic taste sensation.
• Later signs of overdosage are evidenced by polyuria, polydipsia, anorexia, weight loss, nocturia, photophobia, rhinorrhea, pruritus, disorientation, hallucinations, hyperthermia, hypertension, and cardiac arrhythmias.

PRECAUTIONS & CONSIDERATIONS
Caution is necessary with coronary artery disease, kidney stones, and renal impairment. Mineral oil should be avoided during doxercalciferol use. It is unknown if doxercalciferol crosses the placenta or is distributed in breast milk. Safety and efficacy have not been established in children.

There are no age-related precautions noted in the elderly. Consume foods rich in vitamin D including eggs, leafy vegetables, margarine, meats, milk, vegetable oils, and vegetable shortening.

Storage
Store at room temperature. Protect from light.

Administration
Individualize dosing based on serum iPTH levels.

Give oral doxercalciferol without regard to food. Swallow whole and avoid crushing, chewing, or opening the capsules.

For doxercalciferol injection, the recommended initial dose of 4.0 mcg administered as a bolus dose three times weekly at the end of dialysis (approximately every other day). The initial dose should be adjusted, as needed, in order to lower blood iPTH into the range of 150 to 300 pg/mL. The dose may be increased at 8-week intervals by 1.0-2.0 mcg if iPTH is not lowered by 50% and fails to reach the target range. Dosages higher than 18 mcg weekly have not been studied. Drug administration should be suspended if iPTH falls below 100 pg/ml and restarted one week later at a dose which is at least 1.0 mcg lower than the last administered dose. During titration, iPTH, serum calcium, and serum phosphorus levels should be obtained weekly. If hypercalcemia, hyperphosphatemia, or a serum calcium times phosphorus product greater than 70 is noted, the drug should be immediately suspended until these parameters are appropriately lowered. Then, the drug should be restarted at a dose which is 1.0 mcg lower.

Doxycycline
dox-i-sye′kleen
(Adoxa, Apo-Doxy [CAN], Doryx, Doxsig [AUS], Doxy-100, Doxycin [CAN], Doxyhexal [AUS], Doxylin [AUS], Monodox, Periostat, Vibramycin, Vibra-Tabs)
Do not confuse doxycycline with Dicyclomine, doxylamine, or Monopril.

CATEGORY AND SCHEDULE
Pregnancy Risk Category: D

CLASSIFICATION
Antibiotics, tetracyclines

MECHANISM OF ACTION
A tetracycline antibiotic that inhibits bacterial protein synthesis by binding to ribosomes. *Therapeutic Effect:* Bacteriostatic.

AVAILABILITY
Capsules (Doryx): 75 mg, 100 mg.
Capsules (Monodox): 50 mg, 100 mg.
Capsules (Vibramycin): 100 mg.
Oral Suspension (Vibramycin): 25 mg/5 ml.
Syrup (Vibramycin): 50 mg/5 ml.
Tablets (Adoxa): 50 mg, 75 mg, 100 mg.
Tablets (Periostat): 20 mg.
Tablets (Vibra-Tabs): 100 mg.
Injection, Powder for Reconstitution: (Doxy-100) 100 mg.

INDICATIONS AND DOSAGES
▸ **Respiratory, skin, and soft-tissue infections; UTIs; pelvic inflammatory disease (PID); brucellosis; trachoma; Rocky Mountain spotted fever; typhus; Q fever; rickettsia; severe acne (Adoxa); smallpox; psittacosis; ornithosis; granuloma inguinale;**

lymphogranuloma venereum; intestinal amebiasis (adjunctive treatment); prevention of rheumatic fever
PO
Adults, Elderly. Initially, 100 mg q12hr, then 100 mg/day as single dose or 50 mg q12hr for severe infections.
Children 8 yr and older and weighing more than 45 kg. 2-4 mg/kg/day divided q12-24hr. Maximum: 200 mg/day.
IV
Adults, Elderly. Initially, 200 mg as 1-2 infusions; then 100-200 mg/day in 1-2 divided doses.
Children 8 yr and older. 2-4 mg/kg/day divided q12-24hr. Maximum: 200 mg/day.

▸ **Acute gonococcal infections**
PO
Adults. Initially, 200 mg, then 100 mg at bedtime on first day; then 100 mg twice a day for 14 days.

▸ **Syphilis**
PO, IV
Adults. 200 mg/day in divided doses for 14-28 days.

▸ **Traveler's diarrhea**
PO
Adults, Elderly. 100 mg/day during a period of risk (up to 14 days) and for 2 days after returning home.

▸ **Periodontitis**
PO
Adults. 20 mg twice a day.

OFF-LABEL USES
Treatment of atypical mycobacterial infections, rheumatoid arthritis, gonorrhea and malaria; prevention of Lyme disease; prevention or treatment of traveler's diarrhea.

CONTRAINDICATIONS
Children 8 years and younger, hypersensitivity to tetracyclines or sulfites, last half of pregnancy, severe hepatic dysfunction

INTERACTIONS
Drug
Antacids containing aluminum, calcium, or magnesium; laxatives containing magnesium: Decrease doxycycline absorption.
Barbiturates, carbamazepine, phenytoin: May decrease doxycycline blood concentrations.
Cholestyramine, colestipol: May decrease doxycycline absorption.
Oral contraceptives: May decrease the effects of oral contraceptives.
Oral iron preparations: Impair absorption of doxycycline.
Herbal
None known.
Food
None known.

DIAGNOSTIC TEST EFFECTS
May increase serum alkaline phosphatase, amylase, bilirubin, AST (SGOT), and ALT (SGPT) levels. May alter CBC.

▨ IV INCOMPATIBILITIES
Allopurinol (Aloprim), heparin, piperacillin, and tazobactam (Zosyn)

▨ IV Compatibilities
Amiodarone (Cordarone), diltiazem (Cardizem), hydromorphone (Dilaudid), magnesium sulfate, morphine, propofol (Diprivan)

SIDE EFFECTS
Frequent
Anorexia, nausea, vomiting, diarrhea, dysphagia, possibly severe photosensitivity
Occasional
Rash, urticaria

SERIOUS REACTIONS
• Superinfection (especially fungal) and benign intracranial hypertension (headache, visual changes) may occur.

- Hepatoxicity, fatty degeneration of the liver, and pancreatitis occur rarely.

Caution should be used in those who can't avoid sun or ultraviolet exposure, because such exposure may produce a severe photosensitivity reaction.

History of allergies, especially to tetracyclines or sulfites, should be determined before drug therapy. Pattern of daily bowel activity, stool consistency, food intake and tolerance, renal function, and skin for rash should be assessed. Be alert for signs and symptoms of superinfection, such as anal or genital pruritus, diarrhea, and ulceration or changes of the oral mucosa or tongue. LOC should be monitored because of the potential for increased intracranial pressure.

Storage

Store capsules and tablets at room temperature. Store oral suspension for up to 2 weeks at room temperature. After reconstitution, the IV piggyback infusion may be stored for up to 12 hours at room temperature or up to 72 hours if refrigerated. Protect the drug from direct sunlight. Discard it if a precipitate forms.

Administration

Take oral doxycycline with a full glass of fluid. It may also be given with food or milk. Take oral doxycycline 1 to 2 hours before or after antacids that contain aluminum, calcium, or magnesium; laxatives that contain magnesium; or oral iron preparations because these drugs may impair doxycycline absorption. **!** Don't administer doxycycline IM or subcutaneously. Space doses evenly around clock. Reconstitute each 100-mg vial with 10 ml of sterile water for injection to yield a concentration of 10 mg/ml. Further dilute each 100 mg with at least 100 ml of D_5W, 0.9% NaCl, or lactated Ringer's solution. Give the intermittent IV (piggyback) infusion over 1 to 4 hours.

Dronabinol
droe-nab'i-nol
(Marinol)
Do not confuse dronabinol with droperidol.

CATEGORY AND SCHEDULE
Pregnancy Risk Category: C
Controlled Substance
Schedule: III

CLASSIFICATION
Antiemetics/antivertigo

MECHANISM OF ACTION
An antiemetic and appetite stimulant that may act by inhibiting vomiting control mechanisms in the medulla oblongata. *Therapeutic Effect:* Inhibits vomiting and stimulates appetite.

AVAILABILITY
Capsules (Gelatin): 2.5 mg, 5 mg, 10 mg.

INDICATIONS AND DOSAGES
▸ **Prevention of chemotherapy-induced nausea and vomiting**
PO
Adults, Children. Initially, 5 mg/m^2 1-3 hr before chemotherapy, then q2-4hr after chemotherapy for total of 4-6 doses a day. May increase by 2.5 mg/m^2 up to 15 mg/m^2 per dose.

▶ **Appetite stimulant**
PO
Adults. Initially, 2.5 mg twice a day (before lunch and dinner). Range: 2.5-20 mg/day.

CONTRAINDICATIONS
Treatment of nausea and vomiting not caused by chemotherapy

INTERACTIONS
Drug
Alcohol, other CNS depressants: May increase CNS depression.
Herbal
None known.
Food
None known.

DIAGNOSTIC TEST EFFECTS
None known.

SIDE EFFECTS
Frequent (24%-3%)
Euphoria, dizziness, paranoid reaction, somnolence
Occasional (3%-1%)
Asthenia, ataxia, confusion, abnormal thinking, depersonalization
Rare (less than 1%)
Diarrhea, depression, nightmares, speech difficulties, headache, anxiety, tinnitus, flushed skin

SERIOUS REACTIONS
• Mild intoxication may produce increased sensory awareness (including taste, smell, and sound), altered time perception, reddened conjunctiva, dry mouth, and tachycardia.
• Moderate intoxication may produce memory impairment and urine retention.
• Severe intoxication may produce lethargy, decreased motor coordination, slurred speech, and orthostatic hypotension.

PRECAUTIONS & CONSIDERATIONS
Caution is warranted with heart disease, hypertension, depression, mania, and schizophrenia.
    Dronabinol use is not recommended for children. Alcohol, barbiturates, other CNS depressants, and tasks that require mental alertness or motor skills should be avoided. B/P, heart rate, and behavioral and mood reactions should be monitored.
Administration
Take dronabinol before lunch and dinner to stimulate appetite. Relief from nausea and vomiting generally occurs within 15 minutes of drug administration.

Droperidol
droe-pear-'ih-dall
(Inapsine)

CATEGORY AND SCHEDULE
Pregnancy Risk Category: C

CLASSIFICATION
Anesthetics, general, antiemetics/antivertigo, anxiolytics, sedatives/hypnotics

MECHANISM OF ACTION
A general anesthetic and antiemetic agent that antagonizes dopamine neurotransmission at synapses by blocking postsynaptic dopamine receptor sites; partially blocks adrenergic receptor binding sites. *Therapeutic Effect:* Produces tranquilization, antiemetic effect.

PHARMACOKINETICS
Onset of action occurs within 30 minutes. Well absorbed.

Metabolized in liver. Excreted in urine and feces. **Half-life:** 2.3 hrs.

AVAILABILITY
Injection: 2.5 mg/ml (Inapsine).

INDICATIONS AND DOSAGES
▶ **Preoperative**
IM/IV
Adults, Elderly, Children 12 yr and older. 2.5-10 mg 30-60 min before induction of general anesthesia.
Children 2-12 yr. 0.088-0.165 mg/kg.
Adjunct for induction of general anesthesia
IV
Adults, Elderly, Children 12 yr and older. 0.22-0.275 mg/kg.
Children 2-12 yr. 0.088-0.165 mg/kg.
Adjunct for maintenance of general anesthesia
IV
Adults, Elderly. 1.25-2.5 mg.
Diagnostic procedures w/o general anesthesia
IM
Adults, Elderly. 2.5-10 mg 30-60 min before procedure. If needed, may give additional doses of 1.25-2.5 mg (usually by IV injection).

CONTRAINDICATIONS
Known or suspected QT prolongation, hypersensitivity to droperidol or any component of the formulation

INTERACTIONS
Drug
CNS depressants: May increase CNS depressant effect.
Class I, IA, or III antiarrhythmics, cisapride, cyclobenzaprine, phenothiazines, pimozide, quinolone antibiotics, tricyclic antidepressants: May increase risk of QT prolongation.

Hypotensive agents: May increase hypotension.
Herbal
None known.
Food
None known.

SIDE EFFECTS
Frequent
Mild to moderate hypotension
Occasional
Tachycardia, postop drowsiness, dizziness, chills, shivering
Rare
Postop nightmares, facial sweating, bronchospasm

SERIOUS REACTIONS
• Extrapyramidal symptoms may appear as akathisia (motor restlessness) and dystonias: torticollis (neck muscle spasm), opisthotonos (rigidity of back muscles), and oculogyric crisis (rolling back of eyes).
• Overdosage includes symptoms of hypotension, tachycardia, hallucinations, and extrapyramidal symptoms.
• Prolonged QT interval, seizures, and arrhythmias have been reported.

PRECAUTIONS & CONSIDERATIONS
Caution is warranted with impaired hepatic, renal, or cardiac function. Droperidol readily crosses the placenta, and it is unknown if droperidol is distributed in breast milk. Be aware that dystonias are more likely in children. Be aware that elderly patients may be more susceptible to sedative and hypotensive effects.
Change positions slowly to avoid orthostatic hypotension and avoid tasks that require mental alertness or motor skills.
Storage
Store parenteral form at room temperature.

Administration

Be aware that the person must remain recumbent for 30-60 min in head-low position with legs raised, to minimize hypotensive effect.

For IM administration, inject slow and deep into upper outer quadrant of gluteus maximus.

For IV administration, may give undiluted as IV push at a rate of 10 mg or less over 1 min. Dose for high-risk persons should be added to D_5W or lactated Ringer's injection to a concentration of 1 mg/50 ml and given as an IV infusion.

Drotrecogin Alfa
droh-tree-koh′gen
(Xigris)

CATEGORY AND SCHEDULE
Pregnancy Risk Category: C

CLASSIFICATION
Thrombolytics

MECHANISM OF ACTION

A recombinant form of human-activated protein C that exerts an antithrombotic effect by inhibiting Factors Va and VIIIa and may exert an indirect profibrinolytic effect by inhibiting plasminogen activator inhibitor-1 and limiting the generation of activated thrombin-activatable-fibrinolysis-inhibitor. The drug may also exert an anti-inflammatory effect by inhibiting tumor necrosis factor production by monocytes, by blocking leukocyte adhesion to selectins, and by limiting thrombin-induced inflammatory responses. *Therapeutic Effect:* Produces anti-inflammatory, antithrombotic, and profibrinolytic effects.

PHARMACOKINETICS

Inactivated by endogenous plasma protease inhibitors. Clearance occurs within 2 hr of initiating infusion. **Half-life:** 1.6 hr.

AVAILABILITY

Powder for Infusion: 5 mg, 20 mg.

INDICATIONS AND DOSAGES
▸ **Severe sepsis**
IV INFUSION
Adults, Elderly. 24 mcg/kg/hr for 96 hr.

CONTRAINDICATIONS

Active internal bleeding, evidence of cerebral herniation, intracranial neoplasm or mass lesion, presence of an epidural catheter, recent (within the past 3 mo) hemorrhagic stroke, recent (within the past 2 mo) intracranial or intraspinal surgery or severe head trauma, trauma with an increased risk of life-threatening bleeding

INTERACTIONS
Drug
None known.
Herbal
None known.
Food
None known.

DIAGNOSTIC TEST EFFECTS
May prolong aPTT

▨ IV INCOMPATIBILITIES
Don't mix drotrecogin alfa with other medications.
▨ IV Compatibilities
Lactated Ringer's solution, 0.9% NaCl and dextrose are the only solutions that can be administered through the same line.

SIDE EFFECTS
Occasional
Bleeding

SERIOUS REACTIONS
• Bleeding (intrathoracic, retroperi-toneal, GI, GU, intra-abdominal, intracranial) occurs in about 2% of patients.

PRECAUTIONS & CONSIDERATIONS
Caution is warranted with chronic, severe hepatic disease, intracranial aneurysm, platelet count less than 30,000/mm³, or prolonged prothrom-bin time and in those who have had GI bleeding within the past 6 weeks. Caution should be used in those who are using heparin concurrently and in those who have had thrombolytic therapy within the past 3 days or anticoagulant or aspirin therapy within the past 7 days. Caution should also be used when administering other drugs that affect hemostasis. It is unknown if drotrecogin alfa causes fetal harm or is excreted in breast milk. The safety and efficacy of drotrecogin alfa have not been established in children or the elderly.

The following criteria must be met before initiating drotrecogin alfa therapy; age of at least 18 years; weight less than 135 kg; no preg-nancy or breast-feeding; 3 or more systemic inflammatory response criteria (fever, heart rate greater than 90 beats/minute, respiratory rate greater than 20 breaths/minute, increased WBC count); and at least one sepsis-induced organ or system failure (cardiovascular, hepatic, renal, respiratory, or unexplained metabolic acidosis). Monitor for hemorrhagic complications. Bleeding may occur for up to 28 days after treatment. Notify the physician if signs and symptoms of unusual bleeding occur.

Storage
Store unreconstituted vials at room temperature.
Administration
Reconstitute the 5-mg and 20-mg vials by slowly adding 2.5 ml or 10 ml of sterile water for injection, respectively, to yield a concentration of 2 mg/ml. Swirl the vial gently to mix; don't shake or invert it. Add the reconstituted drug to an infusion bag containing 0.9% NaCl, and dilute to a final concentration of 100 to 200 mcg/ml. Direct the stream to the side of the bag to mini-mize agitation. Invert the infusion bag to mix the solution. Start the infusion within 3 hours after recon-stitution. Administer the drug through a dedicated IV line or a dedicated lumen of a multilumen central venous catheter at a rate of 24 mcg/kg/hr for 96 hours. If the infusion is interrupted, restart it at 24 mcg/kg/hr, as prescribed.

Duloxetine
du-lox′uh-teen
(Cymbalta)

CATEGORY AND SCHEDULE
Pregnancy Risk Category: C

CLASSIFICATION
Antidepressants, miscellaneous, serotonin receptor antagonists

MECHANISM OF ACTION
An antidepressant that appears to inhibit serotonin and norepinephrine reuptake at neuronal presynaptic membranes; is a less potent inhibitor

of dopamine reuptake. *Therapeutic Effect:* Relieves depression.

PHARMACOKINETICS
Well absorbed from the GI tract. Protein binding: greater than 90%. Extensively metabolized to active metabolites. Excreted primarily in urine and, to a lesser extent, in feces. **Half-life:** 8-17 hr.

AVAILABILITY
Capsules: 20 mg, 30 mg, 60 mg.

INDICATIONS AND DOSAGES
▶ **Major depressive disorder**
PO
Adults. 20 mg twice a day, increased up to 60 mg/day as a single dose or in 2 divided doses.

CONTRAINDICATIONS
End-stage renal disease (creatinine clearance less than 30 ml/min), severe hepatic impairment, uncontrolled angle-closure glaucoma, use within 14 days of MAOIs

INTERACTIONS
Drug
Alcohol: Increases the risk of hepatic injury.
Fluoxetine, fluvoxamine, paroxetine, quinidine, quinolone antimicrobials: May increase duloxetine plasma concentration.
MAOIs: May cause serotonin syndrome, characterized by autonomic hyperactivity, coma, diaphoresis, excitement, hyperthermia, and rigidity.
Thioridazine: May produce ventricular arrhythmias.
Warfarin: May increase the warfarin plasma concentration.
Herbal
St John's wort: May increase adverse effects.

Food
None known.

DIAGNOSTIC TEST EFFECTS
May increase serum bilirubin, AST (SGOT), and ALT (SGPT) levels.

SIDE EFFECTS
Frequent (20%-11%)
Nausea, dry mouth, constipation, insomnia
Occasional (9%-5%)
Dizziness, fatigue, diarrhea, somnolence, anorexia, diaphoresis, vomiting
Rare (4%-2%)
Blurred vision, erectile dysfunction, delayed or failed ejaculation, anorgasmia, anxiety, decreased libido, hot flashes

SERIOUS REACTIONS
• Duloxetine use may slightly increase the patient's heart rate.
• Colitis, dysphagia, gastritis, and irritable bowel syndrome occur rarely.

PRECAUTIONS & CONSIDERATIONS
Caution is warranted with conditions that may slow gastric emptying, hepatic impairment, history of anemia, history of seizures, renal impairment, and suicidal tendencies. Be aware that duloxetine use in pregnant women may produce neonatal adverse reactions including constant crying, feeding difficulty, hyperreflexia, and irritability. Be aware that it is unknown if duloxetine is distributed in breast milk. Breastfeeding is not recommended. Be aware that the safety and efficacy of duloxetine have not been established in children. Exercise caution when increasing duloxetine doses in the elderly.

Drowsiness and dizziness may occur, so avoid alcohol and tasks that require mental alertness or motor skills. Blood chemistry tests to assess hepatic and renal function should be performed before and periodically during therapy.

Administration
Take without regard to meals. Take with food or milk if GI distress occurs. Do not crush or chew enteric-coated capsules. Do not sprinkle capsule contents on food or mix with liquids. The therapeutic effects of duloxetine will be noted within one to four weeks. Do not abruptly discontinue duloxetine.

Dutasteride
du-tas'tur-ide
(Avodart)

CATEGORY AND SCHEDULE
Pregnancy Risk Category: X

CLASSIFICATION
5-alpha-reductase inhibitors, antiandrogens, hormones/ hormone modifiers

MECHANISM OF ACTION
An androgen hormone inhibitor that inhibits 5-alpha reductase, an intracellular enzyme that converts testosterone into dihydrotestosterone (DHT) in the prostate gland, reducing the serum DHT level.
Therapeutic Effect: Reduces size of the prostate gland.

PHARMACOKINETICS

Route	Onset	Peak	Duration
PO	24 hr	N/A	3-8 wk

Moderately absorbed after PO administration. Widely distributed. Protein binding: 99%. Metabolized

in the liver. Primarily excreted in feces. **Half-life:** Up to 5 wk.

AVAILABILITY
Capsule: 0.5 mg.

INDICATIONS AND DOSAGES
▸ **Benign prostatic hyperplasia (BPH)**
PO
Adults, Elderly. 0.5 mg once a day.

OFF-LABEL USES
Treatment of hair loss

CONTRAINDICATIONS
Females, physical handling of tablets by those who are or may be pregnant

INTERACTIONS
Drug
Calcium channel antagonists, cimetidine: May increase dutasteride concentrations.
Herbal
None known.
Food
None known.

DIAGNOSTIC TEST EFFECTS
Decreases the serum prostate-specific antigen (PSA) level

SIDE EFFECTS
Occasional
Gynecomastia, sexual dysfunction (decreased libido, impotence, and decreased volume of ejaculate)

SERIOUS REACTIONS
• Toxicity may be manifested as rash, diarrhea, and abdominal pain.

PRECAUTIONS & CONSIDERATIONS
Caution is warranted with hepatic impairment, pre-existing sexual dysfunction (such as impotence and decreased libido), and obstructive uropathy. The drug has a pregnancy risk category of X and carries the

risk of causing anomalies in the male fetus.

Dutasteride may cause impotence and decrease ejaculate volume. Serum PSA determinations should be obtained before and periodically during therapy. Intake and output and improvement in BPH signs and symptoms should also be monitored.

Administration

Don't break, crush, or open capsules. Take dutasteride without regard to food. Urinary flow may not improve for up to 6 months after beginning treatment.

Dyphylline
dye′fi-lin
(Dilor, Lufyllin)
Do not confuse with Dilacor.

CATEGORY AND SCHEDULE
Pregnancy Risk Category: C

CLASSIFICATION
Bronchodilators, xanthine derivatives

MECHANISM OF ACTION
A xanthine derivative that acts as a bronchodilator by directly relaxing smooth muscle of the bronchial airway and pulmonary blood vessels similar to theophylline. *Therapeutic Effect:* Relieves bronchospasm, increases vital capacity, produces cardiac and skeletal muscle stimulation.

PHARMACOKINETICS
Rapid absorption after PO administration. Protein binding: unknown. Not metabolized to theophylline in vivo. Excreted in urine. **Half-life:** 2 hr.

AVAILABILITY
Elixir: 100 mg/15 ml (Lufyllin).
Injection: 250 mg/ml (Dilor).
Tablet: 200 mg, 400 mg (Dilor, Lufyllin).

INDICATIONS AND DOSAGES
▶ **Chronic bronchospasm, asthma**
PO
Adults, Elderly. 15 mg/kg 4 times/day.
IM
Adults, Elderly. 250-500 mg. Maximum: 15 mg/kg q6hr.
Children. 4.4-6.6 mg/kg/day in divided doses.
Dosage in renal impairment

Creatinine Clearance	Dosage Percent
50-80 ml/min	Administer 75% of dose
10-50 ml/min	Administer 50% of dose
<10 ml/min	Administer 25% of dose

CONTRAINDICATIONS
Uncontrolled arrhythmias, hyperthyroidism, history of hypersensitivity to dyphylline, related xanthine derivatives, or any component of the formulation

INTERACTIONS
Drug
Beta-blockers: May decrease effects of dyphylline.
Cimetidine, ciprofloxacin, erythromycin, norfloxacin: May increase dyphylline blood concentrations and risk of toxicity.
Glucocorticoids: May produce hypernatremia.
Phenytoin, primidone, rifampin: May increase dyphylline metabolism.
Smoking: May decrease dyphylline blood concentrations.

SIDE EFFECTS
Frequent
Tachycardia, nervousness, restlessness
Occasional
Heartburn, vomiting, headache, mild diuresis, insomnia, nausea

SERIOUS REACTIONS
• Ventricular arrhythmias, hypotension, circulatory failure, seizures, hyperglycemia, and syndrome of inappropriate antidiuretic hormone (SIADH) have been reported.

PRECAUTIONS & CONSIDERATIONS
Caution is necessary with congestive heart failure (CHF), impaired cardiac or renal function, peptic ulcer disease, and seizure disorder. Be aware that dyphylline is equivalent to 70% theophylline.

Serious dosing errors can occur if dyphylline serum levels are monitored by theophylline serum assay. Smoking, charcoal-broiled food, and a high-protein, low-carbohydrate diet may decrease dyphylline level. Caffeine derivatives such as chocolate, coffee, cola, cocoa, and tea should be avoided.

Oxygen depletion may occur and is evident by blue or gray lips, blue or dusky-colored fingernails in light-skinned patients, and gray fingernails in dark-skinned persons.

Storage
Store at room temperature. Discard if solution contains a precipitate.

Administration
Give oral dyphylline with food to avoid gastrointestinal (GI) distress.

Give dyphylline IM injection slowly.

Econazole
e-kone'a-zole
(Ecostatin [CAN], Spectazole)

CATEGORY AND SCHEDULE
Pregnancy Risk Category: C

CLASSIFICATION
Antifungals, topical, dermatologics

MECHANISM OF ACTION
An imidazole derivative that changes the permeability of the fungal cell wall. *Therapeutic Effect:* Inhibits fungal biosynthesis of triglycerides, phospholipids. Fungistatic.

PHARMACOKINETICS
Low systemic absorption. Protein binding: 98%. Metabolized in liver to more than 20 metabolites. Primarily excreted in urine; minimal excretion in feces. Not removed by hemodialysis.

AVAILABILITY
Cream: 1% (Spectazole).

INDICATIONS AND DOSAGES
▸ **Treatment of tinea pedis, tinea cruris, tinea corporis, tinea versicolor**
TOPICAL
Adults, Elderly, Children. Apply once daily to affected area for 2-4 wk.

OFF-LABEL USES
Cutaneous candidiasis, otomycosis

CONTRAINDICATIONS
Hypersensitivity to econazole

INTERACTIONS
Drug
Amphotericin B: May increase antagonism of these agents.

Benzodiazepines: May increase concentrations of benzodiazepines.
Fentanyl: May increase CNS and respiratory depression of fentanyl.
Herbal
None known.
Food
None known.

DIAGNOSTIC TEST EFFECTS
None known.

SIDE EFFECTS
Occasional (10%-1%)
Vulvar/vaginal burning
Rare (less than 1%)
Itching and burning of sexual partner, polyuria, vulvar itching, soreness, edema, discharge

SERIOUS REACTIONS
• None known.

PRECAUTIONS & CONSIDERATIONS
Caution should be used during pregnancy. Econazole should be avoided during the first trimester of pregnancy. Use only if clearly needed in the second and third trimesters.

It is unknown if econazole is distributed in breast milk.
Administration
Apply and rub gently into affected areas once daily. Prolonged therapy over weeks or months may be necessary. Avoid occlusive dressings and wear light clothing for ventilation.

Edetate Calcium Disodium (Calcium EDTA)

ed-eh-tate kal-see-um dye-sow-dee-um

(Calcium Disodium Versenate)

Do not confuse with edetate disodium.

CATEGORY AND SCHEDULE
Pregnancy Risk Category: B

CLASSIFICATION
Antidotes, heavy metal

MECHANISM OF ACTION
A chelating agent that reduces blood concentration of heavy metals, especially lead, forming stable complexes. *Therapeutic Effect:* Allows heavy metal excretion in urine.

PHARMACOKINETICS
Well absorbed after parenteral administration; poorly absorbed from the gastrointestinal (GI) tract. Penetrates to extracellular fluid and slowly diffuses into cerebrospinal fluid (CSF). No metabolism occurs. Excreted in the urine either unchanged or as the metal chelates. **Half-life:** 20-60 min (IV), 1.5 hr (IM).

AVAILABILITY
Injection: 200 mg/ml (Calcium Disodium Versenate).

INDICATIONS AND DOSAGES
▸ **Diagnosis of lead poisoning**
IM/IV
Adults, Elderly. 500 mg/m2. Maximum: 1 g/m2/day divided in equal doses 8-12 hr apart for 5 days, skip 2-4 days and repeat course if needed.
IM
Children. 500 mg/m2 as single dose or 500 mg/m2 each at 12-hr intervals.
IV
Children. 1 g/m2/day IV infusion over 8-12 hr for 5 days, skip 2-4 days and repeat course as needed. Maximum: 75 mg/kg/day
Lead poisoning (without encephalopathy)
IM/IV
Adults, Elderly, Children. 1-1.5 g/m2 daily for 3-5 days (if blood lead concentration >100 mcg/dl, calcium edetate usually given with dimercaprol). Allow at least 2-4 days, up to 2-3 wk between courses of therapy. Adults should not be given more than 2 courses of therapy.
Lead poisoning (with encephalopathy)
IM
Adults, Elderly, Children. Initially, dimercaprol 4 mg/kg; then give dimercaprol 4 mg/kg and calcium EDTA 250 mg/m2; then 4 hr later and q4hr for 5 days.

CONTRAINDICATIONS
Anuria, severe renal disease, hypersensitivity to EDTA or any component of the formulation

INTERACTIONS
Drug
Zinc: May decrease the effects of zinc.
Herbal
None known.
Food
None known.

SIDE EFFECTS
Frequent
Chills, fever, anorexia, headache, histamine-like reaction (sneezing, stuffy nose, watery eyes), decreased blood pressure (B/P), nausea, vomiting, thrombophlebitis
Rare
Frequent urination, secondary gout (severe pain in feet, knees, elbows).

SERIOUS REACTIONS
• Drug may produce same signs of renal damage as severe acute lead poisoning (proteinuria, microscopic hematuria). Transient anemia/bone marrow depression, hypercalcemia (constipation, drowsiness, dry mouth, metallic taste) occurs occasionally.

PRECAUTIONS & CONSIDERATIONS
Edetate calcium disodium is capable of producing toxic effects which can be fatal. Dosage schedules should be followed and at no time should the recommended daily dose be increased. It is unknown whether EDTA is distributed in breast milk. Lead encephalopathy is usually rare in adults, but occurs more often in children. There are no age-related precautions noted in children or the elderly. Edetate calcium disodium may produce the same renal damage as lead poisoning such as proteinuria and microscopic hematuria.

Administration
Be aware that when administering IV, calcium EDTA may be given in 2 divided doses at 12 hr intervals or 12-24 hr infusions; when administered IM and used alone, may be given in divided doses at 8-12 hr intervals; when given IM with dimercaprol in divided doses, administer at 4-hr intervals.

Be aware that total dose is dependent on severity of lead poisoning, patient response and/or tolerance to medication. Consult specific protocols.

For IV administration, dilute with 0.9% NaCl or D_5W. Physically incompatible with $D_{10}W$, LR, and Ringer's injection.

For intermittent IV infusion, administer the dose over at least 1 hour in asymptomatic patients and 2 hours in symptomatic patients.

For IV continuous infusion, dilute to 2-4 mg/ml in 0.9% NaCl or D_5W and infuse over at least 8 hours, usually over 12-24 hours.

Avoid rapid IV infusion (may be lethal due to increased intracranial pressure).

For IM injection, may administer 1 ml of 1% procaine hydrochloride to each ml of EDTA calcium to minimize pain at injection site.

E

Edetate Disodium
ed′eh-tate dye-sow-dee-um
(Disotate, Endrate)
Do not confuse with edetate calcium disodium.

CATEGORY AND SCHEDULE
Pregnancy Risk Category: C

CLASSIFICATION
Antidotes, chelators

MECHANISM OF ACTION
A chelating agent that forms a soluble chelate with calcium, resulting in rapid decrease in plasma calcium concentrations. *Therapeutic Effect:* Allows calcium to be excreted in urine.

PHARMACOKINETICS
Distributed in extracellular fluid and does not appear in red blood cells. No metabolism occurs. Rapidly excreted in the urine. **Half-life:** 1.4-3 hr.

AVAILABILITY
Injection: 150 mg/ml (Disotate, Endrate).

INDICATIONS AND DOSAGES
▸ **Digitalis toxicity, hypercalcemia**

IV
Adults, Elderly. 500 mg/kg/day over
3 hr or more, daily for 5 days, skip
2 days, repeat as needed up to
15 doses. Maximum: 3 g/day.
Children. 40 mg/kg/day over 3 hr
or more, daily for 5 days, skip
5 days, repeat as needed. Maximum:
70 mg/kg/day.

CONTRAINDICATIONS
Anuria, renal impairment, hypersensitivity to EDTA or any component
of the formulation

INTERACTIONS
Drug
Insulin: May increase the effects
of insulin.
Herbal
None known.
Food
None known.

SIDE EFFECTS
Frequent
Abdominal cramps or pain, diarrhea,
nausea, vomiting, circumoral
paresthesia, headache, numbness,
postural hypotension
Rare
Exfoliative dermatitis, toxic skin
and mucous membrane reactions,
thrombophlebitis (at injection site)

SERIOUS REACTIONS
• Nephrotoxicity may occur with
excessive dosages.
• Hypomagnesemia may occur with
prolonged use.

PRECAUTIONS & CONSIDERATIONS
Caution is warranted with diabetes
mellitus, clinical or subclinical
hypokalemia, and limited cardiac
reserve or incipient congestive heart
failure. Be aware that edetate sodium
is recommended only when the
severity of the clinical condition
justifies the aggressive measures
associated with this type of therapy.
It is unknown whether edetate
disodium is distributed in breast
milk. There are no age-related
precautions noted in children or the
elderly.
  Stop edetate sodium immediately
and notify physician if frequent or
sudden urges to urinate occurs.
Administration
Be aware that edetate disodium
is rarely used to treat digitalis-
induced ventricular arrhythmias
since other more effect agents are
available. It should only be used in
emergency situations. It is not for
IM use.
  Dilute solution for injection with
500 ml of D_5W or 0.9% NaCl before
IV administration; in pediatric
patients, concentration should not
exceed 3%. Administer by IV infusion only after dilution. Be aware to
not exceed recommended dose or
rate of administration. A precipitous
drop in serum calcium concentrations may occur. Calcium replacement suitable for intravenous
administration should be instantly
available.

Edrophonium
ed-roe-foe′nee-um
(Enlon, Reversol, Tensilon)

CATEGORY AND SCHEDULE
Pregnancy Risk Category: C

CLASSIFICATION
Cholinesterase inhibitors,
musculoskeletal agents,
stimulants, muscle

MECHANISM OF ACTION
A parasympathetic, anticholinesterase agent that inhibits destruction of acetylcholine by acetylcholinesterase, thus causing accumulation of acetylcholine at cholinergic synapses. Results in an increase in cholinergic responses such as miosis, increased tonus of intestinal and skeletal muscles, bronchial and ureteral constriction, bradycardia and increased salivary and sweat gland secretions. *Therapeutic Effect:* Diagnosis of myasthenia gravis.

PHARMACOKINETICS
Onset of action occurs within 30-60 seconds and has duration of 10 minutes. Rapid absorption after IV administration. Exact method of metabolism is unknown. Rapidly excreted in urine. **Half-life:** 1.8 hr.

AVAILABILITY
Injection: 10 mg/ml (Enlon, Reversol, Tensilon).

INDICATIONS AND DOSAGES
▶ **Diagnosis of myasthenia gravis**
IV
Adults, Elderly. 2 mg test dose over 15-30 seconds. If no reaction in 45 seconds, give additional dose of 8 mg. Test dose may be repeated after 30 minutes.
Children more than 34 kg. Initially, 2 mg over 1 minute. If no reaction in 45 seconds, may repeat at a rate of 1 mg every 30-45 seconds. Maximum cumulative dose: 10 mg.
Children less than 34 kg. Initially, 1 mg over 1 minute. If no reaction in 45 seconds, may repeat at a rate of 1 mg every 30-45 seconds. Maximum cumulative dose: 5 mg.
Infants. 0.5 mg infused over 1 minute.
IM/SC
Adults, Elderly, Children. Initially, 10 mg as a single dose. If no

cholinergic reaction occurs, give 2 mg 30 minutes later to rule out false-negative reaction.
Children more than 34 kg. 5 mg as a single dose.
Children less than 34 kg. 2 mg as a single dose.
Infants. 0.5-1 mg as a single dose.
▶ **Neuromuscular blockade antagonism**
IV
Adults, Elderly. 10 mg over 30-45 seconds. May be repeated as needed until a cholinergic response is detected. Maximum: 40 mg.
IM
Children. 233 mcg/kg as a single dose.
Infants. 145 mcg/kg as a single dose.
Dosage in Renal Impairment
Dose may need to be reduced in patients with chronic renal failure.

CONTRAINDICATIONS
Gastrointestinal (GI) or genitourinary (GU) obstruction, hypersensitivity to edrophonium, sulfites, or any component of the formulation

INTERACTIONS
Drug
Atropine, nondepolarizing muscle relaxants, procainamide, quinidine: May decrease the effects of edrophonium.
Succinylcholine, digoxin, IV acetazolamide, neostigmine, physostigmine: May increase the effects of edrophonium.
Herbal
None known.
Food
None known.

DIAGNOSTIC TEST EFFECTS
May increase serum amylase, SGOT (AST) and SGPT (ALT) levels.

IV Compatibilities
Heparin, hydrocortisone, vitamin B complex with C

SIDE EFFECTS
Frequent
Increase salivation, intestinal secretions, lacrimation, urinary urgency, hyperperistalsis, sweating
Occasional
Bradycardia, hypotension, convulsions, dysphagia, nausea, vomiting, diarrhea
Rare
Bronchoconstriction, cardiac arrest, central respiratory paralysis

SERIOUS REACTIONS
• Overdosage causes symptoms of cholinergic crisis such as muscle weakness, nausea, vomiting, miosis, bronchospasm, and respiratory paralysis.

PRECAUTIONS & CONSIDERATIONS
Caution is warranted with bronchial asthma and those receiving a cardiac glycoside. It is unknown if edrophonium crosses the placenta or is distributed in breast milk. There are no age-related precautions noted in children. Age-related renal impairment may require dose adjustment in the elderly.

If difficulty breathing, dizziness, muscle cramps and spasms, or vomiting occurs, notify the physician immediately. Side effects of edrophonium will not last long because the effects of the drug are short-lived.
Administration
Be aware that atropine should always be readily available as an antagonist for treatment of cholinergic reactions. Intubation and controlled ventilation may also be required if cholinergic crisis occurs.
Be aware that edrophonium is usually administered IV, however, if not possible, IM or subcutaneous may be used.

Efalizumab
(Raptiva)

CATEGORY AND SCHEDULE
Pregnancy Risk Category: C

CLASSIFICATION
Immunosuppressives

MECHANISM OF ACTION
A monoclonal antibody that interferes with lymphocyte activation by binding to the lymphocyte antigen, inhibiting the adhesion of leukocytes to other cell types. *Therapeutic Effect:* Prevents the release of cytokines and the growth and migration of circulating total lymphocytes, predominant in psoriatic lesions.

PHARMACOKINETICS
Clearance is affected by body weight, not by gender or race, after subcutaneous injection. Serum concentration reaches steady state at 4 wk. Mean time to elimination: 25 days.

AVAILABILITY
Powder for Injection: 150 mg, designed to deliver 125 mg/1.25 ml.

INDICATIONS AND DOSAGES
▸ **Psoriasis**
SUBCUTANEOUS
Adults, Elderly. Initially, 0.7 mg/kg followed by weekly doses of 1 mg/kg. Maximum: 200 mg (single dose).

CONTRAINDICATIONS
Concurrent use of immunosuppressive agents

INTERACTIONS
Drug
Immunosuppressive agents:
Increase the risk of infection.
Live-virus vaccines: Decrease the immune response.
Herbal
None known.
Food
None known.

DIAGNOSTIC TEST EFFECTS
May increase the lymphocyte count.

SIDE EFFECTS
Frequent (32%-10%)
Headache, chills, nausea, injection site pain
Occasional (8%-7%)
Myalgia, flu-like symptoms, fever
Rare (4%)
Back pain, acne

SERIOUS REACTIONS
• Hypersensitivity reaction, malignancies, serious infections (abscess, cellulitis, postoperative wound infection, pneumonia), thrombocytopenia, and worsening of psoriasis occur rarely.

PRECAUTIONS & CONSIDERATIONS
Caution is warranted with asthma, chronic infections, a history of allergic reactions, and a history of malignancy. It is unknown if efalizumab is distributed in breast milk. Efalizumab is not indicated for use in children. Age-related increased incidence of infection requires cautious use in the elderly. Phototherapy treatments should be avoided.

Notify the physician of bleeding from gums, bruising or petechiae of the skin, or signs of infection. Skin should be examined throughout therapy and improvement or worsening of psoriasis lesions should be documented. CBC, lymphocyte, and platelet counts should be obtained before beginning therapy and periodically thereafter.

Storage
Refrigerate unopened vials. Reconstituted solution may be stored at room temperature for up to 8 hours.

Administration
For subcutaneous use, slowly inject 1.3 ml of sterile water for injection into the efalizumab vial using the provided prefilled diluent syringe. Swirl the vial gently to dissolve; do not shake it because foaming will occur. Dissolution takes less than 5 minutes. Administer the injection into the abdomen, buttocks, thigh, or upper arm.

E

Efavirenz
e-fahv′er-ins
(Stocrin [AUS], Sustiva)
Do not confuse with Survanta.

CATEGORY AND SCHEDULE
Pregnancy Risk Category: C

CLASSIFICATION
Antivirals, non-nucleoside reverse transcriptase inhibitors

MECHANISM OF ACTION
A nonnucleoside reverse transcriptase inhibitor that inhibits the activity of HIV reverse transcriptase of HIV-1 and the transcription of HIV-1 RNA to DNA. *Therapeutic Effect:* Interrupts HIV replication,

slowing the progression of HIV infection.

PHARMACOKINETICS

Rapidly absorbed after PO administration. Protein binding: 99%. Metabolized to major isoenzymes in the liver. Eliminated in urine and feces. **Half-life:** 40-55 hr.

AVAILABILITY

Capsules: 50 mg, 100 mg, 200 mg.
Tablets: 600 mg.

INDICATIONS AND DOSAGES
▸ **HIV infection (in combination with other antiretrovirals)**
PO
Adults, Elderly, Children 3 yr and older weighing 40 kg or more. 600 mg once a day at bedtime.
Children 3 yr and older weighing 32.5 kg-less than 40 kg. 400 mg once a day.
Children 3 yr and older weighing 25 kg-less than 32.5 kg. 350 mg once a day.
Children 3 yr and older weighing 20 kg-less than 25 kg. 300 mg once a day.
Children 3 yr and older weighing 15 kg-less than 20 kg. 250 mg once a day.
Children 3 yr and older weighing 10 kg-less than 15 kg. 200 mg once a day.

CONTRAINDICATIONS

Concurrent use with ergot derivatives, midazolam, or triazolam; efavirenz as monotherapy; hypersensitivity to efavirenz

INTERACTIONS
Drug
Alcohol, psychoactive drugs: May produce additive CNS effects.
Clarithromycin: Decreases clarithromycin plasma levels.

Ergot derivatives, midazolam, triazolam: May cause serious or life-threatening reactions, such as arrhythmias, prolonged sedation, or respiratory depression.
Indinavir, saquinavir: Decreases the plasma concentrations of these drugs.
Nelfinavir, ritonavir: Increases the plasma concentrations of these drugs.
Phenobarbital, rifabutin, rifampin: Lowers efavirenz plasma concentration.
Warfarin: Alters warfarin plasma concentration.
Herbal
None known.
Food
High-fat meals: May increase drug absorption.

DIAGNOSTIC TEST EFFECTS

May produce false-positive urine test results for cannabinoid and increase total cholesterol, AST (SGOT), ALT (SGPT), and serum triglyceride levels.

SIDE EFFECTS
Frequent (52%)
Mild to severe: Dizziness, vivid dreams, insomnia, confusion, impaired concentration, amnesia, agitation, depersonalization, hallucinations, euphoria, somnolence (mild symptoms don't interfere with daily activities; severe symptoms interrupt daily activities)
Occasional
Mild to moderate: Maculopapular rash (27%); nausea, fatigue, headache, diarrhea, fever, cough (less than 26%) (moderate symptoms may interfere with daily activities)

SERIOUS REACTIONS

• Convulsions and immune reconstitution syndrome rarely occur. Psychiatric symptoms including aggressive behavior, paranoid reactions, severe depression, and manic reactions may occur.

PRECAUTIONS & CONSIDERATIONS

Caution is warranted with a history of liver impairment, mental illness, or substance abuse. Be aware of breast-feeding while taking efavirenz. Be aware that the safety and efficacy of efavirenz have not been established in children younger than 3 years. In children, there may be an increased incidence of rash. There are no age-related precautions noted in the elderly. Efavirenz is not a cure for HIV infection, nor does it reduce risk of transmission to others. Expect to obtain history of all prescription and nonprescription medications before giving the drug because efavirenz interacts with several drugs. Monitor for signs and symptoms of adverse CNS psychological side effects, such as abnormal dreams, dizziness, impaired concentration, insomnia, severe acute depression, including suicidal ideation or attempts, and somnolence. Avoid tasks that require mental alertness or motor skills until response to the drug is established. Be aware that insomnia may begin during the first or second day of therapy and generally resolves in 2 to 4 weeks.

Administration

Take without regard to food. Do not take with high-fat meals because it may decrease drug absorption. For adults and the elderly, take efavirenz at bedtime during the first 2 to 4 weeks because of the increased risk of temporary CNS side effects. Take the medication every day as prescribed. Do not alter the dose or discontinue the medication without first notifying the physician.

Eflornithine
eh-floor-nigh-theen
(Vaniqa)

E

CATEGORY AND SCHEDULE
Pregnancy Risk Category: C

CLASSIFICATION
Antiprotozoals, depilatory agents, dermatologics

MECHANISM OF ACTION
A topical antiprotozoal that inhibits ornithine decarboxylase cell division and synthetic function in the skin. *Therapeutic Effect:* Reduces rate of hair growth.

PHARMACOKINETICS
Absorption is less than 1% from intact skin. Not metabolized. Primarily excreted as unchanged drug in urine. **Half life:** 8 hr.

AVAILABILITY
Cream: 13.9% (Vaniqa).

INDICATIONS AND DOSAGES
▶ **For reduction of unwanted facial hair in women**
TOPICAL
Adults, Elderly. Apply thin layer to affected area of face and adjacent involved areas under chin; rub in thoroughly. Use twice daily at least 8 hr apart. Do not wash area for at least 4 hr.

CONTRAINDICATIONS
Hypersensitivity to eflornithine or any component of the formulation

INTERACTIONS
Drug
None known.

Herbal
None known.
Food
None known.

DIAGNOSTIC TEST EFFECTS
May elevate serum transaminases.

SIDE EFFECTS
Frequent
Acne
Occasional
Headache, stinging/burning skin, dry skin, pruritus, erythema
Rare
Tingling skin, rash, dyspepsia (heartburn, GI distress)

SERIOUS REACTIONS
* Bleeding skin, cheilitis, contact dermatitis, herpes simplex, lip swelling, nausea, numbness, rosacea, and weakness have been reported.

PRECAUTIONS & CONSIDERATIONS
Caution is warranted with pre-existing bone marrow suppression or hematologic abnormalities. It is unknown if eflornithine is distributed in breast milk. Safety and efficacy of eflornithine have not been established in children. There are no age-related precautions noted in the elderly. Transient stinging or burning may occur when applied to broken or abraded skin.
Administration
May continue to use other hair removal techniques in conjunction with eflornithine. Apply eflornithine more than 5 minutes after hair removal. Avoid application on abraded or broken skin. Cosmetics or sunscreen may be applied over treated areas after cream has dried. Therapeutic improvement noted in 4-8 weeks. Condition may return to pre-treatment levels 8 weeks after discontinuing treatment.

Eletriptan
(Relpax)

CATEGORY AND SCHEDULE
Pregnancy Risk Category: C

CLASSIFICATION
Serotonin receptor agonists

MECHANISM OF ACTION
A serotonin receptor agonist that binds selectively to vascular receptors, producing a vasoconstrictive effect on cranial blood vessels. *Therapeutic Effect:* Relieves migraine headache.

PHARMACOKINETICS
Well absorbed after PO administration. Metabolized by the liver to inactive metabolite. Eliminated in urine. **Half-life:** 4.4 hr increased in hepatic impairment and the elderly (older than 65 yr).

AVAILABILITY
Tablets: 20 mg, 40 mg.

INDICATIONS AND DOSAGES
▶ **Acute migraine headache**
PO
Adults, Elderly. 20-40 mg. If headache improves but then returns, dose may be repeated after 2 hr. Maximum: 80 mg/day.

CONTRAINDICATIONS
Arrhythmias associated with conduction disorders, coronary artery disease, ischemic heart disease, severe hepatic impairment, uncontrolled hypertension

INTERACTIONS
Drug
Clarithromycin, itraconazole, ketoconazole, nefazodone, nelfinavir, ritonavir: May decrease eletriptan metabolism.
Ergotamine-containing medications: May produce a vasospastic reaction.
Sibutramine: May produce serotonin syndrome (marked by altered LOC, CNS irritability, motor weakness, myoclonus, and shivering).
Herbal
None known.
Food
None known.

DIAGNOSTIC TEST EFFECTS
None known.

SIDE EFFECTS
Occasional (6%-5%)
Dizziness, somnolence, asthenia, nausea
Rare (3%-2%)
Paresthesia, headache, dry mouth, warm or hot sensation, dyspepsia, dysphagia

SERIOUS REACTIONS
• Cardiac reactions (including ischemia, coronary artery vasospasm, and MI) and noncardiac vasospasm-related reactions (such as hemorrhage and CVA) occur rarely, particularly in patients with hypertension, diabetes, or a strong family history of coronary artery disease; obese patients; smokers; males older than 40 years; and postmenopausal women.

PRECAUTIONS & CONSIDERATIONS
Caution is warranted with controlled hypertension, mild to moderate hepatic or renal impairment, and a history of CVA. Eletriptan is distributed in breast milk and may suppress ovulation. The safety and efficacy of eletriptan have not been established in children younger than 18 years. The elderly are at increased risk for hypertension. Tasks that require mental alertness or motor skills should be avoided.

Notify the physician immediately if palpitations, pain or tightness in the chest or throat, pain or weakness in the extremities, or sudden or severe abdominal pain occurs. B/P for evidence of uncontrolled hypertension should be assessed before treatment. Migraines and associated symptoms, including nausea and vomiting, photophobia, and phonophobia (sound sensitivity) should be assessed before and during treatment.
Administration
! Don't administer clarithromycin, erythromycin, itraconazole, ketoconazole, nefazodone, nelfinavir, or ritonavir during the last 7 days of eletriptan therapy.

Take film-coated tablets whole; don't crush or break them.

Emtricitabine
(Emtriva)

CATEGORY AND SCHEDULE
Pregnancy Risk Category: B

CLASSIFICATION
Antivirals, nucleoside reverse transcriptase inhibitors

MECHANISM OF ACTION
An antiretroviral that inhibits HIV-1 reverse transcriptase by incorporating itself into viral DNA, resulting in chain termination. *Therapeutic Effect:* Interrupts HIV replication,

slowing the progression of HIV infection.

PHARMACOKINETICS
Rapidly and extensively absorbed from the GI tract. Excreted primarily in urine (86%) and, to a lesser extent, in feces (14%); 30% removed by hemodialysis. Unknown if removed by peritoneal dialysis. **Half-life:** 10 hr.

AVAILABILITY
Capsules: 200 mg.

INDICATIONS AND DOSAGES
▸ **HIV infection (in combination with other antiretrovirals)**
PO
Adults, Elderly. 200 mg once a day.
▸ **Dosage in renal impairment**
Dosage and frequency are modified based on creatinine clearance.

Creatinine Clearance	Dosage
30-49 ml/min	200 mg q48hr
15-29 ml/min	200 mg q72hr
Less than 15 ml/min, hemodialysis patients	200 mg q96hr

CONTRAINDICATIONS
None known.

INTERACTIONS
Drug
None known.
Herbal
None known.
Food
None known.

DIAGNOSTIC TEST EFFECTS
May elevate serum amylase, lipase, ALT (SGPT), AST (SGOT), and triglyceride levels. May alter blood glucose levels.

SIDE EFFECTS
Frequent (23%-13%)
Headache, rhinitis, rash, diarrhea, nausea
Occasional (14%-4%)
Cough, vomiting, abdominal pain, insomnia, depression, paresthesia, dizziness, peripheral neuropathy, dyspepsia, myalgia
Rare (3%-2%)
Arthralgia, abnormal dreams

SERIOUS REACTIONS
• Lactic acidosis and hepatomegaly with steatosis occur rarely and may be severe.

PRECAUTIONS & CONSIDERATIONS
Caution is warranted with impaired liver or renal function. Be aware that breast-feeding is not recommended. Be aware that the safety and efficacy of this drug have not been established in children. In the elderly, age-related decreased renal function may require dosage adjustment. Emtricitabine use may cause the redistribution of body fat. Emtricitabine is not a cure for HIV infection, nor does it reduce risk of transmission to others.

Expect to obtain baseline laboratory testing, especially liver function tests and triglycerides before beginning emtricitabine therapy, and at periodic intervals during therapy. Assess for any nausea or vomiting and skin for rash and urticaria. Determine pattern of bowel activity and stool consistency.
Administration
Take without regard to food. Continue emtricitabine therapy for the full length of treatment.

Enalapril

en-al'a-pril

(Alphapril [AUS], Amprace [AUS], Apo-Enalapril [CAN], Auspril [AUS], Renitec [AUS], Vasotec)

Do not confuse with Anafranil, Eldepryl, or ramipril.

CATEGORY AND SCHEDULE

Pregnancy Risk Category: D (C if used in first trimester)

CLASSIFICATION

Angiotensin converting enzyme inhibitors

MECHANISM OF ACTION

This angiotensin-converting enzyme (ACE) inhibitor suppresses the renin-angiotensin-aldosterone system, and prevents conversion of angiotensin I to angiotensin II, a potent vasoconstrictor; may inhibit angiotensin II at local vascular, renal sites. Decreases plasma angiotensin II, increases plasma renin activity, decreases aldosterone secretion. *Therapeutic Effect:* In hypertension, reduces peripheral arterial resistance. In congestive heart failure (CHF), increases cardiac output; decreases peripheral vascular resistance, blood pressure (B/P), pulmonary capillary wedge pressure, heart size.

PHARMACOKINETICS

Route	Onset	Peak	Duration
PO	1 hr	4-6 hr	24 hr
IV	15 min	1-4 hr	6 hr

Readily absorbed from the gastro-intestinal (GI) tract (not affected by food). Protein binding: 50%-60%. Converted to active metabolite. Primarily excreted in urine. Removed by hemodialysis. **Half-life:** 11 hr (half-life is increased in those with impaired renal function).

AVAILABILITY

Tablets: 2.5 mg, 5 mg, 10 mg, 20 mg.
Injection: 1.25 mg/ml.

INDICATIONS AND DOSAGES

▸ **Hypertension alone or in combination with other antihypertensives**
PO
Adults, Elderly. Initially, 2.5-5 mg/day. Range: 10-40 mg/day in 1-2 divided doses.
Children. 0.1 mg/kg/day in 1-2 divided doses. Maximum: 0.5 mg/kg/day.
Neonates. 0.1 mg/kg/day q24hr.
IV
Adults, Elderly. 0.625-1.25 mg q6hr up to 5 mg q6hr.
Children, Neonates. 5-10 mcg/kg/dose q8-24hr.
▸ **Adjunctive therapy for CHF**
PO
Adults, Elderly. Initially, 2.5-5 mg/day. Range: 5-20 mg/day in 2 divided doses.
▸ **Dosage in renal impairment**
Dosage is modified based on creatinine clearance.

Creatinine Clearance	% Usual Dose
10-50 ml/min	75-100
Less than 10 ml/min	50

OFF-LABEL USES

Treatment of diabetic nephropathy or renal crisis in scleroderma

CONTRAINDICATIONS

History of angioedema from previous treatment with ACE inhibitors

E

INTERACTIONS
Drug
Alcohol, antihypertensives, diuretics: May increase the effects of enalapril.
Herbal
None known.
Food
None known.

DIAGNOSTIC TEST EFFECTS
May increase BUN and serum alkaline phosphatase, serum bilirubin, serum creatinine, serum potassium, SGOT (AST), and SGPT (ALT) levels. May decrease serum sodium levels. May cause positive ANA titer.

▓ IV INCOMPATIBILITIES
Amphotericin B (Fungizone), amphotericin B complex (Abelcet, AmBisome, Amphotec), cefepime (Maxipime), phenytoin (Dilantin)

▓ IV Compatibilities
Calcium gluconate, dobutamine (Dobutrex), dopamine (Inotropin), fentanyl (Sublimaze), heparin, lidocaine, magnesium sulfate, morphine, nitroglycerin, potassium chloride, potassium phosphate, propofol (Diprivan)

SIDE EFFECTS
Frequent (7%-5%)
Headache, dizziness
Occasional (3%-2%)
Orthostatic hypotension, fatigue, diarrhea, cough, syncope
Rare (less than 2%)
Angina, abdominal pain, vomiting, nausea, rash, asthenia (loss of strength, energy), syncope

SERIOUS REACTIONS
• Excessive hypotension (first-dose syncope) may occur in patients with CHF and in those who are severely salt or volume depleted.

• Angioedema (swelling of face, lips) and hyperkalemia occur rarely.
• Agranulocytosis and neutropenia may be noted in patients with collagen vascular diseases, including scleroderma and systemic lupus erythematosus, and impaired renal function.
• Nephrotic syndrome may be noted in those with history of renal disease.

PRECAUTIONS & CONSIDERATIONS
Caution is warranted with cerebrovascular and coronary insufficiency, hypovolemia, renal impairment, sodium depletion, and those on dialysis and/or receiving diuretics. Be aware that enalapril crosses the placenta and is distributed in breast milk. Enalapril may cause fetal or neonatal morbidity or mortality. Be aware that the safety and efficacy of enalapril have not been established in children. The elderly may be more susceptible to the hypotensive effects of enalapril.

Dizziness may occur. B/P should be obtained immediately before giving each enalapril dose, in addition to regular monitoring. Be alert to fluctuations in B/P. If an excessive reduction in B/P occurs, place the person in the supine position with legs elevated. CBC and blood chemistry should be obtained before beginning enalapril therapy, then every 2 weeks for the next 3 months, and periodically thereafter in patients with autoimmune disease, or renal impairment, and in those who are taking drugs that affect immune response or leukocyte count. BUN, serum creatinine, and serum potassium should also be monitored in those who are receiving a diuretic.
Administration
Do not skip doses.

Enfuvirtide
en-few'vir-tide
(Fuzeon)
Do not confuse with Furoxone.

CATEGORY AND SCHEDULE
Pregnancy Risk Category: B

CLASSIFICATION
Antivirals, fusion inhibitors

MECHANISM OF ACTION
A fusion inhibitor that interferes with the entry of HIV-1 into CD4+ cells by inhibiting the fusion of viral and cellular membranes. *Therapeutic Effect:* Impairs HIV replication, slowing the progression of HIV infection.

PHARMACOKINETICS
Comparable absorption when injected into subcutaneous tissue of abdomen, arm, or thigh. Protein binding: 92%. Undergoes catabolism to amino acids. **Half-life:** 3.8 hr.

AVAILABILITY
Powder for Injection: 108-mg (approximately 90 mg/ml when reconstituted) vials.

INDICATIONS AND DOSAGES
▶ **HIV infection (in combination with other antiretrovirals)**
SUBCUTANEOUS
Adults, Elderly. 90 mg (1 ml) twice a day.
Children 6-16 yr. 2 mg/kg twice a day. Maximum 90 mg twice a day.

▶ **Pediatric dosing guidelines**

Weight: kg (lb)	Dose: mg (ml)
11-15.5 (24-34)	27 (0.3)
15.6-20 (more than 35-44)	36 (0.4)
20.1-24.5 (more than 45-54)	45 (0.5)
24.6-29 (more than 55-64)	54 (0.6)
29.1-33.5 (more than 65-74)	63 (0.7)
33.6-38 (more than 75-84)	72 (0.8)
38.1-42.5 (more than 85-94)	81 (0.9)
Greater than 42.5 (greater than 94)	90 (1)

CONTRAINDICATIONS
Hypersensitivity to enfuvirtide or any of its components.

INTERACTIONS
Drug
None known.
Herbal
None known.
Food
None known.

DIAGNOSTIC TEST EFFECTS
May elevate blood glucose and serum amylase, CK, lipase, triglyceride, AST (SGOT), and ALT (SGPT) levels. May decrease blood hemoglobin levels and WBC count.

SIDE EFFECTS
Expected (98%)
Local injection site reactions (pain, discomfort, induration, erythema, nodules, cysts, pruritus, ecchymosis)
Frequent (26%-16%)
Diarrhea, nausea, fatigue
Occasional (11%-4%)
Insomnia, peripheral neuropathy, depression, cough, decreased appetite or weight loss, sinusitis, anxiety, asthenia, myalgia, cold sores
Rare (3%-2%)
Constipation, influenza, upper abdominal pain, anorexia, conjunctivitis

SERIOUS REACTIONS
• Enfuvirtide use may potentiate bacterial pneumonia.
• Hypersensitivity (rash, fever, chills, rigors, hypotension), thrombocytopenia, neutropenia, and renal insufficiency or failure may occur rarely.

PRECAUTIONS & CONSIDERATIONS
Caution is warranted with liver function impairment. Breast-feeding is not recommended in this patient population due to the possibility of HIV transmission. Be aware that the safety and efficacy of enfuvirtide have not been established in children younger than 6 years of age. There are no age-related precautions noted in the elderly. Increased rate of bacterial pneumonia has occurred with enfuvirtide and seek medical attention if cough with fever, rapid breathing, or shortness of breath occurs. Enfuvirtide is not a cure for HIV infection, nor does it reduce risk of transmission to others.

Expect to obtain baseline laboratory testing, especially liver function tests and serum triglyceride levels, before beginning enfuvirtide therapy and at periodic intervals during therapy. Assess for hypersensitivity reaction and local injection site reaction, fatigue or nausea, depression, and insomnia.
Storage
Store at room temperature. Refrigerate reconstituted solution; use within 24 hours.

Bring reconstituted solution to room temperature before injection.
Administration
Reconstitute with 1.1 ml sterile water for injection. Visually inspect vial for particulate matter. Solution normally appears clear, colorless. Discard unused portion. Administer subcutaneously into the upper abdomen, anterior thigh, or arm. Administer each injection at a different site than the preceding injection site. Continue taking enfuvirtide for the full length of treatment.

Enoxaparin
e-nox-ah-pair'in
(Klexane [CAN], Lovenox)
Do not confuse Lovenox with Lotronex.

CATEGORY AND SCHEDULE
Pregnancy Risk Category: B

CLASSIFICATION
Anticoagulants

MECHANISM OF ACTION
A low-molecular-weight heparin that potentiates the action of antithrombin III and inactivates coagulation factor Xa. *Therapeutic Effect:* Produces anticoagulation. Does not significantly influence bleeding time, PT, or aPTT.

PHARMACOKINETICS

Route	Onset	Peak	Duration
Subcutaneous	N/A	3-5 hr	12 hr

Well absorbed after subcutaneous administration. Eliminated primarily in urine. Not removed by hemodialysis. **Half-life:** 4.5 hr.

AVAILABILITY
Injection: 30 mg/0.3 ml, 40 mg/0.4 ml, 60 mg/0.6 ml, 80 mg/0.8 ml, 100 mg/ml, 120 mg/0.8 ml, 150 mg/ml in prefilled syringes.

INDICATIONS AND DOSAGES
▸ **Prevention of deep vein thrombosis (DVT) after hip and knee surgery**
SUBCUTANEOUS
Adults, Elderly. 30 mg twice a day, generally for 7-10 days.
▸ **Prevention of DVT after abdominal surgery**
SUBCUTANEOUS
Adults, Elderly. 40 mg a day for 7-10 days.
▸ **Prevention of long-term DVT in nonsurgical acute illness**
SUBCUTANEOUS
Adults, Elderly. 40 mg once a day for 3 wk.
▸ **Prevention of ischemic complications of unstable angina and non-Q-wave MI (with oral aspirin therapy)**
SUBCUTANEOUS
Adults, Elderly. 1 mg/kg q12hr.
▸ **Acute DVT**
SUBCUTANEOUS
Adults, Elderly. 1 mg/kg q12hr or 1.5 mg/kg once daily.
▸ **Usual pediatric dosage**
SUBCUTANEOUS
Children. 0.5 mg/kg q12hr (prophylaxis); 1 mg/kg q12hr (treatment).
▸ **Dosage in renal impairment**
Clearance of enoxaparin is decreased when creatinine clearance is less than 30 ml/min. Monitor patient and adjust dosage as necessary. When enoxaparin is used in abdominal, hip, or knee surgery or acute illness, the dosage in renal impairment is 30 mg once a day. When enoxaparin is used to treat DVT, angina, or MI the dosage in renal impairment is 1 mg/kg once a day.

OFF-LABEL USES
Prevention of DVT following general surgical procedures

CONTRAINDICATIONS
Active major bleeding, concurrent heparin therapy, hypersensitivity to heparin or pork products, thrombocytopenia associated with positive in vitro test for antiplatelet antibodies

INTERACTIONS
Drug
Anticoagulants, platelet inhibitors: May increase bleeding.
Herbal
None known.
Food
None known.

DIAGNOSTIC TEST EFFECTS
Increases (reversible) LDH, serum alkaline phosphatase, AST (SGOT), and ALT (SGPT) levels.

SIDE EFFECTS
Occasional (4%-1%)
Injection site hematoma, nausea, peripheral edema

SERIOUS REACTIONS
• Overdose may lead to bleeding complications ranging from local ecchymoses to major hemorrhage. Antidote: Protamine sulfate (1% solution) equal to the dose of enoxaparin injected. One mg protamine sulfate neutralizes 1 mg enoxaparin. A second dose of 0.5 mg protamine sulfate per 1 mg enoxaparin may be given if aPTT tested 2-4 hr after first injection remains prolonged.

PRECAUTIONS & CONSIDERATIONS
Caution is warranted with conditions associated with increased risk of hemorrhage, history of recent GI ulceration and hemorrhage, history of heparin-induced thrombocytopenia, impaired renal function, uncontrolled arterial hypertension, and in the elderly. Enoxaparin should be used with caution in pregnant women, particularly during the last trimester and immediately postpartum because it increases the risk of

maternal hemorrhage. It is unknown if enoxaparin is excreted in breast milk. Safety and efficacy of enoxaparin have not been established in children. The elderly may be more susceptible to bleeding. Females may experience heavier menstrual flow. Other medications, including OTC drugs, should be avoided. An electric razor and soft toothbrush should be used to prevent bleeding during therapy.

Notify the physician of abdominal or back pain, severe headache, black or red stool, coffee-ground vomitus, dark or red urine, or red-speckled mucus from cough. CBC and stool for occult blood should be periodically monitored. Be aware of signs of bleeding, including bleeding at injection or surgical sites or from gums, blood in stool, bruising, hematuria, and petechiae.

Storage

Store at room temperature.

Administration

! Do not mix with other injections or infusions. Do not give IM. Give initial dose as soon as possible after surgery but not more than 24 hours after surgery.

Parenteral form normally appears clear and colorless to pale yellow. The patient should lie down before administering by deep subcutaneous injection. Inject between the left and right anterolateral and left and right posterolateral abdominal wall. Introduce entire length of needle (one-half inch) into skinfold held between thumb and forefinger, holding skinfold during injection. The usual length of therapy is 7 to 10 days.

Entacapone
en-tak′a-pone
(Comtan)

CATEGORY AND SCHEDULE
Pregnancy Risk Category: C

CLASSIFICATION
Antiparkinson agents, dopaminergics

MECHANISM OF ACTION
An antiparkinson agent that inhibits the enzyme, catechol-*O*-methyltransferase (COMT), potentiating dopamine activity and increasing the duration of action of levodopa. *Therapeutic Effect:* Decreases signs and symptoms of Parkinson's disease.

PHARMACOKINETICS
Rapidly absorbed after PO administration. Protein binding: 98%. Metabolized in the liver. Primarily eliminated by biliary excretion. Not removed by hemodialysis. **Half-life:** 2.4 hr.

AVAILABILITY
Tablets: 200 mg.

INDICATIONS AND DOSAGES
▸ **Adjunctive treatment of Parkinson's disease**
PO
Adults, Elderly. 200 mg concomitantly with each dose of carbidopa and levodopa up to a maximum of 8 times a day (1600 mg).

CONTRAINDICATIONS
Hypersensitivity, use within 14 days of MAOIs

INTERACTIONS
Drug
Ampicillin, cholestyramine, erythromycin, probenecid: May decrease the excretion of entacapone.
Bitolterol, dobutamine, dopamine, epinephrine, isoetharine, isoproterenol, epinephrine, methyldopa, norepinephrine: May increase the risk of arrhythmias and changes in B/P.
Nonselective MAOIs (including phenelzine): May inhibit catecholamine metabolism.
Other CNS depressants: May increase CNS depression.
Herbal
None known.
Food
None known.

DIAGNOSTIC TEST EFFECTS
None known.

SIDE EFFECTS
Frequent (greater than 10%)
Dyskinesia, nausea, dark yellow or orange urine and sweat, diarrhea
Occasional (9%-3%)
Abdominal pain, vomiting, constipation, dry mouth, fatigue, back pain
Rare (less than 2%)
Anxiety, somnolence, agitation, dyspepsia, flatulence, diaphoresis, asthenia, dyspnea

SERIOUS REACTIONS
• None known.

PRECAUTIONS & CONSIDERATIONS
Caution is warranted with hepatic or renal impairment, dyskinesia, orthostatic hypotension, and syncope. It is unknown if entacapone is distributed in breast milk. This drug is not indicated for children. No age-related precautions have been noted in the elderly.

Dizziness, drowsiness, dry mouth, and darkened sweat and urine may occur. Tasks that require mental alertness or motor skills should be avoided. Notify the physician if uncontrolled movement of the hands, arms, legs, eyelids, face, mouth, or tongue occurs. Baseline vital signs should be obtained. Relief of symptoms, such as improvement of masklike facial expression, muscular rigidity, shuffling gait, and resting tremors of the hands and head, should be assessed during treatment. Dyskinesia, diarrhea, and orthostatic hypotension should also be monitored.
Administration
! Always administer entacapone with carbidopa and levodopa.
Take entacapone without regard to food.

Ephedrine
eh-fed′rin
(Pretz-D)
Do not confuse with epinephrine.

CATEGORY AND SCHEDULE
Pregnancy Risk Category: C

CLASSIFICATION
Adrenergic agonists, bronchodilators, decongestants, nasal

MECHANISM OF ACTION
An adrenergic agonist that stimulates alpha-adrenergic receptors causing vasoconstriction and pressor effects, beta$_1$-adrenergic receptors, resulting in cardiac stimulation, and beta$_2$-adrenergic receptors, resulting in bronchial dilation and vasodilation.

Therapeutic Effect: Increases blood pressure (B/P) and pulse rate.

PHARMACOKINETICS
Well absorbed after nasal and parenteral absorption. Metabolized in liver. Excreted in urine. **Half-life:** 3-6 hr.

AVAILABILITY
Capsules: 25 mg.
Injection: 50 mg/ml.
Intranasal spray: 0.25% (Pretz-D).

INDICATIONS AND DOSAGES
▸ **Asthma**
PO
Adults. 25-50 mg q3-4hr as needed.
Children. 3 mg/kg/day in 4 divided doses.
▸ **Hypotension**
IM
Adults. 25-50 mg as a single dose. Maximum 150 mg/day.
Children. 0.2-0.3 mg/kg/dose q4-6hr.
IV
Adults. 5 mg/dose slow IVP as prevention. 10-25 mg/dose slow IVP repeated q5-10min as treatment. Maximum: 150 mg/day.
Children. 0.2-0.3 mg/kg/dose slow IVP q4-6hr
SC
Adults. 25-50 q4-6hr. Maximum 150 mg/day.
Children. 3 mg/kg/day q4-6hr.
▸ **Nasal congestion**
PO
Adults. 25-50 mg q6hr as needed.
Children. 3 mg/kg/day in 4 divided doses.
NASAL
Adults, Children 12 yr and older. 2-3 sprays into each nostril q4hr
Children 6-12 yr. 1-2 sprays into each nostril q4hr

OFF-LABEL USES
Obesity, propofol-induced pain, radiocontrast media reactions

CONTRAINDICATIONS
Anesthesia with cyclopropane or halothane, diabetes (ephedrine injection), hypersensitivity to ephedrine or other sympathomimetic amines, hypertension or other cardiovascular disorders, pregnancy with maternal blood pressure above 130/80, thyrotoxicosis

INTERACTIONS
Drug
Caffeine: May increase cardiac stimulation.
Cardiac glycosides, sympatho-mimetics, theophylline, general anesthetics: May increase toxic cardiac stimulation.
Atropine, MAOIs, oxytocics, tricyclic antidepressants: May increase cardiovascular effects.
Herbal
Ephedra, bitter orange, yohimbe: May increase central nervous system (CNS) and cardiovascular stimulation and effects.
Food
None known.

DIAGNOSTIC TEST EFFECTS
May result in false-positive amphetamine EMIT assay.
Lactic acid serum values may be increased.

▨ IV INCOMPATIBILITIES
Phenobarbital (Luminal), secobarbital (Seconal)
▨ **IV Compatibilities**
Chloramphenicol, fenoldopam (Corlopam), lidocaine, metaraminol (Aramine), nafcillin (Unipen), penicillin G, propofol (Diprivan), tetracycline

SIDE EFFECTS
Frequent
Hypertension, anxiety
Occasional
Nausea, vomiting, palpitations, tremor
Nasal: Burning, stinging, runny nose
Rare
Psychosis, decreased urination, necrosis at injection site from repeated injections

SERIOUS REACTIONS
• Excessive doses may cause hypertension, intracranial hemorrhage, anginal pain, and fatal arrhythmias.
• Prolonged or excessive use may result in metabolic acidosis due to increased serum lactic acid concentrations.
• Observe for disorientation, weakness, hyperventilation, headache, nausea, vomiting, and diarrhea.

PRECAUTIONS & CONSIDERATIONS
Caution is warranted with angina, diabetes, hypoxia (lack of oxygen), heart attack, psychiatric disorders, tachycardia, severe liver or kidney impairment, and in the elderly. Epinephrine crosses the placenta and is distributed in breast milk. Excessive amounts of caffeine such as in chocolate, cocoa, coffee, cola, or tea should be avoided. Changes in vital signs and proper lung function should be monitored. Slight burning or stinging may be experienced when ophthalmic solution is administered to the eye. New symptoms such as dizziness, shortness of breath, or tachycardia (decreased heart rate) experienced with the ophthalmic solution should be reported immediately because they may indicate absorption by the body.
Storage
Injectable and intranasal forms should be stored at room temperature.

Administration
Ampoule should be shaken thoroughly. Solution should not be used if it appears discolored or contains a precipitate (separation of particles from liquid). A tuberculin syringe for subcutaneous injection into lateral deltoid muscle region should be used and injection site massaged. For injection, each 1 mg of 1:1000 solution is diluted with 10 ml 0.9% NaCl to provide 1:10,000 solution, and injected as each 1 mg or fraction thereof over more than 1 minute. For infusion, preparation should be further diluted with 250 to 500 D_5W. Maximum concentration is 64 mg/250 ml, the recommended rate of IV infusion is 1 to 10 mcg/min, adjusted to desired response.

For intranasal administration, before using spray, blow nose gently. Keep head in the upright position and spray into each nostril. Blow nose well 3-5 minutes after using ephedrine. Do not administer more frequently than every 4 hours.

E

Epinastine
(Elestat)

CATEGORY AND SCHEDULE
Pregnancy Risk Category: C

CLASSIFICATION
Antihistamines, H1, ophthalmics

MECHANISM OF ACTION
An ophthalmic H1 receptor antagonist that inhibits the release of histamine from the mast cell. *Therapeutic Effect:* Prevents pruritus associated with allergic conjunctivitis.

PHARMACOKINETICS
Low systemic exposure. Protein binding: 64%. Less than 10% is metabolized. Excreted primarily in urine and, to a lesser extent, in feces. **Half-life:** 12 hr.

AVAILABILITY
Ophthalmic Solution: 0.05%.

INDICATIONS AND DOSAGES
▸ **Allergic conjunctivitis**
OPHTHALMIC
Adults, Elderly, Children 3 yr and older. 1 drop in each eye twice a day. Continue treatment until period of exposure (pollen season, exposure to offending allergen) is over.

CONTRAINDICATIONS
Hypersensitivity to epinastine or any of its components.

INTERACTIONS
Drug
None known.
Herbal
None known.
Food
None known.

DIAGNOSTIC TEST EFFECTS
None known.

SIDE EFFECTS
Occasional
Ocular (10%-1%): Burning sensation in the eye, hyperemia, pruritus
Non-ocular (10%): Cold symptoms, upper respiratory tract infection
Rare (3%-1%)
Headache, rhinitis, sinusitis, increased cough, pharyngitis

SERIOUS REACTIONS
• None known.

PRECAUTIONS & CONSIDERATIONS
It is not known if epinastine is distributed in breast milk. The safety and efficacy of epinastine have not been established in children younger than 3 years. No age-related precautions have been noted in the elderly.

Drowsiness, dizziness, and dry mouth may occur; tolerance usually develops to sedative effects. Therapeutic response should be monitored.

Administration
For ophthalmic use, place a finger on the lower eyelid, and pull it out until a pocket is formed between the eye and lower lid. Don't let the applicator tip touch any surface. Hold the dropper above the pocket, and place the prescribed number of drops in the pocket. Close the affected eye gently so the medication won't squeeze out of the lacrimal sac. Apply gentle pressure to the lacrimal sac at the inner canthus for 1 minute after installation to lessen the risk of systemic absorption. Remove contact lenses before instilling epinastine because the lenses may absorb the drug's preservatives. The lenses may be reinserted 10 minutes after administration unless the treated eye is red.

Epinephrine
ep-i-nef'rin
(Adrenalin, Adrenaline Injection [AUS], EpiPen, Primatene)
Do not confuse epinephrine with ephedrine.

CATEGORY AND SCHEDULE
Pregnancy Risk Category: C

CLASSIFICATION
Adrenergic agonists, bronchodilators, inotropes, ophthalmics

MECHANISM OF ACTION

A sympathomimetic, adrenergic agonist that stimulates alpha-adrenergic receptors causing vaso-constriction and pressor effects, $beta_1$-adrenergic receptors, resulting in cardiac stimulation, and $beta_2$-adrenergic receptors, resulting in bronchial dilation and vasodilation. With ophthalmic form, increases outflow of aqueous humor from anterior eye chamber. *Therapeutic Effect:* Relaxes smooth muscle of the bronchial tree, produces cardiac stimulation, and dilates skeletal muscle vasculature. The ophthalmic form dilates pupils and constricts conjunctival blood vessels.

PHARMACOKINETICS

Route	Onset	Peak	Duration
IM	5-10 min	20 min	1-4 hr
Subcutaneous	5-10 min	20 min	1-4 hr
Inhalation	3-5 min	20 min	1-3 hr
Ophthalmic	1 hr	4-8 hr	12-24 hr

Well absorbed after parenteral administration; minimally absorbed after inhalation. Metabolized in the liver, other tissues, and sympathetic nerve endings. Excreted in urine. The ophthalmic form may be systemically absorbed as a result of drainage into nasal pharyngeal passages. Mydriasis occurs within several min and persists several hr; vasoconstriction occurs within 5 min, and lasts less than 1 hr.

AVAILABILITY

Injection: 0.1 mg/ml, 1 mg/ml.
Injection (Epi-Pen): 0.3 mg/0.3 ml, 0.15 mg/0.3 ml.
Inhalation, aerosol (Primatene Mist): 0.2 mg/inhalation.
Inhalation, solution: 1%, 2.25%.

Ophthalmic solution (Epifrin): 0.5%, 1%, 2%.

INDICATIONS AND DOSAGES

▶ **Asystole**
IV
Adults, Elderly. 1 mg q3-5min up to 0.1 mg/kg q3-5min.
Children. 0.01 mg/kg (0.1 ml/kg of 1:10,000 solution). May repeat q3-5min. Subsequent doses of 0.1 mg/kg (0.1 ml/kg) of a 1:1000 solution q3-5min.

▶ **Bradycardia**
IV INFUSION
Adults, Elderly. 1-10 mcg/min titrated to desired effect.
IV
Children. 0.01 mg/kg (0.1 mg/kg of 1:10,000 solution) q3-5min. Maximum: 1 mg/10 ml.

▶ **Bronchodilation**
IM, SUBCUTANEOUS
Adults, Elderly. 0.1-0.5 mg (1:1000) q10-15min to 4 hr.
SUBCUTANEOUS
Children. 10 mcg/kg (0.01 ml/kg of 1:1000). Maximum: 0.5 mg or suspension (1:200) 0.005 ml/kg/dose (0.025 mg/kg/dose) to a maximum of 0.15 ml (0.75 mg for single dose) q8-12hr.

▶ **Hypersensitivity reaction**
IM, SUBCUTANEOUS
Adults, Elderly. 0.3-0.5 mg q15-20min.
SUBCUTANEOUS
Children. 0.01 mg/kg q15min for 2 doses, then q4hr. Maximum single dose: 0.5 mg.
INHALATION
Adults, Elderly, Children 4 yr and older. 1 inhalation, may repeat in at least 1 min. Give subsequent doses no sooner than 3 hr.
NEBULIZER
Adults, Elderly, Children 4 yr and older. 1-3 deep inhalations. Give subsequent doses no sooner than 3 hr.

E

▸ **Glaucoma**
OPHTHALMIC
Adults, Elderly. 1-2 drops 1-2 times a day.

OFF-LABEL USES
Systemic: Treatment of gingival or pulpal hemorrhage, priapism
Ophthalmic: Treatment of conjunctival congestion during surgery, secondary glaucoma

CONTRAINDICATIONS
Cardiac arrhythmias, cerebrovascular insufficiency, hypertension, hyperthyroidism, ischemic heart disease, narrow-angle glaucoma, shock

INTERACTIONS
Drug
Beta blockers: May decrease the effects of beta blockers.
Digoxin, sympathomimetics: May increase risk of arrhythmias.
Ergonovine, methergine, oxytocin: May increase vasoconstriction.
MAOIs, tricyclic antidepressants: May increase cardiovascular effects.
Herbal
None known.
Food
None known.

DIAGNOSTIC TEST EFFECTS
May decrease serum potassium level.

🔅 IV INCOMPATIBILITIES
Ampicillin (Omnipen, Polycillin)
💉 **IV Compatibilities**
Calcium chloride, calcium gluconate, diltiazem (Cardizem), dobutamine (Dobutrex), dopamine (Intropin), fentanyl (Sublimaze), heparin, hydromorphone (Dilaudid), lorazepam (Ativan), midazolam (Versed), milrinone (Primacor), morphine, nitroglycerin, norepinephrine (Levophed), potassium chloride, propofol (Diprivan)

SIDE EFFECTS
Frequent
Systemic: Tachycardia, palpitations, nervousness
Ophthalmic: Headache, eye irritation, watering of eyes
Occasional
Systemic: Dizziness, lightheadedness, facial flushing, headache, diaphoresis, increased B/P, nausea, trembling, insomnia, vomiting, fatigue
Ophthalmic: Blurred or decreased vision, eye pain
Rare
Systemic: Chest discomfort or pain, arrhythmias, bronchospasm, dry mouth or throat

SERIOUS REACTIONS
• Excessive doses may cause acute hypertension or arrhythmias.
• Prolonged or excessive use may result in metabolic acidosis due to increased serum lactic acid concentrations. Metabolic acidosis may cause disorientation, fatigue, hyperventilation, headache, nausea, vomiting, and diarrhea.

PRECAUTIONS & CONSIDERATIONS
Caution is warranted with angina, diabetes, hypoxia (lack of oxygen), heart attack, psychiatric disorders, tachycardia, severe liver or kidney impairment, and in the elderly. Epinephrine crosses the placenta and is distributed in breast milk. Excessive amounts of caffeine such as in chocolate, cocoa, coffee, cola, or tea should be avoided. Changes in vital signs and proper lung function should be monitored.
    Slight burning or stinging may be experienced when ophthalmic solution is administered to the eye. New symptoms such as dizziness, shortness of breath, or tachycardia (decreased heart rate) experienced with the ophthalmic solution should

be reported immediately because they may indicate absorption by the body.
Storage
Injectable forms should be stored at room temperature.
Administration
Ampoule should be shaken thoroughly. Solution should not be used if it appears discolored or contains a precipitate (separation of particles from liquid). A tuberculin syringe for subcutaneous injection into lateral deltoid muscle region should be used and injection site massaged.

For injection, each 1 mg of 1:1000 solution is diluted with 10 ml 0.9% NaCl to provide 1:10,000 solution, and injected as each 1 mg or fraction thereof over more than 1 minute. For infusion, preparation should be further diluted with 250 to 500 D$_5$W. Maximum concentration is 64 mg/250 ml; the recommended rate of IV infusion is 1 to 10 mcg/min, adjusted to desired response.

Eplerenone
e-plear'a-nown
(Inspra)

CATEGORY AND SCHEDULE
Pregnancy Risk Category: B

CLASSIFICATION
Selective aldosterone receptor antagonist

MECHANISM OF ACTION
An aldosterone receptor antagonist that binds to the mineralocorticoid receptors in the kidney, heart, blood vessels, and brain, blocking the binding of aldosterone. *Therapeutic Effect:* Reduces B/P.

PHARMACOKINETICS
Absorption unaffected by food. Protein binding: 50%. No active metabolites. Excreted in the urine with a lesser amount eliminated in the feces. Not removed by hemodialysis. **Half-life:** 4-6 hr.

AVAILABILITY
Tablets: 25 mg, 50 mg.

INDICATIONS AND DOSAGES
▸ **Hypertension**
PO
Adults, Elderly. 50 mg once a day. If 50 mg once a day produces an inadequate B/P response, may increase dosage to 50 mg twice a day. If patient is concurrently receiving erythromycin, saquinavir, verapamil, or fluconazole, reduce initial dose to 25 mg once a day.
▸ **CHF following MI**
PO
Adults, Elderly. Initially, 25 mg once a day. If tolerated, titrate up to 50 mg once a day within 4 wk.

CONTRAINDICATIONS
Concurrent use of potassium supplements or potassium-sparing diuretics (such as amiloride, spironolactone, and triamterene), or strong inhibitors of the cytochrome P450 3A4 enzyme system (including ketoconazole and itraconazole), creatinine clearance less than 50 ml/min, serum creatinine level greater than 2 mg/dl in males or 1.8 mg/dl in females, serum potassium level greater than 5.5 mEq/L, type 2 diabetes mellitus with microalbuminuria

INTERACTIONS
Drug
ACE inhibitors, angiotensin II antagonists, erythromycin, fluconazole, saquinavir, verapamil: Increases risk of hyperkalemia.

Herbal
St. John's wort: Decreases
eplerenone effectiveness.
Food
Grapefruit juice: Produces small
increase in serum potassium level.

DIAGNOSTIC TEST EFFECTS
May increase serum potassium level.
May decrease serum sodium level.

SIDE EFFECTS
Rare (3%-1%)
Dizziness, diarrhea, cough, fatigue,
flu-like symptoms, abdominal pain

SERIOUS REACTIONS
• Hyperkalemia may occur, particularly in patients with type 2 diabetes
mellitus and microalbuminuria.

PRECAUTIONS & CONSIDERATIONS
Caution is warranted with hyperkalemia and hepatic impairment. It
is unknown if eplerenone crosses the
placenta or is distributed in breast
milk. The safety and efficacy of
eplerenone have not been established
in children. No age-related precautions have been noted in the elderly.
Exercising outside during hot
weather should be avoided because
of the risks of dehydration and
hypotension.
    Dizziness and lightheadedness
may occur. Tasks that require mental
alertness or motor skills should be
avoided. Apical heart rate and B/P
should be obtained immediately
before each dose, in addition to
regular monitoring. Be alert to B/P
fluctuations. If an excessive reduction
in B/P occurs, place in the supine
position with feet slightly elevated,
and notify the physician. Pattern of
daily bowel activity and stool consistency and potassium and sodium
levels should also be monitored.

Administration
Film-coated tablets should not be
broken, crushed, or chewed.

Epoetin Alfa (Erythropoietin)
eh-poh′ee-tin al′fa
(Epogen, Eprex [CAN],
Procrit)
**Do not confuse Epogen with
Neupogen.**

CATEGORY AND SCHEDULE
Pregnancy Risk Category: C

CLASSIFICATION
Hematopoietic agents,
hormones/hormone modifiers

MECHANISM OF ACTION
A glycoprotein that stimulates
division and differentiation of
erythroid progenitor cells in
bone marrow. *Therapeutic Effect:*
Induces erythropoiesis and
releases reticulocytes from bone
marrow.

PHARMACOKINETICS
Well absorbed after subcutaneous
administration. Following administration, an increase in reticulocyte
count occurs within 10 days, and
increases in Hgb, Hct, and RBC
count are seen within 2-6 wk.
Half-life: 4-13 hr.

AVAILABILITY
Injection: 2000 units/ml,
3000 units/ml, 4000 units/ml,
10,000 units/ml, 20,000 units/ml,
40,000 units/ml.

INDICATIONS AND DOSAGES

▶ **Treatment of anemia in chemotherapy patients**
IV, SUBCUTANEOUS
Adults, Elderly, Children.
150 units/kg/dose 3 times a wk.
Maximum: 1200 units/kg/wk.

▶ **Reduction of allogenic blood transfusions in elective surgery**
SUBCUTANEOUS
Adults, Elderly. 300 units/kg/day
10 days before day of, and 4 days after surgery.

▶ **Chronic renal failure**
IV BOLUS, SUBCUTANEOUS
Adults, Elderly. Initially,
50-100 units/kg 3 times a wk.
Target Hct range: 30%-36%. Adjust dosage no earlier than 1-mo intervals unless prescribed. Decrease dosage if Hct is increasing and approaching 36%. Plan to temporarily withhold doses if Hct continues to rise and to reinstate lower dosage when Hct begins to decrease. If Hct increases by more than 4 points in 2 wk, monitor Hct twice a wk for 2-6 wk. Increase dose if Hct does not increase 5-6 points after 8 wk (with adequate iron stores) and if Hct is below target range.
Maintenance: *For patients on dialysis:* 75 units/kg 3 times a wk. Range: 12.5-525 units/kg. *For patients not on dialysis:*
75-150 units/kg/wk.

▶ **HIV infection in patients treated with AZT**
IV, SUBCUTANEOUS
Adults. Initially, 100 units/kg
3 times a wk for 8 wk; may increase by 50-100 units/kg 3 times a wk. Evaluate response q4-8wk thereafter. Adjust dosage by 50-100 units/kg 3 times a wk. If dosages larger than 300 units/kg 3 times a wk are not eliciting response, it is unlikely patient will respond. Maintenance: Titrate to maintain desired Hct.

OFF-LABEL USES
Prevention of anemia in patients donating blood before elective surgery or autologous transfusion, treatment of anemia associated with neoplastic diseases.

CONTRAINDICATIONS
History of sensitivity to mammalian cell-derived products or human albumin, uncontrolled hypertension

INTERACTIONS
Drug
Heparin: An increase in RBC volume may enhance blood clotting. Heparin dosage may need to be increased.
Herbal
None known.
Food
None known.

DIAGNOSTIC TEST EFFECTS
May increase BUN, serum phosphorus, serum potassium, serum creatinine, serum uric acid, and sodium levels. May decrease bleeding time, iron concentration, and serum ferritin levels.

🔹 IV INCOMPATIBILITIES
Do not mix with other medications.

SIDE EFFECTS
Patients receiving chemotherapy
Frequent (20%-17%)
Fever, diarrhea, nausea, vomiting, edema
Occasional (13%-11%)
Asthenia, shortness of breath, paresthesia
Rare (5%-3%)
Dizziness, trunk pain

E

Patients with chronic renal failure
Frequent (24%-11%)
Hypertension, headache, nausea, arthralgia
Occasional (9%-7%)
Fatigue, edema, diarrhea, vomiting, chest pain, skin reactions at administration site, asthenia, dizziness

Patients with HIV infection treated with AZT
Frequent (38%-15%)
Fever, fatigue, headache, cough, diarrhea, rash, nausea
Occasional (14%-9%)
Shortness of breath, asthenia, skin reaction at injection site, dizziness

SERIOUS REACTIONS
• Hypertensive encephalopathy, thrombosis, cerebrovascular accident, MI, and seizures have occurred rarely.
• Hyperkalemia occurs occasionally in patients with chronic renal failure, usually in those who do not conform to medication regimen, dietary guidelines, and frequency of dialysis regimen.

PRECAUTIONS & CONSIDERATIONS
Caution is warranted with a history of seizures and known porphyria (an impairment of erythrocyte formation in bone marrow). It is unknown if epoetin alfa crosses the placenta or is distributed in breast milk. Safety and efficacy of epoetin alfa have not been established in children 12 years of age and younger. No age-related precautions have been noted in the elderly. Avoid potentially hazardous activities during the first 90 days of therapy. There is an increased risk of seizure development in those with chronic renal failure during the first 90 days of therapy.

Notify the physician of severe headache. Hct level should be monitored diligently. The dosage should be reduced if Hct level increases more than 4 points in 2 weeks. CBC should also be monitored before and during therapy. In addition B/P must be monitored aggressively for an increase because 25% of persons taking epoetin alfa require antihypertensive therapy and dietary restrictions. Keep in mind most patients will eventually need supplemental iron therapy. Body temperature, especially in persons receiving chemotherapy and in those with HIV infection treated with zidovudine, and serum BUN, serum phosphorus, serum potassium, serum creatinine, and serum uric acid levels, especially in persons with chronic renal failure.

Storage
Refrigerate vials. Do not shake vials.
Administration
! Avoid excessive agitation of vial; do not shake because it can cause foaming. Also, vigorous shaking may denature medication, rendering it inactive. Patients receiving AZT who have serum erythropoietin levels greater than 500 milliunits are not likely to respond to therapy.

For IV use, reconstitution is not necessary. May be given as an IV bolus.

For subcutaneous administration, use one dose per vial; do not reenter vial. Discard unused portion. May be mixed in a syringe with bacteriostatic 0.9% NaCl with benzyl alcohol 0.9% or bacteriostatic saline at a 1:1 ratio. Benzyl alcohol acts as a local anesthetic and may reduce injection site discomfort.

Epoprostenol (Prostacyclin)

e-poe-pros′ten-ol
(Flolan)

CATEGORY AND SCHEDULE
Pregnancy Risk Category: B

CLASSIFICATION
Platelet inhibitors, vasodilators

MECHANISM OF ACTION
An antihypertensive that directly dilates pulmonary and systemic arterial vascular beds and inhibits platelet aggregation. *Therapeutic Effect:* Reduces right and left ventricular afterload; increases cardiac output and stroke volume.

AVAILABILITY
Injection, Powder for Reconstitution: 0.5 mg, 1.5 mg.

INDICATIONS AND DOSAGES
▶ **Long-term treatment of New York Heart Association Class III and IV primary pulmonary hypertension**
IV infusion
Adults, Elderly. Procedure to determine dose range: Initially, 2 ng/kg/min, increased in increments of 2 ng/kg/min q15min until dose-limiting adverse effects occur. Chronic infusion: Start at 4 ng/kg/min less than the maximum dose rate tolerated during acute dose ranging (or one half of the maximum rate if rate was less than 5 ng/kg/min).

OFF-LABEL USES
Cardiopulmonary bypass surgery; hemodialysis; pulmonary hypertension associated with acute respiratory distress syndrome, systemic lupus erythematosus, or congenital heart disease; neonatal pulmonary hypertension, refractory CHF; severe community-acquired pneumonia

CONTRAINDICATIONS
Long-term use in patients with CHF (severe ventricular systolic dysfunction)

INTERACTIONS
Drug
Acetate in dialysis fluids, other vasodilators: May increase hypotensive effect.
Anticoagulants, antiplatelets: May increase the risk of bleeding.
Vasoconstrictors: May decrease effects of epoprostenol.
Herbal
None known.
Food
None known.

DIAGNOSTIC TEST EFFECTS
None known.

▓ IV INCOMPATIBILITIES
Don't mix epoprostenol with other medications.

SIDE EFFECTS
Frequent
Acute phase: Flushing (58%), headache (49%), nausea (32%), vomiting (32%), hypotension (16%), anxiety (11%), chest pain (11%), dizziness (8%)
Chronic phase (greater than 20%): Dyspnea, asthenia, dizziness, headache, chest pain, nausea, vomiting, palpitations, edema, jaw pain, tachycardia, flushing, myalgia, nonspecific muscle pain, paresthesia, diarrhea, anxiety, chills, fever, or flu-like symptoms
Occasional
Acute phase (5%-2%): Bradycardia, abdominal pain, muscle pain, dyspnea, back pain

Chronic phase (20%-10%): Rash, depression, hypotension, pallor, syncope, bradycardia, ascites

Rare

Acute phase: Paresthesia

Chronic phase (less than 2%): Diaphoresis, dyspepsia, tachycardia

SERIOUS REACTIONS

• Overdose may cause hyperglycemia or ketoacidosis manifested as increased urination, thirst, and fruitlike breath odor.

• Angina, MI, and thrombocytopenia occur rarely.

• Abrupt withdrawal, including a large reduction in dosage or interruption in drug delivery, may produce rebound pulmonary hypertension as evidenced by dyspnea, dizziness, and asthenia.

PRECAUTIONS & CONSIDERATIONS

Interruptions in the IV infusion should be avoided because even a short break in the infusion can result in rebounding pulmonary hypertension. The patient should be closely monitored during initiation of therapy. Use epoprostenol cautiously in the elderly.

Before beginning therapy, a backup infusion pump and IV infusion sets should be obtained to avoid interruptions in therapy. A central venous catheter must be in place. Vital signs should be monitored before and during therapy. Standing and supine B/P should be monitored for several hours after a dosage adjustment. Therapeutic evidence is evidenced by decreased chest pain, dyspnea on exertion, fatigue, pulmonary arterial pressure, pulmonary vascular resistance, and syncope, and improved pulmonary function.

Storage

Store unopened vial at room temperature. Do not freeze. Reconstituted solutions are stable for up to 48 hours if refrigerated.

Administration

❗ Infuse epoprostenol continuously through an indwelling central venous catheter. If necessary and on a temporary basis, infuse through a peripheral vein. Use only the diluent provided by the manufacturer.

Follow instructions of manufacturer for dilution to specific concentrations. Give as pump infusion only.

Eprosartan
eh-pro-sar′tan
(Teveten)

CATEGORY AND SCHEDULE
Pregnancy Risk Category: C (D if used in second or third trimester)

CLASSIFICATION
Angiotensin II receptor antagonists

MECHANISM OF ACTION
An angiotensin II receptor antagonist that blocks the vasoconstrictor and aldosterone-secreting effects of angiotensin II, inhibiting the binding of angiotensin II to the AT_1 receptors. *Therapeutic Effect:* Causes vasodilation, decreases peripheral resistance, and decreases B/P.

PHARMACOKINETICS
Rapidly absorbed after PO administration. Protein binding: 98%. Undergoes first-pass metabolism in the liver to active metabolites. Excreted in urine and biliary system. Minimally removed by hemodialysis. **Half-life:** 5-9 hr.

AVAILABILITY
Tablets: 400 mg, 600 mg.

INDICATIONS AND DOSAGES
▸ **Hypertension**
PO
Adults, Elderly. Initially, 600 mg/day.
Range: 400-800 mg/day.

CONTRAINDICATIONS
Bilateral renal artery stenosis,
hyperaldosteronism

INTERACTIONS
Drug
None known.
Herbal
Licorice, ma huang, yohimbine:
May increase the effectiveness of
eprosartan.
Food
None known.

DIAGNOSTIC TEST EFFECTS
May increase BUN, serum alkaline
phosphatase, serum bilirubin, serum
creatinine, AST (SGOT), and ALT
(SGPT) levels. May decrease blood
Hgb levels.

SIDE EFFECTS
Occasional (5%-2%)
Headache, cough, dizziness
Rare (less than 2%)
Muscle pain, fatigue, diarrhea, upper
respiratory tract infection, dyspepsia

SERIOUS REACTIONS
• Overdosage may manifest as
hypotension and tachycardia.
Bradycardia occurs less often.

PRECAUTIONS & CONSIDERATIONS
Caution is warranted with preexisting renal insufficiency, significant
aortic and mitral stenosis, and unilateral renal artery stenosis. Eprosartan
has caused fetal or neonatal morbidity or mortality. Also, because of the

potential for adverse effects on the
infant, patients taking eprosartan
should not breast-feed. Safety and
efficacy of eprosartan have not been
established in children. No age-related
precautions have been noted in the
elderly. Sodium consumption and
alcohol should be avoided.

Apical pulse and B/P should be
assessed immediately before each
eprosartan dose, and regularly
throughout therapy. Be alert to
fluctuations in apical pulse and B/P.
If an excessive reduction in B/P
occurs, place the person in the
supine position with feet slightly
elevated and notify the physician.
Tasks that require mental alertness
or motor skills should be avoided.
BUN, serum electrolytes, serum
creatinine levels, heart rate for
tachycardia, and urinalysis results
should be obtained before and
during therapy.
Administration
Take eprosartan without regard to
food. Do not crush or break tablets.

Eptifibatide
ep-tih-fib'ah-tide
(Integrilin)

CATEGORY AND SCHEDULE
Pregnancy Risk Category: B

CLASSIFICATION
Platelet inhibitors

MECHANISM OF ACTION
A glycoprotein IIb/IIIa inhibitor that
rapidly inhibits platelet aggregation
by preventing binding of fibrinogen
to receptor sites on platelets.
Therapeutic Effect: Prevents closure
of treated coronary arteries.

Also prevents acute cardiac ischemic complications.

AVAILABILITY
Injection solution: 0.75 mg/ml, 2 mg/ml.

INDICATIONS AND DOSAGES
▸ **Adjunct to percutaneous coronary intervention**
IV BOLUS, IV INFUSION
Adults, Elderly. 180 mcg/kg before PCI initiation; then continuous drip of 2 mcg/kg/min and a second 180 mcg/kg bolus 10 min after the first. Maximum: 15 mg/hr. Continue until hospital discharge or for up to 18-24 hours. Minimum 12 hours is recommended. Concurrent aspirin and heparin therapy is recommended.
▸ **Acute coronary syndrome**
IV BOLUS, IV INFUSION
Adults, Elderly. 180 mcg/kg bolus then 2 mcg/kg/min until discharge or coronary artery bypass graft, up to 72 hr. Maximum: 15 mg/hr. Concurrent aspirin and heparin therapy is recommended.
▸ **Dosage in renal impairment**
Serum creatinine 2-4 mg/dl. Use 180 mcg/kg bolus (maximum 22.6 mg) and 1 mcg/kg/min infusion (maximum: 7.5 mg/hr).

CONTRAINDICATIONS
Active internal bleeding, AV malformation or aneurysm, history of cerebrovascular accident (CVA) within 2 years or CVA with residual neurologic defect, history of vasculitis, intracranial neoplasm, oral anticoagulant use within last 7 days unless PT is less than 1.22 times the control, recent (6 wk or less) GI or GU bleeding, recent (6 wk or less) surgery or trauma, prior IV dextran use before or during PTCA, severe uncontrolled hypertension,

thrombocytopenia (less than 100,000 cells/mcl)

INTERACTIONS
Drug
Anticoagulants, heparin: May increase the risk of hemorrhage.
Dextran, other platelet aggregation inhibitors (such as aspirin), thrombolytic agents: May increase the risk of bleeding.
Herbal
None known.
Food
None known.

DIAGNOSTIC TEST EFFECTS
Increases aPTT, PT, and clotting time. Decreases platelet count.

▓ IV INCOMPATIBILITIES
Administer in separate line; do not add other medications to infusion solution.

SIDE EFFECTS
Occasional (7%)
Hypotension

SERIOUS REACTIONS
• Minor to major bleeding complications may occur, most commonly at arterial access site for cardiac catheterization.

PRECAUTIONS & CONSIDERATIONS
Caution is warranted with PTCA less than 12 hours from the onset of symptoms of acute MI, prolonged PTCA that's greater than 70 minutes, and failed PTCA. Caution should also be used in persons who weigh less than 75 kg, are older than 65 years, have a history of GI disease, or are receiving aspirin, heparin, or thrombolytics. It is unknown if eptifibatide causes fetal harm or can affect reproduction capacity. It is unknown if eptifibatide

is distributed in breast milk. Safety and efficacy of eptifibatide have not been established in children. In the elderly, the risk of major bleeding is increased.

Hgb, Hct, and platelet count should be obtained before treatment. If platelet count is less than 90,000/mm³, additional platelet counts should be obtained routinely to avoid development of thrombocytopenia. NG tube and urinary catheter use should be avoided, if possible.
Storage
Store vials in refrigerator.
Administration
Solution normally appears clear and is colorless. Do not shake. Discard unused portions. Also discard if preparation contains any opaque particles. Withdraw bolus dose from 10-ml vial (2 mg/ml); for IV infusion withdraw from 100-ml vial (0.75 mg/ml). May give IV push and infusion undiluted. Give bolus dose IV push over 1 to 2 minutes.

Ergoloid Mesylates
ur-go-loyd mess-ah-lates
(Gerimal, Hydergine, Hydergine [CAN])

CATEGORY AND SCHEDULE
Pregnancy Risk Category: C

CLASSIFICATION
Ergot alkaloids and derivatives

MECHANISM OF ACTION
An ergot alkaloid that centrally acts and decreases vascular tone, slows heart rate. Peripheral action blocks alpha adrenergic receptors.
Therapeutic Effect: Improved O_2 uptake and improves cerebral metabolism.

PHARMACOKINETICS
Rapidly, incompletely absorbed from GI tract. Metabolized in liver. Eliminated primarily in feces.
Half-life: 2-5 hr.

AVAILABILITY
Capsules: 1 mg (Hydergine).
Oral solution: 1 mg/ml (Hydergine).
Tablets: 1 mg (Germinal, Hydergine).
Tablets, sublingual: 1 mg (Germinal, Hydergine).

INDICATIONS AND DOSAGES
▸ **Age-related decline in mental capacity**
PO
Adults, Elderly. Initially, 1 mg 3 times/day. Range: 1.5-12 mg/day.

CONTRAINDICATIONS
Acute or chronic psychosis (regardless or etiology), hypersensitivity to ergoloid mesylates or any component of the formulation

INTERACTIONS
Drug
Potent CYP450 3A4 inhibitors: May increase risk of ergotism (nausea, vomiting, vasospastic ischemia).
Frovatriptan, naratriptan, rizatriptan, sumatriptan, zolmitriptan: May prolong vasospastic reactions.
Herbal
None known.
Food
Grapefruit juice: May increase risk of ergotism (nausea, vomiting, vasospastic ischemia).

INTERACTIONS
Drug
Potent CYP450 3A4 inhibitors:
May increase risk of ergotism
(nausea, vomiting, vasospastic
ischemia).
Frovatriptan, naratriptan, rizatriptan,
sumatriptan, zolmitriptan: May
prolong vasospastic reactions.
Food
Grapefruit juice: May increase risk
of ergotism (nausea, vomiting,
vasospastic ischemia).

SIDE EFFECTS
Occasional
GI distress, transient nausea, sublin-
gual irritation

SERIOUS REACTIONS
• Overdose may produce blurred
vision, dizziness, syncope, headache,
flushed face, nausea, vomiting,
decreased appetite, stomach cramps,
and stuffy nose.

PRECAUTIONS & CONSIDERATIONS
It is unknown if ergoloid mesylates
crosses the placenta or is distributed
in breast milk. Be aware that the
safety and efficacy of ergoloid
mesylates have not been established
in children. There are no age-related
precautions noted in the elderly.
    Ergoloid mesylates may cause
nausea and GI upset. Elimination of
symptoms is gradual, and results
may not be noted for 3-4 wk.
Storage
Store at room temperature.
Administration
Give with food to avoid GI upset.
Allow sublingual tablets to dissolve
under tongue. Do not swallow tablets
whole.

Ergonovine
er-goe-noe-veen
(Ergotrate)

CATEGORY AND SCHEDULE
Pregnancy Risk Category: X

CLASSIFICATION
Ergot alkaloids and
derivatives, oxytocics,
stimulants, uterine

MECHANISM OF ACTION
An oxytoxic agent that directly
stimulates uterine muscle.
Stimulates alpha adrenergic,
serotonin receptors producing
arterial vasoconstriction. Causes
vasospasm of coronary arteries.
Therapeutic Effect: Increases force
and frequency of contractions.
Induces cervical contractions.

PHARMACOKINETICS
None reported.

AVAILABILITY
Injection: 0.2 mg/ml (Ergotrate).

INDICATIONS AND DOSAGES
▸ **Oxytocic**
IM/IV
Adults. Initially, 0.2 mg. May repeat
no more than q2-4hr for no more
than 5 doses total.

OFF-LABEL USES
Treatment of incomplete abortion,
diagnosis of angina pectoris

CONTRAINDICATIONS
Induction of labor, threatened
spontaneous abortions,
hypersensitivity to ergonovine
maleate or any component of the
formulation

INTERACTIONS
Drug
Vasoconstrictors, vasopressors:
May increase effects of ergonovine maleate.
Herbal
None known.
Food
None known.

DIAGNOSTIC TEST EFFECTS
May decrease prolactin.

▓ IV INCOMPATIBILITIES
Amikacin (Amikin), cephapirin (Cefadyl), procaine, sodium bicarbonate

SIDE EFFECTS
Frequent
Uterine cramping
Occasional
Diarrhea, dizziness, nasal congestion, sweating, ringing in ears
Rare
Headache, nausea, vomiting, allergic reaction

SERIOUS REACTIONS
• Severe hypertensive episodes may result in cerebrovascular accident, serious arrhythmias, seizures; hypertensive effects more frequent with rapid IV administration, concurrent regional anesthesia or vasoconstrictors.
• Peripheral ischemia may lead to gangrene.
• Overdose includes symptoms of angina, bradycardia, confusion, drowsiness, fast, weak pulse; miosis, severe peripheral vasoconstriction (numbness in arms or legs, blue skin color), seizures, tachycardia, thirst, and severe uterine cramping.

PRECAUTIONS & CONSIDERATIONS
Caution is warranted with heart disease, hepatic dysfunction, calcium deficiency, hypertension, mitral valve stenosis, obliterative vascular disease, renal impairment, sepsis, and venoarterial shunts. Ergonovine maleate use is contraindicated during pregnancy, and small amounts of the drug are found in breast milk. There is no information available on ergonovine maleate use in children or the elderly.

Uterine contractions (frequency, strength, duration), bleeding, B/P, and pulse should be monitored every 15 minutes until stable (about 1-2 hours). If uterine cramps occur, notify the physician because dosage reduction may be required.
Storage
Store in refrigerator. Stable for up to 60 days at room temperature. Do not use if discoloration occurs.
Administration
Give IM injection deep in muscle.

Be aware that for intravenous administration, it should only be used with severe uterine bleeding or other life-threatening emergency situations. Administer slowly, over a period of at least 1 minute. May administer undiluted or dilute in 0.9% NaCl to 5 ml.

Ergotamine
er-got′a-meen
(Cafergor [CAN], Ergodryl Mono [AUS], Ergomar, Ergostat, Gynergen)(D.H.E. 45, Dihydergot [AUS], Dihydroergotamine Sandoz [CAN], Migranal)

CATEGORY AND SCHEDULE
Pregnancy Risk Category: X

CLASSIFICATION
Ergot alkaloids and derivatives

MECHANISM OF ACTION
An ergotamine derivative and alpha-adrenergic blocker that directly stimulates vascular smooth muscle, resulting in peripheral and cerebral vasoconstriction. May also have antagonist effects on serotonin. *Therapeutic Effect:* Suppresses vascular headaches.

PHARMACOKINETICS
Slowly and incompletely absorbed from the GI tract; rapidly and extensively absorbed after rectal administration. Protein binding: greater than 90%. Undergoes extensive first-pass metabolism in the liver to active metabolite. Eliminated in feces by the biliary system. **Half-life:** 21 hr.

AVAILABILITY
Tablets (Sublingual [Ergomar]): 2 mg.
Injection (DHE 45): 1 mg/ml.
Nasal Spray (Migranal):
0.5 mg/spray.
Suppositories (ergotamine and caffeine): 2 mg, with 100 mg caffeine.

INDICATIONS AND DOSAGES
▶ **Vascular headaches**
PO (CAFERGOT [FIXED-COMBINATION OF ERGOTAMINE AND CAFFEINE])
Adults, Elderly. 2 mg at onset of headache, then 1-2 mg q30min. Maximum: 6 mg/episode; 10 mg/wk.
SUBLINGUAL
Adults, Elderly. 1 tablet at onset of headache, then 1 tablet q30min. Maximum: 3 tablets/24 hr; 5 tablets/wk.
PO, SUBLINGUAL
Children. 1 mg at onset of headache, then 1 mg q30min. Maximum: 3 mg/episode.
IV
Adults, Elderly. 1 mg at onset of headache; may repeat hourly. Maximum: 2 mg/day; 6 mg/wk.

IM, SUBCUTANEOUS
(DIHYDROERGOTAMINE)
Adults, Elderly. 1 mg at onset of headache; may repeat hourly. Maximum: 3 mg/day; 6 mg/wk.
INTRANASAL
Adults, Elderly. 1 spray (0.5 mg) into each nostril; may repeat in 15 min. Maximum: 4 sprays/day; 8 sprays/wk.
RECTAL
Adults, Elderly. 1 suppository at onset of headache; may repeat dose in 1 hr. Maximum: 2 suppositories/episode; 5 suppositories/wk.

CONTRAINDICATIONS
Coronary artery disease, hypertension, impaired hepatic or renal function, malnutrition, peripheral vascular diseases (such as thromboangiitis obliterans, syphilitic arteritis, severe arteriosclerosis, thrombophlebitis, and Raynaud's disease), sepsis, severe pruritus

INTERACTIONS
Drug
Beta blockers, erythromycin: May increase the risk of vasospasm.
Ergot alkaloids, systemic vasoconstrictors: May increase pressor effect.
Nitroglycerin: May decrease the effects of nitroglycerin.
Herbal
None known.
Food
None known.

DIAGNOSTIC TEST EFFECTS
None known.

SIDE EFFECTS
Occasional (5%-2%)
Cough, dizziness
Rare (less than 2%)
Myalgia, fatigue, diarrhea, upper respiratory tract infection, dyspepsia

SERIOUS REACTIONS
• Prolonged administration or excessive dosage may produce ergotamine poisoning, manifested as nausea and vomiting; paresthesia, muscle pain or weakness; precordial pain; tachycardia or bradycardia; and hypertension or hypotension. Vasoconstriction of peripheral arteries and arterioles may result in localized edema and pruritus. Muscle pain will occur when walking and later, even at rest. Other rare effects include confusion, depression, drowsiness, seizures, and gangrene.

PRECAUTIONS & CONSIDERATIONS
Ergotamine use is contraindicated in pregnancy because it may result in fetal harm and even death. Ergotamine is distributed in breast milk and may inhibit lactation. Ergotamine use may produce diarrhea or vomiting in neonates. Ergotamine may be used safely in children 6 years and older, but only use when unresponsive to other drugs. In the elderly, age-related occlusive peripheral vascular disease increases the risk of peripheral vasoconstriction; in addition, age-related renal impairment may require cautious use.

Notify the physician immediately if the drug does not relieve the headache or if irregular heartbeat, nausea or vomiting, numbness or tingling of the fingers and toes, or pain or weakness of the extremities occurs. Peripheral circulation, including the temperature, color, and strength of pulses in the extremities, should be assessed.
Storage
Don't refrigerate the nasal form.
Administration
For sublingual use, place the sublingual tablet under the tongue, let it dissolve, and then swallow it. Don't administer it with water.

For IV use, administer dihydroergotamine undiluted over 1 minute.

Before nasal administration, prime the pump by squeezing it four times. Discard the drug within 8 hours of opening the container.

Erlotinib
er-low'tih-nib
(Tarceva)

CATEGORY AND SCHEDULE
Pregnancy Risk Category: D

CLASSIFICATION
Antineoplastics, miscellaneous

MECHANISM OF ACTION
A human epidermal growth factor that inhibits tyrosine kinases (TK) associated with transmembrane cell surface receptors found on both normal and cancer cells. One such receptor is epidermal growth factor receptor (EGFR). *Therapeutic Effect:* TK activity appears to be vitally important to cell proliferation and survival.

AVAILABILITY
Tablets: 25 mg, 100 mg, 150 mg.

INDICATIONS AND DOSAGES
▶ Overactive bladder
PO
Adults, Elderly. Initially, 7.5 mg once a day. If response is not adequate after a minimum of 2 weeks, dosage may be increased to 15 mg once daily. Do not exceed 7.5 mg once a day in patients with moderate hepatic impairment.

CONTRAINDICATIONS
Pregnancy

INTERACTIONS
Drug
Aminoglutethimide, carba-mazepine, nafcillin, nevirapine, phenobarbital, phenytoin: May decrease the levels and effects of erlotinib.
Azole antifungals, ciprofloxacin, clarithromycin, diclofenac, doxycycline, erythromycin, imatinib, isoniazid, nefazodone, nicardipine, propofol, protease inhibitors, quinidine, verapamil: May increase the levels and effects of erlotinib.
Ketoconazole: May increase serum erlotinib concentration.
Rifampin: May decrease serum erlotinib concentration.
Herbal
St. John's wort: May increase metabolism and decrease serum erlotinib concentration.
Food
Give erlotinib at least 1 hr before or 2 hr after ingestion of food.

DIAGNOSTIC TEST EFFECTS
May increase hepatic enzyme levels.

SIDE EFFECTS
Frequent (35%-21%)
Dry mouth, constipation
Occasional (8%-4%)
Dyspepsia, headache, nausea, abdominal pain
Rare (3%-2%)
Asthenia, diarrhea, dizziness, ocular dryness

SERIOUS REACTIONS
• Urinary tract infection occurs occasionally.

PRECAUTIONS & CONSIDERATIONS
Caution is warranted with hepatic or severe renal impairment.
Administration
Take erlotinib at least 1 hour before or 2 hours after ingestion of food.

Swallow extended-release tablets whole; do not crush.

Ertapenem
er-ta-pen'em
(Invanz)

CATEGORY AND SCHEDULE
Pregnancy Risk Category: B

CLASSIFICATION
Antibiotics, carbapenems

MECHANISM OF ACTION
A carbapenem that penetrates the bacterial cell wall of microorganisms and binds to penicillin-binding proteins, inhibiting cell wall synthesis. *Therapeutic Effect:* Produces bacterial cell death.

PHARMACOKINETICS
Almost completely absorbed after IM administration. Protein binding: 85%-95%. Widely distributed. Primarily excreted in urine with smaller amount eliminated in feces. Removed by hemodialysis.
Half-life: 4 hr.

AVAILABILITY
Injection Powder for Reconstitution: 1-g.

INDICATIONS AND DOSAGES
▶ **Intra-abdominal infection**
IM, IV
Adults, Elderly. 1 g/day for 5-14 days.
▶ **Skin and skin structure infection**
IM, IV
Adults, Elderly. 1 g/day for 7-14 days.

▸ **Pneumonia, urinary tract infection (UTI)**
IM, IV
Adults, Elderly. 1 g/day for 10-14 days.
▸ **Pelvic infection**
IM, IV
Adults, Elderly. 1 g/day for 3-10 days.
▸ **Dosage in renal impairment**
For adults and elderly patients with creatinine clearance less than 30 ml/min, dosage is 500 mg once a day.

CONTRAINDICATIONS
History of hypersensitivity to beta-lactams (imipenem and cilastin, meropenem), hypersensitivity to amide-type local anesthetics (IM)

INTERACTIONS
Drug
Probenecid: Reduces renal excretion of ertapenem.
Herbal
None known.
Food
None known.

DIAGNOSTIC TEST EFFECTS
May increase serum alkaline phosphatase, AST (SGOT) and ALT (SGPT) levels. May decrease platelet count, blood Hct and Hgb levels, and serum potassium level.

🎐 IV INCOMPATIBILITIES
Do not mix or infuse ertapenem with any other medications. Do not use diluents or IV solutions containing dextrose.
🎐 IV Compatibilities
Water for injection, 0.9% NaCl

SIDE EFFECTS
Frequent (10%-6%)
Diarrhea, nausea, headache

Occasional (5%-2%)
Altered mental status, insomnia, rash, abdominal pain, constipation, vomiting, edema, fever
Rare (less than 2%)
Dizziness, cough, oral candidiasis, anxiety, tachycardia, phlebitis at IV site

SERIOUS REACTIONS
• Antibiotic-associated colitis and other superinfections may occur.
• Anaphylactic reactions have been reported.
• Seizures may occur in those with CNS disorders (including patients with brain lesions or a history of seizures), bacterial meningitis, or severe renal impairment.

PRECAUTIONS & CONSIDERATIONS
Caution is warranted with CNS disorders (particularly with brain lesions or history of seizures), a hypersensitivity to cephalosporins, penicillins, or other allergens, and impaired renal function. Be aware that ertapenem is distributed in breast milk. Be aware that the safety and efficacy of ertapenem have not been established in children younger than 18 years. In the elderly, advanced renal insufficiency and end-stage renal insufficiency may require dosage adjustment.

History of allergies, particularly to beta-lactams, cephalosporins, and penicillins should be obtained before beginning drug therapy. Hydration status, nausea, vomiting, skin for rash, sleep pattern, and mental status should be evaluated. Report any diarrhea, rash, seizures, tremors, or other new symptoms.
Storage
Solution normally appears colorless to yellow (variation in color does not affect potency). Discard if solution contains precipitate. Reconstituted

solution is stable for 6 hours at room temperature, 24 hours if refrigerated.

Administration

For IM use, reconstitute with 3.2 ml 1% lidocaine HCl injection (without epinephrine). Shake vial thoroughly. Give deep IM injections slowly to minimize patient discomfort. To further minimize discomfort, administer IM injections into the gluteus maximus instead of the lateral aspect of the thigh. Administer suspension within 1 hour after preparation.

For IV use, dilute 1-g vial with 10 ml, 0.9% NaCl or bacteriostatic water for injection. Shake well to dissolve. Further dilute with 50 ml 0.9% NaCl. Give by intermittent IV infusion (piggyback). Do not give IV push. Infuse over 20 to 30 minutes.

Erythromycin

er-ith-roe-mye'sin
(A/T/S, Akne-Mycin, Apo-Erythro Base [CAN], EES, Emgel, Eryacne [AUS], Erybid [CAN], Eryc, Eryc LD [AUS], EryDerm, Erygel, EryPed, Ery-Tab, Erythra-Derm, Erythrocin, Erythromid [CAN], PCE)
Do not confuse with Emct, azithromycin, Ethmozine, or Pedialyte.

CATEGORY AND SCHEDULE

Pregnancy Risk Category: B

CLASSIFICATION

Anti-infectives, ophthalmics, topical, antibiotics, macrolides

---

MECHANISM OF ACTION

A macrolide that reversibly binds to bacterial ribosomes, inhibiting bacterial protein synthesis.
Therapeutic Effect: Bacteriostatic.

PHARMACOKINETICS

Variably absorbed from the GI tract (depending on dosage form used). Protein binding: 70%-90%. Widely distributed. Metabolized in the liver. Primarily eliminated in feces by bile. Not removed by hemodialysis.
Half-life: 1.4-2 hr (increased in impaired renal function).

AVAILABILITY

Topical Gel (A/T/S, Emgel, Erygel): 2%.
Injection Powder for Reconstitution (Erythrocin): 500 mg, 1 g.
Ophthalmic Ointment: 5 mg/g.
Topical Ointment (Akne-Mycin): 2%.
Oral Suspension (EryPed, EES): 200 mg/5 ml, 400 mg/5 ml.
Topical Solution (Staticin): 1.5%.
Topical Solution (A/T/S, EryDerm, Erythra-Derm): 2%.
Tablet (Chewable [Ery-Ped]): 200 mg.
Tablets (Ery-Tab): 250 mg, 333 mg, 500 mg.
Tablets (EES): 400 mg.
Tablets (Erythrocin): 250 mg, 500 mg.
Tablets (PCE): 333 mg, 500 mg.

INDICATIONS AND DOSAGES

▸ **Mild to moderate infections of the upper and lower respiratory tract, pharyngitis, skin infections**
PO
Adults, Elderly. 250 mg q6hr, 500 mg q12hr, or 333 mg q8hr. Maximum: 4 g/day.
Children. 30-50 mg/kg/day in divided doses up to 60-100 mg/kg/day for severe infections.
Neonates. 20-40 mg/kg/day in divided doses q6-12hr.

IV
Adults, Elderly, Children. 15-20 mg/
kg/day in divided doses. Maximum:
4 g/day.
▸ **Preoperative intestinal
antisepsis**
PO
Adults, Elderly. 1 g at 1 PM, 2 PM,
and 11 PM on day before surgery
(with neomycin).
Children. 20 mg/kg at 1 PM, 2 PM,
and 11 PM on day before surgery
(with neomycin).
▸ **Acne vulgaris**
TOPICAL
Adults. Apply thin layer to affected
area twice a day.
▸ **Gonococcal ophthalmia neonatorum**
OPHTHALMIC
Neonates. 0.5-2 cm no later than
1 hr after delivery.

OFF-LABEL USES

Systemic: Treatment of acne
vulgaris, chancroid, *Campylobacter*
enteritis, gastroparesis, Lyme disease
Topical: Treatment of minor bacterial
skin infections
Ophthalmic: Treatment of blepharitis,
conjunctivitis, keratitis, chlamydial
trachoma

CONTRAINDICATIONS

Administration of fixed-combination
product, Pediazole, to infants younger
than 2 months; history of hepatitis
due to macrolides; hypersensitivity
to macrolides; pre-existing hepatic
disease.

INTERACTIONS
Drug
**Buspirone, cyclosporine,
felodipine, lovastatin, simvastatin:**
May increase the blood
concentration and toxicity of
these drugs.
Carbamazepine: May inhibit the
metabolism of carbamazepine.

Chloramphenicol, clindamycin:
May decrease the effects of these
drugs.
Hepatotoxic medications:
May increase the risk of
hepatotoxicity.
Theophylline: May increase the
risk of theophylline toxicity.
Warfarin: May increase warfarin's
effects.
Herbal
None known.
Food
None known.

DIAGNOSTIC TEST EFFECTS

May increase serum alkaline phosphatase, bilirubin, AST (SGOT), and
ALT (SGPT) levels.

▧ IV INCOMPATIBILITIES
Fluconazole (Diflucan)
▯ **IV Compatibilities**
Aminophylline, amiodarone
(Cordarone), diltiazem (Cardizem),
heparin, hydromorphone (Dilaudid),
lidocaine, lorazepam (Ativan),
magnesium sulfate, midazolam
(Versed), morphine, multivitamins,
potassium chloride

SIDE EFFECTS
Frequent
IV: Abdominal cramping or discom-
fort, phlebitis or thrombophlebitis
Topical: Dry skin (50%)
Occasional
Nausea, vomiting, diarrhea, rash,
urticaria
Rare
Ophthalmic: Sensitivity reaction
with increased irritation, burning,
itching, and inflammation
Topical: Urticaria

SERIOUS REACTIONS

• Antibiotic-associated colitis
and other superinfections may
occur.

- High dosages in patients with renal impairment may lead to reversible hearing loss.
- Anaphylaxis and hepatotoxicity occur rarely.
- Ventricular arrhythmias and prolonged QT interval occur rarely with the IV drug form.

PRECAUTIONS & CONSIDERATIONS

Caution is warranted with hepatic dysfunction. Caution should also be used with the combination drug Pediazole (erythromycin and sulfisoxazole) cautiously in patients with impaired renal or hepatic function, severe allergies, bronchial asthma, or glucose-6-phosphate dehydrogenase deficiency. Determine if there is a history of hepatitis or allergies to erythromycin or other macrolides before beginning therapy. Erythromycin crosses the placenta and is distributed in breast milk. Erythromycin estolate may increase liver function test results in pregnant women. No age-related precautions have been noted in children or the elderly.

WBC should be monitored to determine if the infection is improving. Diarrhea, GI discomfort, headache, nausea, pattern of daily bowel activity and stool consistency, as well as signs and symptoms of superinfection, including anal or genital pruritus, moderate to severe diarrhea, abdominal cramps, fever, and sore mouth or tongue, should be assessed. Signs of hearing loss should be monitored because high dosages can cause hearing loss with hepatic and renal dysfunction.

Storage

Store capsules and tablets at room temperature. The oral suspension is stable for 14 days at room temperature. Store the parenteral form at room temperature.

The initial reconstituted solution in vial is stable for 24 hours at room temperature and 2 weeks if refrigerated. Diluted IV solutions are stable for 8 hours at room temperature and 24 hours if refrigerated. Discard the solution if a precipitate forms.

Administration

Administer erythromycin base or stearate 1 hour before or 2 hours after a meal. Erythromycin estolate and ethylsuccinate may be given without regard to food, but are absorbed better when given on an empty stomach. Give tablets or capsules with 8 oz of water. If the person has difficulty swallowing, sprinkle the capsule contents in a teaspoonful of applesauce and follow with water. Make to swallow chewable tablets whole.

For IV use, reconstitute each 500-mg vial with 10 ml or each 1-g vial with 20 ml sterile water for injection without a preservative to provide a concentration of 50 mg/ml. Further dilute with 100 to 250 ml D_5W or 0.9% NaCl. Administer intermittent IV infusion (piggyback) over 20 to 60 minutes. Administer continuous infusion over 6 to 24 hours.

For ophthalmic use, place a gloved finger on the lower eyelid and pull it out until a pocket is formed between the eye and the lower lid. Place $1/4$-$1/2$ inch of ointment into the pocket. Close the eye for 1 to 2 minutes and roll the eyeball gently to increase the drug's distribution. Remove excess ointment around the eye with tissue.

Escitalopram
es-sy-tal'oh-pram
(Lexapro)

CATEGORY AND SCHEDULE
Pregnancy Risk Category: C

CLASSIFICATION
Antidepressants, serotonin specific reuptake inhibitors

MECHANISM OF ACTION
A selective serotonin reuptake inhibitor that blocks the uptake of the neurotransmitter serotonin at neuronal presynaptic membranes, increasing its availability at postsynaptic receptor sites. *Therapeutic Effect:* Relieves depression.

PHARMACOKINETICS
Well absorbed after PO administration. Primarily metabolized in the liver. Primarily excreted in feces with a lesser amount eliminated in urine. **Half-life:** 35 hr.

AVAILABILITY
Oral Solution: 5 mg/5 ml.
Tablets: 5 mg, 10 mg, 20 mg.

INDICATIONS AND DOSAGES
▸ **Depression, general anxiety disorder (GAD)**
PO
Adults. Initially, 10 mg once a day in the morning or evening. May increase to 20 mg after a minimum of 1 wk.
Elderly, Patients with hepatic impairment. 10 mg/day.

CONTRAINDICATIONS
Breast-feeding, use within 14 days of MAOIs

INTERACTIONS
Drug
Alcohol, other CNS depressants: May increase CNS depression.
Antifungals, cimetidine, macrolide antibiotics: May increase plasma level of escitalopram.
Carbamazepine: May decrease plasma level of escitalopram.
MAOIs: May cause serotonin syndrome, marked by autonomic hyperactivity, coma, diaphoresis, excitement, hyperthermia, and rigidity, and neuroleptic malignant syndrome.
Metoprolol: Increases plasma level of metoprolol.
Herbal
None known.
Food
None known.

DIAGNOSTIC TEST EFFECTS
May reduce serum sodium level.

SIDE EFFECTS
Frequent (21%-11%)
Nausea, dry mouth, somnolence, insomnia, diaphoresis
Occasional (8%-4%)
Tremor, diarrhea, abnormal ejaculation, dyspepsia, fatigue, anxiety, vomiting, anorexia
Rare (3%-2%)
Sinusitis, sexual dysfunction, menstrual disorder, abdominal pain, agitation, decreased libido

SERIOUS REACTIONS
• Overdose is manifested as dizziness, drowsiness, tachycardia, somnolence, confusion, and seizures.

PRECAUTIONS & CONSIDERATIONS
Caution is warranted with hepatic or renal impairment; those with a history of hypomania, mania, or seizures; and patients concurrently using CNS depressants.

E

Escitalopram is distributed in breast milk. Escitalopram use may increase anticholinergic effects and hyperexcitability in children. The elderly are more sensitive to the drug's anticholinergic effects, such as dry mouth and are more likely to experience confusion, dizziness, hyperexcitability, and sedation. Alcohol and tasks that require mental alertness or motor skills should be avoided. CBC and liver and renal function tests should be performed before and periodically during therapy, especially with long-term use.

Administration
! Make sure at least 14 days elapse between the use of MAOIs and escitalopram.

Take escitalopram without regard to food. Don't crush film-coated tablets. Do not abruptly discontinue escitalopram or increase the dosage.

Esmolol
ess'moe-lol
(Brevibloc)

CATEGORY AND SCHEDULE
Pregnancy Risk Category: C

CLASSIFICATION
Antiadrenergics, beta blocking, antiarrhythmics, class II

MECHANISM OF ACTION
An antiarrhythmic that selectively blocks $beta_1$-adrenergic receptors. *Therapeutic Effect:* Slows sinus heart rate, decreases cardiac output, reducing B/P.

AVAILABILITY
Injection: 10 mg/ml, 250 mg/ml.

INDICATIONS AND DOSAGES
▸ **Arrythmias**
IV
Adults, Elderly. Initially, loading dose of 500 mcg/kg/min for 1 min, followed by 50 mcg/kg/min for 4 min. If optimum response is not attained in 5 min, give second loading dose of 500 mcg/kg/min for 1 min, followed by infusion of 100 mcg/kg/min for 4 min. Additional loading doses can be given and infusion increased by 50 mcg/kg/min, up to 200 mcg/kg/min, for 4 min. Once desired response is attained, cease loading dose and increase infusion by no more than 25 mcg/kg/min. Interval between doses may be increased to 10 min. Infusion usually administered over 24-48 hr in most patients. Range: 50-200 mcg/kg/min, with average dose of 100 mcg/kg/min.

▸ **Intra-operative tachycardia or hypertension (immediate control)**
IV
Adults, Elderly. Initially, 80 mg over 30 seconds, then 150 mcg/kg/min infusion up to 300 mcg/kg/min.

CONTRAINDICATIONS
Cardiogenic shock, overt cardiac failure, second- and third-degree heart block, sinus bradycardia

INTERACTIONS
Drug
Insulin, oral hypoglycemics: May mask symptoms of hypoglycemia and prolong hypoglycemic effect of these drugs.
MAOIs: May cause significant hypertension.
Sympathomimetics, xanthines: May mutually inhibit effects.

Herbal
None known.
Food
None known.

DIAGNOSTIC TEST EFFECTS
None known.

▧ IV INCOMPATIBILITIES
Amphotericin B complex (Abelcet, AmBisome, Amphotec), furosemide (Lasix)
▧ IV Compatibilities
Amiodarone (Cordarone), diltiazem (Cardizem), dopamine (Intropin), heparin, magnesium, midazolam (Versed), potassium chloride, propofol (Diprivan)

SIDE EFFECTS
Esmolol is generally well tolerated, with transient and mild side effects.
Frequent
Hypotension (systolic B/P less than 90 mm Hg) manifested as dizziness, nausea, diaphoresis, headache, cold extremities, fatigue
Occasional
Anxiety, drowsiness, flushed skin, vomiting, confusion, inflammation at injection site, fever

SERIOUS REACTIONS
• Overdose may produce profound hypotension, bradycardia, dizziness, syncope, drowsiness, breathing difficulty, bluish fingernails or palms of hands, and seizures.
• Esmolol administration may potentiate insulin-induced hypoglycemia in diabetic patients.

PRECAUTIONS & CONSIDERATIONS
Caution is warranted with bronchial asthma, bronchitis, CHF, diabetes, emphysema, history of allergy, and impaired renal function.
Notify the physician of cold extremities, dizziness, faintness, or nausea. B/P for hypotension, respiratory status for shortness of breath, pattern of daily bowel activity and stool consistency, EKG for arrhythmias, and pulse for quality, rate and rhythm should be monitored during treatment. If pulse rate is 60 beats/minute or lower or systolic B/P is less than 90 mm Hg, withhold the medication and contact the physician. Signs and symptoms of CHF, such as decreased urine output, distended neck veins, dyspnea (particularly on exertion or lying down), night cough, peripheral edema, and weight gain should also be assessed.
Storage
After dilution, solution is stable for 24 hours.
Administration
! Give esmolol by IV infusion. Avoid using butterfly needles and very small veins.
For IV administration, use only clear and colorless to light yellow solution. Discard solution if it is discolored or if precipitate forms. To prevent vein irritation, dilute the 250-mg/ml ampoule to a final concentration not to exceed 10 mg/ml. Don't administer the drug by direct IV injection. For IV infusion, remove 20 ml from 500-ml container of D_5W, D_5W in Ringer's solution, D_5W in lactated Ringer's solution, D_5W in 0.9% NaCl, D_5W in 0.45% NaCl, 0.9% NaCl, lactated Ringer's solution, or 0.45% NaCl and dilute the prescribed amount of esmolol 250 mg/ml concentration in the remaining 480 ml of solution to provide a concentration of 10 mg/ml. Maximum concentration: 10 g/250 ml (40 mg/ml). Administer by controlled infusion device and titrate according to the patient's tolerance and response. Infuse IV loading dose over 1 to 2 minutes. Monitor the patient for hypotension (a systolic

B/P of less than 90 mm Hg), especially during the first 30 minutes of infusion.

Esomeprazole
es-om-eh-pray'zole
(Nexium)

CATEGORY AND SCHEDULE
Pregnancy Risk Category: B

CLASSIFICATION
Gastrointestinals, proton pump inhibitors

MECHANISM OF ACTION
A proton pump inhibitor that is converted to active metabolites that irreversibly bind to and inhibit hydrogen-potassium adenosine triphosphates, an enzyme on the surface of gastric parietal cells. Inhibits hydrogen ion transport into gastric lumen. *Therapeutic Effect:* Increases gastric pH, reducing gastric acid production.

PHARMACOKINETICS
Well absorbed after oral administration. Protein binding: 97%. Extensively metabolized by the liver. Primarily excreted in urine. **Half-life:** 1-1.5 hr.

AVAILABILITY
Capsules (Delayed-Release): 20 mg, 40 mg.

INDICATIONS AND DOSAGES
▸ **Erosive esophagitis**
PO
Adults, Elderly. 20-40 mg once daily for 4-8 wk.

▸ **To maintain healing of erosive esophagitis**
PO
Adults, Elderly. 20 mg/day.
▸ **Gastroesophageal reflux disease**
PO
Adults, Elderly. 20 mg once a day for 4 wk.
▸ **Duodenal ulcer caused by** *Helicobacter pylori*
PO
Adults, Elderly. 40 mg (esomeprazole) once a day, with amoxicillin 1000 mg and clarithromycin 500 mg twice a day for 10 days.

CONTRAINDICATIONS
None known.

INTERACTIONS
Drug
Digoxin, iron, ketoconazole: May decrease the concentration of digoxin, iron, and ketoconazole.
Herbal
None known.
Food
None known.

DIAGNOSTIC TEST EFFECTS
None known.

SIDE EFFECTS
Frequent (7%)
Headache
Occasional (3%-2%)
Diarrhea, abdominal pain, nausea
Rare (less than 2%)
Dizziness, asthenia or loss of strength, vomiting, constipation, rash, cough

SERIOUS REACTIONS
• Pancreatitis, Stevens-Johnson syndrome, toxic epidermal necrolysis, erythema multiforme occurs rarely.

PRECAUTIONS & CONSIDERATIONS
It is unknown if esomeprazole crosses the placenta or is distributed

in breast milk. Safety and efficacy of esomeprazole have not been established in children. No age-related precautions have been noted in the elderly. Notify the physician if headache, diarrhea, discomfort, or nausea occurs during esomeprazole therapy.

Administration

Take 1 hour or more before eating. Do not crush or open capsule; swallow the capsule whole. May open the capsule and mix pellets with 1 tablespoon of applesauce; swallow the spoonful without chewing.

Estazolam

es-tay-zoe-lam
(ProSom)

CATEGORY AND SCHEDULE

Pregnancy Risk Category: X
Controlled Substance:
Schedule IV

CLASSIFICATION

Sedatives/hypnotics

MECHANISM OF ACTION

A benzodiazepine that enhances action of gamma aminobutyric acid (GABA) neurotransmission in the central nervous system (CNS). *Therapeutic Effect:* Produces depressant effect at all levels of central nervous system (CNS).

PHARMACOKINETICS

Rapidly absorbed from gastrointestinal (GI) tract. Protein binding: 93%. Metabolized in liver. Primarily excreted in urine, minimal in feces.
Half-life: 10-24 hr.

AVAILABILITY

Tablets: 1 mg, 2 mg (ProSom).

INDICATIONS AND DOSAGES

▸ **Insomnia**

PO
Adults (older than 18 yr). 1-2 mg at bedtime.
Elderly, debilitated, liver disease, low serum albumin. 0.5-1 mg at bedtime.

CONTRAINDICATIONS

Pregnancy, hypersensitivity to other benzodiazepines

INTERACTIONS

Drug
Alcohol, CNS depressants: May increase central nervous system (CNS) and respiratory depression, and have hypotensive effects.
Herbal
Kava kava, valerian: May increase CNS depressant effect of alprazolam.
Food
None known.

SIDE EFFECTS

Frequent
Drowsiness, sedation, rebound insomnia (may occur for 1-2 nights after drug is discontinued), dizziness, confusion, euphoria
Occasional
Weakness, anorexia, diarrhea
Rare
Paradoxical CNS excitement, restlessness (particularly noted in elderly/debilitated)

SERIOUS REACTIONS

• Overdosage results in somnolence, confusion, diminished reflexes, and coma.

PRECAUTIONS & CONSIDERATIONS

Caution should be used with impaired renal or liver function.

Be aware that estazolam is contra-indicated in pregnancy. Estazolam crosses the placenta and is distributed in breast milk. Safety and efficacy of estazolam have not been established in children. Use small initial doses and gradually increase them to avoid excessive sedation or ataxia as evidenced by muscular incoordination in the elderly. Rebound insomnia may occur when drug is discontinued after short-term therapy. Avoid alcohol.

Storage
Store at room temperature.

Administration
Take at bedtime. May be taken without regard to meals.

Estradiol

ess-tra-dye′ole
(Aerodil [AUS], Alora, Climara, Delestrogen, Depo-Estradiol, Esclim, Estrace, Estraderm, Estraderm MX [AUS], Estradot [CAN], Estrasorb, Estrogel, Estring, Femring, Kliovance [AUS], Menostar, Oesclim [CAN], Sandrena Gel [AUS], Vagifem, Vivelle, Vivelle Dot, Zumenon [AUS])
Do not confuse Estraderm with Testoderm.

CATEGORY AND SCHEDULE
Pregnancy Risk Category: X

CLASSIFICATION
Estrogens, hormones/hormone modifiers

MECHANISM OF ACTION
An estrogen that increases synthesis of DNA, RNA, and proteins in target tissues; reduces release of gonadotropin-releasing hormone from the hypothalamus; and reduces follicle-stimulating hormone and luteinizing hormone (LH) release from the pituitary. *Therapeutic Effect:* Promotes normal growth, promotes development of female sex organs, and maintains GU function and vasomotor stability. Prevents accelerated bone loss by inhibiting bone resorption, restoring balance of bone resorption and formation. Inhibits LH and decreases serum testosterone concentration.

PHARMACOKINETICS
Well absorbed from the GI tract. Widely distributed. Protein binding: 50%-80%. Metabolized in the liver. Primarily excreted in urine. **Half-life:** Unknown.

AVAILABILITY
Tablets (Estrace): 0.5 mg, 1 mg, 2 mg.
Emulsion (Topical [Estrasorb]): 2.5 mg/g.
Injection (Cypionate [Depo-Estradiol]): 5 mg/ml.
Injection (Valerate [Delestrogen]): 10 mg/ml.
Topical Gel (EstroGel): 1.25 g.
Transdermal System (Alora): twice weekly: 0.025 mg, 0.05 mg, 0.075 mg, 0.1 mg.
Transdermal System (Climara): once weekly: 0.025 mg, 0.0375 mg, 0.05 mg, 0.06 mg, 0.075 mg, 0.1 mg.
Transdermal System (Esclim): twice weekly: 0.025 mg, 0.0375 mg, 0.05 mg, 0.075 mg, 0.1 mg.
Transdermal System (Estraderm): twice weekly: 0.05 mg, 0.1 mg.
Transdermal System (Menostar): once a week: 1 mg.
Transdermal System (Vivelle): twice weekly: 0.025 mg, 0.0375 mg, 0.05 mg, 0.075 mg, 0.1 mg.

Transdermal System (Vivelle Dot):
twice weekly: 0.0375 mg, 0.05 mg,
0.075 mg, 0.1 mg.
Vaginal Cream (Estrace):
0.1 mg/g.
Vaginal Ring (Estring): 2 mg.
Vaginal Ring (Femring):
0.05 mg.
Vaginal Tablet (Vagifem): 25 mcg.

INDICATIONS AND DOSAGES
▶ **Prostate cancer**
IM (VALERATE)
Adults, Elderly. 30 mg or more
q1-2-wk.
PO
Adults, Elderly. 10 mg 3 times a day
for at least 3 mo.
▶ **Breast cancer**
PO
Adults, Elderly. 10 mg 3 times a day
for at least 3 mo.
▶ **Osteoporosis prophylaxis in
post-menopausal females**
PO
Adults, Elderly. 0.5 mg/day cycli-
cally (3 weeks on, 1 week off).
TRANSDERMAL (CLIMARA)
Adults, Elderly. Initially, 0.025 mg
weekly, adjust dose as needed.
TRANSDERMAL (ALORA,
VIVELLE, VIVELLE-DOT)
Adults, Elderly. Initially, 0.025 mg
patch twice weekly, adjust dose as
needed.
TRANSDERMAL (ESTRADERM)
Adults, Elderly. 0.05 mg twice
weekly.
TRANSDERMAL (MENOSTAR)
Adults, Elderly. 1 mg weekly.
▶ **Female hypoestrogenism**
PO
Adults, Elderly. 1-2 mg/day, adjust
dose as needed.
IM (CYPIONATE)
Adults, Elderly. 1.5-2 mg monthly.
IM (VALERATE)
Adults, Elderly. 10-20 mg
q4wk.

▶ **Vasomotor symptoms associated
with menopause**
PO
Adults, Elderly. 1-2 mg/day
cyclically (3 weeks on, 1 week off),
adjust dose as needed.
IM (CYPIONATE)
Adults, Elderly. 1-5 mg q3-4wk.
IM (VALERATE)
Adults, Elderly. 10-20 mg q4wk.
TOPICAL EMULSION
(ESTRASORB)
Adults, Elderly. 3.84 g once a day in
the morning.
TOPICAL GEL (ESTROGEL)
Adults, Elderly. 1.25 g/day.
TRANSDERMAL (CLIMARA)
Adults, Elderly. 0.025 mg weekly.
Adjust dose as needed.
TRANSDERMAL (ALORA,
ESCLIM, ESTRADER,
VIVELLE-DOT)
Adults, Elderly. 0.05 mg twice
a week.
TRANSDERMAL (VIVELLE)
Adults, Elderly. 0.0375 mg twice
a week.
VAGINAL RING (FEMRING)
Adults, Elderly. 0.05 mg. May
increase to 0.1 mg if needed.
▶ **Vaginal atrophy**
VAGINAL RING (ESTRING)
Adults, Elderly. 2 mg.
▶ **Atrophic vaginitis**
VAGINAL TABLET (VAGIFEM)
Adults, Elderly. Initially, 1 tablet/day
for 2 weeks. Maintenance: 1 tablet
twice a week.

OFF-LABEL USES
Treatment of Turner's syndrome

CONTRAINDICATIONS
Abnormal vaginal bleeding, active
arterial thrombosis, blood dyscrasias,
estrogen-dependent cancer, known or
suspected breast cancer, pregnancy,
thrombophlebitis or thromboembolic
disorders, thyroid dysfunction

INTERACTIONS
Drug
Bromocriptine: May interfere with the effects of bromocriptine.
Cyclosporine: May increase blood cyclosporine concentration and the risk of hepatotoxicity and nephrotoxicity.
Hepatotoxic medications: May increase the risk of hepatotoxicity.
Herbal
Saw palmetto: Increases the effects of saw palmetto.
Food
None known.

DIAGNOSTIC TEST EFFECTS
May increase blood glucose, HDL, serum calcium, and triglyceride levels. May decrease serum cholesterol levels and LDH concentrations. May affect metapyrone testing and thyroid function tests.

SIDE EFFECTS
Frequent
Anorexia, nausea, swelling of breasts, peripheral edema marked by swollen ankles and feet
Transdermal: Skin irritation, redness
Occasional
Vomiting, especially with high doses; headache that may be severe; intolerance to contact lenses; hypertension; glucose intolerance; brown spots on exposed skin
Vaginal: Local irritation, vaginal discharge, changes in vaginal bleeding, including spotting, and breakthrough or prolonged bleeding
Rare
Chorea or involuntary movements, hirsutism or abnormal hairiness, loss of scalp hair, depression

SERIOUS REACTIONS
• Prolonged administration increases the risk of gallbladder disease, thromboembolic disease, and breast, cervical, vaginal, endometrial, and hepatic carcinoma.
• Cholestatic jaundice occurs rarely.

PRECAUTIONS & CONSIDERATIONS
Caution is warranted with diseases exacerbated by fluid retention and with hepatic or renal insufficiency. Estradiol is distributed in breast milk and may be harmful to the infant. Estradiol should not be used during breast-feeding. Estradiol should be used cautiously in children whose bone growth is not complete because the drug may accelerate epiphyseal closure. No age-related precautions have been noted in the elderly.

Avoid smoking because of the increased risk of blood clot formation and MI. Limit alcohol and caffeine intake.

Notify the physician of calf or chest pain, depression, numbness or weakness of an extremity, severe abdominal pain, shortness of breath, speech or vision disturbance, sudden headache, unusual bleeding, or vomiting. B/P, weight, blood glucose, hepatic enzyme, and serum calcium levels should be monitored.
Administration
Take oral estradiol at the same time each day.

For IM use, rotate the vial to disperse drug in solution. Give deep IM injection into the gluteus maximus.

For vaginal use, apply estradiol cream at bedtime for best absorption. To administer, insert the end of the filled applicator into the vagina, directing the applicator slightly toward the sacrum; push the plunger down completely. Do not let the cream contact the skin to prevent topical absorption of the drug.

! Transdermal Climara is administered once weekly; other transdermal forms of estradiol are applied twice weekly.

To apply the transdermal system, remove the old patch and select a new site. Consider using the buttocks as an alternative application site. Peel off the protective strip on the patch to expose the adhesive surface. Apply to clean, dry, intact skin on the trunk of the body in an area with as little hair as possible. Press in place for at least 10 seconds. Do not apply the patch to breasts or waistline.

Estrogens, Conjugated

ess'troe-jenz
(Cenestin, C.E.S. [CAN], Congest [CAN], Enjuvia, Premarin, Premarin Créme [AUS])
Do not confuse with Primaxin or Remeron.

CATEGORY AND SCHEDULE
Pregnancy Risk Category: X

CLASSIFICATION
Estrogens, hormones/hormone modifiers

MECHANISM OF ACTION
An estrogen that increases synthesis of DNA, RNA, and various proteins in target tissues; reduces release of gonadotropin-releasing hormone from the hypothalamus; and reduces follicle-stimulating hormone (FSH) and leuteinizing hormone (LH) release from the pituitary gland. *Therapeutic Effect:* Promotes normal growth, promotes development of female sex organs, and maintains GU function and vasomotor stability. Prevents accelerated bone loss by inhibiting bone resorption, restoring balance of bone resorption and formation. Inhibits LH and decreases serum concentration of testosterone.

PHARMACOKINETICS
Well absorbed from the GI tract. Widely distributed. Protein binding: 50%-80%. Metabolized in the liver. Primarily excreted in urine.

AVAILABILITY
Tablets (Cenestin, Premarin): 0.3 mg, 0.45 mg, 0.625 mg, 0.9 mg, 1.25 mg.
Tablets (Enjuvia): 0.625 mg, 1.25 mg.
Injection: 25 mg.
Vaginal Cream. 0.625 mg/g.

INDICATIONS AND DOSAGES
▸ **Vasomotor symptoms associated with menopause, atrophic vaginitis, kraurosis vulvae**
PO
Adults, Elderly. 0.3-0.625 mg/day cyclically (21 days on, 7 days off) or continuously.
INTRAVAGINAL
Adults, Elderly. 0.5-2 g/day cyclically, such as 21 days on and 7 days off.
▸ **Female hypogonadism**
PO
Adults. 0.3-0.625 mg/day in divided doses for 20 days; then a rest period of 10 days.
▸ **Female castration, primary ovarian failure**
PO
Adults. Initially, 1.25 mg/day cyclically. Adjust dosage, upward or downward, according to severity of symptoms and patient response. For maintenance, adjust dosage to lowest level that will provide effective control.

▶ **Osteoporosis**
PO
Adults, Elderly. 0.3-0.625 mg/day, cyclically, such as 25 days on and 5 days off.
▶ **Breast cancer**
PO
Adults, Elderly. 10 mg 3 times a day for at least 3 mo.
▶ **Prostate cancer**
PO
Adults, Elderly. 1.25-2.5 mg 3 times a day.
▶ **Abnormal uterine bleeding**
PO
Adults. 1.25 mg q4hr for 24 hr, then 1.25 mg/day for 7-10 days.
IV, IM
Adults. 25 mg; may repeat once in 6-12 hr.

OFF-LABEL USES
Prevention of estrogen deficiency-induced premenopausal osteoporosis
Cream: Prevention of nosebleeds

CONTRAINDICATIONS
Breast cancer with some exceptions, hepatic disease, thrombophlebitis, undiagnosed vaginal bleeding

INTERACTIONS
Drug
Bromocriptine: May interfere with the effects of bromocriptine.
Cyclosporine: May increase blood cyclosporine concentration and the risk of hepatotoxicity and nephrotoxicity.
Hepatotoxic medications: May increase the risk of hepatotoxicity.
Herbal
None known.
Food
None known.

DIAGNOSTIC TEST EFFECTS
May increase blood glucose, HDL, serum calcium, and triglyceride levels. May decrease serum cholesterol levels and LDH concentrations. May affect serum metapyrone testing and thyroid function tests.

▨ IV INCOMPATIBILITIES
No information available via Y-site administration.

SIDE EFFECTS
Frequent
Vaginal bleeding, such as spotting or breakthrough bleeding; breast pain or tenderness; gynecomastia
Occasional
Headache, hypertension, intolerance to contact lenses
High doses: Anorexia, nausea
Rare
Loss of scalp hair, depression

SERIOUS REACTIONS
• Prolonged administration may increase the risk of gallbladder disease, thromboembolic disease, and breast, cervical, vaginal, endometrial, and hepatic carcinoma.

PRECAUTIONS & CONSIDERATIONS
Caution is warranted with asthma, cardiac dysfunction, diabetes mellitus, epilepsy, migraine headaches, and renal impairment. Conjugated estrogens are distributed in breast milk and may be harmful to the fetus. The drug should be discontinued if the female is pregnant. They should not be used during breast-feeding. Safety and efficacy of conjugated estrogens have not been established in children. No age-related precautions have been noted in the elderly. Avoid smoking because of the increased risk of blood clot formation and MI.
    Notify the physician of weight gain of more than 5 pounds per week,

abnormal vaginal bleeding, depression, or signs and symptoms of blood clots. Also, signs and symptoms of thromboembolic or thrombotic disorders, including loss of coordination, numbness or weakness of an extremity, shortness of breath, speech or vision disturbance, sudden severe headache, and pain in the chest, leg, or groin, should be reported immediately. Breast self-examinations should be made monthly. Weight and B/P should be monitored.

Storage
Refrigerate vials. The reconstituted solution is stable for 60 days refrigerated. Do not use if solution darkens or precipitate forms.

Administration
Take at the same time each day with food or milk if nausea occurs.

For IV and IM use, reconstitute with 5 ml sterile water for injection containing benzyl alcohol (provided). Slowly add diluent, shaking gently. Avoid vigorous shaking. For the IV form, give slowly to prevent flushing.

Estrogens, Esterified

ess′troe-jenz
(Estratab, Menest, Neo-Estrone [CAN])

CATEGORY AND SCHEDULE
Pregnancy Risk Category: X

CLASSIFICATION
Estrogens, hormones/hormone modifiers

MECHANISM OF ACTION
A combination of sodium salts of sulfate esters of estrogenic substances (principle component is estrone) that increases synthesis of DNA, RNA, and various proteins in responsive tissues. Reduces release of gonadotropin-releasing hormone, reducing follicle-stimulating hormone (FSH) and leuteinizing hormone (LH). *Therapeutic Effect:* Promotes vasomotor stability, maintains genitourinary (GU) function, normal growth, development of female sex organs. Prevents accelerated bone loss by inhibiting bone resorption, restoring balance of bone resorption and formation.

PHARMACOKINETICS
Readily absorbed from the gastrointestinal (GI) tract. Widely distributed. Protein binding: 50%-80%. Rapidly metabolized in liver and GI tract to estrone sulfate and conjugated and unconjugated metabolites. Excreted in urine and bile.
Half-life: Unknown.

AVAILABILITY
Tablets: 0.3 mg (Menest), 0.625 mg (Estratab).

INDICATIONS AND DOSAGES
▸ **Vasomotor symptoms associated with menopause, atrophic vaginitis, kraurosis vulvae**
PO
Adults, Elderly. 0.3-1.25 mg/day.
▸ **Female hypogonadism**
PO
Adults. 2.5-7.5 mg/day in divided doses for 20 days; rest 10 days.
▸ **Female castration, primary ovarian failure**
PO
Adults. Initially, 1.25 mg/day cyclically.
▸ **Breast cancer**
PO
Adults, Elderly. 10 mg 3 times/day for at least 3 mo.

▶ **Prostate cancer**
PO
Adults, Elderly. 1.25-2.5 mg
3 times/day.

CONTRAINDICATIONS
Breast cancer with some exceptions, liver disease, thrombophlebitis, undiagnosed vaginal bleeding

INTERACTIONS
Drug
Bromocriptine: May interfere with effects of bromocriptine.
Cyclosporine: May increase blood concentration and liver and nephrotoxicity of cyclosporine.
Liver toxic medications: May increase the risk of liver toxicity.
Herbal
St. John's Wort: May decrease levels of esterified estrogens.
Black cohosh, dong quai: May increase estrogenic activity.
Red clover, saw palmetto, ginseng: May increase hormonal effects.

DIAGNOSTIC TEST EFFECTS
May affect metapyrone testing, thyroid function tests. May decrease serum cholesterol levels and LDH concentrations. May increase blood glucose levels, HDL concentrations, serum calcium and triglyceride levels.

SIDE EFFECTS
Frequent
Change in vaginal bleeding, such as spotting or breakthrough bleeding, breast pain or tenderness, gynecomastia
Occasional
Headache, increased blood pressure (B/P), intolerance to contact lenses, nausea
Rare
Loss of scalp hair, clinical depression

SERIOUS REACTIONS
• Prolonged administration may increase risk of gallbladder, thromboembolic disease, breast, cervical, vaginal, endometrial, and liver carcinoma.

PRECAUTIONS & CONSIDERATIONS
Caution is warranted with asthma, cardiac dysfunction, diabetes mellitus, epilepsy, migraine headaches, and renal impairment. Be aware that esterified estrogen is distributed in breast milk and may be harmful to fetus. Esterified estrogen should not be used during breast-feeding. Be aware that the safety and efficacy of this drug have not been established in children. There are no age-related precautions noted in the elderly. Smoking should be strongly discouraged.

Signs and symptoms of thromboembolic or thrombotic disorders are evident by loss of coordination, numbness or weakness of an extremity, pain in the chest, leg, or groin, shortness of breath, speech or vision disturbance, and sudden severe headache. Abnormal vaginal bleeding, tenderness, and swelling may be signs and symptoms of blood clots.
Administration
Administer at the same time each day. Give esterified estrogen with food or milk if the patient experiences nausea.

Estrone

ess'trone

(Estragyn 5, Estro-A, Estrogenic, Estrogens, Kestrone 5)

CATEGORY AND SCHEDULE

Pregnancy Risk Category: X

CLASSIFICATION

Hormones/hormone modifiers

MECHANISM OF ACTION

An estrogen that increases synthesis of DNA, RNA, proteins in target tissues; reduces release of gonadotropin-releasing hormone from hypothalamus; reduces follicle-stimulating hormone (FSH) and luteinizing hormone (LH) release from the pituitary. *Therapeutic Effect:* Promotes normal growth and development of female sex organs, maintaining genitourinary (GU) function, vasomotor stability. Prevents accelerated bone loss by inhibiting bone resorption, restoring balance of bone resorption and formation. Inhibits LH, decreases serum concentration of testosterone.

PHARMACOKINETICS

Well absorbed from the gastrointestinal (GI) tract. Widely distributed. Protein binding: 50%-80%. Metabolized in liver as well as a certain proportion excreted into the bile and reabsorbed from the intestine. Primarily excreted in urine. **Half-life:** Unknown.

AVAILABILITY

Injection: 2 mg/ml (Estro-A, Estrogenic, Estrogens), 5 mg/ml (Estragyn 5, Kestrone 5).

INDICATIONS AND DOSAGES

▶ **Atrophic vaginitis, female castration, female hypogonadism, Kraurosis vulvae, menopausal symptoms, primary ovarian failure, prostatic carcinoma**

IM

Adults. Initially, 0.1 or 0.5 mg 2-3 times weekly cyclically (21 days on; 7 days off or continuously). When progestin is given concomitantly, begin progestin after 10-13 days of each estrogen cycle.

CONTRAINDICATIONS

Abnormal vaginal bleeding, active arterial thrombosis, blood dyscrasias, estrogen-dependent cancer, known or suspected breast cancer, pregnancy, thrombophlebitis or thromboembolic disorders, hypersensitivity to estrone or any of its components.

INTERACTIONS

Drug

Bromocriptine: May interfere with the effects of bromocriptine.

Cyclosporine: May increase the blood concentration and risk of liver and nephrotoxicity of cyclosporine.

Liver toxic medications: May increase the risk of liver toxicity.

Herbal

Saw palmetto: Increases the effects of saw palmetto.

Food

None known.

DIAGNOSTIC TEST EFFECTS

May affect thyroid function tests, metapyrone, and prothrombin time. May decrease serum cholesterol levels, LDH concentrations. May increase blood glucose levels, HDL concentrations, and triglyceride levels.

SIDE EFFECTS
Frequent
Transient menstrual abnormalities including spotting, change in menstrual flow or cervical secretions, and amenorrhea at initiation of therapy
Occasional
Edema, weight change, breast tenderness, nervousness, insomnia, fatigue, dizziness
Rare
Alopecia, mental depression, dermatologic changes, headache, fever, nausea

SERIOUS REACTIONS
• Thrombophlebitis, pulmonary or cerebral embolism, and retinal thrombosis occur rarely.

PRECAUTIONS & CONSIDERATIONS
Caution should be used with diseases exacerbated by fluid retention and liver or renal insufficiency. Estrone is distributed in breast milk and may be harmful to offspring and should not be used during breast-feeding. Be aware that safety and efficacy have not been established in children. There are no age-related precautions noted in the elderly. Alcohol and caffeine intake should be limited. Smoking should be avoided due to the increased risk of blood clots and myocardial infarction (MI).

Calf or chest pain, mental depression, numbness or weakness of an extremity, severe abdominal pain, shortness of breath, speech or vision disturbance, sudden headache, unusual bleeding, vaginal bleeding, vomiting as well as suspect of pregnancy should be reported immediately.
Administration
Rotate vial to disperse drug in solution. Give deep IM injection into the gluteus maximus.

Estropipate
es-tro-pip′ate
(Genoral [AUS], Ogen, Ortho-Est)

CATEGORY AND SCHEDULE
Pregnancy Risk Category: X

CLASSIFICATION
Estrogens, hormones/hormone modifiers

MECHANISM OF ACTION
An estrogen that increases synthesis of DNA, RNA, and proteins in target tissues; reduces release of gonadotropin-releasing hormone from the hypothalamus; and reduces follicle-stimulating hormone (FSH) and luteinizing hormone (LH) from the pituitary. *Therapeutic Effect:* Promotes normal growth, promotes development of female sex organs, and maintains GU function and vasomotor stability. Prevents accelerated bone loss by inhibiting bone resorption, restoring balance of bone resorption and formation. Inhibits LH and decreases serum testosterone concentration.

AVAILABILITY
Tablets (Ogen, Ortho-Est): 0.625 mg (0.75 mg estropipate), 1.25 mg (1.5 mg estropipate), 2.5 mg (3 mg estropipate).
Vaginal Cream (Ogen): 1.5 mg/g.

INDICATIONS AND DOSAGES
▸ **Vasomotor symptoms, atrophic vaginitis, kraurosis vulvae**
PO
Adults, Elderly. 0.625-5 mg/day cyclically.
▸ **Atrophic vaginitis, kraurosis vulvae**
INTRAVAGINAL
Adults, Elderly. 2-4 g/day cyclically.

‣ **Female hypogonadism, castration, primary ovarian failure**
PO
Adults, Elderly. 1.25-7.5 mg/day for 21 days; then off for 8-10 days. Repeat if bleeding does not occur by end of off cycle.

‣ **Prevention of osteoporosis**
PO
Adults, Elderly. 0.625 mg/day (25 days of 31-day cycle/mo).

CONTRAINDICATIONS
Abnormal vaginal bleeding, active arterial thrombosis, blood dyscrasias, estrogen-dependent cancer, known or suspected breast cancer, pregnancy, thrombophlebitis or thromboembolic disorders, thyroid dysfunction

INTERACTIONS
Drug
Bromocriptine: May interfere with the effects of bromocriptine.
Cyclosporine: May increase blood cyclosporine concentration and the risk of hepatotoxicity and nephrotoxicity.
Hepatotoxic medications: May increase the risk of hepatotoxicity.
Herbal
Saw palmetto: Increases the effects of saw palmetto.
Food
None known.

DIAGNOSTIC TEST EFFECTS
May increase blood glucose, HDL, serum calcium, and triglyceride levels. May decrease serum cholesterol and LDH concentrations. May affect metapyrone testing and thyroid function tests.

SIDE EFFECTS
Frequent
Anorexia, nausea, swelling of breasts, peripheral edema marked by swollen ankles and feet

Occasional
Vomiting, especially with high doses; headache that may be severe; intolerance to contact lenses; hypertension; glucose intolerance; brown spots on exposed skin
Vaginal: Local irritation, vaginal discharge, changes in vaginal bleeding, including spotting, and breakthrough or prolonged bleeding
Rare
Chorea or involuntary movements, hirsutism or abnormal hairiness, loss of scalp hair, depression

SERIOUS REACTIONS
• Prolonged administration increases the risk of gallbladder disease, thromboembolic disease and breast, cervical, vaginal, endometrial, and hepatic carcinoma.
• Cholestatic jaundice occurs rarely.

PRECAUTIONS & CONSIDERATIONS
Caution is warranted with diseases exacerbated by fluid retention and with hepatic or renal insufficiency. Estropipate is distributed in breast milk and may be harmful to the infant. Estropipate should not be used during breast-feeding. Estropipate should be used cautiously in children whose bone growth is not complete because the drug may accelerate epiphyseal closure. No age-related precautions have been noted in the elderly. Avoid smoking because of the increased risk of blood clot formation and MI.

Notify the physician of depression or abnormal vaginal bleeding. Signs and symptoms of thromboembolic or thrombotic disorders, including peripheral paresthesia, shortness of breath, speech or vision disturbance, and sudden headache, should be immediately reported. B/P, weight, and blood glucose, hepatic enzyme,

and serum calcium levels should be monitored.
Storage
Store in a tightly-closed container.
Administration
Take estropipate at the same time each day.

Remain recumbent for at least 30 minutes after vaginal application and do not use tampons during estropipate therapy.

Eszopiclone
es-zoe-pick'lone
(Lunesta)

CATEGORY AND SCHEDULE
Pregnancy Risk Category: C

CLASSIFICATION
Sedatives/hypnotics

MECHANISM OF ACTION
A nonbenzodiazepine that may inter-act with GABA-receptor complexes at binding domains located close to or allosterically coupled to benzodi-azepine receptors. *Therapeutic Effect:* Induces sleep and helps maintain sleep at night.

AVAILABILITY
Tablets (Film-Coated): 1 mg, 2 mg, 3 mg.

INDICATIONS AND DOSAGES
▸ **Insomnia**
PO
Adults. 2 mg before bedtime. Maximum: 3 mg.
Adults using CYP3A4 inhibitors concurrently. 1 mg before bedtime; may be increased to 2 mg if needed.
Elderly. Initially, 1 mg before bedtime. Maximum: 2 mg.
Difficulty maintaining sleep
Adults, Elderly. 2 mg before bedtime.

CONTRAINDICATIONS
None known.

INTERACTIONS
Drug
Alcohol, olanzapine: May lead to decreased psychomotor function.
Aminoglutethimide, carba-mazepine, nafcillin, nevirapine, phenobarbital, phenytoin, rifampicin: May decrease the blood level and effects of eszopiclone.
Clarithromycin, ketoconazole, nefazodone, nelfinavir, ritonavir, traconazole, troleandomycin: May increase the blood level and effects of eszopiclone.
Herbal
Gotu kola, kava kava, St. John's wort, valerian: May increase CNS depression.
Food
Heavy meals: May reduce onset of eszopiclone action if taken with or immediately after a heavy meal.

DIAGNOSTIC TEST EFFECTS
None known.

SIDE EFFECTS
Frequent (34%-21%)
Unpleasant taste, headache
Occasional (10%-4%)
Somnolence, dry mouth, dyspepsia, dizziness, nervousness, nausea, rash, pruritus, depression, diarrhea
Rare (3%-2%)
Hallucinations, anxiety, confusion, abnormal dreams, decreased libido, neuralgia.

SERIOUS REACTIONS
• Chest pain and peripheral edema occur occasionally.

PRECAUTIONS & CONSIDERATIONS
Caution is warranted with clinical depression, hepatic impairment and compromised respiratory function.

Administration
Take immediately before bedtime. Don't take with, or immediately following, a high-fat meal. Don't crush or break tablets.

Etanercept
e-tan′er-cept
(Enbrel)

CATEGORY AND SCHEDULE
Pregnancy Risk Category: B

CLASSIFICATION
Disease modifying antirheumatic drugs, immunomodulators, tumor necrosis factor modulators

MECHANISM OF ACTION
A protein that binds to tumor necrosis factor (TNF), blocking its interaction with cell surface receptors. Elevated levels of TNF, which is involved in inflammatory and immune responses, are found in the synovial fluid of rheumatoid arthritis patients. *Therapeutic Effect:* Relieves symptoms of rheumatoid arthritis.

PHARMACOKINETICS
Well absorbed after subcutaneous administration. **Half-life:** 115 hr.

AVAILABILITY
Powder for Injection: 25 mg.
Prefilled Syringe.

INDICATIONS AND DOSAGES
▸ **Rheumatoid arthritis, psoriatic arthritis, ankylosing spondylitis**
SUBCUTANEOUS
Adults, Elderly. 25 mg twice weekly given 72-96 hr apart.

Alternative weekly dosing: 0.8 mg/kg/dose once a week. Maximum: 50 mg/wk. Maximum: 25 mg/dose.
▸ **Juvenile rheumatoid arthritis**
Children 4-17 yr. 0.4 mg/kg (Maximum: 25 mg dose) twice weekly given 72-96 hr apart. Alternative weekly dosing: 50 mg once weekly. Maximum: 25 mg/dose.
▸ **Plaque psoriasis**
SUBCUTANEOUS
Adults, Elderly. 50 mg twice a week (give 3-4 days apart) for 3 mo. Maintenance: 50 mg once a week.

OFF-LABEL USES
Treatment of Crohn's disease

CONTRAINDICATIONS
Serious active infection or sepsis

INTERACTIONS
Drug
Anakinara: May increase the risk of infection.
Live vaccines: Secondary transmission of infection by the live vaccine may occur.
Herbal
None known.
Food
None known.

DIAGNOSTIC TEST EFFECTS
None known.

SIDE EFFECTS
Frequent (37%)
Injection site erythema, pruritus, pain, and swelling; abdominal pain, vomiting (more common in children than adults)
Occasional (16%-4%)
Headache, rhinitis, dizziness, pharyngitis, cough, asthenia, abdominal pain, dyspepsia
Rare (less than 3%)
Sinusitis, allergic reaction

SERIOUS REACTIONS

• Infections (such as pyelonephritis, cellulitis, osteomyelitis, wound infection, leg ulcer, septic arthritis, diarrhea, bronchitis, and pneumonia), occur in 38%-29% of patients.
• Rare adverse effects include heart failure, hypertension, hypotension, pancreatitis, GI hemorrhage, and dyspnea. The patient also may develop autoimmune antibodies.

PRECAUTIONS & CONSIDERATIONS

Caution is warranted with history of recurrent infections and illnesses that predispose to infection, such as diabetes mellitus. It is unknown if etanercept is excreted in breast milk. No age-related precautions have been noted in the elderly or in children 4 years and older. Avoid receiving live-virus vaccines during treatment. Discontinue therapy and expect to treat with varicella-zoster immune globulin, as prescribed, if the patient experiences significant exposure to varicella virus during treatment.

Notify the physician of bleeding, bruising, pallor, or persistent fever. CBC and erythrocyte sedimentation rate or C-reactive protein level should be monitored. Signs of a therapeutic response, including improved grip strength, increased joint mobility, reduced joint tenderness, and relief of pain, stiffness, and swelling, should be assessed.

Storage

Refrigerate unopened vials. Once reconstituted, the drug may be stored for up to 6 hours in the refrigerator.

Administration

! Don't add other medications to the solution. Don't use a filter during reconstitution or administration.

Reconstitute only with 1 ml sterile bacteriostatic water for injection (containing 0.9% benzyl alcohol).

Don't use other diluents. Slowly inject the diluent into the vial. Some foaming will occur. To avoid excessive foaming, slowly swirl the contents until the powder is dissolved (less than 5 minutes). The reconstituted solution normally appears clear and colorless. Discard the solution if it contains particles or becomes cloudy or discolored. Withdraw all the solution into the syringe. The final volume should be approximately 1 ml. Inject the drug into the abdomen, thigh, or upper arm. Rotate injection sites. Administer each new injection at least 1 inch from an old site, avoiding tender, bruised, hard, or red areas. Injection site reactions generally occur in the first month of treatment and decrease in frequency with continued etanercept therapy.

Ethambutol
e-tham′byoo-tole
(Etibi [CAN], Myambutol)
Do not confuse ethambutol or Myambutol with Nembutal.

CATEGORY AND SCHEDULE
Pregnancy Risk Category: B

CLASSIFICATION
Antimycobacterials

MECHANISM OF ACTION
An isonicotinic acid derivative that interferes with RNA synthesis. *Therapeutic Effect:* Suppresses the multiplication of mycobacteria.

PHARMACOKINETICS
Rapidly and well absorbed from the GI tract. Protein binding: 20%-30%.

Widely distributed. Metabolized in the liver. Primarily excreted in urine. Removed by hemodialysis. **Half-life:** 3-4 hr (increased in impaired renal function).

AVAILABILITY
Tablets: 100 mg, 400 mg.

INDICATIONS AND DOSAGES
▸ **Tuberculosis**
PO
Adults, Elderly, Children. 15-25 mg/kg/day as a single dose or 50 mg/kg 2 times/wk. Maximum: 2.5 g/dose.
▸ **Atypical mycobacterial infections**
PO
Adults, Elderly, Children.
15 mg/kg/day. Maximum: 1 g/day.
▸ **Dosage in renal impairment**
Dosage interval is modified based on creatinine clearance.

Creatinine Clearance	Dosage Interval
10-50 ml/min	q24-36hr
Less than 10 ml/min	q48hr

OFF-LABEL USES
Treatment of atypical mycobacterial infections

CONTRAINDICATIONS
Optic neuritis

INTERACTIONS
Drug
Neurotoxic medications: May increase the risk of neurotoxicity.
Herbal
None known.
Food
None known.

DIAGNOSTIC TEST EFFECTS
May increase serum uric acid levels.

SIDE EFFECTS
Occasional
Acute gouty arthritis (chills, pain, swelling of joints with hot skin), confusion, abdominal pain, nausea, vomiting, anorexia, headache
Rare
Rash, fever, blurred vision, eye pain, red-green color blindness

SERIOUS REACTIONS
• Optic neuritis (more common with high-dosage or long-term ethambutol therapy), peripheral neuritis, thrombocytopenia, and an anaphylactoid reaction occur rarely.

PRECAUTIONS & CONSIDERATIONS
Caution is warranted with cataracts, diabetic retinopathy, gout, recurrent ocular inflammatory conditions, and renal dysfunction. Ethambutol use is not recommended for children younger than 13 years of age. Be aware that ethambutol crosses the placenta and is excreted in breast milk. In the elderly, age-related renal impairment may require dosage adjustment.

Initial complete blood count (CBC) and renal and liver function test results should be evaluated. Uric acid levels should be monitored and signs and symptoms of gout, including hot, painful, or swollen joints, especially in the ankle, big toe, or knee, should be assessed. Signs and symptoms of peripheral neuritis as evidenced by burning, numbness, or tingling of the extremities, should also be assessed. Notify the physician if peripheral neuritis occurs. In addition, notify the physician immediately of any visual problems. Visual effects are generally reversible after ethambutol is discontinued, and in rare cases visual problems may take up to a year to disappear or may become permanent.

E

Administration
Give with food to decrease GI upset.
Do not skip drug doses and take
ethambutol for the full length of therapy, which may be months or years.

Ethinyl Estradiol
ess-tra-dye-ole
(Estinyl)

CATEGORY AND SCHEDULE
Pregnancy Risk Category: X

CLASSIFICATION
Estrogens, hormones/hormone
modifiers

MECHANISM OF ACTION
A synthetic derivative of estradiol
that increases synthesis of DNA,
RNA, proteins in target tissues;
reduces release of gonadotropin-
releasing hormone from hypothalamus; reduces follicle-stimulating
hormone (FSH) and luteinizing
hormone (LH) release from the pituitary. *Therapeutic Effect:* Promotes
normal growth, development of
female sex organs, maintaining genitourinary (GU) function, vasomotor
stability. Prevents accelerated bone
loss by inhibiting bone resorption,
restoring balance of bone resorption
and formation. Inhibits LH,
decreases serum concentration of
testosterone.

PHARMACOKINETICS
Well absorbed from the gastrointestinal (GI) tract. Widely distributed.
Protein binding: 50%-80%. Rapidly
metabolized in liver to estrone and
estriol. Excreted in urine and feces.
Half-life: 8-25 hr.

AVAILABILITY
Tablets: 0.02 mg, 0.05 mg, 0.5 mg
(Estinyl).

INDICATIONS AND DOSAGES
▸ **Female hypogonadism**
PO
Adults. 0.05 mg 1-3 times/day
during the first 2 wk of menstrual
cycle, followed by progesterone
during the last half of cycle for
3-6 mo.
▸ **Menopausal symptoms**
PO
Adults. 0.02-0.05 mg/day cyclically
(3 wk on, 1 wk off).
▸ **Breast cancer**
PO
Adults. 1 mg 3 times/day for at least
3 mo.
▸ **Prostate cancer**
PO
Adults. 0.15-2 mg/day.

CONTRAINDICATIONS
Abnormal vaginal bleeding,
active arterial thrombosis, blood
dyscrasias, estrogen-dependent
cancer, known or suspected breast
cancer, pregnancy, thrombophlebitis
or thromboembolic disorders,
thyroid dysfunction, hypersensitivity
to estrogens

INTERACTIONS
Drug
Bromocriptine: May interfere with
the effects of bromocriptine.
Cyclosporine: May increase the
blood concentration and risk of liver
toxicity and nephrotoxicity of
cyclosporine.
Liver toxic medications: May
increase the risk of liver toxicity.
Herbal
St. John's wort: May decrease
levels of esterified estrogens.
Black cohosh, dong quai: May
increase estrogenic activity.

Red clover, saw palmetto, ginseng:
May increase hormonal effects.

DIAGNOSTIC TEST EFFECTS
May affect metapyrone testing, thyroid function tests. May decrease serum cholesterol levels, LDH concentrations. May increase blood glucose levels, HDL concentrations, serum calcium and triglyceride levels.

SIDE EFFECTS
Frequent
Anorexia, nausea, swelling of breasts, peripheral edema, evidenced by swollen ankles, feet
Occasional
Vomiting, especially with high dosages, headache that may be severe, intolerance to contact lenses, increased blood pressure (B/P), glucose intolerance, brown spots on exposed skin
Rare
Chorea or involuntary movements, hirsutism or abnormal hairiness, loss of scalp hair, depression

SERIOUS REACTIONS
• Prolonged administration increases risk of gallbladder disease, thromboembolic disease, and breast, cervical, vaginal, endometrial, and liver carcinoma.
• Cholestatic jaundice occurs rarely.

PRECAUTIONS & CONSIDERATIONS
Caution is warranted with diseases exacerbated by fluid retention and liver or renal insufficiency. Be aware that ethinyl estradiol is distributed in breast milk and may be harmful to fetus. Ethinyl estradiol should not be used during breast-feeding. Be aware that ethinyl estradiol should be used cautiously in children whose bone growth is not complete as the drug may accelerate epiphyseal closure.

There are no age-related precautions noted in the elderly. Smoking should be strongly discouraged.

Signs and symptoms of thromboembolic or thrombotic disorders are evident by loss of coordination, numbness or weakness of an extremity, pain in the chest, leg, or groin, shortness of breath, speech or vision disturbance, and sudden severe headache. Abnormal vaginal bleeding, tenderness, and swelling may be signs and symptoms of blood clots.
Administration
Administer at the same time each day. Give with food or milk if the patient experiences nausea.

Ethionamide
e-thye-on'am-ide
(Trecator)
Do not confuse with Tricor.

CATEGORY AND SCHEDULE
Pregnancy Risk Category: C

CLASSIFICATION
Antimycobacterials

MECHANISM OF ACTION
An antitubercular agent that inhibits peptide synthesis. *Therapeutic Effect:* Suppresses mycobacterial multiplication. Bactericidal.

PHARMACOKINETICS
Rapidly absorbed from the gastrointestinal (GI) tract. Widely distributed. Protein binding: 10%. Metabolized in liver. Primarily excreted in urine. Removed by hemodialysis. **Half-life:** 2-3 hr (half-life is increased with impaired renal function).

AVAILABILITY
Tablets: 250 mg (Trecator).

INDICATIONS AND DOSAGES
▸ **Tuberculosis**
PO
Adults, Elderly. 500-1000 mg/day as a single to 3 divided doses.
Children. 15-20 mg/kg/day.
Maximum 1 g/day.
▸ **Dosage in renal impairment**
Creatinine clearance less than 50 ml/min, reduce dose by 50%.

OFF-LABEL USES
Treatment of atypical mycobacterial infections

CONTRAINDICATIONS
Severe hepatic impairment, hypersensitivity to ethionamide

INTERACTIONS
Drug
Cycloserine, isoniazid: May increase the risk of toxicity.
Rifampin: May increase the risk of hepatotoxicity.
Herbal
None known.
Food
None known.

DIAGNOSTIC TEST EFFECTS
May increase ALT and AST.

SIDE EFFECTS
Occasional
Abdominal pain, nausea, vomiting, weakness, postural hypotension, psychiatric disturbances, drowsiness, dizziness, headache, confusion, anorexia, headache, metallic taste, diarrhea, stomatitis, peripheral neuritis
Rare
Rash, fever, blurred vision, optic neuritis, seizures, hypothyroidism, hypoglycemia, gynecomastia, thrombocytopenia, jaundice

SERIOUS REACTIONS
• Peripheral neuropathy, anorexia, and joint pain rarely occur.

PRECAUTIONS & CONSIDERATIONS
Caution is warranted in those receiving cycloserine or isoniazid, diabetics, epileptics, and psychiatric illness. Ethionamide crosses the placenta and is excreted in breast milk.

In the elderly, age-related renal impairment may require dosage adjustment.

Stomach upset, loss of appetite, metallic taste, burning, numbness, tingling of the feet or hands, and pain and swelling of joints should be reported.
Administration
Take with food to decrease GI upset.

Ethosuximide
eth-oh-sux′i-mide
(Zarontin)
Do not confuse with Zaroxolyn or Neurontin.

CATEGORY AND SCHEDULE
Pregnancy Risk Category: C

CLASSIFICATION
Anticonvulsants, succinimides

MECHANISM OF ACTION
An anticonvulsant that increases the seizure threshold and suppresses paroxysmal spike-and-wave pattern in absence seizures; depresses nerve transmission in the motor cortex.
Therapeutic Effect: Produces anticonvulsant activity.

PHARMACOKINETICS

Well absorbed from the gastrointestinal (GI) tract. Metabolized in liver. Excreted in urine. Removed by hemodialysis. **Half-life:** 50-60 hr (in adults); 30 hr (in children).

AVAILABILITY

Capsule: 250 mg, 100 mg, 150 mg, 200 mg (Zarontin).
Syrup: 250 mg/5 ml (Zarontin).

INDICATIONS AND DOSAGES

▸ **Absence seizures**
PO
Adults, Elderly, Children older than 6 yr. Initially, 250 mg/day or 15 mg/kg/day in 2 divided doses. Maintenance: 15-40 mg/kg/day in 2 divided doses.
Children 3-6 yr. Initially, 250 mg in 2 divided doses, increased by 250 mg as needed every 4-7 days. Maintenance: 20-40 mg/kg/day in 2 divided doses.
Use with caution in patients with renal impairment.

OFF-LABEL USES

Treatment of learning problems

CONTRAINDICATIONS

Hypersensitivity to succinimides

INTERACTIONS

Drug
Alcohol, central nervous system (CNS) depressants: May increase CNS depression.
Carbamazepine, phenobarbital, phenytoin, primidone, valproic acid: May decrease ethosuximide blood concentration.
Azole antifungals, ciprofloxacin, clarithromycin, isoniazid, quinidine, protease inhibitors, verapamil: May increase ethosuximide blood concentration.

Herbal
Evening primrose oil: May decrease effectiveness of ethosuximide.
Ginkgo: May decrease effectiveness of ethosuximide.
St. John's wort: May decrease ethosuximide blood concentrations.
Food
None known.

DIAGNOSTIC TEST EFFECTS

None known.

SIDE EFFECTS

Occasional
Dizziness, drowsiness, double vision, headache, ataxia, nausea, diarrhea, vomiting, somnolence, urticaria
Rare
Arganulocytosis, gum hypertrophy, leukopenia, myopia, swelling of the tongue, systemic lupus erythematosus, vaginal bleeding

SERIOUS REACTIONS

• Abrupt withdrawal may increase seizure frequency.
• Overdosage results in nausea, vomiting, and CNS depression including coma with respiratory depression.

PRECAUTIONS & CONSIDERATIONS

Caution should be used with renal function impairment. Ethosuximide should be used cautiously when given alone in mixed types of epilepsy. Alcohol and tasks that require mental alertness and motor skills should be avoided until response to the drug is established.

Toxic signs are evident as easy bruising, fever, joint pain, mouth ulcerations, sore throat, and unusual bleeding. Therapeutic serum level for ethosuximide is 40-100 mcg/ml and the toxic serum level for ethosuximide is greater than 150 mcg/ml.

Administration
Take with meals to reduce risk of gastrointestinal (GI) distress. When replacement by another anticonvulsant is necessary, plan to decrease ethosuximide gradually as therapy begins with a low replacement dose.

Etidronate
ee-tid′roe-nate
(Didronel)
Do not confuse etidronate with etidocaine or etomidate.

CATEGORY AND SCHEDULE
Pregnancy Risk Category:
C (parenteral), B (oral)

CLASSIFICATION
Bisphosphonates

MECHANISM OF ACTION
A bisphosphonate that decreases mineral release and matrix in bone and inhibits osteocytic osteolysis. *Therapeutic Effect:* Decreases bone resorption.

AVAILABILITY
Tablets: 200 mg, 400 mg.
Injection: 300-mg ampules (50 mg/ml).

INDICATIONS AND DOSAGES
▸ **Paget's disease**
PO
Adults, Elderly. Initially, 5-10 mg/kg/day not to exceed 6 mo, or 11-20 mg/kg/day not to exceed 3 mo. Repeat only after drug-free period of at least 90 days.

▸ **Heterotopic ossification caused by spinal cord injury**
PO
Adult, Elderly. 20 mg/kg/day for 2 wk; then 10 mg/kg/day for 10 wk.
▸ **Heterotopic ossification complicating total hip replacement**
PO
Adults, Elderly. 20 mg/kg/day for 1 mo before surgery; then 20 mg/kg/day for 3 mo after surgery.
▸ **Hypercalcemia associated with malignancy**
IV
Adults, Elderly. 7.5 mg/kg/day for 3 days. For retreatment, allow 7 days between treatment courses. Follow with oral therapy on day after last infusion. Begin with 20 mg/kg/day for 30 days; may extend up to 90 days.

CONTRAINDICATIONS
Clinically overt osteomalacia

INTERACTIONS
Drug
Antacids containing aluminum, calcium, magnesium mineral supplements: May decrease the absorption of etidronate.
Herbal
None known.
Food
Foods with calcium: May decrease the absorption of etidronate.

DIAGNOSTIC TEST EFFECTS
None known.

▨ IV INCOMPATIBILITIES
Do not mix with other medications.

SIDE EFFECTS
Frequent
Nausea; diarrhea; continuing or more frequent bone pain in patients with Paget's disease

Occasional
Bone fractures, especially of the femur
Parenteral: Metallic, altered taste
Rare
Hypersensitivity reaction

SERIOUS REACTIONS
• Nephrotoxicity, including hematuria, dysuria, and proteinuria, has occurred with parenteral route.

PRECAUTIONS & CONSIDERATIONS
Caution is warranted with hyperphosphatemia, impaired renal function, and restricted calcium and vitamin D intake. Adequate studies have not been done regarding the effect of oral etidronate use during pregnancy. Parenteral etidronate may cause skeletal malformations in the fetus. It is unknown if etidronate is excreted in breast milk. Do not give to women who are breast-feeding. Safety and efficacy of etidronate have not been established in children. The elderly may be prone to overhydration when treated with parenteral etidronate in conjunction with hydration therapy.

Notify the physician of diarrhea. Serum electrolytes, BUN, fluid intake and output should be monitored.

Storage
Store at room temperature.

Administration
Take on an empty stomach. Take etidronate 2 hours before antacids, food, or vitamins. The full therapeutic response may take up to 3 months.

For IV use, must dilute with at least 250 ml 0.9% NaCl or D₅W. Infuse over at least 2 hours.

Etodolac
e-toe-doe′lak
(Apo-Etodolac [CAN], Lodine, Lodine XL, Ultradol [CAN])
Do not confuse Lodine with codeine or iodine.

CATEGORY AND SCHEDULE
Pregnancy Risk Category: C (D if used in third trimester or near delivery)

CLASSIFICATION
Analgesics, non-narcotic, nonsteroidal anti-inflammatory drugs

MECHANISM OF ACTION
An NSAID that produces analgesic and anti-inflammatory effects by inhibiting prostaglandin synthesis. *Therapeutic Effect:* Reduces the inflammatory response and intensity of pain.

PHARMACOKINETICS

Route	Onset	Peak	Duration
PO (analgesic)	30 min	N/A	4-12 hr

Completely absorbed from the GI tract. Protein binding: greater than 99%. Widely distributed. Metabolized in the liver. Primarily excreted in urine. Not removed by hemodialysis. **Half-life:** 6-7 hr.

AVAILABILITY
Capsules (Lodine): 200 mg, 300 mg.
Tablets (Lodine): 400 mg, 500 mg.
Tablets (Extended-Release [Lodine XL]): 400 mg, 500 mg, 600 mg.

INDICATIONS AND DOSAGES
▶ **Osteoarthritis**
PO
Adults, Elderly. Initially,
800-1200 mg/day in 2-4
divided doses. Maintenance:
600-1200 mg/day.
▶ **Rheumatoid arthritis**
PO
Adults, Elderly. Initially, 300 mg
2-3 times a day or 400-500 mg
twice a day. Maintenance:
600-1200 mg/day.
▶ **Analgesia**
PO
Adults, Elderly. 200-400 mg q6-8hr
as needed. Maximum: 1200 mg/day.

OFF-LABEL USES
Treatment of acute gouty arthritis,
vascular headache

CONTRAINDICATIONS
Active peptic ulcer disease, chronic
inflammation of GI tract, GI bleeding
or ulceration, history of hypersensitivity to aspirin or NSAIDs

INTERACTIONS
Drug
Antihypertensives, diuretics:
May decrease the effects of these
drugs.
Aspirin, other salicylates: May
increase the risk of GI side effects
such as bleeding.
Bone marrow depressants: May
increase the risk of hematologic
reactions.
**Heparin, oral anticoagulants,
thrombolytics:** May increase the
effects of these drugs.
Lithium: May increase the blood
concentration and risk of toxicity of
lithium.
Methotrexate: May increase the
risk of methotrexate toxicity.
Probenecid: May increase etodolac
blood concentration.

Herbal
Feverfew, ginkgo biloba: May
increase the risk of bleeding.
Food
None known.

DIAGNOSTIC TEST EFFECTS
May increase bleeding time, liver
function test results, and serum
creatinine level. May decrease serum
uric acid level.

SIDE EFFECTS
Occasional (9%-4%)
Dizziness, headache, abdominal pain
or cramps, bloated feeling, diarrhea,
nausea, indigestion
Rare (3%-1%)
Constipation, rash, pruritus, visual
disturbances, tinnitus

SERIOUS REACTIONS
• Overdose may result in acute
renal failure.
• Rare reactions with long-term use
include peptic ulcer disease, GI
bleeding, gastritis, severe hepatic
reactions (jaundice), nephrotoxicity
(hematuria, dysuria, proteinuria),
and a severe hypersensitivity reaction (bronchospasm, angioedema).

PRECAUTIONS & CONSIDERATIONS
Caution is warranted with hepatic or
renal impairment, a predisposition to
fluid retention, and history of GI
tract disease. It is unknown if
etodolac crosses the placenta or is
distributed in breast milk. Etodolac
should not be used during the last
trimester of pregnancy because it
may cause adverse effects in the
fetus, such as premature closure of
the ductus arteriosus. Notify the
physician if pregnant. The safety and
efficacy of etodolac have not been
established in children. In the elderly,
GI bleeding or ulceration is more
likely to cause serious complications

and age-related renal impairment may increase the risk of hepatotoxicity or renal toxicity; a decreased dosage is recommended. Avoid alcohol and aspirin during therapy because these substances increase the risk of GI bleeding. Tasks that require mental alertness or motor skills should be avoided until response to the drug has been established.

Notify the physician of edema, GI distress, headache, rash, signs of bleeding, or visual disturbances. CBC and blood chemistry studies should be monitored to assess hepatic and renal function. Therapeutic response, such as decreased pain, stiffness, swelling, or tenderness, improved grip strength, and increased joint mobility, should be evaluated.

Administration

! Expect to reduce etodolac dosage for the elderly. Know that the maximum dose for persons weighing 60 kg or less is 20 mg/kg.

Do not crush, open, or break capsules or extended-release tablets. Take etodolac with food or milk, or antacids if GI distress occurs.

Etoposide, VP-16
e-toe-poe'side
(Etopophos, Toposar, VePesid)
Do not confuse VePesid with Pepcid or Versed.

CATEGORY AND SCHEDULE
Pregnancy Risk Category: D

CLASSIFICATION
Antineoplastics, epipodophyllotoxins

MECHANISM OF ACTION
An epipodophyllotoxin that induces single- and double-stranded breaks in DNA. Cell cycle-dependent and phase-specific; most effective in the S and G_2 phases of cell division. *Therapeutic Effect:* Inhibits or alters DNA synthesis.

PHARMACOKINETICS
Variably absorbed from the GI tract. Rapidly distributed, low concentrations in CSF. Protein binding: 97%. Metabolized in the liver. Primarily excreted in urine. Not removed by hemodialysis.
Half-life: 3-12 hr.

AVAILABILITY
Capsules (VePesid): 50 mg.
Injection (Toposar, VePesid): 20 mg/ml.
Injection (Water-soluble [Etopophos]): 100 mg/ml.

INDICATIONS AND DOSAGES
▸ **Refractory testicular tumors**
IV
Adults. 50-100 mg/m^2/day on days 1 to 5, or 100 mg/m^2/day on days 1, 3, 5 (as combination therapy).
▸ **Acute myelocytic leukemia**
IV
Children. 150 mg/m^2/day for 2-3 days and 2-3 cycles.
▸ **Brain tumor**
IV
Children. 150 mg/m^2/day on days 2 and 3 of treatment course.
▸ **Neuroblastoma**
IV
Children. 100 mg/m^2/day on days 1-5 of treatment course; repeated q4wk.
▸ **Small-cell lung carcinoma**
PO
Adults. Twice the IV dose rounded to nearest 50 mg. Give once a day

for doses 400 mg or less, in divided doses for dosages greater than 400 mg.
IV
Adults. 35 mg/m²/day for 4 consecutive days up to 50 mg/m²/day for 5 consecutive days (as combination therapy).
▸ **Leukemia, rhabdomyosarcoma**
Children. 60-150 mg/m²/day for 2-5 days q3-6wk.
▸ **Dosage in renal impairment**
Creatinine clearance 10-50 ml/min. 75% of normal dose.
Creatinine clearance less than 10 ml/min. 50% of normal dose.

OFF-LABEL USES
Treatment of acute myelocytic leukemia, AIDS-associated Kaposi's sarcoma, bladder carcinoma, Ewing's sarcoma, Hodgkin's disease, non-Hodgkin's lymphoma

CONTRAINDICATIONS
Pregnancy

INTERACTIONS
Drug
Bone marrow depressants: May increase myelosuppression.
Live-virus vaccines: May potentiate virus replication, increase vaccine side effects, and decrease the patient's antibody response to the vaccine.
Herbal
None known.
Food
None known.

DIAGNOSTIC TEST EFFECTS
None known.

▩ IV INCOMPATIBILITIES
VePesid: Cefepime (Maxipime), filgrastim (Neupogen), idarubicin (Idamycin).

Etopophos: Amphotericin B (Fungizone), cefepime (Maxipime), chlorpromazine (Thorazine), methylprednisolone (Solu-Medrol), prochlorperazine (Compazine)

🖉 IV Compatibilities
VePesid: Carboplatin (Paraplatin), cisplatin (Platinol), cytarabine (Cytosar), daunorubicin (Cerubidine), doxorubicin (Adriamycin), granisetron (Kytril), mitoxantrone (Novantrone), ondansetron (Zofran)
Etopophos: Carboplatin (Paraplatin), cisplatin (Platinol), cytarabine (Cytosar), dacarbazine (DTIC-Dome), daunorubicin (Cerubidine), dexamethasone (Decadron), diphenhydramine (Benadryl), doxorubicin (Adriamycin), granisetron (Kytril), magnesium sulfate, mannitol, mitoxantrone (Novantrone), ondansetron (Zofran), potassium chloride

SIDE EFFECTS
Frequent (66%-43%)
Mild to moderate nausea and vomiting, alopecia
Occasional (13%-6%)
Diarrhea, anorexia, stomatitis
Rare (2% or less)
Hypotension, peripheral neuropathy

SERIOUS REACTIONS
• Myelosuppression may result in hematologic toxicity, manifested as anemia, leukopenia (occurring 7-14 days after drug administration), thrombocytopenia (occurring 9-16 days after administration and, to lesser extent, pancytopenia. Bone marrow recovery occurs by day 20.
• Hepatotoxicity occurs occasionally.

PRECAUTIONS & CONSIDERATIONS

Caution is warranted with myelosuppression or hepatic or renal impairment. Because of the risk of fetal harm, pregnant women should not take etoposide, especially during the first trimester. Breast-feeding women also should not take this drug. The safety and efficacy of etoposide have not been established in children. In the elderly, age-related renal impairment may require dosage adjustment. Vaccinations and coming in contact with anyone who has recently received a live-virus vaccine should be avoided.

Notify the physician of easy bruising, fever, signs of local infection, sore throat, or unusual bleeding from any site. Hematology test results should be monitored before and frequently during etoposide therapy. WBC counts, Hgb and Hct levels, pattern of daily bowel activity and stool consistency, signs and symptoms of paresthesia and peripheral neuropathy, signs and symptoms of stomatitis should be assessed. Alopecia may occur and is reversible but new hair growth may have a different color or texture.

Storage

Refrigerate gelatin capsules. Store VePesid injection at room temperature before dilution. Reconstituted VePesid solution is stable at room temperature for up to 96 hours at 0.2 mg/ml and 48 hours at 0.4 mg/ml. Discard VePesid solution if crystallization occurs. Refrigerate Etopophos vials. After reconstitution, Etopophos is stable for up to 24 hours at room temperature or refrigerated.

Administration

! Etoposide dosage is individualized based on clinical response and tolerance of the drug's adverse effects.

Treatment is repeated at 3- to 4-week intervals. Administer parenteral etoposide by slow IV infusion. Wear gloves when preparing the solution. If the powder or solution comes in contact with your skin, wash immediately and thoroughly with soap and water. Because etoposide may be carcinogenic, mutagenic, or teratogenic, handle the drug with extreme care during preparation and administration.

VePesid concentrate for injection normally is clear and yellow. For IV use, dilute each 100 mg (5 ml) of VePesid with at least 250 ml D_5W or 0.9% NaCl to provide a concentration of 0.4 mg/ml (or 500 ml for a concentration of 0.2 mg/ml). Infuse VePesid slowly, over 30 to 60 minutes. Rapid IV infusion may produce marked hypotension. Monitor for an anaphylactic reaction manifested as back, chest, or throat pain; chills; diaphoresis; dyspnea; fever; lacrimation; and sneezing.

For IV use (Etopophos), reconstitute each 100 mg of Etopophos with 5 to 10 ml sterile water for injection, D_5W, or 0.9% NaCl to provide a concentration of 20 mg/ml or 10 mg/ml, respectively. Etopophos may be given without further dilution or may be further diluted with 0.9% NaCl or D_5W to a concentration as low as 0.1 mg/ml. Administer Etopophos over 5 to 210 minutes, as appropriate.

Exemestane
ex-uh-mess'tane
(Aromasin)

CATEGORY AND SCHEDULE
Pregnancy Risk Category: D

CLASSIFICATION
Antineoplastics, aromatase inhibitors, hormones/hormone modifiers

MECHANISM OF ACTION
Inactivates aromatase, the principal enzyme that converts androgens to estrogens in both premenopausal and postmenopausal women, thereby lowering the circulating estrogen level. *Therapeutic Effect:* Inhibits the growth of breast cancers that are stimulated by estrogens.

PHARMACOKINETICS
Rapidly absorbed after PO administration. Protein binding: 90%. Distributed extensively into tissues. Metabolized in the liver; eliminated in urine and feces. **Half-life:** 24 hr.

AVAILABILITY
Tablets: 25 mg.

INDICATIONS AND DOSAGES
▶ Breast cancer
PO
Adults, Elderly. 25 mg once a day after a meal.

OFF-LABEL USES
Prevention of prostate cancer

CONTRAINDICATIONS
Hypersensitivity to exemestane

INTERACTIONS
Drug
None known.

Herbal
None known.
Food
None known.

DIAGNOSTIC TEST EFFECTS
May increase serum alkaline phosphatase, AST (SGOT), and ALT (SGPT) levels.

SIDE EFFECTS
Frequent (22%-10%)
Fatigue, nausea, depression, hot flashes, pain, insomnia, anxiety, dyspnea
Occasional (8%-5%)
Headache, dizziness, vomiting, peripheral edema, abdominal pain, anorexia, flu-like symptoms, diaphoresis, constipation, hypertension
Rare (4%)
Diarrhea

SERIOUS REACTIONS
• Myocardial infarction has been reported.

PRECAUTIONS & CONSIDERATIONS
Exemestane is not for premenopausal women. Exemestane is indicated only for postmenopausal women. This drug is not used in children. No age-related precautions have been noted in the elderly.

Potential side effects, including dizziness, headache, insomnia, depression, may occur. Notify the physician if hot flashes or nausea become unmanageable. Nausea and vomiting may be prevented or treated with an antiemetic. Baseline vital signs, especially blood pressure, should be assessed because exemestane may cause hypertension.
Administration
Give oral exemestane after a meal.

Ezetimibe
eh-zet'eh-mibe
(Zetia)
Do not confuse with Zestril.

CATEGORY AND SCHEDULE
Pregnancy Risk Category: C

CLASSIFICATION
Antihyperlipidemics

MECHANISM OF ACTION
An antihyperlipidemic that inhibits cholesterol absorption in the small intestine, leading to a decrease in the delivery of intestinal cholesterol to the liver. *Therapeutic Effect:* Reduces total serum cholesterol, LDL cholesterol, and triglyceride levels; and increases HDL cholesterol concentration.

PHARMACOKINETICS
Well absorbed following oral administration. Protein binding: greater than 90%. Metabolized in the small intestine and liver. Excreted by the kidneys and bile. **Half-life:** 22 hr.

AVAILABILITY
Tablets: 10 mg.

INDICATIONS AND DOSAGES
▸ **Hypercholesterolemia**
PO
Adults, Elderly. Initially, 10 mg once a day, given with or without food. If the patient is also receiving a bile acid sequestrant, give ezetimibe at least 2 hr before or at least 4 hr after the bile acid sequestrant.

CONTRAINDICATIONS
Concurrent use of an HMG-CoA reductase inhibitor (atorvastatin, cerivastatin, fluvastatin, lovastatin, pravastatin, or simvastatin) in patients with active hepatic disease or unexplained persistent elevations in serum transaminase levels, moderate or severe hepatic insufficiency

INTERACTIONS
Drug
Aluminum and magnesium-containing antacids, cyclosporine, fenofibrate, gemfibrozil: Increase ezetimibe plasma concentration.
Cholestyramine: Decreases drug effectiveness.
Herbal
None known.
Food
None known.

DIAGNOSTIC TEST EFFECTS
May increase serum alkaline phosphatase, serum bilirubin, AST (SGOT), and ALT (SGPT) levels.

SIDE EFFECTS
Occasional (4%-3%)
Back pain, diarrhea, arthralgia, sinusitis, abdominal pain
Rare (2%)
Cough, pharyngitis, fatigue

SERIOUS REACTIONS
• None known.

PRECAUTIONS & CONSIDERATIONS
Caution is warranted with chronic renal failure, diabetes, hypothyroidism, liver function impairment, and obstructive liver disease. It is unknown if ezetimibe crosses the placenta or is distributed in breast milk. Safety and efficacy of ezetimibe have not been established in

children 10 years of age and younger. In the elderly, age-related mild hepatic impairment requires dosage adjustment. This drug is not recommended for use in elderly patients with moderate or severe hepatic impairment.

Notify the physician of any abdominal disturbances and back pain. Pattern of daily bowel activity and stool consistency should be assessed. Serum cholesterol and triglyceride levels should be checked at baseline and periodically thereafter.

Administration

Take ezetimibe without regard to food.

Factor IX Complex
(Benefix, Propex T, Konyne)

CATEGORY AND SCHEDULE
Pregnancy Risk Category: C

CLASSIFICATION
Antihemophilic agents, blood
clotting factors

MECHANISM OF ACTION
A blood modifier that raises plasma
levels of factor IX, restoring hemostasis in patients with factor IX deficiency. *Therapeutic Effect:* Increases
blood clotting factors II, VII, IX,
and X.

AVAILABILITY
Injection: Number of units is indicated on each vial.

INDICATIONS AND DOSAGES
▸ **Reversal of anticoagulant effect of
coumarin anticoagulants; bleeding
caused by hemophilia B; bleeding in
patients with hemophilia A who
have factor VIII inhibitors**
IV
Adults, Elderly, Children. Amount
of factor IX required is individualized. Dosage depends on degree of
deficiency, level of each factor
desired, patient's weight, and severity
of bleeding.

CONTRAINDICATIONS
Sensitivity to mouse protein

INTERACTIONS
Drug
Aminocaproic acid: May increase
the risk of thrombosis.
Herbal
None known.
Food
None known.

DIAGNOSTIC TEST EFFECTS
None known.

🖼 IV INCOMPATIBILITIES
Do not mix with other medications.

SIDE EFFECTS
Rare
Mild hypersensitivity reaction marked
by fever, chills, change in BP and
pulse rate, rash, and urticaria

SERIOUS REACTIONS
• There is a high risk of venous
thrombosis during the postoperative
period.
• Acute hypersensitivity reaction or
anaphylactic reaction may occur.
• There is a risk of transmitting
viral hepatitis and other viral
diseases.

PRECAUTIONS & CONSIDERATIONS
Caution is warranted with hepatic
impairment, recent surgery, and sensitivity to factor IX. OTC medications
should be avoided without physician
approval.
 Notify the physician of abdominal
or back pain, gingival bleeding, black
or red stool, coffee-ground emesis,
dark or red urine, or red-speckled
mucus from cough. Intake and output
and vital signs should be monitored.
IV site should be assessed for oozing
every 5 to 15 minutes for 1 to 2 hours
after administration.
Storage
Store in refrigerator. Reconstituted
solution is stable for 12 hours at
room temperature; do not refrigerate.
Administration
Gently agitate vial until powder is
completely dissolved, so that the active
components won't be removed when
the solution is filtered during administration. Filter before administration.
Begin administration within 3 hours
of reconstitution. Administer by slow

IV push or IV infusion. Avoid administering other medications by the IM or subcutaneous route. Infuse slowly, no faster than 3 ml/minute. Too rapid an IV infusion may produce a change in B/P and pulse rate, headache, flushing, and a tingling sensation.

Fenoprofen
fen-oh-proe′fen
(Nalfon)
Do not confuse Nalfon with Naldecon.

CATEGORY AND SCHEDULE
Pregnancy Risk Category: B (D if used in third trimester or near delivery)

CLASSIFICATION
Analgesics, non-narcotic, nonsteroidal anti-inflammatory drugs

MECHANISM OF ACTION
An NSAID that produces analgesic and anti-inflammatory effects by inhibiting prostaglandin synthesis. *Therapeutic Effect:* Reduces the inflammatory response and intensity of pain.

AVAILABILITY
Capsules: 200 mg, 300 mg.
Tablets: 600 mg.

INDICATIONS AND DOSAGES
▸ **Mild to moderate pain**
PO
Adults, Elderly. 200 mg q4-6hr as needed.
▸ **Rheumatoid arthritis, osteoarthritis**
PO
Adults, Elderly. 300-600 mg 3-4 times a day.

OFF-LABEL USES
Treatment of ankylosing spondylitis, psoriatic arthritis, vascular headaches

CONTRAINDICATIONS
Active peptic ulcer disease, chronic inflammation of GI tract, GI bleeding or ulceration, history of hypersensitivity to aspirin or NSAIDs, significant renal impairment

INTERACTIONS
Drug
Antihypertensives, diuretics: May decrease the effects of these drugs.
Aspirin, other salicylates: May increase the risk of GI side effects such as bleeding.
Bone marrow depressants: May increase the risk of hematologic reactions.
Heparin, oral anticoagulants, thrombolytics: May increase the effects of these drugs.
Lithium: May increase the blood concentration and risk of toxicity of lithium.
Methotrexate: May increase the risk of methotrexate toxicity.
Probenecid: May increase fenoprofen blood concentration.
Herbal
None known.
Food
None known.

DIAGNOSTIC TEST EFFECTS
May increase bleeding time, BUN and blood glucose levels, and serum protein, alkaline phosphatase, LDH, creatinine, AST (SGOT), and ALT (SGPT) levels.

SIDE EFFECTS
Frequent (9%-3%)
Headache, somnolence, dyspepsia, nausea, vomiting, constipation

Occasional (2%-1%)
Dizziness, pruritus, nervousness, asthenia, diarrhea, abdominal cramps, flatulence, tinnitus, blurred vision, peripheral edema, and fluid retention

SERIOUS REACTIONS
• Overdose may result in acute hypotension and tachycardia.
• Rare reactions with long-term use include peptic ulcer disease, GI bleeding, gastritis, severe hepatic reaction (jaundice), nephrotoxicity (hematuria, dysuria, proteinuria), and a severe hypersensitivity reaction (bronchospasm, angioedema).

PRECAUTIONS & CONSIDERATIONS
Caution is warranted with hepatic or renal impairment, a predisposition to fluid retention, and history of GI tract disease. Fenoprofen crosses the placenta and is distributed in breast milk. Fenoprofen should not be used during the last trimester of pregnancy because it may cause adverse effects in the fetus, such as premature closure of the ductus arteriosus. The safety and efficacy of fenoprofen have not been established in children. In the elderly, GI bleeding or ulceration is more likely to cause serious complications and age-related renal impairment may increase the risk of hepatotoxicity or renal toxicity; a decreased drug dosage is recommended. Avoid alcohol and aspirin during therapy because these substances increase the risk of GI bleeding. Tasks that require mental alertness or motor skills should be avoided until response to the drug has been established.

Baseline bleeding time, BUN and blood glucose levels, serum alkaline phosphatase, LDH, creatinine,

AST (SGOT), and ALT (SGPT) levels, and urinary protein levels should be obtained at the beginning of therapy. Pattern of daily bowel activity and stool consistency should be assessed during fenoprofen use. Therapeutic response, such as decreased pain, stiffness, swelling, and tenderness, improved grip strength, and increased joint mobility, should be evaluated.

Administration
! Don't exceed a fenoprofen dosage of 3.2 g/day, as prescribed.

Swallow capsules whole; do not crush, open, or break capsules.

F

Fentanyl
fen'ta-nill
(Actig, Duragesic, Sublimaze)
Do not confuse fentanyl with alfentanil.

CATEGORY AND SCHEDULE
Pregnancy Risk Category: C (D if used for prolonged periods or at high dosages at term)
Controlled Substance
Schedule: II

CLASSIFICATION
Analgesics, narcotic, anesthetics, general

MECHANISM OF ACTION
An opioid agonist that binds to opioid receptors in the CNS, reducing stimuli from sensory nerve endings and inhibiting ascending pain pathways. *Therapeutic Effect:* Alters pain reception and increases the pain threshold.

PHARMACOKINETICS

Route	Onset	Peak	Duration
IV	1-2 min	3-5 min	0.5-1 hr
IM	7-15 min	20-30 min	1-2 hr
Trans-dermal	6-8 hr	24 hr	72 hr
Trans-mucosal	5-15 min	20-30 min	1-2 hr

Well absorbed after IM or topical administration. Transmucosal form absorbed through the buccal mucosa and GI tract. Protein binding: 80%-85%. Metabolized in the liver. Primarily eliminated by biliary system. **Half-life:** 2-4 hr IV; 17 hr transdermal; 6.6 hr transmucosal.

AVAILABILITY

Injection (Sublimaze): 50 mcg/ml.
Transdermal Patch (Duragesic): 25 mcg/hr, 50 mcg/hr, 75 mcg/hr, 100 mcg/hr.
Transmucosal Lozenges (Actiq): 200 mcg, 400 mcg, 600 mcg, 800 mcg, 1200 mcg, 1600 mcg.

INDICATIONS AND DOSAGES
▶ **Sedation in minor procedures, analgesia**
IM/IV
Adults, Elderly, Children 12 yr and older. 0.5-1 mcg/kg/dose; may repeat in 30-60 min.
Children 1-11 yr. 1-2 mcg/kg/dose.
Children younger than 1 yr. 1-4 mcg/kg/dose.
▶ **Preoperative sedation, postoperative pain, adjunct to regional anesthesia**
IV, IM
Adults, Elderly, Children 12 yr and older. 50-100 mcg/dose.
▶ **Adjunct to general anesthesia**
IV
Adults, Elderly, Children 12 yr and older. 2-50 mcg/kg.

USUAL TRANSDERMAL DOSE
Adults, Elderly, Children 12 yr and older. Initially, 25 mcg/hr. May increase after 3 days.
USUAL TRANSMUCOSAL DOSE
Adults, Children. 200-400 mcg for breakthrough cancer pain.
USUAL EPIDURAL DOSE
Adults, Elderly. Bolus dose of 100 mcg, followed by continuous infusion of 10 mcg/ml concentration at 4-12 ml/hr.
▶ **Continuous analgesia**
IV
Adults, Elderly, Children 1-12 yr. Bolus dose of 1-2 mcg/kg, followed by continuous infusion of 1 mcg/kg/hr. Range: 1-5 mcg/kg/hr.
Children younger than 1 yr. Bolus dose of 1-2 mcg/kg, followed by continuous infusion of 0.5-1 mcg/kg/hr.
▶ **Dosage in renal impairment**
Dosage is modified based on creatinine clearance.

Creatinine Clearance	Dosage
10-50 ml/min	75% of usual dose
less than 10 ml/min	50% of usual dose

CONTRAINDICATIONS
Increased intracranial pressure, severe hepatic or renal impairment, severe respiratory depression

INTERACTIONS
Drug

Benzodiazepines, CNS depressants: May increase the risk of hypotension and respiratory depression.
Buprenorphine: May decrease the effects of fentanyl.
Herbal
None known.
Food
None known.

DIAGNOSTIC TEST EFFECTS

May increase serum amylase and lipase concentrations.

▓ IV INCOMPATIBILITIES

Phenytoin (Dilantin)

▓ IV Compatibilities

Atropine, bupivacaine (Marcaine, Sensorcaine), clonidine (Duraclon), diltiazem (Cardizem), diphenhydramine (Benadryl), dobutamine (Dobutrex), dopamine (Intropin), droperidol (Inapsine), heparin, hydromorphone (Dilaudid), ketorolac (Toradol), lorazepam (Ativan), metoclopramide (Reglan), midazolam (Versed), milrinone (Primacor), morphine, nitroglycerin, norepinephrine (Levophed), ondansetron (Zofran), potassium chloride, propofol (Diprivan)

SIDE EFFECTS

Frequent

IV: Postoperative drowsiness, nausea, vomiting

Transdermal (10%-3%): Headache, pruritus, nausea, vomiting, diaphoresis, dyspnea, confusion, dizziness, somnolence, diarrhea, constipation, decreased appetite

Occasional

IV: Postoperative confusion, blurred vision, chills, orthostatic hypotension, constipation, difficulty urinating

Transdermal (3%-1%): Chest pain, arrhythmias, erythema, pruritus, swelling of skin, syncope, agitation, tingling or burning of skin

SERIOUS REACTIONS

• Overdose or too rapid IV administration may produce severe respiratory depression and skeletal and thoracic muscle rigidity (which may lead to apnea), laryngospasm, bronchospasm, cold and clammy skin, cyanosis, and coma.

• The patient who uses fentanyl repeatedly may develop a tolerance to the drug's analgesic effect.

PRECAUTIONS & CONSIDERATIONS

Caution is warranted with bradycardia, head injuries, altered LOC, hepatic, renal, or respiratory disease, and concurrent use of MAOIs within 14 days of fentanyl administration. Fentanyl readily crosses the placenta; it is unknown whether fentanyl is distributed in breast milk. Fentanyl may prolong labor if administered in the latent phase of the first stage of labor or before the cervix has dilated 4 to 5 cm. Fentanyl may cause respiratory depression in the neonate if it's given to the mother during labor. The transdermal form of fentanyl is not recommended for children younger than 12 years or children younger than 18 years who weigh less than 50 kg. Neonates and the elderly are more susceptible to the drug's respiratory depressant effects. Age-related renal impairment may require a dosage adjustment in the elderly. Dizziness and drowsiness may occur, so change positions slowly and avoid alcohol, CNS depressants, and tasks that require mental alertness or motor skills until response to the drug is established. B/P, heart rate, respiratory rate, oxygen saturation, pattern of daily bowel activity and stool consistency, and clinical improvement of pain should be monitored.

Storage

Store the parenteral form at room temperature.

Administration

! Keep in mind that fentanyl may be combined with a local anesthetic, such as bupivacaine. Discontinue fentanyl slowly after long-term use. For IV use, make sure resuscitative equipment and an opiate antagonist (naloxone 0.5 mcg/kg) are readily

F

available before administering the drug. For initial anesthesia induction, give a small amount by tuberculin syringe, as prescribed. Give by slow IV push, over 1 to 2 minutes. A too-rapid IV infusion increases the risk of severe adverse reactions, such as anaphylaxis, bronchospasm, laryngospasm, peripheral circulatory collapse, cardiac arrest, and skeletal and thoracic muscle rigidity (which may result in apnea).

For transdermal use, clean the patch site before application; use only water because soap and oils may irritate the skin. Apply the patch to a flat, unirritated, nonhairy area of intact skin on the upper torso. Press the patch onto the skin firmly and evenly for 10 to 20 seconds, ensuring that it comes in full contact with the skin, especially around the edges. Rotate application sites. Carefully fold used patches so that they adhere to themselves, and discard them in the toilet.
For transmucosal use, suck the lozenge vigorously.

Ferrous Salts
fer-rous
(Feostat, Femiron, Ferro-Sequels, Nephro-Fer, Palafer [CAN])
(Apo-Ferrous Gluconate [CAN], Fergon)(Apo-Ferrous Sulfate [CAN], Fer-In-Sol,
Fer-Iron, Ferro-Gradumet [AUS], Slow-Fe)

CATEGORY AND SCHEDULE
Pregnancy Risk Category: A
OTC

CLASSIFICATION
Hematinics

MECHANISM OF ACTION
An enzymatic mineral that is an essential component in the formation of Hgb, myoglobin, and enzymes. Promotes effective erythropoiesis and transport and utilization of oxygen (O_2). *Therapeutic Effect:* Prevents iron deficiency.

PHARMACOKINETICS
Absorbed in the duodenum and upper jejunum. Ten percent absorbed in patients with normal iron stores; increased to 20%-30% in those with inadequate iron stores. Primarily bound to serum transferrin. Excreted in urine, sweat, and sloughing of intestinal mucosa and by menses.
Half-life: 6 hr.

AVAILABILITY
Ferrous fumarate
Tablets (Femiron): 63 mg (20 mg elemental iron).
Tablets (Nephro-Fer): 350 mg (115 mg elemental iron).
Tablets (Chewable [Feostat]): 100 mg (33 mg elemental iron).
Tablet (Timed-Release [Ferro-Sequels]): 150 mg (50 mg elemental iron).
Ferrous gluconate
Tablets: 325 mg (36 mg elemental iron).
Tablets (Fergon): 240 mg (27 mg elemental iron).
Ferrous sulfate
Tablets: 325 mg (65 mg elemental iron).
Tablets (Timed-Release [Slow FE]): 160 mg (50 mg elemental iron).
Elixir: 220 mg/5 ml (44 mg elemental iron per 5 ml).
Oral Drops (Ferr-In-Sol, Fer-Iron): 75 mg/0.6 ml.

INDICATIONS AND DOSAGES
▶ Iron deficiency anemia
Dosage is expressed in terms of milligrams of elemental iron, degree

of anemia, patient weight, and presence of any bleeding. Expect to use periodic hematologic determinations as guide to therapy.
PO (FERROUS FUMARATE)
Adults, Elderly. (ferrous fumarate): 60-100 mg twice a day; (ferrous gluconate): 60 mg 2-4 times a day; (ferrous sulfate): 325 mg 2-4 times a day.
Children. (ferrous fumarate, ferrous gluconate, ferrous sulfate) 3-6 mg/kg/day in 2-3 divided doses.
▸ **Prevention of iron deficiency**
PO
Adults, Elderly. (ferrous fumarate): 60-100 mg/day; (ferrous gluconate): 60 mg/day; (ferrous sulfate): 325 mg/day.
Children. (ferrous fumarate, ferrous gluconate, ferrous sulfate) 1-2 mg/kg/day.

CONTRAINDICATIONS
Hemochromatosis, hemosiderosis, hemolytic anemias, peptic ulcer disease, regional enteritis, ulcerative colitis

INTERACTIONS
Drug
Antacids, calcium supplements, pancreatin, pancrelipase: May decrease the absorption of ferrous fumarate, ferrous gluconate, and ferrous sulfate.
Etidronate, quinolones, tetracyclines: May decrease the absorption of etidronate, quinolones, and tetracyclines.
Herbal
None known.
Food
Eggs, milk: Inhibit ferrous fumarate absorption.

DIAGNOSTIC TEST EFFECTS
May increase serum bilirubin level. May decrease serum calcium level.

May obscure occult blood in stools.

SIDE EFFECTS
Occasional
Mild, transient nausea
Rare
Heartburn, anorexia, constipation, diarrhea

SERIOUS REACTIONS
• Large doses may aggravate existing GI tract disease, such as peptic ulcer disease, regional enteritis, and ulcerative colitis.
• Severe iron poisoning occurs most often in children and is manifested as vomiting, severe abdominal pain, diarrhea, and dehydration, followed by hyperventilation, pallor or cyanosis, and cardiovascular collapse.

PRECAUTIONS & CONSIDERATIONS
Caution is warranted with bronchial asthma and iron hypersensitivity. Ferrous fumarate, ferrous sulfate, and ferrous gluconate cross the placenta and are distributed in breast milk. No age-related precautions have been noted in children or the elderly. Avoid taking the drug with milk or eggs.
Urine may darken in color. Hgb, reticulocyte count, ferritin and serum iron levels, and total iron-binding capacity should be monitored. Daily bowel activity and stool consistency should be assessed. Clinical improvement should also be assessed and relief of iron deficiency symptoms (fatigue, headache, irritability, pallor, and paresthesia of extremities) should be recorded.
Storage
Store all forms, including tablets, capsules, suspension, and drops, at room temperature.

Administration
Take between meals with water unless GI discomfort occurs; if so, give with meals. Use dropper or straw to administer the liquid preparation and allow the drug solution to drop on the back of the patient's tongue, to prevent mucous membrane and teeth staining. To avoid transient staining of mucous membranes and teeth, place liquid on back of tongue with dropper or straw. Do not crush sustained-release form. Avoid simultaneous administration of antacids or tetracycline.

Fexofenadine
fex-oh-fen'eh-deen
(Allegra, Telfast [AUS])

CATEGORY AND SCHEDULE
Pregnancy Risk Category: C

CLASSIFICATION
Antihistamines, H_1

MECHANISM OF ACTION
A piperidine that competes with histamine for H_1-receptor sites on effector cells. *Therapeutic Effect:* Relieves allergic rhinitis symptoms.

PHARMACOKINETICS
Rapidly absorbed after PO administration. Protein binding: 60%-70%. Does not cross the blood-brain barrier. Minimally metabolized. Eliminated in feces and urine. Not removed by hemodialysis. **Half-life:** 14.4 hr (increased in renal impairment).

AVAILABILITY
Tablets: 30 mg, 60 mg, 180 mg.

INDICATIONS AND DOSAGES
▶ **Allergic rhinitis, urticaria**
PO
Adults, Elderly, Children 12 yr and older. 60 mg twice a day or 180 mg once a day.
Children 6-11 yr. 30 mg twice a day.
▶ **Dosage in renal impairment**
For adults, elderly, and children 12 years and older, dosage is reduced to 60 mg once a day. For children 6-11 years, dosage is reduced to 30 mg once a day.

CONTRAINDICATIONS
None known.

INTERACTIONS
Drug
Antacids: May decrease fexofenadine absorption if given within 15 minutes of a fexofenadine dose.
Herbal
None known.
Food
None known.

DIAGNOSTIC TEST EFFECTS
May suppress wheal and flare reactions to antigen skin testing unless drug is discontinued at least 4 days before testing.

SIDE EFFECTS
Rare (less than 2%)
Somnolence, headache, fatigue, nausea, vomiting, abdominal distress, dysmenorrhea

SERIOUS REACTIONS
• None known.

PRECAUTIONS & CONSIDERATIONS
Caution is warranted with severe renal impairment. It is unknown if fexofenadine crosses the placenta or is distributed in breast milk. The safety and efficacy of fexofenadine have not been established in children

younger than 12 years. No age-related precautions have been noted in the elderly. Avoid drinking alcoholic beverages and perfoming tasks that require alertness or motor skills until response to the drug is established.

Drowsiness may occur. Respiratory rate, depth, and rhythm; pulse rate and quality; B/P; and therapeutic response should be monitored.

Administration

Take fexofenadine without regard to food.

Filgrastim
fil-gra′-stim
(Neupogen)
Do not confuse Neupogen with Epogen or Nutramigen.

CATEGORY AND SCHEDULE
Pregnancy Risk Category: C

CLASSIFICATION
Hematopoietic agents, recombinant DNA Origin

MECHANISM OF ACTION
A biologic modifier that stimulates production, maturation, and activation of neutrophils to increase their migration and cytotoxicity. *Therapeutic Effect:* Decreases incidence of infection.

PHARMACOKINETICS
Readily absorbed after subcutaneous administration. Not removed by hemodialysis. **Half-life:** 3.5 hr.

AVAILABILITY
Injection: 300 mcg/ml, 480 mcg/0.8 ml.
Pre-filled syringes (Single Ject): 600 mcg/ml (Neupogen)

INDICATIONS AND DOSAGES
▸ **Myelosuppression**
IV OR SUBCUTANEOUS INFUSION, SUBCUTANEOUS INJECTION
Adults, Elderly. Initially, 5 mcg/kg/day. May increase by 5 mcg/kg for each chemotherapy cycle based on duration or severity of absolute neutrophil count nadir.
▸ **Bone marrow transplant**
IV OR SUBCUTANEOUS INFUSION
Adults, Elderly. 5-10 mcg/kg/day. Adjust dosage daily during period of neutrophil recovery based on neutrophil response.
▸ **Mobilization progenitor cells**
IV OR SUBCUTANEOUS INFUSION
Adults. 10 mcg/kg/day beginning at least 4 days before first leukapheresis and continuing until last leukapheresis.
▸ **Chronic neutropenia, congenital neutropenia**
SUBCUTANEOUS
Adults, Children. 6 mcg/kg/dose twice a day.
▸ **Idiopathic or cyclic neutropenia**
SUBCUTANEOUS
Adults, Children. 5 mcg/kg/dose once a day.

OFF-LABEL USES
Treatment of AIDS-related neutropenia; drug-induced neutropenia; myelodysplastic syndrome

CONTRAINDICATIONS
Hypersensitivity to *Escherichia coli*-derived proteins, 24 hours before or after cytotoxic chemotherapy, concurrent use of other drugs that may result in lowered platelet count

INTERACTIONS
Drug
Lithium: May increase white blood cell count greater than expected.

Topotecan: May prolong the duration of neutropenia.
Herbal
None known.
Food
None known.

DIAGNOSTIC TEST EFFECTS

May increase LDH concentrations, leukocyte alkaline phosphatase (LAP) scores, and serum alkaline phosphatase and uric acid levels.

▓ IV INCOMPATIBILITIES

Amphotericin (Fungizone), cefepime (Maxipime), cefotaxime (Claforan), cefoxitin (Mefoxin), ceftizoxime (Cefizox), ceftriaxone (Rocephin), cefuroxime (Zinacef), clindamycin (Cleocin), dactinomycin (Cosmegen), etoposide (VePesid), fluorouracil, furosemide (Lasix), heparin, mannitol, methylprednisolone (Solu-Medrol), mitomycin (Mutamycin), prochlorperazine (Compazine)

▓ IV Compatibilities

Bumetanide (Bumex), calcium gluconate, hydromorphone (Dilaudid), lorazepam (Ativan), morphine, potassium chloride

SIDE EFFECTS

Frequent
Nausea or vomiting (57%), mild to severe bone pain (22%) that occurs more frequently with high-dose IV form and less frequently with low-dose subcutaneous form; alopecia (18%), diarrhea (14%), fever (12%), fatigue (11%)
Occasional (9%-5%)
Anorexia, dyspnea, headache, cough, rash
Rare (less than 5%)
Psoriasis, hematuria or proteinuria, osteoporosis

SERIOUS REACTIONS

• Long-term administration occasionally produces chronic neutropenia and splenomegaly.
• Thrombocytopenia, MI, and arrhythmias occur rarely.
• Adult respiratory distress syndrome may occur in patients with sepsis.

PRECAUTIONS & CONSIDERATIONS

Caution is warranted with gout, malignancy with myeloid characteristics (because of the potential for granulocyte-colony-stimulating factor potential to act as a growth factor), preexisting cardiac conditions, and psoriasis. It is unknown if filgrastim crosses the placenta or is distributed in breast milk. No age-related precautions have been noted in children or the elderly. Avoid situations that might place risk for contracting an infectious disease, such as influenza.
Notify the physician of chest pain, chills, fever, palpitations, or severe bone pain. B/P should be monitored for a transient decrease. Also, body temperature, Hct, CBC, and hepatic enzyme and serum uric acid levels should be assessed. CBC should be obtained before the start of filgrastim therapy, and twice weekly thereafter. Those with preexisting cardiac conditions should be closely watched. Be alert for adult respiratory distress syndrome in those with sepsis.
Storage
Refrigerate vials for IV use. Filgrastim is stable for up to 24 hours at room temperature, provided vial contents are clear and contain no particulate matter. The drug remains stable if accidentally exposed to freezing temperature. Store vials for subcutaneous use in refrigerator, but remove before use and allow to warm to room temperature.
Administration
! May be given by subcutaneous injection or short IV infusion (15-30 minutes) or by continuous IV infusion. Begin filgrastim therapy at

least 24 hours after last dose of chemotherapy; discontinue at least 24 hours before next dose of chemotherapy. Begin therapy at least 24 hours after bone marrow infusion.

For IV administration, use single-dose vial. Do not reenter vial. Do not shake. Dilute with 10 to 50 ml D_5W to a concentration of 15 mcg/ml or higher. For a concentration from 5 to 14 mcg/ml, add 2 ml of 5% albumin to each 50 ml D_5W to provide a final concentration of 2 mg/ml. Do not dilute to a final concentration of less than 5 mcg/ml. For intermittent infusion (piggyback), infuse over 15 to 30 minutes. For continuous infusion, give single dose over 4 to 24 hours. In all situations, flush IV line with D_5W before and after administration.

For subcutaneous use, aspirate syringe before injecting drug to avoid intra-arterial administration.

Finasteride
feen-as'ter-ide
(Propecia, Proscar)
Do not confuse Proscar with Posicor, ProSom, Prozac, or Psorcon.

CATEGORY AND SCHEDULE
Pregnancy Risk Category: X

CLASSIFICATION
5-alpha-reductase inhibitors, antiandrogens, hormones/hormone modifiers

MECHANISM OF ACTION
An androgen hormone inhibitor that inhibits 5-alpha reductase, an intracellular enzyme that converts testosterone into dihydrotestosterone (DHT) in the prostate gland, resulting in a decreased serum DHT level.

Therapeutic Effect: Reduces size of the prostate gland.

PHARMACOKINETICS

Route	Onset	Peak	Duration
PO	24 hr	1-2 days	5-7 days

Rapidly absorbed from the GI tract. Protein binding: 90%. Widely distributed. Metabolized in the liver. **Half-life:** 6-8 hr. Onset of clinical effect: 3-6 mo of continued therapy.

AVAILABILITY
Tablets (Propecia): 1 mg.
Tablets (Proscar): 5 mg.

INDICATIONS AND DOSAGES
▶ **Benign prostatic hyperplasia (BPH)**
PO
Adults, Elderly. 5 mg once a day (for a minimum of 6 mo).
▶ **Hair loss**
PO
Adults. 1 mg/day.

OFF-LABEL USES
Adjuvant monotherapy after radical prostatectomy in treatment of prostate cancer

CONTRAINDICATIONS
Exposure to the patient's semen or handling of finasteride tablets by those who are or may be pregnant

INTERACTIONS
Drug
None known.
Herbal
None known.
Food
None known.

DIAGNOSTIC TEST EFFECTS
Decreases the serum prostate-specific antigen (PSA) level, even in patients with prostate cancer

SIDE EFFECTS
Rare (4%-2%)
Gynecomastia, sexual dysfunction (impotence, decreased libido, decreased volume of ejaculate)

SERIOUS REACTIONS
• Male breast neoplasia has been reported.

PRECAUTIONS & CONSIDERATIONS
Caution is warranted with hepatic impairment. Women who are or may be pregnant should not handle finasteride tablets because the drug may produce abnormal external genitalia in a male fetus. Finasteride is not indicated for use in children. The efficacy of this drug has not been established in the elderly.

Finasteride may cause impotence and decrease ejaculate volume. Be aware that urinary flow may not improve even if the prostate gland shrinks. Serum PSA determinations should be obtained before and periodically during therapy. Intake and output should also be monitored.

Administration
Don't break or crush film-coated tablets. Take finasteride without regards to food. Full therapeutic effect may take up to 6 months.

Flavocoxid
fla-vo-cox'id
(Limbrel)

CATEGORY AND SCHEDULE
Pregnancy Risk Category: Not classified.

CLASSIFICATION
Nonopioid analgesic

MECHANISM OF ACTION
An oral nutritional supplement that inhibits prostaglandin synthesis and arachidonic acid metabolism, reducing the production of leukotrienes. Also acts through an antioxidant mechanism. *Therapeutic Effect:* Produces anti-inflammatory and analgesic effects and increases mobility.

PHARMACOKINETICS
Undergoes hydrolysis at the gut mucosal border. Food decreases absorption. Little hepatic metabolism.

AVAILABILITY
Capsules: 250 mg.

INDICATIONS AND DOSAGES
▸ **Osteoarthritis**
PO
Adults 18 yr and older, Elderly. One 250-mg capsule q12hr.

CONTRAINDICATIONS
History of peptic ulcer

INTERACTIONS
Drug
None known.
Herbal
None known.
Food
All foods: Decrease the absorption of flavocoxid.

DIAGNOSTIC TEST EFFECTS
None known.

SIDE EFFECTS
Rare (2%)
Increase in varicose veins, psoriasis, mild hypertension

SERIOUS REACTIONS
• GI bleeding, perforation, and ulceration occur rarely in patients

currently or previously treated with NSAIDs or COX-2 inhibitors.

PRECAUTIONS & CONSIDERATIONS

It is unknown if flavocoxid crosses the placenta or is distributed in breast milk. Flavocoxid use is not recommended during pregnancy. The safety and efficacy of flavocoxid have not been established in children younger than 18 years. No age-related precautions have been noted in the elderly.

Therapeutic response, including improved grip strength, increased joint mobility, reduced joint tenderness, and relief of pain, stiffness, and swelling, should be assessed.

Administration

Don't take flavocoxid within 1 hour of eating because food decreases the drug's absorption.

Flavoxate
fla-vox′ate
(Urispas)
Do not confuse Urispas with Urised.

CATEGORY AND SCHEDULE
Pregnancy Risk Category: B

CLASSIFICATION
Anticholinergics, relaxants, urinary tract

MECHANISM OF ACTION
An anticholinergic that relaxes detrusor and other smooth muscle by cholinergic blockade, counteracting muscle spasm in the urinary tract. *Therapeutic Effect:* Produces anticholinergic, local anesthetic, and analgesic effects, relieving urinary symptoms.

AVAILABILITY
Tablets: 100 mg.

INDICATIONS AND DOSAGES
▶ **To relieve symptoms of cystitis, prostatitis, urethritis, urethrocystitis, or urethrotrigonitis**
PO
Adults, Elderly, Adolescents. 100-200 mg 3-4 times a day.

CONTRAINDICATIONS
Duodenal or pyloric obstruction, GI hemorrhage or obstruction, ileus, lower urinary tract obstruction

INTERACTIONS
Drug
None known.
Herbal
None known.
Food
None known.

DIAGNOSTIC TEST EFFECTS
None known.

SIDE EFFECTS
Frequent
Somnolence, dry mouth and throat
Occasional
Constipation, difficult urination, blurred vision, dizziness, headache, increased light sensitivity, nausea, vomiting, abdominal pain
Rare
Confusion (primarily in elderly), hypersensitivity, increased IOP, leukopenia

SERIOUS REACTIONS
• Overdose may produce anticholinergic effects, including unsteadiness, severe dizziness, somnolence, fever, facial flushing, dyspnea, nervousness, and irritability.

F

PRECAUTIONS & CONSIDERATIONS
Caution is warranted with glaucoma.
Avoid tasks that require mental alertness and motor skills until response to
the drug is established. Symptomatic
relief should be assessed. Notify the
physician of symptoms of flavoxate
overdose, including unsteadiness,
severe dizziness, drowsiness, fever,
flushed face, shortness of breath,
nervousness, and irritability.

Administration
Dosage of flavoxate should be reduced
as symptoms improve.

Flecainide
fle′kah-nide
(Tambocor)

CATEGORY AND SCHEDULE
Pregnancy Risk Category: C

CLASSIFICATION
Antiarrhythmics, class IC

MECHANISM OF ACTION
An antiarrhythmic that slows atrial,
AV, His-Purkinje, and intraventricular
conduction. Decreases excitability,
conduction velocity, and automaticity.
Therapeutic Effect: Controls atrial,
supraventricular, and ventricular
arrhythmias.

AVAILABILITY
Tablets: 50 mg, 100 mg.

INDICATIONS AND DOSAGES
▶ **Life-threatening ventricular
arrhythmias, sustained ventricular
tachycardia**
PO
Adults, Elderly. Initially, 100 mg
q12hr, increased by 100 mg (50 mg

twice a day) every 4 days until effective dose or maximum of 400 mg/day
is attained.
▶ **Paroxysmal supraventricular
tachycardias (PSVT), paroxysmal
atrial fibrillation (PAF)**
PO
Adults, Elderly. Initially,
50 mg q12hr, increased by
100 mg (50 mg twice a day)
every 4 days until effective dose or
maximum of 300 mg/day is
attained.

CONTRAINDICATIONS
Cardiogenic shock, pre-existing
second- or third-degree AV
block, right bundle-branch block
(without presence of a
pacemaker)

INTERACTIONS
Drug
Beta blockers: May increase nega-
tive inotropic effects.
Digoxin: May increase blood
concentration of digoxin.
Other antiarrhythmics: May have
additive effects.
Urinary acidifiers: May increase
the excretion of flecainide.
Urinary alkalinizers: May decrease
the excretion of flecainide.
Herbal
None known.
Food
None known.

DIAGNOSTIC TEST EFFECTS
None significant.

SIDE EFFECTS
Frequent (19%-10%)
Dizziness, dyspnea, headache
Occasional (9%-4%)
Nausea, fatigue, palpitations,
chest pain, asthenia (loss of
strength, energy), tremor,
constipation

SERIOUS REACTIONS
- Flecainide may worsen existing arrhythmias or produce new ones.
- CHF may occur or existing CHF may worsen.
- Overdose may increase QRS duration, prolong QT interval, cause conduction disturbances, reduce myocardial contractility, and cause hypotension.

PRECAUTIONS & CONSIDERATIONS
Caution is warranted with CHF, impaired myocardial function, second- and third-degree AV block (with pacemaker), and sick sinus syndrome. Be aware that therapeutic serum level is 0.2 to 1 mcg/ml. Nasal decongestant or OTC cold preparations should be avoided without physician approval.

Side effects of flecainide therapy usually disappear with continued use or decreased dosage. Tasks that require mental alertness or motor skills should be avoided. Continuous cardiac monitoring should be given. EKG measurements, including QRS duration and QT interval should be performed before and periodically during therapy. Pulmonary crackles, weight gain, intake and output, and dyspnea should be monitored in those with CHF.

Administration
Crush scored tablets as needed.

Fluconazole
floo-con'a-zole
(Apo-Fluconazole [CAN], Diflucan)
Do not confuse Diflucan with diclofenac.

CATEGORY AND SCHEDULE
Pregnancy Risk Category: C

CLASSIFICATION
Antifungals

MECHANISM OF ACTION
A fungistatic antifungal that interferes with cytochrome P-450, an enzyme necessary for ergosterol formation. *Therapeutic Effect:* Directly damages fungal membrane, altering its function.

PHARMACOKINETICS
Well absorbed from GI tract. Widely distributed, including to CSF. Protein binding: 11%. Partially metabolized in liver. Excreted unchanged primarily in urine. Partially removed by hemodialysis. **Half-life:** 20-30 hr (increased in impaired renal function).

AVAILABILITY
Tablets: 50 mg, 100 mg, 150 mg, 200 mg.
Powder for Oral Suspension: 10 mg/ml, 40 mg/ml.
Injection: 2 mg/ml (in 100- or 200-ml containers).

INDICATIONS AND DOSAGES
▶ **Oropharyngeal candidiasis**
PO, IV
Adults, Elderly. 200 mg once, then 100 mg/day for at least 14 days.
Children. 6 mg/kg/day once, then 3 mg/kg/day.
▶ **Esophageal candidiasis**
PO, IV

Adults, Elderly. 200 mg once, then 100 mg/day (up to 400 mg/day) for 21 days and at least 14 days following resolution of symptoms.
Children. 6 mg/kg/day once, then 3 mg/kg/day (up to 12 mg/kg/day) for 21 days at least 14 days following resolution of symptoms.

▸ **Vaginal candidiasis**
PO
Adults. 150 mg once.

▸ **Prevention of candidiasis in patients undergoing bone marrow transplantation**
PO
Adults. 400 mg/day.

▸ **Systemic candidiasis**
PO, IV
Adults, Elderly. 400 mg once, then 200 mg/day (up to 400 mg/day) for at least 28 days and at least 14 days following resolution of symptoms.
Children. 6-12 mg/kg/day.

▸ **Cryptococcal meningitis**
PO, IV
Adults, Elderly. 400 mg once, then 200 mg/day (up to 800 mg/day) for 10-12 wk after CSF becomes negative (200 mg/day for suppression of relapse in patients with AIDS).
Children. 12 mg/kg/day once, then 6-12 mg/kg/day (6 mg/kg/day for suppression of relapse in patients with AIDS).

▸ **Onychomycosis**
PO
Adults. 150 mg/wk.

▸ **Dosage in Renal Impairment**
After a loading dose of 400 mg, the daily dosage is based on creatinine clearance:

Creatinine Clearance	% of Recommended Dose
Greater than 50 ml/min	100
21-50 ml/min	50
11-20 ml/min	25
Dialysis	Dose after dialysis

OFF-LABEL USES
Treatment of coccidioidomycosis, cryptococcosis, fungal pneumonia, onychomycosis, ringworm of the hand, septicemia

CONTRAINDICATIONS
None known.

INTERACTIONS
Drug
Cyclosporine: High fluconazole doses increase cyclosporine blood concentration.
Oral antidiabetics: May increase blood concentration and effects of oral antidiabetics.
Phenytoin, warfarin: May decrease the metabolism of these drugs.
Rifampin: May increase fluconazole metabolism.
Herbal
None known.
Food
None known.

DIAGNOSTIC TEST EFFECTS
May increase serum alkaline phosphatase, serum bilirubin, SGOT (AST), and SGPT (ALT) levels.

▨ IV INCOMPATIBILITIES
Amphotericin B (Fungizone), amphotericin B complex (Abelcet, Ambisome, Amphotec), ampicillin (Polycillin), calcium gluconate, cefotaxime (Claforan), ceftazidime (Fortaz), ceftriaxone (Rocephin), cefuroxime (Zinacef), chloramphenicol (Chloromycetin), clindamycin (Cleocin), co-trimoxazole (Bactrim), diazepam (Valium), digoxin (Lanoxin), erythromycin (Erythrocin), furosemide (Lasix), haloperidol (Haldol), hydroxyzine (Vistaril), imipenem and cilastatin (Primaxin)

IV Compatibilities

Diltiazem (Cardizem), dobutamine (Dobutrex), dopamine (Intropin), heparin, lorazepam (Ativan), midazolam (Versed), propofol (Diprivan)

SIDE EFFECTS

Occasional (4%-1%)
Hypersensitivity reaction (including chills, fever, pruritus, and rash), dizziness, drowsiness, headache, constipation, diarrhea, nausea, vomiting, abdominal pain

SERIOUS REACTIONS

• Exfoliative skin disorders, serious hepatic effects, and blood dyscrasias (such as eosinophilia, thrombocytopenia, anemia, and leukopenia) have been reported rarely.

PRECAUTIONS & CONSIDERATIONS

Caution is warranted with liver or renal impairment, hypersensitivity to other triazoles, such as itraconazole or terconazole, or hypersensitivity to imidazoles, such as butoconazole and ketoconazole. Be aware that it is unknown if fluconazole is excreted in breast milk. There are no age-related precautions noted in children. In the elderly, age-related renal impairment may require dosage adjustment.

Expect to monitor the complete blood count (CBC), liver and renal function test results, platelet count, and serum potassium levels. Report any itching or rash promptly. Monitor the temperature daily. Assess daily pattern of bowel activity and stool consistency. Evaluate for dizziness and provide assistance as needed; do not drive or use machinery until response to the drug is established. If dark urine, pale stool, rash with or without itching, or yellow skin or eyes occur, notify the physician. Patients with oropharyngeal

infections should be taught good oral hygiene.

Storage
Store at room temperature.

Administration
Give oral fluconazole without regard to meals. Be aware that PO and IV therapy are equally effective and that IV therapy is for patients intolerant of the drug or unable to take it orally.

For IV administration, do not remove from outer wrap until ready to use. Squeeze inner bag to check for leaks. Do not use parenteral form if the solution is cloudy, a precipitate forms, the seal is not intact, or it is discolored. Do not add another medication to the solution. Do not exceed maximum flow rate 200 mg/hour.

F

Flucytosine
floo-sye'toe-seen
(Ancobon)

CATEGORY AND SCHEDULE
Pregnancy Risk Category: C

CLASSIFICATION
Antifungals

MECHANISM OF ACTION
An antifungal that penetrates fungal cells and is converted to fluorouracil which competes with uracil interfering with fungal RNA and protein synthesis. *Therapeutic Effect:* Damages fungal membrane.

PHARMACOKINETICS
Well absorbed from gastrointestinal (GI) tract. Widely distributed, including cerebrospinal fluid (CSF). Protein binding: 2%-4%. Metabolized in liver.

Partially removed by hemodialysis.
Half-life: 3-8 hr (half-life is increased with impaired renal function).

AVAILABILITY
Capsule: 250 mg, 500 mg.

INDICATIONS AND DOSAGES
▶ **Fungal infections, candidiasis, cryptococcosis**
PO
Adults, Elderly, Children. 50 to 150 mg/kg/day in 4 equally divided doses.
▶ **Dosage in renal function impairment**
Based on creatinine clearance:

Creatinine Clearance	Dosage Interval
20-40 ml/min	q12hr
10-20 ml/min	q24hr
0-10 ml/min	q24-48hr

CONTRAINDICATIONS
Hypersensitivity to flucytosine.

INTERACTIONS
Drug
Amphotericin B: May increase the effects of flucytosine.
Levomethadyl: May increase risk of cardiotoxicity.
Zidovudine: May increase the risk of hematologic toxicity.
Herbal
None known.
Food
None known.

DIAGNOSTIC TEST EFFECTS
May increase creatinine values if determined by the ektachem method.

SIDE EFFECTS
Occasional
Pruritus, rash, photosensitivity, dizziness, drowsiness, headache, diarrhea, nausea, vomiting, abdominal pain, increased liver enzymes, jaundice, increased BUN and creatinine, weakness, hearing loss

SERIOUS REACTIONS
• Hepatic dysfunction and severe bone marrow suppression occur rarely.

PRECAUTIONS & CONSIDERATIONS
Caution is warranted with liver or renal impairment, hematologic disease, or bone marrow suppression. Monotherapy should be avoided. It is unknown if flucytosine is excreted in breast milk. There are no age-related precautions noted in children. In the elderly, age-related renal impairment may require dosage adjustment.

Be alert to bone marrow suppressive symptoms. Unexplained fever, sore throat, rash or hives, trouble breathing, yellow skin or eyes, persistent chest pain, or bloody urine should be reported.
Administration
To avoid GI upset, take a few capsules at a time over 15 minutes with food until full dose is taken. Flucytosine doses should be spaced evenly around the clock to promote less variation in peak and trough blood serum levels. Therapeutic blood serum level is 25-100 mcg/ml. Peak should not exceed 100-120 mcg/ml to avoid bone marrow suppression.

Fludrocortisone
floo-droe-kor'ti-sone
(Florinef)
**Do not confuse Florinef with
Fioricet or Florinal.**

CATEGORY AND SCHEDULE
Pregnancy Risk Category: C

CLASSIFICATION
Corticosteroids

MECHANISM OF ACTION
A mineralocorticoid that acts at distal tubules. *Therapeutic Effect:* Increases potassium and hydrogen ion excretion. Replaces sodium loss and raises blood pressure (with low dosages). Inhibits endogenous adrenal cortical secretion, thymic activity, and secretion of corticotropin by pituitary gland (with higher dosages).

PHARMACOKINETICS
Well absorbed from the GI tract. Protein binding: 42%. Widely distributed. Metabolized in the liver and kidney. Primarily excreted in urine. **Half-life:** 3.5 hr.

AVAILABILITY
Tablets: 0.1 mg.

INDICATIONS AND DOSAGES
▶ **Addison's disease**
PO
Adults, Elderly. 0.05-0.1 mg/day. Range: 0.1 mg 3 times a wk to 0.2 mg/day. Administration with cortisone or hydrocortisone preferred.
▶ **Salt-losing adrenogenital syndrome**
PO
Adults, Elderly. 0.1-0.2 mg/day.
▶ **Usual pediatric dosage**
Children. 0.05-0.1 mg/day.

OFF-LABEL USES
Treatment of acidosis in renal tubular disorders, idiopathic orthostatic hypotension

CONTRAINDICATIONS
CHF, systemic fungal infection

INTERACTIONS
Drug
Digoxin: May increase the risk of digoxin toxicity caused by hypokalemia.
Hepatic enzyme inducers (such as phenytoin): May increase the metabolism of fludrocortisone.
Hypokalemia-causing medications: May increase the effects of fludrocortisone.
Sodium-containing medications: May increase BP, incidence of edema, and serum sodium level.
Herbal
None known.
Food
None known.

DIAGNOSTIC TEST EFFECTS
May increase serum sodium level. May decrease Hct and serum potassium level.

SIDE EFFECTS
Frequent
Increased appetite, exaggerated sense of well-being, abdominal distention, weight gain, insomnia, mood swings
High dosages, prolonged therapy, too rapid withdrawal: Increased susceptibility to infection with masked signs and symptoms, delayed wound healing, hypokalemia, hypocalcemia, GI distress, diarrhea or constipation, hypertension
Occasional
Headache, dizziness, menstrual difficulty or amenorrhea, gastric ulcer development

Rare
Hypersensitivity reaction

SERIOUS REACTIONS
• Long-term therapy may cause muscle wasting (especially in the arms and legs), osteoporosis, spontaneous fractures, amenorrhea, cataracts, glaucoma, peptic ulcer disease, and CHF.
• Abruptly withdrawing the drug after long-term therapy may cause anorexia, nausea, fever, headache, joint pain, rebound inflammation, fatigue, weakness, lethargy, dizziness, and orthostatic hypotension.

PRECAUTIONS & CONSIDERATIONS
Caution is warranted with edema, hypertension, and impaired renal function. It is unknown if fludrocortisone crosses the placenta or is distributed in breast milk. Fludrocortisone use in children may suppress growth and inhibit endogenous steroid production. Effects of fludrocortisone use in the elderly are unknown.

Mood swings, ranging from euphoria to depression, may occur. Notify the physician of fever, muscle aches, sore throat, and sudden weight gain or swelling. Blood glucose level, serum renin, B/P, serum electrolyte levels, height, and weight should be monitored before and during therapy. Be alert to signs and symptoms of infection caused by reduced immune response, including fever, sore throat, and vague symptoms.

Administration
Take fludrocortisone with food or milk. Taper the dosage slowly if fludrocortisone is to be discontinued.

Flumazenil
flew-maz-ah-nil
(Anexate [CAN], Romazicon)

CATEGORY AND SCHEDULE
Pregnancy Risk Category: C

CLASSIFICATION
Antidotes

MECHANISM OF ACTION
An antidote that antagonizes the effect of benzodiazepines on the gamma-aminobutyric acid receptor complex in the CNS. *Therapeutic Effect:* Reverses sedative effect of benzodiazepines.

PHARMACOKINETICS
Route	Onset	Peak	Duration
IV	1-2 min	6-10 min	Less than 1 hr

Duration and degree of benzodiazepine reversal depend on dosage and plasma concentration. Protein binding: 50%. Metabolized by the liver; excreted in urine.

AVAILABILITY
Injection: 0.1 mg/ml.

INDICATIONS AND DOSAGES
▸ **Reversal of conscious sedation or general anesthesia**
IV
Adults, Elderly. Initially, 0.2 mg (2 ml) over 15 sec; may repeat dose in 45 sec; then at 60-sec intervals. Maximum: 1 mg (10-ml) total dose. *Children, Neonates.* Initially, 0.01 mg/kg; may repeat in 45 sec, then at 60-sec intervals. Maximum: 0.2 mg single dose; 0.05 mg/kg or 1 mg cumulative dose.

▶ **Benzodiazepine overdose**
IV
Adults, Elderly. Initially, 0.2 mg
(2 ml) over 30 sec; if desired LOC is
not achieved after 30 sec, 0.3 mg
(3 ml) may be given over 30 sec.
Further doses of 0.5 mg (5 ml) may
be administered over 30 sec at 60-sec
intervals. Maximum: 3 mg (30 ml)
total dose.
Children, Neonates. Initially,
0.01 mg/kg; may repeat in 45 sec, then
at 60-sec intervals. Maximum: 0.2 mg
single dose; 1 mg cumulative dose.

CONTRAINDICATIONS
Anticholinergic signs (such as mydriasis, dry mucosa, and hypoperistal-
sis), arrhythmias, cardiovascular
collapse, history of hypersensitivity
to benzodiazepines, patients with
signs of serious cyclic antidepressant
overdose (such as motor abnormalities), patients who have been given a
benzodiazepine for control of a potentially life-threatening condition (such
as control of status epilepticus or
increased intracranial pressure)

INTERACTIONS
Drug
Tricyclic antidepressants: May
produce seizures and arrhythmias as
flumazenil reverses the sedative
effects of tricyclic antidepressants.
Herbal
None known.
Food
None known.

DIAGNOSTIC TEST EFFECTS
None known.

▨ IV INCOMPATIBILITIES
No information available for Y-site
administration.
▨ IV Compatibilities
Aminophylline, cimetidine
(Tagamet), dobutamine (Dobutrex),

dopamine (Intropin), famotidine
(Pepcid), heparin, lidocaine,
procainamide (Pronestyl), ranitidine
(Zantac)

SIDE EFFECTS
Frequent (11%-4%)
Agitation, anxiety, dry mouth, dys-
pnea, insomnia, palpitations,
tremors, headache, blurred vision,
dizziness, ataxia, nausea, vomiting,
pain at injection site, diaphoresis
Occasional (3%-1%)
Fatigue, flushing, auditory distur-
bances, thrombophlebitis, rash
Rare (less than 1%)
Urticaria, pruritus, hallucinations

SERIOUS REACTIONS
• Toxic effects, such as seizures and
arrhythmias, of other drugs taken in
overdose, especially tricyclic antidepressants, may emerge with reversal
of sedative effect of benzodiazepines.
• Flumazenil may provoke a panic
attack in those with a history of
panic disorder.

PRECAUTIONS & CONSIDERATIONS
Caution is warranted with head
injury, impaired hepatic function,
alcoholism, or drug dependency. Be
aware that it is unknown if flumazenil
crosses the placenta or is distributed
in breast milk. It is not recommended
during labor and delivery. Be aware
that flumazenil is not approved for
infants or neonates. Be aware that
benzodiazepine-induced sedation
tends to be deeper and more
prolonged requiring careful monitoring in the elderly.
    Be aware that flumazenil may wear
off before effects of benzodiazepines.
Arterial blood gases should be
obtained before and at 30-minute
intervals during IV administration.
Prepare to intervene in reestablishing

airway, assisting ventilation. Tasks that require alertness, motor skills, ingestion of alcohol, or taking nonprescription drugs should be avoided until at least 18-24 hours after discharge.

Storage
Store parenteral form at room temperature. Discard after 24 hours once medication is drawn into syringe, is mixed with any solutions, or if particulate or discoloration is noted.

Administration
Be aware that flumazenil is compatible with D_5W, lactated Ringer's, or 0.9% NaCl. Be aware that if resedation occurs, repeat dose at 20-minute intervals. Maximum: 1 mg (given as 0.2 mg/min) at any one time, 3 mg in any 1 hour. Administer through freely running IV infusion into large vein (local injection produces pain, inflammation at injection site). For reverse conscious sedation or general anesthesia, administer over 15 seconds. For benzodiazepine overdose, administer over 30 seconds.

Flunisolide
floo-niss′oh-lide
(AeroBid, Nasalide, Nasarel, Rhinalar [CAN])
Do not confuse flunisolide with fluocinonide, or Nasalide with Nasalcrom.

CATEGORY AND SCHEDULE
Pregnancy Risk Category: C

CLASSIFICATION
Corticosteroids, inhalation

MECHANISM OF ACTION
An adrenocorticosteroid that controls the rate of protein synthesis, depresses migration of polymorphonuclear leukocytes, reverses capillary permeability, and stabilizes lysosomal membranes. *Therapeutic Effect:* Prevents or controls inflammation.

AVAILABILITY
Aerosol (AeroBid): 250 mcg/ activation.
Nasal Spray (Nasalide, Nasarel): 25 mcg/activation.

INDICATIONS AND DOSAGES
▸ **Long-term control of bronchial asthma, assists in reducing or discontinuing oral corticosteroid therapy**
INHALATION
Adults, Elderly. 2 inhalations twice a day, morning and evening.
Maximum: 4 inhalations twice a day.
Children 6-15 yr. 2 inhalations twice a day.
▸ **Relief of symptoms of perennial and seasonal rhinitis**
INTRANASAL
Adults, Elderly. Initially, 2 sprays each nostril twice a day, may increase at 4-7 day intervals to 2 sprays 3 times a day. Maximum: 8 sprays in each nostril daily.
Children 6-14 yr. Initially, 1 spray 3 times a day or 2 sprays twice a day. Maximum: 4 sprays in each nostril daily. Maintenance: 1 spray into each nostril each day.

OFF-LABEL USES
To prevent recurrence of nasal polyps after surgery

CONTRAINDICATIONS
Hypersensitivity to any corticosteroid, persistently positive sputum cultures for *Candida albicans,*

primary treatment of status asthmaticus, systemic fungal infections

INTERACTIONS
Drug
None known.
Herbal
None known.
Food
None known.

DIAGNOSTIC TEST EFFECTS
None known.

SIDE EFFECTS
Frequent
Inhalation (25%-10%): Unpleasant taste, nausea, vomiting, sore throat, diarrhea, upset stomach, cold symptoms, nasal congestion
Occasional
Inhalation (9%-3%): Dizziness, irritability, nervousness, tremors, abdominal pain, heartburn, oropharynx candidiasis, edema
Nasal: Mild nasopharyngeal irritation or dryness, rebound congestion, bronchial asthma, rhinorrhea, altered taste

SERIOUS REACTIONS
• An acute hypersensitivity reaction, marked by urticaria, angioedema, and severe bronchospasm, occurs rarely.
• A transfer from systemic to local steroid therapy may unmask previously suppressed bronchial asthma condition.

PRECAUTIONS & CONSIDERATIONS
Caution is warranted with adrenal insufficiency. Drink plenty of fluids to decrease the thickness of lung secretions.

Pulse rate and quality, ABG levels, and respiratory rate, depth, rhythm, and type should be monitored.

Observe for cyanosis manifested as lips and fingernails with a blue or dusky color in light-skinned patients; a gray color in dark-skinned patients. Notify the physician of nasal irritation or if symptoms, such as sneezing, fail to improve.

Administration
! Expect to see improvement of the symptoms within a few days and relief of symptoms within 3 weeks. Prepare to discontinue the drug after 3 weeks if significant improvement does not occur. Do not abruptly discontinue or change the dosage schedule. The dosage must be tapered gradually under medical supervision.

For inhalation, first shake the container well. Exhale completely and place the mouthpiece between the lips. Inhale and hold breath for as long as possible before exhaling. Allow 1 minute between inhalations to promote deeper bronchial penetration. Rinse mouth with water immediately after inhalation to prevent mouth and throat dryness and oral candidiasis. If using a bronchodilator inhaler concomitantly with a steroid inhaler, use the bronchodilator several minutes before using the corticosteroid to help the steroid penetrate into the bronchial tree.

Clear nasal passages before using flunisolide. This may require the use of a topical nasal decongestant 5 to 15 minutes before flunisolide use. Tilt head slightly forward. Insert spray tip up into the nostril, pointing toward inflamed nasal turbinates, away from the nasal septum. Spray the drug into the nostril while holding the other nostril closed, and at the same time inhale through the nose. Discard opened nasal solution after 3 months.

Fluocinolone Acetonide

floo-oh-sin'oh-lone a-seat'oh-nide
(Capex, Derma-Smooth/FS,
Fluoderm [CAN], Synalar)

CATEGORY AND SCHEDULE
Pregnancy Risk Category: C

CLASSIFICATION
Corticosteriods, topical,
dermatologics

MECHANISM OF ACTION
A fluorinated topical corticosteroid
that controls the rate of protein
synthesis; depresses migration of
polymorphonuclear leukocytes and
fibroblasts; reduces capillary
permeability; prevents or
controls inflammation.
Therapeutic Effect: Decreases
tissue response to inflammatory
process.

PHARMACOKINETICS
Use of occlusive dressings may
increase percutaneous absorption.
Protein binding: more than 90%.
Excreted in urine. **Half-life:**
Unknown.

AVAILABILITY
Cream: 0.01%, 0.025% (Synalar).
Oil: 0.01% (Derma-Smoothe/FS).
Ointment: 0.025% (Synalar).
Shampoo: 0.01% (Capex).
Solution: 0.01% (Synalar).

INDICATIONS AND DOSAGES
▸ Atopic dermatitis
TOPICAL
Adults, Elderly. Apply 3 times/day.
Children 2 yr and older. Apply
2 times/day.

▸ Scalp psoriasis
TOPICAL
Adults, Elderly. Apply to damp or
wet hair and leave on overnight or
for at least 4 hr. Remove by washing
hair with shampoo.
▸ Seborrheic dermatitis, scalp
SHAMPOO
Adults, Elderly. Apply once daily
allowi to remain on scalp for at least
5 min.

OFF-LABEL USES
Vitiligo

CONTRAINDICATIONS
Hypersensitivity to fluocinolone or
other corticosteroids

INTERACTIONS
Drug
None known.
Herbal
None known.
Food
None known.

DIAGNOSTIC TEST EFFECTS
None known.

SIDE EFFECTS
Occasional
Burning, dryness, itching, stinging
Rare
Allergic contact dermatitis, purpura
or blood-containing blisters, thinning
of skin with easy bruising, telangiec-
tasis or raised dark red spots on skin

SERIOUS REACTIONS
• When taken in excessive quantities,
systemic hypercorticism and adrenal
suppression may occur.

PRECAUTIONS & CONSIDERATIONS
It is unknown if fluocinolone crosses
the placenta and is distributed in
breast milk. Be aware that the safety
and efficacy of fluocinolone have

not been established in children younger than 2 years. Be aware that children may absorb larger amounts of topical corticosteroids and should be used sparingly. There are no age-related precautions noted in the elderly. HPA axis suppression should be monitored by urinary free cortisol tests and an ACTH stimulation test.

Administration

Gently cleanse area prior to topical application. Use occlusive dressings only as ordered. Apply sparingly and rub into area thoroughly. When using topical preparation on scalp, massage through dampened hair and scalp. Cover with shower cap. Leave on overnight or for at least 4 hours. Remove by washing hair with shampoo.

When using shampoo preparation, apply to wet hair, massage for 1 minute and allow it to remain on scalp for 5 minutes. Rinse thoroughly.

Fluorescein

flure'e-seen sow-dee-um (AK-Fluor, Angiscein, Diofluor [CAN], Fluor-I-Strip, Fluor-I-Strip-AT, Fluorescite, Fluorets, Ful-Glo)

Do not confuse with fluoride.

CATEGORY AND SCHEDULE

Pregnancy Risk Category: X (parenteral), C (topical)

CLASSIFICATION

Diagnostics, nonradioactive

MECHANISM OF ACTION

An indicator dye used as a diagnostic agent with a low molecular weight, high water solubility, and fluorescence that penetrates any break in epithelial barrier to permit rapid penetration. Emits light at a wavelength of 520 to 530 nanometers (green-yellow) when exposed to light in the blue wavelength (465 to 490 nanometers). *Therapeutic Effect:* Diagnosis of corneal and conjunctival abnormalities.

PHARMACOKINETICS

Rapidly absorbed. Protein binding: 85%. Widely distributed. Metabolized in liver to an active metabolite, fluorescein monoglucuronide. Primarily excreted in urine. **Half-life:** 24 min (parent compound), 4 hr (metabolite).

AVAILABILITY

Injection, solution: 10% (AK-Fluor, Angiscein, Fluorescite), 25% (AK-Fluor, Fluorescite).
Strip, ophthalmic: 0.6 mg (Ful-Glo), 1 mg (Fluorets, Fluor-I-Strip-AT), 9 mg (Fluor-I-Strip).

INDICATIONS AND DOSAGES

▶ **Retinal angiography**
INJECTION
Adults, Elderly. Inject contents of ampule or vial of 10% or 25% solution rapidly into the antecubital vein
▶ **Applanation tonometry**
Ophthlalmic strips
Adults, Elderly. Place strip, which has been moistened with a drop of sterile water, at the fornix in the lower cul-de-sac close to the punctum. Patient should close lid tightly over strip until desired amount of staining is observed or retract upper lid and touch tip of strip to the bulbar conjunctiva on the temporal side until adequate staining is achieved.

CONTRAINDICATIONS

Concomitant soft contact lens use (ophthalmic strips), hypersensitivity to fluorescein or any component of the formulation

INTERACTIONS
Drug
None known.
Herbal
None known.
Food
None known.

DIAGNOSTIC TEST EFFECTS
May interfere with digoxin assay results.

SIDE EFFECTS
Occasional
Ophthalmic: Burning sensation in the eye
Injection: Stinging, bronchospasm, generalized hives and itching, hypersensitivity, headache, gastrointestinal distress, nausea, strong taste, vomiting, hypotension, syncope
Rare
Injection: anaphylaxis, basilar artery ischemia, cardiac arrest, severe shock, convulsions, thrombophlebitis at injection site

SERIOUS REACTIONS
• Anaphylactic reactions have occurred leading to laryngeal edema, bronchospasm, shock, and even death.

PRECAUTIONS & CONSIDERATIONS

Injection preparation should be used cautiously with bronchial asthma or history of allergy. It is unknown if fluorescein crosses the placenta or is distributed in breast milk. Be aware that safety and efficacy have not been established in children. There are no age-related precautions noted in the elderly. Blockages or leakage should be assessed on map location for possible treatment. Normal values will appear normal in size.

Skin and urine may temporarily turn yellow. Abnormal results can mean diabetic or other retinopathy, macular degeneration, cancer, tumors, circulatory problems, inflammation or edema, microaneurysms, or swelling of the optic disc.
Administration
Allow a few seconds for staining when using ophthalmic preparation. Wash out excess with sterile water or irrigating solution. Blink several times after application of strip. For fluorescein injection, inject rapidly into antecubital vein.

Fluoride, Sodium
(Fluor-A-Day, Fluorigard, Fluotic [CAN], Flura-Drops, Luride, NeutroGard, Pediaflor)
Do not confuse with Fludara.

CATEGORY AND SCHEDULE
Pregnancy Risk Category: N/A

CLASSIFICATION
Dental preparations, vitamins/minerals

MECHANISM OF ACTION
A trace element that increases tooth resistance to acid dissolution. *Therapeutic Effect:* Promotes remineralization of decalcified enamel, inhibits dental plaque bacteria, increases resistance to development of caries, maintains bone strength.

AVAILABILITY
Lozenge: 2.2 mg.
Oral Solution Drops: 1.1 mg/ml.
Oral Solution Rinse: 0.05%, 0.2%, 0.44%.

Tablets (Chewable): 0.58 mg,
1.1 mg, 2.2 mg.
Topical Cream: 1.1%.
Topical Gel: 0.4%, 1.1%.
Topical Gel-Drops: 1.1%.

INDICATIONS AND DOSAGES
▸ **Dietary supplement for prevention of dental caries in children**

Fluoride Level in Water	Age	Dosage
Less than 0.3 ppm*	Younger than 2 yr	0.25 mg/day
	2-3 yr	0.5 mg/day
	Older than 3-13 yr	1 mg/day
0.3-0.7 ppm*	Younger than 2 yr	None
	2-3 yr	0.25 mg/day
	Older than 3-13 yr	0.5 mg/day
Greater than 0.7 ppm*	None	None

*ppm = parts per million

CONTRAINDICATIONS
Arthralgia, GI ulceration, severe renal insufficiency

INTERACTIONS
Drug
Aluminum hydroxide, calcium: May decrease the absorption of fluoride.
Herbal
None known.
Food
Dairy products: May decrease fluoride's absorption.

DIAGNOSTIC TEST EFFECTS
May increase serum alkaline phosphatase and AST (SGOT) levels.

SIDE EFFECTS
Rare
Oral mucous membrane ulceration

SERIOUS REACTIONS
• Hypocalcemia, tetany, bone pain (especially in ankles and feet), electrolyte disturbances, and arrhythmias occur rarely.
• Fluoride use may cause skeletal fluorosis, osteomalacia, and osteosclerosis.

F

PRECAUTIONS & CONSIDERATIONS
Fluoride should not be taken with dairy products because they may decrease fluoride's absorption.
Administration
Use gels and rinses at bedtime after brushing and flossing. Expectorate excess fluoride; do not swallow it. Do not drink, eat, or rinse the mouth after application.

Fluoxetine
floo-ox′e-teen
(Auscap [AUS], Fluohexal [AUS], Lovan [AUS], Novo-Fluoxetine [CAN], Prozac, Prozac Weekly, Sarafem, Zactin [AUS])
Do not confuse fluoxetine with fluvastatin; Prozac with Prilosec, Proscar, or ProSom; or Sarafem with Serophene.

CATEGORY AND SCHEDULE
Pregnancy Risk Category: C

CLASSIFICATION
Antidepressants, serotonin specific reuptake inhibitors

MECHANISM OF ACTION
A psychotherapeutic agent that selectively inhibits serotonin uptake in the CNS, enhancing serotonergic function. *Therapeutic Effect:* Relieves depression; reduces obsessive-compulsive and bulimic behavior.

PHARMACOKINETICS
Well absorbed from the GI tract. Crosses the blood-brain barrier. Protein binding: 94%. Metabolized in the liver to active metabolite. Primarily excreted in urine. Not removed by hemodialysis. **Half-life:** 2-3 days; metabolite 7-9 days.

AVAILABILITY
Capsules (Prozac): 10 mg, 20 mg, 40 mg.
Capsules (Sarafem): 10 mg, 20 mg.
Capsules (Delayed-Release[Prozac Weekly]): 90 mg.
Oral Solution (Prozac): 20 mg/5 ml.
Tablets (Prozac): 10 mg, 20 mg.

INDICATIONS AND DOSAGES
▶ **Depression, obsessive-compulsive disorder**
PO
Adults. Initially, 20 mg each morning. If therapeutic improvement does not occur after 2 wk, gradually increase to maximum of 80 mg/day in 2 equally divided doses in morning and at noon. Prozac Weekly: 90 mg/wk, begin 7 days after last dose of 20 mg.
Elderly. Initially, 10 mg/day. May increase by 10-20 mg q2wk.
Children 7-17 yr. Initially, 5-10 mg/day. Titrate upward as needed. Usual dosage is 20 mg/day.
▶ **Panic disorder**
PO
Adults, Elderly. Initially, 10 mg/day. May increase to 20 mg/day after 1 week. Maximum: 60 mg/day.

▶ **Bulimia nervosa**
PO
Adults. 60 mg each morning.
▶ **Premenstrual dysphoric disorder**
PO
Adults. 20 mg/day.

OFF-LABEL USES
Treatment of hot flashes, fibromyalgia, posttraumatic stress disorder

CONTRAINDICATIONS
Use within 14 days of MAOIs

INTERACTIONS
Drug
Alcohol, other CNS depressants: May increase CNS depression.
Highly protein-bound medications (including oral anticoagulants): May increase adverse effects.
MAOIs: May produce serotonin syndrome and neuroleptic malignant syndrome.
Phenytoin: May increase phenytoin blood concentration and risk of toxicity.
Herbal
St. John's wort: May increase fluoxetine's pharmacologic effects and risk of toxicity.
Food
None known.

DIAGNOSTIC TEST EFFECTS
None known.

SIDE EFFECTS
Frequent (more than 10%)
Headache, asthenia, insomnia, anxiety, nervousness, somnolence, nausea, diarrhea, decreased appetite
Occasional (9%-2%)
Dizziness, tremor, fatigue, vomiting, constipation, dry mouth, abdominal pain, nasal congestion, diaphoresis, rash

Rare (less than 2%)
Flushed skin, light-headedness, impaired concentration

SERIOUS REACTIONS
• Overdose may produce seizures, nausea, vomiting, agitation, and restlessness.

PRECAUTIONS & CONSIDERATIONS
Caution is warranted with cardiac dysfunction, diabetes, seizure disorder, and in those at high risk for suicide. It is unknown if fluoxetine crosses the placenta or is distributed in breast milk. Children may be more sensitive to the drug's behavioral side effects, such as insomnia and restlessness. No age-related precautions have been noted in the elderly.

Drowsiness and dizziness may occur, so avoid alcohol and tasks that require mental alertness or motor skills. CBC and liver and renal function tests should be performed before and periodically during long-term therapy. Pattern of daily bowel activity and stool consistency, skin for rash, and blood glucose level should also be assessed.

Administration
! Make sure at least 14 days elapse between the use of MAOIs and fluoxetine. Expect to decrease dosage or frequency in the elderly, those with hepatic or renal impairment or a pre-existing disease, and those who take multiple medications.

Take fluoxetine with food or milk if GI distress occurs. Avoid administration at night. The therapeutic effects of fluoxetine will be noted within one to four weeks. Do not abruptly discontinue fluoxetine.

Fluoxymesterone
floo-ex-ih-mes-te-rone
(Android-F, Halotestin, Halotestin [CAN])

CATEGORY AND SCHEDULE
Pregnancy Risk Category: X
Controlled substance: Schedule III

CLASSIFICATION
Androgens, hormones/hormone modifiers

MECHANISM OF ACTION
An androgen that suppresses gonadotropin-releasing hormone, LH, and FSH. *Therapeutic Effect:* Stimulates spermatogenesis, development of male secondary sex characteristics, and sexual maturation at puberty. Stimulates production of red blood cells (RBCs).

PHARMACOKINETICS
Rapidly absorbed from the gastrointestinal (GI) tract. Protein binding: 98%. Metabolized in liver. Excreted in urine. **Half-life:** 9.2 hr.

AVAILABILITY
Tablets: 2 mg, 5 mg, 10 mg (Halotestin).

INDICATIONS AND DOSAGES
▸ **Males (hypogonadism)**
PO
Adults. 5-20 mg/day.
Males (delayed puberty)
PO
Adults. 2.5-20 mg/day for 4-6 mo.
Females (inoperable breast cancer)
PO
Adults. 10-40 mg/day in divided doses for 1-3 mo.

Females (prevent postpartum breast pain/engorgement)
PO
Adults. Initially, 2.5 mg shortly after delivery, then 5-10 mg/day in divided doses for 4-5 days.

CONTRAINDICATIONS
Serious cardiac, renal, or hepatic dysfunction, men with carcinomas of the breast or prostate, hypersensitivity to fluoxymesterone or any component of the formulation including tartrazine

INTERACTIONS
Drug
Oral anticoagulants: May increase the effect of these drugs.
Hepatotoxic medications: May increase the risk of hepatotoxicity.
Cyclosporine: May increase the risk of cyclosporine toxicity.
Herbal
Chaparral, comfrey, eucalyptus, germander, Jin Bu Huan, kava kava, pennyroyal, skullcap, valerian: May increase the risk of liver damage.
Food
None known.

DIAGNOSTIC TEST EFFECTS
May decrease levels of thyroxine-binding globulin, total T4 serum levels, and resin uptake of T3 and T4. May increase alkaline phosphatase, SGOT (AST), bilirubin, calcium, potassium, sodium, Hgb, Hct, LDL. May decrease HDL.

SIDE EFFECTS
Frequent
Females: Amenorrhea, virilism (e.g., acne, decreased breast size, enlarged clitoris, male pattern baldness), deepening voice
Males: UTI, breast soreness, gynecomastia, priapism, virilism (e.g., acne, early pubic hair growth)

Occasional
Edema, nausea, vomiting, mild acne, diarrhea, stomach pain
Males: Impotence, testicular atrophy

SERIOUS REACTIONS
• Peliosis hepatitis (liver, spleen replaced with blood-filled cysts), hepatic neoplasms, and hepatocellular carcinoma have been associated with prolonged high dosage.

PRECAUTIONS & CONSIDERATIONS
Caution is warranted with impaired renal or liver function, benign prostate hypertrophy, hypercalcemia (may be aggravated in patients with metastatic breast cancer), history of myocardial infarction, and diabetes mellitus. Be aware that fluoxymesterone use is contraindicated during lactation. Safety and efficacy of fluoxymesterone has not been established in children, so use with caution. Be aware that fluoxymesterone use in the elderly may increase the risk of hyperplasia or stimulate growth of occult prostate carcinoma.

Acne, nausea, pedal edema, or vomiting should be reported to the physician. In particular, females should report deepening of voice, hoarseness, and menstrual irregularities; males should report difficulty urinating, frequent erections, and gynecomastia.
Administration
Give with food to minimize GI upset.

Fluphenazine
floo-fen'a-zeen
(Anatensol [AUS], Modecate [AUS], Moditen [CAN], Permitil, Prolixin, Prolixin Decanoate)
Do not confuse Moditen with Modane or Mobidin.

CATEGORY AND SCHEDULE
Pregnancy Risk Category: C

CLASSIFICATION
Antipsychotics, phenothiazines

MECHANISM OF ACTION
A phenothiazine that antagonizes dopamine neurotransmission at synapses by blocking postsynaptic dopaminergic receptors in the brain. *Therapeutic Effect:* Decreases psychotic behavior. Also produces weak anticholinergic, sedative, and antiemetic effects and strong extrapyramidal effects.

AVAILABILITY
Elixir (Prolixin): 2.5 mg/5 ml.
Tablets (Prolixin): 1 mg, 2.5 mg, 5 mg, 10 mg.
Injection (Prolixin): 2.5 mg/ml.
Injection (Prolixin Decanoate): 25 mg/ml.

INDICATIONS AND DOSAGES
▶ Psychosis
PO
Adults, Elderly. 0.5-10 mg/day in divided doses q6-8hr.
IM
Adults, Elderly. 1.5-10 mg/day in divided doses q6-8hr or 12.5 mg (decanoate) q2wk.

OFF-LABEL USES
Treatment of neurogenic pain (adjunct to tricyclic antidepressants)

CONTRAINDICATIONS
Angle-closure glaucoma, myelosuppression, severe cardiac or hepatic disease, severe hypertension or hypotension, subcortical brain damage

INTERACTIONS
Drug
Alcohol, other CNS depressants: May increase hypotensive and CNS and respiratory depressant effects.
Antithyroid agents: May increase the risk of agranulocytosis.
Extrapyramidal symptom-producing medications: May increase extrapyramidal symptoms.
Hypotension-producing medications: May increase hypotension.
Levodopa: May decrease the effects of this drug.
Lithium: May decrease the absorption of fluphenazine and produce adverse neurologic effects.
MAOIs, tricyclic antidepressants: May increase anticholinergic and sedative effects.
Herbal
None known.
Food
None known.

DIAGNOSTIC TEST EFFECTS
May produce false-positive pregnancy and phenylketonuria test results. May cause EKG changes, including Q- and T-wave disturbances.

SIDE EFFECTS
Frequent
Hypotension, dizziness, and syncope (occur frequently after first injection, occasionally after subsequent injections, and rarely with oral doses)
Occasional
Somnolence (during early therapy), dry mouth, blurred vision, lethargy, constipation or diarrhea, nasal congestion, peripheral edema, urine retention

Rare
Ocular changes, altered skin pigmentation (with prolonged use of high doses)

SERIOUS REACTIONS
• Extrapyramidal symptoms appear to be related to high dosages and are divided into 3 categories: akathisia (inability to sit still, tapping of feet), parkinsonian symptoms (such as hypersalivation, masklike facial expression, shuffling gait, and tremors), and acute dystonias (such as torticollis, opisthotonos, and oculogyric crisis).
• Tardive dyskinesia, manifested as tongue protrusion, puffing of the cheeks, and chewing or puckering of the mouth occurs rarely but may be irreversible.
• Abrupt withdrawal after long-term therapy may precipitate dizziness, gastritis, nausea and vomiting, and tremors.
• Blood dyscrasias, particularly agranulocytosis and mild leukopenia, may occur.
• Fluphenazine use may lower the seizure threshold.

PRECAUTIONS & CONSIDERATIONS
Caution is warranted with Parkinson's disease and seizures. Drowsiness may occur, so tasks that require mental alertness or motor skills should be avoided. Exposure to light and sunlight should also be avoided. Signs of tardive dyskinesia such as fine tongue movement and therapeutic response should be monitored. B/P for hypotension, WBC for blood dyscrasias, and therapeutic response should be assessed during therapy.

Administration
May take with food to decrease GI effects. Do not take antacids within 1 hour of trifluoperazine.

For IM use, administer deep injection in large muscle mass.

Fluphenazine Decanoate
(Apo-Fluphenazine [CAN], Modecate [AUS], Prolixin); fluphenazine enanthate (Moditen [CAN], Prolixin); fluphenazine hydrochloride (Prolixin, Permitil)

CATEGORY AND SCHEDULE
Pregnancy Risk Category: C

CLASSIFICATION
Antipsychotics, phenothiazines

MECHANISM OF ACTION
A phenothiazine that blocks dopamine at postsynaptic receptor sites. Possesses weak anticholinergic, sedative and entimetic effects, and strong extrapyramidal activity. *Therapeutic Effect:* Decreases psychotic behavior.

PHARMACOKINETICS
Erratic and variable absorption from the gastrointestinal (GI) tract. Widely distributed. Metabolized in liver. Primarily excreted in urine. **Half-life:** 163-232 hr.

AVAILABILITY
Elixir, as hydrochloride: 2.5 mg/5 ml (Prolixin).
Injection, as decanoate: 25 mg/ml (Prolixin).
Injection, as enanthate: 25 mg/ml (Prolixin).
Injection solution, as hydrochloride: 2.5 mg/ml (Prolixin).
Oral solution, as hydrochloride: 5 mg/ml (Prolixin).

Tablets, as hydrochloride: 1 mg,
2.5 mg, 5 mg, 10 mg (Prolixin).

INDICATIONS AND DOSAGES
▶ **Psychotic disorders**
PO
Adults. Initially, 0.5-10 mg/day
fluphenazine HCl in divided doses
q6-8hr. Increase gradually until ther-
apeutic response is achieved (usually
under 20 mg daily); decrease gradually
to maintenance level (1-5 mg/day).
Elderly. Initially, 1-2.5 mg/day.
IM
Adults. Initially, 1.25 mg, followed
by 2.5-10 mg/day in divided doses
q6-8hr.
▶ **Chronic schizophrenic disorder**
IM
Adults. Initially, 12.5-25 mg of
fluphenazine decanoate q1-6 wk, or
25 mg fluphenazine enanthate q2wk.
Usual elderly dosage (nonpsychotic)
PO
Initially, 1-2.5 mg/day. May increase
by 1-2.5 mg/day q4-7 days.
Maximum: 20 mg/day.

OFF-LABEL USES
Treatment of neurogenic pain (adjunct
to tricyclic antidepressants)

CONTRAINDICATIONS
Severe CNS depression, comatose
states, severe cardiovascular disease,
bone marrow depression, subcortical
brain damage, hypersensitivity to
fluphenazine or any component
of the formulation including
tartrazine

INTERACTIONS
Drug
Alcohol, CNS depressants: May
increase respiratory depression and
the hypotensive effects of
fluphenazine.
Antithyroid agents: May increase
the risk of agranulocytosis.

**Extrapyramidal symptom (EPS)-
producing medications:** May
increase EPS.
Hypotensives: May increase
hypotension.
Levodopa: May decrease the effects
of levodopa.
Lithium: May decrease the absorp-
tion of fluphenazine and produce
adverse neurologic effects.
MAOIs, tricyclic antidepressants:
May increase the anticholinergic and
sedative effects of fluphenazine.
Herbal
**Dong quai, kava kava, gotu kola,
St. John's Wort, valerian:** May
increase risk of photosensitization or
CNS depression.
Food
None known.

DIAGNOSTIC TEST EFFECTS
May produce false-positive pregnancy test, PKU. EKG changes may
occur, including Q and T wave
disturbances.

SIDE EFFECTS
Frequent
Hypotension, dizziness, and fainting
occur frequently after first injection,
occasionally after subsequent injections, and rarely with oral dosage
Occasional
Drowsiness during early therapy,
dry mouth, blurred vision, lethargy,
constipation or diarrhea, nasal
congestion, peripheral edema, urinary
retention
Rare
Ocular changes, skin pigmentation
(those on high doses for prolonged
periods)

SERIOUS REACTIONS
• Extrapyramidal symptoms appear
dose related (particularly high
dosage), divided into 3 categories:
akathisia (inability to sit still, tapping

of feet, urge to move around); parkinsonian symptoms (mask-like face, tremors, shuffling gait, hyper-salivation); and acute dystonias: torticollis (neck muscle spasm), opisthotonos (rigidity of back muscles), and oculogyric crisis (rolling back of eyes).

• Dystonic reaction may also produce profuse sweating, and pallor.

• Tardive dyskinesia (protrusion of tongue, puffing of cheeks, chewing/puckering of the mouth) occurs rarely (may be irreversible).

• Abrupt withdrawal after long-term therapy may precipitate nausea, vomiting, gastritis, dizziness, and tremors.

• Blood dyscrasias, particularly agranulocytosis, or mild leukopenia (sore mouth/gums/throat) may occur.

• May lower seizure threshold

PRECAUTIONS & CONSIDERATIONS

Caution is warranted with impaired respiratory, hepatic, renal and cardiac function, alcohol withdrawal, history of seizures, urinary retention, glaucoma, prostatic hypertrophy, or hypocalcemia (increased susceptibility to dystonias). Withdrawal effects, including severe rhinorrhea, vomiting, respiratory distress, and extrapyramidal effects, have been reported in neonates. Its use should be avoided in pregnant women. Fluphenazine is distributed into breast milk. Children are more likely to develop neuromuscular or extrapyramidal reactions especially dystonias. The elderly may be more susceptible to orthostatic hypotension and exhibit an increased sensitivity to anti-cholinergic and sedative effects.

Visual disturbances should be reported immediately. Dry mouth, constipation, drowsiness, and dizziness are expected to occur. Avoid alcohol and tasks that require mental alertness or motor skills.

Do not abruptly withdraw from long-term therapy.

Storage
Store at room temperature and protect from light.

Administration
Administer IM injection deep into gluteal area. The dosage may be gradually increased as needed and tolerated.

Be aware that the oral dose has been found to be approximately 2 to 3 times higher than the parenteral dose. Take with food or milk to reduce GI irritation.

Flurandrenolide
flure-an-dren´oh-lide
(Cordran, Cordran SP)

CATEGORY AND SCHEDULE
Pregnancy Risk Category: C

CLASSIFICATION
Corticosteroids, topical, dermatologics

MECHANISM OF ACTION
A fluorinated corticosteroid that decreases inflammation by suppression of the migration of polymorphonuclear leukocytes and reversal of increased capillary permeability. *Therapeutic Effect:* Decreases tissue response to inflammatory process.

PHARMACOKINETICS
Repeated applications may lead to percutaneous absorption. Absorption is about 36% from scrotal area, 7% from the forehead, 4% from scalp, and 1% from forearm. Metabolized in liver. Excreted in urine. **Half-life:** Unknown.

AVAILABILITY
Cream: 0.025%, 0.05% (Cordran SP).
Lotion: 0.05% (Cordran).
Ointment: 0.025%, 0.05% (Cordran).
Tape, topical: 4 mcg/cm^2 (Cordran).

INDICATIONS AND DOSAGES
▶ **Anti-inflammatory, immunosuppressant, corticosteroid replacement therapy**
TOPICAL
Adults, Elderly. Apply 2-3 times/day.
Children. Apply 1-2 times/day.

CONTRAINDICATIONS
Hypersensitivity to flurandrenolide or any component of the formulation, viral, fungal, or tubercular skin lesions

INTERACTIONS
Drug
None known.
Herbal
None known.
Food
None known.

DIAGNOSTIC TEST EFFECTS
None known.

SIDE EFFECTS
Occasional
Itching, dry skin, folliculitis
Rare
Intracranial hemorrhage, acne, striae, miliaria, allergic contact dermatitis, telangiectasis, or raised dark red spots on skin

SERIOUS REACTIONS
• When taken in excessive quantities, systemic hypercorticism and adrenal suppression may occur.

PRECAUTIONS & CONSIDERATIONS
Caution should be used over large areas of body, denuded areas, prolonged periods of time, occlusive dressings, and use in small children.

It is unknown if flurandrenolide crosses the placenta or is distributed in breast milk. Be aware that the safety and efficacy of flurandrenolide have not been established in children. Therefore, use the smallest dose necessary to achieve optimal results. Be aware that children are at an increased risk of systemic toxicity and side effects. There are no age-related precautions noted in the elderly. Urinary free cortisol test and ACTH stimulation test should be obtained for suspected HPA axis suppression.
Storage
Store at room temperature.
Administration
Avoid contact with eyes. Gently cleanse area prior to application. Use occlusive dressings only as ordered. Apply sparingly and rub into area thoroughly. Children using flurandrenolide tape should use only once a day.

Flurazepam
flure-az′e-pam
(Apo-Flurazepam [CAN], Dalmane)
Do not confuse with Dialume.

CATEGORY AND SCHEDULE
Pregnancy Risk Category: X
Controlled Substance Schedule: IV

CLASSIFICATION
Benzodiazepines, sedatives/hypnotics

MECHANISM OF ACTION
A benzodiazepine that enhances action of inhibitory neurotransmitter

gamma-aminobutyric acid (GABA). *Therapeutic Effect:* Produces hypnotic effect due to central nervous system (CNS) depression.

PHARMACOKINETICS

Route	Onset	Peak	Duration
PO	15-20 min	3-6 hr	7-8 hr

Well absorbed from the gastrointestinal (GI) tract. Protein binding: 97%. Crosses blood-brain barrier. Widely distributed. Metabolized in liver to active metabolite. Primarily excreted in urine. Not removed by hemodialysis. **Half-life:** 2.3 hr; metabolite: 40-114 hr.

AVAILABILITY

Capsules: 15 mg, 30 mg.

INDICATIONS AND DOSAGES

▶ **Insomnia**
PO
Adults. 15-30 mg at bedtime.
Elderly, debilitated, liver disease, low serum albumin, Children 15 yr and older. 15 mg at bedtime.

CONTRAINDICATIONS

Acute alcohol intoxication, acute angle-closure glaucoma, pregnancy or breast-feeding.

INTERACTIONS

Drug
Alcohol, CNS depressants: May increase CNS depression.
Herbal
Kava kava, valerian: May increase CNS depression.
Food
None known.

DIAGNOSTIC TEST EFFECTS

None known.

SIDE EFFECTS

Frequent
Drowsiness, dizziness, ataxia, sedation Morning drowsiness may occur initially.
Occasional
GI disturbances, nervousness, blurred vision, dry mouth, headache, confusion, skin rash, irritability, slurred speech
Rare
Paradoxical CNS excitement or restlessness, particularly noted in elderly or debilitated

SERIOUS REACTIONS

• Abrupt or too-rapid withdrawal after long-term use may result in pronounced restlessness and irritability, insomnia, hand tremors, abdominal or muscle cramps, vomiting, diaphoresis, and seizures.
• Overdose results in somnolence, confusion, diminished reflexes, and coma.

PRECAUTIONS & CONSIDERATIONS

Caution is warranted with impaired liver or renal function. Be aware that flurazepam crosses the placenta and may be distributed in breast milk. Be aware that chronic flurazepam ingestion during pregnancy may produce withdrawal symptoms and CNS depression in neonates. Be aware that the safety and efficacy of flurazepam have not been established in children younger than 15 years of age. Use small initial doses with gradual dose increases to avoid ataxia or excessive sedation in the elderly. Avoid smoking because it reduces the drug's effectiveness.

Be aware that flurazepam may be habit-forming. B/P, pulse, and respirations should be assessed immediately before beginning flurazepam administration. Disturbed sleep 1 to 2 nights after discontinuing the drug may occur.

Administration
Take flurazepam without regard to
meals. If desired, empty capsules and
mix with food. Do not abruptly
withdraw the medication after long-
term use.

Flutamide
floo'ta-mide
(Euflex [CAN], Eulexin, Flugerel
[AUS], Flutamin [AUS], Fugerel
[AUS], Novo-Flutamide [CAN])
**Do not confuse flutamide with
Flumadine.**

CATEGORY AND SCHEDULE
Pregnancy Risk Category: D

CLASSIFICATION
Antineoplastics, antiandrogens,
hormones/hormone modifiers

MECHANISM OF ACTION
An antiandrogen hormone that
inhibits androgen uptake and prevents
androgen from binding to androgen
receptors in target tissue. Used in
conjuction with leuprolide to inhibit
the stimulant effects of flutamide on
serum testosterone levels. *Therapeutic
Effect:* Suppresses testicular androgen
production and decreases growth of
prostate carcinoma.

PHARMACOKINETICS
Completely absorbed from the
GI tract. Protein binding: 94%-96%.
Metabolized in the liver to active
metabolite. Primarily excreted
in urine. Not removed by
hemodialysis. **Half-life:** 6 hr
(increased in elderly).

AVAILABILITY
Capsules: 125 mg.

INDICATIONS AND DOSAGES
▶ **Prostatic carcinoma (in combina-
tion with leuprolide)**
PO
Adults, Elderly. 250 mg q8hr.

CONTRAINDICATIONS
Severe hepatic impairment;
pregnancy

INTERACTIONS
Drug
Warfarin: May increase risk of
bleeding.
Herbal
**Chaparral, comfrey, eucalyptus,
germander, Jin Bu Huan, kava
kava, pennyroyal, skullcap,
valerian:** May increase the risk of
hepatotoxicity.
Food
None known.

DIAGNOSTIC TEST EFFECTS
May increase blood glucose level
and serum estradiol, testosterone,
bilirubin, creatinine, AST (SGOT),
and ALT (SGPT) levels.

SIDE EFFECTS
Frequent
Hot flashes (50%); decreased libido,
diarrhea (24%); generalized pain
(23%); asthenia (17%); constipation
(12%); nausea, nocturia (11%)
Occasional (8%-6%)
Dizziness, paresthesia, insomnia,
impotence, peripheral edema,
gynecomastia
Rare (5%-4%)
Rash, diaphoresis, hypertension,
hematuria, vomiting, urinary incontinence, headache, flu-like symptoms,
photosensitivity

SERIOUS REACTIONS
• Hepatoxicity, including hepatic
encephalopathy, and hemolytic
anemia may be noted.

F

PRECAUTIONS & CONSIDERATIONS

Flutamide is not used in pregnant women or in children. No age-related precautions have been noted in the elderly. Overexposure to the sun or ultraviolet light should be avoided and protective clothing should be worn outdoors until tolerance of ultraviolet light is determined.

Urine may become amber or yellow-green during flutamide therapy. Liver function test results should be obtained before beginning drug therapy and periodically thereafter.

Administration

Take oral flutamide without regard to food. Do not abruptly discontinue the drug.

Fluticasone

flu-tic′a-zone

(Cutivate, Flixotide Disks [AUS], Flixotide Inhaler [AUS], Flonase, Flovent, Flovent Diskus, Flovent HFA)

CATEGORY AND SCHEDULE

Pregnancy Risk Category: C

CLASSIFICATION

Corticosteroids, inhalation, topical, dermatologics

MECHANISM OF ACTION

A corticosteroid that controls the rate of protein synthesis, depresses migration of polymorphonuclear leukocytes, reverses capillary permeability, and stabilizes lysosomal membranes. *Therapeutic Effect:* Prevents or controls inflammation.

PHARMACOKINETICS

Inhalation/intranasal: Protein binding: 91%. Undergoes extensive first-pass metabolism in liver. Excreted in urine.

Half-life: 3-7.8 hr. Topical: Amount absorbed depends on affected area and skin condition (absorption increased with fever, hydration, inflamed or denuded skin).

AVAILABILITY

Aerosol for Oral Inhalation (Flovent, Flovent HFA): 44 mcg/inhalation, 110 mcg/inhalation, 220 mcg/inhalation.
Powder for Oral Inhalation (Flovent Diskus): 50 mcg, 100 mcg, 250 mcg.
Intranasal Spray (Flonase): 50 mcg/inhalation.
Topical Cream (Cutivate): 0.05%.
Topical Ointment (Cutivate): 0.005%.

INDICATIONS AND DOSAGES

▶ **Allergic Rhinitis**

INTRANASAL

Adults, Elderly. Initially, 200 mcg (2 sprays in each nostril once daily or 1 spray in each nostril q12hr). Maintenance: 1 spray in each nostril once daily. Maximum: 200 mcg/day.
Children older than 4 yr. Initially, 100 mcg (1 spray in each nostril once daily). Maximum: 200 mcg/day.

▶ **Relief of inflammation and pruritus associated with steroid-responsive disorders, such as contact dermatitis and eczema**

TOPICAL

Adults, Elderly, Children older than 3 mo. Apply sparingly to affected area once or twice a day.

▶ **Maintenance treatment for asthma for those previously treated with bronchodilators**

INHALATION POWDER (FLOVENT DISKUS)

Adults, Elderly, Children 12 yr and older. Initially, 100 mcg q12hr. Maximum: 500 mcg/day.

INHALATION (ORAL, FLOVENT)

Adults, Elderly, Children 12 yr and older. 88 mcg twice a day.

Maximum: 440 mcg twice a day.
▸ **Maintenance treatment for asthma for those previously treated with inhaled steroids**
INHALATION POWDER
(FLOVENT DISKUS)
Adults, Elderly, Children 12 yr and older. Initially, 100-250 mcg q12hr.
Maximum: 500 mcg q12hr.
INHALATION, ORAL (FLOVENT)
Adults, Elderly, Children 12 yr and older. 88-220 mcg twice a day.
Maximum: 440 mcg twice a day.
▸ **Maintenance treatment for asthma for those previously treated with oral steroids**
INHALATION POWDER
(FLOVENT DISKUS)
Adults, Elderly, Children 12 yr and older. 500-1000 mcg twice a day.
INHALATION (ORAL, FLOVENT)
Adults, Elderly, Children 12 yr and older. 880 mcg twice a day.

CONTRAINDICATIONS

Primary treatment of status asthmaticus or other acute asthma episodes (inhalation); untreated localized infection of nasal mucosa

INTERACTIONS
Drug
Bupropin: May lower the seizure threshold.
Ketoconazole, ritonavir: May increase plasma fluticason concentrations.
Herbal
None known.
Food
None known.

DIAGNOSTIC TEST EFFECTS
None known.

SIDE EFFECTS
Frequent
Inhalation: Throat irritation, hoarseness, dry mouth, cough, temporary wheezing, oropharyngeal candidiasis (particularly if mouth is not rinsed with water after each administration)
Intranasal: Mild nasopharyngeal irritation; nasal burning, stinging, or dryness; rebound congestion; rhinorrhea; loss of taste
Occasional
Inhalation: Oral candidiasis
Intranasal: Nasal and pharyngeal candidiasis, headache
Topical: Skin burning, pruritus

SERIOUS REACTIONS
• Anaphylaxis, hypersensitivity reactions, and glaucoma *occur* rarely.

PRECAUTIONS & CONSIDERATIONS
Caution is warranted with active or quiescent tuberculosis, ocular herpes simplex infection, and untreated systemic infections (including fungal, bacterial, or viral). It is unknown if fluticasone crosses the placenta or is distributed in breast milk. The safety and efficacy of fluticasone have not been established in children younger than 4 years. Children 4 years and older may experience growth suppression with prolonged or high doses. No age-related precautions have been noted in the elderly. Drink plenty of fluids to decrease the thickness of lung secretions.

Pulse rate and quality, ABG levels, and respiratory rate, depth, rhythm, and type should be monitored. Notify the physician of nasal irritation or if symptoms, such as sneezing, fail to improve.
Administration
For inhalation, first shake the container well. Exhale completely and place the mouthpiece between the lips. Inhale and hold breath for as long as possible before exhaling. Allow 1 minute between inhalations to promote deeper bronchial penetration. Rinse mouth with water immediately after inhalation

to prevent mouth and throat dryness and oral candidiasis. Clears the nasal passages before using fluticasone. May need to use a topical nasal decongestant 5 to 15 minutes before using fluticasone. Tilt head slightly forward. Insert spray tip up into the nostril, pointing toward the inflamed nasal turbinates, away from nasal septum. Spray the drug into the nostril while holding the other nostril closed, and at the same time inhale through the nose.

For topical fluticasone, rub a thin film gently on the affected area. Use the drug only on the prescribed area and for no longer than prescribed. Keep the preparation away from the eyes.

Fluvastatin
floo′va-sta-tin
(Lescol, Lescol XL, Vastin [AUS])
Do not confuse fluvastatin with fluoxetine.

CATEGORY AND SCHEDULE
Pregnancy Risk Category: X

CLASSIFICATION
Antihyperlipidemics, HMG CoA reductase inhibitors

MECHANISM OF ACTION
An antihyperlipidemic that inhibits HMG-CoA reductase, the enzyme that catalyzes the early step in cholesterol synthesis. *Therapeutic Effect:* Decreases LDL cholesterol, VLDL, and plasma triglyceride levels. Slightly increases HDL cholesterol concentration.

PHARMACOKINETICS
Well absorbed from the GI tract and is unaffected by food. Does not cross the blood-brain barrier. Protein binding: greater than 98%. Primarily eliminated in feces. **Half-life:** 1.2 hr.

AVAILABILITY
Capsules (Lescol): 20 mg, 40 mg.
Tablets (Extended-Release [Lescol XL]): 80 mg.

INDICATIONS AND DOSAGES
▶ **Hyperlipoproteinemia**
PO
Adults, Elderly. Initially, 20 mg/day (capsule) in the evening. May increase up to 40 mg/day. Maintenance: 20-40 mg/day in a single dose or divided doses.
Patients requiring more than a 25% decrease in LDL cholesterol. 40 mg (capsule) 1-2 times a day. Or 80-mg tablet once a day.

CONTRAINDICATIONS
Active hepatic disease, unexplained increased serum transaminase levels

INTERACTIONS
Drug
Cyclosporine, erythromycin, gemfibrozil, immunosuppressants, niacin: Increases the risk of acute renal failure and rhabdomyolysis with these drugs.
Herbal
None known.
Food
None known.

DIAGNOSTIC TEST EFFECTS
May increase serum CK and transaminase concentrations

SIDE EFFECTS
Frequent (8%-5%)
Headache, dyspepsia, back pain, myalgia, arthralgia, diarrhea, abdominal cramping, rhinitis

Occasional (4%-2%)
Nausea, vomiting, insomnia, constipation, flatulence, rash, pruritus, fatigue, cough, dizziness

SERIOUS REACTIONS
• Myositis (inflammation of voluntary muscle) with or without increased CK, and muscle weakness, occur rarely. These conditions may progress to frank rhabdomyolysis and renal impairment.

PRECAUTIONS & CONSIDERATIONS
Use fluvastatin cautiously in those who are receiving anticoagulant therapy, have a history of liver disease, or consume substantial amounts of alcohol. Caution is also warranted with hypotension, major surgery, severe acute infection, renal failure secondary to rhabdomyolysis, uncontrolled seizures, and severe electrolyte, endocrine, and metabolic disorders. Expect to discontinue or withhold fluvastatin if these conditions appear. Fluvastatin use is contraindicated in pregnancy, because the suppression of cholesterol biosynthesis may cause fetal toxicity. It is unknown whether fluvastatin is distributed in breast milk; therefore, it is contraindicated during lactation. Safety and efficacy of fluvastatin have not been established in children. No age-related precautions have been noted in the elderly.

Notify the physician of any muscle pain and weakness, especially if accompanied by fever or malaise. Pattern of daily bowel activity and stool consistency should be assessed. Serum lipid cholesterol and triglyceride levels and hepatic function should be checked at baseline and periodically during treatment.

Administration
Take fluvastatin without regard to food.

Fluvoxamine
floo-vox´a-meen
(Faverin [AUS], Luvox)

CATEGORY AND SCHEDULE
Pregnancy Risk Category: C

CLASSIFICATION
Antidepressants, serotonin specific reuptake inhibitors

MECHANISM OF ACTION
An antidepressant and antiobsessive agent that selectively inhibits neuronal reuptake of serotonin. *Therapeutic Effect:* Relieves depression and symptoms of obsessive-compulsive disorder.

AVAILABILITY
Tablets: 25 mg, 50 mg, 100 mg.

INDICATIONS AND DOSAGES
▶ **Obsessive-compulsive disorder**
PO
Adults. 50 mg at bedtime; may increase by 50 mg every 4-7 days. Dosages greater than 100 mg/day given in 2 divided doses. Maximum: 300 mg/day.
Children 8-17 yr. 25 mg at bedtime; may increase by 25 mg every 4-7 days. Dosages greater than 50 mg/day given in 2 divided doses. Maximum: 200 mg/day.

OFF-LABEL USES
Treatment of depression, panic disorder, anxiety disorders in children

CONTRAINDICATIONS
Use within 14 days of MAOIs

INTERACTIONS

Drug
Benzodiazepines, carbamazepine, clozapine, theophylline: May increase the blood concentration and risk of toxicity of these drugs.
Lithium, tryptophan: May enhance fluvoxamine's serotonergic effects.
MAOIs: May produce serious reactions, including hyperthermia, rigidity, and myoclonus.
Tricyclic antidepressants: May increase the fluvoxamine blood concentration.
Warfarin: May increase the effects of warfarin.

Herbal
St. John's wort: May increase fluvoxamine's pharmacologic effects and risk of toxicity.

Food
None known.

DIAGNOSTIC TEST EFFECTS
None known.

SIDE EFFECTS

Frequent
Nausea (40%); headache, somnolence, insomnia (21%-22%)
Occasional (14%-8%)
Nervousness, dizziness, diarrhea, dry mouth, asthenia, weakness, dyspepsia, constipation, abnormal ejaculation
Rare (6%-3%)
Anorexia, anxiety, tremor, vomiting, flatulence, urinary frequency, sexual dysfunction, altered taste

SERIOUS REACTIONS
• Overdose may produce seizures, nausea, vomiting, and extreme agitation and restlessness.

PRECAUTIONS & CONSIDERATIONS
Caution is warranted with impaired hepatic or renal function and in the elderly. Dizziness, somnolence, and dry mouth may occur. Avoid tasks requiring mental alertness or motor skills until response to the drug is established. Baseline blood chemistry tests to assess hepatic function should be performed.

Administration
! Expect to decrease the dosage or dosing frequency for the elderly and those with impaired hepatic function.
Do not abruptly discontinue the drug. Fluvoxamine's maximum therapeutic response may require 4 weeks or more to appear.

Folic Acid
foe'lik
(Apo-Folic [CAN], Folvite, Megafol [AUS]) (Folvite-parenteral)
Do not confuse Folvite with Florvite.

CATEGORY AND SCHEDULE
Pregnancy Risk Category: A (C if used in doses above the recommended daily allowance)
OTC (0.4-mg and 0.8-mg tablets only)

CLASSIFICATION
Hematinics, vitamins/minerals

MECHANISM OF ACTION
A coenzyme that stimulates production of platelets, RBCs, and WBCs. *Therapeutic Effect:* Essential for nucleoprotein synthesis and maintenance of normal erythropoiesis.

PHARMACOKINETICS
PO form almost completely absorbed from the GI tract (upper duodenum). Protein binding: High.

Metabolized in the liver and plasma to active form. Excreted in urine. Removed by hemodialysis.

AVAILABILITY

Tablets: 0.4 mg, 0.8 mg, 1 mg.
Injection: 5 mg/ml.

INDICATIONS AND DOSAGES

▶ **Vitamin B₉ deficiency**
PO, IV, IM, SUBCUTANEOUS
Adults, Elderly, Children 12 yr and older. Initially, 1 mg/day.
Maintenance: 0.5 mg/day.
Children 1-11 yr. Initially 1 mg/day.
Maintenance: 0.1-0.4 mg/day.
Infants. 50 mcg/day.
▶ **Dietary supplement**
PO, IV, IM, SUBCUTANEOUS
Adults, Elderly, Children 4 yr and older. 0.4 mg/day.
Children 1-younger than 4 yr.
0.3 mg/day.
Children younger than 1 yr.
0.1 mg/day.
Pregnant women. 0.8 mg/day.

OFF-LABEL USES

To decrease the risk of colon cancer

CONTRAINDICATIONS

Anemias (aplastic, normocytic, pernicious, refractory)

INTERACTIONS
Drug

Analgesics, carbamazepine, estrogens: May increase folic acid requirements.
Antacids, cholestyramine: May decrease the absorption of folic acid.
Hydantoin anticonvulsants: May decrease the effects of these drugs.
Methotrexate, triamterene, trimethoprim: May antagonize the effects of folic acid.
Herbal
None known.

Food
None known.

DIAGNOSTIC TEST EFFECTS

May decrease vitamin B_{12} concentration.

SIDE EFFECTS

None known.

SERIOUS REACTIONS

• Allergic hypersensitivity occurs rarely with parenteral form. Oral folic acid is nontoxic.

F

PRECAUTIONS & CONSIDERATIONS

Folic acid is distributed in breast milk. No age-related precautions have been noted in children or the elderly. Eating foods rich in folic acid including fruits, vegetables, and organ meats, is encouraged.

Therapeutic improvement, including improved sense of well-being and relief from iron deficiency symptoms, such as fatigue, headache, pallor, dyspnea, and sore tongue, should be assessed. Pernicious anemia should be ruled out with a Schilling test and vitamin B_{12} blood level before beginning folic acid therapy because the signs of pernicious anemia may be masked while irreversible neurologic damage progresses. Be aware that persons with alcoholism, decreased hematopoiesis, or deficiency of vitamin B_6, B_{12}, C, or E and those using antimetabolic drugs may develop a resistance to treatment.
Administration
❗ Parental folic acid is used in acutely ill patients, those receiving enteral or total parenteral nutrition, and patients with malabsorption syndrome who are unresponsive to the oral form. Folic acid dosages greater than 0.1 mg/day may conceal signs of pernicious anemia.

Fomepizole
foe-mep'i-zoll
(Antizol)

CATEGORY AND SCHEDULE
Pregnancy Risk Category: C

CLASSIFICATION
Antidotes

MECHANISM OF ACTION
An alcohol dehydrogenase inhibitor that inhibits the enzyme that catalyzes the metabolism of ethanol, ethylene glycol, and methanol to their toxic metabolites. *Therapeutic Effect:* Inhibits conversion of ethylene glycol and methanol into toxic metabolites.

PHARMACOKINETICS
Protein binding: low. Rapidly distributes to total body water after IV infusion. Extensively metabolized by the liver. Minimal excretion in the urine. Removed by hemodialysis. **Half-life:** 5 hr.

AVAILABILITY
Solution for injection: 1 g/ml (Antizol).

INDICATIONS AND DOSAGES
▸ **Ethylene glycol or methanol intoxication**
IV INFUSION
Adults, Elderly. 15 mg/kg as a loading dose, followed by 10 mg/kg q12hr for 4 doses, then 15 mg/kg q12hr until ethylene glycol or methanol concentrations are below 20 mg/dl. All doses should be administered as a slow IV infusion over 30 minutes.
▸ **Dosage in renal impairment**
During hemodialysis. 15 mg/kg as a loading dose, followed by 10 mg/kg q4hr for 4 doses, then 15 mg/kg q4hr until ethylene glycol or methanol concentrations are below 20 mg/dl.
After hemodialysis. If the time between the last dose and end of hemodialysis is less than 1 hour, do not give dose. If the time between is 1-3 hours, give 50% of next scheduled dose. If time is greater than 3 hours, give next scheduled dose.

OFF-LABEL USES
Butoxyethanol intoxication, diethylene glycol intoxication, ethanol sensitivity

CONTRAINDICATIONS
Hypersensitivity to fomepizole or other pyrazoles

INTERACTIONS
Drug
Alcohol: May reduce elimination of both drugs.
Herbal
None known.
Food
None known.

DIAGNOSTIC TEST EFFECTS
None known.

▨ IV INCOMPATIBILITIES
No drug incompatibilities reported.

SIDE EFFECTS
Frequent
Hypertriglyceridemia, headache, nausea, dizziness
Occasional
Abnormal sense of smell, nystagmus, visual disturbances, ringing in ears, agitation, seizures, anorexia, heartburn, anxiety, vertigo, lightheadedness, altered sense of awareness
Rare
Anuria, disseminated intravascular coagulopathy

SERIOUS REACTIONS
- Mild allergic reactions including rash and eosinophilia occur rarely.
- Overdose may cause nausea, dizziness, and vertigo.

PRECAUTIONS & CONSIDERATIONS
Caution is warranted with liver disease or renal impairment. Dialysis should be considered in addition to fomepizole in cases of renal failure. If less than 6 hours has passed since last dose, do not give dose. If more than 6 hours has passed since last dose, give next scheduled dose. It is unknown if fomepizole crosses the placenta or is distributed in breast milk. Safety and efficacy of fomepizole has not been established in children. Age-related renal impairment may require dosage adjustment in the elderly.

This medication is given to treat antifreeze or windshield wiper fluid ingestion. If not treated, these poisons will cause kidney damage, eye damage, seizures, coma, and possibly death.

Storage
Do not freeze. Store unopened vial at room temperature.

Administration
Dilute at least 100 ml of 0.9% NaCl or D_5W. Administer fomepizole as a slow infusion over 30 minutes. Do not give undiluted or by bolus injection. Adjust dose if the person is receiving dialysis.

Fomivirsen
foh-mih-ver'sen
(Vitravene)

CATEGORY AND SCHEDULE
Pregnancy Risk Category: C

CLASSIFICATION
Antivirals, ophthalmics

MECHANISM OF ACTION
An antiviral that binds to messenger RNA, inhibiting the synthesis of viral proteins. *Therapeutic Effect:* Blocks replication of cytomegalovirus (CMV).

AVAILABILITY
Intravitreal Injection:
6.6 mg/ml.

INDICATIONS AND DOSAGES
▶ CMV retinitis
INTRAVITREAL INJECTION
Adults. 330 mcg (0.05 ml) every other week for 2 doses, then 330 mcg every 4 weeks.

CONTRAINDICATIONS
None significant.

INTERACTIONS
Drug
None significant.
Herbal
None significant.
Food
None significant.

DIAGNOSTIC TEST EFFECTS
May alter liver function test results and serum alkaline phosphatase level. May decrease blood Hgb levels and neutrophil and platelet counts.

SIDE EFFECTS
Frequent (10%-5%)
Fever, headache, nausea, diarrhea, vomiting, abdominal pain, anemia, uveitis, abnormal vision
Occasional (5%-2%)
Chest pain, confusion, dizziness, depression, neuropathy, anorexia, weight loss, pancreatitis, dyspnea, cough

SERIOUS REACTIONS
• Thrombocytopenia may occur. Increased intraocular pressure has been reported.

PRECAUTIONS & CONSIDERATIONS
Caution is warranted with increased intraocular pressure. Be aware that fomivirsen use should be avoided in patients who have received cidofovir within 2 to 4 weeks of fomivirsen therapy.

After fomivirsen injection, evaluate light perception, optic nerve head perfusion, and intraocular pressure. Signs and symptoms of extraocular CMV infection should be monitored, including pneumonitis and colitis.
Administration
Inject directly into eye (in the intravitreal space). Generally, it is administered once every other week for the first two treatments and then every four weeks thereafter.

Fondaparinux
fawn-da-pear'ih-nux
(Arixtra)

CATEGORY AND SCHEDULE
Pregnancy Risk Category: B

CLASSIFICATION
Anticoagulants

MECHANISM OF ACTION
A factor Xa inhibitor and pentasaccharide that selectively binds to antithrombin, and increases its affinity for factor Xa, thereby inhibiting factor Xa and stopping the blood coagulation cascade. *Therapeutic Effect:* Indirectly prevents formation of thrombin and subsequently the fibrin clot.

PHARMACOKINETICS
Well absorbed after subcutaneous administration. Undergoes minimal, if any, metabolism. Highly bound to antithrombin III. Distributed mainly in blood and to a minor extent in extravascular fluid. Excreted unchanged in urine. Removed by hemodialysis. **Half-life:** 17-21 hr (prolonged in patients with impaired renal function).

AVAILABILITY
Injection: 2.5 mg/0.5 ml prefilled syringe.

INDICATIONS AND DOSAGES
▸ **Prevention of venous thromboembolism**
SUBCUTANEOUS
Adults. 2.5 mg once a day for 5-9 days after surgery. Initial dose should be given 6-8 hr after surgery. Dosage should be adjusted in the elderly and in those with renal impairment.

CONTRAINDICATIONS
Active major bleeding, bacterial endocarditis, severe renal impairment (with creatinine clearance less than 30 ml/min), thrombocytopenia associated with antiplatelet antibody formation in the presence of fondaparinux, body weight less than 50 kg.

INTERACTIONS
Drug
Anticoagulants, platelet inhibitors:
May increase bleeding.
Herbal
None known.
Food
None known.

DIAGNOSTIC TEST EFFECTS
Increases reversible serum creatinine, AST (SGOT), and ALT (SGPT) levels. May decrease Hgb, Hct, and platelet count.

SIDE EFFECTS
Occasional (14%)
Fever
Rare (4%-1%)
Injection site hematoma, nausea, peripheral edema

SERIOUS REACTIONS
• Accidental overdose may lead to bleeding complications ranging from local ecchymoses to major hemorrhage.
• Thrombocytopenia occurs rarely.

PRECAUTIONS & CONSIDERATIONS
Caution is warranted with conditions associated with increased risk of hemorrhage, such as concurrent use of antiplatelet agents, GI ulceration, hemophilia, history of cerebrovascular accident, severe uncontrolled hypertension, history of heparin-induced thrombocytopenia, impaired renal function, indwelling epidural catheter or neuraxial anesthesia, and in the elderly. Fondaparinux should be used with caution in pregnant women, particularly during the last trimester and immediately postpartum because it increases the risk of maternal hemorrhage. It is unknown if fondaparinux is excreted in breast milk. Safety and efficacy of fondaparinux have not been established in children. In the elderly, age-related decreased renal function may increase the risk of bleeding. Females may experience heavier menstrual flow. Other medications, including OTC drugs, should be avoided. An electric razor and soft toothbrush should be used to prevent bleeding during therapy.

Notify the physician of bleeding from surgical site, chest pain, dyspnea, severe or sudden headache, swelling in the feet or hands, unusual back pain, bruising, weakness, black or red stool, coffee-ground vomitus, dark or red urine, or red-speckled mucus from cough. CBC, BUN and creatinine levels, B/P, pulse, and stool of occult blood should be monitored. Be aware of signs of bleeding, including bleeding at injection or surgical sites or from gums, blood in stool, bruising, hematuria, and petechiae.

Storage
Store at room temperature. The parenteral form normally appears clear and colorless; discard if discoloration or particulate matter is noted.

Administration
Do not expel the air bubble from the prefilled syringe before injection, to avoid expelling drug. Pinch a fold of the patient's skin at the injection site between the thumb and forefinger. Introduce the entire length of subcutaneous needle into the skinfold. Inject into fatty tissue between the left and right anterolateral or the left and right posterolateral abdominal wall. Rotate injection sites. The usual length of therapy is 5 to 9 days.

F

Formoterol
for-moe'ter-ol
(Foradil Aerolizer, Foradile
[AUS], Oxis [AUS])

CATEGORY AND SCHEDULE
Pregnancy Risk Category: C

CLASSIFICATION
Adrenergic agonists,
bronchodilators

MECHANISM OF ACTION
A long-acting bronchodilator
that stimulates beta$_2$-adrenergic
receptors in the lungs, resulting in
relaxation of bronchial smooth
muscle. Also inhibits release of
mediators from various cells in the
lungs, including mast cells, with
little effect on heart rate.
Therapeutic Effect: Relieves
bronchospasm, reduces airway
resistance. Improves bronchodilation, nighttime asthma control, and
peak flow rates.

PHARMACOKINETICS

Route	Onset	Peak	Duration
Inhalation	1-3 min	0.5-1 hr	12 hr

Absorbed from bronchi after
inhalation. Metabolized in the
liver. Primarily excreted in
urine. Unknown if removed
by hemodialysis.
Half-life: 10 hr.

AVAILABILITY
Inhalation Powder in Capsules:
12 mcg.

INDICATIONS AND DOSAGES
▸ **Asthma, chronic obstructive
pulmonary disease (COPD)**

INHALATION
*Adults, Elderly, Children 5 yr and
older.* 12 mcg capsule q12hr.
▸ **Exercise-induced bronchospasm**
INHALATION
*Adults, Elderly, Children 5 yr and
older.* 12 mcg capsule at least 15 min
before exercise. Do not repeat for
another 12 hr.

CONTRAINDICATIONS
None known.

INTERACTIONS
Drug
Beta blockers: May antagonize
formoterol's bronchodilating effects.
**Diuretics, steroids, xanthine deriv-
atives:** May increase the risk of
hypokalemia.
**Drugs that can prolong QT interval
(including erythromycin, quini-
dine, and thioridazine), MAOIs,
tricyclic antidepressants:** May
potentiate cardiovascular effects.
Herbal
None known.
Food
None known.

DIAGNOSTIC TEST EFFECTS
May decrease serum potassium level.
May increase blood glucose level.

SIDE EFFECTS
Occasional
Tremor, muscle cramps, tachycardia,
insomnia, headache, irritability, irritation of mouth or throat

SERIOUS REACTIONS
• Excessive sympathomimetic stimulation may produce palpitations,
extrasystole, and chest pain.

PRECAUTIONS & CONSIDERATIONS
Caution is warranted with cardiovascular disease, hypertension, a seizure
disorder, and thyrotoxicosis. It is

unknown if formoterol crosses the placenta or is distributed in breast milk. The safety and efficacy of formoterol have not been established in children younger than 5 years. The elderly may be more prone to tachycardia and tremor because of increased sensitivity to sympathomimetics. Drink plenty of fluids to decrease the thickness of lung secretions. Avoid excessive use of caffeinated products, such as chocolate, cocoa, cola, coffee, and tea.

Pulse rate and quality, EKG, respiratory rate, depth, rhythm and type, ABG, and serum potassium levels should be monitored. Keep a log of measurements of peak flow readings.

Administration

Keep capsules in individual blister packs until immediately before use. Don't swallow the capsules. Don't use with a spacer. Pull off the aerolizer inhaler cover, twisting the mouthpiece in the direction of the arrow to open. Place the capsule in the chamber and twist the mouthpiece closed. Press both buttons on the side of the aerolizer only once. This action punctures the capsule. Exhale completely, then place mouth on the mouthpiece and close the lips. Inhale quickly and deeply through the mouth, which causes the capsule to spin and dispense the drug. Hold breath for as long as possible before exhaling slowly. Check the capsule to make sure all the powder is gone. If not, inhale again to receive the rest of the dose. Rinse mouth with water immediately after inhalation to prevent mouth and throat dryness.

Fosamprenavir
fos′am-pren-a-veer
(Lexiva)

CATEGORY AND SCHEDULE
Pregnancy Risk Category: C

CLASSIFICATION
Antivirals, protease inhibitors

F

MECHANISM OF ACTION
An antiretroviral that is rapidly converted to amprenavir, which inhibits HIV-1 protease by binding to the enzyme's active site, thus preventing the processing of viral precursors and resulting in the formation of immature, noninfectious viral particles. *Therapeutic Effect:* Impairs HIV replication and proliferation.

PHARMACOKINETICS
Rapidly absorbed after PO administration. Protein binding: 90%. Metabolized in the liver. Excreted in urine and feces. **Half-life:** 7.7 hr.

AVAILABILITY
Tablets: 700 mg (equivalent to 600 mg amprenavir)

INDICATIONS AND DOSAGES
▸ **HIV infection in patients who have not had previous protease inhibitor therapy**
PO
Adults, Elderly. 1400 mg twice daily without ritonavir; or 1400 mg twice daily plus ritonavir 200 mg once daily; or 700 mg twice daily plus ritonavir 100 mg twice daily.

▶ **HIV infection in patients who have had previous protease inhibitor therapy**
PO
Adults, Elderly. 700 mg twice daily plus ritonavir 100 mg twice daily.
▶ **Concurrent therapy with efavirenz**
PO
Adults, Elderly. In patients receiving fosamprenavir plus once-daily ritonavir in combination with efavirenz, an additional 100 mg/day ritonavir (300 mg total/day) should be given.

CONTRAINDICATIONS
Concurrent use of amprenavir, dihydroergotamine, ergonovine, ergotamine, methylergonovine, pimozide, midazolam, or triazolam. If fosamprenavir is given concurrently with ritonavir, flecainide and propafenone are also contraindicated.

INTERACTIONS
Drug
Amiodarone, bepridil, ergotamine, lidocaine, midazolam, oral contraceptives, quinidine, triazolam, tricyclic antidepressants: May interfere with the metabolism of these drugs.
Antacids, didanosine: May decrease the absorption of fosamprenavir.
Carbamazepine, phenobarbital, phenytoin, rifampin: May decrease the fosamprenavir blood concentration.
Clozapine, HMG-CoA reductase inhibitors (statins), warfarin: May increase the blood concentrations of these drugs.
Herbal
St. John's wort: May decrease the fosamprenavir blood concentration.
Food
None known.

DIAGNOSTIC TEST EFFECTS
May increase serum lipase, triglyceride, AST (SGOT), and ALT (SGPT) levels.

SIDE EFFECTS
Frequent (39%-35%)
Nausea, rash, diarrhea
Occasional (19%-8%)
Headache, vomiting, fatigue, depression
Rare (7%-2%)
Pruritus, abdominal pain, perioral paresthesia

SERIOUS REACTIONS
• Severe and possibly life-threatening dermatologic reactions occur rarely.

PRECAUTIONS & CONSIDERATIONS
Extreme caution should be used with liver impairment. Caution is also warranted with diabetes mellitus, impaired renal function, known sulfonamide allergy and in the elderly. Fosamprenavir is not a cure for HIV infection, nor does it reduce risk of transmission to others.
   Expect to obtain baseline lab values, including blood glucose levels, serum lipase, SGPT (ALT), SGOT (AST), and serum triglyceride levels. Find out which other drugs the person is taking, including ritonavir. Make sure the person is not also taking amprenavir, because it is chemically similar to fosamprenavir. Report any side effects including rash or diarrhea.
Administration
Do not chew, crush, or break film-coated tablets. May take without regard to food.

Foscarnet
foss-car'net
(Foscavir)

CATEGORY AND SCHEDULE
Pregnancy Risk Category: C

CLASSIFICATION
Antivirals

MECHANISM OF ACTION
An antiviral that selectively inhibits binding sites on virus-specific DNA polymerase and reverse transcriptase. *Therapeutic Effect:* Inhibits replication of herpes virus.

PHARMACOKINETICS
Sequestered into bone and cartilage. Protein binding: 14%-17%. Primarily excreted unchanged in urine. Removed by hemodialysis. **Half-life:** 3.3-6.8 hr (increased in impaired renal function).

AVAILABILITY
Injection: 24 mg/ml.

INDICATIONS AND DOSAGES
▸ **Cytomegalovirus (CMV) retinitis**
IV
Adults, Elderly. Initially, 60 mg/kg q8hr or 100 mg/kg q12hr for 2-3 wk. Maintenance: 90-120 mg/kg/day as a single IV infusion.
▸ **Herpes infection**
IV
Adults. 40 mg/kg q8-12hr for 2-3 wk or until healed.
▸ **Dosage in renal impairment**
Dosages are individualized based on creatinine clearance. Refer to the dosing guide provided by the manufacturer.

CONTRAINDICATIONS
None known.

INTERACTIONS
Drug
Nephrotoxic medications: May increase the risk of nephrotoxicity.
Pentamidine (IV): May cause reversible hypocalcemia, hypomagnesemia, and nephrotoxicity.
Zidovudine (AZT): May increase the risk of anemia.
Herbal
None known.
Food
None known.

DIAGNOSTIC TEST EFFECTS
May increase serum alkaline phosphatase, bilirubin, creatinine, AST (SGOT), and ALT (SGPT) levels. May decrease serum magnesium and potassium levels. May alter serum calcium and phosphate concentrations.

▨ IV INCOMPATIBILITIES
Acyclovir (Zovirax), amphotericin B (Fungizone), co-trimoxazole (Bactrim), diazepam (Valium), digoxin (Lanoxin), diphenhydramine (Benadryl), dobutamine (Dobutrex), droperidol (Inapsine), ganciclovir (Cytovene), haloperidol (Haldol), leucovorin (Versed), midazolam (Versed), pentamidine (Pentam IV), prochlorperazine (Compazine), vancomycin (Vancocin)
▨ IV Compatibilities
Dopamine (Intropin), heparin, hydromorphone (Dilaudid), lorazepam (Ativan), morphine, potassium chloride

SIDE EFFECTS
Frequent
Fever (65%); nausea (47%); vomiting, diarrhea (30%)

Occasional (5% or greater)
Anorexia, pain and inflammation at injection site, fever, rigors, malaise, headache, paresthesia, dizziness, rash, diaphoresis, abdominal pain
Rare (5%-1%)
Back or chest pain, edema, flushing, pruritus, constipation, dry mouth

SERIOUS REACTIONS

• Nephrotoxicity occurs to some extent in most patients.
• Seizures and serum mineral or electrolyte imbalances may be life-threatening.

PRECAUTIONS & CONSIDERATIONS

Caution is warranted with altered serum calcium or other serum electrolyte levels, a history of renal impairment, or cardiac or neurologic abnormalities. Be aware that it is unknown if foscarnet is distributed in breast milk. Be aware that the safety and efficacy of foscarnet have not been established in children. In the elderly, age-related renal impairment may require dosage adjustment.

Renal impairment is reduced by ensuring sufficient fluid intake to promote diuresis before and during dosing. Signs and symptoms of anemia such as bleeding, superinfections, and tremors, should be assessed. Institute safety measures for potential seizures. Report numbness in the extremities, paresthesias, or peri-oral tingling, during or after infusion as this may indicate electrolyte abnormalities.

Storage

Store parenteral vials at room temperature. After dilution, foscarnet is stable for 24 hours at room temperature. Do not use if foscarnet solution is discolored or contains particulate material.

Administration

Use the standard 24 mg/ml solution without diluting it when a central venous catheter is used for infusion; the 24 mg/ml solution *must* be diluted to 12 mg/ml when you're giving the drug through a peripheral vein catheter. Use only D_5W or 0.9% NaCl solution for injection for dilution. Because foscarnet dosage is calculated on body weight, remove the unneeded quantity before the start of infusion to avoid overdosage. Use an IV infusion pump to administer foscarnet and prevent accidental overdose. Use aseptic technique and administer the solution within 24 hours of the first entry into the sealed bottle.

! Do not give foscarnet as an IV injection or by rapid infusion because these routes increase the drug's toxicity. Administer foscarnet by IV infusion at a rate not faster than 1 hour for doses up to 60 mg/kg and 2 hours for doses greater than 60 mg/kg. To minimize the risk of phlebitis and toxicity, use central venous lines or veins with an adequate blood flow to permit rapid dilution and dissemination of foscarnet.

Fosfomycin
foss-fo-mye'sin
(Monurol)
Do not confuse Monurol with Monopril.

CATEGORY AND SCHEDULE
Pregnancy Risk Category: B

CLASSIFICATION
Antibiotics, miscellaneous, antiseptics, urinary tract

MECHANISM OF ACTION

An antibiotic that prevents bacterial cell wall formation by inhibiting the synthesis of peptidoglycan. *Therapeutic Effect:* Bactericidal.

AVAILABILITY

Powder for Oral Solution: 3 g.

INDICATIONS AND DOSAGES

▸ **Uncomplicated UTIs in females**
PO
Females. 3 g mixed in 4 oz water as a single dose.
▸ **Uncomplicated UTIs in males**
Males. 3 g/day for 2-3 days.

CONTRAINDICATIONS

None known.

INTERACTIONS

Drug
Metoclopramide: Lowers serum concentration and urinary excretion of fosfomycin.
Herbal
None known.
Food
None known.

DIAGNOSTIC TEST EFFECTS

May increase blood eosinophil count and serum alkaline phosphatase, bilirubin, AST (SGOT), and ALT (SGPT) levels. May alter platelet and WBC counts. May decrease blood Hct and Hgb levels.

SIDE EFFECTS

Occasional (9%-3%)
Diarrhea, nausea, headache, back pain
Rare (less than 2%)
Dysmenorrhea, pharyngitis, abdominal pain, rash

SERIOUS REACTIONS

• None known.

PRECAUTIONS & CONSIDERATIONS
Symptoms should improve 2 to 3 days after the initial dose of fosfomycin
Administration
Take fosfomycin without regard to food. Always mix with water before consuming.

F

Fosinopril

fo-sin'o-pril
(Monopril)
Do not confuse Monopril with Monurol.

CATEGORY AND SCHEDULE

Pregnancy Risk Category: C (D if used in second or third trimester)

CLASSIFICATION

Angiotensin converting enzyme inhibitors

MECHANISM OF ACTION

An ACE inhibitor that suppresses the renin-angiotensin-aldosterone system and prevents conversion of angiotensin I to angiotensin II, a potent vasoconstrictor; may also inhibit angiotensin II at local vascular and renal sites. Decreases plasma angiotensin II, increases plasma renin activity, and decreases aldosterone secretion. *Therapeutic Effect:* Reduces peripheral arterial resistance, pulmonary capillary wedge pressure; improves cardiac output, and exercise tolerance.

PHARMACOKINETICS

Route	Onset	Peak	Duration
PO	1 hr	2-6 hr	24 hr

Slowly absorbed from the GI tract. Protein binding: 97%-98%. Metabolized in the liver and GI mucosa to active metabolite. Primarily excreted in urine. Minimal removal by hemodialysis. **Half-life:** 11.5 hr.

AVAILABILITY

Tablets: 10 mg, 20 mg, 40 mg.

INDICATIONS AND DOSAGES

▸ **Hypertension (monotherapy)**
PO
Adults, Elderly. Initially, 10 mg/day. Maintenance: 20-40 mg/day. Maximum: 80 mg/day.
▸ **Hypertension (with diuretic)**
PO
Adults, Elderly. Initially, 10 mg/day titrated to patient's needs.
▸ **Heart failure**
PO
Adults, Elderly. Initially, 5-10 mg. Maintenance: 20-40 mg/day.

OFF-LABEL USES

Treatment of diabetic and nondiabetic nephropathy, post-myocardial infarction left ventricular dysfunction, renal crisis in scleroderma

CONTRAINDICATIONS

History of angioedema from previous treatment with ACE inhibitors

INTERACTIONS
Drug
Alcohol, antihypertensives, diuretics: May increase the effects of fosinopril.
Lithium: May increase lithium blood concentration and risk of lithium toxicity.

NSAIDs: May decrease the effects of fosinopril.
Potassium-sparing diuretics, potassium supplements: May cause hyperkalemia.
Herbal
None known.
Food
None known.

DIAGNOSTIC TEST EFFECTS

May increase BUN, serum alkaline phosphatase, serum bilirubin, serum creatinine, serum potassium, AST (SGOT), and ALT (SGPT) levels. May decrease serum sodium levels. May cause positive antinuclear antibody titer.

SIDE EFFECTS
Frequent (12%-9%)
Dizziness, cough
Occasional (4%-2%)
Hypotension, nausea, vomiting, upper respiratory tract infection

SERIOUS REACTIONS

• Excessive hypotension (first-dose syncope) may occur in patients with CHF and in those who are severely salt and volume depleted.
• Angioedema (swelling of face and lips) and hyperkalemia occur rarely.
• Agranulocytosis and neutropenia may be noted in those with collagen vascular disease, including scleroderma and systemic lupus erythematosus, and impaired renal function.
• Nephrotic syndrome may be noted in those with history of renal disease.

PRECAUTIONS & CONSIDERATIONS

Caution is warranted with cerebrovascular and coronary insufficiency, hypovolemia, renal impairment, sodium depletion, and those on dialysis and/or receiving diuretics. Fosinopril crosses the placenta, is distributed in breast milk, and may cause fetal or neonatal morbidity or mortality. Safety and efficacy of fosinopril have not been established in children. Neonates and infants may be at increased risk for neurologic abnormalities and oliguria. The elderly may be more sensitive to the hypotensive effects of fosinopril.

Dizziness may occur. B/P should be obtained immediately before giving each fosinopril dose, in addition to regular monitoring. Be alert to fluctuations in B/P. If an excessive reduction in B/P occurs, place the person in the supine position with legs elevated. CBC and blood chemistry should be obtained before beginning fosinopril therapy, then every 2 weeks for the next 3 months, and periodically thereafter in patients with autoimmune disease, or renal impairment, and in those who are taking drugs that affect immune response or leukocyte count. BUN, serum creatinine, and serum potassium should also be monitored in those who are receiving a diuretic. Crackles and wheezes should be assessed for in persons with CHF.

Administration

! Expect to discontinue diuretics 2 to 3 days before beginning fosinopril therapy.

Take fosinopril without regard to food. Crush tablets if necessary.

Fosphenytoin
fos-fen'i-toyn
(Cerebyx)
Do not confuse Cerebyx with Celebrex or Celexa.

CATEGORY AND SCHEDULE
Pregnancy Risk Category: D

CLASSIFICATION
Anticonvulsants, hydantoins

F

MECHANISM OF ACTION
A hydantoin anticonvulsant that stabilizes neuronal membranes by decreasing sodium and calcium ion influx into the neurons. Also decreases post-tetanic potentiation and repetitive discharge. *Therapeutic Effect:* Decreases seizure activity.

PHARMACOKINETICS
Completely absorbed after IM administration. Protein binding: 95%-99%. Rapidly and completely hydrolyzed to phenytoin after IM or IV administration. Time of complete conversion to phenytoin: 4 hr after IM injection; 2 hr after IV infusion. **Half-life:** 8-15 min (for conversion to phenytoin).

AVAILABILITY
Injection: 75 mg/ml (equivalent to 50 mg/ml phenytoin)

INDICATIONS AND DOSAGES
▸ **Status epilepticus**
IV
Adults. Loading dose: 15-20 mg phenytoin equivalent (PE)/kg infused at rate of 100-150 mg PE/min.
▸ **Nonemergent seizures**
IV, IM
Adults. Loading dose: 10-20 mg PE/kg. Maintenance: 4-6 mg PE/kg/day.

▶ **Short term substitution for oral phenytoin**
IM, IV
Adults. May substitute for oral phenytoin at same total daily dose.

CONTRAINDICATIONS
Adams-Stokes syndrome, hypersensitivity to fosphenytoin or phenytoin, second- or third-degree AV block, severe bradycardia, sinoatrial block

INTERACTIONS
Drug
Alcohol, other CNS depressants: May increase CNS depression.
Amiodarone, anticoagulants, cimetidine, disulfiram, fluoxetine, isoniazid, sulfonamides: May increase fosphenytoin blood concentration, effects, and risk of toxicity.
Antacids: May decrease fosphenytoin absorption.
Fluconazole, ketoconazole, miconazole: May increase fosphenytoin blood concentration.
Glucocorticoids: May decrease the effects of glucocorticoids.
Lidocaine, propranolol: May increase cardiac depressant effects.
Valproic acid: May increase the blood concentration and decrease the metabolism of fosphenytoin.
Xanthines: May increase the metabolism of xanthines.
Herbal
None known.
Food
None known.

DIAGNOSTIC TEST EFFECTS
May increase blood glucose, serum GGT, and serum alkaline phosphatase levels.

🖧 IV INCOMPATIBILITIES
Midazolam (Versed)

🖧 IV Compatibilities
Lorazepam (Ativan), phenobarbital, potassium chloride

SIDE EFFECTS
Frequent
Dizziness, paresthesia, tinnitus, pruritus, headache, somnolence
Occasional
Morbilliform rash

SERIOUS REACTIONS
• An elevated fosphenytoin blood concentration may produce ataxia, nystagmus, diplopia, lethargy, slurred speech, nausea, vomiting, and hypotension. As the drug level increases, extreme lethargy may progress to coma.

PRECAUTIONS & CONSIDERATIONS
Caution is warranted with hypoalbuminemia, hypotension, hepatic and renal disease, porphyria, and severe myocardial insufficiency.
Fosphenytoin use during pregnancy may increase the frequency of seizures in the mother and the risk of congenital malformations in the fetus. It is unknown if fosphenytoin is excreted in breast milk. The safety of this drug has not been established in children. A lower fosphenytoin dosage is recommended for the elderly.
    Drowsiness and dizziness may occur, so alcohol and tasks that require mental alertness or motor skills should be avoided. History of the seizure disorder, including the duration, frequency, and intensity of seizures should be assessed. B/P, EKG, and cardiac and respiratory function should be monitored during and for 10-20 minutes after the infusion. Blood level of fosphenytoin should be assessed 2 hours after IV infusion or 4 hours after IM injection.

Storage
Refrigerate unopened vials. Don't store the drug at room temperature for longer than 48 hours; discard vials that contain particulate matter. After dilution, the solution is stable for 8 hours at room temperature or 24 hours if refrigerated.

Administration
! Know that 150 mg fosphenytoin yields 100 mg phenytoin and that the dose, concentration solution, and infusion rate of fosphenytoin are expressed in terms of phenytoin equivalents (PE). Keep in mind that elderly patients may require lower, less frequent dosing and that the drug is not approved for use in children.

For IV use, dilute the drug in D_5W or 0.9% NaCl to a concentration of 1.5 to 25 mg PE/ml. Administer at less than 150 mg PE/minute to decrease the risk of hypotension and arrhythmias. May also be given IM.

Fulvestrant
full'veh-strant
(Faslodex)
Do not confuse with Fosamax.

CATEGORY AND SCHEDULE
Pregnancy Risk Category: D

CLASSIFICATION
Antineoplastics, antiestrogens, hormones/hormone modifiers

MECHANISM OF ACTION
An estrogen antagonist that competes with endogenous estrogen at estrogen receptor binding sites.
Therapeutic Effect: Inhibits tumor growth.

PHARMACOKINETICS
Extensively and rapidly distributed after IM administration. Protein binding: 99%. Metabolized in the liver. Eliminated by hepatobiliary route; excreted in feces. **Half-life:** 40 days in postmenopausal women. Peak serum levels occur in 7-9 days.

AVAILABILITY
Prefilled Syringe: 50 mg/ml in 2.5-ml and 5-ml syringes.

INDICATIONS AND DOSAGES
▸ **Breast cancer**
IM
Adults, Elderly. 250 mg given once monthly.

CONTRAINDICATIONS
Known or suspected pregnancy

INTERACTIONS
Drug
None known.
Herbal
None known.
Food
None known.

DIAGNOSTIC TEST EFFECTS
None known.

SIDE EFFECTS
Frequent (26%-13%)
Nausea, hot flashes, pharyngitis, asthenia, vomiting, vasodilatation, headache
Occasional (12%-5%)
Injection site pain, constipation, diarrhea, abdominal pain, anorexia, dizziness, insomnia, paresthesia, bone or back pain, depression, anxiety, peripheral edema, rash, diaphoresis, fever
Rare (2%-1%)
Vertigo, weight gain

SERIOUS REACTIONS
• UTIs, vaginitis, anemia, thromboembolic phenomena, and leukopenia occur rarely.

PRECAUTIONS & CONSIDERATIONS
Caution should be used in those receiving anticoagulant therapy and those with bleeding diathesis, estrogen receptor-negative breast cancer, hepatic disease or reduced hepatic flow, and thrombocytopenia. Don't administer fulvestrant to pregnant women. It is unknown if fulvestrant is excreted in breast milk. Fulvestrant is not for use in children. No age-related precautions have been noted in the elderly.

Potential side effects, including edema, asthenia, dizziness, headache, nausea and vomiting, may occur. Notify the physician if weakness, hot flashes, or nausea become unmanageable. An estrogen receptor assay test should be performed before therapy; and a computed tomography scan should be performed before and periodically thereafter fulvestrant therapy. Blood chemistry and plasma lipid levels should also be monitored.

Administration
For IM use, administer the drug slowly into the buttock as a single 5-ml injection or two concurrent 2.5-ml injections.

Furosemide
fur-oh'se-mide
(Apo-Furosemide [CAN], Frusehexal [AUS], Frusid [AUS], Lasix, Uremide [AUS], Urex-M [AUS])
Do not confuse Lasix with Lidex, Luvox, or Luxiq, or furosemide with Torsemide.

CATEGORY AND SCHEDULE
Pregnancy Risk Category: C
(D if used in pregnancy-induced hypertension)

CLASSIFICATION
Diuretics, loop

MECHANISM OF ACTION
A loop diuretic that enhances excretion of sodium, chloride, and potassium by direct action at the ascending limb of the loop of Henle.
Therapeutic Effect: Produces diuresis and lower B/P.

PHARMACOKINETICS

Route	Onset	Peak	Duration
PO	30-60 min	1-2 hr	6-8 hr
IV	5 min	20-60 min	2 hr
IM	30 min	N/A	N/A

Well absorbed from the GI tract. Protein binding: 91%-97%. Partially metabolized in the liver. Primarily excreted in urine (nonrenal clearance increases in severe renal impairment). Not removed by hemodialysis.
Half-life: 30-90 min (increased in renal or hepatic impairment, and in neonates).

AVAILABILITY
Oral Solution: 10 mg/ml, 40 mg/5 ml.
Tablets: 20 mg, 40 mg, 80 mg.
Injection: 10 mg/ml.

INDICATIONS AND DOSAGES
▸ **Edema, hypertension**
PO
Adults, Elderly. Initially,
20-80 mg/dose; may increase by
20-40 mg/dose q6-8hr. May titrate
up to 600 mg/day in severe edema-
tous states.
Children. 1-6 mg/kg/day in divided
doses q6-12hr.
IV, IM
Adults, Elderly. 20-40 mg/dose; may
increase by 20 mg/dose q1-2hr.
Children. 1-2 mg/kg/dose q6-12hr.
Neonates. 1-2 mg/kg/dose q12-24hr.
IV INFUSION
Adults, Elderly. Bolus of 0.1 mg/kg,
followed by infusion of 0.1 mg/kg/hr;
may double q2hr. Maximum:
0.4 mg/kg/hr.
Children. 0.05 mg/kg/hr; titrate to
desired effect.

OFF-LABEL USES
Hypercalcemia

CONTRAINDICATIONS
Anuria, hepatic coma, severe electrolyte depletion

INTERACTIONS
Drug
**Amphotericin B, nephrotoxic and
ototoxic medications:** May increase
the risk of nephrotoxicity and
ototoxicity.
Anticoagulants, heparin: May
decrease the effects of these drugs.
Lithium: May increase the risk of
lithium toxicity.
**Other hypokalemia-causing
medications:** May increase the risk
of hypokalemia.

Probenecid: May increase
furosemide blood concentration.
Herbal
None known.
Food
None known.

DIAGNOSTIC TEST EFFECTS
May increase blood glucose, BUN,
and serum uric acid levels. May
decrease serum calcium, chloride,
magnesium, potassium, and sodium
levels.

F

▨ IV INCOMPATIBILITIES
Ciprofloxacin (Cipro), diltiazem
(Cardizem), dobutamine (Dobutrex),
dopamine (Intropin), doxorubicin
(Adriamycin), droperidol (Inapsine),
esmolol (Brevibloc), famotidine
(Pepcid), filgrastim (Neupogen),
fluconazole (Diflucan), gemcitabine
(Gemzar), gentamicin (Garamycin),
idarubicin (Idamycin), labetalol
(Trandate), meperidine (Demerol),
metoclopramide (Reglan), midazo-
lam (Versed), milrinone (Primacor),
nicardipine (Cardene), ondansetron
(Zofran), quinidine, thiopental
(Pentothal), vecuronium (Norcuron),
vinblastine (Velban), vincristine
(Oncovin), vinorelbine (Navelbine)
▨ IV Compatibilities
Aminophylline, amiodarone
(Cordarone), bumetanide (Bumex),
calcium gluconate, cimetidine
(Tagamet), heparin, hydromorphone
(Dilaudid), lidocaine, morphine,
nitroglycerin, norepinephrine
(Levophed), potassium chloride,
propofol (Diprivan)

SIDE EFFECTS
Expected
Increased urinary frequency and
urine volume
Frequent
Nausea, dyspepsia, abdominal

cramps, diarrhea or constipation, electrolyte disturbances

Occasional

Dizziness, light-headedness, headache, blurred vision, paresthesia, photosensitivity, rash, fatigue, bladder spasm, restlessness, diaphoresis

Rare

Flank pain

SERIOUS REACTIONS

• Vigorous diuresis may lead to profound water loss and electrolyte depletion, resulting in hypokalemia, hyponatremia, and dehydration.

• Sudden volume depletion may result in increased risk of thrombosis, circulatory collapse, and sudden death.

• Acute hypotensive episodes may occur, sometimes several days after beginning therapy.

• Ototoxicity—manifested as deafness, vertigo, or tinnitus—may occur, especially in patients with severe renal impairment.

• Furosemide use can exacerbate diabetes mellitus, systemic lupus erythematosus, gout, and pancreatitis.

• Blood dyscrasias have been reported.

PRECAUTIONS & CONSIDERATIONS

Caution is warranted with hepatic cirrhosis. Furosemide crosses the placenta and is distributed in breast milk. Neonates may require an increased dosage interval because the drug's half-life is increased in this age-group. The elderly may be more sensitive to the drug's electrolyte and hypotensive effects, and are at increased risk for circulatory collapse and thromboembolic effects. Age-related renal impairment may require a dosage adjustment in the elderly. Consuming foods high in potassium such as apricots, bananas, legumes, meat, orange juice, raisins, whole grains, including cereals, and white and sweet potatoes, is encouraged. Avoid prolonged exposure to sunlight.

An increase in the frequency and volume of urination and hearing abnormalities, such as a sense of fullness or ringing in the ears, may occur. Blood pressure (B/P), vital signs, electrolytes, intake and output, and weight should be monitored before and during treatment. Be aware of signs of electrolyte disturbances such as hypokalemia or hyponatremia. Hypokalemia may cause arrhythmias, altered mental status, muscle cramps, asthenia, and tremor. Hyponatremia may result in cold and clammy skin, confusion, and thirst.

Administration

Take furosemide with food to avoid GI upset, preferably with breakfast to help prevent nocturia.

The solution for injection normally appears clear and colorless. Discard yellow solutions. Furosemide is compatible with D_5W, 0.9% NaCl, and lactated Ringer's solution, but it may also be given undiluted. Administer each 40 mg or less by IV push over 1 to 2 minutes. Don't exceed an administration rate of 4 mg/minute with renal impairment.

After IM use, monitor for temporary pain at the injection site.

Gabapentin
ga′ba-pen-tin
(Gantin [AUS], Neurontin)
Do not confuse Neurontin with Noroxin.

CATEGORY AND SCHEDULE
Pregnancy Risk Category: C

CLASSIFICATION
Anticonvulsants

MECHANISM OF ACTION
An anticonvulsant and antineuralgic agent whose exact mechanism is unknown. May increase the synthesis or accumulation of gamma-aminobutyric acid by binding to as-yet-undefined receptor sites in brain tissue. *Therapeutic Effect:* Reduces seizure activity and neuropathic pain.

PHARMACOKINETICS
Well absorbed from the GI tract (not affected by food). Protein binding: less than 5%. Widely distributed. Crosses the blood-brain barrier. Primarily excreted unchanged in urine. Removed by hemodialysis. **Half-life:** 5-7 hr (increased in impaired renal function and the elderly).

AVAILABILITY
Capsules: 100 mg, 300 mg, 400 mg.
Oral Solution: 250 mg/5 ml.
Tablets: 600 mg, 800 mg.

INDICATIONS AND DOSAGES
▸ **Adjunctive therapy for seizure control**
PO
Adults, Elderly, Children 12 yr and older. Initially, 300 mg 3 times a day. May titrate dosage.

Range: 900-1800 mg/day in 3 divided doses. Maximum: 3600 mg/day.
Children 3-12 yr. Initially, 10-15 mg/kg/day in 3 divided doses. May titrate up to 25-35 mg/kg/day (for children 5-12 yr) and 40 mg/kg/day (for children 3-4 yr) Maximum: 50 mg/kg/day.
▸ **Adjunctive therapy for neuropathic pain**
PO
Adults, Elderly. Initially, 100 mg 3 times a day; may increase by 300 mg/day at weekly intervals. Maximum: 3600 mg/day in 3 divided doses.
Children. Initially, 5 mg/kg/dose at bedtime, followed by 5 mg/kg/dose for 2 doses on day 2, then 5 mg/kg/dose for 3 doses on day 3. Range: 8-35 mg/kg/day in 3 divided doses.
▸ **Postherpetic neuralgia**
PO
Adults, Elderly. 300 mg on day 1, 300 mg twice a day on day 2, and 300 mg 3 times a day on day 3. Titrate up to 1800 mg/day.
▸ **Dosage in renal impairment**
Dosage and frequency are modified based on creatinine clearance:

Creatinine Clearance	Dosage
60 ml/min or higher	400 mg q8hr
30-59 ml/min	300 mg q12hr
16-29 ml/min	300 mg daily
Less than 16 ml/min	300 mg every other day
Hemodialysis	200-300 mg after each 4-hr hemodialysis session

OFF-LABEL USES
Treatment of essential tremor, hot flashes, hyperhidrosis, migraines, psychiatric disorders

CONTRAINDICATIONS
None known.

G

INTERACTIONS
Drug
Antacids: May decrease gabapentin effectiveness.
Morphine: May increase plasma concentrations of gabapentin.
Herbal
Evening primrose oil, ginkgo: May decrease anticonvulsant effectiveness.
Food
None known.

DIAGNOSTIC TEST EFFECTS
May decrease serum WBC count.

SIDE EFFECTS
Frequent (19%-10%)
Fatigue, somnolence, dizziness, ataxia
Occasional (8%-3%)
Nystagmus, tremor, diplopia, rhinitis, weight gain
Rare (less than 2%)
Nervousness, dysarthria, memory loss, dyspepsia, pharyngitis, myalgia

SERIOUS REACTIONS
• Abrupt withdrawal may increase seizure frequency.
• Overdosage may result in diplopia, slurred speech, drowsiness, lethargy, and diarrhea.

PRECAUTIONS & CONSIDERATIONS
Caution is warranted with renal impairment. It is unknown whether gabapentin is distributed in breast milk. The safety and efficacy of this drug have not been established in children 3 years and younger. In the elderly, age-related renal impairment may require dosage adjustment. Alcohol and tasks requiring mental alertness or motor skills should be avoided.

Seizure disorder, including the onset, duration, frequency, intensity, and type of seizures, should be assessed before and during treatment.

Weight, renal function, and behavior should also be monitored.
Administration
! Keep in mind that the interval between drug doses should not exceed 12 hours.

Gabapentin may be taken with food to reduce GI upset. If gabapentin treatment will be discontinued or another anticonvulsant will be added to the treatment regimen, expect to make the changes gradually over at least 1 week to prevent loss of seizure control.

Galantamine
ga-lan'ta-mene
(Reminyl)
Do not confuse Reminyl with Remeron, Remicade, or Robinul.

CATEGORY AND SCHEDULE
Pregnancy Risk Category: B

CLASSIFICATION
Cholinesterase inhibitors

MECHANISM OF ACTION
A cholinesterase inhibitor that inhibits the enzyme acetylcholinesterase, thus increasing the concentration of acetylcholine at cholinergic synapses and enhancing cholinergic function in the CNS. *Therapeutic Effect:* Slows the progression of Alzheimer's disease.

PHARMACOKINETICS
Rapidly absorbed from the GI tract. Protein binding: 18%. Distributed to blood cells; binds to plasma proteins, mainly albumin. Metabolized in the liver. Excreted in urine. **Half-life:** 7 hr.

AVAILABILITY
Oral Solution: 4 mg/ml.
Tablets: 4 mg, 8 mg, 12 mg.

INDICATIONS AND DOSAGES
▸ **Alzheimer's disease**
PO
Adults, Elderly. Initially, 4 mg twice a day (8 mg/day). After a minimum of 4 wk (if well tolerated), may increase to 8 mg twice a day (16 mg/day). After another 4 wk, may increase to 12 mg twice daily (24 mg/day). Range: 16-24 mg/day in 2 divided doses.
▸ **Dosage in renal impairment**
For moderate impairment, maximum dosage is 16 mg/day. Drug is not recommended for patients with severe impairment.

CONTRAINDICATIONS
Severe hepatic or renal impairment

INTERACTIONS
Drug
Bethanechol, succinylcholine: May interfere with the effects of these drugs.
Cimetidine, erythromycin, ketoconazole, paroxetine: May increase the galantamine blood concentration.
Herbal
None known.
Food
None known.

DIAGNOSTIC TEST EFFECTS
None known.

SIDE EFFECTS
Frequent (17%-5%)
Nausea, vomiting, diarrhea, anorexia, weight loss
Occasional (9%-4%)
Abdominal pain, insomnia, depression, headache, dizziness, fatigue, rhinitis

Rare (less than 3%)
Tremors, constipation, confusion, cough, anxiety, urinary incontinence

SERIOUS REACTIONS
• Overdose may cause cholinergic crisis, characterized by increased salivation, lacrimation, severe nausea and vomiting, bradycardia, respiratory depression, hypotension, and increased muscle weakness. Treatment usually consists of supportive measures and an anticholinergic such as atropine.

G

PRECAUTIONS & CONSIDERATIONS
Caution is warranted with asthma, bladder outflow obstruction, COPD, peptic ulcer disease, history of seizures, moderate hepatic or renal impairment, supraventricular conduction disturbances, and concurrent use of NSAIDs. It is unknown if galantamine crosses the placenta or is distributed in breast milk. Galantamine is not prescribed for children. No age-related precautions have been noted in the elderly, but galantamine is not recommended for those with severe hepatic or renal impairment (creatinine clearance of less than 9 ml/minute). Be aware that galantamine is not a cure for Alzheimer's disease but may slow the progression of its symptoms.
Notify the physician if he or she experiences excessive sweating, tearing, or salivation, depression, dizziness, excessive fatigue, muscle weakness, insomnia, weight loss or persistent GI disturbances occurs. A 12-lead EKG and rhythm strips should be performed periodically. Liver and renal function test results should also be assessed.
Administration
! If galantamine therapy is interrupted for several days or longer, reinstitute therapy as prescribed.
Take galantamine with morning and evening meals.

Ganciclovir
gan-sy′clo-ver
(Cymevene [AUS], Cytovene,
Vitrasert)
**Do not confuse Cytovene with
Cytosar.**

CATEGORY AND SCHEDULE
Pregnancy Risk Category: C

CLASSIFICATION
Antivirals

MECHANISM OF ACTION
This synthetic nucleoside competes
with viral DNA polymerase and is
incorporated into growing viral DNA
chains. *Therapeutic Effect:* Interferes
with synthesis and replication of
viral DNA.

PHARMACOKINETICS
Widely distributed. Protein binding:
1%-2%. Undergoes minimal
metabolism. Excreted unchanged
primarily in urine. Removed by
hemodialysis. **Half-life:** 2.5-3.6 hr
(increased in impaired renal function).

AVAILABILITY
Capsules (Cytovene): 250 mg,
500 mg.
Powder for Injection (Cytovene):
500 mg.
Implant (Vitrasert): 4.5 mg.

INDICATIONS AND DOSAGES
▸ **Cytomegalovirus (CMV) retinitis**
IV
Adults, Children 3 mo and older.
10 mg/kg/day in divided doses q12hr
for 14-21 days, then 5 mg/kg/day as
a single daily dose.
▸ **Prevention of CMV disease in
transplant patients**
IV

Adults, Children. 10 mg/kg/day in
divided doses q12hr for 7-14 days,
then 5 mg/kg/day as a single daily
dose.
▸ **Other CMV infections**
IV
Adults. Initially, 10 mg/kg/day in
divided doses q12hr for 14-21 days,
then 5 mg/kg/day as a single daily
dose. Maintenance: 1000 mg 3 times
a day or 500 mg q3hr (6 times
a day).
Children. Initially, 10 mg/kg/day in
divided doses q12hr for 14-21 days,
then 5 mg/kg/day as a single daily
dose. Maintenance: 30 mg/kg/dose
q8hr.
▸ **Intravitreal implant**
Adults. 1 implant q6-9mo plus oral
ganciclovir.
Children 9 yr and older. 1 implant
q6-9mo plus oral ganciclovir
(30 mg/dose q8hr).
▸ **Adult dosage in renal
impairment**
Dosage and frequency are modified
based on CrCl.

CrCl	Induction Dosage	Mainte-nance Dosage	Oral
50-69 ml/min	2.5 mg/kg q12hr	2.5 mg/kg q24hr	1500 mg/ day
25-49 ml/min day	2.5 mg/kg q24hr	1.25 mg/kg q24hr	1000 mg/ day
10-24 ml/min	1.25 mg/kg q24hr	0.625 mg/kg q24hr	500 mg/ day
Less than 10 ml/min	1.25 mg/ kg 3 times/ wk	0.625 mg/kg 3 times/ wk	500 mg 3 times/ wk

CrCl = creatinine clearance

OFF-LABEL USES
Treatment of other CMV infections,
such as gastroenteritis, hepatitis, and
pneumonitis

CONTRAINDICATIONS

Absolute neutrophil count less than 500/mm³, platelet count less than 25,000/mm³, hypersensitivity to acyclovir or ganciclovir, immunocompetent patients, patients with congenital or neonatal CMV disease.

INTERACTIONS

Drug

Bone marrow depressants: May increase bone marrow depression.
Imipenem and cilastatin: May increase the risk of seizures.
Zidovudine (AZT): May increase the risk of hepatotoxicity.
Herbal
None known.
Food
None known.

DIAGNOSTIC TEST EFFECTS

May increase serum alkaline phosphatase, bilirubin, AST (SGOT), and ALT (SGPT) levels.

IV INCOMPATIBILITIES

Aldesleukin (Proleukin), amifostine (Ethyol), aztreonam (Azactam), cefepime (Maxipime), cytarabine (ARA-C), doxorubicin (Adriamycin), fludarabine (Fludara), foscarnet (Foscavir), gemcitabine (Gemzar), ondansetron (Zofran), piperacillin and tazobactam (Zosyn), sargramostim (Leukine), vinorelbine (Navelbine)

IV Compatibilities

Amphotericin B, enalapril (Vasotec), filgrastim (Neupogen), fluconazole (Diflucan), propofol (Diprivan)

SIDE EFFECTS

Frequent
Diarrhea (41%), fever (40%), nausea (25%), abdominal pain (17%), vomiting (13%)
Occasional (11%-6%)
Diaphoresis, infection, paresthesia, flatulence, pruritus

Rare (4%-2%)
Headache, stomatitis, dyspepsia, phlebitis

SERIOUS REACTIONS

• Hematologic toxicity occurs commonly: leukopenia in 41%-29% of patients and anemia in 25%-19%.
• Intra-ocular insertion occasionally results in visual acuity loss, vitreous hemorrhage, and retinal detachment.
• GI hemorrhage occurs rarely.

PRECAUTIONS & CONSIDERATIONS

Caution should be used in pediatric patients. The long-term safety of this drug has not been determined because of the potential for long-term adverse reproductive and carcinogenic effects. Caution is warranted with impaired renal function, neutropenia, and thrombocytopenia. Be aware that ganciclovir should not be used during pregnancy and breast-feeding should be discontinued during ganciclovir use. Breast-feeding may be resumed no sooner than 72 hours after the last dose of ganciclovir. Be aware that effective contraception should be used during ganciclovir therapy. Be aware that the safety and efficacy of ganciclovir have not been established in children younger than 12 years of age. In the elderly, age-related renal impairment may require dosage adjustment. Ganciclovir may temporarily or permanently inhibit sperm production in males and suppress fertility in females. Barrier contraception should be used during ganciclovir administration and for 90 days after therapy because of mutagenic potential.

Specimens (blood, feces, throat culture, urine) should be obtained for culture and sensitivity testing, as ordered, before giving the drug. Keep in mind that test results are needed to support the differential diagnosis and rule out retinal infection as the result of hematogenous dissemination. Intake and output should be monitored as well as adequate hydration (minimum 1500 ml/24 hours). Hematology reports for decreased platelets, neutropenia, and thrombocytopenia should be evaluated. Altered vision, complications, and therapeutic improvement should be assessed.

Storage

Store vials at room temperature. Do not refrigerate. Reconstituted solution in vial is stable for 12 hours at room temperature. After dilution, refrigerate and use within 24 hours. Discard the solution if precipitate forms or discoloration occurs.

Administration

Give ganciclovir with food. Avoid inhaling the solution. Also avoid solution exposure to the eyes, mucous membranes, or skin. Use latex gloves and safety glasses during preparation and handling of ganciclovir solution. If the solution comes in contact with mucous membranes or the skin, wash the affected area thoroughly with soap and water; rinse eyes thoroughly with plain water.

Reconstitute 500-mg vial with 10 ml sterile water for injection to provide a concentration of 50 mg/ml; do not use bacteriostatic water which contains parabens, and is therefore incompatible with ganciclovir. Further dilute with 100 ml D$_5$W, 0.9% NaCl, lactated Ringer's, or any combination thereof to provide a concentration of 5 mg/ml. Do not give by IV push or rapid IV infusion because these routes increase the risk of ganciclovir toxicity. Administer only by IV infusion over 1 hour. Protect from infiltration because the high pH of this drug causes severe tissue irritation. Use large veins to permit rapid dilution and dissemination of ganciclovir and to minimize the risk of phlebitis. Keep in mind that central venous ports tunneled under subcutaneous tissue may reduce catheter-associated infection.

Gatifloxacin
gah-tee-floks'a-sin
(Tequin, Zymar)

CATEGORY AND SCHEDULE
Pregnancy Risk Category: C

CLASSIFICATION
Antibiotics, quinolones

MECHANISM OF ACTION
A fluoroquinolone that inhibits two enzymes, topoisomerase II and IV, in susceptible microorganisms. *Therapeutic Effect:* Interferes with bacterial DNA replication. Prevents or delays resistance emergence. Bactericidal.

PHARMACOKINETICS
Well absorbed from the gastrointestinal (GI) tract after PO administration. Protein binding: 20%. Widely distributed. Metabolized in liver. Primarily excreted in urine. **Half-life:** 7-14 hr.

AVAILABILITY
Tablets (Tequin): 200 mg, 400 mg.
Injection (Tequin): 200-mg, 400-mg vials.
Ophthalmic Solution (Zymar): 0.3%.

INDICATIONS AND DOSAGES
▶ **Chronic bronchitis, complicated urinary tract infections, pyelonephritis, skin infections**
PO/IV
Adults, Elderly. 400 mg/day for 7-10 days (5 days for chronic bronchitis).

▸ **Sinusitis**
PO/IV
Adults, Elderly. 400 mg/day for
10 days.
▸ **Pneumonia**
PO/IV
Adults, Elderly. 400 mg/day for
7-14 days.
▸ **Cystitis**
PO/IV
Adults, Elderly. 400 mg as a single
dose or 200 mg/day for 3 days.
▸ **Urethral gonorrhea in men and
women, endocervical and rectal
gonorrhea in women**
PO/IV
Adults, Elderly. 400 mg as a single
dose.
▸ **Topical treatment of bacterial
conjunctivitis due to susceptible
strains of bacteria**
OPHTHALMIC
*Adults, Elderly, Children 1 yr and
older.* 1 drop q2hr while awake for
2 days, then 1 drop up to 4 times/day
for days 3-7.
▸ **Dosage in renal impairment**

Creatinine Clearance	Dosage
40 ml/min	400 mg/day
Less than 40 ml/min	Initially, 400 mg/day then 200 mg/day
Hemodialysis	Initially, 400 mg/day then 200 mg/day
Peritoneal dialysis	Initially, 400 mg/day then 200 mg/day

CONTRAINDICATIONS
Hypersensitivity to quinolones

INTERACTIONS
Drug
**Antacids, digoxin, iron prepara-
tions:** May decrease gatifloxacin
plasma concentration and half-life.
Antidiabetic agents: May alter
blood glucose and increase risk of
hypoglycemia or hyperglycemia.
**Cisapride, Class IA and
Class III antiarrhythmic agents,**

**erythromycin, phenothiazines,
TCA antidepressants:** May
increase risk of cardiotoxicity.
Didanosine: May decrease the
effectiveness of gatifloxacin.
Prednisone: May increase blood
glucose and increase risk of hyper-
glycemia.
Probenecid: May increase gati-
floxacin plasma concentration and
half-life.
Warfarin: May increase the risk of
bleeding.
Herbal
None known.
Food
None known.

DIAGNOSTIC TEST EFFECTS
None known.

💉 IV INCOMPATIBILITIES
Amphotericin (Fungizone), potassium phosphate
💉 IV Compatibilities
Aminophylline, calcium gluconate,
hydromorphone (Dilaudid), lidocaine,
lorazepam (Ativan), magnesium
sulfate, methylprednisolone (Solu-
Medrol), metoclopramide (Reglan),
midazolam (Versed), morphine,
nitroglycerin, potassium chloride,
sodium phosphate

SIDE EFFECTS
Occasional (8%-3%)
Nausea, vaginitis, diarrhea,
headache, dizziness
Ophthalmic: conjunctival irritation,
increased tearing, corneal
inflammation
Rare (3%-0.1%)
Abdominal pain, constipation, dyspepsia, stomatitis, edema, insomnia,
abnormal dreams, diaphoresis,
altered taste, rash
Ophthalmic: corneal swelling, dry
eye, eye pain, eyelid swelling,
headache, red eye, reduced visual
acuity, altered taste

G

SERIOUS REACTIONS

• Pseudomembranous colitis as evidenced by severe abdominal pain and cramps, severe watery diarrhea, and fever, may occur.

• Superinfection manifested as genital or anal pruritus, ulceration or changes in oral mucosa, and moderate to severe diarrhea, may occur.

PRECAUTIONS & CONSIDERATIONS

Caution is warranted with cerebral atherosclerosis, central nervous system (CNS) disorders, liver or renal impairment, seizures, those with a prolonged QT interval, and concurrent use of other medications known to prolong the QT interval (e.g., erythromycin, tricyclic antidepressants). Caution should also be used with hypokalemia and those receiving amiodarone, quinidine, procainamide, and sotalol. It is unknown if gatifloxacin is distributed in breast milk. The safety and efficacy of gatifloxacin have not been established in children. Age-related renal impairment may require a dosage adjustment in the elderly.

Dizziness, headache, nausea, signs of infection, and vaginitis should be evaluated. Pattern of daily bowel activity and stool consistency should be assessed. Mental status and white blood cell (WBC) count should also be monitored. History of hypersensitivity to gatifloxacin and other quinolones should be determined before therapy.

Administration

Take oral gatifloxacin without regard to meals. Take 4 hours before giving antacids, buffered tablets or solutions, ferrous sulfate, or multivitamins.

For ophthalmic, tilt head backward and look up. Gently pull the lower eyelid down until a pocket is formed. Hold the dropper above the pocket, and without touching the eyelid or conjunctival sac, place drops into the center of the pocket. Close the eye, and then apply gentle digital pressure to the lacrimal sac at the inner canthus. Remove excess solution around the eye with a tissue.

For IV use, know that the drug is available prediluted and ready for use and that it's also available in 20- and 40-ml vials, which must be diluted in 100-200 ml D5W, 0.9% NaCl. Infuse over 60 minutes. Do not give by rapid or bolus IV.

Gefitinib
ge-fi´tye-nib
(Iressa)

CATEGORY AND SCHEDULE
Pregnancy Risk Category: D

CLASSIFICATION
Antineoplastics, signal transduction inhibitors

MECHANISM OF ACTION

Blocks the signaling pathway that binds to the epidermal growth factor receptor (EGFR) on the surface of normal and cancer cells. EGFR activates the enzyme tyrosine kinase, which sends signals instructing the cells to grow. *Therapeutic Effect:* Inhibits the growth of cancer cells.

PHARMACOKINETICS

Slowly absorbed and extensively distributed throughout the body. Protein binding: 90%. Undergoes extensive metabolism in the liver. Excreted in the feces. **Half-life:** 48 hr.

AVAILABILITY
Tablets: 250 mg.

INDICATIONS AND DOSAGES
▸ **Non–small cell lung cancer**
PO
Adults, Elderly. 250 mg/day;
may increase to 500 mg/day for
patients receiving drugs that
may decrease gefitinib blood
concentrations, such as rifampin
and phenytoin

CONTRAINDICATIONS
None known.

INTERACTIONS
Drug
**Cimetidine, phenytoin,
ranitidine, rifampin, sodium
bicarbonate:** May decrease
gefitinib blood concentration and
effectiveness.
Itraconazole, ketoconazole:
Increases gefitinib blood
concentration.
Metoprolol: Increases the effect of
metoprolol.
Warfarin: Increases the risk of
bleeding.
Herbal
None known.
Food
None known.

DIAGNOSTIC TEST EFFECTS
May increase serum alkaline phos-
phatase, bilirubin, AST (SGOT), and
ALT (SGPT) levels.

SIDE EFFECTS
Frequent (48%-25%)
Diarrhea, rash, acne
Occasional (13%-8%)
Dry skin, nausea, vomiting,
pruritus
Rare (7%-2%)
Anorexia, asthenia, weight loss,
peripheral edema, eye pain

SERIOUS REACTIONS
• Pancreatitis and ocular hemorrhage occur rarely.
• Hypersensitivity reaction
produces angioedema and urticaria.
Interstitial lung disease has been
reported.

PRECAUTIONS & CONSIDERATIONS
Caution is warranted with hepatic
impairment and severe renal impairment. Gefitinib may cause fetal harm
and result in termination of pregnancy. Pregnant or breast-feeding
women should not receive this drug.
Pregnancy should be avoided during
therapy and contraceptive methods
should be used during treatment and
for up to 12 months afterward. The
safety and efficacy of gefitinib have
not been established in children. No
age-related precautions have been
noted in the elderly. Vaccinations
without the physician's approval and
crowds and people with known
infections should be avoided.

Notify the physician of anorexia,
nausea, vomiting, persistent or severe
diarrhea, and signs and symptoms of
infection, including fever and flu-
like symptoms.

Adequate hydration should be
maintained. Bowel sounds for hyperactivity and pattern of daily bowel
activity and stool consistency should
be assessed. Antidiarrheals and
antiemetics should be ordered to help
prevent and treat diarrhea, nausea,
and vomiting. For those who can't
tolerate diarrhea, expect to interrupt
gefitinib therapy for up to
14 days.
Administration
Take gefitinib without regard to
food. Don't crush or break film-
coated tablets.

Gemfibrozil
gem-fi′broe-zil
(Apo-Gemfibrozil [CAN],
Ausgem [AUS], Gemfibromax
[AUS], Jezil [AUS], Lipazil [AUS],
Lopid, Novo-Gemfibrozil [CAN])
**Do not confuse with Lorabid
or Levbid.**

CATEGORY AND SCHEDULE
Pregnancy Risk Category: C

CLASSIFICATION
Antihyperlipidemics, fibric acid
derivatives

MECHANISM OF ACTION
A fibric acid derivative that inhibits
lipolysis of fat in adipose tissue;
decreases liver uptake of free fatty
acids and reduces hepatic triglyceride
production. Inhibits synthesis of
VLDL carrier apolipoprotein B.
Therapeutic Effect: Lowers serum
cholesterol and triglycerides
(decreases VLDL, LDL; increases
HDL).

PHARMACOKINETICS
Well absorbed from the
gastrointestinal (GI) tract. Protein
binding: 99%. Metabolized in liver.
Primarily excreted in urine. Not
removed by hemodialysis. **Half-life:**
1.5 hr.

AVAILABILITY
Tablets: 600 mg.
Capsules: 300 mg.

INDICATIONS AND DOSAGES
▸ **Hyperlipidemia**
PO
Adults, Elderly. 1200 mg/day in
2 divided doses 30 min before
breakfast and dinner.

CONTRAINDICATIONS
Liver dysfunction (including primary
biliary cirrhosis), preexisting gallbladder disease, severe renal
dysfunction

INTERACTIONS
Drug
Lovastatin: May cause rhabdomyol-
ysis, leading to acute renal failure.
**Pioglitazone, repaglinide,
warfarin:** May increase the effect
of these drugs.
Herbal
None known.
Food
None known.

DIAGNOSTIC TEST EFFECTS
May increase serum alkaline phosphatase, serum bilirubin, serum
creatinine kinase, serum LDH
concentrations, and SGOT (AST) and
SGPT (ALT) levels. May decrease
blood Hgb and Hct levels, leukocyte
counts, and serum potassium levels.

SIDE EFFECTS
Frequent (20%)
Dyspepsia
Occasional (10%-2%)
Abdominal pain, diarrhea, nausea,
vomiting, fatigue
Rare (less than 2%)
Constipation, acute appendicitis,
vertigo, headache, rash, pruritus,
altered taste

SERIOUS REACTIONS
• Cholelithiasis, cholecystitis, acute
appendicitis, pancreatitis, and malignancy occur rarely.

PRECAUTIONS & CONSIDERATIONS
Caution is warranted with diabetes
mellitus, receiving estrogen or anticoagulant therapy, and with hypothyroidism. Be aware that it is unknown
if gemfibrozil crosses the placenta or

is distributed in breast milk. Also know that the decision to discontinue breast-feeding or gemfibrozil should be based on the potential for serious adverse effects to the infant. Be aware that gemfibrozil use is not recommended in children younger than 2 years of age because cholesterol is necessary for normal development in this age group. In the elderly, age-related renal impairment may require dosage adjustment.

Notify the physician of any abdominal pain, diarrhea, dizziness, nausea, or vomiting. Pattern of daily bowel activity and stool consistency should be assessed. Serum LDL, VLDL, triglyceride, and cholesterol levels should be checked at baseline and periodically during treatment. Hematology and liver function test results should also be assessed. Blood glucose should be monitored in those receiving insulin or oral antihyperglycemics.

Be aware of the increased risk of developing rhabdomyolysis when coadministered with a statin.

Administration
Take gemfibrozil 30 minutes before morning and evening meals.

Gemifloxacin
gem-ih-flocks'ah-sin
(Factive)

CATEGORY AND SCHEDULE
Pregnancy Risk Category: C

CLASSIFICATION
Antibiotics, quinolones

MECHANISM OF ACTION
A fluoroquinolone that inhibits the enzyme DNA gyrase in susceptible microorganisms, interfering with bacterial cell replication and repair. *Therapeutic Effect:* Bactericidal.

PHARMACOKINETICS
Rapidly and well absorbed from the GI tract. Protein binding: 70%. Widely distributed. Penetrates well into lung tissue and fluid. Undergoes limited metabolism in the liver. Primarily excreted in feces; lesser amount eliminated in urine. Partially removed by hemodialysis. **Half-life:** 4-12 hr.

AVAILABILITY
Tablets: 320 mg.

INDICATIONS AND DOSAGES
▸ **Acute bacterial exacerbation of chronic bronchitis**
PO
Adults, Elderly. 320 mg once a day for 5 days.
▸ **Community-acquired pneumonia**
PO
Adults, Elderly. 320 mg once a day for 7 days.
▸ **Dosage in renal impairment**
Dosage and frequency are modified based on creatinine clearance.

Creatinine Clearance	Dosage
Greater than 40 ml/min	320 mg once a day
40 ml/min or less	160 mg once a day

CONTRAINDICATIONS
Concurrent use of amiodarone, quinidine, procainamide, or sotalol; history of prolonged QTc interval; hypersensitivity to fluoroquinolones; uncorrected electrolyte disorders (such as hypokalemia and hypomagnesemia)

INTERACTIONS
Drug
Aluminum and magnesium-containing antacids, bismuth

subsalicylate, didanosine, iron preparations and other metals, sucralfate, zinc preparations: May decrease the absorption of gemifloxacin.

Antipsychotics, class 1A and class III antiarrhythmics, erythromycin, tricyclic antidepressants: May increase the risk of prolonged QTc interval and life-threatening arrhythmias.

Cyclosporine: Increases the risk of nephrotoxicity.

Probenecid: Increases gemifloxacin serum concentration.

Herbal
None known.

Food
None known.

DIAGNOSTIC TEST EFFECTS

May increase BUN and serum alkaline phosphatase, bilirubin, LDH, creatinine, AST (SGOT), and ALT (SGPT) levels.

SIDE EFFECTS

Occasional (4%-2%)
Diarrhea, rash, nausea
Rare (1% or less)
Headache, abdominal pain, dizziness

SERIOUS REACTIONS

• Antibiotic-associated colitis may result from altered bacterial balance. Hypersensitivity reactions, including photosensitivity (as evidenced by rash, pruritus, blisters, edema, and burning skin), have occurred in patients receiving fluoroquinolones. Tendon ruptures and peripheral neuropathy have been reported.

PRECAUTIONS & CONSIDERATIONS

Caution is warranted with acute myocardial ischemia, clinically significant bradycardia, or impaired hepatic or renal function. Gemifloxacin may be teratogenic. Substitute formula feedings for breast-feeding. The safety and efficacy of gemifloxacin have not been established in children 18 years of age and younger. Age-related renal impairment may require a dosage adjustment in the elderly.

Dizziness, headache, nausea, signs of infection, and skin for rash should be evaluated. Pattern of daily bowel activity and stool consistency should be assessed. Liver function and white blood cell (WBC) count should be monitored. QT and QTc intervals should be checked for prolongation. History of hypersensitivity to gemifloxacin and other quinolones should be determined before therapy.

Administration
Take gemifloxacin without regard to food. Don't crush or break tablets. Take 2 hours before giving antacids, buffered tablets or solutions, ferrous sulfate, or multivitamins.

Gemtuzumab Ozogamicin
gem-too'-ze-mab
(Mylotarg)

CATEGORY AND SCHEDULE
Pregnancy Risk Category: D

CLASSIFICATION
Antineoplastics, monoclonal antibodies, monoclonal antibodies

MECHANISM OF ACTION

Binds to an antigen on the surface of leukemic blast cells, resulting in the formation of a complex that leads to the release of the antibiotic inside the myeloid cells. The antibiotic then binds to DNA, resulting in DNA double-strand breaks and cell death. *Therapeutic Effect:* Inhibits colony formation in cultures of adult leukemic bone marrow cells.

PHARMACOKINETICS
Elimination half-life: 45 hr after first infusion; 60 hr after second infusion

AVAILABILITY
Powder for Injection: 5 mg.

INDICATIONS AND DOSAGES
▸ **CD33 positive acute myeloid leukemia**
IV
Adults 60 yr and older. 9 mg/m² repeated in 14 days for a total of 2 doses.

CONTRAINDICATIONS
None known.

INTERACTIONS
Drug
None known.
Herbal
None known.
Food
None known.

DIAGNOSTIC TEST EFFECTS
May increase serum bilirubin, AST (SGOT), and ALT (SGPT) levels. May decrease blood Hgb and Hct levels, platelet count, WBC count, and serum magnesium and potassium levels.

▨ IV INCOMPATIBILITIES
Don't mix gemtuzumab with any other medications.

SIDE EFFECTS
! Most patients experience a postinfusion symptom complex of fever (85%), chills (73%), nausea (70%), and vomiting (63%) that resolves within 2-4 hours with supportive therapy
Frequent (44%-31%)
Asthenia, diarrhea, abdominal pain, headache, stomatitis, dyspnea, epistaxis

Occasional (25%-15%)
Constipation, neutropenic fever, nonspecific rash, herpes simplex infection, hypertension, hypotension, petechiae, peripheral edema, dizziness, insomnia, back pain
Rare (14%-10%)
Pharyngitis, ecchymosis, dyspepsia, tachycardia, hematuria, rhinitis

SERIOUS REACTIONS
• Severe myelosuppression, characterized by neutropenia, anemia, and thrombocytopenia, occurs in 98% of all patients.
• Sepsis occurs in 25% of patients.
• Hepatotoxicity also may occur.

G

PRECAUTIONS & CONSIDERATIONS
Caution is warranted with hepatic impairment. Pregnant women should not receive gemtuzumab because it may cause fetal harm. It is unknown if gemtuzumab is excreted in breast milk; however, women receiving this drug should not breast-feed. The safety and efficacy of gemtuzumab have not been established in children. No age-related precautions have been noted in the elderly. Vaccinations without the physician's approval and crowds and people with known infections should be avoided.

Notify the physician of bruising, fever, signs of local infection, sore throat, or unusual bleeding from any site. Baseline serum chemistry levels, CBC (to monitor for myelosuppression), B/P, and liver function test results should be obtained before and during therapy. Signs and symptoms for stomatitis (burning or erythema of oral mucosa, ulceration, sore throat, difficulty swallowing), anemia (excessive fatigue and weakness) and myelosuppression (ecchymosis, fever, signs of local infection, sore throat, and unusual bleeding from any site) should be assessed.

Storage
Protect the drug from direct and indirect sunlight and unshielded fluorescent light during preparation and administration. Refrigerate—don't freeze—the powder for injection. After reconstitution, protect the solution from light. The solution is stable for up to 8 hours if refrigerated.

Administration
! Give diphenhydramine 50 mg and acetaminophen 650 to 1000 mg 1 hour before administering gemtuzumab, as prescribed. Follow with acetaminophen 650 to 1000 mg every 4 hours for 2 doses, then every 4 hours as prescribed and as needed. Full recovery from hematologic toxicities is not a requirement for giving the second gemtuzumab dose.

Use strict aseptic technique in preparing the drug to protect the patient from infection. Prepare the drug in a biological safety hood with the fluorescent light off. Before reconstitution, let the vials come to room temperature. Using sterile syringes, reconstitute each vial with 5 ml sterile water for injection to provide a concentration of 1 mg/ml. Gently swirl the vial; then inspect for particulate matter or discoloration. Withdraw the desired volume from each vial and inject into an IV bag containing 100 ml 0.9% NaCl; place the IV bag into an ultraviolet protectant bag. Administer the solution as soon as it has been diluted in 100 ml 0.9% NaCl. Infuse the drug over 2 hours, using a separate peripheral or central line equipped with a low-protein-binding 1.2-micron filter. Don't give gemtuzumab by IV push or bolus.

Gentamicin
jen-ta-mye′sin
(Alcomicin [CAN], Cidomycin [CAN], Garamycin, Genoptic, Gentak, Gentacidin)

CATEGORY AND SCHEDULE
Pregnancy Risk Category: C

CLASSIFICATION
Anti-infectives, ophthalmic, otic, topical, antibiotics, aminoglycosides, dermatologics

MECHANISM OF ACTION
An aminoglycoside antibiotic that irreversibly binds to the protein of bacterial ribosomes. *Therapeutic Effect:* Interferes with protein synthesis of susceptible microorganisms. Bactericidal.

PHARMACOKINETICS
Rapid, complete absorption after IM administration. Protein binding: less than 30%. Widely distributed (doesn't cross the blood-brain barrier, low concentrations in CSF). Excreted unchanged in urine. Removed by hemodialysis. **Half-life:** 2-4 hr (increased in impaired renal function and neonates; decreased in cystic fibrosis and burn or febrile patients).

AVAILABILITY
Injection (Garamycin): 10 mg/ml, 40 mg/ml.
Ophthalmic Solution (Gentacidin, Genoptic, Gentak): 0.3%.
Ophthalmic Ointment (Gentak): 0.3%.
Cream (Garamycin): 0.1%.
Ointment: 0.1%.

INDICATIONS AND DOSAGES
▸ **Acute pelvic, bone, intra-abdominal, joint, respiratory tract, burn wound,**

postoperative, and skin or skin-structure infections; complicated UTIs; septicemia; meningitis
IV, IM
Adults, Elderly. Usual dosage, 3-6 mg/kg/day in divided doses q8hr or 4-6.6 mg/kg once a day.
Children 5-12 yr. Usual dosage 2-2.5 mg/kg/dose q8hr.
Children younger than 5 yr. Usual dosage, 2.5 mg/kg/dose q8hr.
Neonates. Usual dosage 2.5-3.5 mg/kg/dose q8-12hr.
▸ **Hemodialysis**
IV, IM
Adults, Elderly. 0.5-0.7 mg/kg/dose after dialysis.
Children. 1.25-1.75 mg/kg/dose after dialysis.
▸ **Intrathecal**
Adults. 4-8 mg/day.
Children 3 mo-12 yr. 1-2 mg/day.
Neonates. 1 mg/day.
▸ **Superficial eye infections**
OPHTHALMIC OINTMENT
Adults, Elderly. Usual dosage, apply thin strip to conjunctiva 2-3 times a day.
OPHTHALMIC SOLUTION
Adults, Elderly, Children. Usual dosage, 1-2 drops q2-4hr up to 2 drops/hr.
▸ **Superficial skin infections**
TOPICAL
Adults, Elderly. Usual dosage, apply 3-4 times/day.
▸ **Dosage in renal impairment**
Creatinine clearance greater than 40-60 ml/min. Dosage interval q12hr.
Creatinine clearance 20-40 ml/min. Dosage interval q24hr.
Creatinine clearance less than 20 ml/min. Monitor levels to determine dosage interval.

OFF-LABEL USES
Topical: Prophylaxis of minor bacterial skin infections, treatment of dermal ulcer

CONTRAINDICATIONS
Hypersensitivity to gentamicin, other aminoglycosides (cross-sensitivity), or their components. Sulfite sensitivity may result in anaphylaxis, especially in asthmatic patients.

INTERACTIONS
Drug
Nephrotoxic medications, other aminoglycosides, ototoxic medications: May increase the risk of nephrotoxicity or ototoxicity.
Neuromuscular blockers: May increase neuromuscular blockade.
Herbal
None known.
Food
None known.

DIAGNOSTIC TEST EFFECTS
May increase serum creatinine, serum bilirubin, BUN, serum LDH, SGOT (AST), and SGPT (ALT) levels. May decrease serum calcium, magnesium, potassium, and sodium concentrations. Therapeutic peak serum level is 6-10 mcg/ml and trough is 0.5-2 mcg/ml. Toxic peak serum level is greater than 10 mcg/ml, and trough is greater than 2 mcg/ml.

▨ IV INCOMPATIBILITIES
Allopurinol (Aloprim), amphotericin B complex (Abelcet, AmBisome, Amphotec), furosemide (Lasix), heparin, hetastarch (Hespan), idarubicin (Idamycin), indomethacin (Indocin), propofol (Diprivan)

▨ IV Compatibilities
Amiodarone (Cordarone), diltiazem (Cardizem), enalapril (Vasotec), filgrastim (Neupogen), hydromorphone (Dilaudid), insulin, lorazepam (Ativan), magnesium sulfate, midazolam (Versed), morphine, multivitamins

SIDE EFFECTS
Occasional
IM: Pain, induration
IV: Phlebitis, thrombophlebitis,
hypersensitivity reactions (fever,
pruritus, rash, urticaria)
Ophthalmic: Burning, tearing,
itching, blurred vision
Topical: Redness, itching
Rare
Alopecia, hypertension, weakness

SERIOUS REACTIONS
• Nephrotoxicity (as evidenced by
increased BUN and serum creatinine
levels and decreased creatinine clearance) may be reversible if the drug
is stopped at the first sign of
symptoms.
• Irreversible ototoxicity (manifested
as tinnitus, dizziness, ringing or roaring in the ears, and diminished hearing), and neurotoxicity (as evidenced
by headache, dizziness, lethargy,
tremor, and visual disturbances) occur
occasionally. The risk of these effects
increases with higher dosages or
prolonged therapy and when the
solution is applied directly to the
mucosa.
• Superinfections, particularly with
fungal infections, may result from
bacterial imbalance no matter which
administration route is used.
• Ophthalmic application may
cause paresthesia of conjunctiva or
mydriasis.

PRECAUTIONS & CONSIDERATIONS
! Cumulative gentamicin effects may
occur with concurrent systemic
administration and topical application
to large areas. Caution is warranted
with neuromuscular disorders because
of the potential for respiratory
depression, prior hearing loss, renal
impairment, vertigo, and in the
elderly and neonatal patients because
of age-related renal insufficiency

or immaturity. Gentamicin readily
crosses the placenta; it is unknown
if it is distributed in breast milk.
Age-related renal impairment may
require a dosage adjustment in
elderly patients.

Before giving gentamicin, determine if the patient has a history of
allergies, especially to aminoglycosides, sulfites, and parabens (for topical and ophthalmic forms). Expect to
correct dehydration before beginning
parenteral therapy. Establish baseline
hearing acuity before starting therapy. Intake and output and urinalysis
results should be monitored as well
as casts, RBCs, WBCs and decreased
specific gravity. Drink fluids to maintain adequate hydration. Monitor
urinalysis results for casts, RBCs,
WBCs, and decreased specific gravity. Be alert for ototoxic and neurotoxic side effects. If giving ophthalmic
gentamicin, monitor the patient's eye
for burning, itching, redness, and
tearing. If giving topical gentamicin,
monitor for itching and redness.
Be alert for signs and symptoms of
superinfection, particularly changes
in the oral mucosa, diarrhea, and
genital or anal pruritus. Monitor peak
and trough serum drug levels.
Storage
Store ophthalmic preparations and
solution vials for injection at room
temperature. The solution normally
appears clear or slightly yellow.
Intermittent IV infusion or IV piggyback solution is stable for 24 hours
at room temperature. Discard the IV
solution if a precipitate forms.
Administration
! Space parenteral doses evenly
around the clock. Gentamicin dosage
is based on ideal body weight. As
ordered, monitor peak and trough
serum drug levels periodically to
maintain the desired serum concentrations and to minimize the risk

of toxicity. The therapeutic peak serum level is 6 to 10 mcg/ml, and the therapeutic trough level is 0.5 to 2 mcg/ml. The toxic peak serum level is greater than 10 mcg/ml and the toxic trough level is greater than 2 mcg/ml.

For IV administration, dilute with 50 to 200 ml of D_5W or 0.9% NaCl. The amount of diluent for infants and children depends on individual needs. Infuse over 30 to 60 minutes for adults and older children. Infuse over 60 to 120 minutes for infants and young children.

Administer the IM injection slowly and deep in the gluteus maximus rather than the lateral aspect of thigh to minimize injection site pain.

For intrathecal administration, use only 2 mg/ml of the intrathecal preparation without preservative. Mix with 10% of the estimated CSF volume or NaCl. Use the intrathecal form immediately after preparation. Discard any unused portion. Give over 3 to 5 minutes.

For ophthalmic use, place a gloved finger on the lower eyelid and pull it out until a pocket is formed between the eye and lower lid. Hold the dropper above the pocket and place the correct number of drops (or 1/4 to 1/2 inch of ointment) into the pocket. Close the eye gently. After administering ophthalmic solution, apply digital pressure to the lacrimal sac for 1 to 2 minutes to minimize drainage into the nose and throat, thereby reducing the risk of systemic effects. After applying ophthalmic ointment, close the patient's eye for 1 to 2 minutes. Roll the eyeball to increase the drug's contact with the eye. Use tissue to remove excess solution or ointment around the eye.

Glatiramer
gla-teer′a-mer
(Copaxone)
Do not confuse Copaxone with Compazine.

CATEGORY AND SCHEDULE
Pregnancy Risk Category: B

CLASSIFICATION
Immunosuppressives

G

MECHANISM OF ACTION
An immunosuppressive whose exact mechanism is unknown. May act by modifying immune processes thought to be responsible for the pathogenesis of multiple sclerosis (MS). *Therapeutic Effect:* Slows progression of MS.

PHARMACOKINETICS
Substantial fraction of glatiramer is hydrolyzed locally. Some fraction of injected material enters lymphatic circulation, reaching regional lymph nodes; some may enter systemic circulation intact.

AVAILABILITY
Injection: 20 mg/ml in prefilled syringes.

INDICATIONS AND DOSAGES
▸ MS
SUBCUTANEOUS
Adults, Elderly. 20 mg once a day.

CONTRAINDICATIONS
Hypersensitivity to glatiramer or mannitol

INTERACTIONS
Drug
None known.

Herbal
None known.
Food
None known.

DIAGNOSTIC TEST EFFECTS
None known.

SIDE EFFECTS
Expected (73%-40%)
Pain, erythema, inflammation, or
pruritus at injection site; asthenia
Frequent (27%-18%)
Arthralgia, vasodilation, anxiety,
hypertonia, nausea, transient chest
pain, dyspnea, flu-like symptoms,
rash, pruritus
Occasional (17%-10%)
Palpitations, back pain, diaphoresis,
rhinitis, diarrhea, urinary urgency
Rare (8%-6%)
Anorexia, fever, neck pain, periph-
eral edema, ear pain, facial edema,
vertigo, vomiting

SERIOUS REACTIONS
* Infection is a common effect.
* Lymphadenopathy occurs occa-
  sionally.
* Hypertension may occur.
* Transient eosinophilia may occur.

PRECAUTIONS & CONSIDERATIONS
Caution is warranted with an immediate post-injection reaction, including anxiety, chest pain, dyspnea,
flushing, palpitations, and urticaria.
This reaction is usually transient and
self-limiting. Pregnancy should be
avoided during therapy. It is unknown
if glatiramer is distributed in breast
milk. The safety and efficacy of
glatiramer have not been established
in children. No information is available on glatiramer use in the elderly.
   Notify the physician of rash,
weakness, difficulty breathing or
swallowing, or itching or swelling of
the legs. Vital signs, including

temperature, should be obtained at
baseline.
Storage
Refrigerate syringes.
Administration
Administer as subcutaneous injection.

Glimepiride
gly-mep′er-ide
(Amaryl)
**Do not confuse glimepiride
with glipizide or glyburide.**

CATEGORY AND SCHEDULE
Pregnancy Risk Category: C

CLASSIFICATION
Antidiabetic agents, sulfonylureas,
second generation

MECHANISM OF ACTION
A second-generation sulfonylurea
that promotes release of insulin from
beta cells of the pancreas and
increases insulin sensitivity at peripheral sites. *Therapeutic Effect:* Lowers
blood glucose concentration.

PHARMACOKINETICS

Route	Onset	Peak	Duration
PO	N/A	2-3 hr	24 hr

Completely absorbed from the GI
tract. Protein binding: greater than
99%. Metabolized in the liver.
Excreted in urine and eliminated in
feces. **Half-life:** 5-9.2 hr.

AVAILABILITY
Tablets: 1 mg, 2 mg, 4 mg.

INDICATIONS AND DOSAGES
▶ **Diabetes mellitus**
PO
Adults, Elderly. Initially, 1-2 mg
once a day, with breakfast or first

main meal. Maintenance: 1-4 mg once a day. After dose of 2 mg is reached, dosage should be increased in increments of up to 2 mg q1-2wk, based on blood glucose response. Maximum: 8 mg/day.

▸ **Dosage in renal impairment**
PO
Adults. 1 mg once/day.

CONTRAINDICATIONS
Diabetic complications, such as ketosis, acidosis, and diabetic coma; severe hepatic or renal impairment; monotherapy for type 1 diabetes mellitus; stress situations, including severe infection, trauma, and surgery

INTERACTIONS
Drug
Beta-blockers: May increase the hypoglycemic effect of glimepiride and mask signs of hypoglycemia.
Cimetidine, ciprofloxacin, fluconazole, MAOIs, quinidine, ranitidine, large doses of salicylates: May increase the effects of glimepiride.
Corticosteroids, lithium, thiazide diuretics: May decrease the effects of glimepiride.
Oral anticoagulants: May increase the effects of oral anticoagulants.
Herbal
None known.
Food
Hypoglycemia is more likely to occur if alcohol is ingested.

DIAGNOSTIC TEST EFFECTS
May increase BUN and LDH concentrations and serum alkaline phosphatase, creatinine, and AST (SGOT) levels.

SIDE EFFECTS
Frequent
Altered taste sensation, dizziness, somnolence, weight gain, constipation, diarrhea, heartburn, nausea, vomiting, stomach fullness, headache
Occasional
Increased sensitivity of skin to sunlight, peeling of skin, itching, rash

SERIOUS REACTIONS
• Overdose or insufficient food intake may produce hypoglycemia, especially with increased glucose demands.
• GI hemorrhage, cholestatic hepatic jaundice, leukopenia, thrombocytopenia, pancytopenia, agranulocytosis, and aplastic or hemolytic anemia occur rarely.

PRECAUTIONS & CONSIDERATIONS
Caution is warranted with adrenal insufficiency, debilitation, hepatic disease, impaired renal function, intestinal obstruction, malnutrition, pituitary insufficiency, prolonged vomiting, severe diarrhea, and uncontrolled hyperthyroidism. Be alert to conditions that alter blood glucose requirements, such as fever, increased activity, stress, or a surgical procedure. Glimepiride use is not recommended during pregnancy. It is unknown if glimepiride is distributed in breast milk. Safety and efficacy of glimepiride have not been established in children. Hypoglycemia may be difficult to recognize in the elderly. Also, age-related renal impairment may increase sensitivity to glucose-lowering effect. Wear sunscreen and protective eyewear to prevent the effects of light sensitivity.

Food intake and blood glucose should be monitored before and during therapy. Be aware of signs and symptoms of hypoglycemia (anxiety, cool wet skin, diplopia, dizziness, headache, hunger, numbness in mouth, tachycardia, tremors), or hyperglycemia (deep rapid breathing, dim vision, fatigue, nausea,

polydipsia, polyphagia, polyuria, vomiting); carry candy, sugar packets, or other sugar supplements for immediate response to hypoglycemia. Consult the physician when glucose demands are altered (such as with fever, heavy physical activity, infection, stress, trauma). Exercise, good personal hygiene (including foot care), not smoking, and weight control are essential parts of therapy.
Administration
Take glimepiride with breakfast or first main meal.

Glipizide
glip'i-zide
(Glucotrol, Glucotrol XL, Melizide [AUS], Minidiab [AUS])
Do not confuse glipizide with glimepiride or glyburide.

CATEGORY AND SCHEDULE
Pregnancy Risk Category: C

CLASSIFICATION
Antidiabetic agents, sulfonylureas, second generation

MECHANISM OF ACTION
A second-generation sulfonylurea that promotes the release of insulin from beta cells of the pancreas and increases insulin sensitivity at peripheral sites. *Therapeutic Effect:* Lowers blood glucose concentration.

PHARMACOKINETICS

Route	Onset	Peak	Duration
PO	15-30 min	2-3 hr	12-24 hr
Extended-release	2-3 hr	6-12 hr	24 hr

Well absorbed from the GI tract. Protein binding: 99%. Metabolized in the liver. Excreted in urine. **Half-life:** 2-4 hr.

AVAILABILITY
Tablets (Glucotrol): 5 mg, 10 mg.
Tablets (Extended-Release [Glucotrol XL]): 2.5 mg, 5 mg, 10 mg.

INDICATIONS AND DOSAGES
▸ **Diabetes mellitus**
PO
Adults. Initially, 5 mg/day or 2.5 mg in the elderly or those with hepatic disease. Adjust dosage in 2.5- to 5-mg increments at intervals of several days. Maximum single dose: 15 mg. Maximum dose/day: 40 mg. Maintenance (extended-release tablet): 20 mg/day.
Elderly. Initially, 2.5-5 mg/day. May increase by 2.5-5 mg/day q1-2wk.

CONTRAINDICATIONS
Diabetic ketoacidosis with or without coma, type 1 diabetes mellitus

INTERACTIONS
Drug
Beta-blockers: May increase the hypoglycemic effect of glipizide and mask signs of hypoglycemia.
Cimetidine, ciprofloxacin, fluconazole, MAOIs, quinidine, ranitidine, large doses of salicylates: May increase the effects of glipizide.
Corticosteroids, lithium, thiazide diuretics: May decrease the effects of glipizide.
Oral anticoagulants: May increase the effects of oral anticoagulants.
Herbal
None known.
Food
Hypoglycemia is more likely to occur if alcohol is ingested.

DIAGNOSTIC TEST EFFECTS
May increase BUN and LDH concentrations and serum alkaline

phosphatase, creatinine, and AST (SGOT) levels.

SIDE EFFECTS
Frequent
Altered taste sensation, dizziness, somnolence, weight gain, constipation, diarrhea, heartburn, nausea, vomiting, stomach fullness, headache
Occasional
Increased sensitivity of skin to sunlight, peeling of skin, itching, rash

SERIOUS REACTIONS
• Overdose or insufficient food intake may produce hypoglycemia, especially with increased glucose demands.
• GI hemorrhage, cholestatic hepatic jaundice, leukopenia, thrombocytopenia, pancytopenia, agranulocytosis, and aplastic or hemolytic anemia occurs rarely.

PRECAUTIONS & CONSIDERATIONS
Caution is warranted with adrenal or pituitary insufficiency, hypoglycemic reactions, and impaired hepatic or renal function. Be alert to conditions that alter blood glucose requirements, such as fever, increased activity, stress, or a surgical procedure. Insulin is the drug of choice during pregnancy. Glipizide given within 1 month of delivery may produce neonatal hypoglycemia. Glipizide crosses the placenta and is distributed in breast milk. Safety and efficacy of glipizide have not been established in children. Hypoglycemia may be difficult to recognize in the elderly. Also, age-related renal impairment may increase sensitivity to the glucose-lowering effect. Wear sunscreen and protective eyewear to prevent the effects of light sensitivity.

Food intake and blood glucose should be monitored before and during therapy. Be aware of signs and symptoms of hypoglycemia (anxiety, cool wet skin, diplopia, dizziness, headache, hunger, numbness in mouth, tachycardia, tremors), or hyperglycemia (deep rapid breathing, dim vision, fatigue, nausea, polydipsia, polyphagia, polyuria, vomiting); carry candy, sugar packets, or other sugar supplements for immediate response to hypoglycemia. Consult the physician when glucose demands are altered (such as with fever, heavy physical activity, infection, stress, trauma). Exercise, good personal hygiene (including foot care), not smoking, and weight control are essential parts of therapy.
Administration
Take glipizide with food; however the response is better if given 15 to 30 minutes before meals. Do not crush extended-release tablets.

Glucagon Hydrochloride
gloo'ka-gon
(GlucaGen, GlucaGen Diagnostic Kit, Glucagen [AUS], Glucagon, Glucagon Diagnostic Kit, Glucagon Emergency Kit)
Do not confuse glucagon with Glaucon.

CATEGORY AND SCHEDULE
Pregnancy Risk Category: B

CLASSIFICATION
Antihypoglycemics, hormones/hormone modifiers

MECHANISM OF ACTION
A glucose elevating agent that promotes hepatic glycogenolysis,

gluconeogenesis. Stimulates production of cyclic adenosine monophosphate (cAMP), which results in increased plasma glucose concentration, smooth muscle relaxation, and an inotropic myocardial effect. *Therapeutic Effect:* Increases plasma glucose level.

AVAILABILITY
Powder for Injection: 1 mg.

INDICATIONS AND DOSAGES
▸ **Hypoglycemia**
IV, IM, SUBCUTANEOUS
Adults, Elderly, Children weighing more than 20 kg. 0.5-1 mg. May give 1 or 2 additional doses if response is delayed.
Children weighing 20 kg or less. 0.5 mg.
▸ **Diagnostic aid**
IV, IM
Adults, Elderly. 0.25-2 mg 10 min prior to procedure.

OFF-LABEL USES
Treatment of esophageal obstruction due to foreign bodies, toxicity associated with beta blockers or calcium channel blockers

CONTRAINDICATIONS
Hypersensitivity to glucagon or beef or pork proteins, known pheochromocytoma

INTERACTIONS
Drug
Anticoagulants: May increase the effects of these drugs.
Herbal
None known.
Food
None known.

DIAGNOSTIC TEST EFFECTS
May decrease serum potassium level.

▓ IV INCOMPATIBILITIES
Don't mix glucagon with any other medications.

SIDE EFFECTS
Occasional
Nausea, vomiting
Rare
Allergic reaction, such as urticaria, respiratory distress, and hypotension

SERIOUS REACTIONS
• Overdose may produce persistent nausea and vomiting and hypokalemia, marked by severe weakness, decreased appetite, irregular heartbeat, and muscle cramps.

PRECAUTIONS & CONSIDERATIONS
Caution is warranted with a history suggestive of insulinoma or pheochromocytoma. Be aware of how to recognize symptoms of hypoglycemia, including anxiety, increased sweating, difficulty concentrating, headache, hunger, nausea, nervousness, pale and cool skin, shakiness, unusual fatigue, weakness, and unconsciousness. Treat early signs of hypoglycemia with a simple sugar first, such as hard candy, honey, orange juice, sugar cubes, or table sugar dissolved in water or juice, followed by a protein source, such as cheese and crackers, half a sandwich, or a glass of milk.
Storage
Store vials at room temperature. After reconstitution, the solution is stable for 48 hours if refrigerated. If reconstituted with sterile water for injection, use it immediately. Do not use glucagon solution unless it's clear.
Administration
❗ Place the patient on side to avoid

aspiration because glucagon (as well as hypoglycemia) may produce nausea and vomiting. Administer IV dextrose if the patient fails to respond to glucagon.

Reconstitute the powder with the diluent supplied by the manufacturer when preparing doses of 2 mg or less. For doses greater than 2 mg, dilute with sterile water for injection. To provide 1 mg glucagon/ml, reconstitute the 1-mg vial with 1 ml diluent. The patient will usually awaken in 5 to 20 minutes. If the patient fails to respond after 1 or 2 additional doses, give IV glucose as prescribed. When the patient awakens, give oral carbohydrates to restore hepatic glycogen stores and prevent secondary hypoglycemia. If the patient does not awaken within 20 minutes, administer IV dextrose.

Glyburide
glye′byoor-ide
(Daonil [CAN], DiaBeta, Euglucon [CAN], Glimel [AUS], Glynase, Micronase, Semi-Daonil [AUS], Semi-Euglucon [AUS])
Do not confuse glyburide with glimepiride or glipizide, or Micronase with Micro-K, Micronor.

CATEGORY AND SCHEDULE
Pregnancy Risk Category: C

CLASSIFICATION
Antidiabetic agents, sulfonylureas, second generation

MECHANISM OF ACTION
A second-generation sulfonylurea that promotes release of insulin from beta cells of the pancreas and increases insulin sensitivity at peripheral sites. *Therapeutic Effect:* Lowers blood glucose concentration.

PHARMACOKINETICS

Route	Onset	Peak	Duration
PO	0.25-1 hr	1-2 hr	12-24 hr

Well absorbed from the GI tract. Protein binding: 99%. Metabolized in the liver to weakly active metabolite. Primarily excreted in urine. Not removed by hemodialysis. **Half-life:** 1.4-1.8 hr.

AVAILABILITY
Tablets (DiaBeta, Micronase): 1.25 mg, 2.5 mg, 5 mg.
Tablets (Glynase): 1.5 mg, 3 mg, 6 mg.

INDICATIONS AND DOSAGES
▸ **Diabetes mellitus**
PO
Adults. Initially 2.5-5 mg. May increase by 2.5 mg/day at weekly intervals. Maintenance: 1.25-20 mg/day. Maximum: 20 mg/day.
Elderly. Initially, 1.25-2.5 mg/day. May increase by 1.25-2.5 mg/day at 1- to 3-wk intervals.
PO (MICRONIZED TABLETS [GLYNASE])
Adults, Elderly. Initially 0.75-3 mg/day. May increase by 1.5 mg/day at weekly intervals. Maintenance: 0.75-12 mg/day as a single dose or in divided doses.
▸ **Dosage in renal impairment**
Glyburide is not recommended in patients with creatinine clearance less than 50 ml/min.

CONTRAINDICATIONS
Diabetic ketoacidosis with or without coma, monotherapy for type 1 diabetes mellitus

INTERACTIONS
Drug
Beta-blockers: May increase the hypoglycemic effect of glyburide and mask signs of hypoglycemia.
Cimetidine, ciprofloxacin, fluconazole, MAOIs, quinidine, ranitidine, large doses of salicylates: May increase the effects of glyburide.
Corticosteroids, lithium, thiazide diuretics: May decrease the effects of glyburide.
Oral anticoagulants: May increase the effects of oral anticoagulants.
Herbal
None known.
Food
None known.

DIAGNOSTIC TEST EFFECTS
May increase BUN and LDH concentrations and serum alkaline phosphatase, creatinine, and AST (SGOT) levels.

SIDE EFFECTS
Frequent
Altered taste sensation, dizziness, somnolence, weight gain, constipation, diarrhea, heartburn, nausea, vomiting, stomach fullness, headache
Occasional
Increased sensitivity of skin to sunlight, peeling of skin, itching, rash

SERIOUS REACTIONS
• Overdose or insufficient food intake may produce hypoglycemia, especially in patients with increased glucose demands.
• Cholestatic jaundice, leukopenia, thrombocytopenia, pancytopenia, agranulocytosis, and aplastic or hemolytic anemia occur rarely.

PRECAUTIONS & CONSIDERATIONS
Caution is warranted with adrenal or pituitary insufficiency, hypoglycemic reactions, and impaired hepatic or renal function. Be alert to conditions that alter blood glucose requirements, such as fever, increased activity, stress, or a surgical procedure. Insulin is the drug of choice during pregnancy. Glyburide crosses the placenta and is distributed in breast milk. Glyburide use within 2 weeks of delivery may produce neonatal hypoglycemia. Safety and efficacy of glyburide have not been established in children. Hypoglycemia may be difficult to recognize in the elderly. Also, age-related renal impairment may increase sensitivity to the glucose-lowering effect. Wear sunscreen and protective eyewear to prevent the effects of light sensitivity.

Food intake and blood glucose should be monitored before and during therapy. Be aware of signs and symptoms of hypoglycemia (anxiety, cool wet skin, diplopia, dizziness, headache, hunger, numbness in mouth, tachycardia, tremors), or hyperglycemia (deep rapid breathing, dim vision, fatigue, nausea, polydipsia, polyphagia, polyuria, vomiting); carry candy, sugar packets, or other sugar supplements for immediate response to hypoglycemia. Consult the physician when glucose demands are altered (such as with fever, heavy physical activity, infection, stress, trauma). Exercise, good personal hygiene (including foot care), not smoking, and weight control are essential parts of therapy.
Storage
Store at room temperature in a tightly closed container.
Administration
Take glyburide with food to reduce GI symptoms.

Glycerin

gli´ser-in

(Bausch & Lomb Computer Eye Drops, Fleet Bablylax, Fleet Liquid Glycerin Suppositories for Adults and Children, Fleet Maximum-Strength Glycerin Suppositories, Fleet Glycerin Suppositories for Adults, Fleet Glycerin Suppositories for Children, Glyrol, Osmoglyn, Sani-Supp)

CATEGORY AND SCHEDULE

Pregnancy Risk Category: B

OTC (suppositories)

CLASSIFICATION

Ophthalmics

MECHANISM OF ACTION

An osmotic dehydrating agent that increases osmotic pressure and draws fluid into colon and stimulates evacuation of inspissated feces. Lowers both intraocular and intracranial pressure by osmotic dehydrating effects. Increases blood flow to ischemic areas, decreases serum free fatty acids, and increases synthesis of glycerides in the brain.
Therapeutic Effect: Aids in fecal evacuation.

PHARMACOKINETICS

Well absorbed after PO administration but poorly absorbed after rectal administration. Widely distributed to extracellular space. Rapidly metabolized in liver. Primarily excreted in urine. **Half-life:** 30-45 min.

AVAILABILITY

Ophthalmic solution: 1% (Bausch & Lomb Computer Eye Drops).
Oral Solution: 50% (Osmoglyn).
Rectal Solution: 2.3 g (Fleet Babylax), 5.6 g (Fleet Liquid Glycerin Suppositories).
Suppositories: 1 g (Fleet Glycerin Suppositories for Children), 2 g (Fleet Glycerin Suppositories), 3 g (Fleet Maximum-Strength Glycerin Suppositories), 82.5% (Sani-Supp).

INDICATIONS AND DOSAGES

▸ **Constipation**
RECTAL
Adults, Elderly, Children 6 yr and older. 3 g/day.
Children younger than 6 yr. 1-1.5 g/day.
▸ **Ophthalmologic procedures**
OPHTHALMIC
Adults, Elderly, Children. 1 or 2 drops prior to examination q3-4hr.
▸ **Reduction of intracranial pressure**
PO
Adults, Elderly, Children. 1.5 g/kg/day q4hr or 1 g/kg/dose q6hr.
▸ **Reduction of intraocular pressure**
PO
Adults, Elderly, Children. 1-1.8 g/kg 1-1.5 hr preoperatively.

OFF-LABEL USES

Viral meningoencephalitis

CONTRAINDICATIONS

Hypersensitivity to any component in the preparation, well-established anuria, severe dehydration, frank or impending acute pulmonary edema, severe cardiac decompensation

INTERACTIONS

Drug
PO medications: May decrease transit time of concurrently administered oral medication, decreasing absorption.
Herbal
Licorice: May increase risk of hypokalemia

Food
None known.

DIAGNOSTIC TEST EFFECTS
May suppress wheal and flare reactions to antigen skin testing unless antihistamines are discontinued 4 days before testing.

SIDE EFFECTS
Frequent
Oral: Nausea, headache, vomiting
Rectal: Some degree of abdominal discomfort, nausea, mild cramps, headache, vomiting
Occasional
Oral: Diarrhea, dizziness, dry mouth or increased thirst
Ophthalmic: pain and irritation may occur upon instillation
Rectal: faintness, weakness, abdominal pain, bloating

SERIOUS REACTIONS
• Laxative abuse includes symptoms of abdominal pain, weakness, fatigue, thirst, vomiting, edema, bone pain, fluid and electrolyte imbalance, hypoalbuminemia, and syndromes that mimic colitis.

PRECAUTIONS & CONSIDERATIONS
Caution is warranted with diabetes mellitus; hemolytic anemia; altered hydration; cardiac, renal, or hepatic disease. It is unknown if glycerin crosses the placenta or is excreted in breast milk. There are no age-related precautions noted in children. Be aware that glycerin may increase risk of dehydration in the elderly because it reduces water in the body. Unrelieved constipation, dizziness, muscle cramps or pain, rectal bleeding, confusion, irregular heartbeat, and weakness should be reported.
Storage
Discard ophthalmic preparation 6 months after dropper is first placed in the drug solution. Store at room temperature away from damp places like the bathroom or near the kitchen sink as well as heat and direct light because it may cause the medicine to break down.
Administration
Instill ophthalmic drops of solution in each lower conjunctival sac. Gently massage the closed eyelids to help spread the solution to all areas of the conjunctiva. Gently wipe away excess solution from the eyelids and surrounding skin with sterile cotton.

Mix oral glycerin with orange or lemon juice to unflavored 50% oral solution. Pour solution over crushed ice and drink through a straw to improve palatability. May administer doses at 5-hour intervals for reduction of intraocular pressure.

If rectal suppository is too soft, chill for 30 minutes in refrigerator or run cold water over foil wrapper. Moisten suppository with cold water before inserting well into rectum. Lay on left side. Insert suppository high in rectum and retain for 15 minutes. If administering liquid glycerin rectally, gently insert stem with steady pressure at tip pointing toward the navel and squeeze unit until almost all the liquid has been delivered. A small amount of liquid will remain. Withdraw unit.

Increase fluid intake, exercise, and eat a high-fiber diet to promote defecation.

Warn the patient to notify the physician if he or she experiences unrelieved constipation, dizziness, muscle cramps or pain, rectal bleeding, confusion, irregular heartbeat, and weakness.

Tell the patient to lie down during or after oral solution to minimize risk of developing headache.

Glycopyrrolate

glye-koe-pye′roe-late
(Robinul, Robinul Forte, Robinul
Injection [AUS])
Do not confuse with Reminyl.

CATEGORY AND SCHEDULE
Pregnancy Risk Category: B

CLASSIFICATION
Anticholinergics, gastrointestinals

MECHANISM OF ACTION
A quaternary anticholinergic that
inhibits action of acetylcholine at
postganglionic parasympathetic sites
in smooth muscle, secretory glands,
and CNS. *Therapeutic Effect:*
Reduces salivation and excessive
secretions of respiratory tract; reduces
gastric secretions and acidity.

AVAILABILITY
Injection: 0.2 mg/ml.

INDICATIONS AND DOSAGES
▸ **Preoperative inhibition of saliva-
tion and excessive respiratory tract
secretions**
IM
Adults, Elderly. 4.4 mcg/kg
30-60 min before procedure.
Children 2 yr and older. 4.4 mcg/kg.
Children younger than 2 yr.
4.4-8.8 mcg/kg.
▸ **To block effects of anti-
cholinesterase agents**
IV
Adults, Elderly. 0.2 mg for each
1 mg neostigmine or 5 mg pyri-
dostigmine.

CONTRAINDICATIONS
Acute hemorrhage, myasthenia gravis,
narrow-angle glaucoma, obstructive
uropathy, paralytic ileus, tachycardia,
ulcerative colitis, obstructive
diseases of the GI tract

INTERACTIONS
Drug
Antacids, antidiarrheals: May
decrease the absorption of glycopy-
rrolate.
Ketoconazole: May decrease the
absorption of ketoconazole.
Other anticholinergics: May
increase the effects of glycopyrrolate.
Potassium chloride: May increase
the severity of GI lesions with the
wax matrix formulation of potassium
chloride.
Herbal
None known.
Food
None known.

DIAGNOSTIC TEST EFFECTS
May decrease serum uric acid levels.

▓ IV INCOMPATIBILITIES
None known.
🖢 IV Compatibilities
Diphenhydramine (Benadryl),
droperidol (Inapsine), hydromor-
phone (Dilaudid), hydroxyzine
(Vistaril), lidocaine, midazolam
(Versed), morphine, promethazine
(Phenergan)

SIDE EFFECTS
Frequent
Dry mouth, decreased sweating,
constipation
Occasional
Blurred vision, gastric bloating,
urinary hesitancy, somnolence (with
high dosage), headache, intolerance
to light, loss of taste, nervousness,
flushing, insomnia, impotence, mental
confusion or excitement (particularly
in the elderly and children), temporary light-headedness (with
parenteral form), local irritation
(with parenteral form)

G

Rare
Dizziness, faintness

SERIOUS REACTIONS
• Overdose may produce temporary paralysis of ciliary muscle; pupillary dilation; tachycardia; palpitations; hot, dry, or flushed skin; absence of bowel sounds; hyperthermia; increased respiratory rate; EKG abnormalities; nausea; vomiting; rash over face or upper trunk; CNS stimulation; and psychosis (marked by agitation, restlessness, rambling speech, visual hallucinations, paranoid behavior, and delusions, followed by depression).

PRECAUTIONS & CONSIDERATIONS
Caution is warranted with CHF, diarrhea, fever, GI infections, hepatic or renal disease, hypothyroidism, and reflux esophagitis. Avoid hot baths, saunas, and becoming overheated while exercising in hot weather because they may cause heat stroke. Tasks that require mental alertness or motor skills should also be avoided until response to the drug has been established. Antacids or antidiarrheals should not be taken within 1 hour of taking glycopyrrolate because they will decrease glycopyrrolate's effectiveness.

Dry mouth may occur. B/P, body temperature, heart rate, pattern of daily bowel activity and stool consistency, and urine output should be monitored. The person should void before giving the drug to reduce the risk of urine retention.

Administration
For direct injection, administer undiluted through the tubing of a free-flowing compatible IV solution.

For IM use, administer undiluted or diluted with D_5W, $D_{10}W$, or 0.9% NaCl.

Gold Sodium Thiomalate
gold so'dee-um thye-oh-mah'late
(Myochrysine, Myocrisin [AUS])

CATEGORY AND SCHEDULE
Pregnancy Risk Category: C

CLASSIFICATION
Disease modifying antirheumatic drugs, gold compounds

MECHANISM OF ACTION
A gold compound whose mechanism of action is unknown. May decrease prostaglandin synthesis or alter cellular mechanisms by inhibiting sulfhydryl systems. *Therapeutic Effect:* Decreases synovial inflammation, retards cartilage and bone destruction, suppresses or prevents — but does not cure — arthritis and synovitis.

AVAILABILITY
Injection: 50 mg/ml.

INDICATIONS AND DOSAGES
▸ **Rheumatoid arthritis**
IM
Adults, Elderly. Initially, 10 mg, followed by 25 mg for second dose, then 25-50 mg/wk until improvement noted or total of 1 g has been administered. Maintenance: 25-50 mg q2wk for 2-20 wk; if stable, may increase intervals to q3-4wk.
Children. Initially, 10 mg, then 1 mg/kg/wk up to a maximum single dose of 50 mg. Maintenance: 1 mg/kg/dose q2-4wk.
▸ **Dosage in renal impairment**
Dosage is modified based on creatinine clearance.

Creatinine Clearance	Dosage
50-80 ml/min	50% of usual dose
Less than 50 ml/min	Not recommended

OFF-LABEL USES
Treatment of psoriatic arthritis

CONTRAINDICATIONS
Colitis; concurrent use of antimalarials, immunosuppressive agents, penicillamine, or phenylbutazone; CHF; exfoliative dermatitis; history of blood dyscrasias; severe hepatic or renal impairment; systemic lupus erythematosus

INTERACTIONS
Drug
Bone marrow depressants, hepatotoxic and nephrotoxic medications: May increase the risk of toxicity.
Penicillamine: May increase the risk of adverse hematologic or renal effects.
Herbal
None known.
Food
None known.

DIAGNOSTIC TEST EFFECTS
May decrease Hgb level, Hct, and WBC and platelet counts. May increase urine protein level. May alter liver function test results.

SIDE EFFECTS
Frequent
Pruritic dermatitis, stomatitis, diarrhea, abdominal pain, nausea
Occasional
Vomiting, anorexia, flatulence, dyspepsia, conjunctivitis, photosensitivity
Rare
Constipation, urticaria, rash

SERIOUS REACTIONS
• Signs and symptoms of gold toxicity include decreased Hgb level, decreased granulocyte count (less than $150,000/mm^3$), proteinuria, hematuria, blood dyscrasias (anemia, leukopenia [WBC less than $4000 mm^3$], thrombocytopenia, and eosinophilia), glomerulonephritis, nephrotic syndrome, and cholestatic jaundice.

PRECAUTIONS & CONSIDERATIONS   G
Avoid exposure to sunlight, which may turn skin gray or blue. Oral hygiene should be diligently maintained to help prevent stomatitis.
    Pattern of daily bowel activity and stool consistency, urine for hematuria and proteinuria, CBC (particularly Hgb level, Hct, and WBC and platelet counts), renal and liver function tests (especially BUN level and serum alkaline phosphatase, creatinine, AST [SGOT], and ALT [SGPT] levels), skin for rash, and oral mucous membranes for stomatitis should be monitored. Therapeutic response, including improved grip strength, increased joint mobility, reduced joint tenderness, and relief of pain, stiffness, and swelling, should also be assessed.
Administration
! Give gold sodium thiomalate as weekly injections, as prescribed.
    Therapeutic effect may take 6 months or longer to appear.

Gonadorelin Acetate/ Gonadorelin Hydrochloride
goe-nad-oh-rell'-in
(Factrel)

CATEGORY AND SCHEDULE
Pregnancy Risk Category: B

CLASSIFICATION
Hormones/hormone modifiers, stimulants, ovarian

MECHANISM OF ACTION
A synthetic luteinzing hormone that binds to specific transmembrane glycoprotein receptors on gonadotrophic cells of the anterior pituitary which then stimulates synthesis and secretion of gonadotropins through mobilization of intracellular calcium, activation of protein kinase C, and gene transcription. *Therapeutic Effect:* Stimulates synthesis, release of luteinizing hormone (LH), follicle-stimulating hormone (FSH) from anterior pituitary. Stimulates release of gonadotropin-releasing hormone from hypothalamus.

PHARMACOKINETICS
Maximal LH release occurs within 20 minutes. Metabolized in plasma. Excreted in urine as inactive metabolites. **Half-life:** 4 min.

AVAILABILITY
Powder for reconstitution, as hydrochloride: 100 mcg (Factrel).

INDICATIONS AND DOSAGES
▸ **Gonadotropin function evaluation**
IV/SUBCUTANEOUS
Adults. 100 mcg. In females, perform test in early follicular phase of menstrual cycle.

CONTRAINDICATIONS
Any condition exacerbated by pregnancy, patients with ovarian cysts or causes of anovulation other than hypothalamic origin, the presence of a hormonally-dependent tumor, any conditions worsened by an increase of reproductive hormones, hypersensitivity to gonadorelin acetate or hydrochloride

SIDE EFFECTS
Occasional
Swelling, pain, or itching at injection site with subcutanous administration, local or generalized skin rash with chronic subcutaneous administration
Rare
Headache, nausea, lightheadedness, abdominal discomfort, hypersensitivity reactions (bronchospasm, tachycardia, flushing, urticaria), induration at injection site

SERIOUS REACTIONS
• Anaphylactic reaction occurs rarely.

PRECAUTIONS & CONSIDERATIONS
Caution is warranted with pregnancy because gonadorelin could worsen pre-existing conditions like pituitary prolactinemia. Caution should also be used with concurrent use of drugs which directly affect the pituitary secretion of gonadotropin, including androgens, estrogens, progestins, glucocorticoids, spironolactone, levodopa, oral contraceptives, digoxin, phenothiazines and dopamine antagonists which would affect a rise in prolactin. It is unknown if gonadorelin crosses the placenta or is distributed in breast milk. Safety and efficacy have not been established in children. There are no age-related precautions noted in the elderly.
Storage
Store at room temperature. Discard reconstituted product after 24 hours.

Administration
Using standard aseptic technique, add 1 ml of diluent provided to the 100-mcg vial or 2 ml of diluent to the 500-mcg vial. Administer within the early follicular phase of the menstrual cycle, if it can be determined. The solution should be made immediately before use. Unused reconstituted solution and diluent should be discarded.

Goserelin
go'seh-rel-in
(Zoladex, Zoladex Implant [AUS], Zoladex LA)

CATEGORY AND SCHEDULE
Pregnancy Risk Category: D (advanced breast cancer), X (endometriosis, endometrial thinning)

CLASSIFICATION
Antineoplastics, hormones/hormone modifiers, gonadotropin-releasing hormone analogs

MECHANISM OF ACTION
A gonadotropin-releasing hormone analogue and antineoplastic agent that stimulates the release of luteinizing hormone (LH) and follicle-stimulating hormone (FSH) from the anterior pituitary gland. In males, increases testosterone concentrations initially, then suppresses secretion of LH and FSH, resulting in decreased testosterone levels. *Therapeutic Effect:* In females, causes a reduction in ovarian size and function, reduction in uterine and mammary gland size, and regression of sex-hormone-responsive tumors. In males, produces pharmacologic castration and decreases the growth of abnormal prostate tissue.

AVAILABILITY
Implant: 3.6 mg, 10.8 mg.

INDICATIONS AND DOSAGES
▶ **Prostatic carcinoma**
IMPLANT
Adults older than 18 yr, Elderly. 3.6 mg every 28 days or 10.8 mg q12wk subcutaneously into upper abdominal wall.
▶ **Breast carcinoma, endometriosis**
IMPLANT
Adults. 3.6 mg every 28 days subcutaneously into upper abdominal wall.
▶ **Endometrial thinning**
IMPLANT
Adults. 3.6 mg subcutaneously into upper abdominal wall as a single dose or in 2 doses 4 wk apart.

CONTRAINDICATIONS
Pregnancy; hypersensitivity to goserelin products, leutenizing hormone–releasing hormone (LHRH), or LHRH analogues.

INTERACTIONS
Drug
None known.
Herbal
None known.
Food
None known.

DIAGNOSTIC TEST EFFECTS
May increase serum prostatic acid phosphatase and testosterone levels.

SIDE EFFECTS
Frequent
Headache (60%), hot flashes (55%), depression (54%), diaphoresis (45%), sexual dysfunction (21%), decreased erection (18%), lower urinary tract symptoms (13%)
Occasional (10%-5%)
Pain, lethargy, dizziness, insomnia, anorexia, nausea, rash, upper

respiratory tract infection, hirsutism, abdominal pain
Rare
Pruritus

SERIOUS REACTIONS
• Arrhythmias, CHF, and hypertension occur rarely.
• Ureteral obstruction and spinal cord compression have been observed. An immediate orchiectomy may be necessary if these conditions occur.
• Deep vein thrombosis has been reported.

PRECAUTIONS & CONSIDERATIONS
Goserelin crosses the placenta and may cause fetal harm. Women who are or may be pregnant shouldn't use this drug. Pregnancy should be determined before beginning therapy. Females should use nonhormonal contraceptive measures during therapy. It is unknown if goserelin is excreted in breast milk. The safety and efficacy of goserelin have not been established in children. No age-related precautions have been noted in the elderly.

Females should notify the physician if regular menstruation persists or if she becomes pregnant. Breakthrough bleeding may occur if a goserelin dose is missed. Signs and symptoms of worsening of prostatic cancer, especially in the first month, should be monitored.

Administration
For implant, inspect the package for damage before opening. If the package is damaged, don't use the syringe. Remove the sterile syringe from the package immediately before use. Examine the syringe for damage, and check that goserelin is visible in the translucent chamber. Clean an area of skin on the upper abdominal wall with an alcohol swab. Grasp the safety clip tab, pull it out and

away from the needle, and discard it immediately. Then remove the needle cover. Using aseptic technique, stretch or pinch the patient's skin with one hand, and grip the syringe barrel. Insert the needle into the subcutaneous tissue.

! The goserelin syringe should not be used for aspiration. If the needle penetrates a large vessel, you'll see blood instantly in the syringe chamber. If a vessel is penetrated, withdraw the needle and use a new syringe elsewhere.

Direct the needle so that it parallels the abdominal wall. Push the needle in until the barrel hub touches the patient's skin. Withdraw the needle 1 cm to create a space to discharge goserelin. Fully depress the plunger to discharge the drug. Withdraw the needle. Then bandage the site. Confirm the discharge of goserelin by ensuring that the tip of the plunger is visible within the tip of the needle. Dispose of the used needle and syringe in a safe manner.

Granisetron
gra-ni′se-tron
(Kytril)

CATEGORY AND SCHEDULE
Pregnancy Risk Category: B

CLASSIFICATION
Antiemetics/antivertigo, serotonin receptor antagonists

MECHANISM OF ACTION
A 5-HT$_3$ receptor antagonist that acts centrally in the chemoreceptor trigger zone or peripherally at the vagal nerve terminals. *Therapeutic Effect:* Prevents nausea and vomiting.

PHARMACOKINETICS

Route	Onset	Peak	Duration
IV	1-3 min	N/A	24 hr

Rapidly and widely distributed to tissues. Protein binding: 65%. Metabolized in the liver to active metabolite. Eliminated in urine and feces. **Half-life:** 10-12 hr (increased in the elderly).

AVAILABILITY
Oral Solution: 1 mg/5 ml.
Tablets: 1 mg.
Injection: 1 mg/ml.

INDICATIONS AND DOSAGES
▸ **Prevention of chemotherapy-induced nausea and vomiting**
PO
Adults, Elderly. 2 mg once a day up to 1 hr before chemotherapy or 1 mg twice a day.
IV
Adults, Elderly, Children 2 yr and older. 10 mcg/kg/dose (or 1 mg/dose) within 30 min of chemotherapy.
▸ **Prevention of radiation-induced nausea and vomiting**
PO
Adults, Elderly. 2 mg once a day given 1 hr before radiation therapy.
▸ **Postoperative nausea or vomiting**
PO
Adults, Elderly, Children 4 yr and older. 20-40 mcg/kg as a single postoperative dose.
IV
Adults, Elderly. 1 mg as a single postoperative dose.
Children older than 4 yr.
20-40 mcg/kg. Maximum: 1 mg.

OFF-LABEL USES
PO: Prophylaxis of nausea or vomiting associated with radiation therapy

CONTRAINDICATIONS
None known.

INTERACTIONS
Drug
Hepatic enzyme inducers: May decrease the effects of granisetron.
Herbal
None known.
Food
None known.

DIAGNOSTIC TEST EFFECTS
May increase AST (SGOT) and ALT (SGPT) levels.

▨ IV INCOMPATIBILITIES
Amphotericin B (Fungizone)
▨ **IV Compatibilities**
Allopurinol (Aloprim), bumetanide (Bumex), calcium gluconate, carboplatin (Paraplatin), cisplatin (Platinol), cyclophosphamide (Cytoxan), cytarabine (Ara-C), dacarbazine (DTIC-Dome), dexamethasone (Decadron), diphenhydramine (Benadryl), docetaxel (Taxotere), doxorubicin (Adriamycin), etoposide (VePesid), gemcitabine (Gemzar), magnesium, mitoxantrone (Novantrone), paclitaxel (Taxol), potassium

SIDE EFFECTS
Frequent (21%-14%)
Headache, constipation, asthenia
Occasional (8%-6%)
Diarrhea, abdominal pain
Rare (less than 2%)
Altered taste, hypersensitivity reaction

SERIOUS REACTIONS
• None known.

PRECAUTIONS & CONSIDERATIONS
It is unknown if granisetron is distributed in breast milk. The safety and efficacy of granisetron have not been established in children younger than 2 years. Granisetron should be used

G

cautiously in children younger than 2 years. No age-related precautions have been noted in the elderly.

The drug may affect the sense of taste temporarily. Notify the physician if headache occurs. Pattern of daily bowel activity and stool consistency should be assessed.

Storage
Keep the bottle of oral solution tightly closed. Protect the bottle from light and store it in an upright position. Store vials for IV use at room temperature; the solution normally appears clear and colorless; inspect it for particles and discoloration. After dilution, the solution for injection is stable for at least 24 hours at room temperature.

Administration
! Administer only on days of chemotherapy, as prescribed. Administer oral granisetron within 1 hour and the IV form within 30 minutes before starting chemotherapy.

For IV use, administer granisetron undiluted or dilute it with 20 to 50 ml 0.9% NaCl or D_5W. Don't mix it with other medications. Administer the undiluted drug by IV push over 30 seconds. For IV piggyback, infuse over 5 to 20 minutes, depending on the volume of diluent used.

Griseofulvin
griz-ee-oh-full′vin
(Fulvicin P/G, Fulvicin U/F, Grifulvin V, Gris-PEG, Grisovin [AUS])

CATEGORY AND SCHEDULE
Pregnancy Risk Category: C

CLASSIFICATION
Antifungals

MECHANISM OF ACTION
An antifungal that inhibits fungal cell mitosis by disrupting mitotic spindle structure. *Therapeutic Effect:* Fungistatic.

AVAILABILITY
Oral Suspension (Grifulvin V): 125 mg/5 ml.
Tablets (Microsize [Fulvicin-U/F]): 250 mg, 500 mg.
Tablets (Ultramicrosize [Fulvicin P/G]): 125 mg, 165 mg, 250 mg, 330 mg.
Tablets (Ultramicrosize [Gris-PEG]): 125 mg, 250 mg.

INDICATIONS AND DOSAGES
▶ **Tinea capitis, tinea corporis, tinea cruris, tinea pedis, tinea unguium**
MICROSIZE TABLETS, ORAL SUSPENSION
Adults. Usual dosage, 500-1000 mg as a single dose or in divided doses.
Children 2 yr and older. Usual dosage, 10-20 mg/kg/day.
ULTRAMICROSIZE TABLETS
Adults. Usual dosage, 330-750 mg/day as a single dose or in divided doses.
Children 2 yr and older. 5-10 mg/kg/day.

CONTRAINDICATIONS
Hepatocellular failure, porphyria, pregnancy

INTERACTIONS
Drug
Oral contraceptives, warfarin: May decrease the effects of these drugs.
Herbal
None known.
Food
None known.

DIAGNOSTIC TEST EFFECTS
None known.

SIDE EFFECTS

Occasional

Hypersensitivity reaction (including pruritus, rash, and urticaria), headache, nausea, diarrhea, excessive thirst, flatulence, oral thrush, dizziness, insomnia

Rare

Paresthesia of hands or feet, proteinuria, photosensitivity reaction

SERIOUS REACTIONS

• Granulocytopenia occurs rarely.

PRECAUTIONS & CONSIDERATIONS

Caution is warranted with hypersensitivity to penicillins or in those who are exposed to sun or ultraviolet light because photosensitivity may develop. Determine history of allergies, especially to griseofulvin and penicillins, before giving the drug. Avoid alcohol and exposure to sunlight. Maintain good hygiene to help prevent superinfection. Separate personal items that come in direct contact with affected areas.

! Monitor the granulocyte count as appropriate. If granulocytopenia develops, notify the physician and expect to discontinue the drug. If headache occurs, establish and document the headache's location, onset and type. Assess for dizziness. Evaluate skin for rash and therapeutic response to the drug. Assess daily pattern of bowel activity and stool consistency.

Administration

! The duration of treatment depends on the site of infection. Take oral griseofulvin with foods high in fat, such as milk or ice cream, to reduce GI upset and assist in drug absorption. Keep affected areas dry and wear light clothing for ventilation.

Guaifenesin

gwye-fen′e-sin

(Balminil [CAN], Benylin E [CAN], Guiatuss, Humibid LA, Mucinex, Organidin, Robitussin, Tussin)

Do not confuse guaifenesin with guanfacine.

CATEGORY AND SCHEDULE

Pregnancy Risk Category: C

OTC

CLASSIFICATION

Expectorants

MECHANISM OF ACTION

An expectorant that stimulates respiratory tract secretions by decreasing adhesiveness and viscosity of phlegm. *Therapeutic Effect:* Promotes removal of viscous mucus.

PHARMACOKINETICS

Well absorbed from the GI tract. Metabolized in the liver. Excreted in urine.

AVAILABILITY

Tablets (Organidin): 200 mg.
Tablets (Extended-Release [Humibid LA, Mucinex]): 600 mg.
Syrup (Guiatuss, Robitussin, Tussin): 100 mg/5 ml.

INDICATIONS AND DOSAGES

▸ **Expectorant**

PO

Adults, Elderly, Children older than 12 yr. 200-400 mg q4hr.
Children 6-12 yr. 100-200 mg q4hr. Maximum: 1.2 g/day.
Children 2-5 yr. 50-100 mg q4hr.
Children younger than 2 yr.
12 mg/kg/day in 6 divided doses.
PO (EXTENDED-RELEASE)

Adults, Elderly, Children older than 12 yr. 600-1200 mg q12hr. Maximum: 2.4 g/day.
Children 2-5 yr. 600 mg q12hr. Maximum: 600 mg/day.

CONTRAINDICATIONS
None known.

INTERACTIONS
Drug
None known.
Herbal
None known.
Food
None known.

DIAGNOSTIC TEST EFFECTS
None known.

SIDE EFFECTS
Rare
Dizziness, headache, rash, diarrhea, nausea, vomiting, abdominal pain

SERIOUS REACTIONS
• Overdose may produce nausea and vomiting.

PRECAUTIONS & CONSIDERATIONS
It is unknown if guaifenesin crosses the placenta or is distributed in breast milk. No age-related precautions have been noted in children or the elderly. Use guaifenesin cautiously in children younger than 2 years with a persistent cough. Avoid tasks that require mental alertness or motor skills until response to the drug has been established. Fluid intake and environmental humidity should be increased to lower the viscosity of secretions.

Notify the physician of cough that persists or is accompanied by fever, rash, headache, or sore throat. Clinical improvement should be assessed.
Storage
Store syrup, liquid, and capsules at room temperature.

Administration
! Take extended-release capsules at 12-hour intervals, as prescribed.

Take guaifenesin without regard to food. Don't crush or break extended-release capsules. Contents may be sprinkled on soft food and then swallowed without chewing or crushing. Do not take for chronic cough.

Guanabenz
gwan'a-benz
(Wytensin)

CATEGORY AND SCHEDULE
Pregnancy Risk Category: C

CLASSIFICATION
Antiadrenergics, central

MECHANISM OF ACTION
An alpha-adrenergic agonist that stimulates alpha$_2$-adrenergic receptors. Inhibits sympathetic cardioaccelerator and vasoconstrictor center to heart, kidneys, peripheral vasculature. *Therapeutic Effect:* Decreases systolic, diastolic blood pressure (B/P). Chronic use decreases peripheral vascular resistance.

PHARMACOKINETICS
Well absorbed from gastrointestinal (GI) tract. Widely distributed. Protein binding: 90%. Metabolized in liver. Excreted in urine and feces. Not removed by hemodialysis. **Half-life:** 6 hr.

AVAILABILITY
Tablets: 4 mg, 8 mg (Wytensin).

INDICATIONS AND DOSAGES
▸ **Hypertension**

PO
Adults. Initially, 4 mg 2 times/day. Increase by 4-8 mg at 1-2 wk intervals.
Elderly. Initially, 4 mg/day. May increase q1-2 wk. Maintenance: 8-16 mg/day. Maximum: 32 mg/day.

CONTRAINDICATIONS

History of hypersensitivity to guanabenz or any component of the formulation

INTERACTIONS

Drug
Beta-blockers, hypotensive-producing medications: May increase antihypertensive effect.
Herbal
Licorice, yohimbine: May decrease guanabenz effectiveness.
Food
None known.

DIAGNOSTIC TEST EFFECTS

May decrease cholesterol, total triglyceride concentrations.

SIDE EFFECTS

Frequent
Drowsiness, dry mouth, dizziness
Occasional
Weakness, headache, nausea, decreased sexual ability
Rare
Ataxia, sleep disturbances, rash, itching, diarrhea, constipation, altered taste, muscle aches

SERIOUS REACTIONS

• Abrupt withdrawal may result in rebound hypertension manifested as nervousness, agitation, anxiety, insomnia, hand tingling, tremor, flushing, and sweating.
• Overdosage produces hypotension, somnolence, lethargy, irritability, bradycardia, and miosis (pupillary constriction).

PRECAUTIONS & CONSIDERATIONS

Caution is warranted with severe coronary insufficiency, recent MI, cerebrovascular disease, severe hepatic or renal failure. It is unknown if guanabenz crosses the placenta or is distributed in breast milk. Safety and efficacy of guanabenz have not been established in children. There are no age-related precautions noted in the elderly.

Side effects such as dry mouth, drowsiness, dizziness, headache, decreased sexual ability, and GI upset, may occur during the first 2 weeks of therapy but generally diminish during continued therapy. If increased or decreased heartbeat or swollen ankles or feet occurs, notify the physician. Avoid alcohol, and caution should be used driving or operating machinery until tolerance to medication is established. Avoid skipping doses or voluntarily discontinuing drug because it may produce severe, rebound hypertension.
Storage
Store at room temperature and protect from light.
Administration
Give with or without food.

Guanfacine
gwan′fa-seen
(Tenex)

CATEGORY AND SCHEDULE
Pregnancy Risk Category: B

CLASSIFICATION
Antiadrenergics, central

MECHANISM OF ACTION

An alpha-adrenergic agonist that stimulates alpha$_2$-adrenergic receptors and inhibits sympathetic cardioaccelerator and vasoconstrictor center to heart, kidneys, peripheral vasculature. *Therapeutic Effect:* Decreases systolic, diastolic blood pressure (B/P). Chronic use decreases peripheral vascular resistance.

PHARMACOKINETICS

Well absorbed from gastrointestinal (GI) tract. Widely distributed. Protein binding: 71%. Metabolized in liver. Excreted in urine and feces. Not removed by hemodialysis. **Half-life:** 17 hr.

AVAILABILITY

Tablets: 1 mg, 2 mg (Tenex).

INDICATIONS AND DOSAGES

▸ **Hypertension**
PO
Adults, Elderly. Initially, 1 mg/day. Increase by 1 mg/day at intervals of 3-4 wk up to 3 mg/day in single or divided doses.

OFF-LABEL USES

Attention deficit hyperactivity disorder (ADHD), tic disorders

CONTRAINDICATIONS

History of hypersensitivity to guanfacine or any component of the formulation

INTERACTIONS

Drug
Beta-blockers, hypotensive-producing medications: May increase antihypertensive effect.
Bupropion: May increase risk of seizure activity.
Herbal
Licorice, yohimbine: May decrease guanfacine effectiveness.

Ma Huang: May increase blood pressure.
Food
None known.

DIAGNOSTIC TEST EFFECTS

May increase growth hormone concentration. May decrease urinary catecholamine and VMA excretion.

SIDE EFFECTS

Frequent
Dry mouth, somnolence
Occasional
Fatigue, headache, asthenia (loss of strength, energy), dizziness

SERIOUS REACTIONS

• Overdosage may produce difficult breathing, dizziness, faintness, severe drowsiness, bradycardia.

PRECAUTIONS & CONSIDERATIONS

Caution should be used with impaired renal function. It is unknown if guanfacine crosses the placenta or is distributed in breast milk. Be aware that guanfacine is not recommended in treatment of acute hypertension associated with preeclampsia. Safety and efficacy of guanfacine have not been established in children. There are no age-related precautions noted in the elderly.

Therapeutic effect may take 1 week and peak effect should be noted in 1-3 months. Avoid skipping doses or voluntarily discontinuing drug may produce severe, rebound hypertension. Avoid alcohol and caution should be used driving or operating machinery.
Storage
Store at room temperature and protect from light.
Administration
Give guanfacine at bedtime.

Halcinonide
hal-sin'o-nide
(Halog, Halog-E)

CATEGORY AND SCHEDULE
Pregnancy Risk Category: C

CLASSIFICATION
Corticosteroids, topical, dermatologics

MECHANISM OF ACTION
A topical corticosteroid that has anti-inflammatory, antipruritic, and vasoconstrictive properties. The exact mechanism of the anti-inflammatory process is unclear. *Therapeutic Effect:* Reduces or prevents tissue response to the inflammatory process.

PHARMACOKINETICS
Well absorbed systemically. Large variation in absorption among sites. Protein binding: varies. Metabolized in liver. Primarily excreted in urine.

AVAILABILITY
Cream: 0.1% (Halog).
Cream (emollient base): 0.1% (Halog-E).
Ointment: 0.1% (Halog).
Solution: 0.1% (Halog).

INDICATIONS AND DOSAGES
▸ **Dermatoses**
TOPICAL
Adults, Elderly. Apply sparingly 1-3 times/day.

CONTRAINDICATIONS
History of hypersensitivity to halcinonide or other corticosteroids

INTERACTIONS
Drug
None known.
Herbal
None known.
Food
None known.

DIAGNOSTIC TEST EFFECTS
None known.

SIDE EFFECTS
Occasional
Itching, redness, irritation, burning at site of application, dryness, folliculitis, acneiform eruptions, hypopigmentation
Rare
Allergic contact dermatitis, maceration of the skin, secondary infection, skin atrophy

SERIOUS REACTIONS
• The serious reactions of long-term therapy and the addition of occlusive dressings are reversible hypothalamic-pituitary-adrenal (HPA) axis suppression, manifestations of Cushing's syndrome, hyperglycemia, and glucosuria.

PRECAUTIONS & CONSIDERATIONS
Caution should be used over large surface areas and with prolonged use. It is unknown if halcinonide is excreted in breast milk. Halcinonide should not be used during pregnancy because it may cause harmful effects in the neonate. Absorption is more likely with occlusive dressings or extensive application in young children.
Administration
Gently cleanse area before application preferably after bath or shower for best absorption. Use occlusive dressings only as directed. Apply sparingly. Rub into area gently and thoroughly.

Halobetasol
hal-oh-be′ta-sol
(Ultravate)

CATEGORY AND SCHEDULE
Pregnancy Risk Category: C

CLASSIFICATION
Corticosteroids, topical,
dermatologics

MECHANISM OF ACTION
A corticosteroid that inhibits accumulation of inflammatory cells at inflammation sites, phagocytosis, lysosomal enzyme release, and synthesis or release of mediators of inflammation. *Therapeutic Effect:* Decreases or prevents tissue response to inflammatory process.

PHARMACOKINETICS
Variation in absorption among individuals and sites: scrotum 36%, forehead 7%, scalp 4%, forearm 1%.

AVAILABILITY
Cream: 0.05% (Ultravate).
Ointment: 0.05% (Ultravate).

INDICATIONS AND DOSAGES
▸ **Dermatoses, corticosteroid-unresponsive**
TOPICAL
Adults, Elderly, Children more than 12 yr and older. Apply 1-2 times/day. Maximum: 50 g for 2 wk.

CONTRAINDICATIONS
Hypersensitivity to halobetasol or other corticosteroids.

INTERACTIONS
Drug
None known.
Herbal
None known.
Food
None known.

DIAGNOSTIC TEST EFFECTS
None known.

SIDE EFFECTS
Frequent
Burning, stinging, pruritus
Rare
Cushing's syndrome, hyperglycemia, glucosuria, hypothalamic-pituitary-adrenal axis suppression

SERIOUS REACTIONS
• Overdosage can occur from topically applied halobetasol absorbed in sufficient amounts to produce systemic effects producing reversible adrenal suppression, manifestations of Cushing's syndrome, hyperglycemia, and glucosuria in some patients.

PRECAUTIONS & CONSIDERATIONS
Occlusive dressings should be avoided. Halobetasol should only be used for 2 weeks. It is unknown if halobetasol crosses the placenta or is distributed in the breast milk. Safety and efficacy have not been established in children. There are no age-related precautions noted in the elderly.
Administration
Avoid use of occlusive dressings unless otherwise directed by a physician. Apply sparingly to skin or scalp and rub into area thoroughly. Administer for no longer than 2 weeks. Only small areas should be treated at one time. Discontinue treatment when control is achieved. Do not apply on face, groin, or axillae. Avoid contact with eyes.

Haloperidol
ha-loe-per′idole
(Apo-Haloperidol [CAN],
Haldol, Haldol Decanoate,
Novoperidol [CAN], Peridol
[CAN], Serenace [AUS])
**Do not confuse Haldol
with Halcion, Halog,
or Stadol.**

CATEGORY AND SCHEDULE
Pregnancy Risk Category: C

CLASSIFICATION
Antipsychotics

MECHANISM OF ACTION
An antipsychotic, antiemetic, and antidyskinetic agent that competitively blocks postsynaptic dopamine receptors, interrupts nerve impulse movement, and increases turnover of dopamine in the brain. Has strong extrapyramidal and antiemetic effects; weak anticholinergic and sedative effects. *Therapeutic Effect:* Produces tranquilizing effect.

PHARMACOKINETICS
Readily absorbed from the GI tract. Protein binding: 92%. Extensively metabolized in the liver. Primarily excreted in urine. Not removed by hemodialysis. **Half-life:** 12-37 hr PO; 10-19 hr IV; 17-25 hr IM.

AVAILABILITY
Oral Concentrate: 2 mg/ml.
Tablets: 0.5 mg, 1 mg, 2 mg, 5 mg, 10 mg, 20 mg.
Injection (Lactate): 5 mg/ml.
Injection (Decanoate): 50 mg/ml, 100 mg/ml.

INDICATIONS AND DOSAGES
▶ **Treatment of psychotic disorders**
PO
Adults, Children 12 yr and older. Initially, 0.5-5 mg 2-3 times/day. Dosage gradually adjusted as needed.
Elderly. 0.5-2 mg 2-3 times/day. Dosage gradually adjusted as needed.
Children 3-12 yr or weighing 15-40 kg. Initially, 0.05 mg/kg/day in 2-3 divided doses. May increase by 0.5 mg increments at 5-7 day intervals. Maximum: 0.15 mg/kg/day in divided doses.
IM
Adults, Elderly, Children 12 yr and older. Initially, 2-5. May repeat at 1 hour intervals as needed. Maximum: 100 mg/day.
IM (DECANOATE)
Adults, Elderly, Children 12 yr and older. Initially, 10-15 times previous daily oral dose up to maximum initial dose of 100 mg. Maximum: 300 mg/mo.
▶ **Treatment of non-psychotic disorders, Tourette's syndrome**
PO
Children 3-12 yr or weighing 15-40 kg. Initially, 0.05 mg/kg/day in 2-3 divided doses. May increase by 0.5 mg at 5-7 day intervals. Maximum: 0.075 mg/kg/day.

OFF-LABEL USES
Treatment of Huntington's chorea, infantile autism, nausea or vomiting associated with cancer chemotherapy

CONTRAINDICATIONS
Angle-closure glaucoma, CNS depression, myelosuppression, Parkinson's disease, severe cardiac or hepatic disease

INTERACTIONS
Drug
Alcohol, other CNS depressants: May increase CNS depression.

H

Epinephrine: May block alpha-adrenergic effects.
Extrapyramidal symptom-producing medications: May increase extrapyramidal symptoms.
Lithium: May increase neurologic toxicity.
Herbal
None known.
Food
None known.

DIAGNOSTIC TEST EFFECTS

None known. Therapeutic serum drug level is 0.2-1 mcg/ml; toxic serum drug level is greater than 1 mcg/ml.

▓ IV INCOMPATIBILITIES

Allopurinol (Aloprim), amphotericin B complex (Abelcet, AmBisome, Amphotec), cefepime (Maxipime), fluconazole (Diflucan), foscarnet (Foscavir), heparin, nitroprusside (Nipride), piperacillin and tazobactam (Zosyn)
▓ IV Compatibilities
Dobutamine (Dobutrex), dopamine (Intropin), fentanyl (Sublimaze), hydromorphone (Dilaudid), lidocaine, lorazepam (Ativan), midazolam (Versed), morphine, nitroglycerin, norepinephrine (Levophed), propofol (Diprivan)

SIDE EFFECTS

Frequent
Blurred vision, constipation, orthostatic hypotension, dry mouth, swelling or soreness of female breasts, peripheral edema
Occasional
Allergic reaction, difficulty urinating, decreased thirst, dizziness, decreased sexual function, drowsiness, nausea, vomiting, photosensitivity, lethargy

SERIOUS REACTIONS

• Extrapyramidal symptoms appear to be dose-related and typically occur in the first few days of therapy. Marked drowsiness and lethargy, excessive salivation, and fixed stare occur frequently. Less common reactions include severe akathisia (motor restlessness) and acute dystonias (such as torticollis, opisthotonos, and oculogyric crisis).
• Tardive dyskinesia (tongue protrusion, puffing of the cheeks, chewing or puckering of the mouth) may occur during long-term therapy or after discontinuing the drug and may be irreversible. Elderly female patients have a greater risk of developing this reaction.

Caution is warranted with cardiovascular disease, hepatic or renal dysfunction, and a history of seizures. Haloperidol crosses the placenta and is distributed in breast milk. Children are more susceptible to dystonias. Haloperidol use is not recommended for children younger than 3 years. A decreased dosage is recommended for the elderly, who are more susceptible to extrapyramidal and anticholinergic effects, orthostatic hypotension, and sedation. Exposure to sunlight and any conditions that may cause dehydration or overheating should be avoided because they may increase the risk of heat stroke.

Drowsiness may occur but generally subsides with continued therapy. Alcohol and tasks that require mental alertness or motor skills should be avoided. Notify the physician if muscle stiffness occurs. Fine tongue movement, masklike facial expression, rigidity, and tremor should be assessed if it occurs.
Storage
Store vials at room temperature. Protect them from freezing and light. Discard the solution if it

becomes discolored or contains precipitate.

Administration

! Only haloperidol lactate is given IV. Know that the therapeutic serum level for haloperidol is 0.2 to 1 mcg/ml, and the toxic serum level is greater than 1 mcg/ml.

Haloperidol may be given undiluted by IV push. Flush with at least 2 ml 0.9% NaCl before and after administration. To dilute, add the drug to 30 to 50 ml of most solutions; D_5W is preferred. Give IV push at a rate of 5 mg/minute. Infuse IV piggyback over 30 minutes. For IV infusion, administer up to 25 mg/hour, titrating dosage to patient response.

Prepare haloperidol decanoate IM injection using a 21-gauge needle. Don't exceed a volume of 3 ml per IM injection site. Slowly inject the drug deep into the upper outer quadrant of the gluteus maximus. Keep recumbent (head low and legs raised) for 30 to 60 minutes after administration to minimize hypotensive effects.

Take oral haloperidol without regard to food. Crush scored tablets as needed. Full therapeutic effect may take up to 6 weeks to appear. Do not abruptly discontinue the drug after long-term use.

Heparin
hep′a-rin
(Hepalean [CAN], Heparin injection B.P. [AUS], Heparin Leo, Uniparin [AUS])
Do not confuse heparin with Hespan.

CATEGORY AND SCHEDULE
Pregnancy Risk Category: C

CLASSIFICATION
Anticoagulants

MECHANISM OF ACTION
A blood modifier that interferes with blood coagulation by blocking conversion of prothrombin to thrombin and fibrinogen to fibrin. *Therapeutic Effect:* Prevents further extension of existing thrombi or new clot formation. Has no effect on existing clots.

PHARMACOKINETICS
Well absorbed following subcutaneous administration. Protein binding: Very high. Metabolized in the liver. Removed from the circulation via uptake by the reticuloendothelial system. Primarily excreted in urine. Not removed by hemodialysis.
Half-life: 1-6 hr.

AVAILABILITY
Injection: 10 units/ml, 100 units/ml, 1000 units/ml, 2500 units/ml, 5000 units/ml, 7500 units/ml, 10,000 units/ml, 20,000 units/ml, 25,000 units/500 ml infusion.

INDICATIONS AND DOSAGES
▸ **Line flushing**
IV
Adults, Elderly, Children. 100 units q6-8hr.

Infants weighing less than 10 kg.
10 units q6-8hr.
▸ **Treatment of venous thrombosis, pulmonary embolism, peripheral arterial embolism, atrial fibrillation with embolism**
INTERMITTENT IV
Adults, Elderly. Initially, 10,000 units, then 50-70 units/kg (5000-10,000 units) q4-6hr.
Children 1 yr and older. Initially, 50-100 units/kg, then 50-100 units q4hr.
IV INFUSION
Adults, Elderly. Loading dose: 80 units/kg, then 18 units/kg/hr, with adjustments based on aPTT. Range: 10-30 units/kg/hr.
Children 1 yr and older. Loading dose: 75 units/kg, then 20 units/kg/hr with adjustments based on aPTT.
Children younger than 1 yr. Loading dose: 75 units/kg, then 28 units/kg/hr.
▸ **Prevention of venous thrombosis, pulmonary embolism, peripheral arterial embolism, atrial fibrillation with embolism**
SUBCUTANEOUS
Adult, Elderly. 5000 units q8-12hr.

CONTRAINDICATIONS
Intracranial hemorrhage, severe hypotension, severe thrombocytopenia, subacute bacterial endocarditis, uncontrolled bleeding

INTERACTIONS
Drug
Antithyroid medications, cefoperazone, cefotetan, valproic acid: May cause hypoprothrombinemia.
Other anticoagulants, platelet aggregation inhibitors, thrombolytics: May increase the risk of bleeding.
Probenecid: May increase the effects of heparin.

Herbal
Feverfew, ginkgo biloba: May have additive effect.
Food
None known.

DIAGNOSTIC TEST EFFECTS
May increase free fatty acid, AST (SGOT), and ALT (SGPT) levels. May decrease serum cholesterol and triglyceride levels.

▨ IV INCOMPATIBILITIES
Amiodarone (Cordarone), amphotericin B complex (Abelcet, AmBisome, Amphotec), ciprofloxacin (Cipro), dacarbazine (DTIC), diazepam (Valium), dobutamine (Dobutrex), doxorubicin (Adriamycin), droperidol (Inapsine), filgrastim (Neupogen), gentamicin (Garamycin), haloperidol (Haldol), idarubicin (Idamycin), labetalol (Trandate), nicardipine (Cardene), phenytoin (Dilantin), quinidine, tobramycin (Nebcin), vancomycin (Vancocin)

▨ IV Compatibilities
Aminophylline, ampicillin/sulbactam (Unasyn), aztreonam (Azactam), calcium gluconate, cefazolin (Ancef), ceftazidime (Fortaz), ceftriaxone (Rocephin), digoxin (Lanoxin), diltiazem (Cardizem), dopamine (Intropin), enalapril (Vasotec), famotidine (Pepcid), fentanyl (Sublimaze), furosemide (Lasix), hydromorphone (Dilaudid), insulin, lidocaine, lorazepam (Ativan), magnesium sulfate, methylprednisolone (Solu-Medrol), midazolam (Versed), milrinone (Primacor), morphine, nitroglycerin, norepinephrine (Levophed), oxytocin (Pitocin), piperacillin/tazobactam (Zosyn), procainamide (Pronestyl), propofol (Diprivan)

SIDE EFFECTS
Occasional
Itching, burning (particularly on soles of feet) caused by vasospastic reaction
Rare
Pain, cyanosis of extremity 6-10 days after initial therapy lasting 4-6 hours; hypersensitivity reaction, including chills, fever, pruritus, urticaria, asthma, rhinitis, lacrimation, and headache

SERIOUS REACTIONS
• Bleeding complications ranging from local ecchymoses to major hemorrhage occur more frequently in high-dose therapy, intermittent IV infusion, and in women 60 years of age and older.
• Antidote: Protamine sulfate 1-1.5 mg, IV, for every 100 units heparin subcutaneous within 30 minutes of overdose, 0.5-0.75 mg for every 100 units heparin subcutaneous if within 30-60 minutes of overdose, 0.25-0.375 mg for every 100 units heparin subcutaneous if 2 hours have elapsed since overdose, 25-50 mg if heparin was given by IV infusion.

PRECAUTIONS & CONSIDERATIONS
Caution should be used during menstruation in persons receiving IM injections, and in those with peptic ulcer disease, recent invasive or surgical procedures, and severe hepatic or renal disease. Heparin should be used with caution in pregnant women, particularly during the last trimester and immediately postpartum, because it increases the risk of maternal hemorrhage. Heparin does not cross the placenta and is not distributed in breast milk. No age-related precautions have been noted in children. The benzyl alcohol preservative may cause gasping syndrome in infants. The elderly are more susceptible to hemorrhage, and age-related decreased renal function may increase the risk of bleeding. Other medications, including OTC drugs, should be avoided. An electric razor and soft toothbrush should be used to prevent bleeding during therapy.

Notify the physician of bleeding from surgical site, chest pain, dyspnea, severe or sudden headache, swelling in the feet or hands, unusual back pain, bruising, weakness, black or red stool, coffee-ground vomitus, dark or red urine, or red-speckled mucus from cough. CBC, BUN and creatinine levels, B/P, pulse, and stool of occult blood should be monitored. Be aware of signs of bleeding, including bleeding at injection or surgical sites or from gums, blood in stool, bruising, hematuria, and petechiae.

Storage
Store at room temperature.
Administration
! Do not give by IM injection because it may cause pain, hematoma, ulceration, and erythema. The subcutaneous route is used for low-dose therapy.

For subcutaneous use, after withdrawing heparin from the vial, change the needle before injection to prevent leakage along the needle track. Inject the heparin dose above the iliac crest or in abdominal fat layer. Do not inject within 2 inches of umbilicus or scar tissue.

For IV use, dilute IV infusion in isotonic sterile saline, D_5W, or lactated Ringer's solution. Invert IV bag at least 6 times to ensure mixing, and to prevent pooling of the medication. Use constant-rate IV infusion pump.

Hepatitis B Immune Globulin (Human)
hep-ah-tie'tis B ih-mewn' glah'byew-lin
(Bayhep B, H-B-Vax II [AUS], Nabi-HB)

CATEGORY AND SCHEDULE
Pregnancy Risk Category: C

CLASSIFICATION
Immune globulins

MECHANISM OF ACTION
An immune globulin of inactivated hepatitis B virus that provides passive immunity against hepatitis B virus.

AVAILABILITY
Injection: 5-ml vial.

INDICATIONS AND DOSAGES
▶ **Prevention of hepatitis B infection**
IM
Adults, Elderly. Usual 0.06 ml/kg; for acute exposure 3-5 ml. Repeat 28-30 days after exposure.

CONTRAINDICATIONS
Allergies to gamma globulin or thimerosal, IgA deficiency, IM injection in patients with coagulation disorders or thrombocytopenia

INTERACTIONS
Drug
None known.
Herbal
None known.
Food
None known.

DIAGNOSTIC TEST EFFECTS
None known.

SIDE EFFECTS
Frequent
Headache (26%), injection site pain (12%)
Occasional (5%)
Malaise, nausea, myalgia

SERIOUS REACTIONS
• None known.

PRECAUTIONS & CONSIDERATIONS
Caution is warranted with coagulation disorders, thrombocytopenia, IgA deficiency, and allergies to gamma globulin, eggs, chicken, or thimerosal. Notify the physician of any side effects, including headache or injection site pain. Baseline and periodic liver function studies and hepatitis B antibody levels should be obtained.
Storage
Refrigerate this drug; do not freeze it.
Administration
! Avoid giving IM injections to patients with coagulation disorders or thrombocytopenia. This drug is for IM injection only.
    Administer by IM injection only in the gluteal or deltoid area. Complete full course of immunization.

Hetastarch
het'ah-starch
(Hespan, Hextend)

CATEGORY AND SCHEDULE
Pregnancy Risk Category: C

CLASSIFICATION
Plasma expanders

MECHANISM OF ACTION
A plasma volume expander that exerts osmotic pull on tissue fluids. *Therapeutic Effect:* Reduces hemoconcentration and blood viscosity; increases circulating blood volume.

PHARMACOKINETICS
Smaller molecules, less than
50,000 molecular weight, rapidly
excreted by kidneys; larger molecules, 50,000 molecular weight and
greater, slowly degraded to smaller-
sized molecules, then excreted.
Half-life: 17 days.

AVAILABILITY
Injection: 6 g/100 ml 0.9% NaCl
(500 ml infusion container)

INDICATIONS AND DOSAGES
▶ **Plasma volume expansion**
IV
Adults, Elderly. 500-1000 ml/day up
to 1500 ml/day (20 mg/kg) at a rate
up to 20 ml/kg/hr in hemorrhagic
shock and at a slower rate in burns
and septic shock.
▶ **Leukapheresis**
IV
Adults, Elderly. 250-700 ml infused
at a constant rate, usually 1:8 to
venous whole blood.

CONTRAINDICATIONS
Anuria, oliguria, severe bleeding
disorders, severe CHF

INTERACTIONS
Drug
None significant.
Herbal
None known.
Food
None known.

DIAGNOSTIC TEST EFFECTS
May prolong bleeding, and clotting
times, PTT, and PT. May decrease
Hct concentration.

▒ IV INCOMPATIBILITIES
Amikacin (Amikin), ampicillin
(Polycillin), cefazolin (Ancef,
Kefzol), cefotaxime (Claforan),
cefoxitin (Mefoxin), gentamicin

(Garamycin), ranitidine (Zantac),
tobramycin (Nebcin)

SIDE EFFECTS
Rare
Allergic reaction resulting in vomiting, mild temperature elevation,
chills, itching, submaxillary and
parotid gland enlargement, peripheral
edema of lower extremities, mild
flu-like symptoms, headache, muscle
aches

SERIOUS REACTIONS
• Fluid overload may occur
marked by increased B/P and
distended neck veins. Neurologic
changes that may occur include
headache, weakness, blurred vision,
behavioral changes, incoordination,
and isolated muscle twitching.
Pulmonary edema may also
occur, manifested by rapid
breathing, crackles, wheezing, and
coughing.
• Anaphylactic reaction, including
periorbital edema, urticaria, and
wheezing, may occur.

PRECAUTIONS & CONSIDERATIONS
Caution is warranted with CHF,
hepatic disease, pulmonary edema,
sodium-restricted diets, thrombocytopenia, and in the elderly or children.
An electric razor and soft toothbrush
should be used to prevent bleeding
during dextran therapy.
Notify the physician of bleeding
from surgical site, wheezing, itching,
rash, black or red stool, coffee-ground
emesis, dark or red urine, or red-
speckled mucus from cough. Urine
output, vital signs, and laboratory
tests, including coagulation studies
and CBC, should be monitored.
CVP should also be monitored to
detect blood volume overexpansion.
Be aware of signs and symptoms
of fluid overload, such as peripheral

or pulmonary edema, and impending CHF.

Storage
Store solution at room temperature. Solution normally appears clear, pale yellow to amber. Do not use if discolored a deep turbid brown, or if precipitate forms.

Administration
Administer only by IV infusion. Do not add drugs to IV line or mix with other IV fluids. In acute hemorrhagic shock, administer at a rate approaching 1.2 g/kg/hr (20 ml/kg/hr), as prescribed. Expect to use slower rates in burns and septic shock. Monitor CVP when giving by rapid infusion. If CVP rises precipitously, immediately discontinue the drug, as prescribed, to prevent blood volume overexpansion.

Hyaluronan
(Orthovisc Injection)

CATEGORY AND SCHEDULE
Pregnancy Risk Category: NR

CLASSIFICATION
Hyaluronic acid derivatives

MECHANISM OF ACTION
A natural complex sugar of the glycosaminoglycan family that enhances viscoelastic properties of synovial fluid. *Therapeutic Effect:* Produces lubrication for knee joint and relieves pain and increases mobility.

PHARMACOKINETICS
Not known.

AVAILABILITY
Pre-filled syringe: 30 mg hyaluronan/2 ml (Orthovisc).

INDICATIONS AND DOSAGES
▶ **Knee osteoarthritis**
PO
Adults, Elderly. Inject full contents of syringe into one knee weekly for 3 or 4 weeks.

OFF-LABEL USES
Treatment of psoriatic arthritis, vascular headache

CONTRAINDICATIONS
Allergies to avian or avian-derived products (including eggs, feathers, or poultry), skin disease or infection in area of injection site, hypersensitivity to hyaluronate preparations or any one of its components including preservatives

INTERACTIONS
Drug
None known.
Herbal
None known.
Food
None known.

DIAGNOSTIC TEST EFFECTS
None known.

SIDE EFFECTS
Occasional
Arthralgia, back pain, pain at injection site
Rare
Joint stiffness, swelling

SERIOUS REACTIONS
• Transient increases in inflammation in injected knee following hyaluronan injection have been reported in some patients with OA.

PRECAUTIONS & CONSIDERATIONS
Be aware that safety and effectiveness of hyaluronan has not been established in joints other than the knee. Be aware that use of

disinfectants containing quartenary ammonium salts for skin preparation as hyaluronic acid can precipitate in their presence. Safety and efficacy of this drug have not been tested in pregnant, nursing women or children. There are no age-related precautions noted in the elderly. Strenuous activity or weight-bearing activities should be avoided within 48 hours following injection.

Storage
Store syringes at room temperature. Do not freeze.

Administration
Be aware that the pre-filled syringe is for single use only. Discard syringe after administering. Remove the protective rubber cap on tip of syringe, and attach small gauge needle (18-21 gauge) to tip. Inject full contents of syringe into one knee. If treatment is bilateral, use a separate syringe for each knee.

Hydralazine

hye-dral'a-zeen
(Alphapress [AUS], Apresoline, Novohylazin [CAN])
Do not confuse hydralazine with hydroxyzine.

CATEGORY AND SCHEDULE
Pregnancy Risk Category: C

CLASSIFICATION
Vasodilators

MECHANISM OF ACTION
An antihypertensive with direct vasodilating effects on arterioles. *Therapeutic Effect:* Decreases B/P and systemic resistance.

PHARMACOKINETICS

Route	Onset	Peak	Duration
PO	20-30 min	N/A	2-4 hr
IV	5-20 min	N/A	2-6 hr

Well absorbed from the GI tract. Widely distributed. Protein binding: 85%-90%. Metabolized in the liver to active metabolite. Primarily excreted in urine. Not removed by hemodialysis. **Half-life:** 3-7 hr (increased with impaired renal function).

AVAILABILITY
Tablets: 10 mg, 25 mg, 50 mg, 100 mg.
Injection: 20 mg/ml.

INDICATIONS AND DOSAGES
▸ **Moderate to severe hypertension**
PO
Adults. Initially, 10 mg 4 times a day. May increase by 10-25 mg/dose q2-5 days. Maximum: 300 mg/day.
Children. Initially, 0.75-1 mg/kg/day in 2-4 divided doses, not to exceed 25 mg/dose. May increase over 3-4 wk. Maximum: 7.5 mg/kg/day (5 mg/kg/day in infants).
IV, IM
Adults, Elderly. Initially, 10-20 mg/dose q4-6hr. May increase to 40 mg/dose.
Children. Initially, 0.1-0.2 mg/kg/dose (maximum: 20 mg) q4-6hr, as needed, up to 1.7-3.5 mg/kg/day in divided doses q4-6hr.
▸ **Dosage in renal impairment**
Dosage interval is based on creatinine clearance.

Creatinine Clearance	Dosage Interval
10-50 ml/min	q8hr
Less than 10 ml/min	q8-24hr

H

OFF-LABEL USES
Treatment of CHF, hypertension secondary to eclampsia and preeclampsia, primary pulmonary hypertension.

CONTRAINDICATIONS
Coronary artery disease, lupus erythematosus, rheumatic heart disease

INTERACTIONS
Drug
Diuretics, other antihypertensives: May increase hypotensive effect.
Herbal
Licorice, ma huang, yohimbine: May decrease the effectiveness of hydralazine.
Food
None known.

DIAGNOSTIC TEST EFFECTS
May produce positive direct Coombs' test.

▦ IV INCOMPATIBILITIES
Aminophylline, ampicillin (Polycillin), furosemide (Lasix)
▯ IV Compatibilities
Dobutamine (Dobutrex), heparin, hydrocortisone (Solu-Cortef), nitroglycerin, potassium

SIDE EFFECTS
Frequent
Headache, palpitations, tachycardia (generally disappears in 7-10 days)
Occasional
GI disturbance (nausea, vomiting, diarrhea), paresthesia, fluid retention, peripheral edema, dizziness, flushed face, nasal congestion

SERIOUS REACTIONS
• High dosage may produce lupus erythematosus-like reaction, including fever, facial rash, muscle and joint aches, and splenomegaly.

• Severe orthostatic hypotension, skin flushing, severe headache, myocardial ischemia, and cardiac arrhythmias may develop.
• Profound shock may occur with severe overdosage.

PRECAUTIONS & CONSIDERATIONS
Caution is warranted with cerebrovascular disease and impaired renal function. Hydralazine crosses the placenta; it is unknown if it is distributed in breast milk. Hematomas, leukopenia, petechial bleeding, and thrombocytopenia have occurred in newborns; these conditions resolve within 1 to 3 weeks. No age-related precautions have been noted in children. The elderly are more sensitive to the drug's hypotensive effects. In the elderly, age-related renal impairment may require dosage adjustment.

Dizziness and lightheadedness may occur. Rise slowly from a lying to a sitting position and permit legs to dangle from the bed momentarily before standing to reduce the hypotensive effect of hydralazine. Those receiving high doses of hydralazine should notify the physician if fever (lupus-like reaction) or joint and muscle aches occur. Also, notify the physician if headache, palpitations, tachycardia, or peripheral edema of the hands and feet occurs. B/P and pulse should be obtained immediately before each hydralazine dose, in addition to regular B/P monitoring. Be alert for B/P fluctuations. Daily bowel activity and stool consistency should also be monitored.
Storage
Store drug at room temperature.
Administration
Hydralazine is best given with food or regularly spaced meals. Crush tablets if necessary.

For IV use, give undiluted if necessary. Give single dose over 1 minute.

Hydrochlorothiazide
hye-droe-klor-oh-thye′a-zide
(Apo-Hydro [CAN], Aquazide H, Dichlotride [AUS], Dithiazide [AUS], Esidrix, HydroDIURIL, Microzide, Oretic)

CATEGORY AND SCHEDULE
Pregnancy Risk Category: B (D if used in pregnancy-induced hypertension)

CLASSIFICATION
Diuretics, thiazide and derivatives

MECHANISM OF ACTION
A sulfonamide derivative that acts as a thiazide diuretic and antihypertensive. As a diuretic blocks reabsorption of water, sodium, and potassium at the cortical diluting segment of the distal tubule. As an antihypertensive reduces plasma, extracellular fluid volume, and peripheral vascular resistance by direct effect on blood vessels. *Therapeutic Effect:* Promotes diuresis; reduces B/P.

PHARMACOKINETICS

Route	Onset	Peak	Duration
PO (diuretic)	2 hr	4-6 hr	6-12 hr

Variably absorbed from the GI tract. Primarily excreted unchanged in urine. Not removed by hemodialysis. **Half-life:** 5.6-14.8 hr.

AVAILABILITY
Capsules (Microzide): 12.5 mg.
Oral Solution: 50 mg/5 ml.

Tablets (Aquazide, Oretic): 25 mg, 50 mg, 100 mg.

INDICATIONS AND DOSAGES
▸ **Edema, hypertension**
PO
Adults. 12.5-100 mg/day. Maximum: 200 mg/day.
▸ **Usual pediatric dosage**
PO
Children 6 mo-12 yr. 2 mg/kg/day in 2 divided doses. Maximum: 200 mg/day.
Children younger than 6 mo. 2-4 mg/kg/day in 2 divided doses. Maximum: 37.5 mg/day.

OFF-LABEL USES
Treatment of diabetes insipidus, prevention of calcium-containing renal calculi

CONTRAINDICATIONS
Anuria, history of hypersensitivity to sulfonamides or thiazide diuretics, renal decompensation

INTERACTIONS
Drug
Cholestyramine, colestipol: May decrease the absorption and effects of hydrochlorothiazide.
Digitalis glycosides: May increase the risk of digitalis toxicity.
Digoxin: May increase the risk of digoxin toxicity associated with hydrochlorothiazide-induced hypokalemia.
Lithium: May increase the risk of lithium toxicity.
Herbal
Ginkgo biloba: May increase blood pressure.
Licorice: May increase risk of hypokalemia and reduce the effectiveness of hydrochlorothiazide.
Ma huang, yohimbine: May reduce hypotensive effect of hydrochlorothiazide.

H

Food
None known.

DIAGNOSTIC TEST EFFECTS
May increase blood glucose and serum cholesterol, LDL, bilirubin, calcium, creatinine, uric acid, and triglyceride levels. May decrease urinary calcium, and serum magnesium, potassium, and sodium levels.

SIDE EFFECTS
Expected
Increase in urinary frequency and urine volume
Frequent
Potassium depletion
Occasional
Orthostatic hypotension, headache, GI disturbances, photosensitivity

SERIOUS REACTIONS
• Vigorous diuresis may lead to profound water and electrolyte depletion, resulting in hypokalemia, hyponatremia, and dehydration.
• Acute hypotensive episodes may occur.
• Hyperglycemia may occur during prolonged therapy.
• Pancreatitis, blood dyscrasias, pulmonary edema, allergic pneumonitis, and dermatologic reactions occur rarely.
• Overdose can lead to lethargy and coma without changes in electrolytes or hydration.

PRECAUTIONS & CONSIDERATIONS
Caution is warranted with diabetes mellitus, thyroid disorders, hepatic impairment, severe renal disease, and in the elderly and debilitated. Hydrochlorothiazide crosses the placenta and a small amount is distributed in breast milk. Breastfeeding is not recommended. No age-related precautions have been noted in children, except that jaundiced infants may be at risk for hyperbilirubinemia. The elderly may be more sensitive to the drug's electrolyte and hypotensive effects. Age-related renal impairment may require cautious use in the elderly. Consuming foods high in potassium such as apricots, bananas, legumes, meat, orange juice, raisins, whole grains, including cereals, and white and sweet potatoes, is encouraged. Avoid prolonged exposure to sunlight and ultraviolet rays because a photosensitivity reaction may occur.

Dizziness or lightheadedness may occur, so change positions slowly and let legs dangle momentarily before standing. An increase in the frequency and volume of urination may also occur. Blood pressure (B/P), vital signs, electrolytes, intake and output, and weight should be monitored before and during treatment. Be aware of signs of electrolyte disturbances such as hypokalemia or hyponatremia. Hypokalemia may cause arrhythmias, altered mental status, muscle cramps, asthenia, and tremor. Hyponatremia may result in cold and clammy skin, confusion, and thirst.

Administration
Take hydrochlorothiazide with food or milk if GI upset occurs, preferably with breakfast to help prevent nocturia.

Hydrocodone
hye-droe-koe'done
Hydrocodone and acetaminophen,
(Anexsia, Bancap HC, Ceta-Plus,
Co-Gesic, Hydrocet, Hydrogesic,
Lorcet 10/650, Lorcet-HD Lorcet
Plus, Lortab, Margesic H,
Maxidone, Norco, Stagesic,
Vicodin, Vicodin ES, Vicodin HP,
Zydone); hydrocodone and aspirin
(Damason-P); hydrocodone and
chlorpheniramine (Tussionex),
hydrocodone and guaifenesin
(Codiclear DH, Hycosin, Hycotuss,
Kwelcof, Pneumotussin, Vicoden
Tuss, Vitussin); hydrocodone and
homatropin (Hycodan and
Hydromet, Hydropane,
Tussigon); hydrocodone and
ibuprofen, (Vicoprofen);
hydrocodone and pseu-
doephedrine (Detussin, Histussin
D, P-V Tussin); hydrocodone,
chlorpheniramine, phenyle-
phrine, acetaminophen, and
caffeine (Hycomine Compound)

CATEGORY AND SCHEDULE
Pregnancy Risk Category: C, D
if used for prolonged periods,
high dosages at term
Controlled substance: Schedule III

CLASSIFICATION
Antitussive, narcotic analgesic,
opiate derivative, phenathrene
derivative

MECHANISM OF ACTION
Hydrocodone blocks pain perception
in the cerebral cortex by binding to
specific opiate receptors (mu and
kappa) neuronal membranes of
synapses. This binding results in
a decreased synaptic chemical
transmission throughout the CNS
thus inhibiting the flow of pain
sensations into the higher centers
and cause analgesia. *Therapeutic
Effect:* Alters perception of pain and
produces analgesic effect.

PHARMACOKINETICS
Well absorbed. Metabolized in
liver. Excreted in urine. **Half-life:**
3.3-3.4 hr.

AVAILABILITY
Hydrocodone & acetaminophen
Capsules: hydrocodone bitartrate
5 mg and acetaminophen 500 mg
(Bancap HC, Ceta-Plus, Hydrocet,
Hydrogesic, Lorcet-HD, Margesic H,
Stagesic).
Elixir: hydrocodone bitartrate
7.5 mg and acetaminophen 500 mg/
15 ml (Lortab).
Tablets: hydrocodone bitartrate
2.5 mg and acetaminophen 500 mg
(Lortab), hydrocodone bitartrate
5 mg and acetaminophen 325 mg
(Norco), hydrocodone bitartrate
5 mg and acetaminophen 400 mg
(Zydone), hydrocodone bitartrate
5 mg and acetaminophen 500 mg
(Anexsia, Co-Gesic, Lortab 5/500,
Vicodin), hydrocodone bitartrate
7.5 mg and acetaminophen 325 mg
(Norco), hydrocodone bitartrate
5 mg and acetaminophen 400 mg
(Zydone), hydrocodone bitartrate
7.5 mg and acetaminophen 500 mg
(Lortab 7.5/500), hydrocodone
bitartrate 7.5 mg and acetaminophen
650 mg (Anexsia, Lorcet Plus),
hydrocodone bitartrate 7.5 mg and
acetaminophen 750 mg (Vicodin
ES), hydrocodone bitartrate 10 mg
and acetaminophen 325 mg (Norco),
hydrocodone bitartrate 5 mg and
acetaminophen 400 mg (Zydone),
hydrocodone bitartrate 10 mg
and acetaminophen 500 mg

(Lortab 10/500), hydrocodone bitartrate 10 mg and acetaminophen 650 mg (Lorcet 10/650), hydrocodone bitartrate 10 mg and acetaminophen 660 mg (Vicodin HP), hydrocodone bitartrate 10 mg and acetaminophen 750 mg (Maxicodone).

Hydrocodone & aspirin
Tablets: hydrocodone bitartrate 5 mg and aspirin 500 mg (Damason-P).

Hydrocodone & chlorpheniramine
Syrup, extended release: hydrocodone polistirex 10 mg and chlorpheniramine polistirex 8 mg/5 ml (Tussionex).

Hydrocodone & guaifenesin
Liquid: hydrocodone bitartrate 2.5 mg and guaifenesin 200 mg/5 ml (Pneumotussin), hydrocodone bitartrate 5 mg and guaifenesin 100 mg/5 ml (Codiclear DH, Hycosin, Hycotuss, Kwelcof, Vicodin Tuss, Vitussin).
Tablets: hydrocodone bitartrate 2.5 mg and guaifenesin 300 mg (Pneumotussin).

Hydrocodone & homatropine
Syrup: hydrocodone bitartrate 5 mg and homatropine methylbromide 1.5 mg/5 ml (Hycodan, Hydromet, Hydropane)
Tablets: hydrocodone bitartrate 5 mg and homatropine methylbromide 1.5 mg (Hycodan, Tussigon).

Hydrocodone & ibuprofen
Tablets: hydrocodone bitartrate 7.5 mg and aspirin 200 mg (Vicoprofen).

Hydrocodone & pseudoephedrine
Liquid: hydrocodone bitartrate 5 mg and pseudoephedrine 60 mg/5 ml (Detussin, Histussin D).
Tablets: hydrocodone bitartrate 5 mg and pseudoephedrine 60 mg (P-V Tussin).

Hydrocodone, chlorpheniramine, phenylephrine, acetaminophen, & caffeine

Tablets: hydrocodone bitartrate 5 mg, chlorpheniramine maleate 2 mg, phenylephrine hydrochloride 10 mg, acetaminophen 250 mg, and caffeine 30 mg (Hycomine Compound).

INDICATIONS AND DOSAGES
▸ **Hydrocodone & acetaminophen Analgesia**
PO
Adults, Children older than 13 yr or more than 50 kg. 2.5-10 mg q4-6hr. Maximum: 60 mg/day hydrocodone. Maximum dose of acetaminophen: 4 g/day.
Elderly. 2.5-5 mg hydrocodone q4-6hr. Titrate dose to appropriate analgesic effect. Maximum: 4 g/day acetaminophen.
Children 2-13 yr or less than 50 kg. 0.135 mg/kg/dose hydrocodone q4-6hr. Maximum: 6 doses/day of hydrocodone or maximum recommended dose of acetaminophen.

▸ **Hydrocodone & aspirin**
PO
Adults. 2.5-10 mg q4-6hr. Maximum: 60 mg/day hydrocodone. *Elderly.* 2.5-5 mg hydrocodone q4-6hr. Titrate dose to appropriate analgesic effect.
Children 2-13 yr or less than 50 kg. 0.135 mg/kg/dose hydrocodone q4-6hr.

▸ **Hydrocodone & chlorpheniramine**
Adults, Elderly, Children 12 yr and older. 5 ml q12hr. Maximum: 10 ml/24hr.
Children 6-12 yr. 2.5 ml q12hr. Maximum: 5 ml/24hr.

▸ **Hydrocodone & guaifenesin**
Adults, Elderly, Children 12 yr and older. 5 ml q4hr. Maximum: 30 ml/24hr.
Children 2-12 yr. 2.5 ml q4hr.
Children less than 2 yr. 0.3 mg/kg/day (hydrocodone) in 4 divided doses.

▶ **Hydrocodone & homatropine**
Adults, Elderly. 10 mg (hydrocodone)
q4-6hr. A single dose should not
exceed 15 mg and not more
frequently than q4hr.
Children. 0.6 mg/kg/day
(hydrocodone) in 3-4 divided doses.
Do not administer more frequently
than q4hr.
▶ **Hydrocodone & ibuprofen**
Adults. 7.5-15 mg (hydrocodone)
q4-6hr as needed for pain.
Maximum: 5 tablets/day.
▶ **Hydrocodone & pseudoephedrine**
Adults, Elderly. 5 ml 4 times/day.
▶ **Hydrocodone, chlorpheniramine,
phenylephrine, acetaminophen, &
caffeine**
Adults, Elderly. 1 tablet q4hr up to
4 times/day.

CONTRAINDICATIONS
CNS depression, severe respiratory
depression, hypersensitivity to
hydrocodone, or any component of
the formulation

INTERACTIONS
Drug
**Alcohol, central nervous system
(CNS) depressants:** May increase
CNS or respiratory depression, and
hypotension.
**CYP2D6 inhibitors (e.g., chlorpro-
mazine):** May decrease the effects
of hydrocodone.
**Hepatotoxic medications (e.g.,
phenytoin), liver enzyme inducers
(e.g., cimetidine):** May increase
risk of hepatotoxicity associated
with acetaminophen with prolonged
high dose or single toxic dose.
MAOIs, tricyclic antidepressants:
May increase effects of MAOIs and
TCAs and hydrocodone.
Warfarin: May increase the risk of
bleeding with regular use.
Herbal
None known.

Food
None known.

DIAGNOSTIC TEST EFFECTS
None known.

SIDE EFFECTS
Frequent
Dizziness, sedation, drowsiness,
bradycardia
Occasional
Anxiety, dysphoria, euphoria, fear,
lethargy, lightheadedness, malaise,
mental clouding, mental impairment,
mood changes, physiological
dependence, sedation, somnolence,
constipation, bradycardia, heartburn,
nausea, vomiting
Rare
Hypersensitivity reaction, rash

SERIOUS REACTIONS
• Cardiac arrest, circulatory
collapse, coma, hypotension, hypoglycemic coma, ureteral spasm,
urinary retention, vesical sphincter
spasm, agranulocytosis, bleeding
time prolonged, hemolytic anemia,
iron deficiency anemia, occult blood
loss, thrombocytopenia, hepatic
necrosis, hepatits, skeletal muscle
rigidity, renal toxicity, renal tubular
necrosis have been reported.
• Hearing impairment or loss have
been reported with chronic overdose.
• Acute airway obstruction, apnea,
dyspnea, and respiratory depression
occur rarely and are usually dose
related.

PRECAUTIONS & CONSIDERATIONS
Caution is warranted with hypersensitivity reactions to other phenan-
threne derivative opioid agonists
(morphine, hydrocodone, hydromorphone, levorphanol, oxycodone,
oxymorphone). Be aware that tablets
with metabisulfite may cause allergic reactions. Information is not

available for hydrocodone during pregnancy. The manufacturers recommend discontinuing the medication or to discontinue nursing during therapy. Be aware that hydrocodone should be used cautiously in children and the elderly.

Drug dependence or tolerance may occur with prolonged use of high dosages. Avoid alcohol and tasks that require mental alertness or motor skills. Change positions slowly to avoid orthostatic hypotension.

Storage
Store at room temperature.

Administration
Be aware that ambulatory persons and those not in severe pain may experience dizziness, hypotension, nausea, and vomiting more frequently than patients in the supine position or with severe pain. Be aware to expect to reduce the initial dosage in those with hypothyroidism, concurrent CNS depressants, elderly, and debilitated. Take without meals.

Hydrocodone Bitartrate
high-drough-koe′doan
(Hycodan [CAN], Robidone [CAN])

CATEGORY AND SCHEDULE
Pregnancy Risk Category: C
(D if used for prolonged periods or at high dosages at term)
Controlled Substance Schedule: III

CLASSIFICATION
Narcotic (opioid), analgesic

MECHANISM OF ACTION
A narcotic analgesic and antitussive that binds with opioid receptors in the CNS. *Therapeutic Effect:* Alters the perception of and emotional response to pain; suppresses cough reflex.

PHARMACOKINETICS

Route	Onset	Peak	Duration
PO (analgesic)	10-20 min	30-60 min	4-6 hr
PO (antitussive)	N/A	N/A	4-6 hr

Well absorbed from the GI tract. Metabolized in the liver. Primarily excreted in urine. **Half-life:** 3.8 hr (increased in elderly).

INDICATIONS AND DOSAGES
▶ **Analgesia**
PO
Adults, Children older than 12 yr. 5-10 mg q4-6hr.
Elderly. 2.5-5 mg q4-6hr.
▶ **Cough**
PO
Adults. 5-10 mg q4-6hr as needed. Maximum: 15 mg/dose.
Children. 0.6 mg/kg/day in 3-4 divided doses at intervals of at least 4 hr. Maximum single dose: 5 mg (children 2-12 yr), 1.25 mg (children younger than 2 yr).
PO (EXTENDED-RELEASE)
Adults. 10 mg q12hr.
Children 6-12 yr. 5 mg q12hr.

CONTRAINDICATIONS
None known.

INTERACTIONS
Drug
Alcohol, other CNS depressants: May increase CNS or respiratory depression and hypotension.
MAOIs: May produce a severe, sometimes fatal reaction; plan to administer one-quarter of usual hydrocodone dose.
Herbal
None known.

Food
None known.

DIAGNOSTIC TEST EFFECTS
May increase serum amylase and lipase levels.

SIDE EFFECTS
Frequent
Sedation, hypotension, diaphoresis, facial flushing, dizziness, somnolence
Occasional
Urine retention, blurred vision, constipation, dry mouth, headache, nausea, vomiting, difficult or painful urination, euphoria, dysphoria

SERIOUS REACTIONS
• Overdose results in respiratory depression, skeletal muscle flaccidity, cold or clammy skin, cyanosis, and extreme somnolence progressing to seizures, stupor, and coma.
• The patient who uses hydrocodone repeatedly may develop a tolerance to the drug's analgesic effect as well as physical dependence.
• The drug may have a prolonged duration of action and cumulative effect in patients with hepatic or renal impairment.

PRECAUTIONS & CONSIDERATIONS
Extreme caution should be used with acute alcoholism, anoxia, CNS depression, hypercapnia, respiratory depression or dysfunction, seizures, shock, and untreated myxedema. Caution is also warranted with acute abdominal conditions, Addison's disease, COPD, hypothyroidism, hepatic impairment, increased intracranial pressure, benign prostatic hyperplasia, and urethral stricture. Hydrocodone readily crosses the placenta and is distributed in breast milk. Regular use of hydrocodone during pregnancy may produce withdrawal symptoms in the neonate, including irritability, excessive crying, tremors, hyperactive reflexes, fever, vomiting, diarrhea, yawning, sneezing, and seizures. Hydrocodone use may prolong labor if administered in the latent phase of the first stage of labor or before the cervix has dilated 4 to 5 cm. The neonate may develop respiratory depression if the mother receives hydrocodone during labor. Children younger than 2 years may be more susceptible to respiratory depression. The elderly may be more susceptible to respiration depression and paradoxical excitement. In the elderly, age-related renal impairment, benign prostatic hyperplasia, or obstruction may increase the risk of urine retention. A dosage adjustment is recommended.

Dizziness and drowsiness may occur, so change positions slowly and avoid alcohol, CNS depressants, and tasks that require mental alertness or motor skills until response to the drug is established. Notify the physician if constipation, difficulty breathing, nausea, or vomiting occurs during therapy. Vital signs, pattern of daily bowel activity and stool consistency, and clinical improvement of pain should be monitored. The bladder should be palpated for urine retention.

Administration
! Ambulatory patients and those not in severe pain may be more prone to dizziness, hypotension, nausea, and vomiting than patients in the supine position and those in severe pain. Take hydrocodone orally without regard to food. Crush tablets if needed.

Hydrocortisone
hye-dro-kor'ti-sone
(A-HydroCort, Anusol-HC,
Cortaid, Cortef cream [AUS],
Cortic cream [AUS], Cortic DS
[AUS], Cortifoam [AUS],
Cortizone-5, Cortizone-10,
Derm-Aid cream [AUS], Dermaid
[AUS], Dermaid soft cream [AUS],
Egocort cream [AUS], Emcort,
Hycor [AUS], Hycor eye ointment
[AUS], Hysone [AUS], Hytone,
Locoid, Nupercainal
Hydrocortisone Cream,
Preparation H Hydrocortisone,
Protocort, Siquent Hycor [AUS],
Solu-Cortef, Squibb HC [AUS],
WestCort)

CATEGORY AND SCHEDULE
Pregnancy Risk Category: C
(D if used in first trimester)
OTC (Hydrocortisone 0.5%
and 1% Cream, Gel, and
Ointment)

CLASSIFICATION
Corticosteroids, topical,
dermatologics

MECHANISM OF ACTION
An adrenocortical steroid that inhibits
accumulation of inflammatory cells
at inflammation sites, phagocytosis,
lysosomal enzyme release and
synthesis and release of mediators of
inflammation. *Therapeutic Effect:*
Prevents or suppresses cell-mediated
immune reactions. Decreases or
prevents tissue response to inflammatory process.

PHARMACOKINETICS

Route	Onset	Peak	Duration
IV	N/A	4-6 hr	8-12 hr

Well absorbed after IM administration. Widely distributed. Metabolized
in the liver. **Half-life:** Plasma,
1.5-2 hr; biologic, 8-12 hr.

AVAILABILITY
Tablet (Cortef): 5 mg, 10 mg, 20 mg.
*Cream (Rectal [Nupercainal
Hydrocortisone Cream,
Cortizone-10, Preparation H
Hydrocortisone]):* 1%.
Cream (Topical [Cortizone-5]): 0.5%.
*Cream (Topical [Caldecort,
Cortizone-10]):* 1%.
Cream (Topical [Hytone]): 2.5%.
Ointment (Topical [Locoid]): 0.1%.
Ointment (Topical [Westcort]): 0.2%.
Ointment (Topical [Cortizone-5]):
0.5%.
*Ointment (Topical [Anusol-HC,
Cortaid, Cortizone-10]):* 1%.
Ointment (Topical [Hytone]): 2.5%.
Suppositories (Anusol-HC): 25 mg.
Suppositories (Emcort, Protocort):
30 mg.
Injection (A-hydro-Cort, Solu-Cortef):
100 mg, 250 mg, 500 mg, 1 g.

INDICATIONS AND DOSAGES
▸ **Acute adrenal insufficiency**
IV
Adults, Elderly. 100 mg IV bolus;
then 300 mg/day in divided doses q8hr.
Children. 1-2 mg/kg IV bolus; then
150-250 mg/day in divided doses
q6-8hr.
Infants. 1-2 mg/kg/dose IV bolus;
then 25-150 mg/day in divided doses
q6-8hr.
▸ **Anti-inflammation, immunosup-
pression**
IV, IM
Adults, Elderly. 15-240 mg q12hr.
Children. 1-5 mg/kg/day in divided
doses q12hr.
▸ **Physiologic replacement**
PO
Children. 0.5-0.75 mg/kg/day in
divided doses q8hr.

IM
Children. 0.25-0.35 mg/kg/day as a single dose.
▸ **Status asthmaticus**
IV
Adults, Elderly. 100-500 mg q6hr.
Children. 2 mg/kg/dose q6hr.
▸ **Shock**
IV
Adults, Elderly, Children 12 yr and older. 100-500 mg q6hr.
Children younger than 12 yr. 50 mg/kg. May repeat in 4 hr, then q24hr as needed.
▸ **Adjunctive treatment of ulcerative colitis**
RECTAL
Adults, Elderly. 100 mg at bedtime for 21 nights or until clinical and proctologic remission occurs (may require 2-3 mo of therapy).
RECTAL (CORTIFOAM)
Adults, Elderly. 1 applicator 1-2 times a day for 2-3 wk, then every second day until therapy ends.
TOPICAL
Adults, Elderly. Apply sparingly 2-4 times a day.

CONTRAINDICATIONS
Fungal, tuberculosis, or viral skin lesions; serious infections

INTERACTIONS
Drug
Amphotericin: May increase hypokalemia.
Digoxin: May increase the risk of digoxin toxicity caused by hypokalemia.
Diuretics, insulin, oral hypo-glycemics, potassium supplements: May decrease the effects of these drugs.
Hepatic enzyme inducers: May decrease the effects of hydrocorti-sone.
Live virus vaccines: May decrease the patient's antibody response to vaccine, increase vaccine side effects, and potentiate virus replication.
Herbal
None known.
Food
None known.

DIAGNOSTIC TEST EFFECTS
May increase blood glucose and serum lipid, amylase, and sodium levels. May decrease serum calcium, potassium, and thyroxine levels.

▧ IV INCOMPATIBILITIES
Ciprofloxacin (Cipro), diazepam (Valium), idarubicin (Idamycin), mid-azolam (Versed), phenytoin (Dilantin)
▧ IV Compatibilities
Aminophylline, amphotericin, calcium gluconate, cefepime (Maxipime), digoxin (Lanoxin), diltiazem (Cardizem), diphenhy-dramine (Benadryl), dopamine (Intropin), insulin, lidocaine, lorazepam (Ativan), magnesium sulfate, morphine, norepinephrine (Levophed), procainamide (Pronestyl), potassium chloride, propofol (Diprivan)

SIDE EFFECTS
Frequent
Insomnia, heartburn, nervousness, abdominal distention, diaphoresis, acne, mood swings, increased appetite, facial flushing, delayed wound healing, increased suscepti-bility to infection, diarrhea or constipation
Occasional
Headache, edema, change in skin color, frequent urination
Topical: Itching, redness, irritation
Rare
Tachycardia, allergic reaction (such as rash and hives), psychological changes, hallucinations, depression
Topical: Allergic contact dermatitis, purpura

H

Systemic: Absorption more likely with use of occlusive dressings or extensive application in young children

SERIOUS REACTIONS
• Long-term therapy may cause hypocalcemia, hypokalemia, muscle wasting (especially in arms and legs), osteoporosis, spontaneous fractures, amenorrhea, cataracts, glaucoma, peptic ulcer disease, and CHF.
• Abruptly withdrawing the drug after long-term therapy may cause anorexia, nausea, fever, headache, sudden severe joint pain, rebound inflammation, fatigue, weakness, lethargy, dizziness, and orthostatic hypotension.

PRECAUTIONS & CONSIDERATIONS
Caution is warranted with cirrhosis, CHF, diabetes mellitus, hypertension, hyperthyroidism, osteoporosis, peptic ulcer disease, seizure disorders, thromboembolic tendencies, thrombophlebitis, and ulcerative colitis. Hydrocortisone crosses the placenta and is distributed in breast milk. Persons taking hydrocortisone should not breast-feed. Prolonged hydrocortisone use during the first trimester of pregnancy may produce cleft palate in the neonate. Prolonged treatment or high dosages may decrease the cortisol secretion and short-term growth rate in children. The elderly may be more susceptible to developing hypertension or osteoporosis. Dentist or other physicians should be informed of hydrocortisone therapy if taken within the past 12 months. Consult with the physician before taking aspirin or other medications. Avoid alcohol and limit caffeine intake. Hydrocortisone should not be overused for symptomatic relief.

Mood swings, ranging from euphoria to depression, may occur. Notify the physician of fever, muscle aches, sore throat, and sudden weight gain or swelling. Blood glucose level, intake and output, B/P, serum electrolyte levels, height, and weight should be monitored before and during therapy. Be alert to signs and symptoms of infection caused by reduced immune response, including fever, sore throat, and vague symptoms. In long-term therapy, signs and symptoms of hypocalcemia (such as muscle twitching, cramps, and positive Chvostek's or Trousseau's signs) or hypokalemia (such as EKG changes, nausea and vomiting, irritability, weakness and muscle cramps, and numbness or tingling, especially in the lower extremities) should be assessed.

Storage
Store at room temperature. After reconstitution, store hydrocortisone sodium succinate solution at room temperature and use within 72 hours.

Administration
For IV administration, use immediately if further diluted with D_5W, 0.9% NaCl, or other compatible diluent. For hydrocortisone sodium succinate IV push, dilute to 50 mg/ml; for intermittent infusion dilute to 1 mg/ml. Administer hydrocortisone sodium succinate solution IV push over 3 to 5 minutes. Give intermittent infusion over 20 to 30 minutes.

For topical use, gently cleanse area before applying drug; apply topical hydrocortisone valerate after bath or shower for best absorption. Apply sparingly and rub into area thoroughly. Use occlusive dressings only as ordered. Avoid contact with eyes.

For rectal use, shake homogeneous suspension well. Lie on the left side with left leg extended and right leg flexed. Gently insert applicator tip into rectum, pointed slightly toward umbilicus, and slowly instill medication.

Hydroflumethiazide
high-drow-floo-meth-eye'ah-zide
(Diucardin, Saluron)

CATEGORY AND SCHEDULE
Pregnancy Risk Category: C, D if used in pregnancy-induced hypertension

CLASSIFICATION
Diuretics, thiazide and derivatives

MECHANISM OF ACTION
A diuretic that blocks reabsorption of water, the electrolytes sodium and potassium at cortical diluting segment of distal tubule. As an antihypertensive it reduces plasma and extracellular fluid volume and decreases peripheral vascular resistance (PVR) by direct effect on blood vessels. *Therapeutic Effect:* Promotes diuresis, reduces blood pressure (B/P).

PHARMACOKINETICS
Rapidly but incompletely absorbed from the gastrointestinal (GI) tract. Metabolized to metabolite that is extensively bound to red blood cells and has a longer half-life than parent compound. Primarily excreted in urine. Not removed by hemodialysis. **Half-life:** 2-17 hr.

AVAILABILITY
Tablets: 50 mg (Diucardin, Saluron).

INDICATIONS AND DOSAGES
▶ **Edema**
PO
Adults, Elderly. Initially, 50 mg 2 times/day. Maintenance: 25-200 mg/day.
▶ **Hypertension**
Adults, Elderly, Children. 1 mg/kg/day.
Initially, 50 mg 2 times/day. Maintenance: 50-100 mg/day.

OFF-LABEL USES
Treatment of diabetes insipidus

CONTRAINDICATIONS
Anuria, history of hypersensitivity to sulfonamides or thiazide diuretics, renal decompensation, pregnancy

INTERACTIONS
Drug
Ace inhibitors: May increase the risk of postural hypotension.
Beta blockers: May increase hyperglycemic effects in patients with Type 2 diabetes mellitus.
Cylosporine, other thiazides: May increase the risk of gout or renal toxicity.
Cholestyramine, colestipol: May decrease the absorption and effects of hydroflumethiazide.
Digoxin: May increase the risk of toxicity of digoxin caused by hypokalemia.
Lithium: May increase the risk of toxicity of lithium
Neuromuscular blocking agents: May prolong neuromuscular blockade.
NSAIDs: May decrease the effects of hydroflumethiazide.
Herbal
Calcitriol: May increase the risk of hypercalcemia
Ginkgo biloba: May increase blood pressure.

H

Gossypol: May increase the risk of hypokalemia.

Licorice: May increase the risk of hypokalemia and/or reduce effectiveness of hydroflumethiazide.

Ma Huang: May decrease hypotensive effect of hydroflumethiazide.

Yohimbine: May decrease the effects of hydroflumethiazide.

Food

None known.

DIAGNOSTIC TEST EFFECTS

May increase blood glucose levels, serum cholesterol, LDL, bilirubin, calcium, creatinine, uric acid, and triglyceride levels. May decrease urinary calcium, and serum magnesium, potassium, and sodium levels.

▓ IV INCOMPATIBILITIES

None known.

▐ IV Compatibilities

None known.

SIDE EFFECTS

Expected

Increase in urine frequency and volume

Frequent

Potassium depletion

Occasional

Postural hypotension, headache, gastrointestinal (GI) disturbances, photosensitivity reaction

SERIOUS REACTIONS

• Vigorous diuresis may lead to profound water loss and electrolyte depletion, resulting in hypokalemia, hyponatremia, and dehydration.

• Acute hypotensive episodes may occur.

• Hyperglycemia may be noted during prolonged therapy.

• GI upset, pancreatitis, dizziness, paresthesias, headache, blood dyscrasias, pulmonary edema, allergic pneumonitis, and dermatologic reactions occur rarely.

• Overdosage can lead to lethargy and coma without changes in electrolytes or hydration.

PRECAUTIONS & CONSIDERATIONS

Caution is necessary with diabetes mellitus, impaired liver function, severe renal disease, and thyroid disorders. Be aware that hydroflumethiazide crosses the placenta and a small amount is distributed in breast milk. Breast-feeding is not recommended in this patient population. Be aware that safety and efficacy of hydroflumethiazide have not been established in children. Be aware that the elderly may be more sensitive to the drug's electrolyte and hypotensive effects. Age-related renal impairment may require caution in the elderly. Foods high in potassium such as apricots, bananas, legumes, meat, orange juice, white and sweet potatoes, raisins, and whole grains such as cereals should be consumed. Sunlight and ultraviolet rays should be avoided because a photosensitivity reaction can occur.

Hypokalemia may result in change in mental status, muscle cramps, nausea, tachycardia, tremor, vomiting, and weakness. Hyponatremia may result in clammy and cold skin, confusion, and thirst. Be especially alert for potassium depletion in patients taking digoxin, such as cardiac arrhythmias. Frequency and volume of urination is expected to occur.

Administration

Give oral hydroflumethiazide in divided doses when the patient is taking more than 100 mg/day.

Hydromorphone
hye-droe-mor'fone
(Dilaudid, Dilaudid HP,
Hydromorph Contin [CAN],
Palladone)
**Do not confuse with morphine
or Dilantin.**

CATEGORY AND SCHEDULE
Pregnancy Risk Category: B
(D if used for prolonged periods
or at high dosages at term)
Controlled Substance Schedule: II

CLASSIFICATION
Analgesics, narcotic

MECHANISM OF ACTION
An opioid agonist that binds to
opioid receptors in the CNS, reducing the intensity of pain stimuli from
sensory nerve endings. *Therapeutic
Effect:* Alters the perception of and
emotional response to pain;
suppresses cough reflex.

PHARMACOKINETICS

Route	Onset	Peak	Duration
PO	30 min	90-120 min	4 hr
IV	10-15 min	15-30 min	2-3 hr
IM	15 min	30-60 min	4-5 hr
Subcu-taneous	15 min	30-90 min	4 hr
Rectal	15-30 min	N/A	N/A

Well absorbed from the GI tract after
IM administration. Widely distrib-
uted. Metabolized in the liver.
Excreted in urine. **Half-life:** 1-3 hr.

AVAILABILITY
Liquid (Dilaudid): 5 mg/5 ml.
*Capsules (Extended-Release
[Palladone]):* 12 mg, 16 mg, 24 mg,
32 mg.
Tablets (Dilaudid): 2 mg, 3 mg,
4 mg, 8 mg.
Injection (Dilaudid): 1 mg/ml,
2 mg/ml, 4 mg/ml.
Injection (Dilaudid HP): 10 mg/ml.
Suppository (Dilaudid): 3 mg.

INDICATIONS AND DOSAGES
▸ **Analgesia**
PO
*Adults, Elderly, Children weighing
50 kg and more.* 2-4 mg q3-4hr.
Range: 2-8 mg/dose.
*Children older than 6 mo and
weighing less than 50 kg.*
0.03-0.08 mg/kg/dose q3-4hr.
PO (EXTENDED-RELEASE)
Adults, Elderly. 12-32 mg once a day.
IV
*Adults, Elderly, Children weighing
more than 50 kg.* 0.2-0.6 mg q2-3hr.
Children weighing 50 kg or less.
0.015 mg/kg/dose q3-6hr as needed.
RECTAL
Adults, Elderly. 3 mg q4-8hr.
▸ **Patient-controlled analgesia (PCA)**
IV
Adults, Elderly. 0.05-0.5 mg at
5-15 min lockout. Maximum (4-hr):
4-6 mg.
EPIDURAL
Adults, Elderly. Bolus dose of
1-1.5 mg at rate of 0.04-0.4 mg/hr.
Demand dose of 0.15 mg at 30 min
lockout.
▸ **Cough**
PO
*Adults, Elderly, Children older than
12 yr.* 1 mg q3-4hr.
Children 6-12 yr. 0.5 mg q3-4hr.

CONTRAINDICATIONS
Respiratory depression in the
absence of resuscitative equipment,
status asthmatics, depressed
ventilatory function, obstetrical
anesthesia.

H

INTERACTIONS

Drug

Alcohol, other CNS depressants:
May increase CNS or respiratory
depression and hypotension.
MAOIs: May produce a severe,
sometimes fatal reaction; plan to
administer one-quarter of usual
hydromorphone dose.

Herbal
None known.

Food
None known.

DIAGNOSTIC TEST EFFECTS
May increase serum amylase and
lipase concentrations.

🕸 IV INCOMPATIBILITIES
Amphotericin B complex (Abelcet,
AmBisome, Amphotec), cefazolin
(Ancef, Kefzol), diazepam
(Valium), phenobarbital, phenytoin
(Dilantin)

💧 IV Compatibilities
Diltiazem (Cardizem),
diphenhydramine (Benadryl), dobutamine (Dobutrex), dopamine
(Intropin), fentanyl (Sublimaze),
furosemide (Lasix), heparin,
lorazepam (Ativan), magnesium
sulfate, metoclopramide (Reglan),
midazolam (Versed), milrinone
(Primacor), morphine, propofol
(Diprivan)

SIDE EFFECTS

Frequent
Somnolence, dizziness, hypotension
(including orthostatic hypotension),
decreased appetite

Occasional
Confusion, diaphoresis, facial
flushing, urine retention,
constipation, dry mouth, nausea,
vomiting, headache, pain at injection
site

Rare
Allergic reaction, depression

SERIOUS REACTIONS

- Overdose results in respiratory
depression, skeletal muscle flaccidity, cold or clammy skin, cyanosis,
and extreme somnolence progressing
to seizures, stupor, and coma.
- The patient who uses hydromorphone repeatedly may develop a
tolerance to the drug's analgesic
effect as well as physical dependence.
- This drug may have a prolonged
duration of action and cumulative
effect in patients with hepatic or
renal impairment.

PRECAUTIONS & CONSIDERATIONS
Extreme caution should be used with
acute alcoholism, anoxia, CNS
depression, hypercapnia, respiratory
depression or dysfunction, seizures,
shock, and untreated myxedema.
Caution is also warranted with acute
abdominal conditions, Addison's
disease, COPD, hypothyroidism,
hepatic impairment, increased
intracranial pressure, benign prostatic hyperplasia, and urethral stricture. Hydromorphone readily crosses
the placenta; it is unknown if it is
distributed in breast milk. Regular
use of opioids during pregnancy may
produce withdrawal symptoms in the
neonate, including diarrhea, excessive
crying, fever, hyperactive reflexes,
irritability, seizures, sneezing,
tremors, vomiting, and yawning.
Hydromorphone use may prolong
labor if administered in the latent
phase of the first stage of labor or
before cervical dilation of 4 to 5 cm.
The neonate may develop respiratory
depression if the mother receives
hydromorphone during labor.
Children younger than 2 years may
be more susceptible to respiratory
depression. The elderly may be more
susceptible to respiratory depression
and paradoxical excitement. In the

elderly, age-related benign prostatic hyperplasia, obstruction, or renal impairment may increase the risk of urine retention; a dosage adjustment is recommended.

Dizziness and drowsiness may occur, so change positions slowly and avoid alcohol, CNS depressants, and tasks that require mental alertness or motor skills until response to the drug is established. Vital signs, pattern of daily bowel activity and stool consistency, and clinical improvement of pain should be monitored. The drug should be held and the physician should be notified if the respiratory rate is 12 breaths/minute or less in an adult, or 20 breaths/minute or less in a child.

Storage

Store vials at room temperature; protect from light. A slight yellow discoloration of the parenteral form does not indicate a loss of potency. Refrigerate suppositories.

Administration

! Although side effects depend on the dosage and administration route, they occur infrequently when hydromorphone is administered orally as an antitussive. Ambulatory patients and those not in severe pain may be more prone to dizziness, hypotension, nausea, and vomiting than patients in the supine position and those in severe pain.

Take oral hydromorphone without regard to food. Crush tablets, as needed.

! Be aware that a high concentration (10 mg/ml) should be used only in patients currently receiving high doses of another opioid agonist for severe, chronic pain caused by cancer or those who have developed a tolerance to high doses of other opioids.

For IV use, hydromorphone may be given undiluted as IV push over 2 to 5 minutes, or it may be further diluted with 5 ml sterile water for injection or 0.9% NaCl. Be aware that rapid IV administration increases the risk of a severe anaphylactic reaction, marked by apnea, cardiac arrest, and circulatory collapse.

For IM and subcutaneous administration, use a short 25-30-gauge needle for subcutaneous injection. Administer the drug slowly; rotate injection sites. Know that those with circulatory impairment are at increased risk for overdose because of delayed absorption of repeated injections.

For rectal use, moisten the suppository with cold water before inserting it well into the rectum.

Hydroquinone

hye-droe-kwin'one

(Alphaquin HP, Alustra, Claripel, Eldopaque, Eldopaque Forte, Eldoquin, EpiQuin Micro, Esoterica Regular, Glyquin, Lustra, Lustra-AF, Melanex, Melpaque HP, Melquin-3, Melquin HP, NeoStrata AHA, Nuquin HP, Neostrata HQ, Palmer's Skin Success Fade Cream, Solaquin, Solaquin Forte)

CATEGORY AND SCHEDULE

Pregnancy Risk Category: C

CLASSIFICATION

Depigmenting agents, dermatologics

MECHANISM OF ACTION

A depigmenting agent that suppresses melanocyte metabolic

processes of the skin. Inhibits the enzymatic oxidation of tyrosine to DOPA (3,4-dihydroxyphenylalanine). Sun exposure reverses this effect and causes repigmentation. *Therapeutic Effect:* Lighten hyperpigmented areas.

PHARMACOKINETICS

Onset and duration of depigmentation vary among individuals. About 35% is absorbed.

AVAILABILITY

Cream: 2% (Eldopaque, Esoterica Regular, Palmer's Skin Success Fade Cream), 4% (Alphaquin HP, Alustra, EpiQuin Micro, Lustra, Melquin HP, Nuquin HP).
Cream, with sunscreen: 2% (Solaquin), 4% (Claripel, Glyquin, Solaquin, Solaquin Forte, Lustra-AF, Melpaque HP).
Gel: 2% (NeoStrata AHA).
Gel, with sunscreen: 4% (Nuqiun HP, Solaquin Forte)

INDICATIONS AND DOSAGES

▸ Hyperpigmentation, melanin

TOPICAL

Adults, Elderly, Children 12 yr and older. Apply twice daily.

OFF-LABEL USES

None known.

CONTRAINDICATIONS

Hypersensitivity to hydroquinone, sulfites, or any other component of its formulation

INTERACTIONS

Drug
None known.
Herbal
None known.
Food
None known.

DIAGNOSTIC TEST EFFECTS

None known.

IV INCOMPATIBILITIES

None known.

IV Compatibilities
None known.

SIDE EFFECTS

Occasional
Burning, itching, stinging, erythema such as localized contact dermatitis
Rare
Conjunctival changes, fingernail staining

SERIOUS REACTIONS

- Gradual blue-black darkening of skin has been reported.
- Occasional cutaneous hypersensitivity (localized contact dermatitis) may occur.

PRECAUTIONS & CONSIDERATIONS

It is unknown if hydroquinone crosses the placenta or is distributed in breast milk. Caution should be used in pregnant women. Be aware that safety and efficacy of hydroquinone have not been established in children younger than 12 years. There are no age-related precautions noted in the elderly. Sun exposure should be avoided. Protective sunscreen or clothing to cover the skin should be used if sun is unavoidable.

Administration
Hydroquinone is for external use only. Gently cleanse area prior to application. Limit to small areas of the body at one time. Apply sparingly on skin spots and rub into area thoroughly. Avoid contact with eyes.

Hydroxocobalamin (Vitamin B$_{12}$)

hye-drox'oh-co-bal'a-min
(Alphamin, Hydrobexan,
Hydro-Cobex, Hydro-Crysti-12,
Hydroxy-Cobal, LA-12,
Vibal LA)

CATEGORY AND SCHEDULE
Pregnancy Risk Category: A
(C if used at dosages greater than
RDA)

CLASSIFICATION
Vitamins/minerals

MECHANISM OF ACTION
A coenzyme for metabolic functions,
including fat and carbohydrate
metabolism and protein synthesis.
Therapeutic Effect: Necessary for
growth, cell replication,
hematopoiesis, and myelin synthesis.

PHARMACOKINETICS
Rapidly absorbed after IM adminis-
tration. Protein binding: High.
Primarily excreted in urine.
Metabolized in liver. **Half-life:**
6 days.

AVAILABILITY
Injection: 100 mcg/ml (Alphamin),
1000 mcg/ml (Alphamin, Hydrobexan, Hydro-Cobex, Hydro-Crysti-12,
Hydroxy-Cobal, LA-12, Vibal LA).

INDICATIONS AND DOSAGES
▸ Vitamin B$_{12}$ deficiency
IM
Adults, Elderly. 30 mcg/day for
5-10 days then 100-200 mcg
monthly.
Children. 1-5 mg in single doses of
100 mcg over 2 or more weeks, then
30-50 mcg monthly.

CONTRAINDICATIONS
Folate deficient anemia, hereditary
optic nerve atrophy, hypersensitivity
to cobalt, hypersensitivity to hydroxocobalamin or any component of the
formulatioin

INTERACTIONS
Drug
Alcohol, colchicines: May
decrease the absorption of
hydroxocobalamin.
Ascorbic acid: May destroy vitamin
B$_{12}$.
Folic acid (large doses): May
decrease hydroxocobalamin blood
concentration.
Herbal
None known.
Food
None known.

DIAGNOSTIC TEST EFFECTS
None known.

SIDE EFFECTS
Occasional
Diarrhea, itching, pain at injection
site

SERIOUS REACTIONS
• Rare allergic reaction generally
due to impurities in preparation, may
occur.
• May produce peripheral vascular
thrombosis, pulmonary edema,
hypokalemia, and congestive heart
failure (CHF).

PRECAUTIONS & CONSIDERATIONS
Hydroxocobalamin crosses the
placenta and is excreted in breast
milk. There are no age-related
precautions noted in children or the
elderly. Be aware that injection
formulations contain benzoyl alcohol
and should be avoided in premature
infants. Signs and symptoms of CHF
and hypokalemia, especially in those

H

receiving hydroxocobalamin by IM route, and pulmonary edema should be assessed. Foods rich in vitamin B_{12} including clams, dairy products, egg yolks, fermented cheese, herring, muscle meats, organ meats, oysters, and red snapper should be suggested.

Reversal of deficiency symptoms including anorexia, ataxia, fatigue, hyporeflexia, insomnia, irritability, loss of positional sense, pallor, and palpitations on exertion should be evaluated. Serum potassium levels, which normally range between 3.5 to 5 mEq/L, and serum B_{12} levels, which normally range between 200 to 800 mcg/ml should be monitored. Also monitor for a rise in the blood reticulocyte count, which peaks in 5 to 8 days.

Storage

Store at room temperature.

Administration

Administer IM only. May require coadministration of folic acid.

Hydroxychloroquine

hye-drox-ee-klor′oh-kwin
(Apo-Hydroxyquine [CAN],
Plaquenil)
**Do not confuse hydroxychloro-
quine with hydrocortisone or
hydroxyzine.**

CATEGORY AND SCHEDULE

Pregnancy Risk Category: C

CLASSIFICATION

Antiprotozoals, disease modifying antirheumatic drugs

MECHANISM OF ACTION

An antimalarial and antirheumatic that concentrates in parasite acid vesicles, increasing the pH of the vesicles and interfering with parasite protein synthesis. Antirheumatic action may involve suppressing formation of antigens responsible for hypersensitivity reactions.
Therapeutic Effect: Inhibits parasite growth.

AVAILABILITY

Tablets: 200 mg (155 mg base).

INDICATIONS AND DOSAGES

▸ **Treatment of acute attack of
malaria (dosage in mg base)**
PO

Dose	Times	Adults	Children
Initial	Day 1	620 mg	10 mg/kg
Second	6 hr later	310 mg	5 mg/kg
Third	Day 2	310 mg	5 mg/kg
Fourth	Day 3	310 mg	5 mg/kg

▸ **Suppression of malaria**
PO
Adults. 310 mg base weekly on same day each week, beginning 2 wk before entering an endemic area and continuing for 4-6 wk after leaving the area.
Children. 5 mg base/kg/wk, beginning 2 wk before entering an endemic area and continuing for 4-6 wk after leaving the area. If ther-apy is not begun before exposure, administer a loading dose of 10 mg base/kg in 2 equally divided doses 6 hr apart, followed by the ususal dosage regimen.
▸ **Rheumatoid arthritis**
PO
Adults. Initially, 400-600 mg (310-465 mg base) daily for 5-10 days, gradually increased to optimum response level. Maintenance (usually within 4-12 wk): Dosage decreased by 50% and then continued at maintenance dose of 200-400 mg/day. Maximum effect may not be seen for several months.

> **Lupus erythematosus**
PO
Adults. Initially, 400 mg once or twice a day for several weeks or months. Maintenance: 200-400 mg/day.

OFF-LABEL USES
Treatment of juvenile arthritis, sarcoid-associated hypercalcemia

CONTRAINDICATIONS
Long-term therapy for children, porphyria, psoriasis, retinal or visual field changes

INTERACTIONS
Drug
Aurothioglucose: May increase the risk of blood dyscrasias.
Digoxin: May increase serum digoxin concentrations.
Penicillamine: May increase blood penicillamine concentration and the risk of hematologic, renal, or severe skin reactions.
Herbal
None known.
Food
None known.

DIAGNOSTIC TEST EFFECTS
None known.

SIDE EFFECTS
Frequent
Mild, transient headache; anorexia; nausea; vomiting
Occasional
Visual disturbances, nervousness, fatigue, pruritus (especially of palms, soles, and scalp), irritability, personality changes, diarrhea
Rare
Stomatitis, dermatitis, impaired hearing

SERIOUS REACTIONS
• Ocular toxicity, especially retinopathy, may occur and may progress even after drug is discontinued.
• Prolonged therapy may result in peripheral neuritis, neuromyopathy, hypotension, EKG changes, agranulocytosis, aplastic anemia, thrombocytopenia, seizures, and psychosis.
• Overdosage may result in headache, vomiting, visual disturbances, drowsiness, seizures, and hypokalemia followed by cardiovascular collapse and death.

PRECAUTIONS & CONSIDERATIONS H
Caution is warranted with glucose-6-phosphate dehydrogenase deficiency, hepatic disease, alcoholism, and a history of alcohol abuse. Be aware that children are especially susceptible to hydroxychloroquine's fatal effects.
Report decreased hearing, tinnitus, visual difficulties, muscle weakness, or any other new symptoms. Visual disturbances, impaired hearing, and GI distress should be monitored. Liver function should be assessed. The buccal mucosa and skin should be checked for pruritus.
Administration
! Be aware that 200 mg hydroxychloroquine equals 155 mg base. Take the drug dose with food for treatment of malaria.

Hydroxyprogesterone
(progestin derivative, antineoplastic, progestin)
(Gestrol LA)

CATEGORY AND SCHEDULE
Pregnancy Risk Category: D

CLASSIFICATION
Antineoplastic, progestin, progestin derivative

MECHANISM OF ACTION
A hormone that influences prolifera-tive endometrium and transforms into secretory endometrium. Secretion of pituitary gonadotropins is inhibited which prevents follicular maturation and ovulation.
Therapeutic Effect: Facilitates ureteral dilatation associated with hydronephrosis of pregnancy.

AVAILABILITY
Injection: 250 mg/ml (Gestrol LA).

INDICATIONS AND DOSAGES
▸ **Amenorrhea**
IM
Adults. 375 mg given at any point in the menstrual cycle.
▸ **Endogenous estrogen production**
IM
Adults. 125 to 250 mg beginning on the tenth day of cycle and repeated every 7 days until suppression is no longer desired.
▸ **Endometrial carcinoma**
IM
Adults. 1000 mg 1 or more times weekly.
▸ **Abnormal uterine bleeding**
IM
Adults. 5-10 mg for 6 days. When estrogen is given concomitantly, begin progesterone after 2 wk of estrogen therapy; discontinue when menstrual flow begins.
▸ **Prevention of endometrial hyperplasia**
IM
Adults. 200 mg in evening for 12 days per 28-day cycle in combi-nation with daily conjugated estrogen.
▸ **Premature labor**
IM
Adults. 250 to 500 mg once weekly.

OFF-LABEL USES
Alopecia, stress incontinence, menopausal symptoms, preterm delivery, treatment of prostatic hyperplasia, seborrhea, ureteral stones

CONTRAINDICATIONS
Breast cancer, cerebral apoplexy or history of these conditions, missed abortion, severe liver dysfunction, thromboembolic disorders, throm-bophlebitis, undiagnosed vaginal bleeding, genital malignancy, use as a diagnostic test for pregnancy

INTERACTIONS
Drug
Bromocriptine: May interfere with the effects of bromocriptine.
Herbal
None known.
Food
None known.

DIAGNOSTIC TEST EFFECTS
May increase LDL concentrations and serum alkaline phosphatase levels. May decrease glucose tolerance and HDL concentrations. May cause abnormal thyroid, metapyrone, liver and endocrine function tests.

SIDE EFFECTS
Frequent
Breakthrough bleeding or spotting at beginning of therapy, amenorrhea, change in menstrual flow, breast tenderness
Occasional
Edema, weight gain or loss, rash, pruritus, photosensitivity, skin pigmentation
Rare
Pain or swelling at injection site, acne, mental depression, alopecia, hirsutism

SERIOUS REACTIONS
• Thrombophlebitis, cerebrovascu-lar disorders, retinal thrombosis, and pulmonary embolism rarely occur.

Caution is warranted with conditions aggravated by fluid retention, asthma, epilepsy, diabetes mellitus, cardiac or renal dysfunction, or a history of mental depression. Pain, redness, swelling, or warmth in the calf, chest pain, migraine headache, peripheral paresthesia, sudden decrease in vision, and sudden shortness of breath should be reported immediately. Smoking should be avoided during therapy.

Administration
Rotate the vial to disperse drug in solution. Give deep IM injection into the gluteus maximus.

Hydroxyzine
hye-drox′i-zeen
(Apo-Hydroxyzine [CAN], Atarax, Novohydroxyzin [CAN], Vistaril)
Do not confuse hydroxyzine with hydralazine or hydroxyurea.

CATEGORY AND SCHEDULE
Pregnancy Risk Category: C

CLASSIFICATION
Antiemetics/antivertigo, antihistamines, H1, anxiolytics, sedatives/hypnotics

MECHANISM OF ACTION
A piperazine derivative that competes with histamine for receptor sites in the GI tract, blood vessels, and respiratory tract. May exert CNS depressant activity in subcortical areas. Diminishes vestibular stimulation and depresses labyrinthine function. *Therapeutic Effect:* Produces anxiolytic, anticholinergic, antihistaminic, and analgesic effects; relaxes skeletal muscle; controls nausea and vomiting.

PHARMACOKINETICS

Route	Onset	Peak	Duration
PO	15-30 min	N/A	4-6 hr

Well absorbed from the GI tract and after parenteral administration. Metabolized in the liver. Primarily excreted in urine. Not removed by hemodialysis. **Half-life:** 20-25 hr (increased in the elderly).

AVAILABILITY
Capsules (Vistaril): 25 mg, 50 mg, 100 mg.
Oral Suspension (Vistaril): 25 mg/5 ml.
Syrup (Atarax). 10 mg/5 ml.
Tablets (Atarax): 10 mg, 25 mg, 50 mg, 100 mg.
Injection (Vistaril): 25 mg/ml, 50 mg/ml.

INDICATIONS AND DOSAGES
▸ **Anxiety**
PO
Adults, Elderly. 25-100 mg 4 times a day. Maximum: 600 mg/day.
▸ **Nausea and vomiting**
IM
Adults, Elderly. 25-100 mg/dose q4-6hr.
▸ **Pruritus**
PO
Adults, Elderly. 25 mg 3-4 times a day.
▸ **Preoperative sedation**
PO
Adults, Elderly. 50-100 mg.
IM
Adults, Elderly. 25-100 mg.
▸ **Usual pediatric dosage**
PO
Children. 2 mg/kg/day in divided doses q6-8hr.
IM
Children. 0.5-1 mg/kg/dose q4-6hr.

CONTRAINDICATIONS
Early pregnancy.

INTERACTIONS
Drug
Alcohol, other CNS depressants:
May increase CNS depressant
effects.
MAOIs: May increase anticholiner-
gic and CNS depressant effects.
Herbal
None known.
Food
None known.

DIAGNOSTIC TEST EFFECTS
May cause false-positive urine 17-
hydroxycorticosteroid determinations.

SIDE EFFECTS
Side effects are generally mild and
transient.
Frequent
Somnolence, dry mouth, marked
discomfort with IM injection
Occasional
Dizziness, ataxia, asthenia, slurred
speech, headache, agitation,
increased anxiety
Rare
Paradoxical CNS reactions, such as
hyperactivity or nervousness in children and excitement or restlessness
in elderly or debilitated patients
(generally noted during first 2 weeks
of therapy, particularly in presence
of uncontrolled pain)

SERIOUS REACTIONS
• A hypersensitivity reaction,
including wheezing, dyspnea, and
chest tightness, may occur.

PRECAUTIONS & CONSIDERATIONS
Caution is warranted with asthma,
bladder neck obstruction, COPD,
angle-closure glaucoma, and benign
prostatic hyperplasia. It is unknown if
hydroxyzine crosses the placenta or is
distributed in breast milk.
Hydroxyzine use is not recommended
for neonates or premature infants
because they're at increased risk for
anticholinergic effects. Children may
experience paradoxical excitement.
The elderly are at increased risk for
confusion, dizziness, sedation,
hypotension, and hyperexcitability.
Be aware of dehydration which can
occur with severe vomiting.

Drowsiness and dizziness may
occur. Change positions slowly from
recumbent to sitting before standing
to prevent dizziness. Alcohol,
caffeine, and tasks that require
mental alertness or motor skills
should also be avoided. Autonomic
responses, such as cold, clammy
hands and diaphoresis, and motor
responses, such as agitation,
trembling, and tension, should be
assessed. CBC and blood chemistry
tests should be performed periodically in long-term therapy. Breath
sounds, electrolyte levels, and CNS
reactions should also be assessed.
Administration
Crush scored tablets as needed, but
don't crush or break capsules. Shake
the oral suspension thoroughly.
! Don't give hydroxyzine by the
subcutaneous intra-arterial or IV
route because doing so can cause
significant tissue damage, thrombosis, and gangrene.
The IM form may be given undiluted. Inject the drug deep into the
gluteus maximus or midlateral thigh
in adults and the midlateral thigh in
children. Use the Z-track technique
of injection to prevent subcutaneous
infiltration. IM injection may cause
marked discomfort.

Hyoscyamine
hye-oh-sye′a-meen
(Anaspaz, Buscopan [CAN],
Cystospaz, Cystospaz-M,
Hyosine, Levbid, Levsin,
Levsinex, Levsin/SL, NuLev,
Spacol, Spacol T/S, Symax SL,
Symax SR)
**Do not confuse Anaspaz with
Anaprox.**

CATEGORY AND SCHEDULE
Pregnancy Risk Category: C

CLASSIFICATION
Anticholinergics, gastrointestinals

MECHANISM OF ACTION
A GI antispasmodic and anticholinergic agent that inhibits the action of
acetylcholine at post-ganglionic
(muscarinic) receptor sites.
Therapeutic Effect: Decreases
secretions (bronchial, salivary,
sweat gland) and gastric juices and
reduces motility of GI and urinary
tract.

AVAILABILITY
*Tablets (Anaspaz, Cystospaz, Levsin,
Spacol):* 0.125 mg.
*Tablets (Oral-Disintegrating
[NuLev]):* 0.125 mg.
*Tablets (Sublingual [Levsin S/L,
Symax SL]):* 0.125 mg.
*Tablets (Extended-Release
[Levbid, Spacol T/S, Symax SR]):*
0.375 mg.
*Capsules (Extended-Release
[Cystospaz-M, Levsinex]):*
0.375 mg.
Liquid (Hyoscine, Spacol):
0.125 mg/5 ml.
Oral Solution (Hyoscine, Levsin):
0.125 mg/5 ml

INDICATIONS AND DOSAGES
▶ **GI tract disorders**
PO
*Adults, Elderly, Children 12 yr and
older.* 0.125-0.25 mg q4hr as
needed. Extended-release:
0.375-0.75 mg q12hr. Maximum:
1.5 mg/day.
Children 2-11 yr. 0.0625-0.125 mg
q4hr as needed. Extended-release:
0.375 mg q12hr. Maximum:
0.75 mg/day.
IM, IV
*Adults, Elderly, Children 12 yr and
older.* 0.25-0.5 mg q4hr for 1-4 doses.
▶ **Hypermotility of lower urinary
tract**
PO, SUBLINGUAL
Adults, Elderly. 0.15-0.3 mg 4 times
a day; or extended-release 0.375 mg
q12hr.
▶ **Infant colic**
PO
Infants. Individualized drops dosed
q4hr as needed.

CONTRAINDICATIONS
GI or GU obstruction, myasthenia
gravis, narrow-angle glaucoma, paralytic ileus, severe ulcerative colitis

INTERACTIONS
Drug
Antacids, antidiarrheals: May
decrease the absorption of
hyoscyamine.
Ketoconazole: May decrease the
absorption of this drug.
Other anticholinergics: May
increase the effects of hyoscyamine.
Potassium chloride: May increase
the severity of GI lesions with the
matrix formulation of potassium
chloride.
Herbal
None known.
Food
None known.

H

DIAGNOSTIC TEST EFFECTS
None known.

SIDE EFFECTS
Frequent
Dry mouth (sometimes severe), decreased sweating, constipation
Occasional
Blurred vision; bloated feeling; urinary hesitancy; somnolence (with high dosage); headache; intolerance to light; loss of taste; nervousness; flushing; insomnia; impotence; mental confusion or excitement (particularly in the elderly and children); temporary lightheadedness (with parenteral form); local irritation (with parenteral form)
Rare
Dizziness, faintness

SERIOUS REACTIONS
• Overdose may produce temporary paralysis of ciliary muscle; pupillary dilation; tachycardia; palpitations; hot, dry, or flushed skin; absence of bowel sounds; hyperthermia; increased respiratory rate; EKG abnormalities; nausea; vomiting; rash over face or upper trunk; CNS stimulation; and psychosis (marked by agitation, restlessness, rambling speech, visual hallucinations, paranoid behavior, and delusions, followed by depression).

PRECAUTIONS & CONSIDERATIONS
Caution is warranted with cardiac arrhythmias, CHF, chronic lung disease, hyperthyroidism, neuropathy, and prostatic hyperplasia. Avoid hot baths, saunas, and becoming overheated while exercising in hot weather because they may cause heat stroke. Tasks that require mental alertness or motor skills should also be avoided until response to the drug has been established.

Dry mouth may occur, so good oral hygiene should be maintained because the lack of saliva may increase the risk of cavities. Notify the physician of constipation, difficulty urinating, eye pain, or rash. B/P, body temperature, heart rate, pattern of daily bowel activity and stool consistency, and urine output should be monitored. The person should void before giving the drug to reduce the risk of urine retention.

Administration
Give oral hyoscyamine without regard to meals. Crush or have patient chew tablets. Extended-release capsule should be swallowed whole.

For parenteral use, hyoscyamine may be given undiluted.

Ibandronate
eye-band′droh-nate
(Boniva)

CATEGORY AND SCHEDULE
Pregnancy Risk Category: C

CLASSIFICATION
Bisphosphonates

MECHANISM OF ACTION
A bisphosphonate that binds to bone hydroxyapatite (part of the mineral matrix of bone) and inhibits osteoclast activity. *Therapeutic Effect:* Reduces rate of bone turnover and bone resorption, resulting in a net gain in bone mass.

PHARMACOKINETICS
Absorbed in the upper GI tract. Extent of absorption impaired by food or beverages (other than plain water). Rapidly binds to bone. Unabsorbed portion is eliminated in urine. Protein binding: 90%. **Half-life:** 10-60 hr.

AVAILABILITY
Tablets: 2.5 mg

INDICATIONS AND DOSAGES
▶ Osteoporosis
PO
Adults, Elderly. 2.5 mg daily.

CONTRAINDICATIONS
Hypersensitivity to other bisphosphonates, including alendronate, etidronate, pamidronate, risedronate, and tiludronate; inability to stand or sit upright for at least 60 minutes; severe renal impairment with creatinine clearance less than 30 ml/min; uncorrected hypocalcemia

INTERACTIONS
Drug
Antacids containing aluminum, calcium, magnesium; vitamin D: Decrease the absorption of ibandronate.
Herbal
None known.
Food
Beverages other than plain water, dietary supplements, food: Interfere with the absorption of ibandronate.

DIAGNOSTIC TEST EFFECTS
May decrease serum alkaline phosphatase level. May increase blood cholesterol level.

SIDE EFFECTS
Frequent (13%-6%)
Back pain; dyspepsia, including epigastric distress and heartburn; peripheral discomfort; diarrhea; headache; myalgia
Occasional (4%-3%)
Dizziness, arthralgia, asthenia
Rare (2% or less)
Vomiting, hypersensitivity reaction

SERIOUS REACTIONS
• Upper respiratory tract infection occurs occasionally.
• Overdose causes hypocalcemia, hypophosphatemia, and significant GI disturbances

PRECAUTIONS & CONSIDERATIONS
Caution is warranted with GI diseases, including duodenitis, dysphagia, esophagitis, gastritis, and ulcers, and mild to moderate renal impairment. Ibandronate may have teratogenic effects. It is unknown if ibandronate is excreted in breast milk. Breast-feeding is not recommended for female patients taking ibandronate. The safety and efficacy of ibandronate have not been

established in children. No age-related precautions have been noted in the elderly. Avoid taking ibandronate with coffee, mineral water, and orange juice because they significantly reduce the absorption of the drug. Consider beginning weight-bearing exercises, reduce alcohol consumption, and stop cigarette smoking.

Hypocalcemia and vitamin D deficiencies, if present, should be corrected before beginning ibandronate therapy. BUN, creatinine levels, and serum electrolytes, especially calcium and serum alkaline phosphatase levels, should be monitored during therapy.

Administration

Take ibandronate on an empty stomach with 6-8 ounces of plain—not mineral—water 60 minutes before the patient receives his or her first food or beverage of the day. Stay in an upright position while standing or sitting; do not lie down for 60 minutes after drug administration. Do not chew or suck the tablet because of the potential for oropharyngeal ulceration.

Ibuprofen

eye-byoo′pro-fen
(Act-3 [AUS], Advil, Apo-Ibuprofen, Brufen [AUS], Codral Period Pain [AUS], Motrin, Novoprofen [CAN], Nurofen [AUS], Rafen [AUS])

CATEGORY AND SCHEDULE

Pregnancy Risk Category: B (D if used in third trimester or near delivery)
OTC (Tablets: 200 mg, Oral Suspension: 100 mg/5 ml)

CLASSIFICATION

Analgesics, non-narcotic, antipyretics, nonsteroidal anti-inflammatory drugs

MECHANISM OF ACTION

An NSAID that inhibits prostaglandin synthesis. Also produces vasodilation by acting centrally on the heat-regulating center of the hypothalamus. *Therapeutic Effect:* Produces analgesic and anti-inflammatory effects and decreases fever.

PHARMACOKINETICS

Route	Onset	Peak	Duration
PO (anal-gesic)	0.5 hr	N/A	4-6 hr
PO (anti-rheumatic)	2 days	1-2 wk	N/A

Rapidly absorbed from the GI tract. Protein binding: greater than 90%. Metabolized in the liver. Primarily excreted in urine. Not removed by hemodialysis. **Half-life:** 2-4 hr.

AVAILABILITY
Caplets (Advil, Menadol, Motrin): 200 mg.
Capsules (Advil, Advil Migraine): 200 mg.
Gelcaps (Advil, Motrin IB): 200 mg.
Tablets (Advil, Motrin IB): 200 mg.
Tablets (Motin): 400 mg, 600 mg, 800 mg.
Tablets (Chewable [Children's Advil, Children's Motrin]): 50 mg.
Tablets (Chewable [Junior Advil, Junior Strength Motrin]): 100 mg.
Oral Suspension (Children's Advil, Children's Motrin): 100 mg/5 ml.
Oral Drops (Infant Advil, Infant Motrin): 40 mg/ml.

INDICATIONS AND DOSAGES
▸ **Acute or chronic rheumatoid arthritis, osteoarthritis, migraine pain, gouty arthritis**
PO
Adults, Elderly. 400-800 mg 3-4 times a day. Maximum: 3.2 g/day.
▸ **Mild to moderate pain, primary dysmenorrhea**
PO
Adults, Elderly. 200-400 mg q4-6hr as needed. Maximum: 1.6 g/day.
▸ **Fever, minor aches or pain**
PO
Adults, Elderly. 200-400 mg q4-6hr. Maximum: 1.6 g/day.
Children. 5-10 mg/kg/dose q6-8hr. Maximum: 40 mg/kg/day. OTC: 7.5 mg/kg/dose q6-8hr. Maximum: 30 mg/kg/day.
▸ **Juvenile arthritis**
PO
Children. 30-70 mg/kg/day in 3-4 divided doses. Maximum: 400 mg/day in children weighing less than 20 kg, 600 mg/day in children weighing 20-30 kg, 800 mg/day in children weighing greater than 30-40 kg.

OFF-LABEL USES
Treatment of psoriatic arthritis, vascular headaches

CONTRAINDICATIONS
Active peptic ulcer, chronic inflammation of GI tract, GI bleeding disorders or ulceration, history of hypersensitivity to aspirin or NSAIDs

INTERACTIONS
Drug
Antihypertensives, diuretics: May decrease the effects of these drugs.
Aspirin, other salicylates: May increase the risk of GI side effects such as bleeding.
Bone marrow depressants: May increase the risk of hematologic reactions.
Heparin, oral anticoagulants, thrombolytics: May increase the effects of these drugs.
Lithium: May increase the blood concentration and risk of toxicity of lithium.
Methotrexate: May increase the risk of methotrexate toxicity.
Probenecid: May increase the ibuprofen blood concentration.
Herbal
Feverfew: May decrease the effects of feverfew.
Ginkgo biloba: May increase the risk of bleeding.
Food
None known.

DIAGNOSTIC TEST EFFECTS
May prolong bleeding time. May alter blood glucose level. May increase BUN level, and serum creatinine, potassium, AST (SGOT), and ALT (SGPT) levels. May decrease blood Hgb and Hct.

SIDE EFFECTS
Occasional (9%-3%)
Nausea with or without vomiting, dyspepsia, dizziness, rash
Rare (less than 3%)
Diarrhea or constipation, flatulence, abdominal cramps or pain, pruritus

SERIOUS REACTIONS
• Acute overdose may result in metabolic acidosis.
• Rare reactions with long-term use include peptic ulcer disease, GI bleeding, gastritis, a severe hepatic reaction (cholestasis, jaundice), nephrotoxicity (dysuria, hematuria, proteinuria, nephrotic syndrome), and a severe hypersensitivity reaction (particularly in patients with systemic lupus erythematosus or other collagen diseases).

PRECAUTIONS & CONSIDERATIONS
Caution is warranted with CHF, hypertension, dehydration, GI disease (such as GI bleeding or ulcers), hepatic or renal impairment, and concurrent anticoagulant use. It is unknown if ibuprofen crosses the placenta or is distributed in breast milk. Ibuprofen should not be used during the third trimester of pregnancy because it may cause adverse effects in the fetus, such as premature closure of the ductus arteriosus. The safety and efficacy of this drug have not been established in children younger than 6 months. In the elderly, GI bleeding or ulceration is more likely to cause serious complications and age-related renal impairment may increase the risk of hepatotoxicity or renal toxicity; a reduced dosage is recommended. Avoid alcohol and aspirin during therapy because these substances increase the risk of GI bleeding. Tasks that require mental alertness or motor skills should be avoided.

CBC, platelet count, serum alkaline phosphatase, bilirubin, creatinine, AST (SGOT), ALT (SGPT) levels, pattern of daily bowel activity and stool consistency, and skin for rash should be monitored. Therapeutic response, such as decreased pain, stiffness, swelling, and tenderness, improved grip strength, and increased joint mobility, should be evaluated.
Administration
Do not crush or break enteric-coated tablets. Take ibuprofen with food, milk, or antacids.

Ibutilide
eye-byoo'ti-lide
(Corvert)

CATEGORY AND SCHEDULE
Pregnancy Risk Category: C

CLASSIFICATION
Antiarrhythmics, class III

MECHANISM OF ACTION
An antiarrhythmic that prolongs both atrial and ventricular action potential duration and increases the atrial and ventricular refractory period. Activates slow, inward current (mostly of sodium), produces mild slowing of sinus node rate and AV conduction, and causes dose-related prolongation of QT interval. *Therapeutic Effect:* Converts arrhythmias to sinus rhythm.

PHARMACOKINETICS
After IV administration, highly distributed, rapidly cleared.

Protein binding: 40%. Primarily excreted in urine as metabolite.
Half-life: 2-12 hr (average: 6 hr).

AVAILABILITY
Injection: 0.1 mg/ml solution.

INDICATIONS AND DOSAGES
▸ **Rapid conversion of atrial fibrillation or flutter of recent onset to normal sinus rhythm**
IV INFUSION
Adults, Elderly weighing 60 kg or more. One vial (1 mg) given over 10 min. If arrhythmia does not stop within 10 min after end of initial infusion, a second 1 mg/10-min infusion may be given.
Adults, Elderly weighing less than 60 kg. 0.01 mg/kg given over 10 min. If arrhythmia does not stop within 10 min after end of initial infusion, a second 0.01 mg/kg, 10-min infusion may be given.

CONTRAINDICATIONS
None known.

INTERACTIONS
Drug
Class IA antiarrhythmics (disopyramide, moricizine, procainamide, quinidine), Class III antiarrhythmics (amiodarone, bretylium, sotalol): Do not give ibutilide with these drugs or give these drugs within 4 hours after infusing ibutilide.
H₁ receptor antagonists, phenothiazines, tricyclic and tetracyclic antidepressants: May prolong QT interval.
Herbal
None known.
Food
None known.

DIAGNOSTIC TEST EFFECTS
None known.

IV INCOMPATIBILITIES
No information is available for Y-site administration.

SIDE EFFECTS
Ibutilide is generally well tolerated.
Occasional
Ventricular extrasystoles (5.1%), ventricular tachycardia (4.9%), headache (3.6%), hypotension, orthostatic hypotension (2%)
Rare
Bundle-branch block, AV block, bradycardia, hypertension

SERIOUS REACTIONS
• Sustained polymorphic ventricular tachycardia, occasionally with QT prolongation (torsades de pointes) occurs rarely.
• Overdose results in CNS toxicity, including CNS depression, rapid gasping breathing, and seizures.
• Expect prolongation of repolarization may be exaggerated.
• Existing arrhythmias may worsen or new arrhythmias may develop.

PRECAUTIONS & CONSIDERATIONS
Caution is warranted with abnormal hepatic function or heart failure. Because ibutilide is embryocidal and teratogenic in animals, breast-feeding is not recommended during ibutilide therapy. Safety and efficacy of ibutilide have not been established in children. No age-related precautions have been noted in the elderly.
Notify the physician if palpitations or other adverse reactions occur. B/P and EKG should be continuously monitored during therapy. Serum electrolyte levels, especially magnesium and potassium, should be monitored and arrhythmias requiring overdrive cardiac pacing, electrical cardioversion, or defibrillation should be surveyed. Those with atrial fibrillation lasting

more than 3 days should be given an anticoagulant for at least 2 weeks before ibutilide therapy is started. Proarrhythmias may develop.

Storage

Admixtures with diluent are stable at room temperature for up to 24 hours or up to 48 hours if refrigerated.

Administration

Have advanced cardiac life-support equipment, medications, and trained personnel on hand during and after ibutilide administration. Ibutilide is compatible with D_5W and 0.9% NaCl. It is also compatible with polyvinyl chloride plastic and polyolefin bag admixtures. Give undiluted or may dilute in 50 ml diluent. Give over 10 minutes.

Iloprost
eye′low-prost
(Ventavis)

CATEGORY AND SCHEDULE
Pregnancy Risk Category: C

CLASSIFICATION
Miscellaneous respiratory agents

MECHANISM OF ACTION
A prostaglandin that dilates systemic and pulmonary arterial vascular beds, alters pulmonary vascular resistance, and suppresses vascular smooth muscle proliferation.
Therapeutic Effect: Improves symptoms and exercise tolerance in patients with pulmonary hypertension; delays deterioration of condition.

AVAILABILITY
Solution for Oral Inhalation:
10 mcg/ml (2-ml ampule).

INDICATIONS AND DOSAGES
▸ **Pulmonary hypertension in patients with NYHA Class III or IV symptoms**
ORAL INHALATION
Adults. Initially, 2.5 mcg/dose; if tolerated, increased to 5 mcg/dose. Administer 6-9 times a day at intervals of 2 hr or longer while patient is awake. Maintenance: 5 mcg/dose. Maximum daily dose: 45 mcg.

CONTRAINDICATIONS
None known.

INTERACTIONS
Drug
Anticoagulants, antiplatelet agents: May increase the risk of bleeding.
Antihypertensives, other vasodilators: May increase the hypotensive effects of iloprost.
Herbal
None known.
Food
None known.

DIAGNOSTIC TEST EFFECTS
May increase serum alkaline phosphatase and GGT levels.

SIDE EFFECTS
Frequent (39%-27%)
Increased cough, headache, flushing
Occasional (13%-11%)
Flu-like symptoms, nausea, lockjaw, jaw pain, hypotension
Rare (8%-2%)
Insomnia, syncope, palpitations, vomiting, back pain, muscle cramps

SERIOUS REACTIONS
• Hemoptysis and pneumonia occur occasionally.
• CHF, renal failure, dyspnea, and chest pain occur rarely.

PRECAUTIONS & CONSIDERATIONS

Caution is warranted with hepatic impairment and in those who are concurrently taking medications that may increase the risk of syncope.

Administration

Iloprost is administered by inhalation only, using the Prodose ADD system. Transfer the entire contents of the ampoule into the medication chamber. After use, discard any unused portion.

Imatinib
im'a-tin-ib
(Gleevec, Glivec [AUS])

CATEGORY AND SCHEDULE
Pregnancy Risk Category: D

CLASSIFICATION
Antineoplastics, signal transduction inhibitors

MECHANISM OF ACTION

Inhibits Bcr-Abl tyrosine kinase, an enzyme created by the Philadelphia chromosome abnormality found in patients with chronic myeloid leukemia (CML). *Therapeutic Effect:* Suppresses tumor growth during the three stages of CML; blast crisis, accelerated phase, and chronic phase.

PHARMACOKINETICS

Well absorbed after PO administration. Binds to plasma proteins, particularly albumin. Metabolized in the liver. Eliminated mainly in the feces as metabolites. **Half-life:** 18 hr.

AVAILABILITY
Tablets: 100 mg, 400 mg.

INDICATIONS AND DOSAGES
▶ **CML**
PO
Adults, Elderly. 400 mg/day for patients in chronic-phase CML; 600 mg/day for patients in accelerated phase or blast crisis. May increase dosage from 400 to 600 mg/day for patients in chronic phase or from 600 to 800 mg (given as 300-400 mg twice a day) for patients in accelerated phase or blast crisis in the absence of a severe drug reaction or severe neutropenia or thrombocytopenia in the following circumstances: progression of the disease, failure to achieve a satisfactory hematologic response after 3 months or more of treatment, or loss of a previously achieved hematologic response.
Children. 260 mg/m^2 a day as a single daily dose or in 2 divided doses.

CONTRAINDICATIONS
Known hypersensitivity to imatinib

INTERACTIONS
Drug
Carbamazepine, dexamethasone, phenobarbital, phenytoin, rifampicin: Decrease imatinib plasma concentration.
Clarithromycin, erythromycin, itraconazole, ketoconazole: Increase imatinib plasma concentration.
Cyclosporine, pimozide: May alter the therapeutic effects of these drugs.
Dihydropyridine calcium channel blockers, simvastatin, triazolo-benzodiazepines: May increase the blood concentration of these drugs.

Live-virus vaccines: May potentiate viral replication, increase vaccine side effects, and decrease the patient's antibody response to the vaccine.
Warfarin: Reduces the effect of warfarin.
Herbal
St. John's wort: Decreases imatinib concentration.
Food
None known.

DIAGNOSTIC TEST EFFECTS
May increase serum bilirubin AST (SGOT), and ALT (SGPT) levels. May decrease platelet count, WBC count, and serum potassium level.

SIDE EFFECTS
Frequent (68%-24%)
Nausea, diarrhea, vomiting, headache, fluid retention (periorbital, lower extremities), rash, musculoskeletal pain, muscle cramps, arthralgia
Occasional (23%-10%)
Abdominal pain, cough, myalgia, fatigue, fever, anorexia, dyspepsia, constipation, night sweats, pruritus
Rare (less than 10%)
Nasopharyngitis, petechiae, asthenia, epistaxis

SERIOUS REACTIONS
• Severe fluid retention (manifested as pleural effusion, pericardial effusion, pulmonary edema, and ascites) and hepatotoxicity occur rarely.
• Neutropenia and thrombocytopenia are expected responses to the drug.
• Respiratory toxicity, manifested as dyspnea and pneumonia, may occur.

PRECAUTIONS & CONSIDERATIONS
Caution is warranted with hepatic and renal impairment. Because imatinib may cause severe teratogenic effects, female patients should

avoid becoming pregnant and/or breast-feeding while taking this drug. The safety and efficacy of imatinib have not been established in children. The elderly are at increased risk for fluid retention. Vaccinations without the physician's approval, crowds, and contact with people with known infections should be avoided.
Notify the physician of rapid weight gain, fluid retention, nausea, and vomiting. Antiemetics should be ordered to control nausea and vomiting. Pattern of daily bowel activity and stool consistency should be monitored. CBC for evidence of neutropenia and thrombocytopenia and liver function test results for evidence of hepatotoxicity should be assessed. Neutropenia and thrombocytopenia usually last 2 to 4 weeks.
Administration
Give oral imatinib with a meal and a large glass of water.

Imiglucerase
im-i-gloo′-ser-ase
(Cerezyme)
Do not confuse Cerezyme with Cerebyx or Ceredase.

CATEGORY AND SCHEDULE
Pregnancy Risk Category: C

CLASSIFICATION
Enzymes, metabolic, recombinant DNA origin

MECHANISM OF ACTION
An enzyme analogue of the enzyme beta-glucocerebrosidase, which catalyzes hydrolysis of the glycolipid glucocerebroside to glucose and ceramide. *Therapeutic Effect:* Minimizes conditions associated

with Gaucher's disease, such as anemia and bone disease.

AVAILABILITY
Powder for Injection: 212 units (equivalent to a reconstituted withdrawal dose of 200 units), 424 units (equivalent to a reconstituted withdrawal dose of 400 units).

INDICATIONS AND DOSAGES
▶ **Gaucher's disease**
IV
Adults, Elderly, Children. Initially, 2.5 units/kg infused over 1-2 hr 3 times a week up to 60 units/kg/wk. Maintenance: Progressive reduction in dosage while monitoring patient response.

CONTRAINDICATIONS
None known.

INTERACTIONS
Drug
None known.
Herbal
None known.
Food
None known.

DIAGNOSTIC TEST EFFECTS
None known.

▓ IV INCOMPATIBILITIES
Don't mix imiglucerase with any solution other than 0.9% NaCl.

SIDE EFFECTS
Frequent (3%)
Headache
Occasional (less than 3%-1%)
Nausea, abdominal discomfort, dizziness, pruritus, rash, small decrease in B/P, urinary frequency

PRECAUTIONS & CONSIDERATIONS
CBC, platelet count, and liver function test results should be monitored. Notify the physician of headache.

Storage
Refrigerate vials. The reconstituted solution is stable for 24 hours if refrigerated.

Administration
For IV use, reconstitute the 200-unit vial with 5.1 ml sterile water (or the 400-unit vial with 10.2 ml) to provide a concentration of 40 units/ml. Further dilute with 100 to 200 ml 0.9% NaCl. Infuse the solution over 1 to 2 hours.

Imipenem-Cilastatin
i-me-pen'em
(Primaxin)

CATEGORY AND SCHEDULE
Pregnancy Risk Category: C

CLASSIFICATION
Antibiotics, carbapenems

MECHANISM OF ACTION
A fixed-combination carbapenem. Imipenem penetrates the bacterial cell membrane and binds to penicillin-binding proteins, inhibiting cell wall synthesis. Cilastatin competitively inhibits the enzyme dehydropeptidase, preventing renal metabolism of imipenem.
Therapeutic Effect: Produces bacterial cell death.

PHARMACOKINETICS
Readily absorbed after IM administration. Protein binding: 13%-21%. Widely distributed. Metabolized in the kidneys. Primarily excreted in urine. Removed by hemodialysis.
Half-life: 1 hr (increased in impaired renal function).

AVAILABILITY
IV Injection: 250 mg, 500 mg.
IM Injection: 500 mg, 750 mg.

INDICATIONS AND DOSAGES
▶ **Serious respiratory tract, skin and skin-structure, gynecologic, bone, joint, intra-abdominal, nosocomial, and polymicrobic infections; UTIs; endocarditis; septicemia**
IV
Adults, Elderly. 2-4 g/day in divided doses q6hr.
▶ **Mild to moderate respiratory tract, skin and skin-structure, gynecologic, bone, joint, intra-abdominal, and polymicrobic infections; UTIs; endocarditis; septicemia**
IV
Adults, Elderly. 1-2 g/day in divided doses q6-8hr.
Children older than 3 mo-12 yr. 60-100 mg/kg/day in divided doses q6hr. Maximum: 4 g/day.
Children 1-3 mo. 100 mg/kg/day in divided doses q6hr.
Children younger than 1 mo. 20-25 mg/kg/dose q8-24hr.
IM
Adults, Elderly. 500-750 mg q12hr.
▶ **Dosage in renal impairment**
Dosage and frequency are modified based on creatinine clearance and the severity of the infection.

Creatinine Clearance	Dosage (IV)
31-70 ml/min	500 mg q8hr
21-30 ml/min	500 mg q12hr
5-20 ml/min	250 mg q12hr

CONTRAINDICATIONS
None known.

INTERACTIONS
Drug
None known.
Herbal
None known.

Food
None known.

DIAGNOSTIC TEST EFFECTS
May increase BUN level and serum alkaline phosphatase, bilirubin, creatinine, LDH, AST (SGOT) and ALT (SGPT) levels. May decrease blood Hct and Hgb levels.

▓ IV INCOMPATIBILITIES
Allopurinol (Aloprim), amphotericin B complex (Abelcet, AmBisome, Amphotec), fluconazole (Diflucan)
▓ IV Compatibilities
Diltiazem (Cardizem), insulin, propofol (Diprivan)

SIDE EFFECTS
Occasional (3%-2%)
Diarrhea, nausea, vomiting
Rare (2%-1%)
Rash

SERIOUS REACTIONS
• Antibiotic-associated colitis and other superinfections may occur.
• Anaphylactic reactions have been reported.

PRECAUTIONS & CONSIDERATIONS
Caution is warranted with a history of seizures, renal impairment, and/or sensitivity to penicillins. Be aware that imipenem crosses the placenta and is distributed in amniotic fluid, breast milk, and cord blood. This drug may be used safely in children younger than 12 years. In the elderly, age-related renal function impairment may require dosage adjustment. Notify the physician if severe diarrhea occurs but avoid taking antidiarrheals.
Notify the physician of the onset of troublesome or serious adverse reactions, including infusion site pain, redness, or swelling, nausea or vomiting, or skin rash or itching.

History of allergies, particularly to beta-lactams, cephalosporins, and penicillins should be determined before beginning drug therapy.

Storage

Solution normally appears colorless to yellow; discard if solution turns brown. IV infusion (piggyback) is stable for 4 hours at room temperature, 24 hours if refrigerated. Discard if precipitate forms.

Administration

For IM use, prepare with 1% lidocaine without epinephrine, as prescribed; 500-mg vial with 2 ml, 750-mg vial with 3 ml lidocaine HCl. Administer suspension within 1 hour of preparation. Don't mix the suspension with any other medications. Give deep IM injections slowly into a large muscle to minimize patient discomfort. To further minimize discomfort, administer IM injections into the gluteus maximus instead of the lateral aspect of the thigh. Be sure to aspirate with the syringe before injecting the drug to decrease risk of injection into a blood vessel.

For IV use, dilute each 250- or 500-mg vial with 100 ml D_5W; 0.9% NaCl. Give by intermittent IV infusion (piggyback). Do not give IV push. Infuse over 20 to 30 minutes (1-g dose longer than 40 to 60 minutes). Observe the patient during the first 30 minutes of the infusion for possible hypersensitivity reaction.

Imipramine
ih-mih′prah-meen
(Apo-Imipramine [CAN], Melipramine [AUS], Tofranil, Tofranil-PM)
Do not confuse imipramine with desipramine.

CATEGORY AND SCHEDULE
Pregnancy Risk Category: D

CLASSIFICATION
Antidepressants, tricyclic

MECHANISM OF ACTION
A tricyclic antidepressant, antibulimic, anticataplectic, antinarcoleptic, antineuralgic, antineuritic, and antipanic agent that blocks the reuptake of neurotransmitters, such as norepinephrine and serotonin, at presynaptic membranes, increasing their concentration at postsynaptic receptor sites. *Therapeutic Effect:* Relieves depression and controls nocturnal enuresis.

AVAILABILITY
Tablets: 10 mg, 25 mg, 50 mg.
Capsules: 75 mg, 100 mg, 125 mg, 150 mg.

INDICATIONS AND DOSAGES
▶ **Depression**
PO
Adults. Initially, 75-100 mg/day. May gradually increase to 300 mg/day for hospitalized patients, or 200 mg/day for outpatients; then reduce dosage to effective maintenance level, 50-150 mg/day.
Elderly. Initially, 10-25 mg/day at bedtime. May increase by 10-25 mg every 3-7 days. Range: 50-150 mg/day.

Children. 1.5 mg/kg/day. May increase by 1 mg/kg every 3-4 days. Maximum: 5 mg/kg/day.

▸ **Enuresis**
PO
Children older than 6 yr. Initially, 10-25 mg at bedtime. May increase by 25 mg/day. Maximum: 50 mg for children older than 12 yr.

OFF-LABEL USES
Treatment of attention-deficit hyperactivity disorder, cataplexy associated with narcolepsy, neurogenic pain, panic disorder

CONTRAINDICATIONS
Acute recovery period after MI, use within 14 days of MAOIs

INTERACTIONS
Drug
Alcohol, other CNS depressants: May increase the hypotensive effects and CNS and respiratory depression caused by imipramine.
Antithyroid agents: May increase the risk of agranulocytosis.
Cimetidine: May increase imipramine blood concentration and risk of toxicity.
Clonidine, guanadrel: May decrease the effects of these drugs.
MAOIs: May increase the risk of neuroleptic malignant syndrome, hyperpyrexia, hypertensive crisis, and seizures.
Phenothiazines: May increase the anticholinergic and sedative effects of imipramine.
Phenytoin: May decrease the imipramine blood concentration.
Sympathomimetics: May increase the risk of cardiac effects.
Herbal
Ginkgo biloba: May decrease seizure threshold.
St. John's wort: May increase imipramine's pharmacologic effects and risk of toxicity.
Food
None known.

DIAGNOSTIC TEST EFFECTS
May alter blood glucose levels and EKG readings. Therapeutic serum drug level is 225-300 ng/ml; toxic serum drug level is greater than 500 ng/ml.

SIDE EFFECTS
Frequent
Somnolence, fatigue, dry mouth, blurred vision, constipation, delayed micturition, orthostatic hypotension, diaphoresis, impaired concentration, increased appetite, urine retention, photosensitivity.
Occasional
GI disturbances (nausea, metallic taste).
Rare
Paradoxical reactions, (agitation, restlessness, nightmares, insomnia), extrapyramidal symptoms (particularly fine hand tremor).

SERIOUS REACTIONS
• Overdose may produce seizures; cardiovascular effects, such as severe orthostatic hypotension, dizziness, tachycardia, palpitations, and arrhythmias; and altered temperature regulation, including hyperpyrexia or hypothermia.
• Abrupt discontinuation after prolonged therapy may produce headache, malaise, nausea, vomiting, and vivid dreams.

PRECAUTIONS & CONSIDERATIONS
Caution is warranted with cardiac disease, diabetes mellitus, glaucoma, hiatal hernia, history of seizures, history of urinary obstruction or retention, hyperthyroidism, increased

IOP, benign prostatic hyperplasia, renal or hepatic disease, and schizophrenia. Imipramine is minimally distributed in breast milk. Imipramine use is not recommended for children younger than 6 years. Expect to administer a lower dosage to the elderly because they're at increased risk for drug toxicity. Anticholinergic, sedative, and hypotensive effects may occur during early therapy, but tolerance to these effects usually develops. Since dizziness may occur, change positions slowly and avoid alcohol and tasks that require mental alertness or motor skills. Pattern of daily bowel activity, bladder for urine retention, B/P and pulse rate to detect hypotension and arrhythmias, CBC and blood serum chemistry tests to monitor blood glucose level, and liver and renal function tests should be assessed.

Administration
! Make sure at least 14 days elapse between the use of MAOIs and imipramine. Be aware that the therapeutic serum level for imipramine is 225 to 300 ng/ml; the toxic serum level is greater than 500 ng/ml.

Take imipramine with food or milk if GI distress occurs. Don't crush or break film-coated tablets. Improvement may occur 2 to 5 days after starting therapy but the full therapeutic effect will likely occur within 2 to 3 weeks. Do not abruptly discontinue imipramine.

Imiquimod
im-ick'wih-mod
(Aldara)

CATEGORY AND SCHEDULE
Pregnancy Risk Category: C

CLASSIFICATION
Dermatologics, immuno-modulators

MECHANISM OF ACTION
An immune response modifier whose mechanism of action is uknown. *Therapeutic Effect:* Reduces genital and perianal warts.

PHARMACOKINETICS
Minimal absorption after topical administration. Minimal excretion in urine and feces.

AVAILABILITY
Cream: 5% (Aldara).

INDICATIONS AND DOSAGES
▸ **Warts/condyloma acuminata**
TOPICAL
Adults, Elderly, Children 12 yr and older. Apply 3 times/wk before normal sleeping hours; leave on skin 6-10 hr. Remove following treatment period. Continue therapy for maximum of 16 weeks.

CONTRAINDICATIONS
History of hypersensitivity to imiquimod

INTERACTIONS
Drug
None known.
Herbal
None known.
Food
None known.

DIAGNOSTIC TEST EFFECTS
None known.

SIDE EFFECTS
Frequent
Local skin reactions: erythema, itching, burning, erosion, excoriation/flaking, fungal infections (women)
Occasional
Pain, induration, ulceration, scabbing, soreness, headache, flu-like symptoms

SERIOUS REACTIONS
• None reported.

PRECAUTIONS & CONSIDERATIONS
Caution should be used with inflammatory conditions of the skin. Be aware that safety and efficacy have not been established for basal cell nevus syndrome or xeroderma pigmentosum. It is unknown if imiquimod crosses the placenta or is distributed in breast milk. Safety and efficacy of imiquimod have not been established in children younger than 12 years of age. There are no age-related precautions noted in the elderly.

If severe local skin reaction occurs, the cream should be removed by washing the treatment area and may be resumed after the reaction has subsided.

Storage
Store at room temperature.

Administration
Wash application site with soap and water 6-10 hours after applying. Apply a thin layer to affected area. Avoid contact with eyes. Wash hands after application.

Immune Globulin IV (IGIV)
(Baygam [CAN], Carimune, Gamimune N, Gammagard S/D, Gammar-P-IV, Gamunex, Iveegam EN, Octagam, Panglobulin, Polygam S/D, Sandoglobulin [AUS], Venoglobulin-S)
Do not confuse Sandoglobulin with Sandimmune or Sandostatin.

CATEGORY AND SCHEDULE
Pregnancy Risk Category: C

CLASSIFICATION
Immune globulins

MECHANISM OF ACTION
An immune serum that increases antibody titer and antigen-antibody reaction. *Therapeutic Effect:* Provides passive immunity against infection; induces rapid increase in platelet count; produces anti-inflammatory effect.

PHARMACOKINETICS
Evenly distributed between intravascular and extravascular space.
Half-life: 21-23 days.

AVAILABILITY
Injection Solution (Gammune N, Gamunex): 10%.
Injection Solution (Octagam): 5%.
Injection Solution (Venoglobulin S): 5%, 10%.
Injection Powder for Reconstitution (Carimune, Panglobulin): 1 g, 3 g, 6 g, 12 g.
Injection Powder for Reconstitution (Gammagard S/D, Polygam S/D): 2.5 g, 5 g, 10 g.
Injection Powder for Reconstitution (Gammar-P-IV): 1 g, 2.5 g, 5 g, 10 g.

Injection Powder for Reconstitution (Iveegam EN): 0.5 g, 1 g, 2.5 g, 5 g.

INDICATIONS AND DOSAGES
▸ **Primary immunodeficiency syndrome**
IV
Adults, Elderly, Children.
200-400 mg/kg once monthly.
▸ **Idiopathic thrombocytopenic purpura (ITP)**
IV
Adults, Elderly, Children.
400-1000 mg/kg/day for 2-5 days.
▸ **Kawasaki disease**
IV
Adults, Elderly, Children. 2 g/kg as a single dose.
▸ **Chronic lymphocytic leukemia**
IV
Adults, Elderly, Children.
400 mg/kg q3-4wk.
▸ **Bone marrow transplant**
IV
Adults, Elderly, Children. 400-500 mg/kg/dose every week for 12 wk, then every month.

OFF-LABEL USES
Control and prevention of infections in infants and children with immunosuppression due to AIDS or AIDS-related complex; prevention of acute infections in immunosuppressed patients; prevention and treatment of infections in high-risk, preterm, low-birth-weight neonates; treatment of chronic inflammatory demyelinating polyneuropathies and multiple sclerosis

CONTRAINDICATIONS
Allergies to gamma globulin, thimerosal, or anti-IgA antibodies; isolated IgA deficiency

INTERACTIONS
Drug
Live-virus vaccines: May increase vaccine side effects, potentiate virus replication, and decrease the patient's antibody response to the vaccine.
Herbal
None known.
Food
None known.

DIAGNOSTIC TEST EFFECTS
None known.

▩ IV INCOMPATIBILITIES
Do not mix IGIV with any other medications.

SIDE EFFECTS
Frequent
Tachycardia, backache, headache, arthralgia, myalgia
Occasional
Fatigue, wheezing, injection site rash or pain, leg cramps, urticaria, bluish lips and nailbeds, lightheadedness

SERIOUS REACTIONS
• Anaphylactic reactions are rare, but the incidence increases with repeated injections of IGIV. Keep epinephrine readily available.
• Overdose may produce chest tightness, chills, diaphoresis, dizziness, facial flushing, nausea, vomiting, fever, and hypotension.

PRECAUTIONS & CONSIDERATIONS
Caution is warranted with cardiovascular disease, diabetes mellitus, history of thrombosis, impaired renal function, sepsis, or volume depletion and concurrent use of nephrotoxic drugs. It is unknown if IGIV crosses the placenta or is distributed in breast milk. No age-related precautions have been noted in children or the elderly.

Adequate hydration should be maintained before giving IGIV. Notify the physician if dyspnea, decreased urine output, fluid retention, edema, or sudden weight gain occurs. Vital signs and platelet count should be monitored.

Storage

Refer to individual IV preparations for storage requirements and information about stability after reconstitution.

Administration

Reconstitute IGIV only with the diluent provided by the manufacturer. Discard partially used or turbid preparations. Administer IGIV by infusion only through separate tubing. Avoid mixing IGIV with other medications or IV infusion fluids. The infusion rate varies among products. Control the infusion rate carefully. A too-rapid infusion increases the risk of a precipitous drop in B/P, and an anaphylactic reaction, marked by chest tightness, chills, diaphoresis, facial flushing, fever, nausea, and vomiting. Monitor B/P and vital signs diligently during and immediately after IV administration. Stop the infusion immediately if a suspected anaphylactic reaction occurs. Keep epinephrine readily available. A rapid response occurs to therapy, which will last 1 to 3 months.

Inamrinone Lactate
in-am′ri-nohn
(Inamrinone)
Do not confuse with Amiodarone.

CATEGORY AND SCHEDULE
Pregnancy Risk Category: C

CLASSIFICATION
Inotropes, vasodilators

MECHANISM OF ACTION
A positive inotropic agent that inhibits myocardial cyclic adenosine monophosphate (cAMP) phosphodiesterase activity and directly stimulates cardiac contractility. Peripheral vasodilation reduces both preload and afterload. *Therapeutic Effect:* Reduces preload and afterload; increases cardiac output.

PHARMACOKINETICS
After IV administration, rapidly absorbed from the gastrointestinal (GI) tract. Protein binding: 10%-49%. Partially metabolized in liver. Excreted in urine as both inamrinone and its metabolites. **Half-life:** 3-6 hr (half-life increased with congestive heart failure).

AVAILABILITY
Injection: 5 mg/ml (Inamrinone).

INDICATIONS AND DOSAGES
▶ **Short-term management of intractable heart failure**
IV INFUSION (CONTINUOUS)
Adults. Initially, 0.75 mg/kg loading dose over 2-3 minutes followed by a maintenance infusion of 5 and 10 mcg/kg/min. A bolus dose of 0.75 mg/kg may be given 30 minutes after the initiation of therapy. Use within 24 hours and do not dilute with solutions that contain dextrose. Maximum: 10 mg/kg/day.

CONTRAINDICATIONS
Severe aortic or pulmonic valvular disease; hypersensitivity to inamrinone or bisulfites.

INTERACTIONS
Drug
Digitalis: May increase the inotropic effects.
Diuretics: May cause hypovolemia and decrease filling pressure.

Dysopryamide: May cause hypotension.
Herbal
None known.
Food
None known.

DIAGNOSTIC TEST EFFECTS
None known.

▓ IV INCOMPATIBILITIES
Furosemide (Lasix)

SIDE EFFECTS
Occasional
Arrhythmia, nausea, hypotension, thrombocytopenia
Rare
Fever, vomiting, abdominal pain, anorexia, chest pain, decreased tear production hepatotoxicity, and burning at the site of injection, hypersensitivity to inamrinone

SERIOUS REACTIONS
• Overdose may cause severe hypotension.

PRECAUTIONS & CONSIDERATIONS
Blood pressure (B/P) and pulse should be obtained immediately before each inamrinone dose, in addition to regular B/P monitoring. Be alert for B/P fluctuations. The elderly are more sensitive to the drug's hypotensive effects, and age-related renal impairment may require dosage adjustment. Caution should be used in children and the elderly. Cardiac index, stroke volume, systemic vascular resistance, and pulmonary vascular resistance, blood pressure (B/P), heart rate, platelet count, fluid status, and liver and renal function should be monitored.
Storage
Store at room temperature. Store unopened vial at room temperature. Do not freeze.

Administration
Give IV bolus dose undiluted. Reconstituted solutions should be used within 24 hours. Dosage is based on clinical response. Do not dilute with dextrose. Do not administer furosemide in intravenous lines containing inamrinone. Follow instructions of manufacturer for dilution to specific concentrations. Inamrinone is for short-term therapy.

Indapamide
in-dap′a-mide
(Dapa-tabs [AUS], Indahexal [AUS], Insig [AUS], Lozide [CAN], Lozol, Natrilix [AUS], Natrilix SR [AUS])
Do not confuse indapamide with iodamide or iopamidol.

CATEGORY AND SCHEDULE
Pregnancy Risk Category: B (D if used in pregnancy-induced hypertension)

CLASSIFICATION
Diuretics, thiazide and derivatives

MECHANISM OF ACTION
A thiazide-like diuretic that blocks reabsorption of water, sodium, and potassium at the cortical diluting segment of the distal tubule; also reduces plasma and extracellular fluid volume and peripheral vascular resistance by direct effect on blood vessels. *Therapeutic Effect:* Promotes diuresis and reduces B/P.

AVAILABILITY
Tablets: 1.25 mg, 2.5 mg.

INDICATIONS AND DOSAGES
▶ **Edema**
PO
Adults. Initially, 2.5 mg/day, may increase to 5 mg/day after 1 wk.
▶ **Hypertension**
PO
Adults, Elderly. Initially, 1.25 mg, may increase to 2.5 mg/day after 4 wk or 5 mg/day after additional 4 wk.

CONTRAINDICATIONS
None known.

INTERACTIONS
Drug
Digoxin: May increase the risk of digoxin toxicity associated with indapamide-induced hypokalemia.
Lithium: May increase the risk of lithium toxicity.
Herbal
None known.
Food
None known.

DIAGNOSTIC TEST EFFECTS
May increase plasma renin activity. May decrease protein-bound iodine and serum calcium, potassium, and sodium levels.

SIDE EFFECTS
Frequent (5% and greater)
Fatigue, numbness of extremities, tension, irritability, agitation, headache, dizziness, light-headedness, insomnia, muscle cramps
Occasional (less than 5%)
Tingling of extremities, urinary frequency, urticaria, rhinorrhea, flushing, weight loss, orthostatic hypotension, depression, blurred vision, nausea, vomiting, diarrhea or constipation, dry mouth, impotence, rash, pruritus

SERIOUS REACTIONS
• Vigorous diuresis may lead to profound water and electrolyte depletion, resulting in hypokalemia, hyponatremia, and dehydration.
• Acute hypotensive episodes may occur.
• Hyperglycemia may occur during prolonged therapy.
• Pancreatitis, blood dyscrasias, pulmonary edema, allergic pneumonitis, and dermatologic reactions occur rarely.
• Overdose can lead to lethargy and coma without changes in electrolytes or hydration.

PRECAUTIONS & CONSIDERATIONS
Caution is warranted with anuria, diabetes mellitus, a history of hypersensitivity to sulfonamides or thiazide diuretics, hepatic impairment, severe renal disease, thyroid disorders, and in the elderly and debilitated. Consuming foods high in potassium such as apricots, bananas, legumes, meat, orange juice, raisins, whole grains, including cereals, and white and sweet potatoes, is encouraged.

Dizziness or lightheadedness may occur, so change positions slowly and let legs dangle momentarily before standing. An increase in the frequency and volume of urination may occur. Blood pressure (B/P), vital signs, electrolytes, intake and output, and weight should be monitored before and during treatment. Be aware of signs of electrolyte disturbances such as hypokalemia or hyponatremia. Hypokalemia may cause arrhythmias, altered mental status, muscle cramps, asthenia, and tremor. Hyponatremia may result in cold and clammy skin, confusion, and thirst.
Administration
Take indapamide with food or milk if GI upset occurs, preferably with

breakfast to help prevent nocturia. Do not crush or break tablets.

Indinavir
in-din'ah-veer
(Crixivan)
Do not confuse indinavir with Denavir.

CATEGORY AND SCHEDULE
Pregnancy Risk Category: C

CLASSIFICATION
Antivirals, protease inhibitors

MECHANISM OF ACTION
A protease inhibitor that suppresses HIV protease, an enzyme necessary for splitting viral polyprotein precursors into mature and infectious viral particles. *Therapeutic Effect:* Interrupts HIV replication, slowing the progression of HIV infection.

PHARMACOKINETICS
Rapidly absorbed after PO administration. Protein binding: 60%. Metabolized in the liver. Primarily excreted in urine. Unknown if removed by hemodialysis. **Half-life:** 1.8 hr (increased in impaired hepatic function).

AVAILABILITY
Capsules: 100 mg, 200 mg, 333 mg, 400 mg.

INDICATIONS AND DOSAGES
▸ **HIV infection (in combination with other antiretrovirals)**
PO
Adults. 800 mg (two 400-mg capsules) q8hr.

▸ **HIV infection in patients with hepatic insufficiency**
PO
Adults. 600 mg q8hr.

OFF-LABEL USES
Prophylaxis following occupational exposure to HIV

CONTRAINDICATIONS
Hypersensitivity to indinavir; nephrolithiasis

INTERACTIONS
Drug
Midazolam, triazolam: Increases the risk of arrhythmias and prolonged sedation.
Herbal
St. John's wort: May decrease indinavir blood concentration and effect.
Food
Grapefruit: May decrease indinavir blood concentration and effect.
High-fat, high-calorie, and high-protein meals: May decrease indinavir blood concentration.

DIAGNOSTIC TEST EFFECTS
May increase serum bilirubin (in 10% of patients), AST (SGOT), and ALT (SGPT) levels.

SIDE EFFECTS
Frequent
Nausea (12%), abdominal pain (9%), headache (6%), diarrhea (5%)
Occasional
Vomiting, asthenia, fatigue (4%); insomnia; accumulation of fat in waist, abdomen, or back of neck
Rare
Abnormal taste sensation, heartburn, symptomatic urinary tract disease, transient renal dysfunction

SERIOUS REACTIONS
• Nephrolithiasis (flank pain with or without hematuria) occurs in 4% of patients.

PRECAUTIONS & CONSIDERATIONS
Caution is warranted with renal or liver function impairment. Be aware that it is unknown if indinavir is excreted in breast milk. Breast-feeding is not recommended in this population because of the possibility of HIV transmission. Be aware that the safety and efficacy of this drug have not been established in children. There is no information on the effects of this drug's use in the elderly. Avoid St. John's wort and grapefruit or grapefruit juice because they will lower indinavir levels.

! Monitor for signs and symptoms of nephrolithiasis as evidenced by flank pain and hematuria, and notify the physician if symptoms occur. If nephrolithiasis occurs, expect therapy to be interrupted for 1 to 3 days. Establish baseline lab values and monitor renal function before and during therapy, and in particular, evaluate the results of the serum creatinine and urinalysis tests. Maintain adequate hydration and drink 48 oz (1.5 L) of liquid over each 24-hour period during therapy. Assess pattern of daily bowel activity and stool consistency. Evaluate for abdominal discomfort or headache.

Storage
Store drug at room temperature, keep it in the original bottle, and protect it from moisture. Keep in mind that indinavir capsules are sensitive to moisture.

Administration
For optimal drug absorption, take indinavir with water only and without food 1 hour before or 2 hours after a meal. Take indinavir with coffee, juice, skim milk, tea, or water and with a light meal (e.g., dry toast with jelly). Do not take indinavir with meals high in fat, calories, and protein. If indinavir and didanosine are given concurrently, give the drugs at least 1 hour apart on an empty stomach. If a dose is missed, take the next dose at the regularly scheduled time; do not double the dose.

Indomethacin
in-doe-meth′a-sin
(Apo-Indomethacin [CAN], Arthrexin [AUS], Indocid [CAN], Indocin, Indocin-IV, Indocin-SR, Novomethacin [CAN])
Do not confuse with Imodium or Vicodin.

CATEGORY AND SCHEDULE
Pregnancy Risk Category: B
(D if used after 34 weeks′ gestation, close to delivery, or for longer than 48 hours)

CLASSIFICATION
Analgesics, non-narcotic, nonsteroidal anti-inflammatory drugs

MECHANISM OF ACTION
An NSAID that produces analgesic and anti-inflammatory effects by inhibiting prostaglandin synthesis. Also increases the sensitivity of the premature ductus to the dilating effects of prostaglandins. *Therapeutic Effect:* Reduces the inflammatory response and intensity of pain. Closure of the patent ductus arteriosus.

AVAILABILITY
Capsules (Indocin): 25 mg,
50 mg.
*Capsules (Sustained-Release
[Indocin SR]):* 75 mg.
Oral Suspension (Indocin):
25 mg/5 ml.
Powder for Injection (Indocin IV):
1 mg.
Suppository: 50 mg.

INDICATIONS AND DOSAGES
▸ **Moderate to severe rheumatoid arthritis, osteoarthritis, ankylosing spondylitis**
PO
Adults, Elderly. Initially,
25 mg 2-3 times a day;
increased by 25-50 mg/wk up to
150-200 mg/day. Or 75 mg/day
(extended-release) up to 75 mg
twice a day.
Children. 1-2 mg/kg/day.
Maximum: 150-200 mg/day.
▸ **Acute gouty arthritis**
PO
Adults, Elderly. Initially, 100 mg,
then 50 mg 3 times a day.
▸ **Acute shoulder pain**
PO
Adults, Elderly. 75-150 mg/day in
3-4 divided doses.
▸ **Usual rectal dosage**
Adults, Elderly. 50 mg 4 times
a day.
Children. Initially, 1.5-2.5 mg/
kg/day, increased up to 4 mg/kg/day.
Maximum: 150-200 mg/day.
▸ **Patent ductus arteriosus**
IV
Neonates. Initially, 0.2 mg/kg.
Subsequent doses are based on age,
as follows:
Neonates older than 7 days.
0.25 mg/kg for second and third
doses.
Neonates 2-7 days. 0.2 mg/kg for
second and third doses.

Neonates less than 48 hr. 0.1 mg/kg
for second and third doses.

OFF-LABEL USES
Treatment of fever due to malignancy, pericarditis, psoriatic arthritis,
rheumatic complications associated
with Paget's disease of bone, vascular headache

CONTRAINDICATIONS
Active GI bleeding or ulcerations;
hypersensitivity to aspirin,
indomethacin, or other NSAIDs;
renal impairment, thrombocytopenia

INTERACTIONS
Drug
Aminoglycosides: May increase the
blood concentration of these drugs in
neonates.
Antihypertensives, diuretics: May
decrease the effects of these drugs.
Aspirin, other salicylates: May
increase the risk of GI side effects
such as bleeding.
Bone marrow depressants: May
increase the risk of hematologic
reactions.
**Heparin, oral anticoagulants,
thrombolytics:** May increase the
effects of these drugs.
Lithium: May increase the blood
concentration and risk of toxicity of
lithium.
Methotrexate: May increase the
risk of methotrexate toxicity.
Probenecid: May increase the
indomethacin blood concentration.
Triamterene: May potentiate acute
renal failure. Don't give concurrently.
Herbal
Feverfew: May decrease the effects
of feverfew.
Ginkgo biloba: May increase the
risk of bleeding.
Food
None known.

DIAGNOSTIC TEST EFFECTS

May prolong bleeding time. May alter blood glucose level. May increase BUN level, and serum creatinine, potassium, AST (SGOT), and ALT (SGPT) levels. May decrease serum sodium level and platelet count.

▓ IV INCOMPATIBILITIES

Amino acid injection, calcium gluconate, cimetidine (Tagamet), dobutamine (Dobutrex), dopamine (Intropin), gentamicin (Garamycin), tobramycin (Nebcin)

▓ IV Compatibilities

Insulin, potassium

SIDE EFFECTS

Frequent (11%-3%)

Headache, nausea, vomiting, dyspepsia, dizziness

Occasional (less than 3%)

Depression, tinnitus, diaphoresis, somnolence, constipation, diarrhea, bleeding disturbances in patent ductus arteriosus

Rare

Hypertension, confusion, urticaria, pruritus, rash, blurred vision

SERIOUS REACTIONS

• Paralytic ileus and ulceration of the esophagus, stomach, duodenum, or small intestine may occur.
• Patients with impaired renal function may develop hyperkalemia and worsening of renal impairment.
• Indomethacin use may aggravate epilepsy, parkinsonism, and depression or other psychiatric disturbances.
• Nephrotoxicity, including dysuria, hematuria, proteinuria, and nephrotic syndrome, occurs rarely.
• Metabolic acidosis or alkalosis, apnea, and bradycardia occur rarely in patients with patent ductus arteriosus.

PRECAUTIONS & CONSIDERATIONS

Caution is warranted with cardiac dysfunction, hypertension, epilepsy, hepatic or renal impairment and in those receiving anticoagulant therapy concurrently. Avoid alcohol and aspirin during therapy because these substances increase the risk of GI bleeding. Tasks that require mental alertness or motor skills should be avoided.

BUN, serum alkaline phosphatase, bilirubin, creatinine, potassium, AST (SGOT), ALT (SGPT) levels, B/P, EKG, heart rate, platelet count, serum sodium, blood glucose levels, and urine output should be monitored. Therapeutic response, such as decreased pain, stiffness, swelling, and tenderness, improved grip strength, and increased joint mobility, should be evaluated.

Administration

Take oral indomethacin after meals or with food or antacids. Don't crush extended-release capsules.

! IV injection is the preferred route for neonates with patent ductus arteriosus. The drug may also be given orally, by NG tube, or rectally. Administer no more than 3 doses at 12- to 24-hour intervals.

For IV use, reconstitute by adding 1 or 2 ml preservative-free sterile water for injection or 0.9% NaCl to the 1-mg vial to provide a concentration of 1 mg or 0.5 mg/ml, respectively. Don't dilute the solution any further. Administer the IV immediately after reconstitution. The solution normally appears clear; discard if it becomes cloudy or contains precipitate; discard any unused portion. Administer the drug over 5 to 10 seconds. Restrict fluid intake, as ordered.

For rectal use, if suppository is too soft, refrigerate it for 30 minutes or run cold water over the foil wrapper. Moisten the suppository with cold water before inserting it into the rectum.

Infliximab
in-flicks'ih-mab
(Remicade)
Do not confuse Remicade with Reminyl.

CATEGORY AND SCHEDULE
Pregnancy Risk Category: C

CLASSIFICATION
Disease modifying antirheumatic drugs, gastrointestinals, immunomodulators, monoclonal antibodies, tumor necrosis factor modulators

MECHANISM OF ACTION
A monoclonal antibody that binds to tumor necrosis factor (TNF), inhibiting functional activity of TNF. Reduces infiltration of inflammatory cells. *Therapeutic Effect:* Decreases inflamed areas of the intestine.

PHARMACOKINETICS

Route	Onset	Peak	Duration
IV (Crohn's disease)	1-2 wk	N/A	8-48 wk
IV (rheumatoid arthritis [RA])	3-7 days	N/A	6-12 wk

Absorbed into the GI tissue; primarily distributed in the vascular compartment. **Half-life:** 9.5 days.

AVAILABILITY
Powder for Injection: 100 mg.

INDICATIONS AND DOSAGES
▸ **Moderate to severe Crohn's disease**
IV infusion
Adults, Elderly. 5 mg/kg as a single IV infusion.
▸ **Fistulizing Crohn's disease**
IV infusion
Adults, Elderly. Initially, 5 mg/kg followed by additional 5-mg/kg doses at 2 and 6 wk after first infusion.
▸ **RA**
IV infusion
Adults, Elderly. 3 mg/kg; followed by additional doses at 2 and 6 wk after first infusion: Then q8wk.

OFF-LABEL USES
Ankylosing spondylitis, sciatica

CONTRAINDICATIONS
Sensitivity to infliximab or murine proteins, sepsis, serious active infection

INTERACTIONS
Drug
Immunosuppressants: May reduce frequency of infusion reactions and antibodies to infliximab.
Live vaccines: May decrease immune response.
Herbal
None known.
Food
None known.

DIAGNOSTIC TEST EFFECTS
None known.

▦ IV INCOMPATIBILITIES
Do not infuse infliximab in the same IV line with other agents.

SIDE EFFECTS
Frequent (22%-10%)
Headache, nausea, fatigue, fever

Occasional (9%-5%)
Fever or chills during infusion, pharyngitis, vomiting, pain, dizziness, bronchitis, rash, rhinitis, cough, pruritus, sinusitis, myalgia, back pain
Rare (4%-1%)
Hypotension or hypertension, paresthesia, anxiety, depression, insomnia, diarrhea, urinary tract infection

SERIOUS REACTIONS

• Hypersensitivity reaction and lupus-like syndrome may occur.

PRECAUTIONS & CONSIDERATIONS

Caution is warranted with history of recurrent infections. It is unknown if infliximab is distributed in breast milk. Safety and efficacy of infliximab have not been established in children. Use infliximab cautiously in the elderly because of a higher rate of infection in this population.

Follow-up tests, such as ESR, C-reactive protein measurement, and urinalysis, should be obtained. Notify the physician of signs of infection, such as fever. Persons with rheumatoid arthritis should report increase in pain, stiffness, or swelling of joints. Persons with Crohn's disease should report changes in stool color, consistency, or elimination pattern. Hydration status should be assessed before and during therapy.

Storage
Refrigerate vials.

Administration
Reconstitute each vial with 10 ml sterile water for injection, using 21-gauge or smaller needle. Direct the stream of sterile water to the glass wall of the vial. Swirl the vial gently to dissolve the contents. Do not shake. Allow the solution to stand for 5 minutes. Because infliximab is a protein, the solution may develop a few translucent particles; do not use if particles are opaque or foreign particles are present. The solution normally appears colorless to light yellow and opalescent; do not use if discolored. Withdraw and waste a volume of 0.9% NaCl from a 250-ml bag that is equal to the volume of reconstituted solution to be injected into the 250-ml bag (approximately 10 ml). Total dose to be infused should equal 250 ml. Slowly add the reconstituted infliximab solution to the 250 ml infusion bag. Gently mix. Infusion concentration should range between 0.4 and 4 mg/ml. Begin infusion within 3 hours of reconstitution. Administer IV infusion over 2 hours, using set with a low-protein-binding filter.

Insulin
in'sull-in
Rapid acting: Insulin
Lispro (Humalog),
Insulin Aspart (Novolog,
Novorapid [AUS]),
Regular Insulin
(Actrapid [AUS], Humulin R,
Novolin R, Regular Iletin II),
Intermediate acting:
NPH (Humulin N,
Novolin N, Pork), Lente:
(Humulin L, Lente Iletin II,
Monotard [AUS], Novolin L)
NPH/regular mixture
(70%/30%): Humulin 70/30,
Novolin 70/30 NPH/regular
mixture (50%/50%):
Humulin 50/50 NPH/Lispro
mixture (75%/25%): Humalog
Mix 75/25, Novalog Mix
70/30 Long acting: Insulin
Glargine (Lantus)

CATEGORY AND SCHEDULE
Pregnancy Risk Category: B
OTC

CLASSIFICATION
Antidiabetic agents

MECHANISM OF ACTION
An exogenous insulin that
facilitates passage of glucose,
potassium, and magnesium across
the cellular membranes of
skeletal and cardiac muscle and
adipose tissue. Controls storage
and metabolism of carbohydrates,
protein, and fats. Promotes
conversion of glucose to glycogen in
the liver. *Therapeutic Effect:*
Controls glucose levels in
diabetic patients.

PHARMACOKINETICS

Drug Form	Onset (hr)	Peak (hr)	Duration (hr)
Lispro	0.25	0.5-1.5	4-5
Insulin aspart	1/6	1-3	3-5
Regular	0.5-1	2-4	5-7
NPH	1-2	6-14	24+
Lente	1-3	6-14	24+
Insulin glargine	N/A	N/A	24

AVAILABILITY

All insulins are available as
100 units/ml concentrations
Rapid Acting: Humulin R, Novolin R,
Novolog, Humalog, Regular
Iletin II.
Intermediate Acting: Humulin L,
Novolin L, Lente Iletin II, Humulin N,
Novolin N, NPH Illetin II.
Long Acting: Lantus.

INDICATIONS AND DOSAGES
▸ **Treatment of insulin-dependent
type 1 diabetes mellitus and
non-insulin-dependent type 2
diabetes mellitus when diet or
weight control has failed to
maintain satisfactory blood glucose
levels or in event of fever, infection,
pregnancy, surgery, or trauma, or
severe endocrine, hepatic or
renal dysfunction; emergency treatment of ketoacidosis (regular
insulin); to promote passage of
glucose across cell membrane in
hyperalimentation (regular insulin):
to facilitate intracellular shift of
potassium in hyperkalemia (regular
insulin)**
SUBCUTANEOUS
Adults, Elderly, Children.
0.5-1 unit/kg/day.
Adolescents (during growth spurt).
0.8-1.2 unit/kg/day.

CONTRAINDICATIONS
Hypersensitivity or insulin resistance may require change of type or species' source of insulin

INTERACTIONS
Drug
Alcohol: May increase the effects of insulin.
Beta-adrenergic blockers: May increase the risk of hyperglycemia or hypoglycemia; may mask signs and prolong periods of hypoglycemia.
Glucocorticoids, thiazide diuretics: May increase blood glucose level.
Herbal
None known.
Food
None known.

DIAGNOSTIC TEST EFFECTS
May decrease serum magnesium, phosphate, and potassium concentrations.

▧ IV INCOMPATIBILITIES
Diltiazem (Cardizem), dopamine (Intropin), nafcillin (Nafcil)
▦ IV Compatibilities
Amiodarone (Cordarone), ampicillin/sulbactam (Unasyn), cefazolin (Ancef), cimetidine (Tagamet), digoxin (Lanoxin), dobutamine (Dobutrex), famotidine (Pepcid), gentamicin, heparin, magnesium sulfate, metoclopramide (Reglan), midazolam (Versed), milrinone (Primacor), morphine, nitroglycerin, potassium chloride, propofol (Diprivan), vancomycin (Vancocin)

SIDE EFFECTS
Occasional
Localized redness, swelling, and itching caused by improper injection technique or allergy to cleansing solution or insulin

Infrequent
Somogyi effect, including rebound hyperglycemia with chronically excessive insulin dosages: systemic allergic reaction, marked by rash, angioedema, and anaphylaxis; lipodystrophy or depression at injection site due to breakdown of adipose tissue; lipohypertrophy or accumulation of subcutaneous tissue at injection site due to inadequate site rotation
Rare
Insulin resistance

SERIOUS REACTIONS
• Severe hypoglycemia caused by hyperinsulinism may occur with insulin overdose, decrease or delay of food intake, or excessive exercise and in those with brittle diabetes.
• Diabetic ketoacidosis may result from stress, illness, omission of insulin dose, or long-term poor insulin control.

PRECAUTIONS & CONSIDERATIONS
Insulin is the drug of choice for treating diabetes mellitus during pregnancy but close medical supervision is needed. Insulin needs may drop for 24 to 72 hours post partum, then rise to pre-pregnancy levels. Insulin is not secreted in breast milk. Lactation may decrease insulin requirements. No age-related precautions have been noted in children. Decreased vision and shakiness in the elderly may lead to inaccurate insulin self dosing. Be alert to conditions that alter blood glucose requirements, such as fever, increased activity, stress, or a surgical procedure.
  Food intake and blood glucose should be monitored before and during therapy. Be aware of signs and symptoms of hypoglycemia (anxiety, cool wet skin, diplopia,

dizziness, headache, hunger, numbness in mouth, tachycardia, tremors), or hyperglycemia (deep rapid breathing, dim vision, fatigue, nausea, polydipsia, polyphagia, polyuria, vomiting); carry candy, sugar packets, or other sugar supplements for immediate response to hypoglycemia. Consult the physician when glucose demands are altered (such as with fever, heavy physical activity, infection, stress, trauma). Exercise, good personal hygiene (including foot care), not smoking, and weight control are essential parts of therapy.

Storage

Store currently used insulin at room temperature; avoid extreme temperatures and direct sunlight. Store extra vials in refrigerator. Discard unused vials if not used for several weeks. For home situations, prefilled syringes are stable for 1 week when refrigerated, including mixtures once they have stabilized; for example NPH/Regular stabilizes after 15 minutes and Lente/Regular stabilizes after 24 hours. Prefilled syringes should be stored in the vertical or oblique position to avoid plugging.

Administration

! Insulin dosages are individualized and monitored. Adjust dosage, as prescribed, to achieve premeal and bedtime glucose levels of 80 to 140 mg/dl (100 to 200 mg/dl in children younger than 5 years).

Give subcutaneous only. Regular insulin is the only insulin that may be given IV or IM for ketoacidosis or other specific situations. Warm the drug to room temperature; do not give cold insulin. Roll the drug vial gently between hands; do not shake. Regular insulin normally appears clear. Administer insulin approximately 30 minutes before a meal.

Insulin Lispro may be given up to 15 minutes before meals. Check blood glucose concentration before administration. Insulin dosages are highly individualized. Always draw regular insulin first when insulin is mixed. Mixtures must be administered at once because binding can occur within 5 minutes. Humalog may be mixed with Humulin N and Humulin L. Give subcutaneous injections in the abdomen, buttocks, thigh, upper arm, or upper back if there is adequate adipose tissue. Maintain a careful record of rotated injection sites.

To use prefilled syringes, the plunger should be pulled back slightly and the syringe rocked to remix the solution before injection.

For IV administration, use insulin regular and only if solution is clear. May give undiluted.

Insulin Glulisine
in'sull-in
(Apidra)

CATEGORY AND SCHEDULE
Pregnancy Risk Category: C

CLASSIFICATION
Antidiabetic agents, insulins

MECHANISM OF ACTION
A recombinant, rapid-acting insulin analog that facilitates passage of glucose, potassium, magnesium across cellular membranes of skeletal and cardiac muscle, adipose tissue; controls storage and metabolism of carbohydrates, protein, fats. Promotes conversion of glucose to glycogen in liver. *Therapeutic Effect:* Controls glucose levels in diabetic patients.

PHARMACOKINETICS

Drug Form	Onset (min)	Peak (min)	Duration (hrs)
Insulin Glulisine	20 min	55 min	5 hr

AVAILABILITY

Injection: 100 IU/ml (Apidra).

INDICATIONS AND DOSAGES

▶ **Diabetes mellitus (Type 1 and Type 2)**
Subcutaneous, infusion pump
Adults, Elderly, Children.
Individualize per patient needs.

CONTRAINDICATIONS

Current hypoglycemic episode, hypersensitivity or insulin resistance may require change of type or species' source of insulin

INTERACTIONS

Drug
Alcohol: May increase the effects of insulin glulisine.
Beta-adrenergic blockers: May increase the risk of hyperglycemia or hypoglycemia, mask signs of hypoglycemia, and prolong the period of hypoglycemia.
Glucocorticoids, thiazide diuretics: May increase blood glucose.
Herbal
None known.
Food
None known.

DIAGNOSTIC TEST EFFECTS

May decrease serum magnesium, phosphate, and potassium concentrations.

▧ IV INCOMPATIBILITIES

None known.

SIDE EFFECTS

Occasional
Local redness, swelling, itching, caused by improper injection technique or allergy to cleansing solution or insulin
Infrequent
Somogyi effect, including rebound hyperglycemia with chronically excessive insulin doses. Systemic allergic reaction, marked by rash, angioedema, and anaphylaxis, lipodystrophy or depression at injection site due to breakdown of adipose tissue, lipohypertrophy or accumulation of subcutaneous tissue at injection site due to lack of adequate site rotation
Rare
Insulin resistance

SERIOUS REACTIONS

• Severe hypoglycemia caused by hyperinsulinism may occur in overdose of insulin, decrease or delay of food intake, excessive exercise, or those with brittle diabetes.
• Diabetic ketoacidosis may result from stress, illness, omission of insulin dose, or long-term poor insulin control.

PRECAUTIONS & CONSIDERATIONS

Insulin is the drug of choice for treating diabetes mellitus during pregnancy but close medical supervision is needed. Following delivery, insulin needs may drop for 24 to 72 hours, then rise to pre-pregnancy levels. Be aware that insulin is not secreted in breast milk and that lactation may decrease insulin requirements. Be aware that there are no age-related precautions noted in children. Be aware that in the elderly, decreased vision and shakiness may lead to inaccurate dosage administration.

Hypoglycemia including anxiety, cool, wet skin, diplopia, dizziness, headache, hunger, numbness in mouth, tachycardia, and tremors, or hyperglycemia, including deep, rapid breathing, dim vision, fatigue, nausea, polydipsia, polyphagia, polyuria, and vomiting.

Be alert to conditions that alter blood glucose requirements, such as fever, increased activity, stress, or a surgical procedure may occur.

Storage

Store currently used insulin at room temperature, avoiding extreme temperatures and direct sunlight. Store extra vials in refrigerator. Discard unused vials if not used for several weeks. No insulin should have precipitate or discoloration. Candy, sugar packets, or other sugar supplements should be carried at all times for immediate response to hypoglycemia.

Administration

Know that insulin dosages are individualized and monitored. Adjust dosage, as prescribed, to achieve premeal and bedtime glucose level of 80 to 140 mg/dl in adults, and 100 to 200 mg/dl in children younger than 5 years.

Give subcutaneous only. Warm the drug to room temperature—do not give cold insulin. Roll the drug vial gently between hands; do not shake. Regular insulin normally appears clear. No insulin should have precipitate or discoloration. Administer insulin approximately 15 minutes before a meal. Give subcutaneous injections in the abdomen, buttocks, thigh, upper arm, or upper back if there is adequate adipose tissue. Maintain a careful record of rotated injection sites.

Interferon Alfa-2a
inn-ter-fear′on
(Roferon-A)
Do not confuse interferon alfa-2a with interferon alfa-2b.

CATEGORY AND SCHEDULE
Pregnancy Risk Category: C

CLASSIFICATION
Immunologic agents

MECHANISM OF ACTION
A biological response modifier that inhibits viral replication in virus-infected cells, suppresses cell proliferation, increases phagocytic action of macrophage, and augments specific lymphocytic cell toxicity. *Therapeutic Effect:* Prevents rapid growth of malignant cells; inhibits hepatitis virus.

PHARMACOKINETICS
Well absorbed after IM and subcutaneous administration. Undergoes proteolytic degradation during reabsorption in kidneys. **Half-life:** 2 hr (IM); 3 hr (subcutaneous).

AVAILABILITY
Injection, vial: 6 million units/ml.
Injection (Prefilled Syringe): 3 million units/0.5 ml, 6 million units/0.5 ml, 9 million units/ 0.5 ml.
Injection (Single-Dose Vial): 36 million units/ml.

INDICATIONS AND DOSAGES
▸ **Hairy cell leukemia**
IM, SUBCUTANEOUS
Adults. Initially, 3 million units/day for 16-24 wk. Maintenance: 3 million units 3 times a wk. Do not use 36-million-unit vial.

▸ **Chronic myelocytic leukemia**
IM, SUBCUTANEOUS
Adults. 9 million units/day.
▸ **Melanoma**
IM, SUBCUTANEOUS
Adults, Elderly. 12 million units/m²
3 times a week for 3 mo.
▸ **AIDS-related Kaposi's sarcoma**
IM, SUBCUTANEOUS
Adults. Initially, 36 million units/day
for 10-12 wk, may give 3 million
units on day 1, 9 million units on
day 2, 18 million units on day 3,
then 36 million units/day for
remaining of 10-12 wk.
Maintenance: 36 million units/day
3 times a wk.
▸ **Chronic hepatitis C**
IM, SUBCUTANEOUS
Adults, Elderly. 6 million units
3 times a week for 3 mo, then
3 million units 3 times a week for
9 mo.

OFF-LABEL USES
Treatment of active, chronic hepatitis; bladder or renal carcinoma;
malignant melanoma; multiple
myeloma; mycosis fungoides; non-Hodgkin's lymphoma

CONTRAINDICATIONS
None known.

INTERACTIONS
Drug
Bone marrow depressants: May
have increased myelosuppression.
Herbal
None known.
Food
None known.

DIAGNOSTIC TEST EFFECTS
May increase serum LDH, alkaline
phosphatase, AST (SGOT), and
ALT (SGPT) levels. May decrease
Hct, blood Hgb level, and leukocyte
and platelet counts.

SIDE EFFECTS
Frequent (greater than 20%)
Flu-like symptoms, nausea, vomiting, cough, dyspnea, hypotension,
edema, chest pain, dizziness, diarrhea, weight loss, altered taste,
abdominal discomfort, confusion,
paresthesia, depression, visual and
sleep disturbances, diaphoresis,
lethargy
Occasional (20%-5%)
Alopecia (partial), rash, dry throat or
skin, pruritus, flatulence, constipation, hypertension, palpitations,
sinusitis
Rare (less than 5%)
Hot flashes, hypermotility,
Raynaud's syndrome, bronchospasm,
earache, ecchymosis

SERIOUS REACTIONS
• Arrhythmias, CVA, transient
ischemic attacks, CHF, pulmonary
edema, and MI occur rarely.

PRECAUTIONS & CONSIDERATIONS
Caution is warranted with
cardiac diseases or abnormalities,
compromised CNS function, hepatic
or renal impairment, myelosuppression, and seizure disorders.
Interferon alfa-2a should not be
used by pregnant or breast-feeding
women. An effective contraceptive
method should be used during therapy, and the physician should be
notified if the woman becomes or
may be pregnant. The safety and
efficacy of interferon alfa-2a have
not been established in children.
The elderly are more prone to
cardiotoxicity and neurotoxicity.
Age-related renal impairment
may require cautious use of
interferon alfa-2a in the elderly.
Avoid tasks that require mental
alertness or motor skills until
response to the drug has been
established.

Flu-like symptoms may occur but tend to diminish with continued therapy. Notify the physician if nausea and vomiting continues at home. Vital signs, including temperature, should be obtained at baseline. Adequate hydration should be maintained, particularly during early therapy.

Storage
Refrigerate the drug.

Administration
! Subcutaneous administration is preferred for thrombocytopenic patients and other patients at risk for bleeding. Dosage is individualized based on clinical response and tolerance of the drug's adverse effects. When used in combination therapy, expect to consult specific protocols for optimum dosage and sequence of drug administration. If severe adverse reactions occur, modify the dosage or temporarily discontinue the drug, as prescribed. Don't shake the vial.

Administer as IM or subcutaneous injection. The solution normally appears colorless; don't use it if it contains precipitate or becomes discolored. Therapeutic effects may take 1 to 3 months to appear.

Interferon Alfa-2a/2b
inn-ter-fear'on
(Roferon-A)/(Intron-A)

CATEGORY AND SCHEDULE
Pregnancy Risk Category: C

CLASSIFICATION
Immunologic agents

MECHANISM OF ACTION
A biologic response modifier that inhibits viral replication in virus-infected cells. *Therapeutic Effect:* Suppresses cell proliferation; increases phagocytic action of macrophages; augments specific lymphocytic cell toxicity.

PHARMACOKINETICS
Interferon alfa-2a
Well absorbed after IM, subcutaneous administration. Undergoes proteolytic degradation during reabsorption in kidney. **Half-life:** IM: 2 hr; Subcutaneous: 3 hr.
Interferon alfa-2b
Well absorbed after IM, subcutaneous administration. Undergoes proteolytic degradation during reabsorption in kidney. **Half-life:** 2-3 hr.

AVAILABILITY
Interferon alfa-2a
Injection: 3 million units, 6 million units, 9 million units, 36 million units (Roferon-A).
Interferon alfa-2b
Injection Powder for Reconstitution: 3 million units, 5 million units, 6 million units, 10 million units, 18 million units, 25 million units, 50 million units (Intron-A).
Injection, Prefilled Syringes: 3 million units, 5 million units, 6 million units, 10 million units, 18 million units, 25 million units, 50 million units (Intron-A).

INDICATIONS AND DOSAGES
▶ **Hairy cell leukemia**
Interferon alfa-2a
SUBCUTANEOUS/IM
Adults. Initially, 3 million units/day for 16-24 wk. Maintenance: 3 million units 3 times/wk. Do not use 36-million-unit vial.

Interferon alfa-2b
SUBCUTANEOUS/IM
Adults. 2 million units/m^2
3 times/wk. If severe adverse reactions occur, modify dose or temporarily discontinue.

▸ **Chronic myelocytic leukemia (CML)**
Interferon alfa-2a
SUBCUTANEOUS/IM
Adults. 9 million units daily.

▸ **Condylomata acuminate**
Interferon alfa-2b
INTRALESIONAL
Adults. 1 million units/lesion
3 times/wk for 3 wk. Use only
10-million-unit vial, reconstitute with no more than 1 ml diluent. Use tuberculin (TB) syringe with 25- or 26-gauge needle. Give in evening with acetaminophen, which alleviates side effects.

▸ **Melanoma**
Interferon alfa-2a
SUBCUTANEOUS/IM
Adults, Elderly. 12 million units/m^2
3 times/wk for 3 mo.
Interferon alfa-2b
IV
Adults. Initially, 20 million units/m^2
5 times/wk for 4 wk. Maintenance:
10 million units IM/Subcutaneous for 48 wk.

▸ **AIDS-related Kaposi's sarcoma**
Interferon alfa-2a
SUBCUTANEOUS/IM
Adults. Initially, 36 million units/day for 10-12 wk, may give 3 million units on day 1; 9 million units on day 2; 18 million units on day 3; then begin 36 million units/day for remainder of 10-12 wk.
Maintenance: 36 million units/day
3 times/wk.
Interferon alfa-2b
SUBCUTANEOUS/IM
Adults. 30 million units/m^2
3 times/wk. Use only 50-million-unit vials. If severe adverse reactions

occur, modify dose or temporarily discontinue.

▸ **Chronic hepatitis B**
Interferon alfa-2b
SUBCUTANEOUS/IM
Adults. 30-35 million units/wk,
5 million units/day or 10 million units 3 times/wk.

▸ **Chronic hepatitis C**
Interferon alfa-2a
SUBCUTANEOUS/IM
Adults. Initially, 6 million units once a day for 3 wk, then 3 million units 3 times/wk for 6 mo.
Interferon alfa-2b
SUBCUTANEOUS/IM
Adults. 3 million units 3 times/wk for up to 6 mo, for up to 18-24 mo for chronic hepatitis C.

OFF-LABEL USES
Interferon alfa-2a
Treatment of active, chronic hepatitis, bladder or renal carcinoma, malignant melanoma, multiple myeloma, mycosis fungoides, non-Hodgkin's lymphoma
Interferon alfa-2b
Treatment of bladder, cervical, renal carcinoma, chronic myelocytic leukemia, laryngeal papillomatosis, multiple myeloma, mycosis fungoides

CONTRAINDICATIONS
Hypersensitivity to any component of the formulations

INTERACTIONS
Drug
Bone marrow depressants: May have additive effect.
Herbal
None known.
Food
None known.

DIAGNOSTIC TEST EFFECTS
May increase LDH concentration, serum alkaline phosphatase, SGOT

(AST), and SGPT (ALT) levels. May decrease blood Hgb and Hct, and leukocyte and platelet counts.

▓ IV INCOMPATIBILITIES
No information available. Do not mix with other medications via Y-site administration.

SIDE EFFECTS
Frequent
Interferon alfa-2a
Flu-like symptoms, including fever, fatigue, headache, aches, pains, anorexia, and chills, nausea, vomiting, coughing, dyspnea, hypotension, edema, chest pain, dizziness, diarrhea, weight loss, taste change, abdominal discomfort, confusion, paresthesia, depression, visual and sleep disturbances, diaphoresis, lethargy
Interferon alfa-2b
Flu-like symptoms, including fever, fatigue, headache, aches, pains, anorexia, and chills, rash with hairy cell leukemia (Kaposi's sarcoma only)
Kaposi's sarcoma: All previously mentioned side effects plus depression, dyspepsia, dry mouth or thirst, alopecia, rigors
Occasional
Interferon alfa-2a
Partial alopecia, rash, dry throat or skin, pruritus, flatulence, constipation, hypertension, palpitations, sinusitis
Interferon alfa-2b
Dizziness, pruritus, dry skin, dermatitis, alteration in taste
Rare
Interferon alfa-2a
Hot flashes, hypermotility, Raynaud's syndrome, bronchospasm, earache, ecchymosis
Interferon alfa-2b
Confusion, leg cramps, back pain, gingivitis, flushing, tremor, nervousness, eye pain

SERIOUS REACTIONS
• Arrhythmias, stroke, transient ischemic attacks, congestive heart failure (CHF), pulmonary edema, and myocardial infarction (MI) occur rarely with interferon alfa-2a.
• Hypersensitivity reaction occurs rarely with interferon alfa-2b.
• Severe adverse reactions of flu-like symptoms appear dose-related with interferon alfa-2b.

PRECAUTIONS & CONSIDERATIONS
Caution is warranted with cardiac diseases, compromised central nervous system (CNS) function, history of cardiac abnormalities, liver or renal impairment, myelosuppression, and seizure disorders. Be aware that interferon alfa-2a and -2b use should be avoided during pregnancy. Breast-feeding is not recommended in this patient population. Safety and efficacy of interferon alfa-2a and -2b have not been established in children. Be aware that in the elderly, cardiotoxicity and neurotoxicity may occur more frequently. Age-related renal impairment may require cautious use of interferon alfa-2a and -2b in the elderly.

Clinical response may take 1 to 3 months to appear. Flu-like symptoms tend to diminish with continued therapy. Alcohol and tasks that require mental alertness or motor skills should be avoided during drug therapy. Females should use contraception, and to notify the physician if she suspects pregnancy.
Storage
Refrigerate interferon alfa-2a. Stable for 7 days at room temperature. Prepare immediately before use.
Administration
Know that the drug dosage is individualized based on the patient's clinical response and tolerance of the drug's adverse effects. When used in

combination therapy, consult specific protocols for optimum dosage and sequence of drug administration, as prescribed. Remember that side effects are dose-related. Be aware that the subcutaneous route of administration is preferred for thrombocytopenic patients and other patients at risk for bleeding. Remember that the drug dosage is individualized based on the patient's clinical response and tolerance of the drug's adverse effects. When used in combination therapy, expect to consult specific protocols for optimum dosage, and sequence of drug administration. If severe adverse reactions occur, modify the drug dosage or temporarily discontinue the medication, as prescribed.

Do not shake vial. Do not use if precipitate or discoloration occurs; solution normally appears colorless. Give as subcutaneous or IM injection.

Do not give interferon alfa-2b IM if the platelet count is less than 50,000/m^3; instead give subcutaneous.

For hairy cell leukemia, reconstitute each 3-million-unit vial of interferon alfa-2b with 1 ml bacteriostatic water for injection to provide concentration of 3 million units/ml, 1-ml to 5-million-unit vial; 2-ml to 10-million-unit vial; 5-ml to 25-million-unit vial provides concentration of 5 million units/ml.

For condylomata acuminata, reconstitute each 10-million-unit vial of interferon alfa-2b with 1 ml bacteriostatic water for injection to provide concentration of 10 million units/ml.

For acquired immune deficiency syndrome (AIDS)-related Kaposi's sarcoma patients, reconstitute 50-million-unit vial interferon alfa-2b with 1 ml bacteriostatic water for injection to provide concentration of 50 million units/ml.

Agitate the vial gently and withdraw solution with sterile syringe.

For intravenous use, reconstitute interferon alfa-2b with diluent provided by manufacturer. Withdraw desired dose and further dilute with 100 ml 0.9% NaCl to provide final concentration at least 10 million units/100 ml. Administer over 20 minutes.

Interferon Alfa-2b
inn-ter-fear′on
(Intron-A)
Do not confuse interferon alfa-2b with interferon alfa-2a.

CATEGORY AND SCHEDULE
Pregnancy Risk Category: C

CLASSIFICATION
Immunologic agents

MECHANISM OF ACTION
A biological response modifier that inhibits viral replication in virus-infected cells, suppresses cell proliferation, increases phagocytic action of macrophages, and augments specific cytotoxicity of lymphocytes for target cells. *Therapeutic Effect:* Prevents rapid growth of malignant cells; inhibits hepatitis virus.

PHARMACOKINETICS
Well absorbed after IM and subcutaneous administration. Undergoes proteolytic degradation during reabsorption in kidneys. **Half-life:** 2-3 hr.

AVAILABILITY

Injection (Multidose Vial): 6 million units/ml, 10 million units/ml.
Injection (Single-Dose Vial): 3 million units/0.5 ml, 5 million units/0.5 ml, 10 million units/ml.
Injection (Prefilled Solution): 3 million units/0.2 ml, 5 million units/0.2 ml, 10 million units/0.2 ml.

INDICATIONS AND DOSAGES

▸ **Hairy cell leukemia**
IM, SUBCUTANEOUS
Adults. 2 million units/m² 3 times a week. If severe adverse reactions occur, modify dose or temporarily discontinue drug.

▸ **Condyloma acuminatum**
INTRALESIONAL
Adults. 1 million units/lesion 3 times a week for 3 wk. Use only 10-million-unit vial, and reconstitute with no more than 1 ml diluent.

▸ **AIDS-related Kaposi's sarcoma**
IM, SUBCUTANEOUS
Adults. 30 million units/m² 3 times a week. Use only 50-million-unit vials. If severe adverse reactions occur, modify dose or temporarily discontinue drug.

▸ **Chronic hepatitis C**
IM, SUBCUTANEOUS
Adults. 3 million units 3 times a week for up to 6 mo. For patients who tolerate therapy and whose ALT (SGPT) level normalizes within 16 weeks, therapy may be extended for up to 18-24 mo.

▸ **Chronic hepatitis B**
IM, SUBCUTANEOUS
Adults. 30-35 million units weekly, either as 5 million units/day or 10 million units 3 times a week.

▸ **Malignant melanoma**
IV
Adults. Initially, 20 million units/m² 5 times a week for 4 wk. Maintenance: 10 million units IM or subcutaneously 3 times a week for 48 wk.

▸ **Follicular lymphoma**
SUBCUTANEOUS
Adults. 5 million units 3 times a week for up to 18 mo.

OFF-LABEL USES

Treatment of bladder, cervical, or renal carcinoma; chronic myelocytic leukemia; laryngeal papillomatosis; multiple myeloma; mycosis fungoides

CONTRAINDICATIONS

None known.

INTERACTIONS

Drug
Bone marrow depressants: May increase myelosuppression.
Herbal
None known.
Food
None known.

DIAGNOSTIC TEST EFFECTS

May increase PT, aPTT, and serum LDH, alkaline phosphatase, AST (SGOT), and ALT (SGPT) levels. May decrease blood Hgb level, Hct, and leukocyte and platelet counts.

▦ IV INCOMPATIBILITIES

No information available. Do not mix with other medications for Y-site administration.

SIDE EFFECTS

Frequent
Flu-like symptoms, rash (only in patients with hairy cell leukemia Kaposi's sarcoma)
Patients with Kaposi's sarcoma: All previously mentioned side effects plus depression, dyspepsia, dry mouth or thirst, alopecia, rigors
Occasional
Dizziness, pruritus, dry skin, dermatitis, altered taste

Rare

Confusion, leg cramps, back pain, gingivitis, flushing, tremor, nervousness, eye pain

SERIOUS REACTIONS

• Hypersensitivity reactions occur rarely.
• Severe flu-like symptoms may occur at higher doses.

PRECAUTIONS & CONSIDERATIONS

Caution is warranted with cardiac diseases or abnormalities, compromised CNS function, hepatic or renal impairment, myelosuppression, and seizure disorders. Interferon alfa-2b should not be used by pregnant or breast-feeding women. Effective contraceptive measures should be used during therapy and the physician should be notified if the woman is or may be pregnant. The safety and efficacy of interferon alfa-2b have not been established in children. The elderly are more prone to cardiotoxicity and neurotoxicity. Age-related renal impairment may require cautious use of interferon alfa-2b in the elderly. Avoid receiving immunizations without the physician's approval and coming in contact with people who have recently received a live-virus vaccine because interferon alfa-2b lowers the body's resistance. Also, avoid tasks that require mental alertness or motor skills until response to the drug has been established.

Flu-like symptoms may occur but may be minimized by taking the drug at bedtime and tend to diminish with continued therapy. Urinalysis, CBC, platelet count, BUN level, and serum alkaline phosphatase, creatinine, AST (SGOT), and ALT (SGPT) levels should be obtained before and routinely during therapy.

Storage

Refrigerate unopened vials, however, the drug remains stable for 7 days at room temperature.

Administration

! Dosage is individualized based on clinical response and tolerance of the drug's adverse effects. When used in combination therapy, consult specific protocols for optimum dosage and sequence of drug administration, as prescribed. Remember that side effects are dose-related. The drug's therapeutic effect may take 1 to 3 months to appear.

For IV use, prepare the solution immediately before use. Reconstitute with the diluent provided by the manufacturer. Withdraw the desired dose and further dilute with 100 ml 0.9% NaCl to provide final concentration at least 10 million units/ 100 ml. Administer the drug over 20 minutes.

Don't administer interferon alfa-2b by IM injection if platelet count is less than $50,000/m^3$; instead give it subcutaneously.

For hairy cell leukemia, reconstitute as follows: add 1 ml bacteriostatic water for injection to each 3-million-unit vial to provide a concentration of 3 million units/ml, or add 1 ml to each 5-million-unit vial, 2 ml to each 10-million-unit vial, or 5 ml to each 25-million-unit vial to provide a concentration of 5 million units/ml.

For condylomata acuminata, reconstitute each 10-million-unit vial with 1 ml bacteriostatic water for injection to provide a concentration of 10 million units/ml. Use a tuberculin syringe with a 25- or 26-gauge needle. Give the drug in the evening with acetaminophen, which alleviates side effects.

For AIDS-related Kaposi's sarcoma, reconstitute each 50-million-unit vial with 1 ml bacteriostatic water for injection to provide a concentration of 50 million units/ml. Agitate the vial gently and withdraw the solution with a sterile syringe.

Interferon Alfa-n3
in-ter-fear′on
(human leukocyte interferon, antiviral)
(Alferon N)

CATEGORY AND SCHEDULE
Pregnancy Risk Category: C

CLASSIFICATION
Immunologic agents

MECHANISM OF ACTION
A biological response modifier that inhibits viral replication in virus-infected cells, suppresses cell proliferation, increases phagocytic action of macrophages, and augments specific cytotoxicity of lymphocytes for target cells. *Therapeutic Effect:* Inhibits viral growth in condylomata acuminatum.

AVAILABILITY
Injection: 5 million international units/ml.

INDICATIONS AND DOSAGES
▶ **Condyloma acuminatum**
INTRALESIONAL
Adults, Children 18 yr and older. 0.05 ml (250,000 international units) per wart twice a week up to 8 wk. Maximum dose/treatment session: 0.5 ml (2.5 million international units). Do not repeat for 3 mo after initial 8 wk course unless warts enlarge or new warts appear.

OFF-LABEL USES
Treatment of active chronic hepatitis, bladder carcinoma, chronic myelocytic leukemia, laryngeal papillomatosis, malignant melanoma, multiple myeloma, mycosis fungoides, non-Hodgkin's lymphoma

CONTRAINDICATIONS
Previous history of anaphylactic reaction to egg protein, mouse immunoglobulin, or neomycin

INTERACTIONS
Drug
Bone marrow depressants: May increase myelosuppression.
Herbal
None known.
Food
None known.

DIAGNOSTIC TEST EFFECTS
May increase serum LDH, alkaline phosphatase, AST (SGOT), and ALT (SGPT) levels. May decrease blood Hgb level, Hct, and leukocyte and platelet counts.

SIDE EFFECTS
Frequent
Flu-like symptoms
Occasional
Dizziness, pruritus, dry skin, dermatitis, altered taste
Rare
Confusion, leg cramps, back pain, gingivitis, flushing, tremor, nervousness, eye pain

SERIOUS REACTIONS
• Hypersensitivity reaction occurs rarely.
• Severe flu-like symptoms may occur at higher doses.

PRECAUTIONS & CONSIDERATIONS
Caution is warranted with diabetes mellitus and ketoacidosis, hemophilia,

pulmonary embolism, seizure disorders, severe myelosuppression, severe pulmonary disease, thrombophlebitis, uncontrolled CHF, and unstable angina.

Flu-like symptoms may occur but may be minimized by taking the drug at bedtime and tend to diminish with continued therapy. Diagnostic tests, such as CBC, should be obtained before and routinely during therapy.

Storage
Refrigerate vials. Do not freeze or shake them.

Administration
Using a 30-gauge needle, inject the drug into the base of each wart.

Interferon Alfacon-1
in-ter-fear′on
(Infergen)

CATEGORY AND SCHEDULE
Pregnancy Risk Category: C

CLASSIFICATION
Immunologic agents

MECHANISM OF ACTION
A biological response modifier that stimulates the immune system.
Therapeutic Effect: Inhibits hepatitis C virus.

AVAILABILITY
Injection: 9 mcg/0.3 ml, 15 mcg/0.5 ml.

INDICATIONS AND DOSAGES
▸ **Chronic hepatitis C**
SUBCUTANEOUS
Adults. 9 mcg 3 times a week for 24 wk. May increase to 15 mcg

3 times a week in patients who tolerate but fail to respond to 9-mcg dose.

CONTRAINDICATIONS
History of autoimmune hepatitis or severe psychiatric disorders

SIDE EFFECTS
Frequent (greater than 50%)
Headache, fatigue, fever, depression

PRECAUTIONS & CONSIDERATIONS
Caution is warranted with a history of autoimmune disease, cardiac disease, depression, endocrine disorders, hepatic disorders, and myelosuppression. Notify the physician of side effects, including headache or injection site pain, as soon as possible. Serum alkaline phosphatase, AST (SGOT), and ALT (SGPT), hepatitis C virus (HCV) antibody, and HCV-RNA levels should be obtained before and during therapy.

Administration
! Make sure at least 48 hours elapse between doses of interferon alfacon-1.
Administer as subcutaneous injection.

Interferon Beta-1a
in-ter-fear′-on
Do not confuse interferon beta-1a with interferon beta-1b or Avonex with Avelox.

CATEGORY AND SCHEDULE
Pregnancy Risk Category: C

CLASSIFICATION
Immunologic agents

MECHANISM OF ACTION
A biological response modifier that interacts with specific cell receptors

found on the surface of human cells. *Therapeutic Effect:* Produces antiviral and immunoregulatory effects.

PHARMACOKINETICS
Peak serum levels attained 3-15 hr after IM administration. Biological markers increase within 12 hr and remain elevated for 4 days. **Half-life:** 10 hr (Avonex); 69 hr (Rebif).

AVAILABILITY
Injection Solution (Prefilled Syringe [Avonex]): 30 mcg/0.5 ml.
Injection Solution (Prefilled Syringe [Rebif]): 22 mcg/ml, 44 mcg/ml.

INDICATIONS AND DOSAGES
▸ **Relapsing-remitting multiple sclerosis**
IM (Avonex)
Adults. 30 mcg once weekly.
Subcutaneous (Rebif)
Adults. Initially 8.8 mcg 3 times a week, may increase to 44 mcg 3 times a week over 4-6 wk.

OFF-LABEL USES
Treatment of AIDS, AIDS-related Kaposi's sarcoma, malignant melanoma, renal cell carcinoma

CONTRAINDICATIONS
Hypersensitivity to albumin or interferon

INTERACTIONS
Drug
None known.
Herbal
None known.
Food
None known.

DIAGNOSTIC TEST EFFECTS
May increase blood glucose and BUN levels, and serum alkaline phosphatase, bilirubin, calcium, AST (SGOT), and ALT (SGPT) levels.

May decrease blood Hgb level and neutrophil, platelet, and WBC counts.

SIDE EFFECTS
Frequent
Headache (67%), flu-like symptoms (61%), myalgia (34%), upper respiratory tract infection (31%), generalized pain (24%), asthenia, chills (21%), sinusitis (18%), infection (11%)
Occasional
Abdominal pain, arthralgia (9%), chest pain, dyspnea (6%), malaise, syncope (4%)
Rare
Injection site reaction, hypersensitivity reaction (3%)

SERIOUS REACTIONS
• Anemia occurs in 8% of patients.

PRECAUTIONS & CONSIDERATIONS
Caution is warranted with chronic, progressive multiple sclerosis and in children younger than 18 years. Interferon beta-1a may cause spontaneous abortion. It is unknown if interferon beta-1a is distributed in breast milk. Interferon beta-1a should be used cautiously in children because its safety and efficacy have not been established in this age group. No information is available on the use of interferon beta-1a in the elderly.

Notify the physician of flu-like symptoms, headache, or muscle pain or weakness. CBC and serum alkaline phosphatase, AST (SGOT), and ALT (SGPT) levels should be obtained before and during therapy.
Storage
Refrigerate unopened vials of Avonex prefilled syringes; warm vials to room temperature before use; if the drug is not used immediately after reconstitution, refrigerate

it and use it within 6 hours; after 6 hours, discard any unused portion because the drug contains no preservative. Use Avonex prefilled syringe within 12 hours after removal from refrigerator. Refrigerate Rebif prefilled syringes; if refrigeration is unavailable, the drug may be stored at room temperature, away from heat and light, up to 30 days.

Administration

! Gently swirl—do not shake—the vial to dissolve the drug.

For IM use (Avonex powder for injection), reconstitute 30 mcg *MicroPin* (6.6-million-unit) vial with 1.1 ml of the diluent, provided by the manufacturer. Discard it if it becomes discolored or contains a precipitate.

For IM use (Avonex prefilled syringes), allow the drug to warm to room temperature prior to use.

For subcutaneous use (Rebif prefilled syringes), administer the drug at the same time of day 3 days each week. Separate doses by at least 48 hours.

Interferon Beta-1a/b
inn-ter-fear′on
(Avonex, Rebif); (Betaferon, Betaseron)

CATEGORY AND SCHEDULE
Pregnancy Risk Category: C

CLASSIFICATION
Immunologic agents

MECHANISM OF ACTION
A biologic response modifier that interacts with specific cell receptors found on surface of human cells. *Therapeutic Effect:* Possesses antiviral and immunoregulatory activities.

PHARMACOKINETICS
Interferon beta-1a
After IM administration, peak serum levels attained in 3-15 hr. Biologic markers increase within 12 hr and remain elevated for 4 days.
Half-life: 10 hr (IM).
Interferon beta-1b
Half-life: 8 min-4. 3 hr.

AVAILABILITY
Interferon beta-1a
Prefilled Syringes Powder for Injection: 22 mcg (Rebif), 30 mcg (Avonex), 44 mcg (Rebif).
Interferon beta-1b
Powder for Injection: 0. 3 mg (9.6 million units) (Betaseron).

INDICATIONS AND DOSAGES
▶ **Relapsing-remitting multiple sclerosis**
Interferon beta-1a
IM
Adults. 30 mcg Avonex once weekly.
SUBCUTANEOUS
Adults. Initially 8.8 mcg Rebif 3 times/wk, may increase over 4-6 wk to 44 mcg Rebif 3 times/wk.
Interferon beta-1b
SUBCUTANEOUS
Adults. 0.25 mg (8 million units) every other day.

OFF-LABEL USES
Treatment of acquired immune deficiency syndrome (AIDS), AIDS-related Kaposi's sarcoma, malignant melanoma, renal cell carcinoma

CONTRAINDICATIONS
Hypersensitivity to albumin, interferon

INTERACTIONS
Drug
None known.
Herbal
None known.
Food
None known.

DIAGNOSTIC TEST EFFECTS
May increase blood glucose levels, BUN, serum alkaline phosphatase, bilirubin, calcium, SGOT (AST), and SGPT (ALT) levels. May decrease blood Hgb, neutrophil, platelet, and white blood cell (WBC) counts.

SIDE EFFECTS
Frequent
Interferon beta-1a: Headache (67%), flu-like symptoms (61%), myalgia (34%), upper respiratory infection (31%), pain (24%), asthenia, chills (21%), sinusitis (18%), infection (11%)
Interferon beta-1a: Injection site reaction (85%), headache (84%), flu-like symptoms (76%), fever (59%), pain (52%), asthenia (49%), myalgia (44%), sinusitis (36%), diarrhea, dizziness (35%), mental status changes (29%), constipation (24%), diaphoresis (23%), vomiting (21%)
Occasional
Interferon beta-1a: Abdominal pain, arthralgia (9%), chest pain, dyspnea (6%), malaise, syncope (4%)
Interferon beta-1b: Malaise (15%), somnolence (6%), alopecia (4%)
Rare
Interferon beta-1a: Injection site reaction, hypersensitivity reaction (3%)

SERIOUS REACTIONS
• Anemia occurs in 8% of patients taking interferon beta-1a.
• Seizures occur rarely in patients taking interferon beta-1b.

PRECAUTIONS & CONSIDERATIONS
Caution is warranted with children younger than 18 years of age and chronic progressive multiple sclerosis. Be aware that interferon beta-1a has abortifacient potential. Be aware that it is unknown if interferon beta-1a is distributed in breast milk. Be aware that the safety and efficacy of interferon beta-1a have not been established in children. Be aware that there is no information on interferon beta-1a use in the elderly. Be aware that it is unknown if interferon beta-1b is distributed in breast milk. Be aware that the safety and efficacy of interferon beta-1b have not been established in children. Be aware that there is no information available on interferon beta-1b use in the elderly.

Dispose of needles and syringes in the provided puncture-resistant container. Document the type and severity of any injection site reactions; these reactions will not require discontinuation of therapy. Immediately notify the physician if depression or suicidal ideation occurs.
Storage
Refrigerate vials of interferon beta-1a. Following reconstitution of interferon beta-1a, use within 6 hours if refrigerated. Discard if discolored or contains a precipitate.

Store interferon beta-1b vials at room temperature. After reconstitution the solution of interferon beta-1b is stable for 3 hours if refrigerated. Use within 3 hours of reconstitution. Discard the solution if it is discolored or contains a precipitate.
Administration
For IM use of interferon beta-1a, reconstitute 33-mcg (6.6-million-unit) vial with 1.1 ml diluent, which is

supplied by the manufacturer. Gently swirl to dissolve medication; do not shake. Discard unused portion because it contains no preservative. For subcutaneous use of interferon beta-1a, administer drug at the same time of day 3 days each week. Doses should be separated by at least 48 hours.

For subcutaneous use of interferon beta-1b, reconstitute 0.3-mg (9.6-million-unit) vial with 1.2 ml diluent, which is supplied by manufacturer, to provide concentration of 0.25 mg/ml (8 million units/ml). Gently swirl to dissolve medication; do not shake. Withdraw 1 ml solution and inject subcutaneous into the patient's abdomen, arms, hips, or thighs using a 27-gauge needle. Discard unused portion because it contains no preservative.

Interferon Beta-1b
in-ter-fear'-on
(Betaseron)
Do not confuse interferon beta-1b with interferon beta-1a.

CATEGORY AND SCHEDULE
Pregnancy Risk Category: C

CLASSIFICATION
Immunologic agents

MECHANISM OF ACTION
A biological response modifier that interacts with specific cell receptors found on the surface of human cells. *Therapeutic Effect:* Produces antiviral and immunoregulatory effects.

PHARMACOKINETICS
Half-life: 8 min-4.3 hr.

AVAILABILITY
Powder for Injection: 0.3 mg (9.6 million units).

INDICATIONS AND DOSAGES
▶ **Relapsing-remitting multiple sclerosis**
SUBCUTANEOUS
Adults. 0.25 mg (8 million units) every other day.

OFF-LABEL USES
Treatment of acute non-A and non-B hepatitis, AIDS, AIDS-related Kaposi's sarcoma, malignant melanoma, renal cell carcinoma

CONTRAINDICATIONS
Hypersensitivity to albumin or interferon

INTERACTIONS
Drug
None known.
Herbal
None known.
Food
None known.

DIAGNOSTIC TEST EFFECTS
May increase blood glucose and BUN levels, and serum alkaline phosphatase, bilirubin, calcium, AST (SGOT), and ALT (SGPT) levels. May decrease blood Hgb level and neutrophil, platelet, and WBC counts.

SIDE EFFECTS
Frequent
Injection site reaction (85%), headache (84%), flu-like symptoms (76%), fever (59%), asthenia (49%), myalgia (44%), sinusitis (36%), diarrhea, dizziness (35%), mental status changes (29%), constipation (24%), diaphoresis (23%), vomiting (21%)
Occasional
Malaise (15%), somnolence (6%), alopecia (4%)

SERIOUS REACTIONS
• Seizures occur rarely.

PRECAUTIONS & CONSIDERATIONS
Caution is warranted with chronic, progressive multiple sclerosis and in children younger than 18 years. Pregnancy should be avoided. It is unknown if interferon beta-1b is distributed in breast milk. The safety and efficacy of interferon beta-1b have not been established in children. No information is available on the use of interferon beta-1b in the elderly. Sunscreen and protective clothing should be worn when exposed to sunlight or ultraviolet light until the extent of photosensitivity has been determined.

Notify the physician of flu-like symptoms, headache, or muscle pain or weakness. CBC and serum alkaline phosphatase, AST (SGOT), and ALT (SGPT) levels should be obtained before and during therapy. Pattern of daily bowel activity and stool consistency and food intake should be monitored.

Storage
Store vials at room temperature. After reconstitution, the solution is stable for 3 hours if refrigerated. Use the solution within 3 hours of reconstitution.

Administration
! Gently swirl—do not shake—the vial to dissolve the drug.

For subcutaneous injection, reconstitute the 0.3-mg (9.6-million-unit) vial with 1.2 ml of the diluent, supplied by the manufacturer to provide a concentration of 0.25 mg/ml (8 million units/ml). Using a 27-gauge needle, inject 1 ml of the solution subcutaneously into the abdomen, arms, hips, or thighs. Discard the solution if it becomes discolored or contains a precipitate. Discard any unused portion because the solution contains no preservative.

Interferon Gamma-1b
in-ter-fear'on
(Actimmune, Imukin [AUS])

CATEGORY AND SCHEDULE
Pregnancy Risk Category: C

CLASSIFICATION
Immunologic agents

MECHANISM OF ACTION
A biological response modifier that induces activation of macrophages in blood monocytes to phagocytes, which is necessary in the body's cellular immune response to intracellular and extracellular pathogens. Enhances phagocytic function and antimicrobial activity of monocytes. *Therapeutic Effect:* Decreases signs and symptoms of serious infections in chronic granulomatous disease.

PHARMACOKINETICS
Slowly absorbed after subcutaneous administration.

AVAILABILITY
Injection: 100 mcg (2 million units).

INDICATIONS AND DOSAGES
▸ **Chronic granulomatous disease; severe, malignant osteopetrosis**
SUBCUTANEOUS
Adults, Children older than 1 yr.
50 mcg/m^2 (1.5 million units/m^2) in patients with body surface area (BSA) greater than 0.5 m^2; 1.5 mcg/kg/dose in patients with BSA 0.5 m^2 or less. Give 3 times a week.

CONTRAINDICATIONS

Hypersensitivity to *Escherichia coli*-derived products

INTERACTIONS

Drug
Bone marrow depressants: May increase myelosuppression.
Herbal
None known.
Food
None known.

DIAGNOSTIC TEST EFFECTS

None known.

SIDE EFFECTS

Frequent
Fever (52%); headache (33%); rash (17%); chills, fatigue, diarrhea (14%)
Occasional (13%-10%)
Vomiting, nausea
Rare (6%-3%)
Weight loss, myalgia, anorexia

SERIOUS REACTIONS

• Interferon gamma-1b may exacerbate pre-existing CNS disturbances, including decreased mental status, gait disturbance, and dizziness, as well as cardiac disorders.

PRECAUTIONS & CONSIDERATIONS

Caution is warranted with compromised CNS function, myelosuppression, pre-existing cardiac disorders (including arrhythmias, CHF, and myocardial ischemia), and seizure disorders. It is unknown if interferon gamma-1b crosses the placenta or is distributed in breast milk. The safety and efficacy of interferon gamma-1b have not been established in children younger than 1 year. Children are more likely to experience flu-like symptoms. No information is available on the use of interferon gamma-1b in the elderly. Avoid performing tasks that require mental alertness or motor skills until response to the drug has been established.

Notify the physician of flu-like symptoms or rash. CBC, urinalysis, BUN level and serum alkaline phosphatase, creatinine, AST (SGOT), and ALT (SGPT) levels, should be obtained before and every 3 months during therapy.
Storage
Refrigerate unopened vials; don't freeze them. Discard vials kept at room temperature for longer than 12 hours.
Administration
! Avoid excessive agitation of the vial; don't shake it.

Vials come in single doses; discard any unused portion. The solution normally appears clear and colorless. Do not use it if it becomes discolored or contains a precipitate. Administer the drug subcutaneously 3 times a week. Rotate injection sites.

Interleukin-2 (Aldesleukin)
al-des-loo′kin
(IL-2, Proleukin)
Do not confuse interleukin-2 with interferon 2.

CATEGORY AND SCHEDULE

Pregnancy Risk Category: C

CLASSIFICATION

Antineoplastics, biological response modifiers, recombinant DNA origin

MECHANISM OF ACTION

A biological response modifier that acts like human recombinant interleukin-2, promoting proliferation, differentiation, and recruitment of T and B cells, lymphokine-activated and natural cells, and thymocytes. *Therapeutic Effect:* Enhances cytolytic activity in lymphocytes.

PHARMACOKINETICS
Primarily distributed into plasma, lymphocytes, lungs, liver, kidney, and spleen. Metabolized to amino acids in the cells lining the kidneys. **Half-life:** 85 min.

AVAILABILITY
Powder for Injection: 22 million units (1.3 mg).

INDICATIONS AND DOSAGES
▸ **Metastatic melanoma, metastatic renal cell carcinoma**
IV
Adults 18 yr and older.
600,000 units/kg q8hr for 14 doses; followed by 9 days of rest, then another 14 doses for a total of 28 doses per course. Course may be repeated after rest period of at least 7 wk from date of hospital discharge.

OFF-LABEL USES
Treatment of colorectal cancer, Kaposi's sarcoma, non-Hodgkin's lymphoma.

CONTRAINDICATIONS
Abnormal pulmonary function or thallium stress test results, bowel ischemia or perforation, coma or toxic psychosis lasting longer than 48 hr, GI bleeding requiring surgery, intubation lasting more than 72 hr, organ allografts, pericardial tamponade, renal dysfunction requiring dialysis for longer than 72 hr, repetitive or difficult-to-control seizures; retreatment in those who experience any of the following toxicities: angina, MI, recurrent chest pain with

EKG changes, sustained ventricular tachycardia, uncontrolled or unresponsive cardiac rhythm disturbances

INTERACTIONS
Drug
Antihypertensives: May increase hypotensive effect.
Cardiotoxic, hepatotoxic, myelotoxic, or nephrotoxic medications: May increase the risk of toxicity.
Glucocorticoids: May decrease the effects of interleukin.
Herbal
None known.
Food
None known.

DIAGNOSTIC TEST EFFECTS
May increase BUN and serum alkaline phosphatase, bilirubin, creatinine, AST (SGOT), and ALT (SGPT) levels. May decrease serum calcium, magnesium, phosphorus, potassium, and sodium levels.

▨ IV INCOMPATIBILITIES
Ganciclovir (Cytovene), pentamidine (Pentam), prochlorperazine (Compazine), promethazine (Phenergan)
▨ IV Compatibilities
Calcium gluconate, dopamine (Intropin), heparin, lorazepam (Ativan), magnesium, potassium

SIDE EFFECTS
Side effects are generally self-limiting and reversible within 2-3 days after discontinuing therapy.
Frequent (89%-48%)
Fever, chills, nausea, vomiting, hypotension, diarrhea, oliguria or anuria, mental status changes, irritability, confusion, depression, sinus tachycardia, pain (abdominal, chest, back), fatigue, dyspnea, pruritus

Occasional (47%-17%)
Edema, erythema, rash, stomatitis, anorexia, weight gain, infection (UTI, injection site, catheter tip), dizziness
Rare (15%-4%)
Dry skin, sensory disorders (vision, speech, taste), dermatitis, headache, arthralgia, myalgia, weight loss, hematuria, conjunctivitis, proteinuria

SERIOUS REACTIONS

• Anemia, thrombocytopenia, and leukopenia occur commonly.
• GI bleeding and pulmonary edema occur occasionally.
• Capillary leak syndrome results in hypotension (systolic pressure less than 90 mm Hg or a 20 mm Hg drop from baseline systolic pressure), extravasation of plasma proteins and fluid into extravascular space, and loss of vascular tone. It may result in cardiac arrhythmias, angina, MI, and respiratory insufficiency.
• Other rare reactions include fatal malignant hyperthermia, cardiac arrest, CVA, pulmonary emboli, bowel perforation, gangrene, and severe depression leading to suicide.

PRECAUTIONS & CONSIDERATIONS

Extreme caution should be used with a history of cardiac or pulmonary disease even if they have normal thallium stress and pulmonary function test results. Also use the drug cautiously with fixed requirements for large volumes of fluid (such as those with hypercalcemia) or a history of seizures. Interleukin use should be avoided in patients of either sex who don't practice effective contraception. The safety and efficacy of interleukin have not been established in children. The elderly may require cautious use of the drug because of age-related

renal impairment. They are also less able to tolerate drug-related toxicities.

Notify the physician of difficulty urinating, black tarry stools, pinpoint red spots on skin, bruising, fever, signs of local infection, sore throat, or unusual bleeding from any site. Treat persons with bacterial infection and those with indwelling central lines with antibiotic therapy before beginning interleukin therapy. A negative CT scan must be obtained before beginning therapy. Immediately report any symptoms of depression or suicidal ideation. CBC, electrolytes, liver and renal function, amylase concentration, B/P, mental status, intake and output, extravascular fluid accumulation, platelet count, pulse oximetry values, and weight should be assessed.

Storage
Refrigerate—don't freeze—unopened vials. The reconstituted solution is stable for 48 hours at room temperature or refrigerated (refrigerated is preferred).

Administration
! Withhold the drug in patients who exhibit moderate to severe lethargy or somnolence because continued administration may result in coma. Restrict interleukin therapy to patients with normal cardiac and pulmonary function as determined by thallium stress testing and pulmonary function testing. Dosage is individualized based on clinical response and tolerance of the drug's adverse effects.

For IV use, reconstitute the 22-million-unit vial with 1.2 ml sterile water for injection to provide a concentration of 18 million units/ml. Do not use bacteriostatic water for injection or 0.9% NaCl. During reconstitution, direct the diluent at the side of the vial. Swirl the contents gently—do not shake—to avoid foaming. Further dilute the dose in 50 ml D$_5$W and infuse over 15 minutes. Do not use an in-line filter. Warm the solution to room temperature before infusion. Closely monitor the patient for a drop in mean arterial B/P, a sign of capillary leak syndrome. Continued treatment may result in edema, pleural effusion, mental status changes, and significant hypotension (systolic pressure less than 90 mm Hg or a 20 mm Hg drop from baseline systolic pressure).

Iodoquinol
eye-oh-do-kwin'ole
(Yodoxin, Diodoquin [CAN])

CATEGORY AND SCHEDULE
Pregnancy Risk Category: C

CLASSIFICATION
Antiprotozoals

MECHANISM OF ACTION
An antibacterial, antifungal, and antitrichomonal agent that works in the intestinal lumen by an unknown mechanism. *Therapeutic Effect:* Amebicidal.

PHARMACOKINETICS
Partially and irregularly absorbed from the gastrointestinal (GI) tract. Metabolized in liver. Primarily excreted in feces.

AVAILABILITY
Tablets: 210 mg, 650 mg (Yodoxin).
Powder: 25 g, 100 g (Yodoxin).

INDICATIONS AND DOSAGES
▶ **Intestinal amebiasis**
PO
Adults, Elderly. 630-650 mg 3 times a day for 20 days.
Children. 40 mg/kg in 3 divided doses for up to 20 days. Maximum: 650 mg/day.

CONTRAINDICATIONS
Hepatic impairment, renal impairment, chronic diarrhea (especially in children), hypersensitivity to iodine and 8-hydroxyquinolones

INTERACTIONS
Drug
None known.
Herbal
None known.
Food
None known.

DIAGNOSTIC TEST EFFECTS
May result in false-positive ferric chloride test for phenylketonuria. May increase protein-bound serum iodine concentrations reflecting a decrease in 131I uptake.

SIDE EFFECTS
Occasional
Fever, chills, headache, nausea, vomiting, diarrhea, cramps, urticaria, pruritus

SERIOUS REACTIONS
• Optic neuritis, atrophy, and peripheral neuropathy have been reported with high dosages and long-term use.

PRECAUTIONS & CONSIDERATIONS
Caution should be used with thyroid disease and neurologic disorders. It is unknown if iodoquinol is distributed in breast milk. There are no age-related precautions noted in children.

Age-related renal impairment may limit the use of iodoquinol in the elderly.

Nausea, diarrhea, or GI upset may occur. Be aware that iodoquinol may temporarily stain skin, hair, and clothing a yellow-brown color.

Administration

Give after meals. May crush tablets and mix with applesauce. Avoid long term use.

Ipecac
ip'e-kak
(PMS Ipecac Syrup [CAN])

CATEGORY AND SCHEDULE
Pregnancy Risk Category: C

CLASSIFICATION
Vitamins/minerals

MECHANISM OF ACTION
An antidote that acts centrally by stimulating medullary chemoreceptor trigger zone and locally by irritating gastric mucosa. *Therapeutic Effect:* Produces emesis.

PHARMACOKINETICS
Onset of action occurs within 20-30 min. Eliminated very slowly in urine.

AVAILABILITY
Syrup: 70 mg/ml.

INDICATIONS AND DOSAGES
▸ **Poisoning, acute**
PO
Adults, Elderly, Children 12 yr and older. 15-30 ml followed by 200-300 ml of water

Children 6-12 yr. 5-10 ml followed by 10-20 ml/kg.
Children 1-12 yr. 15 ml followed by 10-20 ml/kg.
Children 6 mo-1 yr. 5-10 ml, followed by 10-20 ml/kg.

CONTRAINDICATIONS
Ingestion of petroleum distillate, ingestion of strong acids or bases, ingestion of strychnine, unconsciousness or absence of gag reflex, hypersensitivity to ipecac or any component of the formulation

INTERACTIONS
Drug
Antiemetics: May decrease effect of ipecac.
Herbal
None known.
Food
Carbonated beverages: May cause stomach distention.
Milk or milk products: May decrease effectiveness of ipecac.

DIAGNOSTIC TEST EFFECTS
None known.

SIDE EFFECTS
Expected response
Nausea, vomiting, drowsiness and mild CNS depression after vomiting
Occasional
Diarrhea, lethargy, muscle aching, stomach cramps

SERIOUS REACTIONS
• Cardiotoxicity may occur if ipecac syrup is not vomited (noted as hypotension, tachycardia, precordial chest pain, pulmonary congestion, dyspnea, ventricular tachycardia and fibrillation, cardiac arrest).
• Overdose may produce diarrhea, fast/irregular heartbeat, nausea continuing >30 min, stomach pain,

respiratory difficulty and unusually tired, aching/stiff muscles.

PRECAUTIONS & CONSIDERATIONS

Caution should be used with cardio-vascular disorders. Be aware that the emetic effect may be diminished or delayed if activated charcoal was administered before or concurrently with ipecac syrup. It is unknown if ipecac crosses the placenta or is distributed in breast milk. There are no age-related precautions noted in children or the elderly.

Do not administer to semicon-scious, unconscious, or convulsing person. Gastric lavage, activated charcoal is necessary if vomiting does not occur within 30 minutes of second dosage to avoid drug toxicity (bloody stools, vomitus, abdominal pain, hypotension, dyspnea, shock, cardiac disturbances, seizures, coma). Maintain the person in upright position to enhance emetic effect.

Storage

Store at room temperature.

Administration

Be aware that ipecac fluid extract is 14 times more potent than syrup and should not be used. Be aware if vomiting has not occurred within 20 minutes after first dose, repeat with 15 ml. If vomiting has not occurred within 30 minutes after last dose, initiate gastric lavage, activated charcoal. Administer a large glass of water (no milk or soda) after taking ipecac syrup.

Ipratropium

eye-pra-troep′ee-um
(Apo-Ipravent [CAN], Aproven [AUS], Atrovent, Atrovent Aerosol [AUS], Atrovent Nasal [AUS], Novo-Ipramide [CAN], Nu-Ipratropium [CAN], PMS-Ipratropium [CAN])
Do not confuse Atrovent with Alupent.

CATEGORY AND SCHEDULE

Pregnancy Risk Category: B

CLASSIFICATION

Anticholinergics, bronchodilators

MECHANISM OF ACTION

An anticholinergic that blocks the action of acetylcholine at parasym-pathetic sites in bronchial smooth muscle. *Therapeutic Effect:* Causes bronchodilation and inhibits nasal secretions.

PHARMACOKINETICS

Route	Onset	Peak	Duration
Inhalation	1-3 min	1-2 hr	4 6 hr

Minimal systemic absorption after inhalation. Metabolized in the liver (systemic absorption). Primarily eliminated in feces. **Half-life:** 1.5-4 hr.

AVAILABILITY

Oral Inhalation: 18 mcg/actuation.
Aerosol Solution for Inhalation: 0.02%.
Nasal Spray: 0.03%, 0.06%.

INDICATIONS AND DOSAGES
▶ **Bronchospasm, acute treatment**
INHALATION
Adults, Elderly, Children. 4-8 puffs
as needed.
NEBULIZATION
*Adults, Elderly, Children 12 yr and
older.* 500 mcg q30min for 3 doses,
then q2-4hr as needed.
Children younger than 12 yr.
250 mcg q20min for 3 doses, then
q2-4hr as needed.
▶ **Bronchospasm, maintenance
treatment**
INHALATION
*Adults, Elderly, Children 12 yr and
older.* 2-3 puffs q6hr.
Children younger than 12 yr.
1-2 puffs q6hr.
NEBULIZATION
*Adults, Elderly, Children 12 yr and
older.* 500 mcg q6hr.
Children younger than 12 yr.
250-500 mcg q6hr.
▶ **Rhinorrhea**
INTRANASAL
Adults, Children older than 12 yr.
2 sprays of 0.06% solution 3-4 times
a day.
Adults, Children 6-12 yr. 2 sprays
of (0.03%) solution 2-3 times
a day.

CONTRAINDICATIONS
History of hypersensitivity to
atropine

INTERACTIONS
Drug
Cromolyn inhalation solution:
Avoid mixing these drugs because
they form a precipitate.
Herbal
None known.
Food
None known.

DIAGNOSTIC TEST EFFECTS
None known.

SIDE EFFECTS
Frequent
Inhalation (6%-3%): Cough, dry
mouth, headache, nausea
Nasal: Dry nose and mouth,
headache, nasal irritation
Occasional
Inhalation (2%): Dizziness, transient
increased bronchospasm
Rare (less than 1%)
Inhalation: Hypotension, insomnia,
metallic or unpleasant taste, palpita-
tions, urine retention
Nasal: Diarrhea or constipation, dry
throat, abdominal pain, stuffy nose

SERIOUS REACTIONS
• Worsening of angle-closure glaucoma, acute eye pain, and hypotension occur rarely.

PRECAUTIONS & CONSIDERATIONS
Caution is warranted with bladder
neck obstruction, angle-closure glaucoma, and benign prostatic hyperplasia. It is unknown if ipratropium is
distributed in breast milk. No age-
related precautions have been noted in
children or the elderly. Drink plenty of
fluids to decrease the thickness of
lung secretions. Avoid excessive use
of caffeinated products, such as
chocolate, cocoa, cola, coffee, and tea.
    Pulse rate and quality, respiratory
rate, depth, rhythm and type, ABG
levels, and serum potassium levels
should be monitored. Lips and
fingernails should be examined for a
blue or gray color in light-skinned
patients and a gray color in dark-
skinned patients, which are signs of
hypoxemia. Clinical improvement,
such as cessation of retractions,
quieter and slower respirations, and a
relaxed facial expression should also
be evaluated.
Administration
Shake the container well. Exhale
completely through mouth; then

place the mouthpiece into the mouth and close lips, holding the inhaler upright. Inhale deeply through the mouth while fully depressing the top of the canister. Hold breath for as long as possible before exhaling slowly. Wait 2 minutes before inhaling the second dose to allow for deeper bronchial penetration. Rinse mouth with water immediately after inhalation to prevent mouth and throat dryness. Do not take more than 2 inhalations at a time because excessive use decreases the drug's effectiveness or produces paradoxical bronchoconstriction.

Irbesartan
erb′ba-sar-tan
(Avapro, Karvea [AUS])

CATEGORY AND SCHEDULE
Pregnancy Risk Category: C
(D if used in second or third trimester)

CLASSIFICATION
Angiotensin II receptor antagonists

MECHANISM OF ACTION
An angiotensin II receptor, type AT_1, antagonist that blocks the vasoconstrictor and aldosterone-secreting effects of angiotensin II, inhibiting the binding of angiotensin II to the AT_1 receptors. *Therapeutic Effect:* Causes vasodilation, decreases peripheral resistance, and decreases B/P.

PHARMACOKINETICS
Rapidly and completely absorbed after PO administration.

Protein binding: 90%. Undergoes hepatic metabolism to inactive metabolite. Recovered primarily in feces and, to a lesser extent, in urine. Not removed by hemodialysis.
Half-life: 11-15 hr.

AVAILABILITY
Tablets: 75 mg, 150 mg, 300 mg.

INDICATIONS AND DOSAGES
▸ **Hypertension alone or in combination with other antihypertensives**
PO
Adults, Elderly, Children 13 yr and older. Initially, 75-150 mg/day. May increase to 300 mg/day.
Children 6-12 yr. Initially, 75 mg/day. May increase to 150 mg/day.
▸ **Nephropathy**
PO
Adults, Elderly. Target dose of 300 mg/day.

OFF-LABEL USES
Treatment of heart failure

CONTRAINDICATIONS
Bilateral renal artery stenosis, biliary cirrhosis or obstruction, primary hyperaldosteronism, severe hepatic insufficiency

INTERACTIONS
Drug
Hydrochlorothiazide: Further reduces B/P.
Herbal
None known.
Food
None known.

DIAGNOSTIC TEST EFFECTS
May slightly increase BUN and serum creatinine levels. May decrease blood Hgb level.

SIDE EFFECTS
Occasional (9%-3%)
Upper respiratory tract infection,
fatigue, diarrhea, cough
Rare (2%-1%)
Heartburn, dizziness, headache,
nausea, rash

SERIOUS REACTIONS
• Overdosage may manifest as
hypotension and tachycardia.
Bradycardia occurs less often.

PRECAUTIONS & CONSIDERATIONS

Caution is warranted with CHF,
coronary artery disease, mild to
moderate hepatic dysfunction,
sodium and water depletion, and
unilateral renal artery stenosis. It is
unknown if irbesartan is distributed
in breast milk. Irbesartan may cause
fetal or neonatal morbidity or
mortality. Safety and efficacy of
irbesartan have not been established
in children. No age-related precautions have been noted in the elderly.
Sodium consumption and alcohol
should be avoided.

Apical pulse and B/P should be
assessed immediately before each
irbesartan dose, and regularly
throughout therapy. Be alert to fluctuations in apical pulse and B/P. If
an excessive reduction in B/P
occurs, place the person in the
supine position with feet slightly
elevated and notify the physician.
Tasks that require mental alertness
or motor skills should be avoided.
BUN, serum electrolytes, serum
creatinine levels, heart rate for
tachycardia, and urinalysis results
should be obtained before and
during therapy. Maintain adequate
hydration; exercising outside during
hot weather should be avoided in
order to decrease the risk of dehydration and hypotension.

Administration
! Irbesartan may be given concurrently with other antihypertensives;
if B/P is not controlled by irbesartan
alone, a diuretic may also be
prescribed.

Take irbesartan without regard to
meals.

Irinotecan
eye-ri-noe-tee′kan
(Camptosar)

CATEGORY AND SCHEDULE
Pregnancy Risk Category: C
(first trimester), D (second and
third trimester)

CLASSIFICATION
Antineoplastics, topoisomerase
inhibitors

MECHANISM OF ACTION
A DNA topoisomerase inhibitor that
inhibits the action of topoisomerase I,
an enzyme that allows DNA replication by producing reversible single-
strand breaks in DNA that relieve
torsional strain. Irinotecan prevents
religation of the DNA strand, resulting in damage to double-strand DNA
and cell death. *Therapeutic Effect:*
Kills cancer cells.

PHARMACOKINETICS
Metabolized to active metabolite in
the liver after IV administration.
Protein binding: 95% (metabolite).
Excreted in urine and eliminated by
biliary route. **Half-life:** 6 hr;
metabolite 10 hr.

AVAILABILITY
Injection: 20 mg/ml.

INDICATIONS AND DOSAGES
▶ **Carcinoma of the colon or rectum that has progressed or recurred after treatment with 5-fluorouracil**
IV
Adults, Elderly. Initially, 125 mg/m^2 once weekly for 4 wk, followed by a rest period of 2 wk. Additional courses may be repeated q6wk. Dosage may be adjusted in 25-50 mg/m^2 increments to as high as 150 mg/m^2 or as low as 50 mg/m^2.

CONTRAINDICATIONS
None known.

INTERACTIONS
Drug
Diuretics: May increase the risk of dehydration from vomiting and diarrhea.
Laxatives: May increase the severity of diarrhea.
Live-virus vaccines: May potentiate virus replication, increase vaccine side effects, and decrease the patient's antibody response to the vaccine.
Other bone marrow depressants: May increase the risk of myelosuppression.
Prochlorperazine: May increase akathisia.
Herbal
None known.
Food
None known.

DIAGNOSTIC TEST EFFECTS
May increase serum alkaline phosphatase and AST (SGOT) levels.

▓ IV INCOMPATIBILITIES
Gemcitabine (Gemzar)

SIDE EFFECTS
Expected
Nausea (64%), alopecia (49%), vomiting (45%), diarrhea (32%)

Frequent
Constipation, fatigue (29%); fever (28%); asthenia (25%); skeletal pain (23%); abdominal pain, dyspnea (22%)
Occasional
Anorexia (19%); headache, stomatitis (18%); rash (16%)

SERIOUS REACTIONS
• Myelosuppression characterized as neutropenia occurs in 97% of patients; severe neutropenia—a neutrophil count less than 50/mm^3—occurs in 78% of patients.
• Thrombocytopenia, anemia, and sepsis are common reactions.

PRECAUTIONS & CONSIDERATIONS
Caution is warranted in those who have previously received abdominal or pelvic irradiation because they're at increased risk for myelosuppression and the elderly. Because of the risk of fetal harm, pregnant women should not take irinotecan, especially in the first trimester. It is unknown if irinotecan is distributed in breast milk; however, breast-feeding is not recommended for patients taking this drug. The safety and efficacy of irinotecan have not been established in children. The elderly are at increased risk for diarrhea. Use the drug cautiously in patients older than 65 years. Vaccinations and coming in contact with crowds, people with known infections, and anyone who has recently received a live-virus vaccine should be avoided.

Notify the physician if diarrhea, rash, or inflammation at the infusion site occurs. Hgb levels, CBC, serum electrolytes, and hydration status should be monitored. Hair loss may occur and is reversible but new hair may have a different color or texture.

Storage
Store vials at room temperature, and protect them from light. If the solution is reconstituted in D_5W, it remains stable for up to 24 hours at room temperature or 48 hours if refrigerated. However, because the drug contains no preservative, it should be used within 6 hours if kept at room temperature or within 24 hours if refrigerated. Do not refrigerate the solution if it's diluted with 0.9% NaCl.

Administration
! As prescribed, begin a new irinotecan course when the patient's granulocyte count recovers to at least 1500/mm³, platelet count recovers to at least 100,000/mm³, and treatment-related diarrhea fully resolves.

   Dilute the drug in D_5W (the preferred diluent) or 0.9% NaCl to a concentration of 0.12 to 1.1 mg/ml. Administer all doses by IV infusion over 90 minutes. Assess the patient for signs and symptoms of extravasation. If extravasation occurs, flush the site with sterile water and apply ice.

Iron Dextran
iron dex′tran
(Dexiron [CAN], Infed, Infufer [CAN])

CATEGORY AND SCHEDULE
Pregnancy Risk Category: C

CLASSIFICATION
Hematinics, vitamins/minerals

MECHANISM OF ACTION
A trace element and essential component in the formation of Hgb. Necessary for effective erythropoiesis and transport and utilization of oxygen. Serves as cofactor of several essential enzymes. *Therapeutic Effect:* Replenishes Hgb and depleted iron stores.

PHARMACOKINETICS
Readily absorbed after IM administration. Most absorption occurs within 72 hr; remainder within 3-4 wk. Bound to protein to form hemosiderin, ferritin, or transferrin. No physiologic system of elimination. Small amounts lost daily in shedding of skin, hair, and nails and in feces, urine, and perspiration. **Half-life:** 5-20 hr.

AVAILABILITY
Injection: 50 mg/ml.

INDICATIONS AND DOSAGES
▸ **Iron deficiency anemia (no blood loss)**
Dosage is expressed in terms of milligrams of elemental iron, degree of anemia, patient weight, and presence of any bleeding. Expect to use periodic hematologic determinations as guide to therapy.
IV, IM
Adults, Elderly. Mg iron = 0.66 × weight (kg) × (100 − Hgb [g/dl]/14.8
▸ **Iron replacement secondary to blood loss**
IM, IV
Adults, Elderly. Replacement iron (mg) = blood loss (ml) times Hct.
Maximum daily dosage
Adults weighing more than 50 kg. 100 mg.
Children weighing 10-50 kg. 100 mg.
Children weighing 5-less than 10 kg. 50 mg.
Infants weighing less than 5 kg. 25 mg.

CONTRAINDICATIONS
All anemias except iron deficiency anemia, including pernicious, aplastic, normocytic, and refractory

INTERACTIONS
Drug
None known.
Herbal
None known.
Food
None known.

DIAGNOSTIC TEST EFFECTS
None known.

▓ IV INCOMPATIBILITIES
No information available via Y-site administration.

SIDE EFFECTS
Frequent
Allergic reaction (such as rash and itching), backache, myalgia, chills, dizziness, headache, fever, nausea, vomiting, flushed skin, pain or redness at injection site, brown discoloration of skin, metallic taste

SERIOUS REACTIONS
• Anaphylaxis has occurred during the first few minutes after injection, causing death rarely.
• Leukocytosis and lymphadenopathy occur rarely.

PRECAUTIONS & CONSIDERATIONS
Extreme caution should be used with serious hepatic impairment. Caution is warranted with bronchial asthma, a history of allergies, and rheumatoid arthritis. Iron dextran may cross the placenta in some form and trace amounts of the drug are distributed in breast milk. No age-related precautions have been noted in children and the elderly. Avoid taking oral iron while receiving iron injections.

Stools may become black during iron therapy, but this side effect is harmless unless accompanied by abdominal cramping, pain, or red streaking or sticky consistency of stool. Notify the physician of abdominal cramping or pain, back pain, fever, headache, or red streaking or sticky consistency of stool. Be alert for acute exacerbation of joint pain and swelling in persons with rheumatoid arthritis and iron deficiency anemia.
Storage
Store at room temperature.
Administration
! Plan to discontinue oral iron before administering iron dextran because excessive iron intake may produce excessive iron storage (hemosiderosis). Know that a test dose is generally given before the full dose; stay with the patient for several minutes after injection of the test dose because of the potential for anaphylactic reaction.

For IV use, may give undiluted or dilute in 0.9% NaCl for infusion. Do not exceed an administration rate of 50 mg/min (1 ml/min). A too rapid IV rate may produce flushing, chest pain, shock, hypotension, and tachycardia. The patient should stay recumbent for 30 to 45 minutes after IV administration to minimize orthostatic hypotension.

For IM use, draw up medication with one needle; use new needle for injection, to minimize skin staining. Use Z-tract technique by displacing subcutaneous tissue lateral to injection site before inserting needle, to minimize skin staining. Administer deep into upper outer quadrant of buttock only.

Iron Sucrose
iron su'crose
(Venofer)

CATEGORY AND SCHEDULE
Pregnancy Risk Category: B

CLASSIFICATION
Hematinics, vitamins/minerals

MECHANISM OF ACTION
A trace element that is an essential component in the formation of Hgb. It's necessary for effective erythropoiesis and oxygen transport capacity of blood, and transport and utilization of oxygen, and serves as cofactor of several essential enzymes. *Therapeutic Effect:* Replenishes body iron stores in patients on long-term hemodialysis who have iron deficiency anemia and are receiving erythropoietin.

AVAILABILITY
Injection: 20 mg/ml or 100 mg elemental iron in 5-ml single-dose vial.

INDICATIONS AND DOSAGES
▶ **Iron deficiency anemia**
Dosage is expressed in terms of milligrams of elemental iron.
IV
Adults, Elderly. 5 ml iron sucrose, or 100 mg elemental iron, delivered during dialysis; administer 1-3 times a wk to total dose of 1000 mg in 10 doses. Give no more than 3 times a wk.

OFF-LABEL USES
Treatment of dystrophic epidermolysis bullosa

CONTRAINDICATIONS
All anemias except iron deficiency anemia, including pernicious, aplastic, normocytic, and refractory anemia; evidence of iron overload

INTERACTIONS
Drug
None known.
Herbal
None known.
Food
None known.

DIAGNOSTIC TEST EFFECTS
Increases Hgb and Hct, serum ferritin level, and serum transferrin saturation.

▨ IV INCOMPATIBILITIES
Do not mix with other medications or add to parenteral nutrition solution for IV infusion.

SIDE EFFECTS
Frequent (36%-23%)
Hypotension, leg cramps, diarrhea

SERIOUS REACTIONS
• Too rapid IV administration may produce severe hypotension, headache, vomiting, nausea, dizziness, paresthesia, abdominal and muscle pain, edema, and cardiovascular collapse.
• Hypersensitivity reaction occurs rarely.

PRECAUTIONS & CONSIDERATIONS
Caution is warranted with cardiac dysfunction, bronchial asthma, history of allergies, and hepatic or renal impairment. Notify the physician of leg cramps or diarrhea. Initially, Hct, Hgb, serum ferritin, and serum transferrin levels should be obtained monthly, then every 2 to 3 months as determined by the physician. Serum levels should be obtained 48 hours after iron sucrose administration.

Storage
Store at room temperature.
Administration
! Administer directly into dialysis line during hemodialysis, as prescribed.

May be given as undiluted, slow IV injection. For IV infusion, dilute each vial in maximum of 100 ml 0.9% NaCl immediately before infusion. For IV injection, administer into the dialysis line at a rate of 1 ml, or 20 mg iron, undiluted solution per minute. Allow 5 minutes per vial; do not exceed 1 vial per injection. For IV infusion, administer into dialysis line at a rate of 100 mg iron over at least 15 minutes, to reduce the risk of hypotensive episodes. Expect to monitor the results of treatment.

Isocarboxazid
eye-soe-kar-box′a-zid
(Marplan)

CATEGORY AND SCHEDULE
Pregnancy Risk Category: C

CLASSIFICATION
Antidepressants, monoamine oxidase inhibitors

MECHANISM OF ACTION
An antidepressant that inhibits the MAO enzyme system at central nervous system (CNS) storage sites. The reduced MAO activity causes an increased concentration in epinephrine, norepinephrine, serotonin, and dopamine at neuron receptor sites. *Therapeutic Effect:* Produces antidepressant effect.

AVAILABILITY
Tablets: 10 mg (Marplan).

INDICATIONS AND DOSAGES
▶ **Depression refractory to other antidepressants or electroconvulsive therapy**
PO
Adults, Elderly. Initially, 10 mg 3 times/day. May increase to 60 mg/day.

OFF-LABEL USES
Treatment of panic disorder, vascular or tension headaches

CONTRAINDICATIONS
Cardiovascular disease (CVD), cerebrovascular disease, liver impairment, pheochromocytoma, liver impairment

INTERACTIONS
Drug
Alcohol, CNS depressants: May increase CNS depressant effects.
Buspirone: May increase blood pressure (B/P).
Caffeine-containing medications: May increase cardiac arrhythmias and hypertension.
Carbamazepine, cyclobenzaprine, maprotiline, other MAOIs: May precipitate hypertensive crises.
Fluoxetine, trazodone, tricyclic antidepressants: May cause serotonin syndrome.
Insulin, oral hypoglycemics: May increase effects of insulin and oral hypoglycemics.
Meperidine, other opioid analgesics: May produce coma, convulsions, death, diaphoresis, immediate excitation, rigidity, severe hypertension or hypotension, severe respiratory distress, or vascular collapse.
Methylphenidate: May increase the CNS stimulant effects of methylphenidate.

Sympathomimetics: May increase the cardiac stimulant and vasopressor effects of isocarboxazid.
Tyramine: May cause severe, sudden hypertension.
Herbal
None known.
Food
None known.

DIAGNOSTIC TEST EFFECTS
None known.

SIDE EFFECTS
Frequent (more than 10%)
Postural hypotension, drowsiness, decreased sexual ability, weakness, trembling, visual disturbances
Occasional (10%-1%)
Tachycardia, peripheral edema, nervousness, chills, diarrhea, anorexia, constipation, xerostomia
Rare (less than 1%)
Hepatitis, leukopenia, parkinsonian syndrome

SERIOUS REACTIONS
• Hypertensive crisis, marked by severe hypertension, occipital headache radiating frontally, neck stiffness or soreness, nausea, vomiting, sweating, fever or chilliness, clammy skin, dilated pupils, palpitations, tachycardia or bradycardia, and constricting chest pain.

PRECAUTIONS & CONSIDERATIONS
Caution is warranted in patients with asthma, bronchitis, bipolar disorder, cardiac arrhythmias, cardiovascular disease, diabetes mellitus, epilepsy, headaches, hepatic function impairment, hypertension, hyperthyroidism, Parkinson's disease, renal function impairment, schizophrenia, and those with suicidal tendencies. Foods that require bacteria or molds for their preparation or preservation, or containing tyramine, including avocados, bananas, beer, broad beans, cheese, figs, meat tenderizers, papaya, raisins, sour cream, soy sauce, wine, yeast extracts, yogurt, or excessive amounts of caffeine, such as chocolate, coffee, and tea should be avoided. It is unknown if isocarboxazid crosses the placenta or is distributed in breast milk. Safety and efficacy have not been established in children or the elderly.

Blurred vision, drowsiness, increased sweating, decreased sexual ability, and dizziness may be experienced while taking isocarboxazid. Headache, neck soreness or stiffness should be reported.
Administration
Use the lowest effective dose. Take with or without meals.

Isoetharine Hydrochloride/ Isoetharine Mesylate
eye-soe-eth'a-reen
(Beta-2, Bronkosol, Dey-Lute)
(Bronkometer)

CATEGORY AND SCHEDULE
Pregnancy Risk Category: C

CLASSIFICATION
Adrenergic agonists, bronchodilators

MECHANISM OF ACTION
A sympathomimetic (adrenergic agonist) that stimulates beta2-adrenergic receptors in the lungs, resulting in relaxation of bronchial smooth muscle.

Therapeutic Effect: Relieves bronchospasm, reduces airway resistance.

PHARMACOKINETICS
Rapidly, well absorbed from the gastrointestinal (GI) tract. Extensive metabolism in GI tract. Unknown extent metabolized in liver and lungs. Excreted in urine. **Half-life:** 4 hr.

AVAILABILITY
Metered spray: 0.61% (Brokometer).
Solution for Inhalation: 0.08% (Dey-Lute), 0.1% (Dey-Lute), 0.17% (Dey-Lute), 1% (Beta-2, Brokosol).

INDICATIONS AND DOSAGES
▸ **Bronchospasm**
HAND-BULB NEBULIZER
Adults, Elderly. 4 inhalations (range: 3-7 inhalations) undiluted. May be repeated up to 5 times/day.
▸ **Metered Dose Inhalation**
Adults, Elderly. 1-2 inhalations q4hr. Wait 1 min before administering 2nd inhalation.
▸ **IPPB, Oxygen Aerolization**
Adults, Elderly. 0.5-1 ml of a 0.5% or 0.5 ml of a 1% solution diluted 1:3.

CONTRAINDICATIONS
History of hypersensitivity to sympathomimetics

INTERACTIONS
Drug
Beta-adrenergic blocking agents (beta-blockers): Antagonizes effects of isoetharine.
Digoxin: May increase risk of arrhythmias with digoxin.
MAOIs, tricyclic antidepressants: May potentiate cardiovascular effects.
Herbal
None known.
Food
None known.

DIAGNOSTIC TEST EFFECTS
May decrease serum potassium levels.

SIDE EFFECTS
Occasional
Tremor, nausea, nervousness, palpitations, tachycardia, peripheral vasodilation, dryness of mouth, throat, dizziness, vomiting, headache, increased B/P, insomnia.

SERIOUS REACTIONS
• Excessive sympathomimetic stimulation may produce palpitations, extrasystoles, tachycardia, chest pain, slight increase in B/P followed by a substantial decrease, chills, sweating, and blanching of skin.
• Too frequent or excessive use may lead to loss of bronchodilating effectiveness and severe and paradoxical bronchoconstriction.

PRECAUTIONS & CONSIDERATIONS
Caution is warranted with cardiovascular disease, diabetes mellitus, hypertension, and hyperthyroidism. It is unknown if isoetharine crosses the placenta or is distributed in breast milk. Safety and efficacy have not been established in children. The elderly may be more likely to develop tremors or tachycardia because of the age-related increased sympathetic sensitivity.

Avoid excessive use of caffeine derivatives, such as chocolate, cocoa, coffee, cola, and tea.
Storage
Store at room temperature.
Administration
For inhalation use, shake container well and exhale completely through the mouth. Place the mouthpiece into the mouth and close the lips while holding the inhaler upright. Inhale deeply through the mouth while fully depressing the top of the

canister, and hold breath as long as possible before exhaling slowly. Wait 1 minute before inhaling the second dose because this allows for deeper bronchial penetration. Rinse mouth with water immediately after inhalation to prevent mouth and throat dryness.

For nebulizer use, administer undiluted. May repeat up to 5 times daily.

For oxygen aerolization, administer over a 15-20 minute period of time. Oxygen flow is usually adjusted to 4-6 L/minute. Treatments are usually not repeated more than every 4 hours.

Isoniazid (INH)
eye-soe-nye′a-zid
(INH, Isotamine [CAN], Nydrazid, PMS Isoniazid [CAN])

CATEGORY AND SCHEDULE
Pregnancy Risk Category: C

CLASSIFICATION
Antimycobacterials

MECHANISM OF ACTION
An isonicotinic acid derivative that inhibits mycolic acid synthesis and causes disruption of the bacterial cell wall and loss of acid-fast properties in susceptible mycobacteria. Active only during bacterial cell division. *Therapeutic Effect:* Bactericidal against actively growing intracellular and extracellular susceptible mycobacteria.

PHARMACOKINETICS
Readily absorbed from the GI tract. Protein binding: 10%-15%. Widely distributed (including to CSF).

Metabolized in the liver. Primarily excreted in urine. Removed by hemodialysis. **Half-life:** 0.5-5 hr.

AVAILABILITY
Tablets: 100 mg, 300 mg.
Syrup: 50 mg/5 ml.
Injection: 100 mg/ml.

INDICATIONS AND DOSAGES
▶ **Tuberculosis (in combination with one or more antituberculars)**
PO, IM
Adults, Elderly. 5 mg/kg/day as a single dose. Maximum 300 mg/day.
Children. 10-15 mg/kg/day as a single dose. Maximum 300 mg/day.
▶ **Prevention of tuberculosis**
PO, IM
Adults, Elderly. 300 mg/day as a single dose.
Children. 10 mg/kg/day as a single dose. Maximum 300 mg/day.

CONTRAINDICATIONS
Acute hepatic disease, history of hypersensitivity reactions or hepatic injury with previous isoniazid therapy

INTERACTIONS
Drug
Alcohol: May increase isoniazid metabolism and the risk of hepatotoxicity.
Carbamazepine, phenytoin: May increase the toxicity of these drugs.
Disulfiram: May increase CNS effects.
Hepatotoxic medications: May increase the risk of hepatotoxicity.
Ketoconazole: May decrease ketoconazole blood concentration.
Herbal
None known.
Food
Tyramine-containing foods: May cause a hypertensive crisis.

DIAGNOSTIC TEST EFFECTS

May increase serum bilirubin, AST (SGOT), and ALT (SGPT) levels.

SIDE EFFECTS

Frequent

Nausea, vomiting, diarrhea, abdominal pain

Rare

Pain at injection site, hypersensitivity reaction

SERIOUS REACTIONS

• Rare reactions include neurotoxicity (as evidenced by ataxia and paraesthesia), optic neuritis, and hepatotoxicity.

PRECAUTIONS & CONSIDERATIONS

Caution should be used with alcoholics or chronic liver disease or severe renal impairment because it is more likely cross sensitivity to nicotinic acid or other chemically related medications will occur. Be aware that prophylactic use of isoniazid is usually postponed until after childbirth. Be aware that isoniazid crosses the placenta and is distributed in breast milk. There are no age-related precautions noted in children. The elderly are more susceptible to developing hepatitis. Avoid consuming alcohol during treatment and taking any other medications without first notifying the physician, including antacids. Avoid foods containing tyramine, including aged cheeses, sauerkraut, smoked fish, and tuna because these foods may cause a reaction such as headache, a hot or clammy feeling, lightheadedness, pounding heartbeat, and red or itching skin.

! Determine history of hypersensitivity reactions or liver injury from isoniazid, as well as sensitivity to nicotinic acid or chemically related medications before starting drug therapy. Monitor the patient's liver function test results and assess the patient for signs and symptoms of hepatitis as evidenced by anorexia, dark urine, fatigue, jaundice, nausea, vomiting, and weakness. If hepatitis is suspected, withhold the drug and notify the physician promptly. In addition, assess for burning, numbness, and tingling of the extremities. People at risk for neuropathy, such as alcoholics, those with chronic liver disease, diabetics, the elderly, and malnourished individuals, may receive pyridoxine prophylactically.

Administration

Give 1 hour before or 2 hours after meals. May give with food to decrease GI upset, but this will delay isoniazid absorption. Administer at least 1 hour before antacids, especially those containing aluminum. Do not skip doses and continue taking isoniazid for the full length of therapy (6 to 24 months).

Isoproterenol

eye-soe-proe-ter′e-nole
(Isuprel)

CATEGORY AND SCHEDULE

Pregnancy Risk Category: C

CLASSIFICATION

Adrenergic agonists, bronchodilators

MECHANISM OF ACTION

A sympathomimetic (adrenergic agonist) that stimulates beta1-adrenergic receptors. *Therapeutic Effect:* Increases myocardial contractility, stroke volume, cardiac output.

PHARMACOKINETICS

Readily absorbed. Metabolized in liver. Primarily excreted in urine. **Half-life:** 2.5-5 min.

AVAILABILITY

Injection: 0.02 mg/ml (Isuprel).

INDICATIONS AND DOSAGES

▶ **Arrhythmias**
IV Bolus
Adults, Elderly. Initially, 0.02-0.06 mg (1-3 ml of diluted solution). Subsequent dose range: 0.01-0.2 mg (0.5-10 ml of diluted solution).
IV Infusion
Adults, Elderly. Initially, 5 mcg/min (1.25 ml/min of diluted solution). Subsequent dose range: 2-20 mcg/min.
Children. 2.5 mcg/min or 0.1 mcg/kg per min.
▶ **Complete heart block following closure of ventricular septal defects**
IV
Adults, Elderly. 0.04-0.06 mg (2-3 ml of diluted solution).
Infants. 0.01-0.03 (0.5-1.5 ml of diluted solution).
▶ **Shock**
IV Infusion
Adults, Elderly. Rate of 0.5-5 mcg/min (0.25-2.5 ml of 1:500,000 dilution); rate of infusion based on clinical response (heart rate, central venous pressure, systemic B/P, urine flow measurements).

CONTRAINDICATIONS

Tachycardia due to digitalis toxicity, preexisting arrhythmias, angina, precordial distress, hypersensitivity to isoproterenol or any component of the formulation

INTERACTIONS

Drug
Beta-blockers: May antagonize the effects of isoproterenol.

Digoxin: May increase the risk of arrhythmias.
Tricyclic antidepressants: May increase cardiovascular effects.
Herbal
Ma huang: May increase CNS stimulation.
Food
None known.

DIAGNOSTIC TEST EFFECTS

Decreases serum potassium levels

▨ IV INCOMPATIBILITIES

None known.

SIDE EFFECTS

Frequent
Palpitations, tachycardia, restlessness, nervousness, tremor, insomnia, anxiety
Occasional
Increased sweating, headache, nausea, flushed skin, dizziness, coughing

SERIOUS REACTIONS

• Excessive sympathomimetic stimulation may cause palpitations, extrasystoles, tachycardia, chest pain, slight increase in B/P followed by a substantial decrease, chills, sweating, and blanching of skin.
• Ventricular arrhythmias may occur if heart rate is above 130 beats/min.
• Parotid gland swelling may occur with prolonged use.

PRECAUTIONS & CONSIDERATIONS

Caution is warranted with hypersensitivity to sulfite, elderly/debilitated, hypertension, cardiovascular disease, impaired renal function, hyperthyroidism, diabetes mellitus, prostatic hypertrophy, glaucoma. It is unknown if isoproterenol crosses the placenta or is distributed in breast milk, so it is not administered to pregnant women. Safety and efficacy have not been established in children. Be aware that the elderly may exhibit decreased therapeutic response (decreased heart rate, peripheral vascular response).

If chest pain or palpitations occur, notify the physician.

Storage

Store solution at room temperature. Do not use if solution is pink to brown, contains a precipitate, or appears cloudy. Stability of parenteral admixture at room temperature or at refrigeration is 24 hours.

Administration

Reconstitutite for IV push by diluting 0.2 mg (1 ml) of 1:5000 solution to a volume of 10 ml 0.9% NaCl or D_5W. Give IV push at rate of 1 ml/min.

For IV infusion, dilute 0.2-2 mg (1-10 ml) of 1:5000 solution in 500 ml D_5W to provide a solution of 0.4-4 mcg/ml. Rate of IV infusion determined by the person's heart rate, central venous pressure, systemic B/P, and urine flow measurements. Use microdrip (60 drops/ml) or infusion pump to administer drug.

Regulate by EKG monitoring. If EKG changes occur, heart rate

exceeds 110 beats/minute, or premature beats occur, consider reducing rate of infusion or temporarily stopping infusion.

Isosorbide Dinitrate/Mononitrate

(Apo-ISDN [CAN], Cedocard [CAN], Dilatrate, Isogen [AUS], Isordil, Sorbidin [AUS])(Duride [AUS], Imdur, Imtrate [AUS], ISMO, Monodur Durules [AUS], Monoket)

Do not confuse Isordil with Isuprel or Plendil, or Imdur with Inderal or K-Dur.

CATEGORY AND SCHEDULE

Pregnancy Risk Category: C

CLASSIFICATION

Vasodilators

MECHANISM OF ACTION

A nitrate that stimulates intracellular cyclic guanosine monophosphate. *Therapeutic Effect:* Relaxes vascular smooth muscle of both arterial and venous vasculature. Decreases preload and afterload.

ISOSORBIDE DINITRATE/MONONITRATE PHARMACOKINETICS

	Route	Onset	Peak	Duration
Dinitrate	Sublingual	2-5 min	N/A	1-2 hr
	PO (Chewable)	2-5 min	N/A	1-2 hr
	PO	15-40 min	N/A	4-6 hr
	PO (Sustained-Release)	30 min	N/A	12 hr
Mononitrate	Oral	60 min	N/A	N/A

Dinitrate poorly absorbed and metabolized in the liver to its activate metabolite isosorbide mononitrate. Mononitrate well absorbed after PO administration. Excreted in urine and feces. **Half-life:** Dinitrate, 1-4 hr; mononitrate, 4 hr.

AVAILABILITY

Capsules (Sustained-Release [Dilatrate]): 40 mg.
Tablets (Isordil): 5 mg, 10 mg, 20 mg, 30 mg, 40 mg.
Tablets (Ismo, Monoket): 10 mg, 20 mg.
Tablets (Chewable): 5 mg, 10 mg.
Tablets (Extended-Release [Imdur]): 30 mg, 60 mg, 120 mg.
Tablets (Sublingual [Isordil]): 10 mg.

INDICATIONS AND DOSAGES
▸ **Angina**
PO (isosorbide dinitrate)
Adults, Elderly. 5-40 mg 4 times a day. Sustained-release: 40 mg q8-12hr.
PO (ISOSORBIDE MONONITRATE)
Adults, Elderly. 5-10 mg twice a day given 7 hours apart. Sustained-release: Initially, 30-60 mg/day in morning as a single dose. May increase dose at 3-day intervals. Maximum: 240 mg/day.

OFF-LABEL USES
CHF, dysphagia, pain relief, relief of esophageal spasm with gastroesophageal reflux

CONTRAINDICATIONS
Closed-angle glaucoma, GI hypermotility or malabsorption (extended-release tablets), head trauma, hypersensitivity to nitrates, increased intracranial pressure, orthostatic hypotension, severe anemia (extended-release tablets)

INTERACTIONS
Drug
Antihypertensives, vasodilators: May increase risk of orthostatic hypotension.
Herbal
None known.
Food
Alcohol: May increase risk of orthostatic hypotension.

DIAGNOSTIC TEST EFFECTS
May increase urine catecholamine and urine vanillylmandelic acid levels.

SIDE EFFECTS
Frequent
Burning and tingling at oral point of dissolution (sublingual), headache (possibly severe) occurs mostly in early therapy, diminishes rapidly in intensity, and usually disappears during continued treatment, transient flushing of face and neck, dizziness (especially if patient is standing immobile or is in a warm environment), weakness, orthostatic hypotension, nausea, vomiting, restlessness
Occasional
GI upset, blurred vision, dry mouth

SERIOUS REACTIONS
• Blurred vision or dry mouth may occur (drug should be discontinued).
• Isosorbide administration may cause severe orthostatic hypotension manifested by fainting, pulselessness, cold or clammy skin, and diaphoresis.
• Tolerance may occur with repeated, prolonged therapy, but may not occur with the extended-release form. Minor tolerance may be seen with intermittent use of sublingual tablets.
• High dosage tends to produce severe headache.

Caution is warranted with acute MI, blood volume depletion from therapy, glaucoma (contraindicated in closed-angle glaucoma), hepatic or renal disease, and systolic B/P less than 90 mm Hg. It is unknown if isosorbide crosses the placenta or is distributed in breast milk. The safety and efficacy of isosorbide have not been established in children. The elderly may be more sensitive to the drug's hypotensive effects. In the elderly, age-related decreased renal function may require cautious use. Alcohol should be avoided because it intensifies the drug's hypotensive effect. If alcohol is ingested soon after taking nitrates, an acute hypotensive episode marked by pallor, vertigo, and a drop in B/P may occur.

Dizziness, lightheadedness, and headache may occur. Notify the physician of facial or neck flushing. The onset, type (sharp, dull, or squeezing), radiation, location, intensity, and duration of anginal pain and its precipitating factors, such as exertion and emotional stress should be recorded before therapy begins.

Administration
Best if taken on an empty stomach; however, take oral isosorbide with meals if the headache occurs. Oral tablets, except the extended-release form, may be crushed. Do not crush or break extended-release form. Do not crush chewable form before administering.

For sublingual use, do not crush or chew tablets. Dissolve tablets under tongue without swallowing. Isosorbide should be taken at the first sign or symptom of angina. If angina is not relieved within 5 minutes, dissolve a second tablet under the tongue and then repeat the dosage 5 minutes later if there is no relief. Do not take more than 3 tablets within 15 to 30 minutes.

Isotretinoin
eye-soe-tret′i-noyn
(Accutane, Amnesteem, Claravis, Isotrex [CAN], Sotret)
Do not confuse Accutane with Accupril or Accurbron.

CATEGORY AND SCHEDULE
Pregnancy Risk Category: X

CLASSIFICATION
Retinoids

MECHANISM OF ACTION
Reduces the size of sebaceous glands and inhibits their activity. *Therapeutic Effect:* Decreases sebum production; produces antikeratinizing and anti-inflammatory effects.

PHARMACOKINETICS
Metabolized in the liver; major metabolite active. Eliminated in urine and feces. **Half-life:** 21 hr; metabolite, 21-24 hr.

AVAILABILITY
Capsules: 10 mg, 20 mg, 40 mg.

INDICATIONS AND DOSAGES
▸ **Recalcitrant cystic acne that is unresponsive to conventional acne therapies**
PO
Adults. Initially, 0.5-2 mg/kg/day divided into 2 doses for 15-20 wk. May repeat after at least 2 mo off therapy.

OFF-LABEL USES
Treatment of gram-negative folliculitis, severe keratinization disorders, severe rosacea

CONTRAINDICATIONS
Hypersensitivity to isotretinoin or parabens (component of capsules)

INTERACTIONS
Drug
Etretinate, tretinoin, vitamin A: May increase toxic effects.
Tetracycline: May increase the risk of pseudotumor cerebri.
Herbal
Dong quai, St John's wort: May cause photosensitization.
Food
None known.

DIAGNOSTIC TEST EFFECTS
May increase serum alkaline phosphatase, total cholesterol, LDH, triglyceride, ALT (SGPT), and AST (SGOT) levels; urine uric acid level; erythrocyte sedimentation rate; and fasting blood glucose level. May decrease HDL level.

SIDE EFFECTS
Frequent (90%-20%)
Cheilitis (inflammation of lips), dry skin and mucous membranes, skin fragility, pruritus, epistaxis, dry nose and mouth, conjunctivitis, hypertriglyceridemia, nausea, vomiting, abdominal pain
Occasional (16%-5%)
Musculoskeletal symptoms (including bone pain, arthralgia, generalized myalgia), photosensitivity
Rare
Decreased night vision, depression

SERIOUS REACTIONS
• Inflammatory bowel disease and pseudotumor cerebri (benign intracranial hypertension) have been associated with isotretinoin therapy.

PRECAUTIONS & CONSIDERATIONS
Caution should be used with renal or hepatic dysfunction. Be aware that isotretinoin is contraindicated in pregnancy. There is an extremely high risk of major deformities in infant if pregnancy occurs while taking any amount of isotretinoin, even for short periods. The person must be capable of understanding and carrying out instructions and of complying with mandatory contraception. Be aware that excretion in milk unknown; due to potential for serious adverse effects, it is not recommended during nursing. There are no age-related precautions noted in children or the elderly.

Women must have a negative serum pregnancy test within 2 weeks prior to starting therapy; therapy will begin on the second or third day of the next normal menstrual period. Effective contraception (using 2 reliable forms of contraception simultaneously) must be used for at least 1 month before, during, and for at least 1 month after therapy. Give both oral and written warnings, with the person acknowledging in writing that she understands the warnings and consents to treatment.

Isotretinoin may have decreased tolerance to contact lenses during and after therapy. Notify physician immediately if abdominal pain, severe diarrhea, rectal bleeding (possible inflammatory bowel disease), or headache, nausea and vomiting, visual disturbances (possible pseudotumor cerebri) occur.
Storage
Store at room temperature and protect from light.

Administration
Give isotretinoin with food.

Isradipine
is-rad′i-peen
(DynaCirc, DynaCirc CR)
Do not confuse DynaCirc with Dynabac or Dynacin.

CATEGORY AND SCHEDULE
Pregnancy Risk Category: C

CLASSIFICATION
Calcium channel blockers

MECHANISM OF ACTION
An antihypertensive that inhibits calcium movement across cardiac and vascular smooth-muscle cell membranes. Potent peripheral vasodilator that does not depress SA or AV nodes. *Therapeutic Effect:* Produces relaxation of coronary vascular smooth muscle and coronary vasodilation. Increases myocardial oxygen delivery to those with vasospastic angina.

PHARMACOKINETICS

Route	Onset	Peak	Duration
PO	2-3 hr	2-4 wk (with multiple doses) 8-16 hr (with single dose)	N/A
PO (Controlled-release)	2 hr	8-10 hr	N/A

Well absorbed from the GI tract. Protein binding: 95%. Metabolized in the liver (undergoes first-pass effect). Primarily excreted in urine. Not removed by hemodialysis. **Half-life:** 8 hr.

AVAILABILITY
Capsules (Dynacirc): 2.5 mg, 5 mg.
Capsules (Controlled-Release [Dynacirc-CR]): 5 mg, 10 mg.

INDICATIONS AND DOSAGES
▸ **Hypertension**
PO
Adults, Elderly. Initially 2.5 mg twice a day. May increase by 2.5 mg at 2- to 4-wk intervals. Range: 5-20 mg/day

OFF-LABEL USES
Treatment of chronic angina pectoris, Raynaud's phenomenon

CONTRAINDICATIONS
Cardiogenic shock, CHF, heart block, hypotension, sinus bradycardia, ventricular tachycardia

INTERACTIONS
Drug
Beta blockers: May have additive effect.
Herbal
None known.
Food
Grapefruit, grapefruit juice: May increase the absorption of isradipine.

DIAGNOSTIC TEST EFFECTS
None known.

SIDE EFFECTS
Frequent (7%-4%)
Peripheral edema, palpitations (higher frequency in females)
Occasional (3%)
Facial flushing, cough

Rare (2%-1%)
Angina, tachycardia, rash, pruritus

SERIOUS REACTIONS

• Overdose produces nausea, drowsiness, confusion, and slurred speech.
• CHF occurs rarely.

PRECAUTIONS & CONSIDERATIONS

Caution is warranted with edema, hepatic disease, severe left ventricular dysfunction, sick sinus syndrome and in those concurrently receiving beta blockers or digoxin. It is unknown if isradipine crosses the placenta or is distributed in breast milk. The safety and efficacy of isradipine have not been established in children. In the elderly, age-related renal impairment may require cautious use. Grapefruit juice, which may increase isradipine blood concentration, should be avoided. Tasks that require alertness and motor skills should also be avoided.

Notify the physician if irregular heartbeat, nausea, pronounced dizziness, or shortness of breath occurs. Rise slowly from a lying to a sitting position and wait momentarily before standing to avoid isradipine's hypotensive effect. Apical pulse and B/P should be assessed immediately before beginning isradipine administration. If the pulse rate is 60 beats/minute or lower or systolic B/P is less than 90 mm Hg, withhold the medication and contact the physician. Liver function tests should also be performed before and during therapy. Skin should be assessed for flushing and peripheral edema, especially behind the medial malleolus and the sacral area.

Administration

Do not crush, open, or break capsules. Do not abruptly discontinue isradipine. Compliance is essential to control hypertension.

Itraconazole
it-ra-con'a-zol
(Sporanox)
Do not confuse Sporanox with Suprax.

CATEGORY AND SCHEDULE
Pregnancy Risk Category: C

CLASSIFICATION
Antifungals

MECHANISM OF ACTION
A fungistatic antifungal that inhibits the synthesis of ergosterol, a vital component of fungal cell formation *Therapeutic Effect:* Damages the fungal cell membrane, altering its function.

PHARMACOKINETICS
Moderately absorbed from the GI tract. Absorption is increased if the drug is taken with food. Protein binding: 99%. Widely distributed, primarily in the fatty tissue, liver, and kidneys. Metabolized in the liver to active metabolite. Primarily excreted in urine. Not removed by hemodialysis. **Half-life:** 21 hr; metabolite, 12 hr.

AVAILABILITY
Capsules: 100 mg.
Oral Solution: 10 mg/ml.
Injection: 10 mg/ml
(25-ml ampule).

INDICATIONS AND DOSAGES
▶ **Blastomycosis, histoplasmosis**
PO
Adults, Elderly. Initially, 200 mg once a day. Maximum: 400 mg/day in 2 divided doses.

IV
Adults, Elderly. 200 mg twice a day for 4 doses, then 200 mg once a day.
▸ **Aspergillosis**
PO
Adults, Elderly. 600 mg/day in 3 divided doses for 3-4 days, then 200-400 mg/day in 2 divided doses.
IV
Adults, Elderly. 200 mg twice a day for 4 doses, then 200 mg once a day.
▸ **Esophageal candidiasis**
PO
Adults, Elderly. Swish 10 ml in mouth for several seconds, then swallow. Maximum: 200 mg/day.
▸ **Oropharyngeal candidiasis**
PO
Adults, Elderly. Vigorously swish 10 ml in mouth for several seconds (20 ml total daily dose) once a day.

OFF-LABEL USES
Suppression of histoplasmosis; treatment of disseminated sporotrichosis, fungal pneumonia and septicemia, or ringworm of the hand

CONTRAINDICATIONS
Hypersensitivity to itraconazole, fluconazole, ketoconazole, or miconazole

INTERACTIONS
Drug
Antacids, didanosine, H$_2$ antagonists: May decrease itraconazole absorption.
Buspirone, cyclosporine, digoxin, lovastatin, simvastatin: May increase blood concentration of these drugs.
Oral anticoagulants: May increase the effect of oral anticoagulants.
Phenytoin, rifampin: May decrease itraconazole blood concentration.
Herbal
None known.

Food
Grapefruit juice: May alter itraconazole absorption.

DIAGNOSTIC TEST EFFECTS
May increase serum LDH, serum alkaline phosphatase, serum bilirubin, SGOT (AST), and SGPT (ALT) levels. May decrease serum potassium level.

🔲 IV INCOMPATIBILITIES
! Dilution compatibilities of itraconazole with any solution other than 0.9% NaCl is unknown. Don't mix with D$_5$W or lactated Ringer's solution. Not for IV bolus administration. Don't administer any medication in same bag or through same IV line as itraconazole.

SIDE EFFECTS
Frequent (11%-9%)
Nausea, rash
Occasional (5%-3%)
Vomiting, headache, diarrhea, hypertension, peripheral edema, fatigue, fever
Rare (2% or less)
Abdominal pain, dizziness, anorexia, pruritus

SERIOUS REACTIONS
• Hepatitis (as evidenced by anorexia, abdominal pain, unusual fatigue or weakness, jaundice skin or sclera, and dark urine) occurs rarely.

PRECAUTIONS & CONSIDERATIONS
Caution is warranted with achlorhydria, hepatitis, HIV-infection, hypochlorhydria, or impaired liver function. Be aware that itraconazole is distributed in breast milk. Be aware that the safety and efficacy of itraconazole have not been established in children. In the elderly, age-related renal impairment may require dosage adjustment.

Obtain the baseline temperature, check the liver function test results, as appropriate, and determine if there is a history of allergies before giving the drug. Assess for signs and symptoms of liver dysfunction. Report any anorexia, dark urine, nausea, pale stool, unusual fatigue, yellow skin, or vomiting to the physician. Avoid grapefruit and grapefruit juice as they may alter itraconazole absorption. Therapy will continue for at least 3 months and until lab tests and overall condition indicate that the infection is controlled.

Storage

Store oral formulations and solutions for injection at room temperature. Do not freeze.

Administration

! Doses larger than 200 mg should be given in 2 divided doses. Give capsules with food to increase absorption. Give solution on an empty stomach.

For IV administration, use only components provided by the manufacturer. Do not dilute with any other diluent. Add full contents of amp (250 mg/10 ml) to infusion bag provided (50 ml 0.9% NaCl) and mix gently. Infuse over 60 minutes using the extension line and infusion set provided. After administration, flush infusion set with 15 to 20 ml 0.9% NaCl over 30 seconds to 15 minutes and discard entire infusion line.

Ivermectin
eye-ver-mek'tin
(Stromectol)

CATEGORY AND SCHEDULE
Pregnancy Risk Category: C

CLASSIFICATION
Antihelmintics

MECHANISM OF ACTION

Selectively binds to chloride ion channels in invertebrate nerve/muscle cells, increasing permeability to chloride ions. In general the following organisms are susceptible to ivermectin: *Onchocerca volvulus, Pediculosis capitis, Strongyloides stercoralis, Sarcoptes scabiei,* and *Wuchereria bancrofti. Therapeutic effects:* Causes paralysis/death of parasites.

PHARMACOKINETICS

Does not readily cross the blood-brain barrier. Metabolized in the liver. Excreted in the feces. **Half-life:** 4 hr. Well absorbed with plasma concentrations proportional to the dose.

AVAILABILITY

Tablets: 3 mg, 6 mg

INDICATIONS AND DOSAGES

▸ **Strongyloidiasis**
PO
Adults, Elderly, Children >33 pounds: 200 mcg/kg as a single dose.

▸ **Onchoceriasis**
PO
Adults, Elderly, Children >33 pounds: 150 mcg/kg as a single dose at 3-12-mo intervals.

▶ **Scabies**
PO
Adults. 200 mcg/kg as a single dose and repeat 2 weeks later
▶ **Norwegian Scabies (crusted scabies infection), superinfected scabies, or resistant scabies**
PO
Adults. 200 mcg/kg with repeated treatments or combined with a topical scabicide
▶ **Pediculosis**
PO
Adults. A regimen of 2 doses of 200 mcg/kg with each dose separated by 10 days
▶ **Bancroft's filariasis**
PO
Adults, Children >15 kg. 150 mcg/kg as a single dose. May repeat 1 or 2 more times (each dose a week apart) if larva continues to migrate 1 week after the previous dose.

OFF-LABEL USES
Cutaneous larva migrans, filariasis, pediculosis, scabies, *Wuchereria bancrofti*

CONTRAINDICATIONS
Hypersensitivity to ivermectin or to any one of its components. Should not be used in women who are pregnant or infants.

INTERACTIONS
Drug
Carbamazepine: May decrease the concentration of ivermectin.
CYP 3A4 inducers: Decrease the levels of ivermectin.
CYP 3A4 inhibitors: Increase the levels of ivermectin.

Herbal
None known.
Food
None known.

DIAGNOSTIC TEST EFFECTS
May increase SGOT (AST), SGPT (ALT), alkaline phosphatase, BUN, eosinophil count. May decrease WBC.

SIDE EFFECTS
Occasional
Abdominal pain, anorexia, arthralgia, constipation, diarrhea, dizziness, drowsiness, edema, fatigue, fever, lymphadenopathy, maculopapular or unspecified rash, nausea, vomiting, orthostatic hypotension, pruritis, Stevens-Johnson syndrome, toxic epidermal necrolysis, tremor, urticaria, vertigo, visual impairment, weakness

PRECAUTIONS & CONSIDERATIONS
Caution is warranted with bronchial asthma. Treating Loa loa infection with ivermectin may result in encephalopathy. It is unknown if ivermectin crosses the placenta. Ivermectin is distributed into breast milk. Safety and efficacy have not been established in children or the elderly.

Lightheadedness may occur. Tasks that require mental alertness or motor skills should be avoided. Joint or muscle pain, fever, pain and tender glands in neck, armpits or groin, skin rash or rapid heartbeat may also occur.
Administration
Take with a full glass of water, 1 hour before breakfast.

Kanamycin
kan-a-mye′sin
(Kantrex)

CATEGORY AND SCHEDULE
Pregnancy Risk Category:
Unavailable for irrigating
solution.

CLASSIFICATION
Antibiotics, aminoglycosides

MECHANISM OF ACTION
An aminoglycoside antibiotic that
irreversibly binds to protein on
bacterial ribosomes. *Therapeutic
Effect:* Interferes with protein
synthesis of susceptible
microorganisms.

AVAILABILITY
Injection: 1 g/3 ml.

INDICATIONS AND DOSAGES
▸ **Wound and surgical site
irrigation**
Adults, Elderly. 0.25% solution to
irrigate pleural space, ventricular or
abscess cavities, wounds, or surgical
sites.

CONTRAINDICATIONS
Hypersensitivity to kanamycin, other
aminoglycosides (cross-sensitivity),
or their components.

INTERACTIONS
Drug
None significant.
Herbal
None significant.
Food
None significant.

DIAGNOSTIC TEST EFFECTS
None known.

SIDE EFFECTS
Occasional
Hypersensitivity reactions (fever,
pruritus, rash, urticaria)
Rare
Headache

SERIOUS REACTIONS
• None known.

PRECAUTIONS & CONSIDERATIONS
There is no information available
regarding pregnancy for irrigating
solution. There are no age-related
precautions noted in children
or the elderly. Assess for hypersensitivity to kanamycin or other
aminoglycosides before beginning
therapy.
Administration
Irrigating solution is
administered by all
administration routes.

Kaolin-Pectin
(Donnagel-MB [CAN],
Kao-Spen, Kapectolin)

CATEGORY AND SCHEDULE
Pregnancy Risk Category: NR
OTC

CLASSIFICATION
Antidiarrheal

MECHANISM OF ACTION
An antidiarrheal agent that acts
as an adsorbent and protectant.
Therapeutic Effect: Absorbs
bacteria, toxins, and reduces
water loss.

PHARMACOKINETICS

Not absorbed orally. Up to 90% of pectin decomposed in gastrointestinal (GI) tract.

AVAILABILITY

Suspension: 5.2 g kaolin and 260 mg pectin/30 ml (Kao-Spen), 5.85 g kaolin and 130 mg pectin/30 ml (Kaopectolin).

INDICATIONS AND DOSAGES

▸ Antidiarrheal

PO

Adults, Elderly. 60-120 ml after each loose bowel movement (LBM). *Children 12 yr and older.* 60 ml after each LBM. *Children 6-12 yr.* 30-60 ml after each LBM. *Children 3-6 yr.* 15-30 ml after each LBM.

CONTRAINDICATIONS

Diarrhea secondary to pseudomembranous enterocolitis or toxigenic bacteria, hypersensitivity to kaolin/pectin products

INTERACTIONS

Drug

Chloroquine: May decrease efficacy of chloroquine.
Digoxin: May decrease absorption of digoxin.
HMG-CoA reductase inhibitors: May decrease effectiveness of HMG-CoA reductase inhibitors.
Herbal
None known.
Food
None known.

DIAGNOSTIC TEST EFFECTS

None known.

SIDE EFFECTS

Rare
Constipation

SERIOUS REACTIONS

• Dehydration may occur.

PRECAUTIONS & CONSIDERATIONS

It is unknown if this drug crosses placenta or is distributed in breast milk. Be aware that kaolin/pectin is not recommended in children less than 3 years of age. Be aware that children and the elderly are more sensitive to fluid and electrolyte loss.

To maintain normal bowel habits, it is important to drink plenty of fluids (4 to 6 8 ounce glasses a day), eat foods high in fiber and exercise regularly.
Storage
Store at room temperature.
Administration
Shake suspension well before administration. Kaolin and pectin is usually taken after each loose bowel movement.

Ketamine
(Ketalar)

CATEGORY AND SCHEDULE
Pregnancy Risk Category: B

CLASSIFICATION:
Anesthetics, general

MECHANISM OF ACTION

A rapidly acting general anesthetic that selectively blocks afferent impulses and interacts with CNS transmitter systems. *Therapeutic Effect:* Produces an anesthetic state characterized by profound analgesia and normal pharyngeal-laryngeal reflexes.

K

PHARMACOKINETICS

Route	Onset	Peak	Duration
IM (anesthetic)	3-4 min	N/A	12-25 min
IM (analgesic)	30 min	N/A	15-30 min
IV (anesthetic)	30 sec	N/A	5-10 min
IV (analgesic)	10-15 min	N/A	N/A

Rapidly distributed. Metabolized in the liver. Primarily excreted in urine. **Half-life:** Distribution: 10-15 min, elimination: 2-3 hr.

AVAILABILITY

Injection: 10 mg/ml, 50 mg/ml, 100 mg/ml.

INDICATIONS AND DOSAGES

▸ **Sole anesthetic for short diagnostic and surgical procedures that don't require skeletal muscle relaxation, induction of anesthesia before administering other general anesthetics, supplement to low-potency agents**
IM
Adults, Elderly. 3-8 mg/kg.
Children. 3-7 mg/kg.
IV
Adults, Elderly. 1-4.5 mg/kg.
Children. 0.5-2 mg/kg.

CONTRAINDICATIONS

Aneurysms, angina, CHF, elevated ICP, hypertension, psychotic disorders, thyrotoxicosis

INTERACTIONS

Drug
Antihypertensives, CNS depressants: May increase the risk of hypotension and respiratory depression.
Herbal
None known.
Food
None known.

DIAGNOSTIC TEST EFFECTS

May increase IOP.

▨ IV INCOMPATIBILITIES

No information available for Y-site administration.

▨ IV Compatibilities

Bupivacaine (Marcaine), clonidine (Duraclon), fentanyl (Sublimaze), lidocaine, morphine, propofol (Diprivan)

SIDE EFFECTS

Frequent
Increased BP and pulse rate; emergence reaction (marked by dreamlike state, delirium, hallucinations, and vivid imagery and occasionally accompanied by confusion, excitement, and irrational behavior; lasts from few hours to 24 hours after ketamine administration)
Occasional
Pain at injection site
Rare
Rash

SERIOUS REACTIONS

• Continuous or repeated intermittent infusion may result in extreme somnolence and circulatory or respiratory depression.
• Too-rapid IV administration of ketamine may produce severe hypotension, respiratory depression, and irregular muscle movements.

PRECAUTIONS & CONSIDERATIONS

Caution is warranted with intoxication, chronic alcoholism, a full stomach, gastroesophageal reflux disease, and hepatic impairment. Ketamine is not recommended for pregnant or breast-feeding women. No age-related precautions have been noted in children or the elderly. Avoid tasks requiring mental alertness or motor skills until for 24 hours after anesthesia has been discontinued.

Vital signs should be monitored before and every 3 to 5 minutes during and after ketamine administration until the person has recovered. A barbiturate or hypnotic should be administered in an emergence reaction. Verbal, tactile, and visual stimulation should be minimized during the recovery period.

Administration

Give ketamine by IV push when it's used to induce anesthesia. Dilute the 100 mg/ml vial of ketamine with an equal volume of sterile water for injection, D_5W, or 0.9% NaCl. For a maintenance IV infusion, dilute the 50-mg/ml vial (10 ml) or 100-mg/ml vial (5 ml) of ketamine with 250-500 ml D_5W or 0.9% NaCl to provide a concentration of 1-2 mg/ml. Administer maintenance dose by IV push slowly at a rate of 0.5 mg/kg/minute over 60 seconds. A too-rapid IV administration may result in severe hypotension and respiratory depression.

For IM administration, use the 10-mg/ml vial of ketamine. Do not dilute the 10-mg/ml vial.

Ketoconazole

kee-toe-koe'na-zole
(Apo-Ketocomazole [CAN], Nizoral, Nizoral AD, Sebizole [AUS])
Do not confuse Nizoral with Nasarel.

CATEGORY AND SCHEDULE

Pregnancy Risk Category: C
OTC (1% shampoo only)

CLASSIFICATION

Antifungals, topical, dermatologics

MECHANISM OF ACTION

A fungistatic antifungal that inhibits the synthesis of ergosterol, a vital component of fungal cell formation. *Therapeutic Effect:* Damages the fungal cell membrane, altering its function.

AVAILABILITY

Tablets (Nizoral): 200 mg.
Cream (Nizoral): 2%.
Shampoo (Nizoral AD): 1%.

INDICATIONS AND DOSAGES

▸ **Histoplasmosis, blastomycosis, systemic candidiasis, chronic mucocutaneous candidiasis, coccidioidomycosis, paracoccidioidomycosis, chromomycosis, seborrheic dermatitis, tinea corporis, tinea capitis, tinea manus, tinea cruris, tinea pedis, tinea unguium (onychomycosis), oral thrush, candiduria**
PO
Adults, Elderly. 200-400 mg/day.
Children. 3.3-6.6 mg/kg/day. Maximum: 800 mg/day in 2 divided doses.
TOPICAL
Adults, Elderly. Apply to affected area 1-2 times a day for 2-4 wk.
SHAMPOO
Adults, Elderly. Use twice weekly for 4 wk, allowing at least 3 days between shampooing. Use intermittently to maintain control.

OFF-LABEL USES

Systemic: Treatment of fungal pneumonia, prostate cancer, septicemia

CONTRAINDICATIONS

None known.

K

INTERACTIONS
Drug
Alcohol, hepatotoxic medications: May increase hepatotoxicity of ketoconazole.
Antacids, anticholinergics, H_2 antagonists, omeprazole: May decrease ketoconazole absorption.
Cyclosporine, lovastatin, simvastatin: May increase blood concentration and risk of toxicity of these drugs.
Isoniazid, rifampin: May decrease blood concentration of ketoconazole.
Herbal
Echinacea: May have additive hepatotoxic effects.
Food
None known.

DIAGNOSTIC TEST EFFECTS
May increase serum alkaline phosphatase, serum bilirubin, SGOT (AST), and SGPT (ALT) levels. May decrease serum corticosteroid and testosterone concentrations.

SIDE EFFECTS
Occasional (10%-3%)
Nausea, vomiting
Rare (less than 2%)
Abdominal pain, diarrhea, headache, dizziness, photophobia, pruritus
Topical: itching, burning, irritation

SERIOUS REACTIONS
• Hematologic toxicity (as evidenced by thrombocytopenia, hemolytic anemia, and leukopenia) occurs occasionally.
• Hepatotoxicity may occur within 1 week to several months after starting therapy.
• Anaphylaxis occurs rarely.

PRECAUTIONS & CONSIDERATIONS
Caution is warranted with liver impairment.

Confirm that a culture or histologic test was done for accurate diagnosis; therapy may begin before results are known.

Expect to monitor liver function test results. Be alert for signs and symptoms of hepatotoxicity, including anorexia, dark urine, fatigue, nausea, pale stools, and vomiting, that are unrelieved by giving the medication with food. Monitor complete blood count (CBC) for evidence of hematologic toxicity. Assess daily pattern of bowel activity and stool consistency. Assess for dizziness, provide assistance as needed, and institute safety precautions. Evaluate skin for itching, rash, and urticaria.

Prolonged therapy over weeks or months is usually necessary. Do not miss a dose, and continue therapy for as long as directed. Avoid alcohol to avoid potential liver toxicity. Avoid tasks that require mental alertness or motor skills until response to the drug is established. Take antacids or antiulcer medications at least 2 hours after taking ketoconazole.

If dark urine, increased irritation in topical use, onset of other new symptoms, pale stool, or yellow skin or eyes develop, notify the physician.

Separate personal items that come in direct contact with the affected area.
Administration
Give oral ketoconazole with food to minimize gastrointestinal (GI) irritation.

Tablets may be crushed. Ketoconazole requires acidity; give antacids, anticholinergics, H_2 blockers, and omeprazole at least 2 hours after dosing.

Apply ketoconazole shampoo to wet hair, massage for 1 minute, rinse thoroughly, reapply for 3 minutes, then rinse. Use initially twice weekly for 4 weeks with at least 3 days between shampooing. Further shampooing will be based upon the response to the initial treatment. Apply topical ketoconazole and rub gently into the affected and surrounding area. Avoid drug contact with the eyes, keep the skin clean and dry, and wear light clothing for ventilation.

Ketoprofen

kee-toe-proe'fen
(Apo-Keto [CAN], Novo-Keto-EC, Orudis [AUS], Orudis KT [CAN], Orudis SR [AUS], Oruvail, Oruvail SR [AUS], Rhodis [CAN])

CATEGORY AND SCHEDULE
Pregnancy Risk Category: B
(D if used in third trimester or near delivery)
OTC (tablets)

CLASSIFICATION
Analgesics, non-narcotic, nonsteroidal anti-inflammatory drugs

MECHANISM OF ACTION
An NSAID that produces analgesic and anti-inflammatory effects by inhibiting prostaglandin synthesis. *Therapeutic Effect:* Reduces the inflammatory response and intensity of pain.

AVAILABILITY
Capsules: 50 mg, 75 mg.
Capsules (Extended-Release [Oruvail]): 100 mg, 150 mg, 200 mg.
Tablets (Orudis KT): 12.5 mg (OTC).

INDICATIONS AND DOSAGES
▶ **Acute or chronic rheumatoid arthritis and osteoarthritis**
PO (tablets, capsules)
Adults. Initially, 75 mg 3 times a day or 50 mg 4 times a day.
Elderly. Initially, 25-50 mg 3-4 times a day. Maintenance: 150-300 mg/day in 3-4 divided doses.
PO (Extended-Release)
Adults, Elderly. 100-200 mg once a day.
▶ **Mild to moderate pain, dysmenorrhea**
PO
Adults, Elderly. 25-50 mg q6-8h. Maximum: 300 mg/day.
▶ **Over-the-counter (OTC) dosage**
PO
Adults, Elderly. 12.5 mg q4-6h. Maximum: 6 tabs/day.
▶ **Dosage in renal impairment**
Mild. 150 mg/day maximum.
Severe. 100 mg/day maximum.

OFF-LABEL USES
Treatment of acute gouty arthritis, psoriatic arthritis, ankylosing spondylitis, vascular headache

CONTRAINDICATIONS
Active peptic ulcer disease, chronic inflammation of the GI tract, GI bleeding or ulceration, history of hypersensitivity to aspirin or NSAIDs

INTERACTIONS
Drug
Antihypertensives, diuretics: May decrease the effects of these drugs.
Aspirin, other salicylates: May increase the risk of GI side effects such as bleeding.
Bone marrow depressants: May increase the risk of hematologic reactions.

K

Heparin, oral anticoagulants, thrombolytics: May increase the effects of these drugs.
Lithium: May increase the blood concentration and risk of toxicity of lithium.
Methotrexate: May increase the risk of methotrexate toxicity.
Probenecid: May increase the ketoprofen blood concentration.
Herbal
Feverfew: May decrease the effects of feverfew.
Ginkgo biloba: May increase the risk of bleeding.
Food
None known.

DIAGNOSTIC TEST EFFECTS

May prolong bleeding time. May increase serum alkaline phosphatase levels and liver function test results. May decrease Hct, blood Hgb, and serum sodium levels.

SIDE EFFECTS

Frequent (11%)
Dyspepsia
Occasional (more than 3%)
Nausea, diarrhea or constipation, flatulence, abdominal cramps, headache
Rare (less than 2%)
Anorexia, vomiting, visual disturbances, fluid retention

SERIOUS REACTIONS

• Rare reactions with long-term use include peptic ulcer disease, GI bleeding, gastritis, and severe hepatic reactions (cholestasis, jaundice), nephrotoxicity (dysuria, hematuria, proteinuria, nephrotic syndrome), and severe hypersensitivity reaction (bronchospasm, angioedema).

PRECAUTIONS & CONSIDERATIONS

Caution is warranted with a history of GI tract disease, hepatic or renal impairment, and a predisposition to fluid retention. Avoid alcohol and aspirin during therapy because these substances increase the risk of GI bleeding.

CBC, blood chemistry studies, PT, aPTT, and renal and liver function tests should be obtained at the beginning and throughout therapy. Therapeutic response, such as improved grip strength, increased mobility, improved range of motion, and decreased pain, tenderness, stiffness, and swelling, should be assessed.

Administration

! Don't exceed a ketoprofen dosage of 300 mg/day. Oruvail is not recommended as initial therapy for those older than 75 years, or those with renal impairment.

Take ketoprofen with food, a full glass (8 oz) of water, or milk to minimize GI distress. Don't break, open, or chew extended-release capsules.

Ketorolac

kee-toe'role-ak
(Acular, Acular LS, Acular PF, Toradol)
Do not confuse Acular with Acthar or Ocular.

CATEGORY AND SCHEDULE

Pregnancy Risk Category: C
(D if used in third trimester)

CLASSIFICATION

Analgesics, non-narcotic, nonsteroidal anti-inflammatory drugs, ophthalmics

MECHANISM OF ACTION

An NSAID that inhibits prostaglandin synthesis and reduces prostaglandin levels in the aqueous humor. *Therapeutic Effect:* Relieves pain stimulus and reduces intraocular inflammation.

PHARMACOKINETICS

Route	Onset	Peak	Duration
PO	30-60 min	1.5-4 hr	4-6 hr
IV/IM	30 min	1-2 hr	4-6 hr

Readily absorbed from the GI tract, after IM administration. Protein binding: 99%. Largely metabolized in the liver. Primarily excreted in urine. Not removed by hemodialysis. **Half-life:** 3.8-6.3 hr (increased with impaired renal function and in the elderly).

AVAILABILITY

Tablets (Toradol): 10 mg.
Injection (Toradol): 15 mg/ml, 30 mg/ml.
Ophthalmic Solution (Acular): 0.5%.
Ophthalmic Solution (Acular LS): 0.4%.
Ophthalmic Solution (Acular PF): 0.5%.

INDICATIONS AND DOSAGES

▸ **Short-term relief of mild to moderate pain (multiple doses)**
PO
Adults, Elderly. 10 mg q4-6h. Maximum: 40 mg/24 hr.
IV/IM
Adults younger than 65 yr. 30 mg q6h. Maximum: 120 mg/24 hr.
Adults 65 yr and older, those with renal impairment, those weighing less than 50 kg. 15 mg q6h. Maximum: 60 mg/24 hr.
Children 2-16 yr. 0.5 mg/kg q6h.

▸ **Short-term relief of mild to moderate pain (single dose)**
IV
Adults younger than 65 yr, Children 17 yr and older weighing more than 50 kg. 30 mg.
Adults 65 yr and older, with renal impairment, weighing less than 50 kg. 15 mg.
Children 2-16 yr. 0.5 mg/kg. Maximum: 15 mg.
IM
Adults younger than 65 yr, Children 17 yr and older, weighing more than 50 kg. 60 mg.
Adults 65 yr and older, with renal impairment, weighing less than 50 kg. 30 mg.
Children 2-16 yr. 1 mg/kg. Maximum: 15 kg.
▸ **Allergic conjunctivitis**
OPHTHALMIC
Adults, Elderly, Children 3 yr and older. 1 drop 4 times a day.
▸ **Cataract extraction**
OPHTHALMIC
Adults, Elderly. 1 drop 4 times a day. Begin 24 hr after surgery and continue for 2 wk.
▸ **Refractive surgery**
OPHTHALMIC
Adults, Elderly. 1 drop 4 times a day for 3 days.

OFF-LABEL USES

Prevention or treatment of ocular inflammation (ophthalmic form)

CONTRAINDICATIONS

Active peptic ulcer disease, chronic inflammation of GI tract, GI bleeding or ulceration, history of hypersensitivity to aspirin or NSAIDs

INTERACTIONS

Drug
Antihypertensives, diuretics: May decrease the effects of these drugs.

K

Aspirin, other salicylates: May increase the risk of GI side effects such as bleeding.

Bone marrow depressants: May increase the risk of hematologic reactions.

Heparin, oral anticoagulants, thrombolytics: May increase the effects of these drugs.

Lithium: May increase the blood concentration and risk of toxicity of lithium.

Methotrexate: May increase the risk of methotrexate toxicity.

Probenecid: May increase ketorolac blood concentration.

Herbal

Feverfew: May decrease the effects of feverfew.

Ginkgo biloba: May increase the risk of bleeding.

Food

None known.

DIAGNOSTIC TEST EFFECTS

May prolong bleeding time. May increase liver function test results.

▓ IV INCOMPATIBILITIES

Promethazine (Phenergan)

▓ IV Compatibilities

Fentanyl (Sublimaze), hydromorphone (Dilaudid), morphine, nalbuphine (Nubain)

SIDE EFFECTS

Frequent (17%-12%)

Headache, nausea, abdominal cramps or pain, dyspepsia

Occasional (9%-3%)

Diarrhea

Ophthalmic: Transient stinging and burning

Rare (3%-1%)

Constipation, vomiting, flatulence, stomatitis, dizziness

Ophthalmic: Ocular irritation, allergic reactions, superficial ocular infection, keratitis

SERIOUS REACTIONS

• Rare reactions with long-term use include peptic ulcer disease, GI bleeding, gastritis, severe hepatic reactions (cholestasis, jaundice), nephrotoxicity (glomerular nephritis, interstitial nephritis, nephrotic syndrome), and an acute hypersensitivity reaction (including fever, chills, and joint pain).

PRECAUTIONS & CONSIDERATIONS

Caution is warranted with a history of GI tract disease, hepatic or renal impairment, and a predisposition to fluid retention. It is unknown if ketorolac is excreted in breast milk. Ketorolac should not be used during the third trimester of pregnancy because it may cause adverse effects in the fetus, such as premature closure of the ductus arteriosus. Notify the physician if pregnant. Although the safety and efficacy of ketorolac have not been established in children, doses of 0.5 mg/kg have been used. In the elderly, GI bleeding or ulceration is more likely to cause serious complications and age-related renal impairment may increase the risk of hepatotoxicity or renal toxicity; a decreased dosage is recommended. Avoid alcohol and aspirin during therapy because these substances increase the risk of GI bleeding. Tasks that require mental alertness or motor skills should also be avoided.

CBC, liver and renal function test results, urine output, BUN level, serum alkaline phosphatase, bilirubin, and creatinine levels should be assessed. Be alert for signs of bleeding, which may also occur with ophthalmic use if systemic absorption occurs. Therapeutic response, such as decreased pain, stiffness, swelling, and tenderness, improved grip strength, and increased joint mobility, should be evaluated.

Administration

! Ketorolac should not be administered by any route or combination of routes for more than 5 days. This drug may be given as a single dose, on a schedule, or on an as needed basis, as prescribed.

Take oral ketorolac with food, milk, or antacids if GI distress occurs.

For IV use, administer ketorolac undiluted by IV push over at least 15 seconds.

For IM use, slowly inject the drug deeply and into a large muscle mass.

For ophthalmic use, place a finger on lower eyelid, and pull it out until a pocket is formed between the eye and lower lid. Hold the dropper above the pocket, and place the prescribed number of drops in the pocket. Gently close eye and apply digital pressure to the lacrimal sac for 1 to 2 minutes to minimize drainage into the nose and throat, reducing the risk of systemic effects. Remove excess solution with a tissue.

K

Labetalol
la-bet′a-lole
(Normodyne, Presolol [AUS], Trandate)
Do not confuse Trandate with tramadol or Trental.

CATEGORY AND SCHEDULE
Pregnancy Risk Category: C (D if used in second or third trimester)

CLASSIFICATION
Antiadrenergics, beta blocking

MECHANISM OF ACTION
An antihypertensive that blocks alpha$_1$-, beta$_1$-, and beta$_2$- (large doses) adrenergic receptor sites. Large doses increase airway resistance. *Therapeutic Effect:* Slows sinus heart rate; decreases peripheral vascular resistance, cardiac output, and B/P.

PHARMACOKINETICS

Route	Onset	Peak	Duration
PO	0.5-2 hr	2-4 hr	8-12 hr
IV	2-5 min	5-15 min	2-4 hr

Completely absorbed from the GI tract. Protein binding: 50%. Undergoes first-pass metabolism. Metabolized in the liver. Primarily excreted in urine. Not removed by hemodialysis. **Half-life:** PO, 6-8 hr; IV, 5.5 hr.

AVAILABILITY
Tablets (Normodyne, Trandate): 100 mg, 200 mg, 300 mg.
Injection (Trandate): 5 mg/ml.

INDICATIONS AND DOSAGES
▶ **Hypertension**
PO
Adults. Initially, 100 mg twice a day adjusted in increments of 100 mg twice a day q2-3 days. Maintenance: 200-400 mg twice a day. Maximum: 2.4 g/day.
Elderly. Initially, 100 mg 1-2 times a day. May increase as needed.
▶ **Severe hypertension, hypertensive emergency**
IV
Adults. Initially, 20 mg. Additional doses of 20-80 mg may be given at 10-min intervals, up to total dose of 300 mg.
IV INFUSION
Adults. Initially, 2 mg/min up to total dose of 300 mg.
PO (AFTER IV THERAPY)
Adults. Initially, 200 mg; then, 200-400 mg in 6-12 hr. Increase dose at 1-day intervals to desired level.

OFF-LABEL USES
Control of hypotension during surgery, treatment of chronic angina pectoris

CONTRAINDICATIONS
Bronchial asthma, cardiogenic shock, second- or third-degree heart block, severe bradycardia, uncontrolled CHF

INTERACTIONS
Drug
Diuretics, other antihypertensives: May increase hypotensive effect.
Insulin, oral hypoglycemics: May mask symptoms of hypoglycemia and prolong hypoglycemic effect of these drugs.
MAOIs: May produce hypertension.
Sympathomimetics, xanthines: May mutually inhibit effects.
Herbal
None known.

Food
None known.

DIAGNOSTIC TEST EFFECTS

May increase serum antinuclear antibody titer and BUN, serum LDH, lipoprotein, alkaline phosphatase, bilirubin, creatinine, potassium, triglyceride, uric acid, AST (SGOT), and ALT (SGPT) levels.

▓ IV INCOMPATIBILITIES

Amphotericin B complex (Abelcet, AmBisome, Amphotec), ceftriaxone (Rocephin), furosemide (Lasix), heparin, nafcillin (Nafcil), thiopental

▓ IV Compatibilities

Aminophylline, amiodarone (Cordarone), calcium gluconate, diltiazem (Cardizem), dobutamine (Dobutrex), dopamine (Intropin), enalapril (Vasotec), fentanyl (Sublimaze), hydromorphone (Dilaudid), lidocaine, lorazepam (Ativan), magnesium sulfate, midazolam (Versed), milrinone (Primacor), morphine, nitroglycerin, norepinephrine (Levophed), potassium chloride, potassium phosphate, propofol (Diprivan)

SIDE EFFECTS

Frequent
Drowsiness, difficulty sleeping, unusual fatigue or weakness, diminished sexual ability, transient scalp tingling

Occasional
Dizziness, dyspnea, peripheral edema, depression, anxiety, constipation, diarrhea, nasal congestion, nausea, vomiting, abdominal discomfort

Rare
Altered taste, dry eyes, increased urination, paresthesia

SERIOUS REACTIONS

• Labetolol administration may precipitate or aggravate CHF

because of decreased myocardial stimulation.
• Abrupt withdrawal may precipitate ischemic heart disease, producing sweating, palpitations, headache, and tremor.
• May mask signs and symptoms of acute hypoglycemia (tachycardia, B/P changes) in patients with diabetes.

PRECAUTIONS & CONSIDERATIONS

Caution is warranted with diabetes mellitus, medication-controlled CHF, impaired cardiac or hepatic function, nonallergic bronchospastic disease, including chronic bronchitis and emphysema, and pheochromocytoma. Labetalol crosses the placenta and is distributed in small amounts in breast milk. The safety and efficacy of labetalol have not been established in children. In the elderly, age-related peripheral vascular disease may increase susceptibility to decreased peripheral circulation. Be aware that salt and alcohol intake should be restricted. Nasal decongestants or OTC cold preparations (stimulants) should not be used without physician approval.

Notify the physician of excessive fatigue, headache, prolonged dizziness, shortness of breath, or weight gain. B/P for hypotension, respiratory status for shortness of breath, pattern of daily bowel activity and stool consistency, EKG for arrhythmias, and pulse for quality, rate and rhythm should be monitored during treatment. If pulse rate is 60 beats/minute or lower or systolic B/P is less than 90 mm Hg, withhold the medication and contact the physician. Signs and symptoms of CHF, such as decreased urine output, distended neck veins, dyspnea (particularly on exertion or lying down), night cough, peripheral edema, and weight gain should also be assessed.

L

Storage
Store at room temperature. After dilution, IV solution is stable for 24 hours.

Administration
Labetalol may be taken without regard to meals. Crush tablets if necessary. Do not abruptly discontinue the drug.

! Place the patient in a supine position for IV administration and for 3 hours after receiving the medication. Expect a substantial drop in B/P if the patient stands within 3 hours following drug administration.

The solution for injection normally appears clear and colorless to light yellow; discard solution if precipitate forms or discoloration occurs. For IV infusion, dilute 200 mg in 160 ml dextrose 5% in water, 0.9% NaCl, lactated Ringer's solution, or any combination of these solutions to provide a concentration of 1 mg/ml. For IV push, give over 2 minutes at 10-minute intervals. For IV infusion, administer at a rate of 2 mg/minute (2 ml/minute) initially. Adjust the rate according to the patient's B/P. Monitor the patient's B/P immediately before and every 5 to 10 minutes during IV administration. Maximum effect occurs within 5 minutes.

Lactulose
lak′tyoo-lose
(Acilac [CAN], Actilax [AUS], Cholac, Constilac, Constulose, Duphalac [CAN], Enulose, Generlac, Genlac [AUS], Kristalose, Laxilose [CAN])
Do not confuse Cholac with diclofenac or lactulose with lactose.

CATEGORY AND SCHEDULE
Pregnancy Risk Category: B

CLASSIFICATION
Gastrointestinals, laxatives

MECHANISM OF ACTION
A lactose derivative that retains ammonia in colon and decreases serum ammonia concentration, producing osmotic effect.
Therapeutic Effect: Promotes increased peristalsis and bowel evacuation, which expels ammonia from the colon.

PHARMACOKINETICS

Route	Onset	Peak	Duration
PO	24-48 hr	N/A	N/A
Rectal	30-60 min	N/A	N/A

Poorly absorbed from the GI tract. Acts in the colon. Primarily excreted in feces.

AVAILABILITY
Syrup: 10 g/15 ml.
Packets: 10 g, 20 g.

INDICATIONS AND DOSAGES
▶ **Constipation**
PO
Adults, Elderly. 15-30 ml (10-20 g)/day, up to 60 ml (40 g)/day.

Children. 7.5 ml (5 g)/day after breakfast.

▶ **Portal-systemic encephalopathy**
PO
Adults, Elderly. Initially, 30-45 ml every hr. Then, 30-45 ml (20-30 g) 3-4 times a day. Adjust dose q1-2 days to produce 2-3 soft stools a day.
Children. 40-90 ml/day in divided doses.
Infants. 2.5-10 ml/day in divided doses.
RECTAL (AS RETENTION ENEMA)
Adults, Elderly. 300 ml with 700 ml water or saline solution; patient should retain 30-60 min. Repeat q4-6hr. If evacuation occurs too promptly, repeat immediately.

CONTRAINDICATIONS
Abdominal pain, appendicitis, nausea, patients on a galactose-free diet, vomiting

INTERACTIONS
Drug
Oral medication: May decrease transit time of concurrently administered oral medications, decreasing lactulose absorption.
Herbal
None known.
Food
None known.

DIAGNOSTIC TEST EFFECTS
May decrease serum potassium level.

SIDE EFFECTS
Occasional
Abdominal cramping, flatulence, increased thirst, abdominal discomfort
Rare
Nausea, vomiting

SERIOUS REACTIONS
• Diarrhea indicates overdose.

• Long-term use may result in laxative dependence, chronic constipation, and loss of normal bowel function.

PRECAUTIONS & CONSIDERATIONS
Caution is warranted with diabetes mellitus. It is unknown if lactulose crosses the placenta or is distributed in breast milk. Lactulose use should be avoided in children younger than 6 years of age because this population is usually unable to describe symptoms. No age-related precautions have been noted in the elderly.

Maintain adequate fluid intake. Electrolyte levels and pattern of daily bowel activity and stool consistency should be monitored. Periodic serum ammonia levels should be obtained.
Storage
Store solution at room temperature.
Administration
Oral solution normally appears pale yellow to yellow in color and viscous in consistency. However, cloudy, darkened solution does not indicate potency loss. Drink juice, milk, or water with each dose to aid in stool softening and increase palatability. Evacuation occurs in 24 to 48 hours of the initial drug dose. To promote defecation, increase fluid intake, exercise, and eat a high-fiber diet.

For rectal use, lubricate anus with petroleum jelly before applicator insertion. Insert applicator carefully, to prevent damage to the rectal wall, with nozzle toward navel. Squeeze container until entire dose has been expelled. Retain liquid until definite lower abdominal cramping is felt. Evacuation occurs in 24 to 48 hours of the initial drug dose.

L

Lamivudine (3TC)

la-miv'yoo-deen
(Epivir, Epivir-HBV, Heptovir
[CAN], Zeffix [AUS])
**Do not confuse lamivudine
with lamotrigine.**

CATEGORY AND SCHEDULE
Pregnancy Risk Category: C

CLASSIFICATION
Antivirals, nucleoside reverse
transcriptase inhibitors

MECHANISM OF ACTION
An antiviral that inhibits HIV
reverse transcriptase by viral DNA
chain termination. Also inhibits
RNA- and DNA-dependent DNA
polymerase, an enzyme necessary
for HIV replication. *Therapeutic
Effect:* Interrupts HIV replication,
slowing the progression of HIV
infection.

PHARMACOKINETICS
Rapidly and completely absorbed
from the GI tract. Protein binding:
36%. Widely distributed (crosses
the blood-brain barrier). Primarily
excreted unchanged in urine. Not
removed by hemodialysis or peritoneal dialysis. **Half-life:** 11-15 hr
(intracellular), 2-11 hr (serum, adults),
1.7-2 hr (serum, children) (increased
in impaired renal function).

AVAILABILITY
Oral Solution: (Epivir): 10 mg/ml;
(Epivir-HBV): 5 mg/ml.
Tablets: (Epivir): 150 mg, 300 mg;
(Epivir-HBV): 100 mg.

INDICATIONS AND DOSAGES
▸ **HIV infection (in combination with
other antiretrovirals)**

PO
*Adults, Children 12-16 yr, weighing
more than 50 kg (100 lb).* 150 mg
twice a day or 300 mg once a day.
Adults weighing less than 50 kg.
2 mg/kg twice a day.
Children 3 mo-11 yr. 4 mg/kg twice
a day (up to 150 mg/dose).
▸ **Chronic hepatitis B**
PO
Adults, Children 17 yr and older.
100 mg/day.
Children younger than 17 yr.
3 mg/kg/day. Maximum:
100 mg/day.
▸ **Dosage in renal impairment**
Dosage and frequency are modified
based on creatinine clearance.

Creatinine Clearance (ml/min)	Dosage
50 ml/min or higher	150 mg twice a day
30-49 ml/min	150 mg once a day
15-29 ml/min	150 mg first dose, then 100 mg once a day
5-14 ml/min	150 mg first dose, then 50 mg once a day
Less than 5 ml/min	50 mg first dose, then 25 mg once a day

OFF-LABEL USES
Prophylaxis in health care workers at
risk of acquiring HIV after occupational exposure.

CONTRAINDICATIONS
None known.

INTERACTIONS
Drug
Co-trimoxazole: Increases lamivu-
dine blood concentration.
Herbal
St. John's wort: May decrease
lamivudine blood concentration and
effect.

Food
None known.

DIAGNOSTIC TEST EFFECTS
May increase blood Hgb values, neutrophil count, and serum amylase, AST (SGOT), and ALT (SGPT) levels.

SIDE EFFECTS
Frequent
Headache (35%), nausea (33%), malaise and fatigue (27%), nasal disturbances (20%), diarrhea, cough (18%), musculoskeletal pain, neuropathy (12%), insomnia (11%), anorexia, dizziness, fever or chills (10%)
Occasional
Depression (9%); myalgia (8%); abdominal cramps (6%); dyspepsia, arthralgia (5%)

SERIOUS REACTIONS
• Pancreatitis occurs in 13% of pediatric patients.
• Anemia, neutropenia, and thrombocytopenia occur rarely.

PRECAUTIONS & CONSIDERATIONS
Caution is warranted with impaired renal function, a history of pancreatitis, a history of peripheral neuropathy and in young children. Be aware that lamivudine crosses the placenta and it is unknown if lamivudine is distributed in breast milk. Breastfeeding is not recommended in this population because of the possibility of HIV transmission. Be aware that the safety and efficacy of this drug have not been established in children younger than 3 months. In the elderly, age-related renal impairment may require dosage adjustment. Lamivudine is not a cure for HIV and that he or she may continue to experience illnesses, including opportunistic infections.

Before starting drug therapy, check the baseline lab values, especially renal function. Expect to monitor the serum amylase, BUN, and serum creatinine levels. Assess for altered sleep patterns, cough, dizziness, headache, nausea, and pattern of daily bowel activity and stool consistency. Avoid activities that require mental acuity if dizziness occurs. Modify diet or administer a laxative, if ordered, as needed. Closely monitor children for symptoms of pancreatitis, manifested as clammy skin, hypotension, nausea, severe and steady abdominal pain often radiating to the back, and vomiting accompanying abdominal pain. If pancreatitis in a child occurs, help the child to sit up or flex at the waist to relieve abdominal pain aggravated by movement.
Administration
Give without regard to meals. Take lamivudine for the full length of treatment and evenly space drug doses around the clock.

Lamotrigine
la-moe-trih'jeen
(Lamictal)
Do not confuse lamotrigine with lamivudine.

CATEGORY AND SCHEDULE
Pregnancy Risk Category: C

CLASSIFICATION
Anticonvulsants

MECHANISM OF ACTION
An anticonvulsant whose exact mechanism is unknown. May block voltage-sensitive sodium channels,

thus stabilizing neuronal membranes and regulating presynaptic transmitter release of excitatory amino acids. *Therapeutic Effect:* Reduces seizure activity.

AVAILABILITY

Tablets: 25 mg, 100 mg, 150 mg, 200 mg.
Tablets (Chewable): 2 mg, 5 mg, 25 mg.

INDICATIONS AND DOSAGES

▸ **Seizure control in patients receiving enzyme-inducing antiepileptic drug (EIAEDs), but not valproate acid**
PO
Adults, Elderly, Children 12 yr and older. Recommended as add-on therapy: 50 mg once a day for 2 wk, followed by 100 mg/day in 2 divided doses for 2 wk. Maintenance: Dosage may be increased by 100 mg/day every week, up to 300-500 mg/day in 2 divided doses.
Children 2-12 yr. 0.6 mg/kg/day in 2 divided doses for 2 wk, then 1.2 mg/kg/day in 2 divided doses for wk 3 and 4. Maintenance: 5-15 mg/kg/day. Maximum: 400 mg/day.
▸ **Seizure control in patients receiving combination therapy of EIAEDs and valproic acid**
PO
Adults, Elderly, Children 12 yr and older. 25 mg every other day for 2 wk, followed by 25 mg once a day for 2 wk. Maintenance: Dosage may be increased by 25-50 mg/day q1-2wk, up to 150 mg/day in 2 divided doses.
Children 2-12 yr. 0.15 mg/kg/day in 2 divided doses for 2 wk, then 0.3 mg/kg/day in 2 divided doses for wk 3 and 4. Maintenance: 1-5 mg/kg/day in 2 divided doses. Maximum: 200 mg/day.

▸ **Conversion to monotherapy**
PO
Adults, Children 12 yr and older. Add lamotrigine 50 mg/day for 2 wk; then 100 mg/day during wk 3 and 4. Increase by 100 mg/day q1-2wk until maintenance dosage (300-500 mg/day in 2 divided doses) is achieved. Gradually discontinue other EIAEDs over 4 wk once maintenance dose is achieved.
▸ **Bipolar disorder**
PO
Adults, Elderly. Initially, 25 mg/day. May double dose after wk 2, 4, and 5. Target dose: 200 mg/day.
▸ **Discontinuation therapy**
Adults, Children older than 12 yr. A dosage reduction of approximately 50% per week over at least 2 wk is recommended.

CONTRAINDICATIONS
None known.

INTERACTIONS
Drug
Carbamazepine, phenobarbital, phenytoin, primidone, valproic acid: Decrease lamotrigine blood concentration.
Carbamazepine, valproic acid: May increase serum levels of these drugs.
Herbal
None known.
Food
None known.

DIAGNOSTIC TEST EFFECTS
None known.

SIDE EFFECTS
Frequent
Dizziness (38%), diplopia (28%), headache (29%), ataxia (22%), nausea (19%), blurred vision (16%), somnolence, rhinitis (14%)

Occasional (10%-5%)
Rash, pharyngitis, vomiting, cough, flu-like symptoms, diarrhea, dysmenorrhea, fever, insomnia, dyspepsia
Rare
Constipation, tremor, anxiety, pruritus, vaginitis, hypersensitivity reaction

SERIOUS REACTIONS
• Abrupt withdrawal may increase seizure frequency.

PRECAUTIONS & CONSIDERATIONS
Caution is warranted with cardiac, hepatic, and renal impairment. Exposure to sunlight and artificial light should be avoided.

Drowsiness and dizziness may occur, so alcohol and tasks requiring mental alertness or motor skills should be avoided. Notify the physician if fever, rash, or swollen glands occur. Seizure disorder, including the onset, duration, frequency, intensity, and type of seizures, should be assessed before and during treatment.
Administration
! If the patient is currently taking valproic acid, expect to reduce the lamotrigine dosage to less than half the normal dosage. Be aware that a decreased dosage may be effective in patients with significant renal impairment.

Take lamotrigine without regard to food. Do not discontinue the drug abruptly after long-term therapy. Strict maintenance of drug therapy is essential for seizure control.

Lansoprazole
lan-soe′pray-zole
(Prevacid, Prevacid IV, Prevacid Solu-Tab, Zoton [AUS])
Do not confuse Prevacid with Pepcid, Pravachol, or Prevpac.

CATEGORY AND SCHEDULE
Pregnancy Risk Category: B

CLASSIFICATION
Gastrointestinals, proton pump inhibitors

MECHANISM OF ACTION
A proton pump inhibitor that selectively inhibits the parietal cell membrane enzyme system (hydrogen-potassium adenosine triphosphatase) or proton pump. *Therapeutic Effect:* Suppresses gastric acid secretion.

PHARMACOKINETICS

Route	Onset	Peak	Duration
PO (15 mg)	2-3 hr	N/A	24 hr
PO (30 mg)	1-2 hr	N/A	Longer than 24 hr

Rapid and complete absorption (food may decrease absorption) once drug has left stomach. Protein binding: 97%. Distributed primarily to gastric parietal cells and converted to two active metabolites. Extensively metabolized in the liver. Eliminated in bile and urine. Not removed by hemodialysis. **Half-life:** 1.5 hr (increased in the elderly and in those with hepatic impairment).

AVAILABILITY
Capsules (Extended-Release [Prevacid]): 15 mg, 30 mg.
Granules for Oral Suspension

(Prevacid): 15 mg/pack; 30 mg/pack.
*Injection Powder for Reconstitution
(Prevacid IV):* 30 mg.
*Oral-disintegrating Tablets (Prevacid
Solu-Tab):* 15 mg, 30 mg.

INDICATIONS AND DOSAGES
▸ **Duodenal ulcer**
PO
Adults, Elderly. 15 mg/day, before
eating, preferably in the morning, for
up to 4 wk.
▸ **Erosive esophagitis**
PO
Adults, Elderly. 30 mg/day, before
eating, for up to 8 wk. If healing
does not occur within 8 wk (in
5%-10% of cases), may give for
additional 8 wk. Maintenance:
15 mg/day.
IV
Adults, Elderly. 30 mg once a day
for up to 7 days. Switch to oral
lansoprazole therapy as soon as
patient can tolerate oral route.
▸ **Gastric ulcer**
PO
Adults. 30 mg/day for up to 8 wk.
▸ **NSAID gastric ulcer**
PO
Adults, Elderly. (Healing): 30 mg/day
for up to 8 wk. (Prevention):
15 mg/day for up to 12 wk.
▸ **Healed duodenal ulcer,
gastroesophageal reflux disease**
PO
Adults. 15 mg/day.
▸ **Usual pediatric dosage**
*Children 3 mo-14 yr, weighing more
than 20 kg.* 30 mg once daily.
*Children 3 mo-14 yr, weighing
10-20 kg.* 15 mg once daily.
*Children 3 mo-14 yr, weighing
less than 10 kg.* 7.5 mg once
daily.
▸ *Helicobacter pylori* **infection**
PO
Adults. 30 mg twice a day for 10 days
(with amoxicillin and clarithromycin).

▸ **Pathologic hypersecretory
conditions (including Zollinger-
Ellison syndrome)**
PO
Adults, Elderly. 60 mg/day.
Individualize dosage according
to patient needs and for as long
as clinically indicated. May
increase to 120 mg/day in divided
doses.

CONTRAINDICATIONS
None known.

INTERACTIONS
Drug
**Ampicillin, digoxin, iron
salts, ketoconazole:** May
interfere with the absorption of
ampicillin, digoxin, iron salts, and
ketoconazole.
Sucralfate: May delay the absorption
of lansoprazole.
Herbal
None known.
Food
None known.

DIAGNOSTIC TEST EFFECTS
May increase LDH, serum alkaline
phosphatase, bilirubin, cholesterol,
creatinine, AST (SGOT), ALT
(SGPT), triglyceride, and uric acid
levels. May produce abnormal
albumin/globulin ratio, electrolyte
balance, and platelet, RBC, and
WBC counts. May increase Hgb
and Hct.

SIDE EFFECTS
Occasional (3%-2%)
Diarrhea, abdominal pain, rash,
pruritus, altered appetite
Rare (1%)
Nausea, headache

SERIOUS REACTIONS
• Bilirubinemia, eosinophilia, and
hyperlipemia occur rarely.

PRECAUTIONS & CONSIDERATIONS

Caution is warranted with impaired hepatic function. It is unknown if lansoprazole is distributed in breast milk. Safety and efficacy of lansoprazole have not been established in children. No age-related precautions have been noted in the elderly, but doses larger than 30 mg are not recommended in this population. Laboratory values, including CBC and blood chemistry, should be obtained before and periodically during therapy.

Storage
Store drug at room temperature.

Administration
Take lansoprazole capsules while fasting or before meals because food diminishes absorption. Do not chew or crush delayed-release capsules. May open capsules and sprinkle granules on 1 tablespoon of applesauce; swallow immediately. Take lansoprazole 30 minutes before sucralfate because sucralfate may delay lansoprazole absorption.

May give solu-tabs with oral syringe or NG tube. May dissolve in 4 ml water (15 mg) or 10 ml water (30 mg).

For IV use, infuse over 30 minutes.

Lanthanum Carbonate

lan-than′um car-bo′nate
(Fosrenol)

CATEGORY AND SCHEDULE
Pregnancy Risk Category: C

CLASSIFICATION
Chelators

MECHANISM OF ACTION

A phosphate regulator that dissociates in the acidic environment of the upper GI tract to lanthanum ions, which bind to dietary phosphate released from food during digestion, forming highly insoluble lanthanum phosphate complexes. *Therapeutic Effect:* Reduces phosphate absorption.

PHARMACOKINETICS

Phosphate complexes are eliminated in urine.

AVAILABILITY

Tablets (Chewable): 250 mg, 500 mg.

INDICATIONS AND DOSAGES
▶ **Reduce serum phosphate in end-stage renal disease**
PO
Adults, Elderly. 750 mg-1500 mg in divided doses, taken with or immediately after a meal. Dosage may be titrated in 750-mg increments q2-3wk based on serum phosphate levels.

CONTRAINDICATIONS

None known.

INTERACTIONS
Drug
Antacids: Interact with lanthanum; separate administration by 2 hours.
Herbal
None known.
Food
All foods: Enhance lanthanum's effect and reduce phosphate absorption.

DIAGNOSTIC TEST EFFECTS

None known.

SIDE EFFECTS
Frequent
Nausea (11%), vomiting (9%), dialysis graft occlusion (8%), abdominal pain (5%)

SERIOUS REACTIONS
• None known.

PRECAUTIONS & CONSIDERATIONS
Caution is warranted with acute peptic ulcer disease, bowel obstruction, Crohn's disease, and ulcerative colitis. Side effects of nausea and vomiting should decrease over time.
Administration
Chew the tablets thoroughly before swallowing. Take the drug with or immediately after a meal. Take lanthanum within 2 hours of antacids.

Laronidase
lair-oh'-ni-days
(Aldurazyme)

CATEGORY AND SCHEDULE
Pregnancy Risk Category: B

CLASSIFICATION
Enzymes, metabolic

MECHANISM OF ACTION
An enzyme that increases the catabolism of glycosaminoglycans in those with a deficiency of the lysosomal enzymes required for glycosaminoglycan catabolism. *Therapeutic Effect:* Prevents glycosaminoglycans from causing widespread cellular, tissue, and organ dysfunction.

AVAILABILITY
Injection: 2.9 mg/5 ml.

INDICATIONS AND DOSAGES
▶ **Mucopolysaccharidosis**
IV
Adults, Elderly. 0.58 mg/kg infused once weekly.

CONTRAINDICATIONS
None known.

INTERACTIONS
Drug
None known.
Herbal
None known.
Food
None known.

DIAGNOSTIC TEST EFFECTS
None known.

SIDE EFFECTS
Frequent (36%-18%)
Infusion-related reactions, such as facial flushing, rash, fever, and headache
Occasional (9%)
Cough, bronchospasm, urticaria, pruritus, angioedema, dependent edema, hypotension, hyperreflexia

SERIOUS REACTIONS
• Upper respiratory tract infection occurs commonly.
• Anaphylactic reactions, such as angioedema, severe bronchospasm, and dyspnea, occur rarely.

PRECAUTIONS & CONSIDERATIONS
Closely monitor for infusion-related reactions. Slowing the infusion rate, temporarily stopping the infusion, or administering additional antipyretics and antihistamines may ameliorate such reactions.
Storage
Refrigerate vials. Once reconstituted, the solution should be used immediately. If this isn't possible, refrigerate the solution for no longer than 36 hours from the time of preparation to completion of administration.
Administration
Pre-treat with antipyretics and antihistamines, as prescribed, 60 minutes before starting the IV infusion. The total volume of the infusion is determined by the patient's weight.

Persons who weigh 20 kg or less should receive a total volume of 100 ml. Persons who weigh more than 20 kg should receive a total volume of 250 ml. Dilute with 0.1% albumin (human) in 0.9% NaCl. Take care not to shake the solution. Administer using a 0.2-micrometer filter. Begin the infusion at a rate of 10 mcg/kg/hour, and increase it in 15-minute increments to 20 mcg/kg/hour, then 50 mcg/kg/hour, and then 100 mcg/kg/hour during the first hour, as prescribed. Give the remainder of the infusion at 200 mcg/kg/hour over 2 to 3 hours for a total infusion time of 3 to 4 hours.

Leflunomide
le-flu'na-mide
(Arava)

CATEGORY AND SCHEDULE
Pregnancy Risk Category: X

CLASSIFICATION
Disease modifying antirheumatic drugs, immunomodulators

MECHANISM OF ACTION
An immunomodulatory agent that inhibits dihydroorotate dehydrogenase, the enzyme involved in autoimmune process that leads to rheumatoid arthritis. *Therapeutic Effect:* Reduces signs and symptoms of rheumatoid arthritis and slows structural damage.

PHARMACOKINETICS
Well absorbed after PO administration. Protein binding: greater than 99%. Metabolized to active metabolite in the GI wall and liver. Excreted through both renal and biliary systems. Not removed by hemodialysis. **Half-life:** 16 days.

AVAILABILITY
Tablets: 10 mg, 20 mg.

INDICATIONS AND DOSAGES
▶ **Rheumatoid arthritis**
PO
Adults, Elderly. Initially, 100 mg/day for 3 days, then 10-20 mg/day.

CONTRAINDICATIONS
Pregnancy or plans to become pregnant

INTERACTIONS
Drug
Rifampin: Increases the blood concentration of leflunomide.
Warfarin: May increase the effects of warfarin.
Herbal
None known.
Food
None known.

DIAGNOSTIC TEST EFFECTS
May increase hepatic enzyme levels, especially AST (SGOT), and ALT (SGPT).

SIDE EFFECTS
Frequent (20%-10%)
Diarrhea, respiratory tract infection, alopecia, rash, nausea

SERIOUS REACTIONS
• Transient thrombocytopenia and leukopenia occur rarely.

PRECAUTIONS & CONSIDERATIONS
Caution is warranted with immunodeficiency, bone marrow dysplasia, impaired hepatic or renal function, and positive serology for hepatitis B or C. Leflunomide may cause fetal harm. Avoid becoming pregnant. Although it is not known whether

leflunomide is excreted in breast milk, the drug is not recommended for breast-feeding women. The safety and efficacy of leflunomide have not been established in children younger than 18 years. No age-related precautions have been noted in the elderly.

Liver function test results should be monitored. Symptomatic relief of rheumatoid arthritis, including relief of pain and improved range of motion, grip strength, and mobility, should be assessed.

Administration
Take leflunomide without regard to food. Therapeutic effect may take longer than 8 weeks to appear.

Lepirudin
leh-peer′u-din
(Refludan)

CATEGORY AND SCHEDULE
Pregnancy Risk Category: B

CLASSIFICATION
Anticoagulants, thrombin inhibitors

MECHANISM OF ACTION
An anticoagulant that inhibits thrombogenic action of thrombin (independent of antithrombin II and not inhibited by platelet factor 4). One molecule of lepirudin binds to one molecule of thrombin. *Therapeutic Effect:* Produces dose-dependent increases of aPTT.

PHARMACOKINETICS
Distributed primarily in extra-cellular fluid. Primarily eliminated by the kidneys. **Half-life:** 1.3 hr (increased in impaired renal function).

AVAILABILITY
Powder for Injection: 50 mg.

INDICATIONS AND DOSAGES
▸ **Heparin-induced thrombocytopenia and associated thromboembolic disease to prevent further thromboembolic complications**
IV, IV INFUSION
Adults, Elderly. 0.2-0.4 mg/kg, IV slowly over 15-20 sec, followed by IV infusion of 0.1-0.15 mg/kg/hr for 2-10 days or longer.
▸ **Dosage in renal impairment**
Initial dose is decreased to 0.2 mg/kg, with infusion rate adjusted based on creatinine clearance.

Creatinine Clearance (ml/min)	% of Standard Infusion Rate	Infusion Rate (mg/kg/hr)
45-60	50	0.075
30-44	30	0.045
15-29	15	0.0225

CONTRAINDICATIONS
None known.

INTERACTIONS
Drug
Platelet aggregation inhibitors, thrombolytics, warfarin: May increase the risk of bleeding complications.
Herbal
Ginkgo biloba: May increase the risk of bleeding.
Food
None known.

DIAGNOSTIC TEST EFFECTS
Increases aPTT and thrombin time.

▒ IV INCOMPATIBILITIES
Do not mix with other medications.

SIDE EFFECTS
Frequent (14%-5%)
Bleeding from gums, puncture sites or wounds, hematuria, fever, GI and rectal bleeding
Occasional (3%-1%)
Epistaxis; allergic reaction, such as rash and pruritus; vaginal bleeding

SERIOUS REACTIONS
- Overdose is characterized by excessively high aPTT.
- Intracranial bleeding occurs rarely.
- Abnormal hepatic function occurs in 6% of patients.

PRECAUTIONS & CONSIDERATIONS
Caution is warranted with conditions associated with increased risk of bleeding, such as bacterial endocarditis, cerebrovascular accident, hemorrhagic diathesis, intracerebral surgery, recent major bleeding, recent major surgery, severe hypertension, severe hepatic or renal impairment, and stroke. It is unknown if lepirudin crosses the placenta or is distributed in breast milk. Safety and efficacy of lepirudin have not been established in children. In the elderly, age-related renal impairment may require dosage adjustment. Females may experience a heavier menstrual flow. Other medications, including OTC drugs, should be avoided. An electric razor and soft toothbrush should be used to prevent bleeding during therapy.

Notify the physician of bleeding, breathing difficulty, bruising, dizziness, edema, fever, itching, lightheadedness, rash, black or red stool, coffee-ground vomitus, dark or red urine, or red-speckled mucus from cough. CBC, B/P, pulse rate, Hct, platelet count, renal function, BUN, serum creatinine, AST and ALT levels, and stool and urine specimen for occult blood should be monitored before and during therapy. Be aware of signs of bleeding, including bleeding at injection or surgical sites or from gums, blood in stool, bruising, hematuria, and petechiae.

Storage
Store unreconstituted vials at room temperature. Reconstituted solution should be used immediately, but the IV infusion is stable for up to 24 hours at room temperature.

Administration
! Give initial dose as soon as possible after surgery but not more than 24 hours after surgery. Dosage adjusted according to aPTT ratio with target range of 1.5 to 2.5 normal. For patients weighing more than 110 kg, the maximum initial dose is 44 mg, with maximum rate of 16.5 mg/hr.

To reconstitute, add 1 ml sterile water for injection or 0.9% NaCl to 50-mg vial and shake gently. Be aware that reconstitution normally produces a clear, colorless solution; do not use if solution is cloudy. For IV push, further dilute by transferring to syringe and adding sufficient sterile water for injection, 0.9% NaCl, or D_5W to produce a concentration of 5 mg/ml. For IV infusion, add contents of 2 vials (100 mg) to 250 or 500 ml 0.9% NaCl or D_5W, providing a concentration of 0.4 or 0.2 mg/ml, respectively. Give IV push over 15 to 20 seconds. Expect to adjust IV infusion based on aPTT or patient's body weight.

Letrozole
le'tro-zole
(Femara)
Do not confuse with Femhrt.

CATEGORY AND SCHEDULE
Pregnancy Risk Category: D

CLASSIFICATION
Antineoplastics, aromatase inhibitors, hormones/hormone modifiers

MECHANISM OF ACTION
Decreases the level of circulating estrogen by inhibiting aromatase, an enzyme that catalyzes the final step in estrogen production. *Therapeutic Effect:* Inhibits the growth of breast cancers that are stimulated by estrogens.

PHARMACOKINETICS
Rapidly and completely absorbed. Metabolized in the liver. Primarily eliminated by the kidneys. Unknown if removed by hemodialysis. **Half-life:** Approximately 2 days.

AVAILABILITY
Tablets: 2.5 mg.

INDICATIONS AND DOSAGES
▶ **Breast cancer**
PO
Adults, Elderly. 2.5 mg/day. Continue until tumor progression is evident.

CONTRAINDICATIONS
None known.

INTERACTIONS
Drug
None known.

Herbal
None known.
Food
None known.

DIAGNOSTIC TEST EFFECTS
May increase serum calcium, cholesterol, GGT, AST (SGOT), and ALT (SGPT) levels.

SIDE EFFECTS
Frequent (21%-9%)
Musculoskeletal pain (back, arm, leg), nausea, headache
Occasional (8%-5%)
Constipation, arthralgia, fatigue, vomiting, hot flashes, diarrhea, abdominal pain, cough, rash, anorexia, hypertension, peripheral edema
Rare (4%-1%)
Asthenia, somnolence, dyspepsia, weight gain, pruritus

SERIOUS REACTIONS
• None known.

PRECAUTIONS & CONSIDERATIONS
Caution is warranted with hepatic and renal impairment. Women who are or may be pregnant shouldn't use this drug. Pregnancy should be determined before beginning therapy. It is unknown if letrozole is distributed in breast milk. The safety and efficacy of letrozole have not been established in children. No age-related precautions have been noted in the elderly.

Potential side effects, including asthenia, dizziness, headache, nausea, vomiting, and musculoskeletal pain, may occur. Notify the physician if weakness, hot flashes, or nausea become unmanageable. Vital signs, especially blood pressures, should be assessed before therapy begins because letrozole may cause hypertension. CBC, serum electrolyte

levels, thyroid function, and liver and renal function tests should be monitored during therapy.
Administration
Take oral letrozole without regard to food.

Leucovorin
loo-koe-vor'in
(Calcium Leucovorin [AUS], Wellcovorin)
Do not confuse Wellcovorin with Wellbutrin or Wellferon.

CATEGORY AND SCHEDULE
Pregnancy Risk Category: C

CLASSIFICATION
Antidotes, vitamins/minerals

MECHANISM OF ACTION
An antidote to folic acid antagonists that may limit methotrexate action on normal cells by competing with methotrexate for the same transport processes into the cells. *Therapeutic Effect:* Reverses toxic effects of folic acid antagonists. Reverses folic acid deficiency.

PHARMACOKINETICS
Readily absorbed from the GI tract. Widely distributed. Primarily concentrated in the liver. Metabolized in the liver and intestinal mucosa to active metabolite. Primarily excreted in urine.
Half-life: 15 min; metabolite, 30-35 min.

AVAILABILITY
Tablets: 5 mg, 10 mg, 15 mg, 25 mg.
Injection: 10 mg/ml.
Powder for Injection: 50 mg, 100 mg, 200 mg, 350 mg.

INDICATIONS AND DOSAGES
▶ **Conventional rescue dosage in high-dose methotrexate therapy**
PO, IV, IM
Adults, Elderly, Children. 10 mg/m^2 IM or IV one time, then PO q6hr until serum methotrexate level is less than 10^{-8} M. If 24-hr serum creatinine level increases by 50% or greater over baseline or methotrexate level exceeds 5×10^{-6} M or 48-hr level exceeds 9×10^{-7} M, increase to 100 mg/m^2 IV q3hr until methotrexate level is less than 10^{-8} M.
▶ **Folic acid antagonist overdose**
PO
Adults, Elderly, Children. 2-15 mg/day for 3 days or 5 mg every 3 days.
▶ **Megaloblastic anemia**
IM
Adults, Elderly, Children. 3-6 mg/day.
▶ **Megaloblastic anemia secondary to folate deficiency**
IM
Adults, Elderly, Children. 1 mg/day.
▶ **Prevention of hematologic toxicity (for toxoplasmosis), with sulfadiazine**
PO, IV
Adults, Elderly, Children. 5-10 mg/day, repeat every 3 days.
▶ **Prevention of hematologic toxicity with pyrimethamine, PCP**
PO, IV
Adults, Children. 25 mg once weekly.

OFF-LABEL USES
Treatment of Ewing's sarcoma, gestational trophoblastic neoplasms, or non-Hodgkin's lymphoma; treatment adjunct for head and neck carcinoma

CONTRAINDICATIONS
Pernicious anemia, other megaloblastic anemias secondary to vitamin B$_{12}$ deficiency

INTERACTIONS
Drug
Anticonvulsants: May decrease the effects of anticonvulsants.
Chemotherapeutic agents: May increase the effects and toxicity of these drugs when taken in combination.
Herbal
None known.
Food
None known.

DIAGNOSTIC TEST EFFECTS
None known.

▓ IV INCOMPATIBILITIES
Amphotericin B complex (Abelcet, AmBisome, Amphotec), droperidol (Inapsine), foscarnet (Foscavir)
▓ IV Compatibilities
Cisplatin (Platinol AQ), cyclophosphamide (Cytoxan), doxorubicin (Adriamycin), etoposide (VePesid), filgrastim (Neupogen), 5-fluorouracil, gemcitabine (Gemzar), granisetron (Kytril), heparin, methotrexate, metoclopramide (Reglan), mitomycin (Mutamycin), piperacillin and tazobactam (Zosyn), vinblastine (Velban), vincristine (Oncovin)

SIDE EFFECTS
Frequent
When combined with chemotherapeutic agents: Diarrhea, stomatitis, nausea, vomiting, lethargy or malaise or fatigue, alopecia, anorexia
Occasional
Urticaria, dermatitis

SERIOUS REACTIONS
• Excessive dosage may negate chemotherapeutic effects of folic acid antagonists.
• Anaphylaxis occurs rarely.
• Diarrhea may cause rapid clinical deterioration.

PRECAUTIONS & CONSIDERATIONS
Caution is warranted with bronchial asthma and history of allergies. Caution should also be used with 5-fluorouracil in persons with GI toxicities. It is unknown if leucovorin crosses the placenta or is distributed in breast milk. Leucovorin use in children may increase the risk of seizures by counteracting the anticonvulsant effects of barbiturates and hydantoins. Age-related renal impairment may require a dosage adjustment for the elderly receiving drug for rescue from effects of high-dose methotrexate therapy. Consuming foods with folic acid, including dried beans, meat proteins, and green leafy vegetables, is encouraged in those with folic acid deficiency.

CBC, BUN and serum creatinine levels (important in leucovorin rescue) should be monitored. Electrolyte levels and liver function test results in those receiving chemotherapeutic agents in combination with leucovorin should be assessed. For treatment of accidental overdosage of folic acid antagonists, leucovorin should be given as soon as possible (preferably within 1 hour), as prescribed.
Storage
Store vials for parenteral use at room temperature. Use the solution immediately if reconstituted with sterile water for injection and within 7 days if reconstituted with bacteriostatic water for injection.
Administration
Scored tablets may be crushed. The injection solution normally appears clear and yellowish. Reconstitute each 50-mg vial with 5 ml sterile water for injection or bacteriostatic water for injection (containing benzyl alcohol) to provide a concentration of 10 mg/ml. Reconstitute doses greater than

10 mg/m² with sterile water for injection. Further dilute with D₅W or 0.9% NaCl. Don't exceed an infusion rate of 160 mg/minute (because of drug's calcium content).

Leuprolide
loo′proe-lide
(Eligard, Lucrin [AUS], Lucrin Depot Inj [AUS], Lupron, Lupron Depot, Lupron Depot Ped, Viadur)
Do not confuse leuprolide or Lupron with Lopurin or Nuprin.

CATEGORY AND SCHEDULE
Pregnancy Risk Category: X

CLASSIFICATION
Antineoplastics, hormones/hormone modifiers, gonadotropin-releasing hormone analogs

MECHANISM OF ACTION
A gonadotropin-releasing hormone analogue and antineoplastic agent that stimulates the release of luteinizing hormone (LH) and follicle-stimulating hormone (FSH) from the anterior pituitary gland. *Therapeutic Effect:* Produces pharmacologic castration and decreases the growth of abnormal prostate tissue in males; causes endometrial tissue to become inactive and atrophic in females; and decreases the rate of pubertal development in children with central precocious puberty.

PHARMACOKINETICS
Rapidly and well absorbed after subcutaneous administration. Absorbed slowly after IM administration. Protein binding: 43%-49%. **Half-life:** 3-4 hr.

AVAILABILITY
Implant (Viadur): 65 mg.
Injection Depot Formulation (Eligard): 7.5 mg, 22.5 mg, 30 mg.
Injection Depot Formulation (Leupron Depot): 3.75 mg, 7.5 mg, 11.25 mg, 22.5 mg, 30 mg.
Injection Depot Formulation (Lupron Depot-Ped): 7.5 mg, 11.25 mg, 15 mg.
Injection solution (Lupron): 5 mg/ml.

INDICATIONS AND DOSAGES
▸ **Advanced prostatic carcinoma**
IM
Adults, Elderly. (Lupron Depot) 7.5 mg every month or 22.5 mg every 3 months or 30 mg every 4 months.
SUBCUTANEOUS
Adults, Elderly. (Eligard) 7.5 mg every month or 22.5 mg every 3 months or 30 mg every 4 months; (Lupron) 1 mg/day; (Viadur) 65 mg implanted every 12 months.
▸ **Endometriosis**
IM
Adults, Elderly. (Lupron Depot) 3.75 mg/mo for up to 6 months or 11.25 mg every 3 months for up to 2 doses.
▸ **Uterine leiomyomata**
IM (WITH IRON)
Adults, Elderly. (Lupron Depot) 3.75 mg/mo for up to 3 months or 11.25 mg as a single injection.
▸ **Precocious puberty**
IM
Children. (Lupron Depot) 0.3 mg/kg/dose every 28 days. Minimum: 7.5 mg. If down regulation is not achieved, titrate upward in 3.75-mg increments q4wk.
SUBCUTANEOUS
Children. (Lupron) 20-45 mcg/kg/day. Titrate upward by 10 mcg/kg/day if down regulation is not achieved.

CONTRAINDICATIONS
Pernicious anemia, pregnancy

INTERACTIONS
Drug
None known.
Herbal
None known.
Food
None known.

DIAGNOSTIC TEST EFFECTS
May increase serum prostatic acid phosphatase (PAP) levels. Initially increases, then decreases, serum testosterone concentration.

SIDE EFFECTS
Frequent
Hot flashes (ranging from mild flushing to diaphoresis)
Females: Amenorrhea, spotting
Occasional
Arrhythmias; palpitations; blurred vision; dizziness; edema; headache; burning or itching, or swelling at injection site; nausea; insomnia; weight gain
Females: Deepening voice, hirsutism, decreased libido, increased breast tenderness, vaginitis, altered mood
Males: Constipation, decreased testicle size, gynecomastia, impotence, decreased appetite, angina
Rare
Males: Thrombophlebitis

SERIOUS REACTIONS
• Signs and symptoms of metastatic prostatic carcinoma (such as bone pain, dysuria or hematuria, and weakness or paresthesia of the lower extremities) occasionally worsen 1 to 2 weeks after the initial dose but then subside with continued therapy.
• Pulmonary embolism and MI occur rarely.

PRECAUTIONS & CONSIDERATIONS
Caution is warranted with children receiving long-term therapy. Leuprolide use is contraindicated in pregnancy because the drug may cause spontaneous abortion. Pregnancy should be determined before therapy. Nonhormonal contraceptives should be used during leuprolide use. The long-term safety of leuprolide in children has not been established. No age-related precautions have been noted in the elderly.

Potential side effects, including dizziness, nausea, and vomiting, may occur. Females should notify the physician if regular menstruation persists or pregnancy occurs. The person should be assessed for peripheral edema, arrhythmias and palpitations, sleep pattern changes, and visual difficulties. Serum testosterone and PAP levels should be obtained periodically during leuprolide therapy. Be aware that serum testosterone and PAP levels should increase during the first week of therapy. The testosterone level should decrease to baseline level or less within 2 weeks, and the PAP level should decrease within 4 weeks.
Storage
Refrigerate Lupron vials. Store Lupron Depot at room temperature; do not freeze and protect from light and heat. Store Eligard in the refrigerator.
Administration
! Because leuprolide may be carcinogenic, mutagenic, or teratogenic, handle it with extreme care during preparation and administration.

For subcutaneous (Lupron) use, the injection should appear clear and colorless. Discard the solution if it appears discolored or contains precipitate. Administer the drug undiluted into the abdomen, anterior thigh, or deltoid muscle.

For IM (Lupron Depot) use, reconstitute only with the diluent provided. Follow mixing instructions provided by the manufacturer. Use the reconstituted solution immediately. Do not use needles smaller than 22 gauge; use syringes provided by the manufacturer (0.5 ml low-dose insulin syringes may be used as an alternative).

For IM (Eligard) use, allow drug to warm to room temperature before reconstitution. Follow mixing instructions provided by the manufacturer. Administer the drug within 30 minutes after reconstitution.

Levalbuterol
lee-val-byoo′ter-ole
(Xopenex)
Do not confuse Xopenex with Xanax.

CATEGORY AND SCHEDULE
Pregnancy Risk Category: C

CLASSIFICATION
Adrenergic agonists, bronchodilators

MECHANISM OF ACTION
A sympathomimetic that stimulates beta$_2$-adrenergic receptors in the lungs resulting in relaxation of bronchial smooth muscle. *Therapeutic Effect:* Relieves bronchospasm and reduces airway resistance.

PHARMACOKINETICS

Route	Onset	Peak	Duration
Inhalation	10-17 min	1.5 hr	5-6 hr

Metabolized in the liver to inactive metabolite. **Half-life:** 3.3-4 hr.

AVAILABILITY
Solution for Nebulization: 0.31 in 3-ml vials, 0.63 mg in 3-ml vials, 1.25 mg in 3-ml vials.

INDICATIONS AND DOSAGES
▶ **Treatment and prevention of bronchospasm**
NEBULIZATION
Adults, Elderly, Children 12 yr and older. Initially, 0.63 mg 3 times a day 6-8 hr apart. May increase to 1.25 mg 3 times a day with dose monitoring.
Children 3-11 yr. Initially 0.31 mg 3 times a day. Maximum: 0.63 mg 3 times a day.

CONTRAINDICATIONS
History of hypersensitivity to sympathomimetics

INTERACTIONS
Drug
Beta blockers: Antagonize the effects of levalbuterol.
Digoxin: May increase the risk of arrhythmias.
MAOIs, tricyclic antidepressants: May potentiate cardiovascular effects.
Herbal
None known.
Food
None known.

DIAGNOSTIC TEST EFFECTS
May increase serum potassium level.

SIDE EFFECTS
Frequent
Tremor, nervousness, headache, throat dryness and irritation
Occasional
Cough, bronchial irritation
Rare
Somnolence, diarrhea, dry mouth, flushing, diaphoresis, anorexia

SERIOUS REACTIONS
• Excessive sympathomimetic stimulation may produce palpitations, extrasystoles, tachycardia, chest pain, a slight increase in B/P followed by a substantial decrease, chills, diaphoresis, and blanching of skin.
• Too-frequent or excessive use may lead to decreased bronchodilating effectiveness and severe, paradoxical bronchoconstriction.

PRECAUTIONS & CONSIDERATIONS
Caution is warranted with cardiovascular disorders (such as arrhythmias), diabetes mellitus, hypertension, and seizures. Levalbuterol crosses the placenta. It is unknown if the drug is distributed in breast milk. The safety and efficacy of levalbuterol have not been established in children younger than 12 years. A lower initial dosage is recommended for the elderly. Drink plenty of fluids to decrease the thickness of lung secretions. Avoid excessive use of caffeinated products, such as chocolate, cocoa, cola, coffee, and tea.

Pulse rate and quality, respiratory rate, depth, rhythm and type, EKG, ABG levels, and serum potassium levels should be monitored.
Storage
Protect the solution from light and excessive heat. Store it at room temperature.

Administration
For nebulization, use the solution within 2 weeks of opening the foil. Discard the solution if it's not colorless. Don't dilute the solution. Don't mix levalbuterol with other medications. Administer levalbuterol over 5 to 15 minutes.

Levetiracetam
leva-tir-ass'eh-tam
(Keppra)
Do not confuse Keppra with Kaletra.

CATEGORY AND SCHEDULE
Pregnancy Risk Category: C

CLASSIFICATION
Anticonvulsants

MECHANISM OF ACTION
An anticonvulsant that inhibits burst firing without affecting normal neuronal excitability. *Therapeutic Effect:* Prevents seizure activity.

AVAILABILITY
Liquid: 100 mg/ml.
Tablets: 250 mg, 500 mg, 750 mg.

INDICATIONS AND DOSAGES
▶ **Partial-onset seizures**
PO
Adults, Elderly. Initially, 500 mg q12hr. May increase by 1000 mg/day q2wk. Maximum: 3000 mg/day.
Children 4-16 yr. 10-20 mg/kg/day in 2 divided doses. May increase at weekly intervals by 10-20 mg/kg. Maximum: 60 mg/kg.

▸ **Dosage in renal impairment**
Dosage is modified based on
creatinine clearance.

Creatinine Clearance (ml/min)	Dosage
Higher than 80 ml/min	500-1500 mg q12hr
50-80 ml/min	500-1000 mg q12hr
30-50 ml/min	250-750 mg q12hr
Less than 30 ml/min	250-500 mg q12hr
End stage renal disease using dialysis	500-1000 mg q12hr, after dialysis, a 250- to 500-mg supplemental dose is recommended

CONTRAINDICATIONS
Hypersensitivity reaction

INTERACTIONS
Drug
None known.
Herbal
None known.
Food
None significant.

DIAGNOSTIC TEST EFFECTS
May increase blood Hgb level,
Hct, and RBC and WBC
counts.

SIDE EFFECTS
Frequent (15%-10%)
Somnolence, asthenia, headache,
infection
Occasional (9%-3%)
Dizziness, pharyngitis, pain, depres-
sion, nervousness, vertigo, rhinitis,
anorexia
Rare (less than 3%)
Amnesia, anxiety, emotional
lability, cough, sinusitis, anorexia,
diplopia

SERIOUS REACTIONS
• None known.

PRECAUTIONS & CONSIDERATIONS
Caution is warranted with renal
impairment. Drowsiness and dizziness may occur, so alcohol and tasks
requiring mental alertness or motor
skills should be avoided. Seizure
disorder, including the onset, duration, frequency, intensity, and type of
seizures, should be assessed before
and during treatment.
Administration
! If the patient is currently taking
valproic acid, expect to reduce the
levetiracetam dosage to less than half
the normal dosage. Be aware that a
decreased dosage may be effective
in patients with significant renal
impairment.
　　Take levetiracetam without regard
to food. Do not discontinue the drug
abruptly after long-term therapy.
Strict maintenance of drug therapy
is essential for seizure control.

Levocabastine
levo-cab'a-steen
(Livostin)

CATEGORY AND SCHEDULE
Pregnancy Risk Category: C

CLASSIFICATION
Antihistamines, H1 ophthalmics

MECHANISM OF ACTION
An antiallergic agent that selectively
antagonizes H1 receptor. *Therapeutic
Effect:* Blocks histamine-associated
symptoms of seasonal allergic
conjunctivitis.

PHARMACOKINETICS
Duration of action is about 2 hours.
Minimal systemic absorption.

L

AVAILABILITY
Ophthalmic Suspension: 0.05%
(Livostin).

INDICATIONS AND DOSAGES
▶ **Allergic conjunctivitis**
OPHTHALMIC
*Adults, Elderly, Children 12 yr or
older.* 1 drop 4 times/day, for up to
2 wk.

CONTRAINDICATIONS
Wearing of soft contact lenses (product contains benzalkonium chloride),
hypersensitivity to levocabastine or
any component of the formulation

INTERACTIONS
Drug
None known.
Herbal
None known.
Food
None known.

DIAGNOSTIC TEST EFFECTS
None known.

SIDE EFFECTS
Frequent
Transient stinging, burning, discom-
fort, headache
Occasional
Dry mouth, fatigue, eye dryness,
lacrimation/discharge, eyelid edema
Rare
Rash, erythema, nausea, dyspnea

SERIOUS REACTIONS
• None reported.

PRECAUTIONS & CONSIDERATIONS
Be aware that levocabastine is for
ophthalmic use only. Not for injection. It is unknown if levocabastine
crosses the placenta or is distributed
in breast milk. Safety and efficacy
of levocabastine has not been established in children younger than

12 years old. There are no age-related
precautions noted in the elderly.
Mild transitory burning and stinging
may occur upon instillation.
Storage
Store at room temperature. Do not
use if suspension is discolored.
Administration
First shake suspension well. Then
place finger on lower eyelid and pull
out until pocket is formed between
eye and lower lid. Hold dropper
above pocket and place prescribed
number of drops in pocket. Close
eyes gently so medication will not be
squeezed out of sac. Apply gentle
finger pressure to the lacrimal sac at
inner canthus for 1 minute following
installation (lessens risk of systemic
absorption). Do not wear soft
contact lenses during therapy.
Therapy may last up to 2 weeks.

Levodopa
lev-oh-dope-ah
(Dopar, Larodopa)

CATEGORY AND SCHEDULE
Pregnancy Risk Category: C

CLASSIFICATION
Antiparkinson agents,
dopaminergics

MECHANISM OF ACTION
A dopamine prodrug that is
converted to dopamine in basal
ganglia. Increases dopamine concentrations in the brain, inhibiting
hyperactive cholinergic activity.
Therapeutic Effect: Decreases signs
and symptoms of Parkinson's disease.

PHARMACOKINETICS
About 30% absorbed. May be
reduced with high-protein meal.

Protein binding: minimal.
Crosses blood-brain barrier.
Converted to dopamine.
Eliminated primarily in urine
and to a lesser amount in feces
and expired air. Not removed by
hemodialysis. **Half-life:** 0.75-1.5 hr.

AVAILABILITY
Capsules: 100 mg, 250 mg, 500 mg
(Dopar).
Tablets: 100 mg, 250 mg, 500 mg
(Larodopa).

INDICATIONS AND DOSAGES
▶ **Parkinsonism**
PO
Adults, Elderly. Initially, 0.5-1 g
2-4 times/day. May increase in
increments not exceeding 0.75 g
every 3-7 days, up to a maximum of
8 g/day.

CONTRAINDICATIONS
Nonselective MAOI therapy,
hypersensitivity to levodopa or
any component of its formulation.

INTERACTIONS
Drug
Alcohol: May increase the risk of
CNS depression.
**Anticonvulsants, benzodiazepines,
bromperidol, droperidol, haloperidol, phenothiazines:** May decrease
the effects of levodopa.
Bupropion: May increase risk
of nausea, vomiting, excitation,
restlessness, and postural tremor.
Cisapride: May increase risk of
levodopa adverse effects.
Ferric ammonium citrate: May
decrease the effects of levodopa.
Indinavir: May increase dyskinesias.
Iron: May decrease the effects of
levodopa.
Isoniazide: May increase symptomatic deterioration of Parkinson's
disease.

MAOIs: May increase risk of
hypertensive crises.
Metoclopramide: May increase
bioavailability and increase incidence
of extrapyramidal symptoms.
Phenytoin: May decrease the
effects of levodopa.
Selegiline: May increase dyskinesias,
nausea, orthostatic hypotension,
confusion, hallucinations.
Herbal
Kava kava: May decrease the
effects of levodopa.
Pyridoxine: May decrease the
effects of levodopa.
Food
High protein meals: May decrease
peak levodopa concentrations.

DIAGNOSTIC TEST EFFECTS
May increase BUN, LDH concentrations, serum alkaline phosphatase
and bilirubin, SGOT (AST), and
SGPT (ALT) levels. May falsely
increase acetaminophen levels. May
result in false positive urine glucose
measurements.

SIDE EFFECTS
Frequent
Uncontrolled body movements
of the face, tongue, arms and
upper body, nausea and vomiting,
anorexia
Occasional
Depression, anxiety, confusion,
nervousness, difficulty urinating,
irregular heartbeats, hiccoughs,
dizziness, lightheadedness,
decreased appetite, blurred vision,
constipation, dry mouth, flushed
skin, headache, insomnia, diarrhea,
unusual tiredness, darkening of
urine, discolored sweat
Rare
Hypertension, ulcer, hemolytic
anemia, marked by tiredness or
weakness.

SERIOUS REACTIONS

• High incidence of involuntary dystonic, and dyskinetic movements may be noted in patients on long-term therapy.

• Mental changes, such as paranoid ideation, psychotic episodes and depression, may be noted.

• Numerous mild to severe central nervous system (CNS) psychiatric disturbances may include reduced attention span, anxiety, nightmares, daytime somnolence, euphoria, fatigue, paranoia, and hallucinations.

PRECAUTIONS & CONSIDERATIONS

Caution is warranted with active peptic ulcer, underlying depression or psychosis, asthma, history of melanoma, concurrent pyridoxine use, diabetes mellitus, history of myocardial infarction (MI), severe cardiac, liver, pulmonary, and renal impairment, and treated open-angle glaucoma. It is unknown if levodopa crosses the placenta or is distributed in breast milk. Know that levodopa may inhibit lactation. Do not breast-feed while taking this drug. Be aware that the safety and efficacy of levodopa have not been established in children younger than 18 years. The elderly are more sensitive to the effects of levodopa and may require lower doses. Alcohol and tasks that require mental alertness or motor skills should be avoided. High protein meals may delay the effects of levodopa.

Clinical reversal of symptoms, such as improvement of masklike facial expression, muscular rigidity, shuffling gait, and resting tremors of hands and head should be assessed. Difficulty urinating, irregular heartbeats, mental changes, severe nausea or vomiting, or uncontrolled movement of arms, eyelids, face, hands, mouth, legs, or tongue should be reported.

Administration

Levodopa should be given with a dopa decarboxylase inhibitor such as carbidopa. In rare cases when one is intolerant to carbidopa, levodopa monotherapy is given. May be given with meals if GI upset occurs but it is preferred to be taken on an empty stomach for best absorption. When discontinuing levodopa therapy, gradually taper dose to prevent the occurrence of a condition resembling neuroleptic malignant syndrome (NMS).

Levofloxacin
levo-flox′a-sin
(Iquix, Levaquin, Quixin)

CATEGORY AND SCHEDULE
Pregnancy Risk Category: C

CLASSIFICATION
Anti-infectives, ophthalmics, antibiotics, quinolones

MECHANISM OF ACTION
A fluoroquinolone that inhibits the enzyme DNA gyrase in susceptible microorganisms, interfering with bacterial cell replication and repair. *Therapeutic Effect:* Bactericidal.

PHARMACOKINETICS
Well absorbed after both PO and IV administration. Protein binding: 8%-24%. Penetrates rapidly and extensively into leukocytes, epithelial cells, and macrophages. Lung concentrations are 2-5 times higher than those of plasma. Eliminated unchanged in the urine. Partially removed by hemodialysis.
Half-life: 8 hr.

AVAILABILITY
Tablets (Levaquin): 250 mg, 500 mg, 750 mg.
Injection (Levaquin): 500-mg/20-ml vials.
Premixed Solution (Levaquin): 250 mg/50 ml, 500 mg/100 ml, 750 mg/150 ml.
Ophthalmic Solution (Quixin): 1.5%
Ophthalmic Solution (Iquix): 0.5%.

INDICATIONS AND DOSAGES
▸ **Bronchitis**
PO, IV
Adults, Elderly. 500 mg q24hr for 7 days.
▸ **Community-acquired pneumonia**
PO
Adults, Elderly. 750 mg/day for 5 days.
▸ **Pneumonia**
PO, IV
Adults, Elderly. 500 mg q24hr for 7-14 days.
▸ **Acute maxillary sinusitis**
PO, IV
Adults, Elderly. 500 mg q24hr for 10-14 days.
▸ **Skin and skin-structure infections**
PO, IV
Adults, Elderly. 500 mg q24hr for 7-10 days.
▸ **UTIs, acute pyelonephritis**
PO, IV
Adults, Elderly. 250 mg q24hr for 10 days.
▸ **Bacterial conjunctivitis**
OPHTHALMIC
Adults, Elderly, Children 1 yr and older. 1-2 drops q2hr for 2 days (up to 8 times a day), then 1-2 drops q4hr for 5 days.
▸ **Corneal ulcer**
OPHTHALMIC
Adults, Elderly, Children older than 5 yr. Days 1-3: Instill 1-2 drops q30min to 2 hours while awake and 4-6 hours after retiring. Days 4 through completion: 1-2 drops q1-4hr while awake.
▸ **Dosage in renal impairment**
For bronchitis, pneumonia, sinusitis, and skin and skin-structure infections, dosage and frequency are modified based on creatinine clearance.

Creatinine Clearance	Dosage
50-80 ml/min	No change
20-49 ml/min	500 mg initially, then 250 mg q24hr
10-19 ml/min	500 mg initially, then 250 mg q48hr

Dialysis 500 mg initially, then 250 mg q48hr
For UTIs and pyelonephritis, dosage and frequency are modified based on creatinine clearance.

Creatinine Clearance	Dosage
20 ml/min	No change
10-19 ml/min	250 mg initially, then 250 mg q48hr

CONTRAINDICATIONS
Hypersensitivity to levofloxacin, other fluoroquinolones, or nalidixic acid

INTERACTIONS
Drug
Antacids, iron preparations, sucralfate, zinc: Decrease levofloxacin absorption.
NSAIDs: May increase the risk of CNS stimulation or seizures.
Herbal
None known.
Food
None known.

DIAGNOSTIC TEST EFFECTS
May alter blood glucose levels.

▨ IV INCOMPATIBILITIES

Furosemide (Lasix), heparin, insulin, nitroglycerin, propofol (Diprivan)

▨ IV Compatibilities

Aminophylline, dobutamine (Dobutrex), dopamine (Intron), fentanyl (Sublimaze), lidocaine, lorazepam (Ativan), morphine

SIDE EFFECTS

Occasional (3%-1%)
Diarrhea, nausea, abdominal pain, dizziness, drowsiness, headache, lightheadedness
Ophthalmic: Local burning or discomfort, margin crusting, crystals or scales, foreign body sensation, ocular itching, altered taste
Rare (less than 1%)
Flatulence; altered taste; pain; inflammation or swelling in calves, hands, or shoulder; chest pain; difficulty breathing; palpitations; edema; tendon pain
Ophthalmic: Corneal staining, keratitis, allergic reaction, eyelid swelling, tearing, reduced visual acuity

SERIOUS REACTIONS

• Antibiotic-associated colitis and other superinfections may occur from altered bacterial balance. Hypersensitivity reactions, including photosensitivity (as evidenced by rash, pruritus, blisters, edema, and burning skin), have occurred in patients receiving fluoroquinolones.

PRECAUTIONS & CONSIDERATIONS

Caution is warranted with bradycardia, cardiomyopathy, hypokalemia, hypomagnesemia, impaired renal function, seizure disorders, or suspected CNS disorder. Levofloxacin is excreted in breast milk and should be avoided during pregnancy. The safety and efficacy of levofloxacin have not been established in children younger than 18 years. Age-related renal impairment may require a dosage adjustment in the elderly.

Chest pain, difficulty breathing, palpitations, edema, tendon pain as well as hypersensitivity reactions, including photosensitivity, pruritus, skin rash, and urticaria, should be reported immediately. Be alert for signs and symptoms of superinfection, such as moderate to severe diarrhea, new or increased fever, and ulceration or changes in the oral mucosa. Symptomatic relief should be provided for nausea. Blood glucose levels, liver and renal function, and white blood cell (WBC) count should be monitored. History of hypersensitivity to levofloxacin and other quinolones should be determined before therapy.

Administration

Take levofloxacin without regard to food. Don't take antacids (containing aluminum or magnesium), sucralfate, iron preparations, or multivitamins containing zinc within 2 hours of levofloxacin because these drugs significantly reduce levofloxacin absorption. Consume citrus fruits and cranberry juice to acidify urine.

For IV use, levofloxacin is available in single-dose 20-ml (500-mg) vials and as a premixed (with D_5W), ready-to-infuse solution. For infusion using the single-dose vial, withdraw the desired amount (10 ml for 250 mg, 20 ml for 500 mg). Dilute each 10 ml (250 mg) with at least 40 ml 0.9% NaCl or D_5W. Administer the drug slowly, over not less than 60 minutes.

For ophthalmic use, place a gloved finger on the lower eyelid, and pull it out until a pocket is formed between the eye and lower lid. Hold the dropper above the pocket, and place the correct number of drops into the pocket. Close the eye gently. Apply digital pressure to the lacrimal sac for 1 to 2 minutes to minimize drainage of the medication into the patient's nose and throat, reducing the risk of systemic effects.

Levonorgestrel
lee-voe-nor-jes'trel
(Ange 28 [JAPAN], duofem [GERMANY], ECEEZ [INDIA], Levonelle [NEW ZEALAND], Microlut [COLOMBIA], Microval [COLOMBIA], Mirena [CHINA, COLOMBIA, GERMANY, HONG KONG, ISRAEL, KOREA, PHILIPPINES, SOUTH AFRICA, THAILAND], Norlevo [FRANCE, SOUTH AFRICA], Norplant, Norplant 36 [ISRAEL], Plan B, Postinor-2 [ISRAEL, NEW ZEALAND, SINGAPORE], Vikela [FRANCE])

CATEGORY AND SCHEDULE
Pregnancy Risk Category: X

CLASSIFICATION
Contraceptives, hormones/ hormone modifiers, progestins

MECHANISM OF ACTION
A contraceptive hormone that causes thickening of cervical mucus, inhibition of ovulation and inhibition of implantation. *Therapeutic Effect:* Prevents ovulation or fertilization.

PHARMACOKINETICS
Levonorgestrel is rapidly and completely absorbed after oral administration. Maximum serum concentrations of approximately 15 ng/ml occur at an average of 2 hours. Does not appear to be extensively metabolized by the liver. Protein binding: 97.5%.

Primarily excreted in the urine, with smaller amounts recovered in the feces.

AVAILABILITY
Tablet: 0.75 mg
Intrauterine: 20 mcg/day

INDICATIONS AND DOSAGES
▸ **Long-term prevention of pregnancy**
INTRAUTERINE
Adults, Elderly: Insert 1 system into uterine cavity within 7 days of onset of menstruation or immediately after first trimester abortion. Releases 20 mcg levonorgestrel daily over 5 years.
▸ **Emergency contraception**
PO
Adults, Elderly. One 0.75 mg tablet as soon as possible within 72 hours of unprotected sexual intercourse. A second 0.75 mg tablet 12 hours after the first dose.

CONTRAINDICATIONS
Active thrombophlebitis or thromboembolic disorders, undiagnosed abnormal genital bleeding, known or suspected pregnancy, acute liver disease; benign or malignant liver tumors, known or suspected carcinoma of the breast, history of idiopathic intracranial hypertension, hypersensitivity to levonorgestrel or any of the components of the levonorgestrel implants.

INTERACTIONS
Drug
CYP3A4 inducers: May decrease effects of levonorgestrel.
Phenytoin, Carbamazepine: May decrease efficacy of levonorgestrel through increased metabolism.

Herbal
St. John's wort: May decrease levonorgestrel serum levels.
Food
None known.

DIAGNOSTIC TEST EFFECTS
Decreased concentrations of sex hormone-binding globulin; decreased thyroxine concentrations; increased triiodothyronine uptake.

SIDE EFFECTS
Occassional
Hypertension, headache, depression, nervousness, breast pain, dysmenorrheal, decreased libidoabdominal pain, nausea, weight gain, leucorrhea, vaginitis.
Rare
Alopecia, anemia, cervicitis, dyspareunia, eczema, failed insertion, migraine, sepsis, vomiting.

SERIOUS REACTIONS
• None known.

PRECAUTIONS & CONSIDERATIONS
Caution is necessary with coagulopathy or concomitant anticoagulant use, vaginitis or cervicitis, valvular or congenital heart disease and surgically constructed systemic-pulmonary shunts, conditions aggravated by fluid retention, diabetes mellitus, and a history of mental depression. Levonorgestrel is contraindicated in pregnancy and is in breast milk and may be harmful to fetus. Levonorgestrel should not be used during breast-feeding. Safety and efficacy of this drug have not been established in children. There are no age-related precautions noted in the elderly. Avoid smoking while taking levonorgestrel.

Menstrual spotting may occur between periods. Pain, redness, swelling, or warmth in the calf, chest pain, migraine headache, peripheral paresthesia, sudden decrease in vision, and sudden shortness of breath should be reported immediately.

Storage
Store at room temepature away from heat and moisture.
Administration
As post-coital contraception, take tablets as soon as possible within 72 hours after unprotected intercourse. The second dose must be taken 12 hours later.

Usually, one set of six implants is surgically inserted every 5 years. Do not insert intrauterine device until 6 weeks postpartum or until involution of the uterus is complete.

Levorphanol
lee-vor′fa-nole
(Levo-Dromoran)

CATEGORY AND SCHEDULE
Pregnancy Risk Category: C
Controlled substance: Schedule II

CLASSIFICATION
Analgesics, narcotic

MECHANISM OF ACTION
An opioid agonist that binds at opiate receptor sites in central nervous system (CNS). *Therapeutic Effect:* Reduced intensity of pain stimuli incoming from sensory nerve endings, altering pain perception and emotional response to pain.

PHARMACOKINETICS
Rapidly absorbed. Protein binding: 40%-50%. Extensively distributed. Metabolized in liver. Excreted in urine. **Half-life:** 11 hr.

AVAILABILITY
Tablets: 2 mg (Levo-Dromoran).
Injection: 2 mg/ml (Levo-Dromoran).

INDICATIONS AND DOSAGES
▶ **Pain**
PO
Adults, Elderly. 2 mg. May be increased to 3 mg, if needed.
IM/SUBCUTANEOUS
Adults, Elderly. 1-2 mg as a single dose. May repeat in 6-8 hr as needed. Maximum: 3-8 mg/day.
IV
Adults. Up to 1 mg injection in divided doses. May repeat in 3-6 hr as needed. Maximum: 4-8 mg/day.
▶ **Preoperative**
IM/SUBCUTANEOUS
Adults, Elderly. 1-2 mg as a single dose 60-90 min before surgery.

CONTRAINDICATIONS
Hypersensitivity to levorphanol or any component of the formulation

INTERACTIONS
Drug
Alcohol, central nervous system (CNS) depressants: May increase CNS or respiratory depression, and hypotension.
MAOIs: May produce severe, fatal reaction unless dosage reduced by one quarter.
Herbal
None known.
Food
None known.

DIAGNOSTIC TEST EFFECTS
May increase serum amylase and lipase levels.

SIDE EFFECTS
Effects are dependent on dosage amount, route of administration. Ambulatory patients and those not in severe pain may experience dizziness, nausea, vomiting, hypotension more frequently than those in supine position or having severe pain
Frequent
Dizziness, drowsiness, hypotension, nausea, vomiting
Occasional
Shortness of breath, confusion, decreased urination, stomach cramps, altered vision, constipation, dry mouth, headache, difficult or painful urination
Rare
Allergic reaction (rash, itching), histamine reaction (decreased B/P, increased sweating, flushed face, wheezing)

SERIOUS REACTIONS
• Overdosage results in respiratory depression, skeletal muscle flaccidity, cold clammy skin, cyanosis, extreme somnolence progressing to convulsions, stupor, coma.
• Tolerance to analgesic effect, physical dependence may occur with repeated use.
• Paralytic ileus may occur with prolonged use.

PRECAUTIONS & CONSIDERATIONS
Extreme caution should be used with acute alcoholism, anoxia, central nervous system (CNS) depression, hypercapnia, respiratory depression, respiratory dysfunction, seizures, shock, and untreated myxedema. Caution is also warranted with acute abdominal conditions, Addison's disease, chronic obstructive pulmonary disease (COPD), hypothyroidism, impaired liver function, increased intracranial pressure, prostatic hypertrophy, and urethral stricture; be aware to expect to reduce the initial dosage in these conditions.

Vital signs should be taken before giving medication. If respirations are 12/min or lower (20/min or lower in children), withhold medication, contact physician. Vital signs should be monitored after administration as well.

Be aware that ambulatory persons and those not in severe pain may experience dizziness, hypotension, nausea, and vomiting more frequently than persons in the supine position or with severe pain. Avoid alcohol and tasks that require mental alertness or motor skills. Change positions slowly to avoid orthostatic hypotension.

Storage
Store at room temperature.

Administration
Dosage should be individualized based on degree of pain and physical condition of the person. May be administered IV, IM, or subcutaneous.

Levothyroxine
lee-voe-thye-rox′een
(Droxine [AUS], Eltroxin [CAN], Eutroxsig [AUS], Levothroid, Levoxyl, Novothyrox [CAN], Oroxine [AUS], Synthroid, Unithroid)
Do not confuse levothyroxine with liothyronine.

CATEGORY AND SCHEDULE
Pregnancy Risk Category: A

CLASSIFICATION
Hormones/hormone modifiers, thyroid agents

MECHANISM OF ACTION
A synthetic isomer of thyroxine involved in normal metabolism, growth, and development, especially of the CNS in infants. Possesses catabolic and anabolic effects.
Therapeutic Effect: Increases basal metabolic rate, enhances gluconeogenesis and stimulates protein synthesis.

PHARMACOKINETICS
Variable, incomplete absorption from the GI tract. Protein binding: 99%. Widely distributed. Deiodinated in peripheral tissues, minimal metabolism in the liver. Eliminated by biliary excretion.
Half-life: 6-7 days.

AVAILABILITY
Tablets (Levo-T, Levothroid, Levoxyl, Synthroid, Unithroid): 0.025 mg, 0.05 mg, 0.075 mg, 0.088 mg, 0.1 mg, 0.112 mg, 0.125 mg, 0.137 mg, 0.15 mg, 0.175 mg, 0.2 mg, 0.3 mg.
Injection (Synthroid): 200 mcg, 500 mcg.

INDICATIONS AND DOSAGES
▸ **Hypothyroidism**
PO
Adults, Elderly. Initially,
12.5-50 mcg. May increase by
25-50 mcg/day q2-4wk.
Maintenance: 100-200 mcg/day.
Children 13 yr and older.
150 mcg/day.
Children 6-12 yr. 100-125 mcg/day.
Children 1-5 yr. 75-100 mcg/day.
Children 7-11 mo. 50-75 mcg/day.
Children 3-6 mo. 25-50 mcg/day.
Children 3 mo and younger.
10-15 mcg/day.
▸ **Thyroid suppression therapy**
PO
Adults, Elderly. 2-6 mcg/kg/day for
7-10 days.
▸ **Thyroid stimulating hormone
suppression in thyroid cancer,
nodules, euthyroid goiters**
PO
Adults, Elderly. 2-6 mcg/kg/day for
7-10 days.
IV
Adults, Elderly, Children. Initial
dosage approximately half the
previously established oral
dosage.

CONTRAINDICATIONS
Hypersensitivity to tablet components, such as tartrazine; allergy
to aspirin; lactose intolerance; MI
and thyrotoxicosis uncomplicated
by hypothyroidism; treatment of
obesity

INTERACTIONS
Drug
Cholestyramine, colestipol: May
decrease the absorption of levothyroxine.
Oral anticoagulants: May alter the
effects of oral anticoagulants
Sympathomimetics: May increase
the risk of coronary insufficiency
and the effects of levothyroxine.

Herbal
None known.
Food
None known.

DIAGNOSTIC TEST EFFECTS
None known.

▨ IV INCOMPATIBILITIES
Do not use or mix with other IV
solutions.

SIDE EFFECTS
Occasional
Reversible hair loss at the start of
therapy (in children)
Rare
Dry skin, GI intolerance, rash, hives,
pseudotumor cerebri or severe
headache in children

SERIOUS REACTIONS
• Excessive dosage produces signs
and symptoms of hyperthyroidism,
including weight loss, palpitations,
increased appetite, tremors, nervousness, tachycardia, hypertension,
headache, insomnia, and menstrual
irregularities.
• Cardiac arrhythmias occur rarely.

PRECAUTIONS & CONSIDERATIONS
Caution is warranted with angina
pectoris, hypertension, other cardiovascular disease, and in the elderly.
Levothyroxine does not cross the
placenta and is minimally excreted
in breast milk. No age-related
precautions have been noted in children. Use caution in interpreting
thyroid function tests in neonates.
The elderly may be more sensitive to
thyroid effects. Individualized
dosages are recommended for this
population.
Reversible hair loss or increased
aggressiveness may occur during
the first few months of therapy.
Notify the physician of chest pain,

insomnia, nervousness, tremors, weight loss, or a pulse rate of 100 beats/minute or more. Weight and vital signs, especially pulse rate and rhythm, should be monitored. Keep in mind levothyroxine may intensify the signs and symptoms of adrenal insufficiency, diabetes insipidus, diabetes mellitus, and hypopituitarism. Also, know that adrenocortical steroids should be prescribed before thyroid therapy in persons with coexisting hypoadrenalism and hypothyroidism.

Storage
Store vials at room temperature.

Administration
! Do not use different brands of levothyroxine interchangeably because of problems with bioequivalence among manufacturers. Begin therapy with small doses and increase the dosage gradually, as prescribed.

Take oral levothyroxine at same time each day to maintain hormone levels. Take before breakfast to prevent insomnia. Full therapeutic effect of the drug may take 1 to 3 weeks to appear. Crush tablets, as needed. Do not discontinue this drug; replacement therapy for hypothyroidism is life-long.

For IV use, reconstitute 200- or 500-mcg vial with 5 ml 0.9% NaCl to provide a concentration of 40 or 100 mcg/ml, respectively; shake until clear. Use immediately, and discard unused portion. Give each 100 mcg or less over 1 minute.

Lidocaine (Systemic)
lye′doe-kane
(Lidoderm, Lignocaine Gel [AUS], Xylocaine, Xylocaine Aerosol [AUS], Xylocaine Ointment [AUS], Xylocaine Viscous Topical Solution [AUS], Xylocard [CAN], Zilactin-L [CAN])

CATEGORY AND SCHEDULE
Pregnancy Risk Category: B

CLASSIFICATION
Anesthetics, local, topical, antiarrhythmics, class IB, dermatologics

MECHANISM OF ACTION
An amide anesthetic that inhibits conduction of nerve impulses. *Therapeutic Effect:* Causes temporary loss of feeling and sensation. Also an antiarrhythmic that decreases depolarization, automaticity, excitability of the ventricle during diastole by direct action. *Therapeutic Effect:* Inhibits ventricular arrhythmias.

PHARMACOKINETICS

Route	Onset	Peak	Duration
IV	30-90 sec	N/A	10-20 min
Local anesthetic	2.5 min	N/A	30-60 min

Completely absorbed after IM administration. Protein binding: 60% to 80%. Widely distributed. Metabolized in the liver. Primarily excreted in urine. Minimally removed by hemodialysis.
Half-life: 1-2 hr.

AVAILABILITY
IM Injection: 300 mg/3 ml.
Direct IV Injection: 10 mg/ml,
20 mg/ml.
IV Admixture Injection: 40 mg/ml,
100 mg/ml, 200 mg/ml.
IV Infusion: 2 mg/ml, 4 mg/ml,
8 mg/ml.
Injection (anesthesia): 0.5%, 1%,
1.5%, 2%, 4%.
Liquid: 2.5%, 5%.
Ointment: 2.5%, 5%.
Cream: 0.5%.
Gel: 0.5%, 2.5%.
Topical Spray: 0.5%.
Topical Solution: 2%, 4%.
Topical Jelly: 2%.
Dermal Patch: 5%.

INDICATIONS AND DOSAGES
▸ **Rapid control of acute ventricular arrhythmias after an MI, cardiac catheterization, cardiac surgery, or digitalis-induced ventricular arrhythmias**
IM
Adults, Elderly. 300 mg (or
4.3 mg/kg). May repeat in
60-90 min.
IV
Adults, Elderly. Initially, 50-100 mg
(1 mg/kg) IV bolus at rate of
25-50 mg/min. May repeat in 5 min.
Give no more than 200-300 mg in
1 hr. Maintenance: 20-50 mcg/
kg/min (1-4 mg/min) as IV infusion.
Children, Infants. Initially,
0.5-1 mg/kg IV bolus; may repeat
but total dose not to exceed
3-5 mg/kg. Maintenance: 10-50 mcg/
kg/min as IV infusion.
▸ **Dental or surgical procedures, childbirth**
Infiltration or nerve block
Adults. Local anesthetic dosage
varies with procedure, degree of
anesthesia, vascularity, duration.
Maximum dose: 4.5 mg/kg. Do not
repeat within 2 hr.

▸ **Local skin disorders (minor burns, insect bites, prickly heat, skin manifestations of chickenpox, abrasions), and mucous membrane disorders (local anesthesia of oral, nasal, and laryngeal mucous membranes; local anesthesia of respiratory, urinary tract; relief of discomfort of pruritus ani, hemorrhoids, pruritus vulvae)**
TOPICAL
Adults, Elderly. Apply to affected
areas as needed.
▸ **Treatment of shingles-related skin pain**
TOPICAL (DERMAL PATCH)
Adults, Elderly. Apply to intact skin
over most painful area (up to 3 applications once for up to 12 hr in a
24-hr period).

CONTRAINDICATIONS
Adams-Stokes syndrome,
hypersensitivity to amide-type
local anesthetics, septicemia
(spinal anesthesia), supraventricular
arrhythmias, Wolff-Parkinson-White
syndrome

INTERACTIONS
Drug
Anticonvulsants: May increase
cardiac depressant effects.
Beta-adrenergic blockers: May
increase risk of toxicity.
Other antiarrhythmics: May
increase cardiac effects.
Herbal
None known.
Food
None known.

DIAGNOSTIC TEST EFFECTS
IM lidocaine may increase
creatine kinase level (used to
diagnose acute MI). Therapeutic
blood level is 1.5 to 6 mcg/ml;
toxic blood level is greater than
6 mcg/ml.

▓ IV INCOMPATIBILITIES

Amphotericin B complex (Abelcet, AmBisome, Amphotec), thiopental

▓ IV Compatibilities

Aminophylline, amiodarone (Cordarone), calcium gluconate, digoxin (Lanoxin), diltiazem (Cardizem), dobutamine (Dobutrex), dopamine (Intropin), enalapril (Vasotec), furosemide (Lasix), heparin, insulin, nitroglycerin, potassium chloride

SIDE EFFECTS

CNS effects are generally dose-related and of short duration.

Occasional

IM: Pain at injection site
Topical: Burning, stinging, tenderness at application site

Rare

Generally with high dose:
Drowsiness; dizziness; disorientation; lightheadedness; tremors; apprehension; euphoria; sensation of heat, cold, or numbness; blurred or double vision; ringing or roaring in ears (tinnitus); nausea

SERIOUS REACTIONS

• Although serious adverse reactions to lidocaine are uncommon, high dosage by any route may produce cardiovascular depression, bradycardia, hypotension, arrhythmias, heart block, cardiovascular collapse, and cardiac arrest.

• Potential for malignant hyperthermia.

• CNS toxicity may occur, especially with regional anesthesia use, progressing rapidly from mild side effects to tremors, somnolence, seizures, vomiting, and respiratory depression.

• Methemoglobinemia (evidenced by cyanosis) has occurred following topical application of lidocaine for teething discomfort and laryngeal anesthetic spray.

PRECAUTIONS & CONSIDERATIONS

Caution is warranted with atrial fibrillation, bradycardia, heart block, hypovolemia, liver disease, marked hypoxia, and severe respiratory depression. Be aware that lidocaine crosses the placenta and is distributed in breast milk. There are no age-related precautions noted in children. The elderly are more sensitive to the adverse effects of lidocaine. Lidocaine dose and rate of infusion should be reduced in the elderly. In the elderly, age-related renal impairment may require dosage adjustment. Chewing gum, drinking, or eating for 1 hour after oral mucous membrane lidocaine application should be avoided; the swallowing reflex may be impaired, increasing risk of aspiration, and numbness of tongue or buccal mucosa may lead to trauma.

A loss of feeling or sensation will occur, and patients will need protection from trauma until anesthetic wears off. Hypersensitivity to amide anesthetics and lidocaine should be determined before beginning drug therapy. B/P, pulse, respirations, EKG, and serum electrolytes should be obtained at baseline and periodically thereafter.

Storage

Store at room temperature.

Administration

! Keep resuscitative equipment and drugs, including O_2, readily available when administering lidocaine by any route. Know that lidocaine's therapeutic serum level is 1.5-6 mcg/ml and the toxic serum level is greater than 6 mcg/ml.

For IM administration, use 10% (100 mg/ml) and clearly identify that the lidocaine preparation. Give injection in deltoid muscle because the blood level will be significantly higher than if the injection is given in gluteus muscle or lateral thigh. For transdermal use, may cut patch to size before removing adhesive backing.

! Use only lidocaine without preservative, clearly marked for IV use.

For IV infusion, prepare solution by adding 1 g to 1 L D₅W to provide concentration of 1 mg/ml (0.1%). Know that commercially available preparations of 0.2%, 0.4%, and 0.8% may be used for IV infusion. Be aware that the maximum concentration is 4 g/250 ml. For IV push, use 1% (10 mg/ml) or 2% (20 mg/ml). Administer IV push at rate of 25 to 50 mg/min. Administer for IV infusion at rate of 1 to 4 mg/min (1 to 4 ml) and use a volume control IV set.

For topical use, be aware that this form is not for ophthalmic use. For skin disorders, apply directly to affected area or put on a gauze or bandage, which is then applied to the skin. For mucous membrane use, apply to desired area as per manufacturer's insert. Administer the lowest dosage possible that still provides anesthesia.

Lindane (Gamma Benzene Hexachloride)

lin′dane
(Lindane, Hexit [CAN], PMS-Lindane [CAN])
Do not confuse lidocaine.

CATEGORY AND SCHEDULE
Pregnancy Risk Category: B

CLASSIFICATION
Anti-infectives, topical, dermatologics, scabicides/pediculicides

MECHANISM OF ACTION
A scabicidal agent that is directly absorbed by parasites and ova through the exoskeleton. *Therapeutic Effect:* Stimulates the nervous system resulting in seizures and death of parasitic arthropods.

PHARMACOKINETICS
May be absorbed systemically. Metabolized in liver. Excreted in the urine and feces. **Half-life:** 17-22 hr.

AVAILABILITY
Lotion: 1% (Lindane).
Shampoo: 1% (Lindane).

INDICATIONS AND DOSAGES
▶ **Treatment of scabies**
TOPICAL
Adults, Elderly, Children. Apply thin layer. Massage on skin from neck to the toes. Bathe and remove drug after 8-12 hr.
▶ **Head lice, crab lice**
TOPICAL
Adults, Elderly, Children. Apply about 30 ml of shampoo to dry hair and massage into hair for 4 min. Add small amounts of water to hair until lather forms, then rinse hair thoroughly and comb with a fine-tooth comb to remove nits.
Maximum: 60 ml of shampoo.

CONTRAINDICATIONS
Hypersensitivity to lindane or any component of the formulation, uncontrolled seizure disorders, crusted (Norwegian) scabies, acutely-inflamed skin or raw, weeping surfaces, or other skin conditions which may increase systemic absorption

INTERACTIONS
Drug
None known.

L

Herbal
None known.
Food
None known.

DIAGNOSTIC TEST EFFECTS
None known.

SIDE EFFECTS
Rare (less than 1%)
Burning, stinging, cardiac arrhythmia, ataxia, dizziness, headache, restlessness, seizures, pain, alopecia, contact dermatitis, skin and adipose tissue may act as repositories, eczematous eruptions, pruritus, urticaria, nausea, vomiting, aplastic anemia, hepatitis, paresthesias, hematuria, pulmonary edema

SERIOUS REACTIONS
• Seizures rarely occur.

PRECAUTIONS & CONSIDERATIONS
Lindane is second-line choice because of the potential for systemic absorption and CNS side effects. Caution should be used in people taking medications for seizures. It is unknown if lindane is excreted in breast milk. Avoid using on infants. There are no age-related precautions noted in the elderly. Clothing and bedding should be washed in hot water or by dry cleaning to kill the scabies mite.
Administration
Apply lotion immediately after a hot, soapy bath. Skin should be clean and free of any lotions, creams, or oils prior to lindane application. Apply a thin layer and massage onto clean, dry skin from the neck to the toes. Wait at least 8-12 hours after bathing or showering. Avoid contact with eyes or face.
Apply shampoo to clean, dry hair. Wait at least 1 hour after washing hair before applying lindane shampoo. Hair should be washed with a shampoo not containing conditioner. Hair should be free of any lotions, oils, or creams prior to lindane application.

Linezolid
li-nee′zoh-lid
(Zyvox, Zyvoxam)
Do not confuse Zoverax or Vioxx.

CATEGORY AND SCHEDULE
Pregnancy Risk Category: C

CLASSIFICATION
Antibiotics, oxalodinones

MECHANISM OF ACTION
An oxalodinone anti-infective that binds to a site on bacterial 23S ribosomal RNA, preventing the formation of a complex that is essential for bacterial translation. *Therapeutic Effect:* Bacteriostatic against enterococci and staphylococci; bactericidal against streptococci.

PHARMACOKINETICS
Rapidly and extensively absorbed after PO administration. Protein binding: 31%. Metabolized in the liver by oxidation. Excreted in urine. **Half-life:** 4-5.4 hr.

AVAILABILITY
Powder for Oral Suspension: 100 mg/5 ml.
Tablets: 400 mg, 600 mg.
Injection: 2 mg/ml in 100-ml, 200-ml, 300-ml bags.

INDICATIONS AND DOSAGES
▸ **Vancomycin-resistant infections**
PO, IV
Adults, Elderly, Children older

than 11 yr. 600 mg q12hr for
14-28 days.
▸ **Pneumonia, complicated skin and
skin structure infections**
PO, IV
*Adults, Elderly, Children older than
11 yr.* 600 mg q12hr for 10-14 days.
▸ **Uncomplicated skin and skin
structure infections**
PO
Adults, Elderly. 400 mg q12hr for
10-14 days.
Children older than 11 yr. 600 mg
q12hr for 10-14 days.
Children 5-11 yr. 10 mg/kg/dose
q12hr for 10-14 days.
▸ **Usual neonate dosage**
PO, IV
Neonates. 10 mg/kg/dose q8-12hr.

CONTRAINDICATIONS
None known.

INTERACTIONS
Drug
**Adrenergic agents (sympathomimet-
ics):** Increase the effects of linezolid.
MAOIs: Decrease the effects of
MAOIs.
Herbal
None known.
Food
**Tyramine-containing foods and
beverages:** Excessive amounts may
cause significant hypertension.

DIAGNOSTIC TEST EFFECTS
May decrease blood Hgb, platelet
count, WBC count, and ALT (SGPT)
levels.

▦ IV INCOMPATIBILITIES
Amphotericin B complex (Abelcet,
AmBisome, Amphotec), chlorpro-
mazine (Thorazine), co-trimoxazole
(Bactrim), diazepam (Valium),
erythromycin (Erythrocin), pentami-
dine (Pentam IV), phenytoin
(Dilantin)

SIDE EFFECTS
Occasional (5%-2%)
Diarrhea, nausea, headache
Rare (less than 2%)
Altered taste, vaginal candidiasis,
fungal infection, dizziness, tongue
discoloration

SERIOUS REACTIONS
• Thrombocytopenia and myelosuppression occur rarely.
• Antibiotic-associated colitis and
other superinfections may result
from altered bacterial balance.

PRECAUTIONS & CONSIDERATIONS
Caution is warranted with carcinoid
syndrome, pheochromocytoma,
severe renal or hepatic impairment,
uncontrolled hypertension, or
untreated hyperthyroidism. It is
unknown if linezolid is distributed in
breast milk. The safety and efficacy
of linezolid have not been established
in children. No age-related precautions have been noted in the elderly.
Avoid excessive amounts of tyramine-
containing foods (such as aged
cheese and red wine) as these foods
may cause severe reactions including
diaphoresis, neck stiffness, palpitations, and severe headache.
Mild GI effects may be tolerable,
but severe symptoms may indicate the
onset of antibiotic-associated colitis.
Pattern of daily bowel activity and
stool consistency should be monitored. Be alert for signs and symptoms of superinfection, including
abdominal pain, moderate to severe
diarrhea, severe anal or genital pruritus, and severe mouth soreness. CBC
should be monitored weekly.
Storage
Use the oral suspension within
21 days of reconstitution. Store the
drug at room temperature and
protect it from light. A yellow color
does not affect potency.

L

Administration
Take linezolid without regard to food. May take with food or milk if GI upset occurs. Space drug doses evenly around the clock and continue linezolid therapy for the full course of treatment.
! Don't mix linezolid for IV use with other medications. If the same line is used to administer another drug, flush it with a compatible fluid (D$_5$W, 0.9% NaCl, lactated Ringer's). Infuse the drug over 30 to 120 minutes.

Liothyronine T$_3$
lye-oh-thye′roe-neen
(Cytomel, Tertroxin [AUS], Triostat)
Do not confuse liothyronine with levothyroxine.

CATEGORY AND SCHEDULE
Pregnancy Risk Category: A

CLASSIFICATION
Hormones/hormone modifiers, thyroid agents

MECHANISM OF ACTION
A synthetic form of triiodothyronine (T$_3$), a thyroid hormone involved in normal metabolism, growth, and development, especially of the CNS in infants. Possesses catabolic and anabolic effects.
Therapeutic Effect: Increases basal metabolic rate, enhances gluconeogenesis, and stimulates protein synthesis.

AVAILABILITY
Tablets (Cytomel): 5 mcg, 25 mcg, 50 mcg.
Injection (Triostat): 10 mcg/ml.

INDICATIONS AND DOSAGES
▸ **Hypothyroidism**
PO
Adults, Elderly. Initially, 25 mcg/day. May increase in increments of 12.5-25 mcg/day q1-2wk. Maximum: 100 mcg/day.
Children. Initially, 5 mcg/day. May increase by 5 mcg/day q3-4wk. Maintenance: 100 mcg/day (children older than 3 yr); 50 mcg/day (children 1-3 yr); 20 mcg/day (infants).
▸ **Myxedema**
PO
Adults, Elderly. Initially, 5 mcg/day. Increase by 5-10 mcg q1-2wk (after 25 mcg/day has been reached, may increase in 12.5-mcg increments). Maintenance: 50-100 mcg/day.
▸ **Nontoxic goiter**
PO
Adults, Elderly. Initially, 5 mcg/day. Increase by 5-10 mcg/day q1-2wk. When 25 mcg/day has been reached, may increase by 12.5-25 mcg/day q1-2wk. Maintenance: 75 mcg/day.
Children. 5 mcg/day. May increase by 5 mcg q1-2wk. Maintenance: 15-20 mcg/day.
▸ **Congenital hypothyroidism**
PO
Children. Initially, 5 mcg/day. Increase by 5 mcg/day q3-4 days. Maintenance: Full adult dosage (children older than 3 yr); 50 mcg/day (children 1-3 yr); 20 mcg/day (infants).
▸ **T$_3$ suppression test**
PO
Adults, Elderly. 75-100 mcg/day for 7 days; then repeat I^{131} thyroid uptake test.

▶ **Myxedema coma, precoma**
IV
Adults, Elderly. Initially, 25-50 mcg (10-20 mcg in patients with cardiovascular disease). Total dose at least 65 mcg/day.

CONTRAINDICATIONS
MI and thyrotoxicosis uncomplicated by hypothyroidism; obesity

INTERACTIONS
Drug
Cholestyramine, colestipol: May decrease the absorption of liothyronine.
Oral anticoagulants: May alter the effects of these drugs.
Sympathomimetics: May increase the risk of coronary insufficiency and the effects of liothyronine.
Herbal
None known.
Food
None known.

DIAGNOSTIC TEST EFFECTS
None known.

SIDE EFFECTS
Occasional
Reversible hair loss at start of therapy (in children)
Rare
Dry skin, GI intolerance, rash, hives, pseudotumor cerebri or severe headache in children

SERIOUS REACTIONS
• Excessive dosage produces signs and symptoms of hyperthyroidism, including weight loss, palpitations, increased appetite, tremors, nervousness, tachycardia, hypertension, headache, insomnia, and menstrual irregularities.
• Cardiac arrhythmias occur rarely.

PRECAUTIONS & CONSIDERATIONS
Caution is warranted with adrenal insufficiency, cardiovascular disease, coronary artery disease, diabetes insipidus, and diabetes mellitus. Liothyronine does not cross the placenta and is minimally excreted in breast milk. No age-related precautions have been noted in children. Use caution in interpreting thyroid function test results in neonates. The elderly may be more sensitive to thyroid effects. Individualized dosages are recommended for this population. Reversible hair loss or increased aggressiveness may occur during the first few months of therapy. Notify the physician of chest pain, insomnia, nervousness, tremors, weight loss, or a pulse rate of 100 beats/ minute or more. Weight and vital signs, especially pulse rate and rhythm, should be monitored. Keep in mind liothyronine may intensify the signs and symptoms of adrenal insufficiency, diabetes insipidus, diabetes mellitus, and hypopituitarism. Also, know that adrenocortical steroids should be prescribed before thyroid therapy in persons with coexisting hypoadrenalism and hypothyroidism.
Administration
! Initial and subsequent dosages are based on the clinical status and response. Do not use different brands of liothyronine interchangeably because of problems with bioequivalence among manufacturers.
    Take at the same time each day, preferably in the morning. Do not abruptly discontinue the drug; replacement therapy for hypothyroidism is life-long.
    Administer IV dose over 4 hours but no longer than 12 hours apart.

Lisinopril

ly-sin'oh-pril
(Apo-Lisinopril [CAN], Fibsol
[AUS], Lisodur [AUS], Prinivil,
Zestril)
**Do not confuse with Desyrel,
fosinopril, Lioresal, Plendil,
Prilosec, Proventil, Restoril, or
Zostrix.**

CATEGORY AND SCHEDULE

Pregnancy Risk Category: C
(D if used in second or third
trimester)

CLASSIFICATION

Angiotensin converting enzyme
inhibitors

MECHANISM OF ACTION

This angiotensin-converting
enzyme (ACE) inhibitor suppresses
the renin-angiotensin-aldosterone
system and prevents conversion of
angiotensin I to angiotensin II, a
potent vasoconstrictor; may also
inhibit angiotensin II at local
vascular and renal sites.
Decreases plasma angiotensin II,
increases plasma renin activity,
and decreases aldosterone
secretion. *Therapeutic Effect:*
Reduces peripheral arterial resistance, blood pressure (B/P), afterload, pulmonary capillary wedge
pressure (preload), pulmonary
vascular resistance. In those
with heart failure, also
decreases heart size, increases
cardiac output, and exercise
tolerance time.

PHARMACOKINETICS

Route	Onset	Peak	Duration
PO	1 hr	6 hr	24 hr

Incompletely absorbed from
the gastrointestinal (GI) tract.
Protein binding: 25%. Primarily
excreted unchanged in urine.
Removed by hemodialysis.
Half-life: 12 hr (half-life is
prolonged in those with impaired
renal function).

AVAILABILITY

Tablets (Prinivil, Zestril): 2.5 mg,
5 mg, 10 mg, 20 mg, 30 mg,
40 mg.

INDICATIONS AND DOSAGES

▶ **Hypertension (used alone)**
PO
Adults. Initially, 10 mg/day.
May increase by 5-10 mcg/day at
1-2 wk intervals. Maximum:
40 mg/day.
Elderly. Initially, 2.5-5 mg/day.
May increase by 2.5-5 mg/day at
1- to 2-wk intervals. Maximum:
40 mg/day.
▶ **Hypertension (used in
combination with other
antihypertensives)**
PO
Adults. Initially, 2.5-5 mg/day
titrated to patient's needs.
▶ **Adjunctive therapy for management
of heart failure**
PO
Adults, Elderly. Initially,
2.5-5 mg/day. May increase by no
more than 10 mg/day at intervals
of at least 2 wk. Maintenance:
5-40 mg/day.
▶ **Improve survival in patients
after a myocardial
infarction (MI)**
PO
Adults, Elderly. Initially, 5 mg, then
5 mg after 24 hr, 10 mg after 48 hr,
then 10 mg/day for 6 wk. For
patients with low systolic B/P, give
2.5 mg/day for 3 days, then
2.5-5 mg/day.

▶ **Dosage in renal impairment**
Titrate to patient's needs after giving the following initial dose:

Creatinine Clearance	% Normal Dose
10-50 ml/min	50-75
Less than 10 ml/min	25-50

OFF-LABEL USES
Treatment of hypertension or renal crises with scleroderma

CONTRAINDICATIONS
History of angioedema from previous treatment with ACE inhibitors

INTERACTIONS
Drug
Alcohol, diuretics, hypotensive agents: May increase the effects of lisinopril.
Lithium: May increase lithium blood concentration and risk of toxicity.
NSAIDs: May decrease the effects of lisinopril.
Potassium-sparing diuretics, potassium supplements: May cause hyperkalemia.
Herbal
None known.
Food
None known.

DIAGNOSTIC TEST EFFECTS
May increase BUN, serum alkaline phosphatase, serum bilirubin, serum creatinine, serum potassium, SGOT (AST), and SGPT (ALT) levels. May decrease serum sodium levels. May cause positive ANA titer.

SIDE EFFECTS
Frequent (12%-5%)
Headache, dizziness, postural hypotension

Occasional (4%-2%)
Chest discomfort, fatigue, rash, abdominal pain, nausea, diarrhea, upper respiratory infection
Rare (1% or less)
Palpitations, tachycardia, peripheral edema, insomnia, paresthesia, confusion, constipation, dry mouth, muscle cramps

SERIOUS REACTIONS
• Excessive hypotension ("first-dose syncope") may occur in patients with congestive heart failure (CHF) and severe salt and volume depletion.
• Angioedema (swelling of face and lips) and hyperkalemia occurs rarely.
• Agranulocytosis and neutropenia may be noted in patients with collagen vascular disease, including scleroderma and systemic lupus erythematosus, and impaired renal function.
• Nephrotic syndrome may be noted in patients with history of renal disease.

PRECAUTIONS & CONSIDERATIONS
Caution is warranted with cerebrovascular and coronary insufficiency, hypovolemia, renal impairment, sodium depletion, and those on dialysis and/or receiving diuretics. Be aware that lisinopril crosses the placenta and that it is unknown if lisinopril is distributed in breast milk. Lisinopril has caused fetal or neonatal morbidity or mortality. Be aware that the safety and efficacy of lisinopril have not been established in children. The elderly may be more sensitive to the hypotensive effects of lisinopril.
Dizziness may occur. B/P should be obtained immediately before giving each lisinopril dose, in addition to regular monitoring. Be alert to fluctuations in B/P. If an excessive reduction in B/P occurs, place the

person in the supine position with legs elevated. CBC and blood chemistry should be obtained before beginning lisinopril therapy, then every 2 weeks for the next 3 months, and periodically thereafter in patients with autoimmune disease, or renal impairment, and in those who are taking drugs that affect immune response or leukocyte count. BUN, serum creatinine, serum potassium, renal function, and white blood cell count (WBC) should also be monitored. Lungs should be auscultated for rales. Pattern of daily bowel activity and stool consistency should be assessed.

Administration

! Expect to discontinue diuretics 2 to 3 days before beginning lisinopril therapy.

Take lisinopril without regard to food. Crush tablets if necessary.

Lithium

lith´ee-um
(Duralith [CAN], Eskalith, Lithicarb [AUS], Lithobid, Quilonum SR [AUS]) (Cibalith-S)
Do not confuse Lithobid with Levbid, Lithostat, or Lithotabs.

CATEGORY AND SCHEDULE
Pregnancy Risk Category: D

CLASSIFICATION
Antipsychotics

MECHANISM OF ACTION

A psychotherapeutic agent that affects the storage, release, and reuptake of neurotransmitters. Antimanic effect may result from increased norepinephrine reuptake and serotonin receptor sensitivity.

Therapeutic Effect: Produces antimanic and antidepressant effects.

PHARMACOKINETICS

Rapidly and completely absorbed from the GI tract. Primarily excreted unchanged in urine. Removed by hemodialysis. **Half-life:** 18-24 hr (increased in elderly).

AVAILABILITY

Capsules: 150 mg, 300 mg, 600 mg.
Syrup: 300 mg/ml.
Tablets: 300 mg.
Tablets (controlled release): 450 mg.
Tablets (slow release): 300 mg.

INDICATIONS AND DOSAGES

! During acute phase, a therapeutic serum lithium concentration of 1-1.4 mEq/L is required. For long-term control, the desired level is 0.5-1.3 mEq/L. Monitor serum drug concentration and clinical response to determine proper dosage.

▸ **Prevention or treatment of acute mania, manic phase of bipolar disorder (manic-depressive illness)**
PO
Adults. 300 mg 3-4 times a day or 450-900 mg slow-release form twice a day. Maximum: 2.4 g/day.
Elderly. 300 mg twice a day. May increase by 300 mg/day q1wk. Maintenance: 900-1200 mg/day.
Children 12 yr and older. 600-1800 mg/day in 3-4 divided doses (2 doses/day for slow-release).
Children younger than 12 yr. 15-60 mg/kg/day in 3-4 divided doses.

OFF-LABEL USES

Prevention of vascular headache; treatment of depression, neutropenia

CONTRAINDICATIONS

Debilitated patients, severe cardiovascular disease, severe dehydration, severe renal disease, severe sodium depletion

INTERACTIONS
Drug
Antithyroid medications, iodinated glycerol, potassium iodide: May increase the effects of these drugs.
Diuretics, NSAIDs: May increase lithium serum concentration and risk of toxicity.
Haloperidol: May increase extrapyramidal symptoms and the risk of neurologic toxicity.
Molindone: May increase the risk of neurotoxicity.
Phenothiazines: May decrease the absorption of phenothiazines, increase the intracellular concentration and renal excretion of lithium, and increase delirium and extrapyramidal symptoms. Antiemetic effect of some phenothiazines may mask early signs of lithium toxicity.
Herbal
None known.
Food
None known.

DIAGNOSTIC TEST EFFECTS
May increase blood glucose, immunoreactive parathyroid hormone, and serum calcium levels. Therapeutic lithium serum level is 0.6-1.2 mEq/L; toxic serum level is greater than 1.5 mEq/L.

SIDE EFFECTS
! Side effects are dose related and seldom occur at lithium serum levels less than 1.5 mEq/L.
Occasional
Fine hand tremor, polydipsia, polyuria, mild nausea
Rare
Weight gain, bradycardia or tachycardia, acne, rash, muscle twitching, cold and cyanotic extremities, pseudotumor cerebri

(eye pain, headache, tinnitus, vision disturbances)

SERIOUS REACTIONS
• A lithium serum concentration of 1.5-2.0 mEq/L may produce vomiting, diarrhea, drowsiness, confusion, incoordination, coarse hand tremor, muscle twitching, and T-wave depression on EKG.
• A lithium serum concentration of 2.0-2.5 mEq/L may result in ataxia, giddiness, tinnitus, blurred vision, clonic movements, and severe hypotension.
• Acute toxicity may be characterized by seizures, oliguria, circulatory failure, coma, and death.

PRECAUTIONS & CONSIDERATIONS
Caution is warranted with thyroid disease, renal impairment, or cardiovascular disease as well as those receiving medications which alter sodium such as diuretics, ACE inhibitors, and NSAIDs. Caution should also be used if there is a risk of suicide. Lithium crosses the placenta and is excreted in breast milk. Children and elderly are more sensitive to an increased drug dosage and have a higher risk for toxicity. Steady salt and fluid intake should be maintained especially during summer months.

Lithium concentrations should be monitored. Therapeutic serum levels are 0.6-1.2 mEq/ml. The toxic serum level for lithium is greater than 1.5 mEq/ml. Adverse effects are seen at levels about 1.5 mEq/ml. Serum lithium should be monitored every 4-5 days during initial therapy, then every 1-3 months when stable. Draw lithium serum concentrations 8-12 hours after dose. Closely supervise patients at risk for committing suicide during early therapy.

Administration
Take with food or milk if gastrointestinal (GI) distress occurs. Slow release tablets must be swallowed whole. Do not crush or chew. Drink 2-3 L of water daily.

Lodoxamide
loe-dox'a-mide
(Alomide)

CATEGORY AND SCHEDULE
Pregnancy Risk Category: B

CLASSIFICATION
Mast cell stabilizers, ophthalmics

MECHANISM OF ACTION
A mast cell stabilizer that prevents increase in cutaneous vascular permeability, antigen-stimulated histamine release and may prevent calcium influx into mast cells. *Therapeutic Effect:* Inhibits sensitivity reaction.

PHARMACOKINETICS
Non-detectable absorption.
Half-life: 8.5 hr.

AVAILABILITY
Ophthalmic Solution: 0.1% (Alomide).

INDICATIONS AND DOSAGES
▶ **Treatment of vernal keratoconjunctivitis, conjunctivitis, and keratitis**
OPHTHALMIC
Adults, Elderly, Children 2 yr or older. 1-2 drops 4 times/day, for up to 3 mo.

CONTRAINDICATIONS
Wearing soft contact lenses (product contains benzalkonium chloride), hypersensitivity to lodoxamide tromethamine or any component of the formulation

INTERACTIONS
Drug
None known.
Herbal
None known.
Food
None known.

DIAGNOSTIC TEST EFFECTS
None known.

SIDE EFFECTS
Frequent
Transient stinging, burning, instillation discomfort
Occasional
Ocular itching, blurred vision, dry eye, tearing/discharge/foreign body sensation, headache
Rare
Scales on lid/lash, ocular swelling, sticky sensation, dizziness, somnolence, nausea, sneezing, dry nose, rash

SERIOUS REACTIONS
• None reported.

PRECAUTIONS & CONSIDERATIONS
Be aware that lodoxamide tromethamine is for ophthalmic use only. Not for injection. It is unknown if lodoxamide tromethamine crosses the placenta or is distributed in breast milk. Be aware that the safety and efficacy of lodoxamide tromethamine have not been established in children younger than 2 years old. There are no age-related precautions noted in the elderly.
Storage
Store at room temperature.

Administration
Tilt the patient's head back; place solution in conjunctival sac. Close eyes, then press gently on the lacrimal sac for 1 minute. Do not wear soft contact lenses during therapy. Therapy may last up to 3 months.

Lomefloxacin
low-meh-flocks'ah-sin
(Maxaquin)

CATEGORY AND SCHEDULE
Pregnancy Risk Category: C

CLASSIFICATION
Antibiotics, quinolones

MECHANISM OF ACTION
A quinolone that inhibits the enzyme DNA gyrase in susceptible microorganisms, interfering with bacterial cell replication and repair.
Therapeutic Effect: Bactericidal.

PHARMACOKINETICS
Well absorbed from the GI tract. Protein binding: 10%. Widely distributed. Metabolized in the liver. Primarily excreted in urine. Not removed by hemodialysis.
Half-life: 4-6 hr (increased with impaired renal function and in the elderly).

AVAILABILITY
Tablets: 400 mg.

INDICATIONS AND DOSAGES
▸ **Complicated UTIs**
PO
Adults, Elderly. 400 mg/day for 10-14 days.

▸ **Uncomplicated UTIs**
PO
Adults (females). 400 mg/day for 3 days.
▸ **Lower respiratory tract infections**
PO
Adults, Elderly. 400 mg/day for 10 days.
▸ **Surgical prophylaxis**
PO
Adults, Elderly. 400 mg 2-6 hr before surgery.
▸ **Dosage in renal impairment**
Dosage and frequency are modified based on creatinine clearance.

Creatinine Clearance	Dosage
41 ml/min and higher	No change
10-40 ml/min	400 mg initially, then 200 mg/day for 10-14 days

CONTRAINDICATIONS
Hypersensitivity to quinolones

INTERACTIONS
Drug
Antacids, iron preparations, sucralfate: May decrease lomefloxacin absorption.
Caffeine, oral anticoagulants: May increase the effects of these drugs.
Theophylline: Decreases clearance and may increase blood concentration and risk of toxicity of theophylline.
Herbal
None known.
Food
None known.

DIAGNOSTIC TEST EFFECTS
May increase BUN and serum alkaline phosphatase, bilirubin, creatinine, LDH, AST (SGOT), and ALT (SGPT) levels.

L

SIDE EFFECTS
Occasional (3%-2%)
Nausea, headache, photosensitivity, dizziness
Rare (1%)
Diarrhea

SERIOUS REACTIONS
• Antibiotic-associated colitis and other superinfections may result from altered bacterial balance.
• Hypersensitivity reactions, including photosensitivity (as evidenced by rash, pruritus, blisters, edema, and burning skin), have occurred in patients receiving fluoroquinolones.
• Arthropathy may occur if the drug is given to children younger than 18 years.

PRECAUTIONS & CONSIDERATIONS
Caution is warranted with CNS disorders, renal impairment, or seizures, and those taking caffeine or theophylline. It is unknown if lomefloxacin is distributed in breast milk. If possible, pregnant or breast-feeding women should avoid taking the drug because of the risk of arthropathy in the fetus or infant. The safety and efficacy of lomefloxacin have not been established in children. Age-related renal impairment may require a dosage adjustment in the elderly. Avoid exposure to sunlight and ultraviolet light and wear sunscreen and protective clothing if photosensitivity develops.

Dizziness, headache, and signs and symptoms of infections should be assessed. Mental status and WBC count should be monitored. Be alert for signs and symptoms of superinfection, such as anal or genital pruritus, fever, oral candidiasis, and vaginitis. History of hypersensitivity to lomefloxacin and other quinolones should be determined before therapy.

Administration
Take lomefloxacin without regard to food, but the preferred administration time is 2 hours after a meal. Don't take antacids containing aluminum or magnesium within 2 hours of lomefloxacin. Consume citrus fruits and cranberry juice to acidify urine. Continue for full course of therapy and do not skip doses.

Loperamide
loe-per′a-mide
(Apo-Loperamide [CAN], Gastro-Stop [AUS], Imodium [AUS], Imodium A-D, Loperacap [CAN], Novo-Loperamide [CAN])
Do not confuse Imodium with Indocin or Ionamin.

CATEGORY AND SCHEDULE
Pregnancy Risk Category: B
OTC liquid, tablets

CLASSIFICATION
Antidiarrheals, gastrointestinals

MECHANISM OF ACTION
An antidiarrheal that directly affects the intestinal wall muscles. *Therapeutic Effect:* Slows intestinal motility and prolongs transit time of intestinal contents by reducing fecal volume, diminishing loss of fluid and electrolytes, and increasing viscosity and bulk of stool.

PHARMACOKINETICS
Poorly absorbed from the GI tract. Protein binding: 97%. Metabolized in the liver. Eliminated in feces and excreted in urine. Not removed by hemodialysis. **Half-life:** 9.1-14.4 hr.

AVAILABILITY
Capsules: 2 mg.
Liquid: 1 mg/5 ml (OTC).
Tablets: 2 mg (OTC).

INDICATIONS AND DOSAGES
▶ **Acute diarrhea**
PO (CAPSULES)
Adults, Elderly. Initially, 4 mg; then 2 mg after each unformed stool. Maximum: 16 mg/day.
Children 9-12 yr, weighing more than 30 kg. Initially, 2 mg 3 times a day for 24 hr.
Children 6-8 yr, weighing 20-30 kg. Initially, 2 mg twice a day for 24 hr.
Children 2 5 yr, weighing 13-20 kg. Initially, 1 mg 3 times/day for 24 hr. Maintenance: 1 mg/10 kg only after loose stool.
▶ **Chronic diarrhea**
PO
Adults, Elderly. Initially, 4 mg; then 2 mg after each unformed stool until diarrhea is controlled.
Children. 0.08-0.24 mg/kg/day in 2-3 divided doses. Maximum: 2 mg/dose.
▶ **Traveler's diarrhea**
PO
Adults, Elderly. Initially, 4 mg; then 2 mg after each loose bowel movement (LBM). Maximum: 8 mg/day for 2 days.
Children 9-11 yr. Initially, 2 mg; then 1 mg after each LBM. Maximum: 6 mg/day for 2 days.
Children 6-8 yr. Initially, 1 mg; then 1 mg after each LBM. Maximum: 4 mg/day for 2 days.

CONTRAINDICATIONS
Acute ulcerative colitis (may produce toxic megacolon), diarrhea associated with pseudomembranous enterocolitis due to broad-spectrum antibiotics or to organisms that invade intestinal mucosa (such as *Escherichia coli*, shigella, and salmonella), patients who must avoid constipation

INTERACTIONS
Drug
Opioid (narcotic) analgesics: May increase the risk of constipation.
Herbal
None known.
Food
None known.

DIAGNOSTIC TEST EFFECTS
None known.

SIDE EFFECTS
Rare
Dry mouth, somnolence, abdominal discomfort, allergic reaction (such as rash and itching)

SERIOUS REACTIONS
• Toxicity results in constipation, GI irritation, including nausea and vomiting, and CNS depression. Activated charcoal is used to treat loperamide toxicity.

PRECAUTIONS & CONSIDERATIONS
Caution is warranted with fluid and electrolyte depletion and hepatic impairment. It is unknown if loperamide crosses the placenta or is distributed in breast milk. Loperamide use is not recommended in children younger than 6 years of age. Infants younger than 3 months of age are more susceptible to CNS effects. Loperamide use in the elderly may mask dehydration and electrolyte depletion. Tasks that require mental alertness or motor skills should be avoided until response to the drug has been established. Alcohol should also be avoided during drug therapy. Dry mouth may occur. Notify the physician if abdominal distention and pain, diarrhea that does not stop within 3 days, or fever occurs.

Pattern of daily bowel activity and stool consistency and hydration status should be monitored.

Administration

Do not give if bloody diarrhea is present or temperature is greater than 101° F. When administering the oral liquid to children, use the accompanying plastic dropper to measure the liquid.

Lopinavir/Ritonavir
lop-in'a-veer/rit-on'a-veer
(Kaletra)
Do not confuse Kaletra with Keppra.

CATEGORY AND SCHEDULE
Pregnancy Risk Category: C

CLASSIFICATION
Antivirals, protease inhibitors

MECHANISM OF ACTION
A protease inhibitor combination drug in which lopinavir inhibits the activity of the enzyme protease late in the HIV replication process and ritonavir increases plasma levels of lopinavir. *Therapeutic Effect:* Formation of immature, noninfectious viral particles.

PHARMACOKINETICS
Readily absorbed after PO administration (absorption increased when taken with food). Protein binding: 98%-99%. Metabolized in the liver. Eliminated primarily in feces. Not removed by hemodialysis. **Half-life:** 5-6 hr.

AVAILABILITY
Capsules: 133.3 mg lopinavir/33.3 mg ritonavir.

Oral Solution: 80 mg/ml lopinavir/20 mg/ml ritonavir.

INDICATIONS AND DOSAGES
▶ **HIV infection**
PO
Adults. 3 capsules (400 mg lopinavir/ 100 mg ritonavir) or 5 ml twice a day. Increase to 4 capsules (533 mg lopinavir/133 mg ritonavir) or 6.5 ml when taken with efavirenz or nevirapine.
Children weighing 15-40 kg who are not taking efavirenz or nevirapine. 10 mg/kg twice a day.
Children weighing 7-14 kg who are not taking Alprenavir, efavirenz, nelfinavir, nevirapine. 12 mg/kg twice a day.
Children weighing 15-40 kg who are taking efavirenz or nevirapine. 11 mg/kg twice a day.
Children weighing 7-14 kg who are taking efavirenz or nevirapine. 13 mg/kg twice a day.

CONTRAINDICATIONS
Concomitant use of ergot derivatives (causes peripheral ischemia of extremities and vasospasm), flecainide, midazolam, pimozide, propafenone (increases the risk of serious cardiac arrhythmias), or triazolam (increases sedation or respiratory depression); hypersensitivity to lopinavir or ritonavir

INTERACTIONS
Drug
Atorvastatin: May increase lopinavir and ritonavir blood concentration and risk of myopathy.
Atovaquone, methadone, oral contraceptives: May decrease blood concentration and effects of these drugs.
Carbamazepine, corticosteroids, efavirenz, nevirapine, phenobarbital, phenytoin, rifampin: May decrease

blood concentration and effects of lopinavir and ritonavir.
Clarithromycin, felodipine, immunosuppressants, nicardipine, nifedipine, rifabutin: May increase blood concentration and effects of these drugs.
Itraconazole, ketoconazole: May increase blood concentration of these drugs.
Metronidazole: May produce a disulfiram-like reaction.
Herbal
St. John's wort: May decrease blood concentration and effects of lopinavir and ritonavir.
Food
None known.

DIAGNOSTIC TEST EFFECTS

May increase blood glucose, GGT, total cholesterol, and serum uric acid, AST (SGOT), ALT (SGPT), and triglyceride levels.

SIDE EFFECTS

Frequent (14%)
Mild to moderate diarrhea
Occasional (6%-2%)
Nausea, asthenia, abdominal pain, headache, vomiting
Rare (less than 2%)
Insomnia, rash

SERIOUS REACTIONS

• Anemia, leukopenia, lymphadenopathy, deep vein thrombosis, Cushing's syndrome, pancreatitis, and hemorrhagic colitis occur rarely.

PRECAUTIONS & CONSIDERATIONS

! High-doses of itraconazole or ketoconazole are not recommended in persons taking lopinavir/ritonavir. Lopinavir/ritonavir oral solution contains alcohol and should not be given to those receiving metronidazole because this combination may cause a disulfiram-type reaction. Caution is warranted with hepatitis B or C or impaired liver function. Be aware that it is unknown if lopinavir/ritonavir is excreted in breast milk. Breast-feeding is not recommended in this population because of the possibility of HIV transmission. Be aware that the safety and efficacy of lopinavir/ritonavir have not been established in children younger than 6 months. In the elderly, age-related cardiac function, renal, or liver impairment requires caution. Lopinavir/ritonavir is not a cure for HIV infection, nor does it reduce risk of transmission to others.

Expect to establish baseline values for complete blood count (CBC), renal and liver function tests, and weight. Assess for nausea and vomiting, pattern of daily bowel activity and stool consistency, and signs and symptoms of pancreatitis as evidenced by abdominal pain, nausea, and vomiting. Eat small, frequent meals to offset nausea or vomiting. Evaluate for signs and symptoms of opportunistic infections as evidenced by cough, onset of fever, oral mucosa changes, or other respiratory symptoms. Check the weight at least twice a week.
Storage
Refrigerate until dispensed and avoid exposure to excessive heat. If stored at room temperature, use within 2 months.
Administration
Take with food.

Loratadine
loer-at′ah-deen
(Alavert, Claritin, Claritin
RediTab, Dimetapp, Tavist ND)

CATEGORY AND SCHEDULE
Pregnancy Risk Category: B

CLASSIFICATION
Antihistamines, H1

MECHANISM OF ACTION
A long-acting antihistamine that
competes with histamine for H_1
receptor sites on effector cells.
Therapeutic Effect: Prevents allergic
responses mediated by histamine,
such as rhinitis, urticaria, and
pruritus.

PHARMACOKINETICS

Route	Onset	Peak	Duration
PO	1-3 hr	8-12 hr	Longer than 24 hr

Rapidly and almost completely
absorbed from the GI tract.
Protein binding: 97%; metabolite,
73%-77%. Distributed mainly
to the liver, lungs, GI tract, and
bile. Metabolized in the liver to
active metabolite; undergoes
extensive first-pass metabolism.
Eliminated in urine and feces.
Not removed by hemodialysis.
Half-life: 8.4 hr; metabolite, 28 hr
(increased in elderly and hepatic
impairment).

AVAILABILITY
Syrup (Claritin): 10 mg/10 ml.
*Tablets (Alavert, Claritin, Tavist
ND):* 10 mg.
*Tablets (Rapid-Disintegrating
[Alavert, Claritin RediTab]):* 10 mg.

INDICATIONS AND DOSAGES
▸ **Allergic rhinitis, urticaria**
PO
*Adults, Elderly, Children 6 yr and
older.* 10 mg once a day.
Children 2-5 yr. 5 mg once
a day.
▸ **Dosage in hepatic impairment**
For adults, elderly, and
children 6 years and older
dosage is reduced to 10 mg
every other day.

OFF-LABEL USES
Adjunct treatment of bronchial
asthma

CONTRAINDICATIONS
Hypersensitivity to loratadine or its
ingredients

INTERACTIONS
Drug
**Clarithromycin, erythromycin,
fluconazole, ketoconazole:** May
increase the loratadine blood
concentration.
Herbal
None known.
Food
All foods: Delay the absorption of
loratadine.

DIAGNOSTIC TEST EFFECTS
May suppress wheal and flare
reactions to antigen skin testing
unless the drug is discontinued
4 days before testing.

SIDE EFFECTS
Frequent (12%-8%)
Headache, fatigue, somnolence
Occasional (3%)
Dry mouth, nose, or throat
Rare
Photosensitivity

SERIOUS REACTIONS
• None known.

PRECAUTIONS & CONSIDERATIONS

Caution should be used in breast-feeding women, children, and with hepatic impairment. Loratadine is excreted in breast milk. Children and the elderly are more sensitive to the drug's anticholinergic effects, such as dry mouth, nose, and throat. Avoid exposure to sunlight, drinking alcoholic beverages and tasks that require alertness or motor skills until response to the drug is established.

Drowsiness and dry mouth may occur. Respiratory rate, depth, and rhythm, pulse rate and quality, B/P, and therapeutic response should be monitored.

Administration

Take loratadine on an empty stomach because food delays its absorption.

Lorazepam

lor-a'ze-pam
(Apo-Lorazepam [CAN], Ativan, Lorazepam Intensol, Novolorazepam [CAN])
Do not confuse lorazepam with Alprazolam.

CATEGORY AND SCHEDULE

Pregnancy Risk Category: D
Controlled Substance
Schedule: IV

CLASSIFICATION

Anxiolytics, benzodiazepines

MECHANISM OF ACTION

A benzodiazepine that enhances the action of the inhibitory neuro-transmitter gamma-aminobutyric acid in the CNS, affecting memory, as well as motor, sensory, and cognitive function. *Therapeutic Effect:* Produces anxiolytic, anticon-vulsant, sedative, muscle relaxant, and antiemetic effects.

PHARMACOKINETICS

Route	Onset	Peak	Duration
PO	60 min	N/A	8-12 hr
IV	15-30 min	N/A	8-12 hr
IM	30-60 min	N/A	8-12 hr

Well absorbed after PO and IM administration. Protein binding: 85%. Widely distributed. Metabolized in the liver. Primarily excreted in urine. Not removed by hemodialysis. **Half-life:** 10-20 hr.

AVAILABILITY

Tablets (Ativan): 0.5 mg, 1 mg, 2 mg.
Injection (Ativan): 2 mg/ml, 4 mg/ml.
Oral solution (Lorazepam Intensol): 2 mg/ml.

INDICATIONS AND DOSAGES

▸ **Anxiety**
PO
Adults. 1-10 mg/day in 2-3 divided doses. Average: 2-6 mg/day.
Elderly. Initially, 0.5-1 mg/day. May increase gradually. Range: 0.5-4 mg.
IV
Adults, Elderly. 0.02-0.06 mg/kg q2-6hr.
IV INFUSION
Adults, Elderly. 0.01-0.1 mg/kg/hr.
PO, IV
Children. 0.05 mg/kg/dose q4-8hr. Range: 0.02-0.1 mg/kg. Maximum: 2 mg/dose.
▸ **Insomnia due to anxiety**
PO
Adults. 2-4 mg at bedtime.
Elderly. 0.5-1 mg at bedtime.

▸ **Preoperative sedation**
IV
Adults, Elderly. 0.044 mg/kg
15-20 min before surgery. Maximum
total dose: 2 mg.
IM
Adults, Elderly. 0.05 mg/kg 2 hr
before procedure. Maximum total
dose: 4 mg.
▸ **Status epilepticus**
IV
Adults, Elderly. 4 mg over 2-5 min.
May repeat in 10-15 min. Maximum:
8 mg in 12-hr period.
Children. 0.1 mg/kg over 2-5 min.
May give second dose of 0.05 mg/kg
in 15-20 min. Maximum: 4 mg.
Neonates. 0.05 mg/kg. May repeat
in 10-15 min.

OFF-LABEL USES
Treatment of alcohol withdrawal,
panic disorders, skeletal muscle
spasms, chemotherapy-induced
nausea or vomiting, tension headache,
tremors; adjunctive treatment before
endoscopic procedures (diminishes
patient recall)

CONTRAINDICATIONS
Angle-closure glaucoma; pre-existing
CNS depression; severe hypotension;
severe uncontrolled pain

INTERACTIONS
Drug
Alcohol, other CNS depressants:
May increase CNS depression.
Herbal
Kava kava, valerian: May increase
CNS depression.
Food
None known.

DIAGNOSTIC TEST EFFECTS
None known. Therapeutic
serum drug level is 50-240 ng/ml;
toxic serum drug level is
unknown.

▨ IV INCOMPATIBILITIES
Aldesleukin (Proleukin), aztreonam
(Azactam), idarubicin (Idamycin),
ondansetron (Zofran), sufentanil
(Sufenta)
▨ IV Compatibilities
Bumetanide (Bumex), cefepime
(Maxipime), diltiazem (Cardizem),
dobutamine (Dobutrex), dopamine
(Intropin), heparin, labetalol
(Normodyne, Trandate), milrinone
(Primacor), norepinephrine
(Levophed), piperacillin and
tazobactam (Zosyn), potassium,
propofol (Diprivan)

SIDE EFFECTS
Frequent
Somnolence (initially in the morning),
ataxia, confusion
Occasional
Blurred vision, slurred speech,
hypotension, headache
Rare
Paradoxical CNS restlessness or
excitement in elderly or debilitated

SERIOUS REACTIONS
• Abrupt or too-rapid withdrawal
may result in pronounced restlessness, irritability, insomnia, hand
tremor, abdominal or muscle cramps,
diaphoresis, vomiting, and seizures.
• Overdose results in somnolence,
confusion, diminished reflexes, and
coma.

PRECAUTIONS & CONSIDERATIONS
Caution is warranted with pulmonary,
hepatic, renal impairment, and in
those using other CNS depressants
concurrently. Lorazepam may cross
the placenta and be distributed in
breast milk. Lorazepam may increase
the risk of fetal abnormalities if
administered during the first trimester
of pregnancy. Females on long-term
therapy should use effective contraception during therapy and notify the

physician immediately if she becomes or may be pregnant. Chronic lorazepam use during pregnancy may produce withdrawal symptoms in the patient and CNS depression in the neonate. The safety and efficacy of this drug have not been established in children younger than 12 years. In the elderly, expect to give small doses initially and to increase dosage gradually to avoid ataxia and excessive sedation.

Drowsiness and dizziness may occur. Change positions slowly from recumbent, to sitting, before standing to prevent dizziness. Alcohol, caffeine, and tasks that require mental alertness or motor skills should also be avoided. B/P, heart rate, respiratory rate, CBC with differential, and hepatic and renal function should be monitored.

Storage
Refrigerate—don't freeze—parenteral form.

Administration
Take oral lorazepam with food. Crush tablets as needed.

Don't use the solution for injection if it appears discolored or contains a precipitate. Dilute with an equal volume of sterile water for injection, 0.9% NaCl, or D_5W. To dilute a prefilled syringe, remove air from a half-filled syringe, aspirate an equal volume of diluent, pull the plunger back slightly to allow for mixing, and gently invert the syringe several times—don't shake vigorously. Give by IV push into the tubing of a free-flowing IV infusion of 0.9% NaCl or D_5W at a rate not exceeding 2 mg/minute. Stay recumbent for up to 8 hours after parenteral administration to reduce the drug's hypotensive effect. The therapeutic serum level for lorazepam is 50-240 ng/ml; the toxic serum level is unknown.

For IM use, inject the drug deep into a large muscle mass, such as gluteus maximus.

Losartan
lo-sar'tan
(Cozaar)
Do not confuse Cozaar with Zocor.

CATEGORY AND SCHEDULE
Pregnancy Risk Category: C
(D if used in second or third trimesters)

CLASSIFICATION
Angiotensin II receptor antagonists

MECHANISM OF ACTION
An angiotensin II receptor, type AT_1, antagonist that blocks vasoconstrictor and aldosterone-secreting effects of angiotensin II, inhibiting the binding of angiotensin II to the AT_1 receptors. *Therapeutic Effect:* Causes vasodilation, decreases peripheral resistance, and decreases BP.

PHARMACOKINETICS
Route	Onset	Peak	Duration
PO	N/A	6 hr	24 hr

Well absorbed after PO administration. Protein binding: 98%. Undergoes first-pass metabolism in the liver to active metabolites. Excreted in urine and via the biliary system. Not removed by hemodialysis. **Half-life:** 2 hr, metabolite: 6-9 hr.

AVAILABILITY
Tablets: 25 mg, 50 mg, 100 mg.

INDICATIONS AND DOSAGES
▸ **Hypertension**
PO
Adults, Elderly. Initially, 50 mg once a day. Maximum: May be given once or twice a day, with total daily doses ranging from 25-100 mg.
▸ **Nephropathy**
PO
Adults, Elderly. Initially, 50 mg/day. May increase to 100 mg/day based on B/P response.
▸ **Stroke reduction**
PO
Adults, Elderly. 50 mg/day. Maximum: 100 mg/day.
▸ **Hypertension in patients with impaired hepatic function**
PO
Adults, Elderly. Initially, 25 mg/day.

CONTRAINDICATIONS
None known.

INTERACTIONS
Drug
Cimetidine: May increase the effects of losartan.
Ketoconazole, troleandomycin: May inhibit the effects of these drugs.
Lithium: May increase lithium blood concentration and risk of lithium toxicity.
Phenobarbital, rifampin: May decrease the effects of losartan.
Herbal
None known.
Food
Grapefruit juice: May alter the absorption of losartan.

DIAGNOSTIC TEST EFFECTS
May increase BUN, serum alkaline phosphatase, serum bilirubin, serum creatinine, AST (SGOT), and ALT (SGPT) levels. May decrease blood Hgb and Hct levels.

SIDE EFFECTS
Frequent (8%)
Upper respiratory tract infection
Occasional (4%-2%)
Dizziness, diarrhea, cough
Rare (1% or less)
Insomnia, dyspepsia, heartburn, back and leg pain, muscle cramps, myalgia, nasal congestion, sinusitis

SERIOUS REACTIONS
• Overdosage may manifest as hypotension and tachycardia. Bradycardia occurs less often.

PRECAUTIONS & CONSIDERATIONS
Caution is warranted with hepatic and renal impairment and renal arterial stenosis. Losartan has caused fetal or neonatal morbidity or mortality and may adversely affect the breast-fed infant. Patients should not breast-feed while taking losartan. Safety and efficacy of losartan have not been established in children. No age-related precautions have been noted in the elderly.

Apical pulse and B/P should be assessed immediately before each losartan dose, and regularly throughout therapy. Be alert to fluctuations in apical pulse and B/P. If an excessive reduction in B/P occurs, place the person in the supine position with feet slightly elevated and notify the physician. Tasks that require mental alertness or motor skills should be avoided. BUN, serum electrolytes, serum creatinine levels, heart rate, urinalysis, and pattern of daily bowel activity and stool consistency should be assessed. Maintain adequate hydration; exercising outside during hot weather should be avoided in order to decrease the risk of dehydration and hypotension.
Administration
Take losartan without regard to food. Do not crush or break tablets.

Lovastatin
lo'va-sta-tin
(Altoprev, Lotrel, Mevacor)
Do not confuse with Leustatin, Livostin, or Mivacron.

CATEGORY AND SCHEDULE
Pregnancy Risk Category: X

CLASSIFICATION
Antihyperlipidemics, HMG CoA reductase inhibitors

MECHANISM OF ACTION
An antihyperlipidemic that inhibits HMG-CoA reductase, the enzyme that catalyzes the early step in cholesterol synthesis. *Therapeutic Effect:* Decreases LDL cholesterol, VLDL cholesterol, plasma triglycerides; increases HDL cholesterol.

PHARMACOKINETICS

Route	Onset	Peak	Duration
PO	3 days	4-6 wk	N/A

Incompletely absorbed from the GI tract (increased on empty stomach). Protein binding: 95%. Hydrolyzed in the liver to active metabolite. Primarily eliminated in feces. Not removed by hemodialysis. **Half-life:** 1.1-1.7 hr.

AVAILABILITY
Tablets (Mevacor): 10 mg, 20 mg, 40 mg.
Tablets (Extended-Release [Altoprev]): 20 mg, 40 mg, 60 mg.

INDICATIONS AND DOSAGES
▸ **Hyperlipoproteinemia, primary prevention of coronary artery disease**
PO
Adults, Elderly. Initially, 20-40 mg/day with evening meal. Increase at 4-wk intervals up to maximum of 80 mg/day. Maintenance: 20-80 mg/day in single or divided doses.
PO (EXTENDED RELEASE)
Adults, Elderly. Initially, 20 mg/day. May increase at 4-wk intervals up to 60 mg/day.
Children 10-17 yr. 10-40 mg/day with evening meal.
▸ **Heterozygous familial hypercholesterolemia**
PO
Children 10-17 yr. Initially, 10 mg/day. May increase to 20 mg/day after 8 wk and 40 mg/day after 16 wk if needed.

CONTRAINDICATIONS
Active liver disease, pregnancy, unexplained elevated liver function tests

INTERACTIONS
Drug
Cyclosporine, erythromycin, gemfibrozil, immunosuppressants, niacin: Increases the risk of acute renal failure and rhabdomyolysis.
Erythromycin, itraconazole, ketoconazole: May increase lovastatin blood concentration causing severe muscle inflammation, myalgia, and weakness.
Herbal
None known.
Food
Grapefruit juice: Large amounts of grapefruit juice may increase risk of side effects, such as myalgia and weakness.

DIAGNOSTIC TEST EFFECTS
May increase serum creatine kinase and serum transaminase concentrations.

SIDE EFFECTS
Generally well tolerated. Side effects usually mild and transient.

Frequent (9%-5%)
Headache, flatulence, diarrhea, abdominal pain or cramps, rash and pruritus
Occasional (4%-3%)
Nausea, vomiting, constipation, dyspepsia
Rare (2%-1%)
Dizziness, heartburn, myalgia, blurred vision, eye irritation

SERIOUS REACTIONS
• There is a potential for cataract development.

PRECAUTIONS & CONSIDERATIONS
Caution is warranted with history of heavy or chronic alcohol use, renal impairment, and those who use cyclosporine, fibrates, and niacin. Be aware that lovastatin use is contraindicated in pregnancy, because the suppression of cholesterol biosynthesis may cause fetal toxicity, and lactation. Be aware that it is unknown if lovastatin is distributed in breast milk. Be aware that the safety and efficacy of lovastatin have not been established in children. There are no age-related precautions noted in the elderly. Be aware that grapefruit juice should be avoided.

Notify the physician of changes in the color of stool or urine, muscle weakness, myalgia, severe gastric upset, rash, unusual bruising, vision changes, or yellowing of eyes or skin. Pattern of daily bowel activity and stool consistency should be assessed. Serum lipid cholesterol and triglyceride levels and hepatic function should be checked at baseline and periodically during treatment.
Administration
Take lovastatin with meals.

Loxapine
lox′a-peen
(Apo-Loxapine [CAN], Loxapac [CAN], Loxitane)

CATEGORY AND SCHEDULE
Pregnancy Risk Category: C

CLASSIFICATION
Antipsychotics

MECHANISM OF ACTION
A dibenzodiazepine derivative that interferes with the binding of dopamine at postsynaptic receptor sites in brain. Strong anticholinergic effects. *Therapeutic Effect:* Suppresses locomotor activity, produces tranquilization.

PHARMACOKINETICS
Onset of action occurs within 1 hour. Metabolized to active metabolites 8-hydroxyloxapine, 7-hydroxyloxapine, and 8-hydroxyamoxapine. Excreted in urine. **Half-life:** 4 hr.

AVAILABILITY
Capsules: 5 mg, 10 mg, 25 mg, 50 mg (Loxitane).

INDICATIONS AND DOSAGES
▸ **Psychotic disorders**
PO
Adults. 10 mg 2 times/day. Increase dosage rapidly during first week to 50 mg, if needed. Usual therapeutic, maintenance range: 60-100 mg daily in 2-4 divided doses. Maximum: 250 mg/day.

CONTRAINDICATIONS
Severe central nervous system (CNS) depression, comatose states,

hypersensivitiy to loxapine or any component of the formulation

INTERACTIONS
Drug
Alcohol, CNS depressants: May increase CNS depressant effects.
Antacids, antidiarrheals: May decrease absorption of loxapine.
Extrapyramidal symptom (EPS)-producing medications: May increase risk of EPS.
Herbal
None known.
Food
None known.

DIAGNOSTIC TEST EFFECTS
None known.

SIDE EFFECTS
Frequent
Blurred vision, confusion, drowsiness, dry mouth, dizziness, lightheadedness
Occasional
Allergic reaction (rash, itching), decreased urination, constipation, decreased sexual ability, enlarged breasts, headache, photosensitivity, nausea, vomiting, insomnia, weight gain

SERIOUS REACTIONS
• Extrapyramidal symptoms frequently noted are akathisia (motor restlessness, anxiety). Less frequently noted are akinesia (rigidity, tremor, salivation, mask-like facial expression, reduced voluntary movements). Infrequently noted dystonias: torticollis (neck muscle spasm), opisthotonos (rigidity of back muscles), and oculogyric crisis (rolling back of eyes). Tardive dyskinesia (protrusion of tongue, puffing of cheeks, chewing/puckering of mouth) occurs rarely but may be irreversible. Risk is greater in female elderly patients.

Extreme caution should be used with history of seizures. Caution is also warranted with cardiovascular disease, glaucoma, history of seizures, prostatic hypertrophy, and urinary retention. It is unknown if loxapine crosses the placenta or is distributed in breast milk. Safety and efficacy of loxapine have not been established in children. The elderly are more susceptible to anticholinergic effects and sedation, increased risk for extrapyramidal effects, and orthostatic hypotension. A decreased dosage is recommended in the elderly. Avoid alcohol and tasks that require mental alertness or motor skills.
Storage
Store at room temperature.
Administration
Give loxapine with food or a full glass of water or milk to decrease GI irritation. The full therapeutic effect may take up to 6 weeks. Do not abruptly discontinue loxapine.

Lymphocyte Immune Globulin N
lym′phow-site
(Atgam)
Do not confuse Atgam with Ativan.

CATEGORY AND SCHEDULE
Pregnancy Risk Category: C

CLASSIFICATION
Immune globulins, immunosuppressives

MECHANISM OF ACTION
A biological response modifier that acts as a lymphocyte selective

immunosuppressant, reducing the number and altering the function of T lymphocytes, which are responsible for cell-mediated and humoral immunity. Lymphocyte immune globulin N also stimulates the release of hematopoietic growth factors. *Therapeutic Effect:* Prevents allograft rejection; treats aplastic anemia.

AVAILABILITY
Injection: 250 mg/5 ml.

INDICATIONS AND DOSAGES
▶ **To delay onset of renal allograft rejection**
IV
Adults, Elderly, Children. 15 mg/kg/day for 14 days, then every other day for 14 days. First dose within 24 hr before or after transplantation.
▶ **Treatment of renal allograft rejection**
IV
Adults, Elderly, Children. 10-15 mg/kg/day for 14 days, then every other day for 14 more days. Maximum: 21 doses.
▶ **Aplastic anemia**
IV
Adults, Elderly, Children. 10-20 mg/kg once a day for 8-14 days, then every other day. Maximum: 21 doses.

OFF-LABEL USES
Immunosuppressant in bone marrow, heart, and liver transplants, treatment of pure red cell aplasia, multiple sclerosis, myasthenia gravis, and scleroderma

CONTRAINDICATIONS
Systemic hypersensitivity reaction to previous injection of lymphocyte immune globulin N

INTERACTIONS
Drug
None known.

Herbal
None known.
Food
None known.

DIAGNOSTIC TEST EFFECTS
May alter renal function test results.

▩ IV INCOMPATIBILITIES
No information is available for Y-site administration.

SIDE EFFECTS
Frequent
Fever (51%), thrombocytopenia (30%), rash (2%), chills (16%), leukopenia (14%), systemic infection (13%)
Occasional (10%-5%)
Serum sickness-like reaction, dyspnea, apnea, arthralgia, chest pain, back pain, flank pain, nausea, vomiting, diarrhea, phlebitis.

SERIOUS REACTIONS
• Thrombocytopenia may occur but is generally transient.
• A severe hypersensitivity reaction, including anaphylaxis, occurs rarely.

PRECAUTIONS & CONSIDERATIONS
Caution is warranted with concurrent immunosuppressive therapy. Immediately notify the physician of chest pain, rapid or irregular heartbeat, shortness of breath, wheezing, or swelling of the face or throat, which may occur during the IV infusion. Avoid exposure to people with colds or infections and notify the physician as soon as signs or symptoms of infection develop.
Storage
Keep the drug refrigerated before and after dilution. Discard the diluted solution after 24 hours.
Administration
For IV use, dilute the total daily dose with 0.9% NaCl, as prescribed, to a

final concentration of no more than 4 mg/ml. Gently rotate the diluted solution; avoid shaking it. Use a 0.2- to 1-micron filter, and infuse the total daily dose over at least 4 hours. To prevent chemical phlebitis, avoid using a peripheral vein for IV infusion. Instead, expect to use a central venous catheter, a Groshong catheter, or a peripherally inserted central catheter. Expect to monitor frequently for chills, fever, erythema, and pruritus. An order for prophylactic antihistamines or corticosteroids should be obtained to treat these potential side effects.

L

Mafenide
ma'fe-nide
(Sulfamylon)

CATEGORY AND SCHEDULE
Pregnancy Risk Category: C

CLASSIFICATION
Anti-infectives, topical,
dermatologics

MECHANISM OF ACTION
A topical anti-infective that
decreases number of bacteria
avascular tissue of second- and
third-degree burns. *Therapeutic
Effect:* Bacteriostatic. Promotes
spontaneous healing of deep
partial-thickness burns.

PHARMACOKINETICS
Absorbed through devascularized
areas into systemic circulation
following topical administration.
Excreted in the form of its metabolite rho-carboxybenzenesulfonamide

AVAILABILITY
Cream: 85 mg base/g (Sulfamylon).

INDICATIONS AND DOSAGES
▸ **Burns**
TOPICAL
Adults, Elderly, Children. Apply
1-2 times/day.

CONTRAINDICATIONS
Hypersensitivity to mafenide or
sulfite or any other component of
the formulation

INTERACTIONS
Drug
None known.
Herbal
None known.

Food
None known.

DIAGNOSTIC TEST EFFECTS
None known.

SIDE EFFECTS
Difficult to distinguish side effects
and effects of severe burn
Frequent
Pain, burning upon application
Occasional
Allergic reaction (usually 10-14 days
after initiation): itching, rash, facial
edema, swelling; unexplained
syndrome of marked hyperventila-
tion with respiratory alkalosis
Rare
Delay in eschar separation, excoria-
tion of new skin

SERIOUS REACTIONS
• Hemolytic anemia, porphyria,
bone marrow depression, superinfections (especially with fungi),
metabolic acidosis occurs rarely.

PRECAUTIONS & CONSIDERATIONS
Caution is warranted with impaired
renal function because of risk of
metabolic acidosis. Be aware that
cross-sensitivity to sulfonamides is
not certain. It is unknown if mafenide
crosses the placenta or is distributed
in breast milk. Be aware that mafenide
is not recommended in newborn
infants since sulfonamides may cause
kernicterus. There are no age-related
precautions noted in the elderly.

Signs/symptoms of metabolic
acidosis should be monitored such as
Kussmaul's respirations, nausea,
vomiting, diarrhea, headache, tremors,
weakness, and cardiac arrhythmias
(due to associated hyperkalemia),
sensorium changes, decreased PCO_2,
blood pH, and HCO_3.
Storage
Store at room temperature.

Administration
Mafenide is for external use only.
Apply mafenide with gloved hands.
Burned area should be kept covered
with mafenide at all times. Bathe
burn area daily.

Magaldrate
(Iosopan Plus, Lowsium Plus,
Riopan Plus)

CATEGORY AND SCHEDULE
Pregnancy Risk Category: C

CLASSIFICATION
Aluminum and magnesium
hydroxide acid sulfate mixture,
antacid

MECHANISM OF ACTION
An antacid that causes less hydrogen
ion available for diffusion thru the
gastrointestinal (GI) mucosa.
Therapeutic Effect: Reduces and
neutralizes gastric acid.

AVAILABILITY
Suspension: magaldrate 540 mg and
simethicone 20 mg/5 ml, magaldrate
540 mg and simethicone 40 mg/5 ml,
magaldrate 1080 mg and simethicone
40 mg/5 ml.
Tablets (chewable): magaldrate
540 mg and simethicone 20 mg,
magaldrate 1080 mg and simethicone
20 mg.

INDICATIONS AND DOSAGES
▸ **Hyperacidity and gas**
PO
Adults, Elderly. 540 to 1080 mg
between meals and at bedtime.

CONTRAINDICATIONS
Hypersensitivity to magaldrate,
colostomy or ileostomy, appendicitis,
ulcerative colitis, diverticulits

INTERACTIONS
Drug
Fluoroquinolones: May decrease
the effects of fluoroquinolones.
Ketoconazole, methenamine: May
decrease the effects of ketoconazole
or methenamine. Mecamylamine:
May increase the effects of
mecamylamine.
**Sodium polystyrene sulfonate
resin:** May decrease the effects of
antacids.
Tetracyclines: May decrease the
effects of both tetracyclines and
antacids.
Herbal
None known.
Food
None known.

SIDE EFFECTS
Rare
Constipation, diarrhea, fluid
retention, dizziness or lightheadedness, continuing discomfort,
irregular heartbeat, loss of appetite,
mood or mental changes, muscle
weakness, unusual tiredness or
weakness, weight loss, chalky
taste

SERIOUS REACTIONS
• None known.

PRECAUTIONS & CONSIDERATIONS
Caution should be used with congestive heart failure. Diarrhea should be
reported.
Administration
Drink several glasses of water a day
to help reduce possible constipation.
Take other medications at least
2 hours before or after taking with
magaldrate.

Magnesium
(Mag-Delay SR, Slow-Mag)
(Citrate of Magnesia, Citro-Mag
[CAN]) (Phillips Milk of Magnesia)
(Mag-Ox 400, Uro-Mag)
**Do not confuse magnesium
sulfate with manganese sulfate.**

CATEGORY AND SCHEDULE
Pregnancy Risk Category: B

CLASSIFICATION
Laxatives

MECHANISM OF ACTION
An antacid, laxative, electrolyte, and
anticonvulsant. As an antacid acts in
the stomach to neutralize gastric acid.
Therapeutic Effect: Increases pH.
As a laxative has an osmotic effect,
primarily in the small intestine, and
draws water into the intestinal lumen.
Produces distention and promotes
peristalsis and bowel evacuation. As
a systemic dietary supplement and
electrolyte replacement, is found
primarily in intracellular fluids and
is essential for enzyme activity, nerve
conduction, and muscle contraction.
As an anticonvulsant, blocks neuromuscular transmission and the amount
of acetylcholine released at the motor
end plate. Controls seizure. Maintains
and restores magnesium levels.

PHARMACOKINETICS
Antacid, laxative: Minimal
absorption through the intestine.
Absorbed dose primarily excreted in
urine. Systemic: Widely distributed.
Primarily excreted in urine.

AVAILABILITY
Magnesium chloride
Tablets (Slo-Mag, Mag Delay SR):
64 mg.

Magnesium citrate
Oral Solution (Citrate of Magnesia):
290 mg/5 ml.
Magnesium hydroxide
*Oral Liquid (Phillips Milk of
Magnesia):* 400 mg/5 ml,
800 mg/5 ml.
*Chewable Tablets (Phillips Milk of
Magnesia):* 311 mg.
Magnesium oxide
Tablets (Mag-Ox 400): 400 mg.
Capsules (Uro-Mag): 140 mg.
Magnesium sulfate
Premix Infusion Solution:
10 mg/ml, 20 mg/ml, 40 mg/ml,
80 mg/ml.
Injection: 125 mg/ml,
500 mg/ml.

INDICATIONS AND DOSAGES
▸ **Hypomagnesemia (magnesium
sulfate)**
PO
Adults, Elderly. 3 g q6hr for 4 doses
as needed.
IV, IM
Adults, Elderly. 1-12 g/day in
divided doses.
Children. 25-50 mg/kg/dose
q4-6hr for 3-4 doses. Maintenance:
30-60 mg/kg/day.
▸ **Hypertension, seizures (magnesium
sulfate)**
IV, IM
Children. 20-100 mg/kg/dose q4-6hr
as needed.
IV
Adults. Initially, 4 g then 1-4 g/hr by
continuous infusion.
▸ **Arrhythmias (magnesium sulfate)**
IV
Adults, Elderly. Initially, 1-2 g then
infusion of 1-2 g/hr.
▸ **Treat constipation (magnesium
sulfate)**
PO
*Adults, Elderly, Children older
than 11 yr.* 10-30 g/day in
divided doses.

Children 6-11 yr. 5-10 g/day in divided doses.
Children 2-5 yr. 2.5-5 g/kg/day in divided doses.

▸ **Treat constipation (magnesium hydroxide)**
PO
Adults, Elderly, Children older than 11 yr. 6-8 tablets or 30-60 ml/day.
Children 6-11 yr. 3-4 tablets or 7.5-15 ml/day.
Children 2-5 yr. 1-2 tablets or 2.5-7.5 ml/day.

▸ **Treatment of hyperacidity (magnesium hydroxide)**
PO
Adults, Elderly. 2-4 tablets or 5-15 ml as needed up to 4 times a day.
Children 7-14 yr. 1 tablet or 2.5-5 ml as needed up to 4 times a day.

▸ **Magnesium deficiency (magnesium oxide)**
PO
Adults, Elderly. 1-2 tablets 2-3 times/day.

▸ **Dietary supplement (magnesium chloride)**
PO
Adults, Elderly. 54-483 mg/day in 2-4 divided doses.

▸ **Cathartic (magnesium citrate)**
PO
Adults, Elderly, Children 12 yr and older. 120-300 ml.
Children 6-11 yr. 100-150 ml.
Children younger than 6 yr. 0.5 ml/kg up to maximum of 200 ml.

CONTRAINDICATIONS

Antacid: Appendicitis or symptoms of appendicitis, ileostomy, intestinal obstruction, severe renal impairment
Laxative: Appendicitis, CHF, colostomy, hypersensitivity, ileostomy, intestinal obstruction, undiagnosed rectal bleeding

Systemic: Heart block, myocardial damage, renal failure

INTERACTIONS
Drug
Antacid
Ketoconazole, tetracyclines: May decrease the absorption of ketoconazole and tetracyclines.
Methenamine: May decrease the effects of methenamine.
Antacid, laxative
Digoxin, oral anticoagulants, phenothiazines: May decrease the effects of these drugs.
Tetracyclines: May form nonabsorbable complex with tetracyclines.
Systemic (dietary supplement, electrolyte replacement)
Calcium: May neutralize the effects of magnesium.
CNS depression-producing medications: May increase CNS depression.
Digoxin: May cause changes in cardiac conduction or heart block with digoxin.
Herbal
None known.
Food
None known.

DIAGNOSTIC TEST EFFECTS

Antacid: May increase gastrin production and pH.
Laxative: May decrease serum potassium level.
Systemic (dietary supplement, electrolyte replacement): None known.

🕸 IV INCOMPATIBILITIES
Amphotericin B complex (Abelcet, AmBisome, Amphotec), cefepime (Maxipime)

⬛ IV Compatibilities
Amikacin (Amikin), cefazolin (Ancef), ciprofloxacin (Cipro), dobutamine (Dobutrex), enalapril (Vasotec), gentamicin, heparin,

M

hydromorphone (Dilaudid), insulin, milrinone (Primacor), morphine, piperacillin/tazobactam (Zosyn), potassium chloride, propofol (Diprivan), tobramycin (Nebcin), vancomycin (Vancocin)

SIDE EFFECTS
Frequent
Antacid: Chalky taste, diarrhea, laxative effect
Occasional
Antacid: Nausea, vomiting, stomach cramps
Antacid, laxative: With prolonged use or large doses in renal impairment, possible hypermagnesemia, marked by dizziness, irregular heartbeat, mental changes, fatigue, and weakness
Laxative: Cramping, diarrhea, increased thirst, flatulence
Systemic (dietary supplement, electrolyte replacement): Reduced respiratory rate, decreased reflexes, flushing, hypotension, decreased heart rate

SERIOUS REACTIONS
• Magnesium as an antacid or laxative has no known serious reactions.
• Systemic use of magnesium may produce prolonged PR interval and widening of QRS interval.
• Magnesium toxicity may cause loss of deep tendon reflexes, heart block, respiratory paralysis, and cardiac arrest. The antidote for toxicity is 10-20 ml 10% calcium gluconate (5-10 mEq of calcium).

PRECAUTIONS & CONSIDERATIONS
Magnesium antacids should be used cautiously with chronic diarrhea, colostomy, diverticulitis, ulcerative colitis, and undiagnosed GI and rectal bleeding. The laxative form should be used cautiously with diabetes mellitus and in those on a low-salt diet because some magnesium supplements contain sugar or sodium. When magnesium is given for systemic use, it should be used cautiously in severe renal impairment. It is unknown if antacid forms of magnesium are distributed in breast milk. Parenteral magnesium readily crosses the placenta and is distributed in breast milk for 24 hours after therapy has been discontinued. Continuous IV infusion of magnesium increases the risk of magnesium toxicity in the neonate. Magnesium should not be administered IV during the 2 hours preceding delivery. Magnesium should be used cautiously in children younger than 6 years of age because safety is unknown. The elderly are at increased risk for developing magnesium deficiency, because of decreased magnesium absorption, other medications they may be taking, and poor diet.

Adequate hydration should be maintained. Notify the physician if signs and symptoms of hypermagnesemia occur, including confusion, cramping, dizziness, irregular heartbeat, lightheadedness, or unusual fatigue or weakness. EKG, BUN, serum creatinine and magnesium levels should be monitored in those receiving systemic form. Patellar reflexes should be tested before giving repeat parenteral doses of systemic magnesium to assess for CNS depression. Know that suppressed reflexes may indicate impending respiratory arrest. That patellar reflexes should be present and respiratory rate should be greater than 16 breaths/minute, before each parenteral dose.
Storage
Refrigerate citrate of magnesia to retain potency and improve palatability. Store parenteral formulation at room temperature.

Administration

! Keep in mind that antacids may be given up to 4 times a day.

When using antacids, shake suspension well before use. Make sure that chewable tablets are chewed thoroughly before swallowing and are followed by a full glass of water. Take magnesium antacids at least 2 hours before or 2 hours after other medications. Do not take magnesium antacids for longer than 2 weeks, unless directed by the physician. Those with peptic ulcer disease should take magnesium antacids 1 and 3 hours after meals and at bedtime for 4 to 6 weeks.

When using laxatives, drink a full glass of liquid (8 oz) with each dose to prevent dehydration. Follow dose with citrus carbonated beverage or fruit juice to improve flavor. Magnesium laxatives are for short-term use only.

For IV use, the solution must be diluted to avoid exceeding 20 mg/ml concentration. For infusion, do not exceed magnesium sulfate concentration of 200 mg/ml (20%). Do not exceed infusion rate of 150 mg/minute.

For IM use, for adults and the elderly, use 250 mg/ml (25%) or 500 mg/ml (50%) magnesium sulfate concentration, as prescribed. For children and infants, do not exceed 200 mg/ml (20%) as prescribed.

Magnesium Salicylate
(Backache Pain Relief Extra Strength, Doan's Original, Extra Strength Doan's, Keygesic-10, Mobidin, Momentum)

CATEGORY AND SCHEDULE
Pregnancy Risk Category: NR
OTC

CLASSIFICATION
Analgesics, non-narcotic, salicylates

MECHANISM OF ACTION
A nonsteroidal anti-inflammatory that inhibits cyclooxygenase and suppresses prostaglandin synthesis. *Therapeutic Effect:* Produces analgesic and anti-inflammatory effect.

PHARMACOKINETICS
Rapidly absorbed from the gastrointestinal (GI) tract. Widely distributed. Protein binding: 80%-90%. Metabolized in liver. Primarily excreted in urine. Removed by hemodialysis. **Half-life:** 2-3 hr.

AVAILABILITY
Tablets: 467 mg (Backache Pain Relief Extra Strength, Momentum), 325 mg (Doan's Original), 500 mg (Extra Strength Doan's), 650 mg (Keygesic-10), 600 mg (Mobidin).

INDICATIONS AND DOSAGES
▸ **Arthritis, inflammation, musculoskeletal disorders (backache)**
PO
Adults, Elderly. 650 mg times/day or 1090 mg 3 times/day. May increase to 3.6-4.8 g/day in 3-4 divided doses.

CONTRAINDICATIONS
Severe renal impairment, hypersensitivity to magnesium salicylate or any component of the formulation

INTERACTIONS
Drug
Heparin, oral anticoagulants, thrombolytics: May increase the risk of bleeding.
Probenecid: May increase magnesium salicylate blood concentration.
Varicella virus vaccine: May increase risk of developing Reye's syndrome.
Herbal
Tamarind: May increase salicylate toxicity.
Tan-shen: May increase salicylate concentrations and decrease tan-shen concentrations.
Food
None known.

DIAGNOSTIC TEST EFFECTS
May cause false increases in acetaminophen levels.

SIDE EFFECTS
Occasional
Gastric mucosal irritation, bleeding

SERIOUS REACTIONS
• Overdosage may cause tinnitus.
• Toxic levels may be reached quickly in dehydrated, febrile children. Marked toxicity is manifested as hyperthermia, restlessness, abnormal breathing patterns, convulsions, respiratory failure, and coma.

PRECAUTIONS & CONSIDERATIONS
Caution is warranted with acute or chronic renal or hepatic insufficiency, gastritis, peptic ulcer disease, and chronic alcoholism. It is unknown if magnesium salicylate crosses the placenta or is distributed in breast milk. Be aware that magnesium salicylate use should be avoided during the last trimester of pregnancy because the drug may adversely affect the fetal cardiovascular system causing premature closure of ductus arteriosus. Use caution in giving this drug to children with acute febrile illness because this increases the risk of developing Reye's syndrome. Magnesium salicylate should not be given to children or teenagers who have the chickenpox or flu as this increases the risk of developing Reye's syndrome. Be aware that lower aspirin dosages are recommended in the elderly because this age group may be more susceptible to toxicity.
Storage
Store at room temperature.
Administration
May give with food, milk, or antacids if GI distress occurs. If pain is not relieved within 10 days, fever within 3 days, or sore throat within 2 days, notify the physician.

Mannitol
man'i-tall
(Osmitrol)

CATEGORY AND SCHEDULE
Pregnancy Risk Category: C

CLASSIFICATION
Diuretics, osmotic

MECHANISM OF ACTION
An osmotic diuretic, antiglaucoma, and antihemolytic agent that elevates osmotic pressure of the glomerular filtrate, inhibiting tubular reabsorption of water and electrolytes, resulting in increased flow of water into interstitial fluid and plasma. *Therapeutic Effect:* Produces diuresis;

reduces IOP; reduces ICP and cerebral edema.

PHARMACOKINETICS

Route	Onset	Peak	Duration
IV (diuresis)	15-30 min	N/A	2-8 hr
IV (Reduced ICP)	15-30 min	N/A	3-8 hr
IV (Reduced IOP)	N/A	30-60 min	4-8 hr

Remains in extracellular fluid. Primarily excreted in urine. Removed by hemodialysis. **Half-life:** 100 min.

AVAILABILITY
Injection: 5%, 10%, 15%, 20%, 25%.

INDICATIONS AND DOSAGES
▸ **Prevention and treatment of oliguric phase of acute renal failure; to promote urinary excretion of toxic substances (such as aspirin, barbiturates, bromides, and imipramine); to reduce increased ICP due to cerebral edema or edema of injured spinal cord; to reduce increased IOP due to acute glaucoma**
IV
Adults, Elderly, Children. Initially, 0.5-1 g/kg, then 0.25-0.5 g/kg q4-6hr.

CONTRAINDICATIONS
Dehydration, intracranial bleeding, severe pulmonary edema and congestion, severe renal disease

INTERACTIONS
Drug
Digoxin: May increase the risk of digoxin toxicity associated with mannitol-induced hypokalemia.
Herbal
None known.
Food
None known.

DIAGNOSTIC TEST EFFECTS
May decrease serum phosphate, potassium, and sodium levels.

🗟 IV INCOMPATIBILITIES
Cefepime (Maxipime), doxorubicin liposomal (Doxil), filgrastim (Neupogen)
🗟 IV Compatibilities
Cisplatin (Platinol), ondansetron (Zofran), propofol (Diprivan)

SIDE EFFECTS
Frequent
Dry mouth, thirst
Occasional
Blurred vision, increased urinary frequency and urine volume, headache, arm pain, backache, nausea, vomiting, urticaria, dizziness, hypotension or hypertension, tachycardia, fever, angina-like chest pain

SERIOUS REACTIONS
• Fluid and electrolyte imbalance may occur from rapid administration of large doses or inadequate urine output resulting in overexpansion of extracellular fluid.
• Circulatory overload may produce pulmonary edema and CHF.
• Excessive diuresis may produce hypokalemia and hyponatremia.
• Fluid loss in excess of electrolyte excretion may produce hypernatremia and hyperkalemia.

PRECAUTIONS & CONSIDERATIONS
It is unknown if mannitol crosses the placenta or is distributed in breast milk. The safety and efficacy of mannitol have not been established in children younger than 12 years. Age-related renal impairment may require cautious use in the elderly.
    Dry mouth and an increase in the frequency and volume of urination may occur. Blood pressure (B/P), BUN, liver function test results,

M

electrolytes, and urine output should be assessed before and during treatment. Weight should be monitored daily. Be aware of signs of electrolyte disturbances such as hypokalemia or hyponatremia. Hypokalemia may cause arrhythmias, altered mental status, muscle cramps, asthenia, and tremor. Hyponatremia may result in cold and clammy skin, confusion, and thirst.

Storage
Store the drug at room temperature.

Administration
! Assess the IV site for patency before administering each dose. Pain and thrombosis are noted with extravasation. With suspected renal insufficiency or marked oliguria, a test dose should be given. The test dose is 12.5 g for adults (200 mg/kg for children) over 3 to 5 minutes to produce a urine flow of at least 30 to 50 ml/hour (1 ml/kg/hour for children) over 2 to 3 hours.

If the solution crystallizes, warm the bottle in hot water and shake it vigorously at intervals. Don't use the solution if crystals remain after the warming procedure. Cool the solution to body temperature before administration. Use an in-line filter (less than 5 microns) for drug concentrations greater than 20%. The test dose for oliguria is IV push over 3 to 5 minutes. The test dose for cerebral edema or elevated ICP is IV over 20 to 30 minutes. Maximum concentration is 25%. Don't add potassium chloride or sodium chloride to mannitol with a concentration of 20% or greater. Don't add mannitol to whole blood for transfusion.

Maprotiline
mah-pro′tih-leen
(Ludiomil)

CATEGORY AND SCHEDULE
Pregnancy Risk Category: B

CLASSIFICATION
Antidepressants, tetracyclic

MECHANISM OF ACTION
A tetracyclic compound that blocks reuptake norepinephrine by CNS presynaptic neuronal membranes, increasing availability at postsynaptic neuronal receptor sites, and enhances synaptic activity. *Therapeutic Effect:* Produces antidepressant effect, with prominent sedative effects and low anticholinergic activity.

PHARMACOKINETICS
Slowly and completely absorbed after PO administration. Protein binding: 88%. Metabolized in liver by hydroxylation and oxidative modification. Excreted in urine. Unknown if removed by hemodialysis. **Half-life:** 27-58 hr.

AVAILABILITY
Tablets: 25 mg, 50 mg, 75 mg (Ludiomil).

INDICATIONS AND DOSAGES
▸ **Mild to moderate depression**
PO
Adults. 75 mg/day to start, in 1-4 divided doses. *Elderly:* 50-75 mg/day. In 2 weeks, increase dosage gradually in 25-mg increments until therapeutic response is achieved. Reduce to lowest effective maintenance level.
Severe depression
PO
Adults. 100-150 mg/day in 1-4

divided doses. May increase
gradually to maximum
225 mg/day.
Usual elderly dosage
PO
Initially, 25 mg at bedtime. May
increase by 25 mg q3-7 days.
Maintenance: 50-75 mg/day.

CONTRAINDICATIONS
Acute recovery period following
myocardial infarction (MI),
within 14 days of MAOI ingestion,
known or suspected seizure
disorder, hypersensitivity to
maprotiline or any component of
the formulation

INTERACTIONS
Drug
MAOIs: May increase risk of
hypertensive crisis and severe
convulsions.
Sympathomimetics: May
increase cardiovascular effects
(arrhythmias, tachycardias,
severe hypertension).
Herbal
None known.
Food
None known.

DIAGNOSTIC TEST EFFECTS
None known.

🖾 IV INCOMPATIBILITIES
None known.
🍵 **IV Compatibilities**
None known.

SIDE EFFECTS
Frequent
Drowsiness, fatigue, dry mouth,
blurred vision, constipation,
delayed micturition, postural
hypotension, excessive sweating,
disturbed concentration,
increased appetite, urinary
retention

Occasional
GI disturbances (nausea, GI distress,
metallic taste sensation), photosensitivity
Rare
Paradoxical reaction (agitation,
restlessness, nightmares,
insomnia), extrapyramidal
symptoms (particularly fine
hand tremor)

SERIOUS REACTIONS
• Higher incidence of
seizures than with tricyclic
antidepressants, especially
in those with no previous
history of seizures.
• High dosage may produce cardiovascular effects, such as severe
postural hypotension, dizziness,
tachycardia, palpitations, and
arrhythmias.
• May also result in altered temperature regulation (hyperpyrexia or
hypothermia).
• Abrupt withdrawal from
prolonged therapy may
produce headache, malaise,
nausea, vomiting, and
vivid dreams.

PRECAUTIONS & CONSIDERATIONS
Caution is warranted with prostatic
hypertrophy, history of urinary
retention or obstruction, glaucoma,
diabetes mellitus, history of seizures,
hyperthyroidism, cardiac/hepatic/
renal disease, schizophrenia,
increased intraocular pressure, and
hiatal hernia. Be aware that maprotiline is distributed in breast milk.
Be aware that the safety and efficacy
of this drug have not been established in children. In the elderly,
age-related renal impairment
may require cautious use.
Tolerance usually develops to
postural hypotension, sedative,
and anticholinergic effects.

M

Avoid alcohol and tasks that require mental alertness and motor skills. Visual disturbances should be reported immediately.

Storage

Store at room temperature.

Administration and Handling

Take maprotiline without food. Be aware to make sure at least 14 days elapse between discontinuing MAOIs and instituting maprotiline therapy. Also, plan to allow at least 14 days to pass after discontinuing maprotiline and instituting MAOI therapy.

Mazindol

may-zin-doll

(Sanorex)

CATEGORY AND SCHEDULE

Pregnancy Risk Category: C

CLASSIFICATION

Anorexiants, stimulants, central nervous system

MECHANISM OF ACTION

An isoindole that stimulates the central nervous system and primarily exerting its effect on the limbic system. *Therapeutic Effect:* Stimulates the hypothalamus to reduce appetite.

PHARMACOKINETICS

Slow but complete absorption. Protein binding: greater than 99%. Metabolized in liver to metabolites. Primarily excreted in urine as well as feces. Unknown if removed by hemodialysis.

Half-life: 30-50 hr.

AVAILABILITY

Tablets: 1 mg, 2 mg (Sanorex).

INDICATIONS AND DOSAGES

▸ **Obesity**

PO

Adults. 1 mg/day. Maximum: 3 mg/day.

OFF-LABEL USES

Narcolepsy

CONTRAINDICATIONS

Agitated states, glaucoma, history of drug abuse, symptomatic cardiovascular disease (arrhythmias), coadministration with or within 14 days of MAOI therapy, hypersensitivity to mazindol

INTERACTIONS

Drug

Guanethidine: May decrease the hypotensive effects of guanethidine.

MAOIs: May increase the risk of hypertensive crisis

Sibutramine, sympathomimetics, tricyclic antidepressants: May increase the risk of hypertension and tachycardia.

Herbal

None known.

Food

None known.

DIAGNOSTIC TEST EFFECTS

None known.

▨ IV INCOMPATIBILITIES

None known.

▨ **IV Compatibilities**

None known.

SIDE EFFECTS

Occasional

Insomnia, headache, tachycardia, palpitations, tremors, nervousness, restlessness, dry mouth, constipation

Rare
Blurred vision, impotence, insulin sensitivity, rash, sweating, weakness

SERIOUS REACTIONS
• Overdosage includes symptoms of irritability, agitation, hyperactivity, tachycardia, arrhythmia, tachypnea.

PRECAUTIONS & CONSIDERATIONS
Caution is necessary with hypertension, heart disease, and diabetes mellitus. It is unknown if mazindol is excreted in breast milk. Mazindol use is not recommended during pregnancy or in breast-feeding women. Be aware that the safety and efficacy of mazindol has not been established in children. There are no age-related precautions noted in the elderly. A nutritionally balanced, reduced-calorie diet and exercise is recommended.

Unpleasant side effects, such as restlessness and increased heart rate may occur.

Administration
Tolerance may develop after a few weeks of mazindol use. Mazindol should be discontinued if tolerance develops. Give with food. Mazindol is not for long-term use. Mazindol should be discontinued after 4-6 weeks.

Mebendazole
meh-ben'dah-zole
(Vermox)

CATEGORY AND SCHEDULE
Pregnancy Risk Category: C

CLASSIFICATION
Antihelmintics

MECHANISM OF ACTION
A synthetic benzimidazole derivative that degrades parasite cytoplasmic microtubules and irreversibly blocks glucose uptake in helminthes and larvae. Vermicidal. *Therapeutic Effect:* depletes glycogen, decreases ATP, causes helminth death.

PHARMACOKINETICS
Poorly absorbed from GI tract (absorption increases with food). Metabolized in liver. Primarily eliminated in feces. **Half-life:** 2.5-9 hr (half life increased with impaired renal function).

AVAILABILITY
Tablets, chewable: 100 mg (Vermox).

INDICATIONS AND DOSAGES
▶ **Trichuriasis, ascariasis, hookworm**
PO
Adults, Elderly, Children older than 2 yr. 1 tablet in morning and at bedtime for 3 days.
▶ **Enterobiasis**
PO
Adults, Elderly, Children older than 2 yr. 1 tablet one time.

OFF-LABEL USES
Ancylostoma duodenale or Necator americanus

CONTRAINDICATIONS
Hypersensitivity to mebendazole or any component of the formulation

INTERACTIONS
Drug
Carbamazepine: May decrease concentrations of mebendazole.
Herbal
None known.
Food
None known.

M

DIAGNOSTIC TEST EFFECTS
May increase SGOT (AST), SGPT (ALT), alkaline phosphatase, BUN. May decrease Hgb.

IV INCOMPATIBILITIES
None known.
IV Compatibilities
None known.

SIDE EFFECTS
Occasional
Nausea, vomiting, headache, dizziness, transient abdominal pain, diarrhea with massive infection and expulsion of helminths
Rare
Fever

SERIOUS REACTIONS
* High dosage may produce reversible myelosuppression (granulocytopenia, leukopenia, neutropenia).

PRECAUTIONS & CONSIDERATIONS
Be aware that mebendazole is ineffective in hydatid disease. It is unknown if mebendazole crosses the placenta or is distributed in breast milk. Safety and efficacy has not been established in children 2 years and younger. There are no age-related precautions noted in the elderly. Avoid walking barefoot (larval entry into system). Change and launder underclothing, pajamas, bedding, towels, and washcloths daily. Due to high transmission of pinworm infections, all family members should be treated simultaneously; the infected person should sleep alone, and shower frequently.
Storage
Store at room temperature.
Administration
For high dosages, take with food. Tablets may be crushed, swallowed, or mixed with food. Take and continue iron supplements as long as ordered (may be 6 months after treatment) for anemia associated with whipworm and hookworm.

Mecamylamine
mek-a-mil′a-meen hye-droe-klor-ide
(ganglionic blocker, antihypertensive, ganglionic blocker)
(Inversine)

CATEGORY AND SCHEDULE
Pregnancy Risk Category: C

CLASSIFICATION
Antiadrenergics, peripheral

MECHANISM OF ACTION
A ganglionic blocker that inhibits acetylcholine at the autonomic ganglia. Blocks central nicotinic cholinergic receptors, which inhibits effects of nicotine. *Therapeutic Effect:* Reduces blood pressure; decreases desire to smoke.

PHARMACOKINETICS
Completely absorbed following PO administration. Widely distributed. Excreted in urine. **Half-life:** 24 hr.

AVAILABILITY
Tablets: 2.5 mg (Inversine).

INDICATIONS AND DOSAGES
▸ Hypertension
PO
Adults. Initially, 2.5 mg q12hr for 2 days, then increase by 2.5 mg increments at more than 2 day intervals until desired blood pressure is achieved. The average daily dose is 25 mg in 3 divided doses.

▶ **Smoking cessation**
PO
Adults. Initially, 2.5 mg q12hr for 2 days, then increase by 2.5 mg increments during the first week of therapy. Range: 10-20 mg in divided doses.

OFF-LABEL USES
Tourette's syndrome, hyperreflexia

CONTRAINDICATIONS
Coronary insufficiency, pyloric stenosis, glaucoma, uremia, recent myocardial infarction, unreliable patients

INTERACTIONS
Drug
Sulfonamides, antibiotics: May increase the effect of mecamylamine.
Herbal
None known.
Food
None known.

DIAGNOSTIC TEST EFFECTS
None known.

▓ IV INCOMPATIBILITIES
None known.
🍶 **IV Compatibilities**
None known.

SIDE EFFECTS
Occasional
Nausea, diarrhea, orthostatic hypotension, tachycardia, drowsiness, urinary retention, blurred vision, dilated pupils, confusion, mental depression, decreased sexual ability, loss of appetite
Rare
Pulmonary edema, pulmonary fibrosis, paresthesias

SERIOUS REACTIONS
• Overdosage includes symptoms such as hypotension, nausea, vomiting, urinary retention, and constipation.

PRECAUTIONS & CONSIDERATIONS
Caution should be used in the elderly and with renal impairment. Caution is also warranted with CNS abnormalities, prostatic hyperplasia, bladder obstruction or urethral strictive as well as people under general anesthesia. It is unknown if mecamylamine crosses the placenta or is distributed in breast milk. Safety and efficacy of mecamylamine have not been established in children. Blood pressure (B/P) should be taken immediately before each mecamylamine dose and regularly monitor throughout therapy.
Be alert to fluctuations in B/P.
Administration
Take after the same meal each day. Do not abruptly discontinue mecamylamine.

M

Meclizine
mek′li-zeen
(Antivert, Bonamine [CAN], Bonine)
Do not confuse with Axert.

CATEGORY AND SCHEDULE
Pregnancy Risk Category: B

CLASSIFICATION
Antiemetics/antivertigo, antihistamines, H1

MECHANISM OF ACTION
An anticholinergic that reduces labyrinthine excitability and diminishes vestibular stimulation of the labyrinth, affecting the chemoreceptor trigger zone. *Therapeutic Effect:* Reduces nausea, vomiting, and vertigo.

PHARMACOKINETICS

Route	Onset	Peak	Duration
PO	30-60 min	N/A	12-24 hr

Well absorbed from the GI tract. Widely distributed. Metabolized in the liver. Primarily excreted in urine. **Half-life:** 6 hr.

AVAILABILITY

Tablets (Antivert): 12.5 mg, 25 mg, 50 mg.
Tablets, chewable (Bonine): 25 mg.

INDICATIONS AND DOSAGES

▸ **Motion sickness**
PO
Adults, Elderly, Children 12 yr and older. 12.5-25 mg 1 hr before travel. May repeat q12-24hr. May require a dose of 50 mg.
▸ **Vertigo**
PO
Adults, Elderly, Children 12 yr and older. 25-100 mg/day in divided doses, as needed.

CONTRAINDICATIONS

None known.

INTERACTIONS

Drug
Alcohol, CNS depression-producing medications: May increase CNS depressant effect.
Herbal
None known.
Food
None known.

DIAGNOSTIC TEST EFFECTS

May produce false-negative results in antigen skin testing unless meclizine is discontinued 4 days before testing.

SIDE EFFECTS

Frequent
Drowsiness

Occasional
Blurred vision; dry mouth, nose, or throat

SERIOUS REACTIONS

• A hypersensitivity reaction, marked by eczema, pruritus, rash, cardiac disturbances, and photosensitivity, may occur.
• Overdose may produce CNS depression (manifested as sedation, apnea, cardiovascular collapse, or death) or severe paradoxical reactions (such as hallucinations, tremor, and seizures).
• Children may experience paradoxical reactions, including restlessness, insomnia, euphoria, nervousness, and tremors.
• Overdose in children may result in hallucinations, seizures, and death.

PRECAUTIONS & CONSIDERATIONS

Caution is warranted with angle-closure glaucoma and obstructive diseases of the GI or GU tract. It is unknown if meclizine crosses the placenta or is distributed in breast milk. Meclizine use may produce irritability in breast-feeding infants. Children and the elderly may be more sensitive to the drug's anticholinergic effects, such as dry mouth. Alcohol and tasks that require mental alertness or motor skills should be avoided.

Dizziness, drowsiness, and dry mouth may occur. B/P, electrolytes, and skin should be assessed.
Administration
! The elderly (older than 60 years) are at increased risk for developing agitation, disorientation, dizziness, sedation, hypotension, confusion, and psychotic-like symptoms.

Take meclizine orally without regard to food. Crush scored tablets if needed.

Meclofenamate
me′kloe-fen′a-mate soe-dee-um
(Meclomen [CAN])
Do not confuse with meclizine.

CATEGORY AND SCHEDULE
Pregnancy Risk Category: B
(D if used in third trimester or
near delivery)

CLASSIFICATION
Analgesics, non-narcotic, nonsteroidal anti-inflammatory drugs

MECHANISM OF ACTION
A nonsteroidal anti-inflammatory
drug that inhibits prostaglandin
synthesis by decreasing activity
of the enzyme, cyclooxygenase,
which results in decreased formation
of prostaglandin precursors.
Therapeutic Effect: Reduces
inflammatory response and
intensity of pain stimulus reaching
sensory nerve endings.

PHARMACOKINETICS
PO route, onset 15 minutes, peak
0.5-1.5 hours, duration 2-4 hours.
Completely absorbed from the
gastrointestinal (GI) tract. Widely
distributed. Protein binding:
greater than 99%. Metabolized
in liver. Primarily excreted in
urine and feces as metabolites.
Not removed by hemodialysis.
Half-life: 2-3.3 hr.

AVAILABILITY
Capsules: 50 mg, 100 mg.

INDICATIONS AND DOSAGES
▸ **Mild to moderate pain**
PO
Adults, Elderly. 50 mg q4-6hr as
needed.

▸ **Excessive menstrual blood loss
and primary dysmenorrhea**
PO
Adults, Elderly. 100 mg 3 times/day
for 6 days, starting at the onset of
menstrual flow.
▸ **Rheumatoid arthritis,
osteoarthritis**
PO
Adults, Elderly. 200-400 mg
3-4 times/day.

CONTRAINDICATIONS
Active peptic ulcer disease, chronic
inflammation of GI tract, GI bleeding disorders, GI ulceration, history
of hypersensitivity to aspirin or
NSAIDs

INTERACTIONS
Drug
Antihypertensives, diuretics: May
decrease the effects of antihypertensives and diuretics.
Aspirin, salicylates: May increase
the risk of GI bleeding and side
effects.
Bone marrow depressants: May
increase the risk of hematologic
reactions.
**Heparin, oral anticoagulants,
thrombolytics:** May increase the
effects of heparin, oral anticoagulants, and thrombolytics.
Lithium: May increase the blood
concentration and risk of toxicity of
lithium.
Methotrexate: May increase
the risk of toxicity with
methotrexate.
Probenecid: May increase meclofenamate blood concentration.
Herbal
Feverfew: May increase the risk of
bleeding.
Ginkgo biloba: May increase the
risk of bleeding.
Food
None known.

DIAGNOSTIC TEST EFFECTS

May increase chloride and sodium test results. May increase BUN, serum LDH concentration, serum alkaline phosphatase, serum creatinine, potassium, and transaminase levels, and urine protein levels. May decrease serum uric acid levels.

SIDE EFFECTS

Frequent (33%-10%)
Diarrhea, nausea, abdominal cramping/pain, dyspepsia (heartburn, indigestion, epigastric pain)
Occasional (9%-1%)
Flatulence, rash, dizziness
Rare (less than 1%)
Constipation, anorexia, stomatitis, headache, ringing in the ears, rash

SERIOUS REACTIONS

• Overdosage may result in headache, seizure, vomiting, and cerebral edema.
• Peptic ulcer disease, GI bleeding, gastritis, severe hepatic reactions, such as jaundice, nephrotoxicity, marked by hematuria, dysuria, proteinuria, and severe hypersensitivity reaction, including bronchospasm, and facial edema occur rarely.

PRECAUTIONS & CONSIDERATIONS

Caution is warranted with a history of GI tract disease, impaired liver or renal function, and predisposition to fluid retention. Pregnancy should be reported immediately. It is unknown if meclofenamate crosses the placenta or is distributed in breast milk. Meclofenamate use should be avoided during the last trimester of pregnancy as the drug may adversely affect the fetal cardiovascular system. Safety and efficacy have not been established in children. GI bleeding and ulceration is more

likely to cause serious adverse effects in elderly patients.
Age-related renal impairment may increase risk of liver or renal toxicity and a decreased dosage is recommended.
Administration
Do not crush, open, or break capsules. May give with antacids, food, or milk if the patient experiences GI distress. Dose should be reduced in the elderly.

Medroxyprogesterone

me-drox´ee-proe-jess´te-rone
(Depo-Provera, Depo-Provera Contraceptive, Novo-Medrone [CAN], Provera, Ralovera [AUS])
Do not confuse medroxyprogesterone with hydroxyprogesterone, methylprednisolone, or methyltestosterone.

CATEGORY AND SCHEDULE

Pregnancy Risk Category: X

CLASSIFICATION

Antineoplastics, hormones/hormone modifiers, contraceptives, progestins

MECHANISM OF ACTION

A hormone that transforms endometrium from proliferative to secretory in an estrogen-primed endometrium. Inhibits secretion of pituitary gonadotropins.
Therapeutic Effect: Prevents follicular maturation and ovulation. Stimulates growth of mammary alveolar tissue and relaxes uterine smooth muscle. Corrects hormonal imbalance.

PHARMACOKINETICS

Slowly absorbed after IM administration. Protein binding: 90%. Metabolized in the liver. Primarily excreted in urine. **Half-life:** 30 days.

AVAILABILITY

Tablets (Provera): 2.5 mg, 5 mg, 10 mg.
Injection (Depo-Provera Contraceptive): 150 mg/ml.
Injection (Depo-Provera): 400 mg/ml.

INDICATIONS AND DOSAGES
▸ **Endometrial hyperplasia**
PO
Adults. 2.5-10 mg/day for 14 days.
▸ **Secondary amenorrhea**
PO
Adults. 5-10 mg/day for 5-10 days, beginning at any time during menstrual cycle or 2.5 mg/day.
▸ **Abnormal uterine bleeding**
PO
Adults. 5-10 mg/day for 5-10 days, beginning on calculated day 16 or day 21 of menstrual cycle.
▸ **Endometrial, renal carcinoma**
IM
Adults, Elderly. Initially, 400-1000 mg; repeat at 1-wk intervals. If improvement occurs and disease is stabilized, begin maintenance with as little as 400 mg/mo.
▸ **Prevention of pregnancy**
IM
Adults. 150 mg q3mo.

OFF-LABEL USES

Hormone replacement therapy in estrogen-treated menopausal women, treatment of endometriosis

CONTRAINDICATIONS

Carcinoma of breast; estrogen-dependent neoplasm; history of or active thrombotic disorders, such as cerebral apoplexy, thrombophlebitis, or thromboembolic disorders; hypersensitivity to progestins; known or suspected pregnancy; missed abortion; severe hepatic dysfunction; undiagnosed abnormal genital bleeding; use as pregnancy test

INTERACTIONS
Drug
Bromocriptine: May interfere with the effects of bromocriptine.
Herbal
None known.
Food
None known.

DIAGNOSTIC TEST EFFECTS

May alter results for serum thyroid and liver function tests, prothrombin time, and metapyrone test

SIDE EFFECTS
Frequent
Transient menstrual abnormalities (including spotting, change in menstrual flow or cervical secretions, and amenorrhea) at initiation of therapy
Occasional
Edema, weight change, breast tenderness, nervousness, insomnia, fatigue, dizziness
Rare
Alopecia, depression, dermatologic changes, headache, fever, nausea

SERIOUS REACTIONS
• Thrombophlebitis, pulmonary or cerebral embolism, and retinal thrombosis occur rarely.

PRECAUTIONS & CONSIDERATIONS

Caution is warranted with conditions aggravated by fluid retention, including asthma, seizures, migraine, cardiac or renal dysfunction, and in those with diabetes mellitus or history of depression. Medroxyprogesterone use should be avoided during pregnancy, especially in the first 4 months

M

because the drug may cause congenital heart and limb reduction defects in the neonate. Medroxyprogesterone is distributed in breast milk. Safety and efficacy of medroxyprogesterone have not been established in children. No age-related precautions have been noted in the elderly. Avoid smoking because of the increased risk of blood clot formation and MI.

Notify the physician of chest pain, blood-tinged expectorants, hemoptysis, numbness in the arm or leg, severe headache, severe pain or swelling in the calf, severe abdominal pain or tenderness, sudden loss of vision, or unusually heavy vaginal bleeding. B/P, weight, blood glucose, hepatic enzyme, and serum calcium levels should be monitored.

Administration

Take oral medroxyprogesterone without regard to meals.

For IM use, shake vial immediately before administering to ensure complete suspension. Inject IM only in upper arm or upper outer aspect of buttock. Rarely, a residual lump, change in skin color, or sterile abscess occurs at injection site.

Mefenamic Acid

me-fe-nam'ik
(Apo-Mefenamic [CAN],
Nu-Mefenamic [CAN],
PMS-Mefenamic Acid [CAN],
Ponstan [CAN], Ponstel)

CATEGORY AND SCHEDULE

Pregnancy Risk Category: C
(D if used in third trimester or near delivery)

CLASSIFICATION

Analgesics, non-narcotic, non-steroidal anti-inflammatory drugs

MECHANISM OF ACTION

A nonsteroidal anti-inflammatory that produces analgesic and anti-inflammatory effect by inhibiting prostaglandin synthesis. *Therapeutic Effect:* Reduces inflammatory response and intensity of pain stimulus reaching sensory nerve endings.

PHARMACOKINETICS

Rapidly absorbed from the gastrointestinal (GI) tract. Protein binding: high. Metabolized in liver. Partially excreted in urine and partially in the feces. Not removed by hemodialysis. **Half-life:** 3.5 hr.

AVAILABILITY

Capsules: 250 mg (Ponstel).

INDICATIONS AND DOSAGES
▶ **Mild to moderate pain, lower back pain, dysmenorrhea**
PO
Adults, Elderly, Children 14 yr and older. Initially, 500 mg to start, then 250 mg q4hr as needed. Maximum: 1 week of therapy.

OFF-LABEL USES
Cataract prevention, menorrhagia, osteoarthritis, premenstrual syndrome, rheumatoid arthritis

CONTRAINDICATIONS
History of hypersensitivity to aspirin or NSAIDs, pregnancy

INTERACTIONS
Drug
Antihypertensives, diuretics: May decrease the effects of antihypertensives and diuretics.
Aspirin, salicylates: May increase the risk of GI bleeding and side effects.
Bone marrow depressants: May increase the risk of hematologic reactions.
Heparin, oral anticoagulants, thrombolytics: May increase the effects of heparin, oral anticoagulants, and thrombolytics.
Lithium: May increase the blood concentration and risk of toxicity of lithium.
Methotrexate: May increase the risk of toxicity of methotrexate.
Probenecid: May increase mefenamic acid blood concentration.

DIAGNOSTIC TEST EFFECTS
May increase chloride and sodium levels. May prolong bleeding time. May increase liver function tests.

SIDE EFFECTS
Occasional (10%-1%)
Dyspepsia, including heartburn, indigestion, flatulence, abdominal cramping, constipation, nausea, diarrhea, epigastric pain, vomiting, headache, nervousness, dizziness, bleeding, elevated liver function tests, tinnitus
Rare (less than 1%)
Fluid retention, arrhythmias, tachycardia, confusion, drowsiness, rash, dry eyes, blurred vision, hot flashes

SERIOUS REACTIONS
• Peptic ulcer, GI bleeding, gastritis, and severe hepatic reaction, such as cholestasis and jaundice, occur rarely.
• Nephrotoxicity, including dysuria, hematuria, proteinuria, and nephrotic syndrome and severe hypersensitivity reaction, marked by bronchospasm, and angioedema occur rarely.

PRECAUTIONS & CONSIDERATIONS
Caution is warranted with asthma, congestive heart failure (CHF), dehydration, hemostatic disease, history of GI disease, such as ulcers, hypertension, impaired liver or renal function as well as concurrent use of anticoagulants. Report pregnancy or suspicion of pregnancy. Mefenamic acid is excreted in breast milk. Safety and efficacy of mefenamic acid have not been established in children younger than 14 years old. In the elderly, age-related renal impairment may require dosage adjustment. Be aware that the elderly are more susceptible to GI toxicity and a lower dosage of the drug is recommended for this patient population. Alcohol and aspirin should be avoided during therapy due to an increased risk of GI bleeding.
Administration
Take mefenamic acid with regard to meals. Do not to chew or crush capsules. Antacids, food, or milk may be taken if GI distress occurs.

M

Mefloquine
me'flow-quine
(Lariam)
Do not confuse with Librium.

CATEGORY AND SCHEDULE
Pregnancy Risk Category: C

CLASSIFICATION
Antiprotozoals

MECHANISM OF ACTION
A quinolone-methanol compound
structurally similar to quinine
that destroys the asexual blood
forms of malarial pathogens,
Plasmodium falciparum,
P. vivax, P. malariae, P. ovale.
Therapeutic Effect: Inhibits
parasite growth.

PHARMACOKINETICS
Well absorbed from the gastrointesti-
nal (GI) tract. Protein binding: 98%.
Widely distributed, including
cerebrospinal fluid (CSF).
Metabolized in liver.
Primarily excreted in urine.
Half-life: 21-22 days.

AVAILABILITY
Tablets: 250 mg.

INDICATIONS AND DOSAGES
▶ **Suppression of malaria**
PO
Adults. 250 mg base weekly
starting 1 week before travel,
continuing weekly during
travel and for 4 weeks after
leaving endemic area.
Children more than 45 kg. 250 mg
weekly starting 1 week before
travel, continuing weekly during
travel and for 4 weeks after
leaving endemic area.

Children 45-31 kg. 187.5 mg
($3/4$ tablet) weekly starting 1 week
before travel, continuing weekly
during travel and for 4 weeks after
leaving endemic area.
Children 30-20 kg. 125 mg
($1/2$ tablet) weekly starting 1 week
before travel, continuing weekly
during travel and for 4 weeks after
leaving endemic area.
Children 19-15 kg. 62.5 mg
($1/4$ tablet) weekly starting 1 week
before travel, continuing weekly
during travel and for 4 weeks after
leaving endemic area.
▶ **Treatment of malaria**
PO
Adults. 1250 mg as a single dose.
Children. 15-25 mg/kg in a single
dose. Maximum: 1250 mg.

CONTRAINDICATIONS
Cardiac abnormalities, severe psychiatric disorders, epilepsy, history of
hypersensitivity to mefloquine

INTERACTIONS
Drug
Cytochrome P450 effect: Inhibits
CYP 3A4.
Beta-blockers: May increase brady-
cardia with beta-blockers.
Chloroquine, quinine, quinidine:
May increase the risk of toxicity
with these drugs.
Valproic acid: May decrease the
effect of valproic acid.
Herbal
None known.
Food
None known.

DIAGNOSTIC TEST EFFECTS
None known.

SIDE EFFECTS
Occasional
Mild transient headache, diffi-
culty concentrating, insomnia,

lightheadedness, vertigo, diarrhea, nausea, vomiting, visual disturbances, tinnitus

Rare
Aggressive behavior, anxiety, brady-cardia, depression, hallucinations, hypotension, panic attacks, paranoia, psychosis, syncope, tremor

SERIOUS REACTIONS
• Prolonged therapy may result in peripheral neuritis, neuromyopathy, hypotension, electrocardiogram (EKG) changes, agranulocytosis, aplastic anemia, thrombocytopenia, seizures, and psychosis.
• Overdosage may result in headache, vomiting, visual distur-bance, drowsiness, and seizures.

PRECAUTIONS & CONSIDERATIONS
Caution is warranted with history of depression, liver diseases as well as people who pilot airplanes and oper-ate machines since dizziness and disturbed sense of balance are side effects. It is unknown if mefloquine crosses the placenta or is excreted in breast milk. There are no age-related precautions noted in the children or the elderly.

Any new symptoms of anxiety, confusion, depression, restlessness, tinnitus, and visual difficulties should be reported.

Administration
Begin therapy before and continue after trip. Take mefloquine with regard to food and at least 8 oz. of water. Tablets may be crushed and mixed with water for oral adminis-tration. Continue taking mefloquine for the full length of treatment.

Megestrol
me-jess'trole
(Apo-Megestrol [CAN], Megace, Megostat [AUS])

CATEGORY AND SCHEDULE
Pregnancy Risk Category: X (for suspension), D (for tablets)

CLASSIFICATION
Progestin derivative, antineoplastic, appetite stimulant

MECHANISM OF ACTION
A hormone and antineoplastic agent that suppresses the release of luteinizing hormone from the anterior pituitary gland by inhibiting pituitary function. *Therapeutic Effect:* Shrinks tumors. Also increases appetite by an unknown mechanism.

PHARMACOKINETICS
Well absorbed from the GI tract. Metabolized in the liver; excreted in urine.

AVAILABILITY
Tablets: 20 mg, 40 mg.
Suspension: 40 mg/ml.

INDICATIONS AND DOSAGES
▸ **Palliative treatment of advanced breast cancer**
PO
Adults, Elderly. 160 mg/day in 4 equally divided doses.
▸ **Palliative treatment of advanced endometrial carcinoma**
PO
Adults, Elderly. 40-320 mg/day in divided doses. Maximum: 800 mg/day in 1-4 divided doses.

M

▸ **Anorexia, cachexia, weight loss**
PO
Adults, Elderly. 800 mg (20 ml)/day.

OFF-LABEL USES

Appetite stimulant, treatment of hormone-dependent or advanced prostate carcinoma

CONTRAINDICATIONS

None known.

INTERACTIONS

Drug
None known.
Herbal
None known.
Food
None known.

DIAGNOSTIC TEST EFFECTS

May increase blood glucose level.

SIDE EFFECTS

Frequent
Weight gain secondary to increased appetite
Occasional
Nausea, breakthrough bleeding, backache, headache, breast tenderness, carpal tunnel syndrome
Rare
Feeling of coldness

SERIOUS REACTIONS

• Thrombophlebitis and pulmonary embolism occur rarely.

PRECAUTIONS & CONSIDERATIONS

Caution is warranted with a history of thrombophlebitis. Megestrol use should be avoided during pregnancy, if possible, especially in the first 4 months. Pregnancy should be determined before initiating megestrol therapy. Megestrol has a pregnancy risk category of X in suspension form and D in tablet form. Contraception is imperative

during therapy. Breast-feeding is not recommended for patients taking this drug. The safety and efficacy of megestrol have not been established in children. No age-related precautions have been noted in the elderly. Potential side effects, including backache, breast tenderness, headache, nausea and vomiting, may occur. Notify the physician if calf pain, difficulty breathing, or vaginal bleeding develops.
Administration
Shake suspension well before using.

Meloxicam
mel-oks′i-kam
(Mobic)

CATEGORY AND SCHEDULE

Pregnancy Risk Category: C (D if used in third trimester or near delivery)

CLASSIFICATION

Analgesics, non-narcotic, non-steroidal anti-inflammatory drugs

MECHANISM OF ACTION

An NSAID that produces analgesic and anti-inflammatory effects by inhibiting prostaglandin synthesis. *Therapeutic Effect:* Reduces the inflammatory response and intensity of pain.

PHARMACOKINETICS

Route	Onset	Peak	Duration
PO (analgesic)	30 min	4-5 hr	N/A

Well absorbed after PO administration. Protein binding: 99%.

Metabolized in the liver. Eliminated in urine and feces. Not removed by hemodialysis. **Half-life:** 15-20 hr.

AVAILABILITY
Tablets: 7.5 mg, 15 mg.

INDICATIONS AND DOSAGES
▶ **Osteoarthritis, rheumatoid arthritis**
PO
Adults. Initially, 7.5 mg/day. Maximum: 15 mg/day.

CONTRAINDICATIONS
Aspirin-induced nasal polyps associated with bronchospasm

INTERACTIONS
Drug
Aspirin: May increase the risk of epigastric distress, such as heartburn and indigestion.
Lithium: May increase the plasma concentration and risk of toxicity of lithium.
Herbal
Ginkgo biloba: May increase the risk of bleeding.
Food
None known.

DIAGNOSTIC TEST EFFECTS
May increase serum creatinine, AST (SGOT), and ALT (SGPT) levels.

SIDE EFFECTS
Frequent (9%-7%)
Dyspepsia, headache, diarrhea, nausea
Occasional (4%-3%)
Dizziness, insomnia, rash, pruritus, flatulence, constipation, vomiting
Rare (less than 2%)
Somnolence, urticaria, photosensitivity, tinnitus

SERIOUS REACTIONS
• Rare reactions with long-term use include peptic ulcer disease, GI bleeding, gastritis, severe hepatic reaction (jaundice), nephrotoxicity (hematuria, dysuria, proteinuria), and a severe hypersensitivity reaction (bronchospasm, angioedema).

PRECAUTIONS & CONSIDERATIONS
Caution is warranted with asthma, CHF, hypertension, dehydration, hemostatic disease, hepatic or renal impairment, a history of GI disorders (such as ulcers), and concurrent anticoagulant use. Meloxicam should not be used during pregnancy because it may cause fetal harm. Meloxicam is excreted in breast milk. The safety and efficacy of meloxicam have not been established in children. The elderly require a dosage adjustment because of age-related renal impairment and increased susceptibility to GI toxicity. Avoid alcohol and aspirin during therapy because these substances increase the risk of GI bleeding. Tasks that require mental alertness or motor skills should also be avoided.

Notify the physician if chest pain, difficulty breathing, palpitations, peripheral edema, persistent abdominal cramps or pain, rash, ringing in the ears, severe nausea or vomiting, or unusual bleeding or ecchymosis occurs. CBC, BUN level, and serum alkaline phosphatase, bilirubin, creatinine, AST (SGOT), and ALT (SGPT) levels should be assessed during therapy. Therapeutic response, such as decreased pain, stiffness, swelling, and tenderness, improved grip strength, and increased joint mobility, should be evaluated.
Administration
Take meloxicam without regard to food.

M

Memantine
meh-man'teen
(Namenda)

CATEGORY AND SCHEDULE
Pregnancy Risk Category: B

CLASSIFICATION
NMDA receptor antagonists

MECHANISM OF ACTION
A neurotransmitter inhibitor that decreases the effects of glutamate, the principle excitatory neurotransmitter in the brain. Persistent CNS excitation by glutamate is thought to cause the symptoms of Alzheimer's disease. *Therapeutic Effect:* May reduce clinical deterioration in moderate to severe Alzheimer's disease.

PHARMACOKINETICS
Rapidly and completely absorbed after PO administration. Protein binding: 45%. Undergoes little metabolism; most of the dose is excreted unchanged in urine.
Half-life: 60-80 hr.

AVAILABILITY
Tablets: 5 mg, 10 mg.

INDICATIONS AND DOSAGES
▸ **Alzheimer's disease**
PO
Adults, Elderly. Initially, 5 mg once a day. May increase dosage at intervals of at least 1 wk in 5-mg increments to 10 mg/day (5 mg twice a day), then 15 mg/day (5 mg and 10 mg as separate doses), and finally 20 mg/day (10 mg twice a day). Target dose: 20 mg/day.

CONTRAINDICATIONS
Severe renal impairment

INTERACTIONS
Drug
Carbonic anhydrase inhibitors, sodium bicarbonate: May decrease the renal elimination of memantine.
Herbal
None known.
Food
None known.

DIAGNOSTIC TEST EFFECTS
None known.

SIDE EFFECTS
Occasional (7%-4%)
Dizziness, headache, confusion, constipation, hypertension, cough
Rare (3%-2%)
Back pain, nausea, fatigue, anxiety, peripheral edema, arthralgia, insomnia

SERIOUS REACTIONS
• None known.

PRECAUTIONS & CONSIDERATIONS
Caution is warranted with moderate renal impairment. It is unknown if memantine crosses the placenta or is distributed in breast milk. Memantine is not prescribed for use in children. No age-related precautions have been noted in the elderly, but memantine is not recommended for the elderly with severe renal impairment (creatinine clearance less than 9 ml/minute). Be aware that memantine is not a cure for Alzheimer's disease but may slow the progression of its symptoms. Adequate fluid intake should be maintained. Renal function and urine pH should be monitored; alkaline urine may lead to an accumulation of the drug and a possible increase in side effects.
Administration
Take memantine without regard to food. Do not abruptly discontinue or adjust the drug dosage. If therapy is interrupted for several days, restart

the drug at the lowest dose and increase the dosage at intervals of at least 1 week to the most recent dose, as prescribed.

Menotropins
men-oh-troe'-pins
(Humegon, Pergonal, Repronex)

CATEGORY AND SCHEDULE
Pregnancy Risk Category: X

CLASSIFICATION
Hormones/hormone modifiers, stimulants, ovarian

MECHANISM OF ACTION
A mixture of equal activity of follicle stimulating hormone (FSH) and lutenizing hormone (LH) that are isolated from the urine of post-menopausal women and are necessary for the development, maturation, and release of ova from ovaries and for spermatogenesis in the testes. *Therapeutic Effect:* Promotes ovulation and pregnancy in infertile women.

PHARMACOKINETICS
Not absorbed from the gastrointestinal (GI) tract. Cleared from circulation by glomular filtration. Degraded in proximal tubule or excreted unchanged in urine. **Half-life:** 2.2-2.9 hr.

AVAILABILITY
Injection: 75 units FSH activity and 150 units LH activity/2 ml ampule (Humegon, Pergonal, Repronex), 150 units FSH activity and 150 units LH activity/2 ml ampule (Humegon, Pergonal, Repronex)

INDICATIONS AND DOSAGES
▸ **Follicle maturation, ovulation and pregnancy induction**
IM
Adults. Initially, 75 International Units (IU) daily for 7-12 days followed by hCG, 5000-10,000 units one day after the last dose of menotropins. Treat until indices of estrogen activity are equivalent to or greater than those of the normal individual. If signs of ovulation are present but pregnancy does not occur, repeat this dosage regime for at least two more courses before increasing the dose of menotropins.
▸ **Follicle maturation, ovulation and pregnancy induction**
IM
Adults. After three course failures at 75 IU, increase dose to 150 IU daily for 7-12 days followed by 5000-10,000 units of hCG one day after the last dose of menotropins. If signs of ovulation are present but pregnancy does not develop, repeat the same dose for two more courses.
▸ **Stimulation of spermatogenesis**
IM
Adults. Pretreatment with 5000 units hCG 3 times weekly is required prior to initiating concomitant therapy with menotropins. Continue pretreatment until serum testosterone levels are in the normal range and masculinization is reached (may require 4-6 months); then initiate therapy with menotropins 75 IU 3 times weekly and 2000 units hCG twice weekly for a minimum of 4 months. If the patient has not responded after 4 months, continue treatment with 75 IU menotropins 3 times weekly or increase dose to 150 IU 3 times weekly, keeping the dose for hCG the same

CONTRAINDICATIONS
Prior hypersensitivity to menotropins

M

Women: Known or suspected pregnancy, high FSH level indicating primary ovarian failure, abnormal bleeding of undetermined origin, an organic intracranial lesion such as a pituitary tumor, elevated gonadotropin levels indicating primary testicular failure, presence of any cause of infertility other than anovulation, unless they are candidates for in vitro fertilization, ovarian cysts or enlargement not due to polycystic ovary syndrome, uncontrolled thyroid and adrenal dysfunction

Men: infertility disorders other than hypogonadotropic hypogonadism, normal gonadotropin levels indicating normal pituitary function

INTERACTIONS
Drug
None known.
Herbal
None known.
Food
None known.

DIAGNOSTIC TEST EFFECTS
None known.

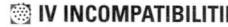 IV INCOMPATIBILITIES
None known.
IV Compatibilities
None known.

SIDE EFFECTS
Occasional
Women: Abdominal pain, bloating, diarrhea, nausea, vomiting, body rash, dizziness, dyspnea, tachypnea, ovarian cysts, ovarian enlargement, pain, rash, swelling at injection site, tachycardia
Men: Gynecomastia

SERIOUS REACTIONS
• Acute respiratory distress syndrome, atelectasis, pulmonary embolism, pulmonary infarction, arterial occlusion, cerebral vascular occlusion, venous thrombophlebitis, congenital abnormalities, ectopic pregnancy, and ovarian hyperstimulation syndrome have been reported.

PRECAUTIONS & CONSIDERATIONS
Be aware that menotropins should be discontinued if the ovaries become enlarged or abdominal pain occurs. Be aware that multiple births can occur with menotropin use for ovulation induction. Be aware that menotropins are contraindicated in pregnancy and unknown if distributed in breast milk. Be aware that the safety and efficacy of this drug have not been established in children and the elderly.

Storage
Lyophilized powder may be refrigerated or stored at room temperature. After reconstitution, inject immediately. Discard any unused portion. Protect from light.

Administration
Be aware that doses larger than 150 IU are not routinely recommended. Be aware that doses to produce maturation of the follicle must be individualized for each person. Single courses of therapy in women should not exceed 12 days.

Be aware if the ovaries are abnormally enlarged on the last day of menotropins therapy, hCG should be withheld. Stop administration of menotropins if the ovaries become abnormally enlarged or abdominal pain occurs.

Be aware that the couple should have intercourse daily, beginning on the day prior to the administration of hCG until ovulation becomes apparent.

Mix Pergonal with NaCl available with the medication and allow to completely dissolve.

Repronex may be administered IM or subcutaneous. Administer in lower abdomen, alternating sides, for subcutaneous administration.

Meperidine
me-per'i-deen
(Demerol, Pethidine Injection [AUS])
Do not confuse with Demulen or Dymelor.

CATEGORY AND SCHEDULE
Pregnancy Risk Category: B (D if used for prolonged periods or at high dosages at term)
Controlled Substance Schedule: II

CLASSIFICATION
Analgesics, narcotic, preanesthetics

MECHANISM OF ACTION
An opioid agonist that binds to opioid receptors in the CNS. *Therapeutic Effect:* Alters the perception of and emotional response to pain.

PHARMACOKINETICS

Route	Onset	Peak	Duration
PO	15 min	60 min	2-4 hr
IV	Less than 5 min	5-7 min	2-3 hr
IM	10-15 min	30-50 min	2-4 hr
Subcutaneous	10-15 min	30-50 min	2-4 hr

Variably absorbed from the GI tract; well absorbed after IM administration. Protein binding: 60%-80%. Widely distributed. Metabolized in the liver to active metabolite. Primarily excreted in urine. Not removed by hemodialysis. **Half-life:** 2.4-4 hr; metabolite 8-16 hr (increased in hepatic impairment and disease).

AVAILABILITY
Syrup: 50 mg/5 ml.
Tablets: 50 mg, 100 mg.
Injection: 25 mg/ml, 50 mg/ml, 75 mg/ml, 100 mg/ml.

INDICATIONS AND DOSAGES
▶ **Analgesia**
PO, IM, SUBCUTANEOUS
Adults, Elderly. 50-150 mg q3-4hr.
Children. 1.1-1.5 mg/kg q3-4hr. Don't exceed single dose of 100 mg.
▶ **Patient-controlled analgesia (PCA)**
IV
Adults. Loading dose: 50-100 mg. Intermittent bolus: 5-30 mg. Lockout interval: 10-20 min. Continuous infusion: 5-40 mg/hr. Maximum (4-hr): 200-300 mg.
▶ **Dosage in renal impairment**
Dosage is based on creatinine clearance.

Creatinine Clearance	Dosage
10-50 ml/min	75% of usual dose
Less than 10 ml/min	50% of usual dose

CONTRAINDICATIONS
Delivery of premature infant, diarrhea due to poisoning, use within 14 days of MAOIs

INTERACTIONS
Drug
Alcohol, other CNS depressants: May increase CNS or respiratory depression and hypotension.
MAOIs: May produce a severe, sometimes fatal reaction. Meperidine use is contraindicated.
Herbal
Valerian: May increase CNS depression.
Food
None known.

M

DIAGNOSTIC TEST EFFECTS

May increase serum amylase and lipase levels. Therapeutic serum level is 100-550 ng/ml; toxic serum level is greater than 1000 ng/ml.

🞂 IV INCOMPATIBILITIES

Allopurinol (Aloprim), amphotericin B complex (Abelcet, AmBisome, Amphotec), cefepime (Maxipime), cefoperazone (Cefobid), doxorubicin liposomal (Doxil), furosemide (Lasix), idarubicin (Idamycin), nafcillin (Nafcil)

🞂 IV Compatibilities

Bumetanide (Bumex), diltiazem (Cardizem), dobutamine (Dobutrex), dopamine (Intropin), heparin, insulin, lidocaine, magnesium, oxytocin (Pitocin), potassium

SIDE EFFECTS

Frequent
Sedation, hypotension (including orthostatic hypotension), diaphoresis, facial flushing, dizziness, nausea, vomiting, constipation

Occasional
Confusion, arrhythmias, tremors, urine retention, abdominal pain, dry mouth, headache, irritation at injection site, euphoria, dysphoria

Rare
Allergic reaction (rash, pruritus), insomnia

SERIOUS REACTIONS

• Overdose results in respiratory depression, skeletal muscle flaccidity, cold or clammy skin, cyanosis, and extreme somnolence progressing to seizures, stupor, and coma. The antidote is 0.4 mg naloxone.

• The patient who uses meperidine repeatedly may develop a tolerance to the drug's analgesic effect and physical dependence.

PRECAUTIONS & CONSIDERATIONS

Caution is warranted with acute abdominal conditions, cor pulmonale, history of seizures, increased intracranial pressure, hepatic or renal impairment, respiratory abnormalities, supraventricular tachycardia, and in the debilitated or elderly. Be aware that with renal impairment, meperidine's metabolite may increase and cause seizures, tremors, and twitching. Meperidine crosses the placenta and is distributed in breast milk. Regular use of opiates during pregnancy may produce withdrawal symptoms in the neonate, such as diarrhea, excessive crying, fever, hyperactive reflexes, irritability, seizures, sneezing, tremors, vomiting, and yawning. The neonate may develop respiratory depression if the mother receives meperidine during labor. Children are more prone to develop paradoxical excitement. Children younger than 2 years and the elderly are more susceptible to the drug's respiratory depressant effects. In the elderly, age-related renal impairment may increase the risk of urine retention. Be aware that drug dependence and tolerance may occur with prolonged use of high doses.

Dizziness and drowsiness may occur, so change positions slowly and avoid alcohol, CNS depressants, and tasks that require mental alertness or motor skills until response to the drug is established. Vital signs, pattern of daily bowel activity and stool consistency, and clinical improvement of pain should be monitored. The drug should be withheld and the physician should be notified if the respiratory rate is 12 breaths/minute or less in an adult, or 20 breaths/ minute or less in a child. Vital signs should be monitored for 15 to 30 minutes after an IM or subcutaneous dose and for 5 to 10 minutes after an IV dose.

Be alert for decreased B/P, as well as a change in quality and rate of pulse.
Storage
Store vials at room temperature.
Administration
! Be aware that meperidine's side effects are dependent on the dosage and route of administration. Know that ambulatory patients and those not in severe pain may be more prone to dizziness, nausea, and vomiting than those in the supine position and those in severe pain.

Take oral meperidine without regard to food. Dilute the syrup in a glass of water to prevent an anesthetic effect on mucous membranes.
! Give meperidine by slow IV push or IV infusion. Know that therapeutic serum drug level is 100 to 550 ng/ml; toxic serum drug level is greater than 1000 ng/ml.

Meperidine may be given undiluted or may be diluted in D_5W, Ringer's solution, lactated Ringer's solution, a dextrose-saline combination (such as 2.5%, 5%, or 10% dextrose and 0.45% or 0.9% NaCl), or Molar (M/6) Sodium Lactate Injection for IV injection or infusion. Place the patient in a recumbent position before administering parenteral meperidine. Administer IV push very slowly, over 2 to 3 minutes. Rapid IV administration increases the risk of a severe anaphylactic reaction, marked by apnea, cardiac arrest, and circulatory collapse.
! The IM route is preferred over the subcutaneous route because subcutaneous injection can produce induration, local irritation, and pain.

For IM use, inject the drug slowly. Know that patients with circulatory impairment are at increased risk for overdose because of delayed absorption of repeated injections.

Mephobarbital
me'foe-bar'bi-tal
(Mebaral)

CATEGORY AND SCHEDULE
Controlled substance:
Schedule IV

CLASSIFICATION
Anticonvulsants, barbiturates, sedatives/ hypnotics

MECHANISM OF ACTION
A barbiturate that increases seizure threshold in the motor cortex. *Therapeutic Effect:* Depresses monosynaptic and polysynaptic transmission in the central nervous system (CNS).

PHARMACOKINETICS
PO route onset 20-60 minutes, peak N/A, duration 6-8 hours. Well absorbed after PO administration. Widely distributed. Metabolized in liver to active metabolite, a form of phenobarbital. Minimally excreted in urine. Removed by hemodialysis.
Half-life: 34 hr.

AVAILABILITY
Tablets: 32 mg, 50 mg, 100 mg (Mebaral).

INDICATIONS AND DOSAGES
▶ **Epilepsy**
PO
Adults, Elderly. 400-600 mg/day in divided doses or at bedtime.
Children more than 5 yr. 32-64 mg 3 or 4 times/day.
Children less than 5 yr. 16-32 mg 3 or 4 times/day.

▶ **Sedation**
PO
Adults, Elderly. 32-100 mg/day in
3-4 divided doses.
Children. 16-32 mg in 3-4 divided
doses.

CONTRAINDICATIONS
Porphyria, history of hypersensitivity to mephobarbital or other
barbituates

INTERACTIONS
Drug
Alcohol, CNS depressants: May
increase the effects of mephobarbital.
Carbamazepine: May increase the
metabolism of carbamazepine.
**Digoxin, glucocorticoids, metro-
nidazole, oral anticoagulants,
quinidine, tricyclic antidepressants:** May decrease the effects of
these medications.
Pyridoxine: May decrease the
effectiveness of mephobarbital.
Valproic acid: Decreases the
metabolism and increases the
concentration and risk of toxicity of
mephobarbital.
Herbal
Catnip oil: May increase the CNS
effects of mephobarbital.
Eucalyptol: May decrease the
effectiveness of mephobarbital.
Evening primrose oil: May
decrease the anticonvulsant effectiveness of mephobarbital.
Ginkgo biloba: May decrease the
anticonvulsant effectiveness of
mephobarbital.
Kava kava: May increase the CNS
effects of mephobarbital.
Passion flower: May increase the
CNS effects of mephobarbital.
St. John's Wort: May decrease
CNS depressive effects of
mephobarbital.
Valerian: May increase the CNS
effects of mephobarbital.

Food
None known.

DIAGNOSTIC TEST EFFECTS
None known.

SIDE EFFECTS
Frequent
Dizziness, lightheadedness,
somnolence
Occasional
Confusion, headache, insomnia,
mental depression, nervousness,
nightmares, unusual excitement
Rare
Rash, paradoxical CNS hyperactivity
or nervousness in children, excitement or restlessness in elderly,
generally noted during first 2 weeks
of therapy, particularly noted in
presence of uncontrolled pain

SERIOUS REACTIONS
• Abrupt withdrawal after prolonged
therapy may produce effects including
markedly increased dreaming, nightmares or insomnia, tremor, sweating,
vomiting, hallucinations, delirium,
seizures, and status epilepticus.
• Skin eruptions appear as hypersensitivity reaction.
• Blood dyscrasias, liver disease,
and hypocalcemia occur rarely.
• Overdosage produces cold
or clammy skin, hypothermia,
severe CNS depression, cyanosis,
rapid pulse, and Cheyne-Stokes
respirations.
• Toxicity may result in severe renal
impairment.

PRECAUTIONS & CONSIDERATIONS
Caution should be used with liver or
renal impairment. Mephobarbital
readily crosses the placenta and is
distributed in breast milk. Withdrawal
symptoms may appear in neonates
born to women receiving barbiturates
during last trimester of pregnancy.

Mephobarbital use may cause paradoxical excitement in children. The elderly may exhibit confusion, excitement, and mental depression while taking mephobarbital. Alcohol should be avoided and caffeine intake should be limited. Tasks that require mental alertness or motor skills should be avoided because mephobarbital may cause dizziness and drowsiness.

Administration

Take mephobarbital without regard to meals. Crush tablets as needed. Do not discontinue the drug abruptly.

Meprobamate
me-proe'ba-mate
(Miltown, Novo-Mepro [CAN])

CATEGORY AND SCHEDULE
Pregnancy Risk Category: D

CLASSIFICATION
Anxiolytics

MECHANISM OF ACTION
A carbamate derivative that affects the thalamus and limbic system. Appears to inhibit multi-neuronal spinal reflexes. *Therapeutic Effect:* Relieves pain or muscle spasms.

PHARMACOKINETICS
Slowly absorbed from the gastrointestinal (GI) tract. Protein binding: 0%-30%. Metabolized in liver. Excreted in urine and feces. Moderately dialyzable. **Half-life:** 10 hr.

AVAILABILITY
Tablets: 200 mg, 400 mg, 600 mg (Miltown).

INDICATIONS AND DOSAGES
▶ **Anxiety disorders**
PO
Adults, Children 12 yr and older.
400 mg 3-4 times. Maximum: 2400 mg/day.
Children 6-12 yr. 100-200 mg 2-3 times/day.
Elderly. Use lowest effective dose. 200 mg 2-3 times/day
▶ **Dosage in renal impairment**

Creatinine Clearance	Dosage Interval
10-50 ml/min	Every 9-12 hr
Less than 10 ml/min	Every 12-18 hr

OFF-LABEL USES
Muscle contraction, headache, premenstrual tension, external sphincter spasticity, muscle rigidity, opisthotonos-associated with tetanus

CONTRAINDICATIONS
Acute intermittent porphyria, hypersensitivity to meprobamate or related compounds

INTERACTIONS
Drug
Alcohol, central nervous system (CNS) depressants: May increase CNS depression.
Herbal
Gotu kola, kava kava, St. John's wort: May increase CNS depression.
Food
None known.

DIAGNOSTIC TEST EFFECTS
None known.

SIDE EFFECTS
Frequent
Drowsiness, dizziness
Occasional
Tachycardia, palpitations, headache, lightheadedness, dermatitis, diarrhea, nausea, vomiting, dyspnea,

rash, weakness, blurred vision, wheezing.

SERIOUS REACTIONS
• Agranulocytosis, aplastic anemia, leukopenia, anaphylaxis, cardiac arrhythmias, hypotensive crisis, syncope, Stevens-Johnson syndrome and bullous dermatitis have been reported.
• Overdose may cause CNS depression, ataxia, coma, shock, hypotension, and death.

PRECAUTIONS & CONSIDERATIONS
Caution is warranted with the elderly as well as those with liver or renal impairment and those who use alcohol, psychotropic drugs, or other CNS depressants. Prolonged use of meprobamate may produce dependence. Meprobamate crosses the placenta and is distributed in breast milk. Be aware that the safety and efficacy of meprobamate has not been established in children younger than 6 years. In the elderly, there is an increased risk of central nervous system (CNS) toxicity, manifested as confusion, hallucinations, mental depression, and sedation. Age-related renal impairment may require a decreased dosage in the elderly.

Complete blood count (CBC), renal function tests, BUN, serum creatinine, liver function tests including aspartate amino transferase (AST) and alanine amino transferase (ALT) and alkaline phosphatase should be monitored as well as blood concentrations of meprobamate. Therapeutic levels range between 6-12 ng/ml. Toxic signs are CNS manifestations (drowsiness, lethargy, coma, shock) and cardiovascular disturbances (arrhythmias, tachycardia, bradycardia, persistent and profound hypotension).

Dizziness and drowsiness are expected side effects with meprobamate. Avoid alcohol and sudden changes in posture to help prevent hypotensive effects.
Administration
May give without regard to meals. Give last dose at bedtime. Avoid abrupt discontinuation in patients with prolonged use of meprobamate.

Meropenem
mear-ro-pen′em
(Merrem IV)

CATEGORY AND SCHEDULE
Pregnancy Risk Category: B

CLASSIFICATION
Antibiotics, carbapenems

MECHANISM OF ACTION
A carbapenem that binds to penicillin-binding proteins and inhibits bacterial cell wall synthesis. *Therapeutic Effect:* Produces bacterial cell death.

PHARMACOKINETICS
After IV administration, widely distributed into tissues and body fluids, including CSF. Protein binding: 2%. Primarily excreted unchanged in urine. Removed by hemodialysis. **Half-life:** 1 hr.

AVAILABILITY
Powder for Injection: 500 mg, 1 g.

INDICATIONS AND DOSAGES
▸ **Mild to moderate infections**
IV
Adults, Elderly. 0.5-1 g q8hr.
Children 3 mo and older.
20 mg/kg/dose q8hr.

Children younger than 3 mo. 20 mg/kg/dose q8-12hr.

▸ **Meningitis**

IV

Adults, Elderly, Children weighing 50 kg or more. 2 g q8hr.

Children 3 mo and older weighing less than 50 kg. 40 mg/kg q8hr. Maximum: 2 g/dose.

▸ **Dosage in renal impairment**

Dosage and frequency are modified based on creatinine clearance.

Creatinine Clearance	Dosage	Interval
26-49 ml/min	Recommended dose (1000 mg)	q12hr
10-25 ml/min	¹/₂ of recommended dose	q12hr
Less than 10 ml/min	¹/₂ of recommended dose	q24hr

OFF-LABEL USES

Lower respiratory tract infections, febrile neutropenia, gynecologic and obstetric infections, sepsis

CONTRAINDICATIONS

None known.

INTERACTIONS

Drug

Probenecid: Reduces renal excretion of meropenem.

Herbal

None known.

Food

None known.

DIAGNOSTIC TEST EFFECTS

May increase BUN level and serum alkaline phosphatase, bilirubin, creatinine, LDH, AST (SGOT), and ALT (SGPT) levels. May decrease blood Hct and Hgb levels and serum potassium levels.

IV INCOMPATIBILITIES

Acyclovir (Zovirax), amphotericin B (Fungizone), diazepam (Valium), doxycycline (Vibramycin), metronidazole (Flagyl), ondansetron (Zofran)

IV Compatibilities

Dobutamine (Dobutrex), dopamine (Intropin), heparin, magnesium

SIDE EFFECTS

Frequent (5%-3%)

Diarrhea, nausea, vomiting, headache, inflammation at injection site

Occasional (2%)

Oral candidiasis, rash, pruritus

Rare (less than 2%)

Constipation, glossitis

SERIOUS REACTIONS

• Antibiotic-associated colitis and other superinfections may occur.

• Anaphylactic reactions have been reported.

• Seizures may occur in those with CNS disorders (including brain lesions and a history of seizures), bacterial meningitis, or impaired renal function.

M

PRECAUTIONS & CONSIDERATIONS

Caution is warranted with CNS disorders (particularly a history of seizures), hypersensitivity to cephalosporins, penicillins, or other allergens, and renal function impairment. Be aware that it is unknown if meropenem is distributed in breast milk. Be aware that the safety and efficacy of meropenem have not been established in children younger than 3 months. In the elderly, age-related renal impairment may require dosage adjustment. Notify the physician if severe diarrhea occurs but avoid taking antidiarrheals.

Notify the physician of the onset of troublesome or serious adverse reactions, including infusion site pain, redness, or swelling, nausea or vomiting, or skin rash or itching. Electrolytes (especially potassium), intake and output, and renal function test results should be monitored. Blood pressure, temperature, and mental status should be monitored.

Storage
Store vials at room temperature. After reconstitution with 0.9% NaCl, solution is stable for 2 hours at room temperature, 18 hours if refrigerated (with D_5W, stable for 1 hour at room temperature, 8 hours if refrigerated).

Administration
! Space drug doses evenly around the clock.

For IV use, reconstitute each 500 mg with 10 ml sterile water for injection to provide a concentration of 50 mg/ml. Shake to dissolve until clear. May further dilute with 100 ml 0.9% NaCl or D_5W. May give by IV push or IV intermittent infusion (piggyback). If administering as IV intermittent infusion (piggyback), give over 15 to 30 minutes; if administered by IV push (5 to 20 ml), give over 3 to 5 minutes.

Mesalamine
mez-al′a-meen
(Asacol, Fiv-Canasa, Mesasal [CAN], Pentasa, Rowasa, Salofalk [CAN])
Do not confuse Asacol with Os-Cal.

CATEGORY AND SCHEDULE
Pregnancy Risk Category: B

CLASSIFICATION
Gastrointestinals, salicylates

MECHANISM OF ACTION
A salicylic acid derivative that locally inhibits arachidonic acid metabolite production, which is increased in patients with chronic inflammatory bowel disease. *Therapeutic Effect:* Blocks prostaglandin production and diminishes inflammation in the colon.

PHARMACOKINETICS
Poorly absorbed from the colon. Moderately absorbed from the GI tract. Metabolized in the liver to active metabolite. Unabsorbed portion eliminated in feces; absorbed portion excreted in urine. Unknown if removed by hemodialysis. **Half-life:** 0.5-1.5 hr; metabolite, 5-10 hr.

AVAILABILITY
Tablets (Delayed-Release [Asacol]): 400 mg.
Capsules (Controlled-Release [Pentasa]): 250 mg.
Rectal Suspension (Rowasa): 4 g/60 ml.
Suppositories (Canasa): 500 mg.

INDICATIONS AND DOSAGES
▸ **Ulcerative colitis, proctosigmoiditis, proctitis**
PO (ASACOL)
Adults, Elderly. 800 mg 3 times a day for 6 wk.
Children. 50 mg/kg/day q8-12hr.
PO (PENTASA)
Adults, Elderly. 1 g 4 times a day for 8 wk.
Children. 50 mg/kg/day q6-12hr.
RECTAL (RETENTION ENEMA)
Adults, Elderly. 60 ml (4 g) at bedtime; retain overnight (about 8 hr) for 3-6 wk.
RECTAL (SUPPOSITORY)
Adults, Elderly. 1 suppository (500 mg) twice a day, retain 1-3 hr for 3-6 wk.

▶ **To maintain remission in ulcerative colitis**

PO (ASACOL)
Adults, Elderly. 1.6 g/day in divided doses.

PO (PENTASA)
Adults, Elderly. 1 g 4 times a day.

CONTRAINDICATIONS
None known.

INTERACTIONS
Drug
None known.
Herbal
None known.
Food
None known.

DIAGNOSTIC TEST EFFECTS
May increase BUN, serum alkaline phosphatase, creatinine, AST (SGOT), and ALT (SGPT) levels.

SIDE EFFECTS
Mesalamine is generally well tolerated, with only mild and transient effects.

Frequent (greater than 6%)
PO: Abdominal cramps or pain, diarrhea, dizziness, headache, nausea, vomiting, rhinitis, unusual fatigue
Rectal: Abdominal or stomach cramps, flatulence, headache, nausea
Occasional (6%-2%)
PO: Hair loss, decreased appetite, back or joint pain, flatulence, acne
Rectal: Hair loss
Rare (less than 2%)
Rectal: Anal irritation

SERIOUS REACTIONS
• Sulfite sensitivity may occur in susceptible patients, manifested by cramping, headache, diarrhea, fever, rash, hives, itching, and wheezing. Discontinue drug immediately.
• Hepatitis, pancreatitis, and pericarditis occur rarely with oral forms.

PRECAUTIONS & CONSIDERATIONS
Caution is warranted with preexisting renal disease and sulfasalazine sensitivity. It is unknown if mesalamine crosses the placenta or is distributed in breast milk. Safety and efficacy of mesalamine have not been established in children. In the elderly, age-related renal impairment may require cautious use. Avoid tasks that require mental alertness or motor skills until response to the drug has been established.

Be aware that mesalamine use may discolor urine yellow-brown; mesalamine suppositories stain fabrics. Adequate fluid intake should be maintained. Daily bowel activity and stool consistency and skin for rash should be assessed. Mesalamine should be discontinued if cramping, diarrhea, fever, or rash occurs.

Storage
Store rectal suspension, suppositories, and oral forms at room temperature.

Administration
For oral use, do not break outer coating of tablet; swallow whole. Take mesalamine without regard to food.

For rectal use, shake bottle well. Lie on left side with lower leg extended, upper leg flexed forward, or to assume the knee-chest position. Insert applicator tip into rectum, pointing toward umbilicus. Squeeze bottle steadily until contents are emptied. Retain the enema for as long as tolerable, preferably for a minimum of 8 hours.

M

Mesoridazine
mez-oh-rid'a-zeen
(Serentil)
**Do not confuse Serentil
with Proventil, Serevent, or
sertraline.**

CATEGORY AND SCHEDULE
Pregnancy Risk Category: C

CLASSIFICATION
Antipsychotics, phenothiazines

MECHANISM OF ACTION
A phenothiazine that blocks
dopamine at postsynaptic receptor
sites in the brain. *Therapeutic Effect:*
Diminishes schizophrenic behavior.
Also has anticholinergic and sedative
effects.

AVAILABILITY
Oral Solution: 25 mg/ml.
Tablets: 10 mg, 25 mg, 50 mg,
100 mg.
Injection: 25 mg/ml.

INDICATIONS AND DOSAGES
▶ **Schizophrenia**
PO
Adults, Elderly. 25-50 mg 3 times a
day. Maximum: 400 mg/day.
IM
Adults, Elderly. Initially, 25 mg.
May repeat in 30-60 min. Range:
25-200 mg.
▶ **Severe behavioral problems
(combativeness or explosive,
hyperexcitable behavior)
associated with neurologic
diseases**
PO
Elderly. Initially, 10 mg once or
twice a day. May increase
at 4-7 day intervals.
Maximum: 250 mg.

IM
Adults, Elderly. Initially, 25 mg.
May repeat in 30-60 min. Range:
25-200 mg.

CONTRAINDICATIONS
Coma, myelosuppression, severe
cardiovascular disease, severe CNS
depression, subcortical brain damage

INTERACTIONS
Drug
Alcohol, other CNS depressants:
May increase CNS and respiratory
depression and the hypotensive
effects of mesoridazine.
Antithyroid agents: May increase
the risk of agranulocytosis.
**Extrapyramidal symptom produc-
ing medications:** May increase
extrapyramidal symptoms.
**Hypotension-producing medica-
tions:** May increase hypotension.
Levodopa: May decrease the effects
of levodopa.
Lithium: May decrease mesoridazine
absorption and produce adverse
neurologic effects.
MAOIs, tricyclic antidepressants:
May increase the anticholinergic and
sedative effects of mesoridazine.
Herbal
None known.
Food
None known.

DIAGNOSTIC TEST EFFECTS
May produce false-positive pregnancy and phenylketonuria test
results. May produce EKG changes,
including prolonged QT and QTc
intervals and T-wave depression or
inversion.

SIDE EFFECTS
Frequent
Orthostatic hypotension, dizziness,
syncope (occur frequently after
first injection, occasionally after

subsequent injections, and rarely with oral form)

Occasional

Somnolence (during early therapy), dry mouth, blurred vision, lethargy, constipation or diarrhea, nasal congestion, peripheral edema, urine retention

Rare

Ocular changes, altered skin pigmentation (in those taking high doses for prolonged periods), darkening of urine

SERIOUS REACTIONS

• Abrupt withdrawal after long-term therapy may precipitate nausea, vomiting, gastritis, dizziness, and tremors.

• Blood dyscrasias, particularly agranulocytosis and mild leukopenia may occur.

• Mesoridazine use may lower the seizure threshold.

PRECAUTIONS & CONSIDERATIONS

Caution is warranted with alcohol withdrawal, glaucoma, history of seizures, benign prostatic hyperplasia, myocarditis, urine retention, and impaired cardiac, hepatic, renal, and respiratory function.

Urine may darken. Drowsiness may occur but generally subsides with continued therapy. Alcohol and tasks that require mental alertness or motor skills should be avoided. Notify the physician if visual disturbances occur. A baseline EKG should be performed before therapy. Pattern of daily bowel activity and stool consistency should be assessed.

Administration

Skin contact with the oral solution should be avoided because it may cause contact dermatitis. Full therapeutic effect may take up to 6 weeks to appear. Do not abruptly discontinue after long-term use.

Metaproterenol

met-a-proe-ter′e-nole
(Alupent)

Do not confuse metaproterenol with metipranolol or metoprolol, or Alupent with Atrovent.

CATEGORY AND SCHEDULE

Pregnancy Risk Category: C

CLASSIFICATION

Adrenergic agonists, bronchodilators

MECHANISM OF ACTION

A sympathomimetic that stimulates beta$_2$-adrenergic receptors, resulting in relaxation of bronchial smooth muscle. *Therapeutic Effect:* Relieves bronchospasm and reduces airway resistance.

M

AVAILABILITY

Syrup: 10 mg/5 ml.
Tablets: 10 mg, 20 mg.
Aerosol Oral Inhalation (Alupent): 0.65 mg/inhalation.
Solution for Oral Inhalation: 0.4%, 0.6%, 5%.

INDICATIONS AND DOSAGES

▸ **Treatment of bronchospasm**

PO

Adults, Children older than 9 yr. 20 mg 3-4 times a day.
Elderly. 10 mg 3-4 times a day. May increase to 20 mg/dose.
Children 6-9 yr. 10 mg 3-4 times a day.
Children 2-5 yr. 1.3-2.6 mg/kg/day in 3-4 divided doses.
Children younger than 2 yr. 0.4 mg/kg 3-4 times a day.
INHALATION
Adults, Elderly, Children 12 yr

and older. 2-3 inhalations q3-4hr.
Maximum: 12 inhalations/24 hr.
NEBULIZATION
Adults, Elderly, Children 12 yr and older. 10-15 mg (0.2-0.3 ml) of 5% q4-6hr.
Children younger than 12 yr, Infants. 0.5-1 mg/kg (0.01-0.02 ml/kg) of 5% q4-6hr.

CONTRAINDICATIONS
Angle-closure glaucoma, preexisting arrhythmias associated with tachycardia

INTERACTIONS
Drug
Beta blockers: May decrease the effects of beta blockers.
Digoxin, other sympathomimetics: May increase the risk of arrhythmias.
MAOIs: May increase the risk of hypertensive crisis.
Tricyclic antidepressants: May increase cardiovascular effects.
Herbal
None known.
Food
None known.

DIAGNOSTIC TEST EFFECTS
May decrease serum potassium level.

SIDE EFFECTS
Frequent (over 10%)
Rigors, tremors, anxiety, nausea, dry mouth
Occasional (9%-1%)
Dizziness, vertigo, asthenia, headache, GI distress, vomiting, cough, dry throat
Rare (less than 1%)
Somnolence, diarrhea, altered taste

SERIOUS REACTIONS
• Excessive sympathomimetic stimulation may cause palpitations, extrasystoles, tachycardia, chest pain, a slight increase in B/P followed by a substantial decrease, chills, diaphoresis, and blanching of skin.
• Too-frequent or excessive use may lead to decreased drug effectiveness and severe, paradoxical bronchoconstriction.

PRECAUTIONS & CONSIDERATIONS
Caution is warranted with arrhythmias, CHF, ischemic heart disease, diabetes mellitus, hypertension, hyperthyroidism, and a seizure disorder. Drink plenty of fluids to decrease the thickness of lung secretions. Avoid excessive use of caffeinated products, such as chocolate, cocoa, cola, coffee, and tea.
    Anxiety, insomnia, and restlessness may occur. Notify the physician of chest pain, difficulty breathing, dizziness, flushing, headache, palpitations, tachycardia, or tremors. Pulse rate and quality, respiratory rate, depth, rhythm and type, EKG, ABG levels, pulmonary function, and clinical improvement should be monitored. Evidence of cyanosis, a blue or a dusky color in light-skinned patients and a gray color in dark-skinned patients, should also be assessed.
Administration
Do not exceed the recommended dosage.

Metaraminol
met-ar-am'e-nol
(Aramine)

CATEGORY AND SCHEDULE
Pregnancy Risk Category: D

CLASSIFICATION
Adrenergic agonists

MECHANISM OF ACTION
An alpha-adrenergic receptor agonist that causes vasoconstriction, reflex bradycardia, inhibits GI smooth muscle and vascular smooth muscle supplying skeletal muscle and increases heart rate and force of heart muscle contraction. *Therapeutic Effect:* Increases both systolic and diastolic pressure.

PHARMACOKINETICS

Route	Onset	Peak	Duration
IM (pressor effect)	10 min	N/A	20-60 min
IV	1-2 min	N/A	
SC	5-20 min	N/A	

Metabolized in the liver. Excreted in the urine and the bile.

AVAILABILITY
Injection: 10 mg/ml (Aramine).

INDICATIONS AND DOSAGES
▸ **Prevention of hypotension**
IM/SC
Adults, Elderly. 2-10 mg as a single dose.
Children. 0.01 mg/kg as a single dose.
▸ **Adjunctive treatment of hypotension**
IV
Adults, Elderly. 15-100 mg IV infusion, administered at a rate to maintain the desired blood pressure.
▸ **Severe shock**
IV
Adults, Elderly. 0.5-5 mg direct IV injection followed by 15-100 mg IV infusion in 250-500 ml fluid for control of blood pressure.

CONTRAINDICATIONS
Cyclopropane or halothane anesthesia, use of MAOIs, pregnancy, hypersensitivity to metaraminol

INTERACTIONS
Drug
Cyclopropane, halothane, MAOIs, digoxin, oxytocin, reserpine: May increase the risk of metaraminol toxicity.
Tricyclic antidepressants: May decrease the effect of metaraminol.
Herbal
None known.
Food
None known.

DIAGNOSTIC TEST EFFECTS
None known.

▨ IV INCOMPATIBILITIES
Amphotericin B, dexamethasone, erythromycin, hydrocortisone, methicillin, penicillin G, prednisolone, thiopental (Pentothal)

▨ IV Compatibilities
Amikacin (Amikin), amiodarone (Cordarone), cephalothin (Ceporacin), cephapirin (Cefadyl), chloramphenicol, cimetidine (Tagamet), cyanocobalamin, dexamethasone, dobutamine (Dobutrex), ephedrine, hydrocortisone, inamrinone, lidocaine, oxytocin (Pitocin), potassium, procainamide, promazine

M

(Sparine), secobarbital (Seconal),
sodium bicarbonate, sulfisoxazole
(Gantrisin), tetracycline, verapamil

SIDE EFFECTS
Occasional
Tachycardia, hypertension, cardiac
arrhythmias, flushing, palpitations,
hypotension, angina, tremors,
nervousness, headache, dizziness,
weakness, sloughing of skin, nausea,
abscess formation, diaphoresis

SERIOUS REACTIONS
• Overdosage produces hypertension, cerebral hemorrhage, cardiac
arrest, and seizures.

PRECAUTIONS & CONSIDERATIONS
Caution should be used with
previous myocardial infarction,
hypertension, and hyperthyroidism.
Metaraminol crosses the placenta
and is distributed in breast milk.
Use metaraminol with caution in
children. In the elderly, age-related
renal impairment may require dosage
adjustment. Increased heart rate or
palpitations should be reported.
Administration
For IM and subcutaneous injection,
in order to prevent necrosis, infiltrate
area with 10-15 ml of saline containing 5-10 mg of phentolamine.
 For IV injection, as adjunctive
treatment of hypotension or severe
shock, mix 15-100 mg in 250-500 ml
NS or D_5W. For severe shock,
metaraminol may also be administered endotracheally. Prolonged use
may produce cumulative effects.

Metaxalone
me-tax′a-lone
(Skelaxin)

CATEGORY AND SCHEDULE
Pregnancy Risk Category: C

CLASSIFICATION
Musculoskeletal agents,
relaxants, skeletal muscle

MECHANISM OF ACTION
A central depressant whose exact
mechanism is unknown. Many
effects due to its central depressant
actions. *Therapeutic Effect:* Relieves
pain or muscle spasms.

PHARMACOKINETICS
PO route onset 1 hour, peak 3 hours,
duration 4-6 hours. Well absorbed
from the gastrointestinal (GI) tract.
Metabolized in liver. Primarily
excreted in urine. **Half-life:** 9 hr.

AVAILABILITY
Tablets: 400 mg, 800 mg (Skelaxin).

INDICATIONS AND DOSAGES
▸ **Muscle relaxant**
PO
*Adults, Elderly, Children older than
12 yr.* 800 mg 3-4 times/day.

CONTRAINDICATIONS
Impaired renal or hepatic function,
history of drug-induced hemolytic
anemias or other anemias,
history of hypersensitivity
to metaxalone

INTERACTIONS
Drug
**Alcohol, central nervous system
(CNS) depression-producing
medications, tricyclic antidepres-
sants:** May increase CNS depression.

MAOIs: May increase the risk of hypertensive crisis and severe seizures.
Herbal
None known.
Food
None known.

DIAGNOSTIC TEST EFFECTS
May give false-positive Benedict's test.

SIDE EFFECTS
Occasional
Drowsiness, headache, lightheadedness, dermatitis, nausea, vomiting, stomach cramps, dyspnea

SERIOUS REACTIONS
• Overdose may cause CNS depression, coma, shock, and respiratory depression.

PRECAUTIONS & CONSIDERATIONS
Caution should be used with impaired liver or renal function. It is unknown if metaxalone crosses the placenta or is distributed in breast milk. Safety and efficacy of metaxalone have not been established in children younger than 12 years. In the elderly, there is an increased risk of central nervous system (CNS) toxicity, manifested as confusion, hallucinations, mental depression, and sedation. Age-related renal impairment may require a decreased dosage in the elderly. Alcohol as well as tasks that require mental alertness or motor skills should be avoided during therapy.
Administration
Take metaxalone without regard to food.

Metformin
met-for'min
(Fortamet, Glucophage, Glucophage XL, Glycon [CAN], Novo-Metformin [CAN], Riomet)

CATEGORY AND SCHEDULE
Pregnancy Risk Category: B

CLASSIFICATION
Antidiabetic agents, biguanides

MECHANISM OF ACTION
An antihyperglycemic that decreases hepatic production of glucose. Decreases absorption of glucose and improves insulin sensitivity. *Therapeutic Effect:* Improves glycemic control, stabilizes or decreases body weight, and improves lipid profile.

PHARMACOKINETICS
Slowly, incompletely absorbed after oral administration. Food delays or decreases the extent of absorption. Protein binding: Negligible. Primarily distributed to intestinal mucosa and salivary glands. Primarily excreted unchanged in urine. Removed by hemodialysis. **Half-life:** 3-6 hr.

AVAILABILITY
Oral Solution (Riomet): 100 mg/ml.
Tablets (Glucophage): 500 mg, 850 mg, 1000 mg.
Tablets (Extended-Release [Glucophage XL]): 500 mg, 750 mg.
Tablets (Extended-Release [Fortamet]): 500 mg, 1000 mg.

INDICATIONS AND DOSAGES
▸ **Diabetes mellitus**
PO (500-mg, 1000-mg Tablet)
Adults, Elderly. Initially, 500 mg twice a day, with morning and

M

evening meals. May increase in 500-mg increments every week, in divided doses. May give twice a day up to 2000 mg/day (for example, 1000 mg twice a day [with morning and evening meals]). If 2500 mg/day is required, give 3 times a day with meals. Maximum: 2500 mg/day.
Children 10-16 yr. Initially, 500 mg twice a day. May increase by 500 mg/day at weekly intervals. Maximum: 2000 mg/day.
PO (850-mg Tablet)
Adults, Elderly. Initially, 850 mg/day, with morning meal. May increase dosage in 850-mg increments every other week, in divided doses. Maintenance: 850 mg twice a day, with morning and evening meals. Maximum: 2550 mg/day (850 mg 3 times a day).
PO (Extended-release Tablets)
Adults, Elderly. Initially, 500 mg once a day. May increase by 500 mg/day at weekly intervals. Maximum: 2000 mg once a day.
▸ **Adjunct to insulin therapy**
PO
Adults, Elderly. Initially, 500 mg/day. May increase by 500 mg at 7-day intervals. Maximum: 2500 mg/day (2000 mg/day for extended-release form).

OFF-LABEL USES
Treatment of metabolic complications of AIDS, prediabetes, weight reduction

CONTRAINDICATIONS
Acute CHF, MI, cardiovascular collapse, renal disease or dysfunction, respiratory failure, septicemia

INTERACTIONS
Drug
Alcohol, amiloride, cimetidine, digoxin, furosemide, morphine, **nifedipine, procainamide, quinidine, quinine, ranitidine, triamterene, trimethoprim, vancomycin:** Increase metformin blood concentration.
Furosemide, hypoglycemia-causing medications: May require a decrease in metformin dosage.
Iodinated contrast studies: May cause acute renal failure and increased risk of lactic acidosis.
Herbal
None known.
Food
None known.

DIAGNOSTIC TEST EFFECTS
None known.

SIDE EFFECTS
Occasional (greater than 3%)
GI disturbances (including diarrhea, nausea, vomiting, abdominal bloating, flatulence, and anorexia) that are transient and resolve spontaneously during therapy.
Rare (3%-1%)
Unpleasant or metallic taste that resolves spontaneously during therapy.

SERIOUS REACTIONS
• Lactic acidosis occurs rarely but is a fatal complication in 50% of cases. Lactic acidosis is characterized by an increase in blood lactate levels (greater than 5 mmol/L), a decrease in blood pH, and electrolyte disturbances. Signs and symptoms of lactic acidosis include unexplained hyperventilation, myalgia, malaise, and somnolence, which may advance to cardiovascular collapse (shock), acute CHF, acute MI, and prerenal azotemia.

PRECAUTIONS & CONSIDERATIONS
Caution is warranted with CHF, chronic respiratory difficulty, and uncontrolled hyperthyroidism or

hypothyroidism, hepatic impairment, concurrent use of drugs that affect renal function, conditions that cause hyperglycemia or hypoglycemia, or delay food absorption, such as diarrhea, high fever, malnutrition, gastroparesis, and vomiting, and in the elderly, debilitated, or malnourished with renal impairment. Caution should also be used in those who consume excessive amounts of alcohol; alcohol should be avoided during therapy. Insulin is the drug of choice during pregnancy. Metformin is distributed in breast milk in animals. Safety and efficacy of metformin have not been established in children. In the elderly, age-related renal impairment or peripheral vascular disease may require dosage adjustment or discontinuation of drug.

Notify the physician of diarrhea, easy bleeding or bruising, change in color of stool or urine, headache, nausea, persistent rash, and vomiting. Hgb and Hct, RBC count, and serum creatinine level should be obtained before beginning metformin therapy and annually thereafter. Food intake, blood glucose level, glycosylated Hgb, folic acid level, and renal function should also be monitored. Be aware of signs and symptoms of hypoglycemia (anxiety, cool wet skin, diplopia, dizziness, headache, hunger, numbness in mouth, tachycardia, tremors), or hyperglycemia (deep rapid breathing, dim vision, fatigue, nausea, polydipsia, polyphagia, polyuria, vomiting) especially in persons also taking oral sulfonylureas; carry candy, sugar packets, or other sugar supplements for immediate response to hypoglycemia. Consult the physician when glucose demands are altered (such as with fever, heavy physical activity, infection, stress, trauma). Exercise, good personal hygiene (including foot care), not

smoking, and weight control are essential parts of therapy.

Administration
! Lactic acidosis is a rare but potentially severe consequence of metformin therapy. Expect to withhold metformin in patients with conditions that may predispose to lactic acidosis, such as dehydration, hypoperfusion, hypoxemia, and sepsis.

Take metformin orally with meals. Do not crush film-coated tablets.

Methacholine
meth-a-ko′leen
(Provocholine)

CATEGORY AND SCHEDULE
Pregnancy Risk Category: C

CLASSIFICATION
Cholinergics, diagnostics, nonradioactive

M

MECHANISM OF ACTION
A cholinergic, parasympathomimetic, synthetic analogue of acetylcholine that stimulates muscarinic, postganglionic parasympathetic receptors. *Therapeutic Effect:* Results in smooth muscle contraction of the airways and increased tracheobronchial secretions.

PHARMACOKINETICS
PO route onset rapid, peak 1-4 minutes, duration 15-75 minutes or 5 minutes if methacholine challenge is followed with a beta-agonist agent. Undergoes rapid hydrolysis in the plasma by acetylcholinesterase.

AVAILABILITY
Powder for oral inhalation:
100-mg/5 ml (Provocholine).

INDICATIONS AND DOSAGES
▸ **Asthma diagnosis**
INHALATION
Challenge test: Before inhalation challenge, perform baseline pulmonary function tests; the patient must have an FEV1 of at least 70% of the predicted value. The following is a suggested schedule for administration of methacholine challenge. Calculate cumulative units by multiplying number of breaths by concentration given. Total cumulative units are the sum of cumulative units for each concentration given.
Vial E:
* Serial concentration: 0.025 mg/ml
* No. of breaths: 5
* Cumulative units per concentration: 0.125
* Total cumulative units: 0.125
Vial D:
* Serial concentration: 0.25 mg/ml
* No. of breaths: 5
* Cumulative units per concentration: 1.25
* Total cumulative units: 1.375
Vial C:
* Serial concentration: 2.5 mg/ml
* No. of breaths: 5
* Cumulative units per concentration: 12.5
* Total cumulative units: 13.88
Vial B:
* Serial concentration: 10 mg/ml
* No. of breaths: 5
* Cumulative units per concentration: 50
* Total cumulative units: 63.88
Vial A:
* Serial concentration: 25 mg/ml
* No. of breaths: 5
* Cumulative units per concentration: 125
* Total cumulative units: 188.88
Determine FEV1 within 5 minutes of challenge, a positive challenge is a 20% reduction in FEV1.

OFF-LABEL USES
Adie syndrome diagnosis, familial dysautonomia diagnosis, peripheral ischemia, parotitis

CONTRAINDICATIONS
Asthma, wheezing, or very low baseline pulmonary function tests, concomitant use of beta-blockers, hypersensitivity to the drug; because of the potential for severe bronchoconstriction

INTERACTIONS
Drug
Beta-blockers: May increase risk of prolonged bronchoconstriction.
Herbal
None known.
Food
None known.

DIAGNOSTIC TEST EFFECTS
None known.

SIDE EFFECTS
Occasional
Headache, lightheadedness, itching, throat irritation, wheezing

SERIOUS REACTIONS
* Severe bronchoconstriction and reduction in respiratory function can result. Patients with severe hyperreactivity of the airways can experience bronchoconstriction at a dosage as low as 0.025 mg/ml (0.125 cumulative units). If severe bronchoconstriction occurs, reverse immediately by administration of a rapid-acting inhaled bronchodilator (beta-agonist).

PRECAUTIONS & CONSIDERATIONS
Caution is warranted with liver function impairment, pulmonary disease, and significant cardiovascular disease. Safety and efficacy of methacholine have not been established in children. Chest, dyspnea,

coughing, and wheezing indicate a positive response.

Administration

Methacholine challenge may be administered nasally to measure hyperactivity of the nasal area in the diagnosis of perennial rhinitis.

The following are guidelines for reconstitution and further dilution of methacholine chloride powder for a single-patient testing:

All dilutions should be made with 0.9% NaCl injection containing 0.4% phenol (pH 7). Add 4 ml of 0.9% NaCl injection to the 5-ml vial containing 100 mg of methacholine chloride (vial A). The final concentration will be 25 mg/ml (vial A). Remove 1 ml of solution from vial A and add 1.5 ml of 0.9% NaCl injection (vial B). The final concentration will be 10 mg/ml. Remove 1 ml of solution from vial A and transfer to another vial with an additional 9 ml of 0.9% NaCl injection. The final concentration will be 2.5 mg/ml (vial C). Remove 1 ml of solution from vial C and transfer to another vial with an additional 9 ml of 0.9% NaCl injection. The final concentration will be 0.25 mg/ml (vial D). Remove 1 ml of solution from vial D and transfer to another vial with an additional 9 ml of 0.9% NaCl injection. The final concentration will be 0.025 mg/ml (vial E). A 0.22-micron filter should be used when transferring the solutions from each vial to a nebulizer.

The solutions in vials A through D may be refrigerated for a maximum of 2 weeks. Vial E must be prepared on the day of challenge.

Methadone
meth'a-done
(Dolophine, Metadol [CAN], Methadone Intensol, Methadose, Physeptone [AUS])

CATEGORY AND SCHEDULE
Pregnancy Risk Category: B (D if used for prolonged periods or at high dosages at term) Controlled Substance Schedule: II

CLASSIFICATION
Analgesics, narcotic

MECHANISM OF ACTION
An opioid agonist that binds with opioid receptors in the CNS. *Therapeutic Effect:* Alters the perception of and emotional response to pain; reduces withdrawal symptoms from other opioid drugs.

PHARMACOKINETICS

Route	Onset	Peak	Duration
Oral	0.5-1 hr	1.5-2 hr	6-8 hr
IM	10-20 min	1-2 hr	4-5 hr
IV	N/A	15-30 min	3-4 hr

Well absorbed after IM injection. Protein binding: 80%-85%. Metabolized in the liver. Primarily excreted in urine. Not removed by hemodialysis. **Half-life:** 15-25 hr.

AVAILABILITY
Oral Concentrate (Methadone Intensol, Methadose): 10 mg/ml.
Oral Solution: 5 mg/5 ml, 10 mg/5 ml.
Tablets (Dolophine, Methadose): 5 mg, 10 mg.
Tablets (Dispersible [Methadose]): 40 mg.
Injection (Dolophine): 10 mg/ml.

INDICATIONS AND DOSAGES
▸ **Analgesia**
PO, IV, IM, SUBCUTANEOUS
Adults. 2.5-10 mg q3-8hr as needed up to 5-20 mg q6-8hr.
Elderly. 2.5 mg q8-12hr.
Children. Initially, 0.1 mg/kg/dose q4hr for 2-3 doses, then q6-12hr. Maximum: 10 mg/dose.
▸ **Detoxification**
PO
Adults, Elderly. 15-40 mg/day.
▸ **Temporary maintenance treatment of narcotic abstinence syndrome**
PO
Adults, Elderly. 20-120 mg/day.

CONTRAINDICATIONS
Delivery of premature infant, diarrhea due to poisoning, hypersensitivity to narcotics, labor

INTERACTIONS
Drug
Alcohol, other CNS depressants: May increase CNS or respiratory depression and hypotension.
MAOIs: May produce a severe, sometimes fatal reaction; plan to administer one-quarter of usual methadone dose.
Herbal
Valerian: May increase CNS depression.
Food
None known.

DIAGNOSTIC TEST EFFECTS
May increase serum amylase and lipase levels.

SIDE EFFECTS
Frequent
Sedation, decreased B/P (including orthostatic hypotension), diaphoresis, facial flushing, constipation, dizziness, nausea, vomiting

Occasional
Confusion, urine retention, palpitations, abdominal cramps, visual changes, dry mouth, headache, decreased appetite, anxiety, insomnia
Rare
Allergic reaction (rash, pruritus)

SERIOUS REACTIONS
• Overdose results in respiratory depression, skeletal muscle flaccidity, cold or clammy skin, cyanosis, and extreme somnolence progressing to seizures, stupor, and coma. The antidote is 0.4 mg naloxone.
• The patient who uses methadone long-term may develop a tolerance to the drug's analgesic effect and physical dependence.

PRECAUTIONS & CONSIDERATIONS
Caution is warranted with acute abdominal conditions, cor pulmonale, history of seizures, impaired hepatic or renal function, increased intracranial pressure, respiratory abnormalities, supraventricular tachycardia, and in the debilitated or elderly. Methadone crosses the placenta and is distributed in breast milk. Regular use of opioids during pregnancy may produce withdrawal symptoms in the neonate, such as diarrhea, excessive crying, fever, hyperactive reflexes, irritability, seizures, sneezing, tremors, vomiting, and yawning. The neonate may develop respiratory depression if the mother receives methadone during labor. Children are more prone to experience paradoxical excitement. Children younger than 2 years and the elderly are more susceptible to the drug's respiratory depressant effects. Age-related renal impairment may increase the risk of urine retention in the elderly.
    Dizziness and drowsiness may occur, so change positions slowly and avoid alcohol, CNS depressants, and

tasks that require mental alertness or motor skills until response to the drug is established. Vital signs should be monitored for 15 to 30 minutes after an IM or subcutaneous dose and for 5 to 10 minutes after an IV dose. Clinical improvement should be monitored. The drug should be withheld and the physician should be notified if the respiratory rate is
12 breaths/minute or less in an adult or 20 breaths/minute or less in a child.

Storage
Store vials at room temperature.

Administration
Know that oral methadone is one-half as potent as parenteral methadone. Take methadone without regard to food. Dilute the syrup in a glass of water to prevent an anesthetic effect on mucous membranes.

! Be aware that the IM route is preferred over the subcutaneous route because the subcutaneous route may produce induration, local irritation, and pain.

For IM and subcutaneous, don't use the solution if it appears cloudy or contains a precipitate. Place the patient in the recumbent position before giving parenteral methadone. Inject the drug slowly. Know that patients with circulatory impairment are at increased risk for overdose because of delayed absorption of repeated injections.

Methamphetamine
meth-am-fet′a-meen
(Desoxyn, Gradumet)
Do not confuse with Dextran, dextromethorphan, or Excedrin.

CATEGORY AND SCHEDULE
Pregnancy Risk Category: C
Controlled substance: Schedule II

CLASSIFICATION
Adrenergic agonists, amphetamines, anorexiants, stimulants, central nervous system

MECHANISM OF ACTION
A sympathomimetic amine related to amphetamine and ephedrine that enhances CNS stimulant activity. Peripheral actions include elevation of systolic and diastolic blood pressure and weak bronchodilator and respiratory stimulant action. *Therapeutic Effect:* Increases motor activity, mental alertness; decreases drowsiness, fatigue.

PHARMACOKINETICS
Rapidly absorbed from the gastrointestinal (GI) tract. Metabolized in liver. Primarily excreted in the urine. Unknown if removed by hemodialysis. **Half-life:** 4-5 hr.

AVAILABILITY
Tablets: 5 mg.
Tablets (extended-release): 5 mg, 10 mg, 15 mg (Desoxyn, Gradumet).

INDICATIONS AND DOSAGES
▶ **Attention deficit/hyperactivity disorder (ADHD)**
PO
Adults, Children 6 yr and older.
Initially, 2.5-5 mg 1-2 times/day.

Increase by 5 mg/day at weekly intervals until therapeutic response is achieved.

▶ **Appetite suppressant**
PO
Adults, Children 12 yr and older.
5 mg daily, given 30 min before meals. Extended-release 10-15 mg in the morning.

OFF-LABEL USES
Narcolepsy

CONTRAINDICATIONS
Advanced arteriosclerosis, agitated states, glaucoma, history of drug abuse, history of hypersensitivity to sympathomimetic amines, hyperthyroidism, moderate to severe hypertension, symptomatic cardiovascular disease, within 14 days following discontinuation of an MAOI

INTERACTIONS
Drug
Beta-blockers: May increase risk of bradycardia, heart block, and hypertension.
Central nervous system (CNS) stimulants: May increase the effects of methamphetamine.
Digoxin: May increase the risk of arrhythmias with this drug.
MAOIs: May prolong and intensify the effects of methamphetamine.
Meperidine: May increase the risk of hypotension, respiratory depression, seizures, and vascular collapse.
Tricyclic antidepressants: May increase cardiovascular effects.
Herbal
Ephedra: May cause arrhythmias and hypertension.
Food
None known.

DIAGNOSTIC TEST EFFECTS
May increase plasma corticosteroid concentrations.

SIDE EFFECTS
Frequent
Irregular pulse, increased motor activity, talkativeness, nervousness, mild euphoria, insomnia
Occasional
Headache, chills, dry mouth, gastrointestinal (GI) distress, worsening depression in patients who are clinically depressed, tachycardia, palpitations, chest pain

SERIOUS REACTIONS
• Overdose may produce skin pallor, flushing, arrhythmias, and psychosis.
• Abrupt withdrawal following prolonged administration of high dosage may produce lethargy which may last for weeks.
• Prolonged administration to children with ADHD may produce a temporary suppression of normal weight and height patterns.

PRECAUTIONS & CONSIDERATIONS
Caution is warranted with bipolar disorder, diabetes mellitus, cardiovascular disease, seizure disorders, insomnia, or mild hypertension. It is unknown if methamphetamine crosses the placenta or is excreted in breast milk. Children may be more susceptible to develop abdominal pain, anorexia, decreased weight, and insomnia. Chronic methamphetamine use may inhibit growth in children. There are no age-related precautions noted in the elderly.

Decreased appetite, dizziness, dry mouth, or pronounced nervousness may occur and should be reported to the physician.
Administration
Do not take methamphetamine in afternoon or evening because the drug can cause insomnia. Take dose 30 to 45 minutes before meals.

Do not abruptly discontinue methamphetamine in patients who have received the drug for prolonged periods.

Methazolamide
meth-ah-zole'ah-mide
(Apo-Methazolamide [CAN],
Glauctabs, Neptazane)
Do not confuse with nefazodone.

CATEGORY AND SCHEDULE
Pregnancy Risk Category: C

CLASSIFICATION
Carbonic anhydrase inhibitors

MECHANISM OF ACTION
A noncompetitive inhibitor of carbonic anhydrase that inhibits the enzyme at the luminal border of cells of the proximal tubule. Increases urine volume and changes to an alkaline pH with subsequent decreases in the excretion of titratable acid and ammonia. *Therapeutic Effect:* Produces a diuretic and antiglaucoma effect.

PHARMACOKINETICS
PO route onset 2-4 hr, peak 6-8 hr, duration 10-18 hr. Well absorbed slowly from the GI tract. Protein binding: 55%. Distributed into the tissues (including CSF). Metabolized slowly from the gastrointestinal (GI) tract. Partially excreted in urine. Not removed by hemodialysis. **Half-life:** 14 hr.

AVAILABILITY
Tablets: 25 mg, 50 mg.

INDICATIONS AND DOSAGES
▸ **Glaucoma**
PO
Adults, Elderly. 50-100 mg/day 2-3 times/day.

OFF-LABEL USES
Motion sickness, essential tremor

CONTRAINDICATIONS
Kidney or liver dysfunction, severe pulmonary obstruction, hypersensitivity to methazolamide or any component of the formulation

INTERACTIONS
Drug
Amphetamines, quinidine, procainamide, methenamine, phenobarbital, salicylates: May increase the excretion of these drugs.
Aspirin: May increase the risk for anorexia, tachypnea, lethargy, coma and death have been reported when receiving high-dose aspirin and methazolamide concomitantly.
Diuretics: May increase the risk of hypokalemia.
Lithium: May increase the excretion of lithium.
Memantine: May decrease the clearance of memantine.
Steroids: May increase the risk of hypokalemia.
Topiramate: May increase the risk of nephrolithiasis.
Herbal
None known.
Food
None known.

DIAGNOSTIC TEST EFFECTS
None known.

SIDE EFFECTS
Occasional
Paresthesias, hearing dysfunction or tinnitus, fatigue, malaise, loss of appetite, taste alteration, nausea,

M

vomiting, diarrhea, polyuria, drowsiness, confusion, hypokalemia

Rare

Metabolic acidosis, electrolyte imbalance, transient myopia, urticaria, melena, hematuria, glycosuria, hepatic insufficiency, flaccid paralysis, photosensitivity, convulsions, and rarely, crystalluria, renal calculi

SERIOUS REACTIONS

• Malaise and complaints of tiredness and myalgia are signs of excessive dosing and acidosis in the elderly.

• Stevens-Johnson syndrome, toxic epidermal necrolysis, fulminant hepatic necrosis, agranulocytosis, aplastic anemia, and other blood dyscrasias have been reported and have caused fatalities.

PRECAUTIONS & CONSIDERATIONS

Caution should be used with allergies to sulfonamides, sulfonylureas, carbonic anhydrase inhibitors, thiazides, and loop diuretics (except ethacrynic acid) due to a risk of cross-reaction. Anorexia, tachypnea, lethargy, coma, and death have been reported with concomitant use of high-dose aspirin and methazolamide. Caution is also warranted with respiratory acidosis, diabetes mellitus, or mental impairment. It is unknown if methazolamide crosses the placenta and is excreted in breast milk. Safety and efficacy of this drug has not been established in children. The elderly may be at an increased risk for developing hypokalemia.

Hypokalemia may result in cardiac arrhythmias, changes in mental status and muscle strength, muscle cramps, and tremor. Potassium should be assessed before and during treatment. Frequency and volume of urination is expected to increase.

Administration

Take methazolamide with food to avoid GI upset.

Methenamine

(Dehydral [CAN], Hiprex, Hip-Rex [CAN], Mandelamine, Urasal [CAN], Urex)

CATEGORY AND SCHEDULE

Pregnancy Risk Category: C

CLASSIFICATION

Anti-infectives, urinary

MECHANISM OF ACTION

A hippuric acid salt that hydrolyzes to formaldehyde and ammonia in acidic urine. *Therapeutic Effect:* Formaldehyde has antibacterial action. Bacteriocidal.

PHARMACOKINETICS

Readily absorbed from the gastrointestinal (GI) tract. Partially metabolized by hydrolysis (unless protected by enteric coating) and partially by the liver. Primarily excreted in urine. **Half-life:** 3-6 hr.

AVAILABILITY

Oral Suspension, as mandelate: 0.5 g/5 ml.

Tablets, as hippurate: 1 g (Urex, Hiprex).

Tablets, enteric coated, as mandelate: 500 mg, 1 g (Mandelamine).

INDICATIONS AND DOSAGES

▸ **Urinary tract infection (UTI)**

PO

Adults, Elderly. 1 g 2 times/day (as hippurate). 1 g 4 times/day (as mandelate)

Children 6-12 yr. 25-50 mg/kg/day q12hr (as hippurate). 50-75 mg/kg/day q6hr (as mandelate).

OFF-LABEL USES
Hyperhidrosis

CONTRAINDICATIONS
Moderate to severe renal impairment, hepatic impairment (hippurate salt), tartrazine sensitivity (Hiprex contains tartrazine), hypersensitivity to methenamine or any of its components

INTERACTIONS
Drug
Acetazolamide, sodium bicarbonate: May decrease effect secondary to alkalinization of urine.
Antacids: May decrease the effectiveness of methenamine.
Dichlorphenamide: May inhibit the action of methenamine to alkalinize the urine.
Sulfamethizole: May increase the risk of crystalluria.
Herbal
None known.
Food
None known.

DIAGNOSTIC TEST EFFECTS
Formaldehyde, the active form of methenamine, interferes with fluorometric procedures for the determination of urinary catecholamines and vanillylmandelic acid (VMA), causing false high results.

SIDE EFFECTS
Occasional
Rash, nausea, dyspepsia, difficulty urinating
Rare
Bladder irritation, increased liver enzymes

SERIOUS REACTIONS
• Crystalluria can occur when methenamine is given in large doses.

PRECAUTIONS & CONSIDERATIONS
Caution should be used with hepatic impairment. Be aware that Hiprex contains tartrazine. It is unknown if methenamine crosses the placenta and is excreted in breast milk. There are no age-related precautions noted in children older than 6 years of age. Avoid using in the elderly with age-related renal impairment. Antacids should be avoided. Sun and ultraviolet light should be avoided. If it is not avoidable, sunscreens and protective clothing should be worn. Urine pH should be monitored.
Administration
Take methenamine with food or milk to reduce GI upset. Take with cranberry juice or ascorbic acid to acidify urine.

Methimazole
meth-im'a-zole
(Tapazole)

CATEGORY AND SCHEDULE
Pregnancy Risk Category: D

CLASSIFICATION
Antithyroid agents, hormones/hormone modifiers

MECHANISM OF ACTION
A thiomidazole derivative that inhibits synthesis of thyroid hormone by interfering with the incorporation of iodine into tyrosyl residues.
Therapeutic Effect: Effectively treats

hyperthyroidism by decreasing thyroid hormone levels.

AVAILABILITY
Tablets: 5 mg, 10 mg.

INDICATIONS AND DOSAGES
▸ **Hyperthyroidism**
PO
Adults, Elderly. Initially, 15-60 mg/day in 3 divided doses. Maintenance: 5-15 mg/day.
Children. Initially, 0.4 mg/kg/day in 3 divided doses. Maintenance: One-half the initial dose.

CONTRAINDICATIONS
None known.

INTERACTIONS
Drug
Amiodarone, iodinated glycerol, iodine, potassium iodide: May decrease response to methimazole.
Digoxin: May increase the blood concentration of digoxin as patient becomes euthyroid.
I^{131}: May decrease thyroid uptake of I^{131}.
Oral anticoagulants: May decrease the effects of oral anticoagulants.
Herbal
None known.
Food
None known.

DIAGNOSTIC TEST EFFECTS
May increase LDH, serum alkaline phosphatase, bilirubin, AST (SGOT), and ALT (SGPT) levels and prothrombin time. May decrease prothrombin level and WBC count.

SIDE EFFECTS
Frequent (5%-4%)
Fever, rash, pruritus
Occasional (3%-1%)
Dizziness, loss of taste, nausea, vomiting, stomach pain, peripheral neuropathy or numbness in fingers, toes, face
Rare (less than 1%)
Swollen lymph nodes or salivary glands

SERIOUS REACTIONS
• Agranulocytosis as long as 4 months after therapy, pancytopenia, and hepatitis have occurred.

PRECAUTIONS & CONSIDERATIONS
Caution is warranted with concurrent use of other agranulocytosis-inducing drugs, impaired hepatic function, and in persons older than 40 years of age. Methimazole crosses the placenta and should be avoided during pregnancy. Methimazole should be avoided in patients who are breast-feeding. Restrict the consumption of iodine products and seafood.

Notify the physician of illness, unusual bleeding or bruising, or rash. Weight, pulse, CBC, prothrombin time, thyroid function, and serum hepatic enzymes should be monitored.
Storage
Store at room temperature in a light-resistant container.
Administration
Take with food if GI symptoms occur. Space doses evenly around the clock.

Methocarbamol
meth-oh-kar′ba-mole
(Carbacot, Robaxin)

CATEGORY AND SCHEDULE
Pregnancy Risk Category: C

CLASSIFICATION
Musculoskeletal agents,
relaxants, skeletal muscle

MECHANISM OF ACTION
A carbamate derivative of guaifenesin
that causes skeletal muscle relaxation by general CNS depression.
Therapeutic Effect: Relieves muscle
spasticity.

PHARMACOKINETICS
Rapidly and almost completely
absorbed from the gastrointestinal
(GI) tract. Protein binding: 46%-50%.
Metabolized in liver by dealkylation
and hydroxylation. Primarily excreted
in urine as metabolites. **Half-life:**
1-2 hr.

AVAILABILITY
Injection: 100 mg/ml (Robaxin).
Tablets: 325 mg, 500 mg
(Carbacot, Robaxin), 750 mg
(Carbacot).

INDICATIONS AND DOSAGES
▶ **Musculoskeletal spasm**
IM/IV
Adults, Children 16 yr and older.
1 g q8hr for no more than 3 consecutive days. May repeat course of
therapy after a drug-free interval of
48 hr.
PO
Adults, Children 16 yr and older.
1.5 g 4 times/day for 2-3 days (up to
8 g/day may be given in severe
conditions). Decrease to 4-4.5 g/day
in 3-6 divided doses.

Elderly. Initially, 500 mg 4 times
a day. May gradually increase
dosage.
▶ **Tetanus spasm**
IV
Adults. 1-3 g q6hr until oral dosing
is possible. Injection should be used
no more than 3 consecutive days.
Children. 15 mg/kg/dose or 500 mg/
m^2/dose q6hr as needed. Maximum:
1.8 g/m^2/day for 3 days only.

CONTRAINDICATIONS
Hypersensitivity to methocarbamol
or any component of the formulation, renal impairment (injection
formulation)

INTERACTIONS
Drug
**CNS depressants, including
alcohol:** May potentiate effects
when used with other CNS depres-
sants, including alcohol.
Herbal
**Gotu kola, kava kava, St. John's
wort:** May increase CNS depression.
Food
None known.

DIAGNOSTIC TEST EFFECTS
None known.

SIDE EFFECTS
Frequent
Transient drowsiness, weakness,
dizziness, lightheadedness, nausea,
vomiting.
Occasional
Headache, constipation, anorexia,
hypotension, confusion, blurred
vision, vertigo, facial flushing,
rash
Rare
Paradoxical CNS excitement and
restlessness, slurred speech, tremor,
dry mouth, diarrhea, nocturia, impotence, bradycardia, hypotension,
syncope

M

SERIOUS REACTIONS

• Anaphylactoid reactions, leukopenia, and seizures (intravenous form) have been reported.
• Methocarbamol overdosage results in cardiac arrhythmias, nausea, vomiting, drowsiness, and coma.

PRECAUTIONS & CONSIDERATIONS

Caution is necessary with oral formulation and with renal or hepatic impairment. Use injectable formulation cautiously with a history of seizures or hepatic impairment. It is unknown if methocarbamol crosses the placenta or is distributed in breast milk. Be aware that the safety and efficacy of methocarbamol has not been established in children younger than 16 years. In the elderly, there is an increased risk of central nervous system (CNS) toxicity, manifested as confusion, hallucinations, mental depression, and sedation.

Age-related renal impairment may require a decreased dosage in the elderly.

Administration

Maximum of 5 ml can be administered into each gluteal region with IM injection.

IV injection may be administered undiluted as a direct intravenous bolus at a maximum rate of 3 ml/minute. Solution should be hypertonic. May dilute 1 g of methocarbamol to no more than 250 ml with IV solutions. Do not use for more than 3 consecutive days. Administer IV while in recumbent position. Maintain position for 15-30 minutes following infusion.

Give oral formulation without regard to meals. Tablets may be crushed and mixed with food or liquid if needed. May crush tablets and give by nasogastric (NG) tube if necessary.

Methoxsalen
meth-ox'a-len
(8-MOP, Oxsoralen, Oxsoralen-Ultra, Ultramop [CAN], Uvadex)
Do not confuse with methsuximide or methotrexate.

CATEGORY AND SCHEDULE
Pregnancy Risk Category: C

CLASSIFICATION
Photosensitizers, psoralens

MECHANISM OF ACTION

A member of the family of psoralens that induces an augmented sunburn reaction followed by hyperpigmentation in the presence of long-wave ultraviolet radiation. Bonds covalently to pyrimidine bases in DNA, inhibits the synthesis of DNA, and suppresses cell division. The augmented sunburn reaction involves excitation of the methoxsalen molecule by radiation in the long-wave ultraviolet light (UVA), resulting in transference of energy to the methoxsalen molecule producing an excited state or "triplet electronic state". The molecule, in this "triplet state", then reacts with cutaneous DNA. *Therapeutic Effect:* Results in symptomatic control of severe, recalcitrant disabling psoriasis, repigmentation of idiopathic vitiligo, palliative treatment of skin manifestations of cutaneous T-cell lymphoma (CTCL), repigmentation of idiopathic vitiligo, and palliative treatment of skin manifestations of CTCL.

PHARMACOKINETICS

Absorption varies. Food increases peak serum levels. Reversibly bound to albumin. Metabolized in the liver.

Excreted in the urine. **Half-life:** 2 hr.

AVAILABILITY
Capsule: 10 mg (8-MOP).
Gelcap: 10 mg (Oxsoralen-Ultra).
Lotion: 1% (Oxsoralen).
Solution: 20 mcg/ml (Uvadex).

INDICATIONS AND DOSAGES
▸ **Psoriasis**
PO
Adults, Elderly. 10-70 mg 1.5-2 hr before exposure to UVA light, repeated 2-3 times/week. Give at least 48 hours apart. Dosage is based upon patient's body weight and skin type: *Less than 30 kg:* 10 mg, *30-50 kg:* 20 mg, *51-65 kg:* 30 mg, *66-80 kg:* 40 mg, *81-90 kg:* 50 mg, *91-115 kg:* 60 mg, *more than 115 kg:* 70 mg.
▸ **Vitiligo**
PO
Adults, Elderly, Children older than 12 yr. 20 mg 2-4 hr before exposure to UVA light. Give at least 48 hr apart.
TOPICAL
Adults, Elderly, Children older than 12 yr. Apply 1-2 hr. before exposure to UVA light, no more than once weekly.
▸ **CTCL**
EXTRACORPOREAL
Adults, Elderly. Inject 200 mcg into the photoactivation bag during collection cycle using the UVAR photopheresis system, 2 consecutive days every 4 weeks for a minimum of 7 treatment cycles.

OFF-LABEL USES
Dermographism, eczema, hypereosinophilic syndrome, hypopigmented sarcoidosis, ichthyosis linearis circumflexa, lymphomatoid papulosis, mycosis fungoides, palmoplantar pustulosis, pruritus, scleromyxedema, systemic sclerosis

CONTRAINDICATIONS
Cataract, invasive squamous cell cancer, aphakia, melanoma, pregnancy (Uvadex), diseases associated with photosensitivity, hypersensitivity to methoxsalen (psoralens) or any component of the formulation

INTERACTIONS
Drug
Caffeine: May inhibit caffeine metabolism.
Phenytoin, fosphenytoin: May decrease the effectiveness of methoxsalen.
Herbal
None known.
Food
None known.

SIDE EFFECTS
Occasional
Nausea, pruritus, edema, hypotension, nervousness, vertigo, depression, dizziness, headache, malaise, painful blistering, burning, rash, urticaria, loss of muscle coordination, leg cramps

SERIOUS REACTIONS
• Hypersensitivity reaction, such as nausea and severe burns, may occur.

PRECAUTIONS & CONSIDERATIONS
Caution should be used with renal disease and with other agents that may cause photosensitivity. Methoxsalen crosses the placenta but it is unknown if it is excreted in breast milk. Safety and efficacy have not been determined in children younger than 12 years old. There are no age-related precautions in the elderly. Hematocrit, white blood cell count differential, platelets, serum bilirubin, SGOT, alkaline phosphatase, LDH, uric acid, BUN, serum creatinine, ANA, and urinalysis should be monitored at 6 months, 1 year, and yearly thereafter.

Ophthalmologic evaluation should be given at 6 months, 1 year, and yearly thereafter. Histopathologic exams should be performed for any skin lesion suspected of being malignant at any time during therapy. Burning or blistering or intractable pruritus must be reported. Direct and indirect sunlight should be avoided for 8 hours after oral and 12-48 hours after topical therapy. If sunlight cannot be avoided, protective clothing and/or sunscreens should be worn. Sunbathing should be avoided for at least 24 hours prior to therapy or 48 hours after PUVA therapy.

Administration

Take oral methoxsalen with food or in 2 divided doses 30 minutes apart to reduce nausea.

Hands and fingers of the person applying the lotion should be protected to prevent possible photosensitization and burns. Administer in conjunction with scheduled controlled doses of UVA radiation.

Methscopolamine
meth-scoe-pol-a-meen
(Pamine, Pamine Forte)

CATEGORY AND SCHEDULE
Pregnancy Risk Category: C

CLASSIFICATION
Anticholinergics, gastrointestinals

MECHANISM OF ACTION
A peripheral anticholinergic agent that has limited ability to cross the blood-brain barrier and provides a peripheral blockade of muscarinic receptors. *Therapeutic Effect:* Reduces the volume and the total acid content of gastric secretions, inhibits salivation, and reduces gastrointestinal motility.

PHARMACOKINETICS
Poorly and unreliably absorbed from the gastrointestinal (GI) tract. Limited ability to cross the blood brain barrier. Primarily excreted in the urine and the bile. The effects of methscopolamine appear to occur within 1 hour and last for 4-6 hours. Primarily excreted in urine. **Half-life:** unknown.

AVAILABILITY
Tablets: 2.5 mg (Pamine), 5 mg (Pamine Forte).

INDICATIONS AND DOSAGES
▸ **Peptic ulcer**
Adults, Elderly. Initially, 2.5 mg 30 minutes before meals and 2.5-5 mg at bedtime. May increase dose to 5 mg every 12 hours

OFF-LABEL USES
Gastrointestinal spasm

CONTRAINDICATIONS
Reflux esophagitis; glaucoma, obstructed uropathy, obstructed disease of the GI tract (pyloroduodenal stenosis), paralytic ileus, intestinal atony of elderly or debilitated individuals, unstable cardiovascular status in acute hemorrhage, severe ulcerative colitis, toxic megacolon, complicated ulcerative colitis, myasthenia gravis, hypersensitivity to methscopolamine, any component of the formulation, or related drugs

INTERACTIONS
Drug
Antacids: May decrease absorption of methscopolamine.
Antipsychotic agents: May produce additive anticholinergic effects.

Tricyclic antidepressants: May produce additive anticholinergic effects.
Herbal
None known.
Food
None known.

DIAGNOSTIC TEST EFFECTS
None known.

SIDE EFFECTS
Occasional
Dry mouth, throat, and nose, urinary hesitancy and/or retention, constipation, tachycardia, palpitations, headache, insomnia, dry skin, urticaria, weakness

SERIOUS REACTIONS
• Overdosage may vary from CNS depression, including sedation, apnea, hypotension, cardiovascular collapse, or death to severe paradoxical reaction (such as hallucinations, tremor, and seizures).

PRECAUTIONS & CONSIDERATIONS
Caution is necessary with diarrhea, since it may be an early symptom of incomplete intestinal obstruction. Large doses should be used cautiously because methscopolamine may suppress intestinal motility, causing paralytic ileus and precipitate or aggravate toxic megacolon. Caution is also warranted with autonomic neuropathy, BPH, hyperthyroidism, ulcerative colitis, hepatic or renal dysfunction, arrhythmias, cardiovascular disease, CHF, hypertension, or in the elderly. The elderly are at an increased risk of developing confusion, dizziness, hyperexcitability, hypotension, and sedation. It is unknown if methscopolamine crosses the placenta or is excreted in breast milk. Safety and efficacy have not been established in children.

Peptic ulcers should be monitored while under treatment of methscopolamine by upper gastrointestinal contrast radiology or endoscopy to insure healing.
Expected responses to the drug include dizziness, drowsiness, and dry mouth. Tasks that require mental alertness or motor skills should be avoided. Blood in stool should be reported to the physician.
Administration
Take methscopolamine 30 minutes before food.

Methsuximide
meth-sux′i-mide
(Celontin)
Do not confuse with methoxsalen.

CATEGORY AND SCHEDULE
Pregnancy Risk Category: C

CLASSIFICATION
Anticonvulsants, succinimides

MECHANISM OF ACTION
An anticonvulsant agent that increases the seizure threshold, suppresses paroxysmal spike-and-wave pattern in absence seizures and depresses nerve transmission in the motor cortex. *Therapeutic Effect:* Controls absence (petit mal) seizures.

PHARMACOKINETICS
Rapidly metabolized in liver to active metabolite, N-desmethylmethsuximide. Primarily excreted in urine. Unknown if removed by hemodialysis. **Half-life:** 1.4 hr.

AVAILABILITY
Capsules: 150 mg, 300 mg
(Celontin).

INDICATIONS AND DOSAGES
▸ **Absence seizures**
PO
Adults, Elderly. Initially, 300 mg/day
for the first week. Increase dosage
by 300 mg/day at weekly intervals
until response is attained.
Maintenance: 1200 mg/day at
2-4 times/day. Do not exceed
1000 mg/day in children 12-15 yr,
1200 mg/day in patients older than
15 yr.
Children. Initially, 10-15 mg/
kg/day 3-4 times/day. Increase at
weekly intervals. Maximum:
30 mg/kg/day.

OFF-LABEL USES
Partial complex (psychomotor)
seizures

CONTRAINDICATIONS
Hypersensitivity to succinimides or
any component of the formulation

INTERACTIONS
Drug
**Alcohol, benzodiazepines, barbitu-
rates, and other CNS depressants:**
May cause increased sedative
effects.
Anticonvulsants: May increase
plasma concentrations of other anti-
convulsants.
Cyclosporine: May decrease
cyclosporine blood levels by increas-
ing its metabolism.
Herbal
Evening primrose oil: May
decrease the effects of methsux-
imide.
Ginkgo biloba: May decrease the
effects of methsuximide.
Food
None known.

DIAGNOSTIC TEST EFFECTS
None known.

SIDE EFFECTS
Frequent
Drowsiness, dizziness, nausea,
vomiting
Occasional
Visual abnormalities, such as spots
before eyes, difficulty focusing,
blurred vision, dry mouth or pharynx,
tongue irritation, nervousness,
insomnia, headache, constipation
or diarrhea, rash, weight loss,
proteinuria, edema

SERIOUS REACTIONS
• Toxic reactions appear as blood
dyscrasias, including aplastic
anemia, agranulocytosis, thrombocytopenia, leukopenia, leukocytosis,
eosinophilia, cardiovascular disturbances, such as congestive heart
failure (CHF), hypotension or hypertension, thrombophlebitis, arrhythmias, and dermatologic effects,
such as rash, urticaria, pruritus,
photosensitivity.
• Abrupt withdrawal may precipitate
status epilepticus.

PRECAUTIONS & CONSIDERATIONS
Caution is warranted with impaired
cardiac, liver, or renal function.
Caution should be used in any
seizure type. Methsuximide is not
first-line therapy. It is unknown
if methsuximide crosses the
placenta and is distributed in
breast milk. Behavioral changes are
more likely to occur in children
taking methsuximide. The elderly
are more susceptible to agitation,
atrioventricular (AV) block, bradycardia, and confusion. Blood tests
should be repeated frequently
during first 3 months of therapy
and at monthly intervals thereafter
for 2-3 years.

Drowsiness usually disappears during therapy. Tasks that require mental alertness and motor skills should be avoided.

Administration

Take with meals to reduce risk of gastrointestinal (GI) distress. Be aware when replacement by another anticonvulsant is necessary, plan to decrease methsuximide gradually as therapy begins with a low replacement dose. Abrupt withdrawal of the drug may precipitate absence status. Methsuximide must be used in combination with other anticonvulsants in patients with both absence and tonic-clonic seizures

---

Methyclothiazide
meth-i-kloe-thye′ah-zide
(Aquatensen, Enduron)

CATEGORY AND SCHEDULE
Pregnancy Risk Category: B
(D if used in pregnancy-induced hypertension)

CLASSIFICATION
Diuretics, thiazide and derivatives

MECHANISM OF ACTION
A sulfonamide derivative that acts as a thiazide diuretic and antihypertensive. As a diuretic it blocks the reabsorption of water, sodium, and potassium at cortical diluting segment of distal tubule. As an antihypertensive it reduces plasma and extracellular fluid volume and decreases peripheral vascular resistance (PVR) by direct effect on blood vessels. *Therapeutic Effect:* Promotes diuresis, reduces blood pressure (B/P).

PHARMACOKINETICS
Variably absorbed from the gastrointestinal (GI) tract. Primarily excreted unchanged in urine. Not removed by hemodialysis. **Half-life:** 24 hr.

AVAILABILITY
Tablets: 2.5 mg, 5 mg (Aquatensen, Enduron).

INDICATIONS AND DOSAGES
▸ **Edema**
PO
Adults. 2.5-10 mg/day.
HYPERTENSION
PO
Adults. 2.5-5 mg/day.

OFF-LABEL USES
Treatment of diabetes insipidus, prevention of calcium-containing renal stones

CONTRAINDICATIONS
Anuria, history of hypersensitivity to sulfonamides or thiazide diuretics, renal decompensation

INTERACTIONS
Drug
Ace inhibitors: May increase the risk of postural hypotension.
Beta blockers: May increase hyperglycemic effects in patients with Type 2 diabetes mellitus.
Cylosporine, other thiazides: May increase the risk of gout or renal toxicity.
Cholestyramine, colestipol: May decrease the absorption and effects of methyclothiazide.
Digoxin: May increase the risk of toxicity of digoxin caused by hypokalemia.
Lithium: May increase the risk of toxicity of lithium
Neuromuscular blocking agents: May prolong neuromuscular blockade.

M

NSAIDs: May decrease the effects of methylchlothiazide.
Herbal
Dong quai, St. John's wort: May cause photosensitization.
Garlic: May increase antihypertensive effect.
Ginkgo biloba: May increase blood pressure.
Gossypol: May increase the risk of hypokalemia.
Licorice: May increase the risk of hypokalemia and/or reduce effectiveness of methychlorthiazide.
Ma Huang: May decrease hypotensive effect of methychlothiazide.
Ephedra, ginseng, yohimbine: May decrease the effects of methychlothiazide.
Food
None known.

DIAGNOSTIC TEST EFFECTS

May increase blood glucose levels, serum cholesterol, LDL, bilirubin, calcium, creatinine, uric acid, and triglyceride levels. May decrease urinary calcium, and serum magnesium, potassium, and sodium levels.

⚙ IV INCOMPATIBILITIES
None known.
⚙ IV Compatibilities
None known.

SIDE EFFECTS
Expected
Increase in urinary frequency and volume
Frequent
Potassium depletion
Occasional
Postural hypotension, headache, gastrointestinal (GI) disturbances, photosensitivity reaction, anorexia

SERIOUS REACTIONS
• Vigorous diuresis may lead to profound water loss and electrolyte

depletion leading to hypokalemia, hyponatremia, and dehydration.
• Acute hypotensive episodes may occur.
• Hyperglycemia may be noted during prolonged therapy.
• GI upset, pancreatitis, dizziness, paresthesias, headache, blood dyscrasias, pulmonary edema, allergic pneumonitis, and dermatologic reactions occur rarely.
• Overdosage can lead to lethargy and coma without changes in electrolytes or hydration.

PRECAUTIONS & CONSIDERATIONS

Caution is necessary with debilitated and elderly persons. Caution is warranted with diabetes mellitus, impaired liver function, severe renal disease, electrolyte disturbances, history of gout, and thyroid disorders. Methyclothiazide crosses the placenta and a small amount is distributed in breast milk. Breast-feeding is not recommended in this patient population. There are no age-related precautions noted in children, except that jaundiced infants may be at risk for hyperbilirubinemia. Be aware that the elderly may be more sensitive to the drug's electrolyte and hypotensive effects. In the elderly, age-related renal impairment may require dosage adjustment.

Frequency and volume of urination is expected to increase. Be aware that methyclothiazide may aggravate digitalis toxicity. Be aware that sensitivity reactions may occur with or without history of allergy or asthma. Skin should be protected from sunlight.

Hypokalemia may result in change in mental status, muscle cramps, nausea, tachycardia, tremor, vomiting, and weakness. Hyponatremia may result in clammy and cold skin, confusion, and thirst. Be especially alert for potassium depletion in persons taking digoxin, such as cardiac arrhythmias. Foods high in potassium such as apricots, bananas, legumes, meat, orange juice, white and sweet potatoes, raisins, and whole grains, such as cereals should be eaten during treatment.

Administration

May give methychlothiazide with food or milk if GI upset occurs, preferably with breakfast to help prevent nocturia.

Methylcellulose
meth-ill-cell'you-los
(Citrucel, Cologel)
Do not confuse Citrucel with Citracal.

CATEGORY AND SCHEDULE
Pregnancy Risk Category: C
OTC

CLASSIFICATION
Laxatives

MECHANISM OF ACTION
A bulk-forming laxative that dissolves and expands in water. *Therapeutic Effect:* Provides increased bulk and moisture content in stool, increasing peristalsis and bowel motility.

PHARMACOKINETICS

Route	Onset	Peak	Duration
PO	12-24 hr	N/A	N/A

Acts in small and large intestines. Full effect may not be evident for 2-3 days.

AVAILABILITY
Powder.

INDICATIONS AND DOSAGES
▶ **Constipation**
PO
Adults, Elderly. 1 tbsp (15 ml) in 8 oz water 1-3 times a day.
Children 6-12 yr. 1 tsp (5 ml) in 4 oz water 3-4 times a day.

CONTRAINDICATIONS
Abdominal pain, dysphagia, nausea, partial bowel obstruction, symptoms of appendicitis, vomiting

INTERACTIONS
Drug
Digoxin, oral anticoagulants, salicylates: May decrease the effects of digoxin, oral anticoagulants, and salicylates by decreasing absorption of these drugs.
Potassium-sparing diuretics, potassium supplements: May interfere with the effects of potassium-sparing diuretics and potassium supplements.
Herbal
None known.
Food
None known.

DIAGNOSTIC TEST EFFECTS
May increase blood glucose level.
May decrease serum potassium level.

SIDE EFFECTS
Rare
Some degree of abdominal discomfort, nausea, mild cramps, griping, faintness

SERIOUS REACTIONS
• Esophageal or bowel obstruction may occur if administered with less than 250 ml or 1 full glass of liquid.

PRECAUTIONS & CONSIDERATIONS
Methylcellulose may be used safely in pregnancy. Safety and efficacy of methylcellulose have not been

established in children younger than 6 years of age. Methylcellulose use is not recommended in this age-group. No age-related precautions have been noted in the elderly. Pattern of daily bowel activity and stool consistency and serum electrolyte levels should be monitored.

Administration

Drink 6 to 8 glasses of water a day to aid in stool softening. Drug should not be swallowed in dry form but should be mixed with at least 1 full glass (8 oz) of liquid. A full glass of water should be taken with each dose; an inadequate amount of fluid may cause choking or swelling in the throat. To promote defecation, increase fluid intake, exercise, and eat a high-fiber diet.

Methyldopa

meth-ill-doe′pa
(Aldomet, Apo-Methyldopa [CAN], Hydopa [AUS], Novomedopa [CAN], Nudopa [AUS])
Do not confuse Aldomet with Anzemet.

CATEGORY AND SCHEDULE

Pregnancy Risk Category: B

CLASSIFICATION

Antiadrenergics, central

MECHANISM OF ACTION

An antihypertensive agent that stimulates central inhibitory alpha-adrenergic receptors, lowers arterial pressure, and reduces plasma renin activity. *Therapeutic Effect:* Reduces B/P.

AVAILABILITY

Tablets: 250 mg, 500 mg.
Injection: 50 mg/ml.

INDICATIONS AND DOSAGES
▸ **Moderate to severe hypertension**
PO
Adults. Initially, 250 mg 2-3 times a day for 2 days. Adjust dosage at intervals of 2 days (minimum).
Elderly. Initially, 125 mg 1-2 times a day. May increase by 125 mg q2-3 days. Maintenance: 500 mg to 2 g/day in 2-4 divided doses.
Children. Initially, 10 mg/kg/day in 2-4 divided doses. Adjust dosage at intervals of 2 days (minimum). Maximum: 65 mg/kg/day or 3 g/day, whichever is less.
IV
Adults. 250-1000 mg q6-8hr. Maximum: 4 g/day.
Children. Initially, 2-4 mg/kg/dose. May increase to 5-10 mg/kg/dose in 4-6h if no response. Maximum: 65 mg/kg/day or 3 g/day, whichever is less.

CONTRAINDICATIONS

Hepatic disease, pheochromocytoma

INTERACTIONS
Drug
Hypotensive-producing medications, such as antihypertensives and diuretics: May increase the effects of methyldopa.
Lithium: May increase the risk of lithium toxicity.
MAOIs: May cause hyperexcitability.
NSAIDs, tricyclic antidepressants: May decrease the effects of methyldopa.
Other sympathomimetics: May decrease the effects of sympathomimetics.
Herbal
None known.

Food
None known.

DIAGNOSTIC TEST EFFECTS
May increase BUN and serum prolactin, alkaline phosphatase, bilirubin, creatinine, potassium, sodium, uric acid, AST (SGOT), and ALT (SGPT) levels. May produce false-positive Coombs' test and prolong prothrombin time.

SIDE EFFECTS
Frequent
Peripheral edema, somnolence, headache, dry mouth
Occasional
Mental changes (such as anxiety, depression), decreased sexual function or libido, diarrhea, swelling of breasts, nausea, vomiting, lightheadedness, paraesthesia, rhinitis

SERIOUS REACTIONS
• Hepatotoxicity (abnormal liver function test results, jaundice, hepatitis), hemolytic anemia, unexplained fever, and flu-like symptoms may occur. If these conditions appear, discontinue the medication and contact the physician.

PRECAUTIONS & CONSIDERATIONS
Caution is warranted with renal impairment. Dizziness and lightheadedness may occur. Tasks requiring mental alertness and motor skills should be avoided. B/P, pulse, weight, and liver function tests should be monitored before and during therapy. B/P and pulse should be monitored every 30 minutes until stabilized.
Administration
Inspect the drug vial for particulate matter and discoloration and discard if present. For IV infusion, add the prescribed dose to 100 ml D_5W and infuse over 30-60 minutes. Alternatively, add the prescribed

dose to D_5W to make a final concentration of 100 mg per 10 ml and infuse over 30-60 minutes.

Methylergonovine
meth-ill-er-goe-noe'veen
(Methergine)

CATEGORY AND SCHEDULE
Pregnancy Risk Category: C

CLASSIFICATION
Ergot alkaloids and derivatives, oxytocics, stimulants, uterine

MECHANISM OF ACTION
An ergot alkaloid that stimulates alpha-adrenergic and serotonin receptors, producing arterial vasoconstriction. Causes vasospasm of coronary arteries and directly stimulates uterine muscle. *Therapeutic Effect:* Increases strength and frequency of uterine contractions. Decreases uterine bleeding.

PHARMACOKINETICS

Route	Onset	Peak	Duration
PO	5-10 min	N/A	N/A
IV	Immediate	N/A	3 hr
IM	2-5 min	N/A	N/A

Rapidly absorbed from the GI tract after IM administration. Distributed rapidly to plasma, extracellular fluid, and tissues. Metabolized in the liver and undergoes first-pass effect. Primarily excreted in urine. **Half-life:** IV (alpha phase), 2-3 min or less; IV (beta phase), 20-30 min or longer.

AVAILABILITY
Tablets: 0.2 mg.
Injection: 0.2 mg/ml.

M

INDICATIONS AND DOSAGES

▶ **Prevention and treatment of postpartum and postabortion hemorrhage due to atony or involution**

PO

Adults. 0.2 mg 3-4 times a day. Continue for up to 7 days.

IV, IM

Adults. Initially, 0.2 mg. May repeat q2-4hr for no more than a total of 5 doses.

OFF-LABEL USES

Treatment of incomplete abortion

CONTRAINDICATIONS

Hypertension, pregnancy, toxemia, untreated hypocalcemia

INTERACTIONS

Drug

Vasoconstrictors, vasopressors: May increase the effects of methylergonovine.

Herbal

None known.

Food

None known.

DIAGNOSTIC TEST EFFECTS

May decrease serum prolactin concentration.

🔲 IV INCOMPATIBILITIES

No information available for Y-site administration.

🔲 IV Compatibilities

Heparin, potassium

SIDE EFFECTS

Frequent

Nausea, uterine cramping, vomiting

Occasional

Abdominal pain, diarrhea, dizziness, diaphoresis, tinnitus, bradycardia, chest pain

Rare

Allergic reaction, such as rash and itching; dyspnea; severe or sudden hypertension

SERIOUS REACTIONS

• Severe hypertensive episodes may result in CVA, serious arrhythmias, and seizures. Hypertensive effects are more frequent with patient susceptibility, rapid IV administration, and concurrent use of regional anesthesia or vasoconstrictors.

• Peripheral ischemia may lead to gangrene.

PRECAUTIONS & CONSIDERATIONS

Caution is warranted with coronary artery disease, hepatic or renal impairment, occlusive peripheral vascular disease, and sepsis. Methylergonovine use is contraindicated during pregnancy. Small amounts of the drug are distributed in breast milk. Safety and efficacy of methylergonovine use in children or the elderly are unknown. Avoid smoking because of added effects of vasoconstriction.

Notify the physician of chest pain, increased bleeding, cold or pale feet or hands, cramping, or foul-smelling lochia. Be aware that the drug may diminish circulation. B/P, pulse rate, and uterine tone should be monitored every 15 minutes until stable for 1 to 2 hours.

Storage

Refrigerate ampoules.

Administration

❗ Methylergonovine should never be used for induction or augmentation of labor.

May give PO, IV, or IM. Initial dose may be given parenterally, followed by an oral regimen.

Use IV route in life-threatening situations only, as prescribed. Dilute drug with 0.9% NaCl to a volume of 5 ml. Give over at least 1 minute, carefully monitoring B/P.

Methylphenidate
meth-ill-fen′i-date
(Attenta [AUS], Concerta, Metadate CD, Metadate ER, Methylin, Methylin ER, PMS-Methylphenidate [CAN], Riphenidate [CAN], Ritalin, Ritalin LA, Ritalin SR)
Do not confuse Ritalin with Rifadin.

CATEGORY AND SCHEDULE
Pregnancy Risk Category: C
Controlled Substance Schedule: II

CLASSIFICATION
Stimulants, central nervous system

MECHANISM OF ACTION
A CNS stimulant that blocks the reuptake of norepinephrine and dopamine into presynaptic neurons. *Therapeutic Effect:* Decreases motor restlessness and fatigue; increases motor activity, attention span, and mental alertness; produces mild euphoria.

PHARMACOKINETICS

Onset	Peak	Duration
Immediate-release	2 hr	3-5 hr
Sustained-release	4-7 hr	3-8 hr
Extended-release	N/A	8-12 hr

Slowly and incompletely absorbed from the GI tract. Protein binding: 15%. Metabolized in the liver. Eliminated in urine and in feces by biliary system. Unknown if removed by hemodialysis.
Half-life: 2-4 hr.

AVAILABILITY
Capsules (Extended-Release [Metadate CD]): 10 mg, 20 mg, 30 mg.
Capsules (Extended-Release [Ritalin LA]): 20 mg, 30 mg, 40 mg.
Tablets (Ritalin): 5 mg, 10 mg, 20 mg.
Tablets (Extended-Release [Mentadate ER, Methylin ER]): 10 mg, 20 mg.
Tablets (Extended-Release [Concerta]): 18 mg, 27 mg, 36 mg, 54 mg.
Tablets (Sustained-Release [Ritalin SR]): 20 mg.
Tablets (Chewable [Methylin]): 2.5 mg, 5 mg, 10 mg.
Oral Solution (Methylin): 5 mg/5 ml, 10 mg/5 ml.

INDICATIONS AND DOSAGES
▸ **Attention deficit hyperactivity disorder (ADHD)**
PO
Children 6 yr and older. Immediate release: Initially, 2.5-5 mg before breakfast and lunch. May increase by 5-10 mg/day at weekly intervals. Maximum: 60 mg/day.
PO (CONCERTA)
Children 6 yr and older. Initially, 18 mg once a day; may increase by 18 mg/day at weekly intervals. Maximum: 54 mg/day.
PO (METADATE CD)
Children 6 yr and older. Initially, 20 mg/day. May increase by 20 mg/day at weekly intervals. Maximum: 60 mg/day.
PO (RITALIN LA)
Children 6 yr and older. Initially, 20 mg/day. May increase by 10 mg/day at weekly intervals. Maximum: 60 mg/day.
▸ **Narcolepsy**
PO
Adults, Elderly. 10 mg 2-3 times a day. Range: 10-60 mg/day.

M

OFF-LABEL USES
Treatment of secondary mental depression

CONTRAINDICATIONS
Use within 14 days of MAOIs

INTERACTIONS
Drug
MAOIs: May increase the effects of methylphenidate.
Other CNS stimulants: May have an additive effect.
Herbal
None known.
Food
None known.

DIAGNOSTIC TEST EFFECTS
None known.

SIDE EFFECTS
Frequent
Anxiety, insomnia, anorexia
Occasional
Dizziness, drowsiness, headache, nausea, abdominal pain, fever, rash, arthralgia, vomiting
Rare
Blurred vision, Tourette syndrome (marked by uncontrolled vocal outbursts, repetitive body movements, and tics), palpitations

SERIOUS REACTIONS
• Prolonged administration to children with ADHD may delay growth.
• Overdose may produce tachycardia, palpitations, arrhythmias, chest pain, psychotic episode, seizures, and coma.
• Hypersensitivity reactions and blood dyscrasias occur rarely.

PRECAUTIONS & CONSIDERATIONS

Caution is warranted with hypertension, seizures, acute stress reaction, emotional instability, and a history of drug dependence. It is unknown if methylphenidate crosses the placenta or is distributed in breast milk. Children are more prone to develop abdominal pain, anorexia, weight loss, and insomnia. Long-term methylphenidate use may inhibit growth in children. No age-related precautions have been noted in the elderly. Caffeinated beverages should be avoided during therapy.

Tasks that require mental alertness and motor skills should be avoided until response to the drug is established. Notify the physician if fever, anxiety, palpitations, a rash, vomiting or, for those with a seizure disorder, an increase in the number of seizures, occurs. CBC, WBC count with differential, and platelet should be monitored. Baseline height and weight should be obtained at the beginning and periodically throughout therapy.

Administration
! Sustained- and extended-release tablets may be given in place of regular tablets once the daily dose is titrated using regular tablets and if the titrated dosage corresponds to the sustained- or extended-release tablet strength.

Take methylphenidate 30 to 45 minutes before meals (usually before breakfast and lunch). Take the last dose before 6 PM to help prevent insomnia. Crush tablets as needed, but don't crush or break extended-release capsules. Open the Metadate CD capsule and sprinkle the pellets on applesauce, if desired.

Methylprednisolone

meth-il-pred-niss'oh-lone
(Medrol) (Depo-Medrol, Depo-
Nisolone [AUS]) (A-Methapred,
Solu-Medrol)
**Do not confuse methylpred-
nisolone with medroxyproges-
terone or Medrol with
Mebaral.**

CATEGORY AND SCHEDULE
Pregnancy Risk Category: C

CLASSIFICATION
Corticosteroids

MECHANISM OF ACTION
An adrenocortical steroid that
suppresses migration of polymorphonuclear leukocytes and reverses
increased capillary permeability.
Therapeutic Effect: Decreases
inflammation.

PHARMACOKINETICS

Route	Onset	Peak	Duration
PO	N/A	1-2 hr	30-36 hr
IM	N/A	4-8 days	1-4 wk

Well absorbed from the GI tract
after IM administration. Widely
distributed. Metabolized in
the liver. Excreted in urine.
Removed by hemodialysis.
Half-life: 3.5 hr.

AVAILABILITY
Tablets (Medrol): 2 mg, 4 mg, 8 mg,
16 mg, 32 mg.
*Injection Powder for Reconstitution
(A-Methapred, Solu-Medrol):* 40 mg,
125 mg, 500 mg, 1 g.
Injection Suspension (Depo-Medrol):
20 mg/ml, 40 mg/ml, 80 mg/ml.

INDICATIONS AND DOSAGES
▶ **Substitution therapy for deficiency
states: acute or chronic adrenal
insufficiency, adrenal insufficiency
secondary to pituitary insufficiency,
and congenital adrenal hyperplasia;
nonendocrine disorders: allergic,
collagen, hepatic, intestinal tract,
ocular, renal, and skin diseases;
arthritis; bronchial asthma; cerebral
edema; malignancies; and rheumatic
carditis**
PO
Adults, Elderly. Initially, 4-48 mg/day.
IV (METHYLPREDNISOLONE
SODIUM SUCCINATE)
Adults, Elderly. 40-250 mg q4-6hr.
High dosage: 30 mg/kg over
at least 30 min. Repeat q4-6hr for
48-72 hr.
▶ **Spinal cord injury**
IV BOLUS
Adults, Elderly. 30 mg/kg over
15 min. Maintenance dose: 5.4 mg/
kg/h for 23 hr, to be given within
45 min of bolus dose.
IM (METHYLPREDNISOLONE
ACETATE)
Adults, Elderly. 10-80 mg/day.
Intra-articular, intralesional
Adults, Elderly. 4-40 mg, up to
80 mg q1-5wk.

CONTRAINDICATIONS
Administration of live virus
vaccines, systemic fungal infection

INTERACTIONS
Drug
Amphotericin: May increase
hypokalemia.
Digoxin: May increase the risk of
digoxin toxicity caused by
hypokalemia
**Diuretics, insulin, oral hypo-
glycemics, potassium supplements:**
May decrease the effects of these
drugs.

M

Hepatic enzyme inducers: May decrease the effects of methylprednisolone.

Live virus vaccines: May decrease the patient's antibody response to vaccine, increase vaccine side effects, and potentiate virus replication.

Herbal
None known.

Food
None known.

DIAGNOSTIC TEST EFFECTS

May increase blood cholesterol, glucose and serum lipid, amylase, and sodium levels. May decrease serum calcium, potassium, and thyroxine levels.

▓ IV INCOMPATIBILITIES

Ciprofloxacin (Cipro), diltiazem (Cardizem), docetaxel (Taxotere), etoposide (VePesid), filgrastim (Neupogen), gemcitabine (Gemzar), paclitaxel (Taxol), potassium chloride, propofol (Diprivan), vinorelbine (Navelbine)

▓ IV Compatibilities

Dopamine (Intropin), heparin, midazolam (Versed), theophylline

SIDE EFFECTS

Frequent
Insomnia, heartburn, anxiety, abdominal distention, diaphoresis, acne, mood swings, increased appetite, facial flushing, GI distress, delayed wound healing, increased susceptibility to infection, diarrhea or constipation

Occasional
Headache, edema, tachycardia, change in skin color, frequent urination, depression

Rare
Psychosis, increased blood coagulability, hallucinations

SERIOUS REACTIONS

• Long-term therapy may cause hypocalcemia, hypokalemia, muscle wasting (especially in arms and legs), osteoporosis, spontaneous fractures, amenorrhea, cataracts, glaucoma, peptic ulcer disease, and CHF.

• Abruptly withdrawing the drug after long-term therapy may cause anorexia, nausea, fever, headache, sudden severe myalgia, rebound inflammation, fatigue, weakness, lethargy, dizziness, and orthostatic hypotension.

PRECAUTIONS & CONSIDERATIONS

Caution is warranted with cirrhosis, CHF, diabetes mellitus, hypertension, hypothyroidism, thromboembolic disorders, and ulcerative colitis. Methylprednisolone crosses the placenta and is distributed in breast milk. Women taking methylprednisolone should not breast-feed. Prolonged methylprednisolone use in the first trimester of pregnancy may cause cleft palate in the neonate. Prolonged treatment or high dosages may decrease cortisol secretion and short-term growth rate in children. No age-related precautions have been noted in the elderly. Severe stress, including serious infection, surgery, or trauma, may require an increase in methylprednisolone dosage. Dentist or other physician should be informed of methylprednisolone therapy if taken within the past 12 months.

Mood swings, ranging from euphoria to depression, may occur. Notify the physician of fever, muscle aches, sore throat, and sudden weight gain or swelling. Blood glucose level, intake and output, B/P, serum electrolyte levels, pattern of daily bowel activity, height, and weight should be monitored before and during therapy.

Be alert to signs and symptoms of infection caused by reduced immune response, including fever, sore throat, and vague symptoms. In long-term therapy, signs and symptoms of hypocalcemia (such as muscle twitching, cramps, and positive Chvostek's or Trousseau's signs) or hypokalemia (such as EKG changes, nausea and vomiting, irritability, weakness and muscle cramps, and numbness or tingling, especially in the lower extremities) should be assessed.

Storage
Store vials for injection at room temperature.

Administration
! Individualize dosage based on the disease, person, and response.

Take oral methylprednisolone with food or milk. Take single doses before 9 AM; give multiple doses at evenly spaced intervals. Do not abruptly discontinue the drug or change the dosage or schedule; the drug must be withdrawn gradually under medical supervision.

For IV use, follow directions with Mix-o-vial. For infusion, add to D_5W or 0.9% NaCl. Give IV push over 2 to 3 minutes. Give IV piggyback over 10 to 20 minutes. Do not give methylprednisolone acetate via IV line.

For IM use, methylprednisolone acetate should not be further diluted. Reconstitute methylprednisolone sodium succinate with bacteriostatic water for injection. Give deep IM injection into gluteus maximus.

Methyltestosterone
meth-il-tes-tos′te-rone
(Android, Android-10, Android-25, Oreton Methyl, Testred, Virilon)
Do not confuse with methylprednisolone.

CATEGORY AND SCHEDULE
Pregnancy Risk Category: X
Controlled substance: Schedule III

CLASSIFICATION
Androgens, hormones/hormone modifiers

MECHANISM OF ACTION
A synthetic testosterone derivative with androgen activity that promotes growth and development of male sex organs and maintains secondary sex characteristics in androgen-deficient males. Therapeutic Effect: Treats hypogonadism and delayed puberty in males.

PHARMACOKINETICS
Well absorbed from the gastrointestinal (GI) tract. Protein binding: 98%. Metabolized in liver. Primarily excreted in urine. Unknown if removed by hemodialysis. **Half-life:** 10-100 min.

AVAILABILITY
Capsules: 10 mg (Android, Testred, Virilon).
Tablets: 10 mg (Android-10, Oreton Methyl), 25 mg (Android-25).

INDICATIONS AND DOSAGES
▸ **Breast cancer**
PO
Adults, Elderly. 50-200 mg/day.

▶ **Delayed puberty**
PO
Adults. 10-50 mg/day.
Adults, Elderly. 50-200 mg/day.
▶ **Hypogonadism**
PO
Adults. 10-50 mg/day.

OFF-LABEL USES
Hereditary angiodema

CONTRAINDICATIONS
Pregnancy, prostatic or breast cancer in males, hypersensitivity to methyltestosterone or any other component of its formulation

INTERACTIONS
Drug
Bupropion: May increase the risk of seizures by decreasing seizure threshold.
Cyclosporine: May increase risk of cyclosporine toxicity.
Liver toxic medications: May increase liver toxicity.
Oral anticoagulants: May increase the effects of oral anticoagulants.
Herbal
None known.
Food
None known.

DIAGNOSTIC TEST EFFECTS
May increase blood Hgb and Hct, LDL concentrations, serum alkaline phosphatase, bilirubin, calcium, potassium, SGOT (AST) levels, and sodium levels. May decrease HDL concentrations.

▓ IV INCOMPATIBILITIES
None known.
▓ IV Compatibilities
None known.

SIDE EFFECTS
Frequent
Gynecomastia, acne, amenorrhea or other menstrual irregularities
Females: Hirsutism, deepening of voice, clitoral enlargement that may not be reversible when drug is discontinued.
Occasional
Edema, nausea, insomnia, oligospermia, priapism, male pattern of baldness, bladder irritability, hypercalcemia in immobilized patients or those with breast cancer, hypercholesterolemia
Rare
Polycythemia

SERIOUS REACTIONS
• Cholestatic jaundice, hepatocellular neoplasms, peliosis hepatitis, edema with or without congestive heart failure and suppression of clotting factors II, V, VII, and X have been reported.

PRECAUTIONS & CONSIDERATIONS
Caution is warranted with diabetes, congestive heart failure of preexisting cardiac, liver or renal disease, epilepsy, history of migraine, other conditions that may be aggravated by fluid retention, and hypertension due to the risk of increased blood pressure. Methyltestosterone use is contraindicated during lactation. Safety and efficacy of methyltestosterone have not been established in children, so use with caution. Be aware that methyltestosterone use in the elderly may increase the risk of hyperplasia or stimulate growth of occult prostate carcinoma. Adequate calories and protein should be consumed.

Acne, nausea, pedal edema, or vomiting may occur. Women should report deepening of voice, hoarseness, and menstrual irregularities. Men should report difficulty urinating, frequent erections, and gynecomastia. Weight should be obtained each day. Weekly weight gains of more than 5 pounds should be reported.

Storage
Store at room temperature.

Administration
Give methyltestosterone with meals.

Metoclopramide
met'oh-kloe-pra'mide
(Apo-Metoclop [CAN], Maxolon [AUS], Pramin [AUS], Reglan)
Do not confuse Reglan with Renagel.

CATEGORY AND SCHEDULE
Pregnancy Risk Category: B

CLASSIFICATION
Antiemetics/antivertigo, gastrointestinals, stimulants, gastrointestinal

MECHANISM OF ACTION
A dopamine receptor antagonist that stimulates motility of the upper GI tract and decreases reflux into the esophagus. Also raises the threshold of activity in the chemoreceptor trigger zone. *Therapeutic Effect:* Accelerates intestinal transit and gastric emptying; relieves nausea and vomiting.

PHARMACOKINETICS

Route	Onset	Peak	Duration
PO	30-60 min	N/A	N/A
IV	1-3 min	N/A	N/A
IM	10-15 min	N/A	N/A

Well absorbed from the GI tract. Metabolized in the liver. Protein binding: 30%. Primarily excreted in urine. Not removed by hemodialysis. **Half-life:** 4-6 hr.

AVAILABILITY
Syrup: 5 mg/5 ml.
Tablets: 5 mg, 10 mg.
Injection: 5 mg/ml.

INDICATIONS AND DOSAGES
▶ **Prevention of chemotherapy-induced nausea and vomiting**
IV
Adults, Elderly, Children. 1-2 mg/kg 30 min before chemotherapy; repeat q2hr for 2 doses, then q3hr as needed.
▶ **Postoperative nausea and vomiting**
IV
Adults, Elderly, Children 15 yr and older. 10 mg; repeat q6-8hr as needed.
Children 14 yr and younger. 0.1-0.2 mg/kg/dose; repeat q6-8hr as needed.
▶ **Diabetic gastroparesis**
PO, IV
Adults. 10 mg 30 min before meals and at bedtime for 2-8 wk.
PO
Elderly. Initially, 5 mg 30 min before meals and at bedtime. May increase to 10 mg.
IV
Elderly. 5 mg over 1-2 min. May increase to 10 mg.
▶ **Symptomatic gastroesophageal reflux**
PO
Adults. 10-15 mg up to 4 times a day, or single doses up to 20 mg as needed.
Elderly. Initially, 5 mg 4 times a day. May increase to 10 mg.
Children. 0.4-0.8 mg/kg/day in 4 divided doses.

M

▸ **To facilitate small bowel intubation (single dose)**
IV
Adults, Elderly. 10 mg as a single dose.
Children 6-14 yr. 2.5-5 mg as a single dose.
Children younger than 6 yr. 0.1 mg/kg as a single dose.
▸ **Dosage in renal impairment**
Dosage is modified based on creatinine clearance.

Creatinine Clearance	% of Normal Dose
40-50 ml/min	75%
10-40 ml/min	50%
Less than 10 ml/min	25%-50%

OFF-LABEL USES
Prevention of aspiration pneumonia; treatment of drug-related postoperative nausea and vomiting, persistent hiccups, slow gastric emptying, vascular headaches

CONTRAINDICATIONS
Concurrent use of medications likely to produce extrapyramidal reactions, GI hemorrhage, GI obstruction or perforation, history of seizure disorders, pheochromocytoma

INTERACTIONS
Drug
Alcohol, other CNS suppressants: May increase CNS depressant effect.
Herbal
None known.
Food
None known.

DIAGNOSTIC TEST EFFECTS
May increase serum aldosterone and prolactin concentrations.

▨ IV INCOMPATIBILITIES
Allopurinol (Aloprim), cefepime (Maxipime), doxorubicin liposomal (Doxil), furosemide (Lasix), propofol (Diprivan)
▨ IV Compatibilities
Dexamethasone, diltiazem (Cardizem), diphenhydramine (Benadryl), fentanyl (Sublimaze), heparin, hydromorphone (Dilaudid), morphine, potassium chloride

SIDE EFFECTS
Frequent (10%)
Somnolence, restlessness, fatigue, lethargy
Occasional (3%)
Dizziness, anxiety, headache, insomnia, breast tenderness, altered menstruation, constipation, rash, dry mouth, galactorrhea, gynecomastia
Rare (less than 3%)
Hypotension or hypertension, tachycardia

SERIOUS REACTIONS
• Extrapyramidal reactions occur most commonly in children and young adults (18-30 years) receiving large doses (2 mg/kg) during chemotherapy and are usually limited to akathisia (involuntary limb movement and facial grimacing).

PRECAUTIONS & CONSIDERATIONS
Caution is warranted with cirrhosis, CHF, and renal impairment. Metoclopramide crosses the placenta and is distributed in breast milk. Children are more susceptible to dystonic reactions. The elderly are more likely to have parkinsonian reactions and dyskinesias after long-term therapy. Alcohol and tasks that require mental alertness or motor skills should be avoided.
Dizziness, drowsiness, and dry mouth may occur. Notify the physician if involuntary eye, facial, or limb movement occurs. B/P, heart rate, renal function, skin for rash, and pattern

of daily bowel activity and stool consistency should be monitored.

Storage
Store vials at room temperature. After dilution, IV piggyback infusion is stable for 48 hours.

Administration
! Metoclopramide may be given by PO and IM routes and by IV push or IV infusion. Doses of 2 mg/kg or more or prolonged therapy may increase the incidence of side effects.

Take oral metoclopramide 30 minutes before meals and at bedtime. Crush tablets as needed.

For IV use, dilute doses greater than 10 mg in 50 ml D_5W, 0.9% NaCl, or lactated Ringer's solution. Infuse over 15 minutes. Give slow IV push of 10 mg over 1 to 2 minutes. Too-rapid IV injection may produce intense anxiety or restlessness, followed by drowsiness.

Metolazone
met-tole′a-zone
(Mykrox, Zaroxolyn)
Do not confuse metolazone with methazolamide, or metoprolol, or Zaroxolyn with Zarontin.

CATEGORY AND SCHEDULE
Pregnancy Risk Category: B, D if used in pregnancy-induced hypertension

CLASSIFICATION
Diuretics, thiazide and derivatives

MECHANISM OF ACTION
A thiazide-like diuretic and antihypertensive. As a diuretic, blocks reabsorption of sodium, potassium, and chloride at the distal convoluted tubule, increasing renal excretion of sodium and water. As an antihypertensive, reduces plasma and extracellular fluid volume and peripheral vascular resistance. *Therapeutic Effect:* Promotes diuresis and reduces B/P.

PHARMACOKINETICS

Route	Onset	Peak	Duration
PO (diuretic)	1 hr	2 hr	12-24 hr

Incompletely absorbed from the GI tract. Protein binding: 95%. Primarily excreted unchanged in urine. Not removed by hemodialysis.
Half-life: 14 hr.

AVAILABILITY
Tablets (Prompt-Release [Mykrox]): 0.5 mg.
Tablets (Extended-Release [Zaroxolyn]): 2.5 mg, 5 mg, 10 mg.

INDICATIONS AND DOSAGES
▶ **Edema**
PO
Adults, Elderly. 5-10 mg/day. May increase to 20 mg/day in edema associated with renal disease or heart failure.
Children. 0.2-0.4 mg/kg/day in 1-2 divided doses.
▶ **Hypertension**
PO (ZAROXOLYN)
Adults, Elderly. 2.4-5 mg/day.
PO (MYDROX)
Adults, Elderly. Initially, 0.5 mg/day. May increase up to 1 mg/day.
▶ **Usual elderly dosage (Zaroxolyn)**
PO
• *Elderly.* Initially, 2.5 mg/day or every other day.

CONTRAINDICATIONS
Anuria, hepatic coma or precoma, history of hypersensitivity to

M

sulfonamides or thiazide diuretics, renal decompensation

INTERACTIONS
Drug
Cholestyramine, colestipol: May decrease the absorption and effects of metolazone.
Digoxin: May increase the risk of digoxin toxicity associated with metolazone-induced hypokalemia.
Lithium: May increase the risk of lithium toxicity.
Herbal
None known.
Food
None known.

DIAGNOSTIC TEST EFFECTS
May increase blood glucose and serum cholesterol, LDL, bilirubin, calcium, creatinine, uric acid, and triglyceride levels. May decrease urinary calcium, and serum magnesium, potassium, and sodium levels.

SIDE EFFECTS
Expected
Increase in urinary frequency and urine volume
Frequent (10%-9%)
Dizziness, lightheadedness, headache
Occasional (6%-4%)
Muscle cramps and spasm, fatigue, lethargy
Rare (less than 2%)
Asthenia, palpitations, depression, nausea, vomiting, abdominal bloating, constipation, diarrhea, urticaria

SERIOUS REACTIONS
• Vigorous diuresis may lead to profound water and electrolyte depletion, resulting in hypokalemia, hyponatremia, and dehydration.
• Acute hypotensive episodes may occur.
• Hyperglycemia may occur during prolonged therapy.

• Pancreatitis, paresthesia, blood dyscrasias, pulmonary edema, allergic pneumonitis, and dermatologic reactions occur rarely.
• Overdose can lead to lethargy and coma without changes in electrolytes or hydration.

PRECAUTIONS & CONSIDERATIONS
Caution is warranted with diabetes, elevated cholesterol and triglyceride levels, gout, hepatic impairment, lupus erythematosus, and severe renal disease. Metolazone crosses the placenta and a small amount is distributed in breast milk. Breast-feeding is not recommended for patients taking this drug. No age-related precautions have been noted in children. The elderly may be more sensitive to the drug's electrolyte and hypotensive effects. Age-related renal impairment may require cautious use in the elderly. Consuming foods high in potassium such as apricots, bananas, legumes, meat, orange juice, raisins, whole grains, including cereals, and white and sweet potatoes, is encouraged.

An increase in the frequency and volume of urination may occur. Blood pressure (B/P), vital signs, electrolytes, intake and output, and weight should be monitored before and during treatment. Be aware of signs of electrolyte disturbances such as hypokalemia or hyponatremia. Hypokalemia may cause arrhythmias, altered mental status, muscle cramps, asthenia, and tremor. Hyponatremia may result in cold and clammy skin, confusion, and thirst.
Administration
Take metolazone with food or milk if GI upset occurs, preferably with breakfast to help prevent nocturia.

Metoprolol

me-toe′pro-lole
(Apo-Metoprolol [CAN], Betaloc
[CAN], Lopresor [AUS],
Lopressor, Metohexal [AUS],
Metolol [AUS], Minax [AUS], Nu-
Metop [CAN], PMS-Metoprolol
[CAN], Toprol XL)
**Do not confuse metoprolol with
metaproterenol or metolazone.**

CATEGORY AND SCHEDULE

Pregnancy Risk Category: C (D if
used in second or third trimester)

CLASSIFICATION

Antiadrenergics, beta blocking

MECHANISM OF ACTION

An antianginal, antihypertensive,
and MI adjunct that selectively
blocks beta$_1$-adrenergic receptors;
high dosages may block
beta$_2$-adrenergic receptors.
Decreases oxygen requirements.
Large doses increase airway
resistance. *Therapeutic Effect:*
Slows sinus node heart rate,
decreases cardiac output, and
reduces B/P. Also decreases
myocardial ischemia severity.

PHARMACOKINETICS

Route	Onset	Peak	Duration
PO	10-15 min	N/A	6 hr
PO (extended release)	N/A	6-12 hr	24 hr
IV	Immediate	20 min	5-8 hr

Well absorbed from the GI tract.
Protein binding: 12%. Widely
distributed. Metabolized in the liver
(undergoes significant first-pass
metabolism). Primarily excreted in
urine. Removed by hemodialysis.
Half-life: 3-7 hr.

AVAILABILITY

Tablets (Lopressor): 25 mg, 50 mg,
100 mg.
*Tablets (Extended-Release [Toprol
XL]):* 25 mg, 50 mg, 100 mg,
200 mg.
Injection (Lopressor): 1 mg/ml.

INDICATIONS AND DOSAGES

▸ **Mild to moderate hypertension**
PO
Adults. Initially, 100 mg/day as
single or divided dose. Increase at
weekly (or longer) intervals.
Maintenance: 100-450 mg/day.
Elderly. Initially, 25 mg/day. Range:
25-300 mg/day.
PO (Extended-release Tablets)
Adults. 50-100 mg/day as single
dose. May increase at least at
weekly intervals until optimum
B/P attained. Maximum:
200 mg/day.
▸ **Chronic, stable angina
pectoris**
PO
Adults. Initially, 100 mg/day as
single or divided dose. Increase at
weekly (or longer) intervals.
Maintenance: 100-450 mg/day.
PO (Extended-release Tablets)
Adults. Initially, 100 mg/day as
single dose. May increase at least
at weekly intervals until optimum
clinical response achieved.
Maximum: 200 mg/day.
▸ **Congestive heart failure**
PO (Extended-release Tablets)
Adults. Initially, 25 mg/day. May
double dose q2wk. Maximum:
200 mg/day.
▸ **Early treatment of MI**
IV
Adults. 5 mg q2min for 3 doses,
followed by 50 mg orally q6hr for
48 hr. Begin oral dose 15 min after

M

last IV dose. Or, in patients who do not tolerate full IV dose, give 25-50 mg orally q6hr, 15 min after last IV dose.

▸ **Late treatment and maintenance after an MI**
PO
Adults. 100 mg twice a day for at least 3 mo.

OFF-LABEL USES
To increase survival rate in diabetic patients with coronary artery disease (CAD); treatment or prevention of anxiety; cardiac arrhythmias; hypertrophic cardiomyopathy; mitral valve prolapse syndrome; pheochromocytoma; tremors; thyrotoxicosis; vascular headache

CONTRAINDICATIONS
Cardiogenic shock, MI with a heart rate less than 45 beats/minute or systolic BP less than 100 mm Hg, overt heart failure, second- or third-degree heart block, sinus bradycardia

INTERACTIONS
Drug
Cimetidine: May increase metoprolol blood concentration.
Diuretics, other antihypertensives: May increase hypotensive effect.
Insulin, oral hypoglycemics: May mask symptoms of hypoglycemia and prolong hypoglycemic effect of these drugs.
NSAIDs: May decrease antihypertensive effect.
Sympathomimetics, xanthines: May mutually inhibit effects.
Herbal
None known.
Food
None known.

DIAGNOSTIC TEST EFFECTS
May increase serum antinuclear antibody titer and BUN, serum lipoprotein, serum LDH, serum alkaline phosphatase, serum bilirubin, serum creatinine, serum potassium, serum uric acid, AST (SGOT), ALT (SGPT), and serum triglyceride levels.

IV INCOMPATIBILITIES
Amphotericin B complex (Abelcet, AmBisome, Amphotec)
IV Compatibilities
Alteplase (Activase)

SIDE EFFECTS
Metoprolol is generally well tolerated, with transient and mild side effects.
Frequent
Diminished sexual function, drowsiness, insomnia, unusual fatigue or weakness
Occasional
Anxiety, nervousness, diarrhea, constipation, nausea, vomiting, nasal congestion, abdominal discomfort, dizziness, difficulty breathing, cold hands or feet
Rare
Altered taste, dry eyes, nightmares, paraesthesia, allergic reaction (rash, pruritus)

SERIOUS REACTIONS
• Overdose may produce profound bradycardia, hypotension, and bronchospasm.
• Abrupt withdrawal of metoprolol may result in diaphoresis, palpitations, headache, tremulousness, exacerbation of angina, MI, and ventricular arrhythmias.
• Metoprolol administration may precipitate CHF and MI in patients with heart disease; thyroid storm in those with thyrotoxicosis; and peripheral ischemia in those with existing peripheral vascular disease.
• Hypoglycemia may occur in patients with previously controlled diabetes.

PRECAUTIONS & CONSIDERATIONS

Caution is warranted with bronchospastic disease, diabetes, hyperthyroidism, impaired renal function, inadequate cardiac function, and peripheral vascular disease. Metoprolol crosses the placenta and is distributed in breast milk. Metoprolol use should be avoided in pregnant women after the first trimester because it may result in low-birth-weight infants. The drug may also produce apnea, bradycardia, hypoglycemia, or hypothermia during childbirth. The safety and efficacy of metoprolol have not been established in children. In the elderly, age-related peripheral vascular disease may increase susceptibility to decreased peripheral circulation. Be aware that salt and alcohol intake should be restricted. Nasal decongestants or OTC cold preparations (stimulants) should not be used without physician approval.

Notify the physician of excessive fatigue, headache, prolonged dizziness, shortness of breath, or weight gain. B/P for hypotension, respiratory status for shortness of breath, pattern of daily bowel activity and stool consistency, EKG for arrhythmias, and pulse for quality, rate and rhythm should be monitored during treatment. If pulse rate is 60 beats/minute or lower or systolic B/P is less than 90 mm Hg, withhold the medication and contact the physician. In those receiving metoprolol for treatment of angina, the onset, type (sharp, dull, squeezing), radiation, location, intensity, and duration of anginal pain and its precipitating factors, including exertion and emotional stress should be recorded. Signs and symptoms of CHF, such as decreased urine output, distended neck veins, dyspnea (particularly on exertion or lying down), night cough, peripheral edema, and weight gain should also be assessed.

Storage

Store at room temperature.

Administration

Crush tablets if necessary; do not crush or break extended-release tablets. Take at same time each day. Take with or immediately after meals to enhance absorption.

For IV use, give undiluted as necessary. Administer IV injection over 1 minute. Monitor the patient's EKG and B/P during administration.

Metronidazole

me-troe-ni′da-zole
(Apo-Metronidazole [CAN], Flagyl, Flagyl ER, MetroCream, MetroGel, Metrogyl [AUS], MetroLotion, Metronidazole IV [AUS], Metronide [AUS], NidaGel [CAN], Noritate, Novonidazol [CAN], Rozex [AUS])

CATEGORY AND SCHEDULE

Pregnancy Risk Category: B

CLASSIFICATION

Anti-infectives, topical, antibiotics, miscellaneous, antiprotozoals, dermatologics

MECHANISM OF ACTION

A nitroimidazole derivative that disrupts bacterial and protozoal DNA, inhibiting nucleic acid synthesis. *Therapeutic Effect:* Produces bactericidal, antiprotozoal, amebicidal, and trichomonacidal effects. Produces anti-inflammatory and immunosuppressive effects when applied topically.

PHARMACOKINETICS

Well absorbed from the GI tract; minimally absorbed after topical application. Protein binding: less than 20%. Widely distributed; crosses blood-brain barrier. Metabolized in the liver to active metabolite. Primarily excreted in urine; partially eliminated in feces. Removed by hemodialysis.
Half-life: 8 hr (increased in alcoholic hepatic disease and in neonates).

AVAILABILITY

Capsules (Flagyl): 375 mg.
Tablets (Flagyl): 250 mg, 500 mg.
Tablets (Extended-Release [Flagyl ER]): 750 mg.
Injection (Infusion): 500 mg/100 ml.
Lotion: 0.75%.
Topical Gel (MetroGel): 0.75%.
Topical Cream (MetroCream): 0.75%.
Topical Cream (Noritate): 1%.
Vaginal Gel (MetroGel-Vaginal): 0.75%.

INDICATIONS AND DOSAGES
▸ **Amebiasis**
PO
Adults, Elderly. 500-750 mg q8hr.
Children. 35-50 mg/kg/day in divided doses q8hr.
▸ **Trichomoniasis**
PO
Adults, Elderly. 250 mg q8hr or 2 g as a single dose.
Children. 15-30 mg/kg/day in divided doses q8hr.
▸ **Anaerobic skin and skin-structure, CNS, lower respiratory tract, bone, joint, intra-abdominal, and gynecologic infections; endocarditis; septicemia**
PO, IV
Adults, Elderly, Children. 30 mg/kg/day in divided doses q6hr.
Maximum: 4 g/day.

▸ **Antibiotic-associated pseudomembranous colitis**
PO
Adults, Elderly. 250-500 mg 3-4 times a day for 10-14 days.
Children. 30 mg/kg/day in divided doses q6hr for 7-10 days.
▸ **Helicobacter pylori infections**
PO
Adults, Elderly. 250-500 mg 3 times a day (in combination).
Children. 15-20 mg/kg/day in 2 divided doses.
▸ **Bacterial vaginosis**
PO
Adults. 750 mg at bedtime for 7 days.
▸ **Intravaginal**
Adults. One applicatorful twice a day or once a day at bedtime for 5 days.
▸ **Rosacea**
TOPICAL
Adults. Apply thin layer of lotion to affected area twice a day or cream once a day.

OFF-LABEL USES

Treatment of bacterial vaginosis, grade III-IV decubitus ulcers with anaerobic infection, *H. pylori*-associated gastritis and duodenal ulcer, inflammatory bowel disease; topical treatment of acne rosacea

CONTRAINDICATIONS

Hypersensitivity to metronidazole or other nitroimidazole derivatives (also parabens with topical application)

INTERACTIONS
Drug
Alcohol: May cause a disulfiram-type reaction.
Disulfiram: May increase the risk of toxicity.
Oral anticoagulants: May increase the effects of these drugs.
Herbal
None known.

Food
None known.

DIAGNOSTIC TEST EFFECTS
May increase serum LDH, AST (SGOT), and ALT (SGPT) levels.

▓ IV INCOMPATIBILITIES
Amphotericin B complex (Abelcet, AmBisome, Amphotec), filgrastim (Neupogen)

▓ IV Compatibilities
Diltiazem (Cardizem), dopamine (Intropin), heparin, hydromorphone (Dilaudid), lorazepam (Ativan), magnesium sulfate, midazolam (Versed), morphine

SIDE EFFECTS
Frequent
Systemic: Anorexia, nausea, dry mouth, metallic taste
Vaginal: Symptomatic cervicitis and vaginitis, abdominal cramps, uterine pain
Occasional
Systemic: Diarrhea or constipation, vomiting, dizziness, erythematous rash, urticaria, reddish brown urine
Topical: Transient erythema, mild dryness, burning, irritation, stinging, tearing when applied too close to eyes
Vaginal: Vaginal, perineal, or vulvar itching; vulvar swelling
Rare
Mild, transient leukopenia; thrombophlebitis with IV therapy

SERIOUS REACTIONS
- Oral therapy may result in furry tongue, glossitis, cystitis, dysuria, pancreatitis, and flattening of T waves on EKG readings.
- Peripheral neuropathy, manifested as numbness and tingling in hands or feet, is usually reversible if treatment is stopped immediately after neurologic symptoms appear.
- Seizures occur occasionally.

PRECAUTIONS & CONSIDERATIONS
Caution is warranted with blood dyscrasias, CNS disorders, severe hepatic dysfunction, predisposition to edema, and in those receiving corticosteroid therapy concurrently. Metronidazole readily crosses the placenta and is distributed in breast milk. Metronidazole use is contraindicated during the first trimester of pregnancy in women with trichomoniasis. Topical use during pregnancy or breast-feeding is discouraged. No age-related precautions have been noted in children; however, the safety and efficacy of topical administration in those younger than 21 years have not been established. Age-related hepatic impairment may require a dosage adjustment in the elderly. Prolonged indwelling catheters should be avoided. Avoid alcohol and alcohol-containing preparations (such as cough syrups and elixirs) during and for at least 3 to 5 days post-therapy, excessive sunlight, exposure to very hot and cold temperatures, and hot and spicy foods while taking metronidazole. Avoid sexual intercourse, if taking metronidazole for trichomoniasis, until the full treatment is completed.

Urine may become reddish brown during therapy. Skin should be examined for rash and urticaria. Pattern of daily bowel activity and stool consistency should be monitored; document the number and characteristics of stools in those with amebiasis. Be alert for signs and symptoms of superinfection, including abdominal pain, moderate to severe diarrhea, severe anal or genital pruritus, and severe mouth soreness. In addition, be alert for neurologic symptoms such as dizziness and paresthesia. Avoid tasks requiring mental alertness or motor skills until the drug is established. Metronidazole acts on

M

papules, pustules, and erythema, but has no effect on ocular problems (conjunctivitis, keratitis, blepharitis), rhinophyma (hypertrophy of nose), or telangiectasia.

Storage
Store ready-to-use infusion bags at room temperature.

Administration
Take oral metronidazole without regard to food. However, give it with food if GI upset occurs.

For IV use, infuse metronidazole over 30 to 60 minutes. Don't give as an IV bolus injection.

Metyrosine
me-tye′roe-seen
(Demser)

CATEGORY AND SCHEDULE
Pregnancy Risk Category: C

CLASSIFICATION
Antihypertensives

MECHANISM OF ACTION
A tyrosine hydroxylase inhibitor that blocks conversion of tyrosine to dihydroxyphenylalanine, the rate limiting step in the biosynthetic pathway of catecholamines. *Therapeutic Effect:* Reduces levels of endogenous catecholamines.

PHARMACOKINETICS
Well absorbed from the gastrointestinal (GI) tract. Metabolized in the liver. Excreted primarily in the urine. **Half-life:** 7.2 hr.

AVAILABILITY
Capsule: 250 mg (Demser).

INDICATIONS AND DOSAGES
▸ **Pheochromocytoma (preoperative)**
PO
Adults, Elderly. Initially, 250 mg 4 times/day. Increase by 250-500 mg/day up to 4 g/day. Maintenance: 2-4 g/day in 4 divided doses for 5-7 days.

OFF-LABEL USES
Tourette syndrome

CONTRAINDICATIONS
Hypertension of unknown etiology, hypersensitivity to metyrosine or any component of the formulation

INTERACTIONS
Drug
Alcohol: May increase CNS depression.
Phenothiazines, haloperidol: May potentiate extrapyramidal symptoms (EPS).
Herbal
None known.
Food
None known.

DIAGNOSTIC TEST EFFECTS
None known.

SIDE EFFECTS
Frequent
Drowsiness, extrapyramidal symptoms, diarrhea
Occasional
Galactorrhea, edema of the breasts, nausea, vomiting, dry mouth, impotence, nasal congestion
Rare
Lower extremity edema, urinary problems, urticaria, anemia, depression, disorientation

SERIOUS REACTIONS
• Serious or life-threatening allergic reaction characterized hallucinations,

hematuria, hyperstimulation after withdrawal, severe lower extremity edema, and parkinsonism.

PRECAUTIONS & CONSIDERATIONS
Caution should be used with impaired liver or renal function. It is unknown if metyrosine is distributed in breast milk. Safety and efficacy of metyrosine have not been established in children younger than 12 years old. The elderly with impaired renal function may need dose adjustment. Alcoholic beverages should be avoided during therapy.
Administration
Take with regard to food. Increase fluid intake.

Mexiletine
mex-il′e-teen
(Mexitil)

CATEGORY AND SCHEDULE
Pregnancy Risk Category: C

CLASSIFICATION
Antiarrhythmics, class IB

MECHANISM OF ACTION
An antiarrhythmic that shortens duration of action potential and decreases effective refractory period in the His-Purkinje system of the myocardium by blocking sodium transport across myocardial cell membranes. *Therapeutic Effect:* Suppresses ventricular arrhythmias.

AVAILABILITY
Capsules: 150 mg, 200 mg, 250 mg.

INDICATIONS AND DOSAGES
▶ **Arrhythmias**
PO
Adults, Elderly. Initially, 200 mg q8hr. Adjust dosage by 50-100 mg at 2- to 3-day intervals. Maximum: 1200 mg/day.

OFF-LABEL USES
Treatment of diabetic neuropathy

CONTRAINDICATIONS
Cardiogenic shock, pre-existing second- or third-degree AV block, right bundle-branch block without presence of pacemaker

INTERACTIONS
Drug
Antacids: May reduce mexiletine absorption.
Cimetidine: May increase mexiletine blood concentration.
Metoclopramide: May increase mexiletine absorption.
Phenobarbital, phenytoin, rifampin: May decrease mexiletine blood concentration.
Herbal
None known.
Food
None known.

DIAGNOSTIC TEST EFFECTS
May increase liver enzymes, such as ALT and AST. May decrease WBCs and thrombocytes.

SIDE EFFECTS
Frequent (greater than 10%)
GI distress, including nausea, vomiting, and heartburn; dizziness; lightheadedness; tremor
Occasional (10%-1%)
Nervousness, change in sleep habits, headache, visual disturbances, paresthesia, diarrhea or constipation, palpitations, chest pain, rash, respiratory difficulty, edema

SERIOUS REACTIONS
• Mexiletine has the ability to worsen existing arrhythmias or produce new ones.
• CHF may occur and existing CHF may worsen.

PRECAUTIONS & CONSIDERATIONS
Caution is warranted with CHF, impaired myocardial function, second- and third-degree AV block, with pacemaker, and sick sinus syndrome. Nasal decongestants and over-the-counter cold preparations should be avoided without physician approval. Alcohol and salt intake should be restricted.

Notify the physician if dark urine, cough, generalized fatigue, nausea, pale stools, severe or persistent abdominal pain, shortness of breath, unexplained sore throat or fever, vomiting, or yellowing of the eyes or skin occurs. EKG and vital signs should be monitored before and during therapy. Pulse for irregular rate and quality, GI disturbances, pattern of daily bowel activity and stool consistency, dizziness and syncope, hand movement for evidence of tremor, and signs and symptoms of CHF should be assessed.

Administration
If 300 mg every 8 hours or less controls arrhythmias, may take dose every 12 hours. Do not crush, open, or break capsules.

Miconazole
mih-kon'ah-zole
(Femizol-M, Micatin, Micozole [CAN], Monistat [CAN], Monistat-3, Monistat-7, Monistat-Derm)

CATEGORY AND SCHEDULE
Pregnancy Risk Category: C

CLASSIFICATION
Antifungals, topical, dermatologics

MECHANISM OF ACTION
An imidazole derivative that inhibits synthesis of ergosterol (vital component of fungal cell formation), damaging cell membrane. *Therapeutic Effect:* Fungistatic; may be fungicidal, depending on concentration.

PHARMACOKINETICS
Parenteral: Widely distributed in tissues. Metabolized in liver. Primarily excreted in urine. **Half-life:** 24 hr. Topical: No systemic absorption following application to intact skin. Intravaginally: Small amount absorbed systemically.

AVAILABILITY
Injection: 10 mg/ml.
Vaginal Suppository: 100 mg (Monistat-7), 200 mg (Monistat-3).
Topical Cream: 2% (Micatin, Monistat-Derm).
Vaginal Cream: 2% (Femizol-M).
Topical Powder: 2% (Micatin).
Topical Spray: 2% (Lotrimin-AF).

INDICATIONS AND DOSAGES
▶ Coccidioidomycosis
IV
Adults, Elderly. 1.8-3.6 g/day for 3-20 wk or longer.

▸ **Cryptococcosis**
IV
Adults, Elderly. 1.2-2.4 g/day for
3-12 wk or longer.
▸ **Petriellidiosis**
IV
Adults, Elderly. 0.6-3.0 g/day for
5-20 wk or longer.
▸ **Candidiasis**
IV
Adults, Elderly. 0.6-1.8 g/day for
1-20 wk or longer.
▸ **Paracoccidioidomycosis**
IV
Adults, Elderly. 0.2-1.2 g/day for
2-16 wk or longer.
Usual dosage for children
IV
20-40 mg/kg/day in 3 divided doses.
(Do not exceed 15 mg/kg for any
1 infusion).
▸ **Vulvovaginal candidiasis**
INTRAVAGINALLY
Adults, Elderly. One 200 mg supposi-
tory at bedtime for 3 days; one
100 mg suppository or one applica-
torful at bedtime for 7 days.
Topical fungal infections, cutaneous
candidiasis
TOPICAL
*Adults, Elderly, Children 2 yr and
older.* Apply liberally 2 times/day,
morning and evening.

CONTRAINDICATIONS
Children younger than 1 year old,
hypersensitivity to miconazole
or any component of the
formulation
Topically: Children younger than
2 years old

INTERACTIONS
Drug
**Oral anticoagulants, oral hypo-
glycemics:** May increase effects of
these drugs.
Isoniazid, rifampin: May decrease
concentrations.

Herbal
None known.
Food
None known.

DIAGNOSTIC TEST EFFECTS
None known.

▨ IV INCOMPATIBILITIES
Do not administer other medications
via Y-site.

SIDE EFFECTS
Frequent
Phlebitis, fever, chills, rash, itching,
nausea, vomiting
Occasional
Dizziness, drowsiness, headache,
flushed face, abdominal pain, consti-
pation, diarrhea, decreased appetite
Topical: Itching, burning, stinging,
erythema, urticaria
Vaginal: Vulvovaginal burning, itch-
ing, irritation, headache, skin rash

SERIOUS REACTIONS
• Anemia, thrombocytopenia, and
liver toxicity occur rarely

PRECAUTIONS & CONSIDERATIONS
Caution should be used with liver
impairment. It is unknown if
miconazole crosses the placenta or
is excreted in breast milk. There are
no age-related precautions noted in
children or the elderly.
Storage
Store at room temperature.
Administration
Be aware that IV doses may be
divided over 3 IV infusions.
After reconstitution, IV solution is
stable for 24 hr at room temperature
with D_5W or 0.9% NaCl. Dilute each
200 mg ampoule with at least 200 ml
D_5W or 0.9% NaCl to provide maximum concentration of 1 mg/ml. Give
IV infusion (piggyback) over at least
30-60 min (rapid administration may

M

cause arrhythmias). Initial treatment should be performed in hospital with physician in attendance for first 200 mg dose.

For intravaginal use, insert high in vagina. Be aware that the base in the vaginal preparation interacts with certain latex products such as contraceptive diaphragm.

For topical administration, wash and dry area before applying medication. Apply a thin layer on affected area. Avoid contact with eyes. Keep areas clean, dry; wear light clothing for ventilation. Separate personal items in contact with affected areas.

Midazolam
mid-az′zoe-lam
(Apo-Midazolam [CAN], Hypnovel [AUS], Versed)
Do not confuse Versed with VePesid.

CATEGORY AND SCHEDULE
Pregnancy Risk Category: D
Controlled substance:
Schedule IV

CLASSIFICATION
Benzodiazepines, preanesthetics, sedatives/hypnotics

MECHANISM OF ACTION
A benzodiazepine that enhances the action of gamma-aminobutyric acid, one of the major inhibitory neurotransmitters in the brain. *Therapeutic Effect:* Produces anxiolytic, hypnotic, anticonvulsant, muscle relaxant, and amnestic effects.

PHARMACOKINETICS

Route	Onset	Peak	Duration
PO	10-20 min	N/A	N/A
IV	1-5 min	5-7 min	20-30 min
IM	5-15 min	15-60 min	2-6 hr

Well absorbed after IM administration. Protein binding: 97%. Metabolized in the liver to active metabolite. Primarily excreted in urine. Not removed by hemodialysis. **Half-life:** 1-5 hr.

AVAILABILITY
Syrup: 2 mg/ml.
Injection: 1 mg/ml, 5 mg/ml.

INDICATIONS AND DOSAGES
▸ **Preoperative sedation**
PO
Children. 0.25-0.5 mg/kg.
Maximum: 20 mg.
IV
Children 6-12 yr. 0.025-0.05 mg/kg.
Children 6 mo-5 yr. 0.05-0.1 mg/kg.
IM
Adults, Elderly. 0.07-0.08 mg/kg 30-60 min before surgery.
Children. 0.1-0.15 mg/kg 30-60 min before surgery. Maximum: 10 mg.
▸ **Conscious sedation for diagnostic, therapeutic, and endoscopic procedures**
IV
Adults, Elderly. 1-2.5 mg over 2 min. Titrate as needed. Maximum total dose: 2.5-5 mg.
▸ **Conscious sedation during mechanical ventilation**
IV
Adults, Elderly. 0.01-0.05 mg/kg; may repeat q10-15min until adequately sedated. Then continuous infusion at initial rate of 0.02-0.1 mg/kg/hr (1-7 mg/hr).
Children older than 32 wk. Initially, 1 mcg/kg/min as continuous infusion.

Children 32 wk and younger.
Initially, 0.5 mcg/kg/min as continuous infusion.

▶ **Status epilepticus**
IV
Children older than 2 mo. Loading dose of 0.15 mg/kg followed by continuous infusion of 1 mcg/kg/min. Titrate as needed. Range: 1-18 mcg/kg/min.

CONTRAINDICATIONS
Acute alcohol intoxication, acute angle-closure glaucoma, coma, shock

INTERACTIONS
Drug
Alcohol, other CNS depressants: May increase CNS and respiratory depression and hypotensive effects of midazolam.
Hypotension-producing medications: May increase hypotensive effects of midazolam.
Herbal
Kava kava, valerian: May increase CNS depression.
Food
Grapefruit juice: Increases the oral absorption and systemic availability of midazolam.

DIAGNOSTIC TEST EFFECTS
None known.

🟦 IV INCOMPATIBILITIES
Albumin, ampicillin and sulbactam (Unasyn), amphotericin B complex (Abelcet, AmBisome, Amphotec), ampicillin (Polycillin), bumetanide (Bumex), co-trimoxazole (Bactrim), dexamethasone (Decadron), fosphenytoin (Cerebyx), furosemide (Lasix), hydrocortisone (Solu-Cortef), methotrexate, nafcillin (Nafcil), sodium bicarbonate, sodium pentothal (Thiopental)

🟦 IV Compatibilities
Amiodarone (Cordarone), calcium gluconate, diltiazem (Cardizem), dobutamine (Dobutrex), dopamine (Intropin), etomidate (Amidate), fentanyl (Sublimaze), heparin, hydromorphone (Dilaudid), insulin, lorazepam (Ativan), milrinone (Primacor), morphine, nitroglycerin, norepinephrine (Levophed), potassium chloride, propofol (Diprivan)

SIDE EFFECTS
Frequent (10%-4%)
Decreased respiratory rate, tenderness at IM or IV injection site, pain during injection, oxygen desaturation, hiccups
Occasional (3%-2%)
Hypotension, paradoxical CNS reaction
Rare (less than 2%)
Nausea, vomiting, headache, coughing

SERIOUS REACTIONS
• Inadequate or excessive dosage or improper administration may result in cerebral hypoxia, agitation, involuntary movements, hyperactivity, and combativeness.
• A too-rapid IV rate, excessive doses, or a single large dose increases the risk of respiratory depression or arrest.
• Respiratory depression or apnea may produce hypoxia and cardiac arrest.

PRECAUTIONS & CONSIDERATIONS
Caution is warranted with acute illness, CHF, pulmonary, renal, or hepatic impairment, severe fluid and electrolyte imbalance, and treated angle-closure glaucoma. Midazolam crosses the placenta; it is unknown if midazolam is distributed in breast milk. Females on long-term therapy should use effective contraception

M

during therapy and notify the physician immediately if she becomes or may be pregnant. Neonates are more likely to experience respiratory depression. In the elderly, age-related renal impairment may require dosage adjustment.

Midazolam produces an amnesic effect. Vital signs should be obtained before and after administering midazolam. Respiratory rate and oxygen saturation should be monitored continuously during parenteral administration to detect apnea and respiratory depression. Sedation should be assessed every 3 to 5 minutes.

Storage
Store vials at room temperature.

Administration
! Midazolam dosage is individualized based on age, underlying disease, and medications and on the desired effect.

Midazolam may be given undiluted or as an infusion. Ensure that resuscitative supplies, such as endotracheal tubes, suction equipment, and oxygen, are readily available. Administer the drug by slow IV injection in incremental doses. Give each incremental dose over 2 minutes or more and wait at least 2 minutes between doses. Reduce the IV rate in patients older than 60 years, debilitated patients, and those with chronic diseases or impaired pulmonary function. A too-rapid IV rate, excessive doses, or a single large dose increases the risk of respiratory depression or arrest.

For IM use, inject the drug deep into a large muscle mass, such as the gluteus maximus.

Midodrine
mid′o-dreen
(Amatine, ProAmatine)
Do not confuse ProAmantine with Amantadine or protamine.

CATEGORY AND SCHEDULE
Pregnancy Risk Category: C

CLASSIFICATION
Adrenergic agonists

MECHANISM OF ACTION
A vasopressor that forms the active metabolite desglymidodrine, an alpha$_1$-agonist, activating alpha receptors of the arteriolar and venous vasculature. *Therapeutic Effect:* Increases vascular tone and B/P.

AVAILABILITY
Tablets: 2.5 mg, 5 mg, 10 mg.

INDICATIONS AND DOSAGES
▸ **Orthostatic hypotension**
PO
Adults, Elderly. 10 mg 3 times a day. Give during the day when patient is upright, such as upon arising, midday, and late afternoon. Do not give later than 6 PM.
▸ **Dosage in renal impairment**
For adults and elderly patients, give 2.5 mg 3 times a day; increase gradually, as tolerated.

CONTRAINDICATIONS
Acute renal function impairment, persistent hypertension, pheochromocytoma, severe cardiac disease, thyrotoxicosis, urine retention

INTERACTIONS
Drug
Digoxin: May have additive brady-
cardia effects.
**Sodium-retaining steroids (such as
fludrocortisone):** May increase
sodium retention.
Vasoconstrictors: May have an
additive vasoconstricting effect.
Herbal
None known.
Food
None known.

DIAGNOSTIC TEST EFFECTS
None known.

SIDE EFFECTS
Frequent (20%-7%)
Paresthesia, piloerection, pruritus,
dysuria, supine hypertension
Occasional (less than 7%-1%)
Pain, rash, chills, headache, facial
flushing, confusion, dry mouth,
anxiety

SERIOUS REACTIONS
• None known.

PRECAUTIONS & CONSIDERATIONS
Caution is warranted with a history
of vision problems and renal and
hepatic impairment. B/P and liver
and renal function test results should
be monitored. OTC medications,
such as cough, cold, and diet
preparations should be avoided
because they may affect B/P.
Administration
Do not take the last dose of the
day after the evening meal or less
than 4 hours before bedtime. Do not
take the medication while lying
down.

Mifepristone
miff-eh-pris'tone
(Mifeprex)
**Do not confuse Mifeprex with
Mirapex or mifepristone with
misoprostol.**

CATEGORY AND SCHEDULE
Pregnancy Risk Category: X

CLASSIFICATION
Abortifacients, oxazolidinediones,
stimulants, uterine

MECHANISM OF ACTION
An abortifacient that has anti-
progestational activity resulting
from competitive interaction with
progesterone. Inhibits the activity of
endogenous or exogenous progesterone. Also has antiglucocorticoid
and weak antiandrogenic activity.
Therapeutic Effect: Terminates
pregnancy.

AVAILABILITY
Tablets: 200 mg.

INDICATIONS AND DOSAGES
▸ **Termination of pregnancy**
PO
Adults. Day 1: 600 mg as single
dose. Day 3: 400 mcg misoprostol.
Day 14: Post-treatment
examination.

OFF-LABEL USES
Cushing's syndrome, endometriosis,
intrauterine fetal death or nonviable
early pregnancy, postcoital contraception or contragestation, unresectable
meningioma

CONTRAINDICATIONS
Chronic adrenal failure, concurrent
long-term steroid or anticoagulant

M

therapy, confirmed or suspected ectopic pregnancy, intrauterine device (IUD) in place, hemorrhagic disorders, inherited porphyria

INTERACTIONS
Drug
Carbamazepine, phenobarbital, phenytoin, rifampin: May increase the metabolism of mifepristone.
Erythromycin, itraconazole, ketoconazole: May inhibit the metabolism of mifepristone.
Herbal
St. John's wort: May increase the metabolism of mifepristone.
Food
Grapefruit: May inhibit the metabolism of mifepristone.

DIAGNOSTIC TEST EFFECTS
May decrease Hgb level and Hct and RBC count.

SIDE EFFECTS
Frequent (greater than 10%)
Headache, dizziness, abdominal pain, nausea, vomiting, diarrhea, fatigue
Occasional (10%-3%)
Uterine hemorrhage, insomnia, vaginitis, dyspepsia, back pain, fever, viral infections, rigors
Rare (2%-1%)
Anxiety, syncope, anemia, asthenia, leg pain, sinusitis, leukorrhea

SERIOUS REACTIONS
• None known.

PRECAUTIONS & CONSIDERATIONS
Caution is warranted with cardiovascular disease, diabetes, hepatic or renal impairment, hypertension, severe anemia, and in persons older than 35 years of age or who smoke more than 10 cigarettes a day. Be aware anticonvulsants, erythromycin, itraconazole, ketoconazole, and

rifampin may inhibit the metabolism of mifepristone. Uterine cramping and vaginal bleeding may occur. Hgb level and Hct should be monitored. An IUD, if in place, should be removed before therapy begins.
Storage
Refrigerate ampoules.
Administration
! Treatment with mifepristone and misoprostol requires three office visits.

Miglitol
mig-lee'tall
(Glyset)

CATEGORY AND SCHEDULE
Pregnancy Risk Category: B

CLASSIFICATION
Alpha glucosidase inhibitors, antidiabetic agents

MECHANISM OF ACTION
An alpha-glucosidase inhibitor that delays the digestion of ingested carbohydrates into simple sugars such as glucose. *Therapeutic Effect:* Produces smaller rise in blood glucose concentration after meals.

AVAILABILITY
Tablets: 25 mg, 50 mg, 100 mg.

INDICATIONS AND DOSAGES
▸ **Diabetes mellitus**
PO
Adults, Elderly. Initially, 25 mg 3 times a day with first bite of each main meal. Maintenance: 50 mg 3 times a day. Maximum: 100 mg 3 times a day.

CONTRAINDICATIONS
Colonic ulceration, diabetic ketoacidosis, hypersensitivity to miglitol, inflammatory bowel disease, partial intestinal obstruction

INTERACTIONS
Drug
Digoxin, propranolol, ranitidine: May decrease the blood concentrations and effects of these drugs.
Herbal
None known.
Food
None known.

DIAGNOSTIC TEST EFFECTS
None known.

SIDE EFFECTS
Frequent (40%-10%)
Flatulence, loose stools, diarrhea, abdominal pain
Occasional (5%)
Rash

PRECAUTIONS & CONSIDERATIONS
Caution is warranted with renal impairment. Adequate studies have not been done in pregnant women. Miglitol is distributed in breast milk; breast-feeding is not recommended during miglitol therapy. Safety and efficacy have not been established in children.

Food intake and blood glucose should be monitored before and during therapy. Be aware of signs and symptoms of hypoglycemia (anxiety, cool wet skin, diplopia, dizziness, headache, hunger, numbness in mouth, tachycardia, tremors), or hyperglycemia (deep rapid breathing, dim vision, fatigue, nausea, polydipsia, polyphagia, polyuria, vomiting); carry candy, sugar packets, or other sugar supplements for immediate response to hypoglycemia. Consult the physician when glucose demands are altered (such as with fever, heavy physical activity, infection, stress, trauma). Exercise, good personal hygiene (including foot care), not smoking, and weight control are essential parts of therapy.
Administration
Take with the first bite of each main meal.

Miglustat
mig-lew´stat
(Zavesca)

CATEGORY AND SCHEDULE
Pregnancy Risk Category: X

CLASSIFICATION
Metabolics

M

MECHANISM OF ACTION
A Gaucher disease agent that inhibits the enzyme, glucosylceramide synthase, reducing the rate of synthesis of most glycosphingolipids. Allows the residual activity of the deficient enzyme, glucocerebrosidase, to be more effective in degrading lysosomal storage within tissues. *Therapeutic Effect:* Minimizes conditions associated with Gaucher's disease, such as anemia and bone disease.

AVAILABILITY
Capsules: 100 mg.

INDICATIONS AND DOSAGES
▸ **Gaucher's disease**
PO
Adults, Elderly. One 100-mg capsule 3 times a day at regular intervals.

▸ **Dosage in renal impairment**
For patients with creatinine clearance of 50-70 ml/min, dosage is reduced to 100 mg twice a day.
For patients with creatinine clearance of 30-49 ml/min dosage is 100 mg once a day.

CONTRAINDICATIONS
Women who are or may become pregnant

INTERACTIONS
Drug
Imiglucerase: May decrease the effects of imiglucerase.
Herbal
None known.
Food
None known.

DIAGNOSTIC TEST EFFECTS
None known.

SIDE EFFECTS
Expected (89%-65%)
Diarrhea, weight loss
Frequent (39%-11%)
Hand tremor, flatulence, headache, abdominal pain, nausea
Occasional (7%-4%)
Paresthesia, anorexia, dyspepsia, leg cramps, vomiting

SERIOUS REACTIONS
• Thrombocytopenia occurs in 7% of patients.
• Overdose produces dizziness and neutropenia.

PRECAUTIONS & CONSIDERATIONS
Caution is warranted with impaired fertility and renal function. Reliable contraceptive methods are necessary during miglustat treatment and for 3 months afterward. Notify the physician and plan to stop miglustat therapy before trying to conceive. Avoid high-carbohydrate foods during miglustat treatment if diarrhea occurs.
    Notify the physician of hand tremor. Adequate hydration should be maintained. Baseline neurologic evaluation should be performed, with follow-up evaluations every 6 months throughout treatment. Pattern of daily bowel activity and stool consistency and weight should be monitored.
Administration
Take miglustat without regard to food. Don't open, crush, or break capsules.

Milrinone
mill're-none
(Primacor)

CATEGORY AND SCHEDULE
Pregnancy Risk Category: C

CLASSIFICATION
Inotropes, vasodilators

MECHANISM OF ACTION
A cardiac inotropic agent that inhibits phosphodiesterase, which increases cyclic adenosine monophosphate and potentiates the delivery of calcium to myocardial contractile systems. *Therapeutic Effect:* Relaxes vascular muscle, causing vasodilation. Increases cardiac output; decreases pulmonary capillary wedge pressure and vascular resistance.

PHARMACOKINETICS

Route	Onset	Peak	Duration
IV	5-15 min	N/A	N/A

Protein binding: 70%. Primarily excreted unchanged in urine.
Half-life: 2.4 hr.

AVAILABILITY
Injection: 1 mg/ml, 10-ml single-dose vial, 20-mg single-dose vial, 50-ml single-dose vial, 5-ml sterile cartridge unit.
Injection (Premix): 200 mcg/ml.

INDICATIONS AND DOSAGES
▸ **Short-term management of CHF**
IV
Adults. Initially, 50 mcg/kg over 10 min. Continue with maintenance infusion rate of 0.375-0.75 mcg/kg/min based on hemodynamic and clinical response. Total daily dosage: 0.59-1.13 mg/kg.
▸ **Dosage in renal impairment**
For patients with severe renal impairment, reduce dosage to 0.2-0.43 mcg/kg/min.

CONTRAINDICATIONS
None known.

INTERACTIONS
Drug
Other cardiac glycosides:
Produces additive inotropic effects.
Herbal
None known.
Food
None known.

DIAGNOSTIC TEST EFFECTS
None known.

📖 IV INCOMPATIBILITIES
Furosemide (Lasix)
🜄 **IV Compatibilities**
Calcium gluconate, digoxin (Lanoxin), diltiazem (Cardizem), dobutamine (Dobutrex), dopamine (Intropin), heparin, lidocaine, magnesium, midazolam (Versed), nitroglycerin, potassium, propofol (Diprivan)

SIDE EFFECTS
Occasional (3%-1%)
Headache, hypotension
Rare (less than 1%)
Angina, chest pain

SERIOUS REACTIONS
• Supraventricular and ventricular arrhythmias (12%), nonsustained ventricular tachycardia (2%), and sustained ventricular tachycardia (1%) may occur.

PRECAUTIONS & CONSIDERATIONS
Caution is warranted with atrial fibrillation or flutter, history of ventricular arrhythmias, impaired renal function, and severe obstructive aortic or pulmonic valvular disease. It is unknown if milrinone crosses the placenta or is distributed in breast milk. The safety and efficacy of milrinone have not been established in children. In the elderly, age-related renal impairment may require dosage adjustment.

Notify the physician if palpitations or chest pain occurs. Cardiac output, heart rate, B/P, renal function, and serum potassium levels should be assessed before beginning treatment and during IV therapy. Breath sounds for crackles and rhonchi and skin for edema should also be assessed.
Storage
Store at room temperature.
Administration
For IV infusion, dilute 20-mg (20-ml) vial with 80 or 180 ml diluent (0.9% NaCl, D_5W) or 10-mg (10-ml) vial with 40 or 90 ml diluent to provide concentration of 200 or 100 mcg/ml, respectively. Maximum concentration: 100 mg/250 ml. For a loading dose IV injection, administer milrinone undiluted slowly over 10 minutes. Monitor for arrhythmias and hypotension during IV therapy. If one or both of these conditions

M

occur, reduce or temporarily discontinue infusion until condition stabilizes.

Minocycline
mi-noe-sye'kleen
(Akamin [AUS], Dynacin, Minocin, Minomycin [AUS], Myrac, Novo Minocycline [CAN])
Do not confuse Dynacin with Dynabac or Minocin with Mithracin or niacin.

CATEGORY AND SCHEDULE
Pregnancy Risk Category: D

CLASSIFICATION
Antibiotics, tetracyclines

MECHANISM OF ACTION
A tetracycline antibiotic that inhibits bacterial protein synthesis by binding to ribosomes. *Therapeutic Effects:* Bacteriostatic.

AVAILABILITY
Capsules (Dynacin, Minocin): 50 mg, 75 mg, 100 mg.
Capsules, pellet-filled (Minocin): 50 mg, 100 mg.
Tablets (Minocin, Myrac): 50 mg, 75 mg, 100 mg.
Powder for Injection (Minocin, Myrac): 100 mg.

INDICATIONS AND DOSAGES
▶ **Mild, moderate, or severe prostate, urinary tract, and CNS infections (excluding meningitis); uncomplicated gonorrhea; inflammatory acne; brucellosis; skin granulomas; cholera; trachoma; nocardiasis; yaws; and syphilis when penicillins are contraindicated**
PO
Adults, Elderly. Initially, 100-200 mg, then 100 mg q12hr or 50 mg q6hr.
IV
Adults, Elderly. Initially, 200 mg, then 100 mg q12hr up to 400 mg/day.
PO, IV
Children older than 8 yr. Initially, 4 mg/kg, then 2 mg/kg q12hr.

OFF-LABEL USES
Treatment of atypical mycobacterial infections, rheumatoid arthritis, scleroderma

CONTRAINDICATIONS
Children younger than 8 years, hypersensitivity to tetracyclines, last half of pregnancy

INTERACTIONS
Drug
Carbamazepine, phenytoin: May decrease minocycline blood concentration.
Cholestyramine, colestipol: May decrease minocycline absorption.
Oral contraceptives: May decrease the effects of oral contraceptives.
Herbal
St. John's wort: May increase the risk of photosensitivity.
Food
None known.

DIAGNOSTIC TEST EFFECTS
May increase serum alkaline phosphatase, amylase, bilirubin, AST (SGOT), and ALT (SGPT) levels.

▧ IV INCOMPATIBILITIES
Piperacillin and tazobactam (Zosyn)
▧ IV Compatibilities
Heparin, magnesium, potassium

SIDE EFFECTS
Frequent
Dizziness, lightheadedness, diarrhea, nausea, vomiting, abdominal cramps, possibly severe photosensitivity, drowsiness, vertigo
Occasional
Altered pigmentation of skin or mucous membranes, rectal or genital pruritus, stomatitis

SERIOUS REACTIONS
• Superinfection (especially fungal), anaphylaxis, and benign intracranial hypertension may occur.
• Bulging fontanelles occur rarely in infants.

PRECAUTIONS & CONSIDERATIONS
Caution is warranted with renal impairment and in those who can't avoid sun or ultraviolet exposure because such exposure may produce a severe photosensitivity reaction.

History of allergies, especially to tetracyclines or sulfites, should be determined before drug therapy. Dizziness, drowsiness, and vertigo may occur while taking minocycline. Avoid tasks that require mental alertness or motor skills until response to the drug is established. Pattern of daily bowel activity, stool consistency, food intake and tolerance, renal function, skin for rash should be assessed. Be alert for signs and symptoms of superinfection, such as anal or genital pruritus, diarrhea, and ulceration or changes of the oral mucosa or tongue. B/P and LOC should be monitored because of the potential for increased intracranial pressure.
Storage
Store the oral drug at room temperature. The IV solution may be stored for up to 24 hours at room temperature.

Discard the solution if a precipitate forms.
Administration
Take capsules and tablets with a full glass of water. Space drug doses evenly around the clock.

For intermittent IV (piggyback) infusion, reconstitute each 100-mg vial with 5 to 10 ml of sterile water for injection to provide a concentration of 20 or 10 mg/ml, respectively. Further dilute with 500 to 1000 ml D_5W or 0.9% NaCl. Administer the piggyback IV infusion immediately after reconstitution. Infuse it over 6 hours.

Minoxidil
min-nox′i-dill
(Apo-Gain [CAN], Loniten, Milnox [CAN], Regaine [AUS], Rogaine, Rogaine Extra Strength)
Do not confuse Loniten with Lotensin.

CATEGORY AND SCHEDULE
Pregnancy Risk Category: C
OTC (topical solution)

CLASSIFICATION
Vasodilators

MECHANISM OF ACTION
An antihypertensive and hair growth stimulant that has direct action on vascular smooth muscle, producing vasodilation of arterioles. *Therapeutic Effect:* Decreases peripheral vascular resistance and B/P; increases cutaneous blood flow; stimulates hair follicle epithelium and hair follicle growth.

PHARMACOKINETICS

Route	Onset	Peak	Duration
PO	0.5 hr	2-8 hr	2-5 days

Well absorbed from the GI tract; minimal absorption after topical application. Protein binding: None. Widely distributed. Metabolized in the liver to active metabolite. Primarily excreted in urine. Removed by hemodialysis. **Half-life:** 4.2 hr.

AVAILABILITY

Tablets (Loniten): 2.5 mg, 10 mg.
Topical Solution (Rogaine): 2% (20 mg/ml).
Topical Solution (Rogaine ExtraStrength): 5% (50 mg/ml).

INDICATIONS AND DOSAGES

▶ **Severe symptomatic hypertension, hypertension associated with organ damage, hypertension that has failed to respond to maximal therapeutic dosages of a diuretic or two other antihypertensives**
PO
Adults. Initially, 5 mg/day. Increase with at least 3-day intervals to 10 mg, then 20 mg, then up to 40 mg/day in 1-2 doses.
Elderly. Initially, 2.5 mg/day. May increase gradually. Maintenance: 10-40 mg/day. Maximum: 100 mg/day.
Children. Initially, 0.1-0.2 mg/kg (5 mg maximum) daily. Gradually increase at minimum 3-day intervals. Maintenance: 0.25-1 mg/kg/day in 1-2 doses. Maximum: 50 mg/day.
▶ **Hair regrowth**
TOPICAL
Adults. 1 ml to affected areas of scalp 2 times a day. Total daily dose not to exceed 2 ml.

CONTRAINDICATIONS

Pheochromocytoma

INTERACTIONS

Drug
Parenteral antihypertensives: May increase hypotensive effect.
NSAIDs: May decrease the hypotensive effects of minoxidil.
Herbal
None known.
Food
None known.

DIAGNOSTIC TEST EFFECTS

May increase plasma renin activity and BUN, serum alkaline phosphatase, serum creatinine, and serum sodium levels. May decrease blood Hgb and Hct levels and erythrocyte count.

SIDE EFFECTS

Frequent
PO: Edema with concurrent weight gain, hypertrichosis (elongation, thickening, increased pigmentation of fine body hair; develops in 80% of patients within 3-6 weeks after beginning therapy)
Occasional
PO: T-wave changes (usually revert to pretreatment state with continued therapy or drug withdrawal)
Topical: Pruritus, rash, dry or flaking skin, erythema
Rare
PO: Breast tenderness, headache, photosensitivity reaction
Topical: Allergic reaction, alopecia, burning sensation at scalp, soreness at hair root, headache, visual disturbances

SERIOUS REACTIONS

• Tachycardia and angina pectoris may occur because of increased oxygen demands associated with increased heart rate and cardiac output.
• Fluid and electrolyte imbalance and CHF may occur, especially if a

diuretic is not given concurrently with minoxidil.

• Too rapid reduction in B/P may result in syncope, CVA, MI, and ocular or vestibular ischemia.

• Pericardial effusion and tamponade may be seen in patients with impaired renal function who are not on dialysis.

PRECAUTIONS & CONSIDERATIONS

Caution is warranted with chronic CHF, coronary artery disease, recent MI (within 1 month), and severe renal impairment. Minoxidil crosses the placenta and is distributed in breast milk. No age-related precautions have been noted in children. The elderly are more sensitive to the drug's hypotensive effects. In the elderly, age-related renal impairment may require dosage adjustment. Exposure to sunlight and artificial light sources should be avoided.

B/P should be assessed on both arms and take the patient's pulse for 1 full minute immediately before giving the medication. If pulse rate increases 20 beats/minute or more over baseline, or systolic or diastolic B/P decreases more than 20 mm Hg, withhold minoxidil and contact the physician. Weight and electrolytes should also be monitored during therapy.

Administration

Take oral minoxidil without regard to food. Can take with food if GI upset occurs. Crush tablets if necessary. Maximum B/P response occurs 3 to 7 days after initiation of minoxidil therapy and reversible growth of fine body hair may begin 3 to 6 weeks after the start of treatment. For topical use, shampoo and dry hair before applying medication. Wash hands immediately after application. Do not use a hair dryer

to dry the hair after application (reduces effectiveness). Treatment must continue on a permanent basis and any cessation of treatment will reverse new hair growth.

Mirtazapine
mir-taz′a-peen
(Avanza [AUS], Remeron, Remeron Soltab)
Do not confuse Remeron with Premarin.

CATEGORY AND SCHEDULE
Pregnancy Risk Category: C

CLASSIFICATION
Antidepressants, tetracyclic

MECHANISM OF ACTION
A tetracyclic compound that acts as an antagonist at presynaptic alpha$_2$-adrenergic receptors, increasing both norepinephrine and serotonin neurotransmission. Has low anticholinergic activity. *Therapeutic Effect:* Relieves depression and produces sedative effects.

PHARMACOKINETICS
Rapidly and completely absorbed after PO administration; absorption not affected by food. Protein binding: 85%. Metabolized in the liver. Primarily excreted in urine. Unknown if removed by hemodialysis. **Half-life:** 20-40 hr (longer in males [37 hr] than females [26 hr]).

AVAILABILITY
Tablets: 7.5 mg, 15 mg, 30 mg, 45 mg.
Tablets (Disintegrating): 15 mg, 30 mg, 45 mg.

INDICATIONS AND DOSAGES
▸ **Depression**
PO
Adults. Initially, 15 mg at bedtime.
May increase by 15 mg/day q1-2wk.
Maximum: 45 mg/day.
Elderly. Initially, 7.5 mg at bedtime.
May increase by 7.5-15 mg/day
q1-2wk. Maximum: 45 mg/day.

CONTRAINDICATIONS
Use within 14 days of MAOIs

INTERACTIONS
Drug
Alcohol, diazepam: May increase
impairment of cognition and motor
skills.
MAOIs: May increase the risk of
neuroleptic malignant syndrome,
hypertensive crisis, and severe
seizures.
Herbal
None known.
Food
None known.

DIAGNOSTIC TEST EFFECTS
May increase serum cholesterol,
triglyceride, AST (SGOT), and ALT
(SGPT) levels.

SIDE EFFECTS
Frequent
Somnolence (54%), dry mouth (25%),
increased appetite (17%), constipation (13%), weight gain (12%)
Occasional
Asthenia (8%), dizziness (7%),
flu-like symptoms (5%), abnormal
dreams (4%)
Rare
Abdominal discomfort, vasodilation,
paresthesia, acne, dry skin, thirst,
arthralgia

SERIOUS REACTIONS
• Mirtazapine poses a higher risk of
seizures than tricyclic antidepressants,
especially in those with no previous
history of seizures.
• Overdose may produce cardiovascular effects, such as severe
orthostatic hypotension, dizziness,
tachycardia, palpitations, and
arrhythmias.
• Abrupt discontinuation after
prolonged therapy may produce
headache, malaise, nausea, vomiting,
and vivid dreams.
• Agranulocytosis occurs rarely.

PRECAUTIONS & CONSIDERATIONS
Caution is warranted with cardiovascular disorders, GI disorders, angle-
closure glaucoma, benign prostatic
hyperplasia, hepatic or renal impairment, and urine retention. It is
unknown if mirtazapine is distributed in breast milk. The safety and
efficacy of this drug have not been
established in children. In the
elderly, age-related renal impairment
may require cautious use.
Drowsiness and dizziness may
occur, so avoid alcohol and tasks that
require mental alertness or motor
skills. CBC, serum alkaline phosphatase, bilirubin, AST (SGOT), and
ALT (SGPT) levels should be
assessed before and periodically
during therapy to assess hepatic and
renal function in patients on long-
term therapy. EKG should also be
performed to assess for arrhythmias.
Administration
! Make sure at least 14 days elapse
between the use of MAOIs and
mirtazapine.
Take mirtazapine at bedtime without regard to food. Scored tablets
may be crushed or broken if needed.

Misoprostol
mis-oh-pros-toll
(Cytotec)
Do not confuse with Cytomel.

CATEGORY AND SCHEDULE
Pregnancy Risk Category: X

CLASSIFICATION
Abortifacients, gastrointestinals, oxazolidinediones, oxytocics, prostaglandins, stimulants, uterine

MECHANISM OF ACTION
A prostaglandin that inhibits basal, nocturnal gastric acid secretion via direct action on parietal cells. *Therapeutic Effect:* Increases production of protective gastric mucus.

PHARMACOKINETICS
Rapidly absorbed from gastrointestinal (GI) tract. Rapidly converted to active metabolite. Primarily excreted in urine. **Half-life:** 20-40 min.

AVAILABILITY
Tablets: 100 mcg, 200 mcg (Cytotec).

INDICATIONS AND DOSAGES
▶ **Prevention of NSAID-induced gastric ulcer**
PO
Adults. 200 mcg 4 times/day with food (last dose at bedtime). Continue for duration of NSAID therapy. May reduce dosage to 100 mcg if 200 mcg dose is not tolerable.
Elderly: 100-200 mcg 4 times/day with food.

OFF-LABEL USES
Treatment of duodenal ulcer

CONTRAINDICATIONS
Pregnancy (produces uterine contractions), hypersensitivity to misoprostol or any component of the formulation

INTERACTIONS
Drug
Antacids: May decrease misoprostol effectiveness.
Phenylbutazone: May increase neurosensory effects (headache, dizziness, ataxia).
Herbal
None known.
Food
None known.

DIAGNOSTIC TEST EFFECTS
None known.

SIDE EFFECTS
Frequent
Abdominal pain, diarrhea
Occasional
Nausea, flatulence, dyspepsia, headache
Rare
Vomiting, constipation

SERIOUS REACTIONS
• Overdosage may produce sedation, tremor, convulsions, dyspnea, palpitations, hypotension, and bradycardia.

PRECAUTIONS & CONSIDERATIONS
Caution is warranted with renal impairment and women of childbearing age. Be aware that misoprostol is contraindicated in pregnancy and will produce uterine contractions, uterine bleeding, and expulsion of products of conception. Be aware that it is unknown if misoprostol is distributed in breast milk. Safety and efficacy of the drug have not been established in children. There are no age-related precautions noted in the elderly.

Storage
Store at room temperature.
Administration
Take with or after meals to minimize diarrhea.

Mitotane
mye′toe-tane
(Lysodren)

CATEGORY AND SCHEDULE
Pregnancy Risk Category: C

CLASSIFICATION
Antineoplastics, miscellaneous

MECHANISM OF ACTION
A hormonal agent that inhibits activity of the adrenal cortex. *Therapeutic Effect:* Suppresses functional and nonfunctional adrenocortical neoplasms by direct cytoxic effect.

AVAILABILITY
Tablets: 500 mg.

INDICATIONS AND DOSAGES
▸ **Adrenocortical carcinomas**
PO
Adults, Elderly. Initially, 2-6 g/day in 3-4 divided doses. Increase by 2-4 g/day every 3-7 days up to 9-10 g/day. Range: 2-16 g/day.

OFF-LABEL USES
Treatment of Cushing's syndrome

CONTRAINDICATIONS
Known hypersensitivity to mitotane

INTERACTIONS
Drug
CNS depressants: May increase CNS depression.
Herbal
None known.

Food
None known.

DIAGNOSTIC TEST EFFECTS
May decrease levels of plasma cortisol, urinary 17-hydroxycorticosteroids, protein-bound iodine, and serum uric acid.

SIDE EFFECTS
Frequent (greater than 15%)
Anorexia, nausea, vomiting, diarrhea, lethargy, somnolence, adrenocortical insufficiency, dizziness, vertigo, maculopapular rash, hypouricemia
Occasional (less than 15%)
Blurred or double vision, retinopathy, hearing loss, excessive salivation, urine abnormalities (hematuria, cystitis, albuminuria), hypertension, orthostatic hypotension, flushing, wheezing, dyspnea, generalized aching, fever

SERIOUS REACTIONS
• Brain damage and functional impairment may occur with long-term, high-dosage therapy.

PRECAUTIONS & CONSIDERATIONS
Caution is warranted with impaired hepatic function. Vaccinations and coming in contact with crowds, people with known infections, and anyone who has recently received a live-virus vaccine should be avoided.
   Dizziness and drowsiness may occur; tasks that require mental alertness or motor skills should be avoided. Notify the physician if darkening of the skin, diarrhea, depression, loss of appetite, nausea and vomiting, or rash occurs. Adequate hydration should be maintained to prevent urinary side effects. The drug should be discontinued immediately after shock or trauma, as prescribed, because it produces adrenal suppression. Liver function

test results, serum uric acid levels, and urine tests, including urine chemistry and urinalysis should be assessed. Be aware that neurologic and behavioral assessments are performed periodically on those receiving prolonged therapy (over 2 years).

Administration

❗ Mitotane may be carcinogenic, mutagenic, or teratogenic; handle it with extreme care during administration.

Mitoxantrone
mye-toe-zan′trone
(Novantrone, Onkotrone [AUS])

CATEGORY AND SCHEDULE
Pregnancy Risk Category: D

CLASSIFICATION
Antineoplastics, miscellaneous

MECHANISM OF ACTION
An anthracenedione that inhibits B-cell, T-cell, and macrophage proliferation and DNA and RNA synthesis. Active throughout the entire cell cycle. *Therapeutic Effect:* Causes cell death.

PHARMACOKINETICS
Protein binding: 78%. Widely distributed. Metabolized in the liver. Primarily eliminated in feces by the biliary system. Not removed by hemodialysis. **Half-life:** 2.3-13 days.

AVAILABILITY
Injection: 2 mg/ml.

INDICATIONS AND DOSAGES
▸ **Leukemias**
IV
Adults, Elderly, Children 2 yr and older. 12 mg/m^2 once a day for 2-3 days.

Children younger than 2 yr. 0.4 mg/kg once a day for 3-5 days.
▸ **Acute leukemia in relapse**
IV
Adults, Elderly, Children older than 2 yr. 8-12 mg/m^2 once a day for 4-5 days.
▸ **Acute nonlymphocytic leukemia**
IV
Adults, Elderly, Children older than 2 yr. 10 mg/m^2 once a day for 3-5 days.
▸ **Solid tumors**
IV
Adults, Elderly. 12-14 mg/m^2 once q3-4wk.
Children. 18-20 mg/m^2 once q3-4wk.
▸ **Prostate cancer**
IV
Adults, Elderly. 12-14 mg/m^2 every 21 days.
▸ **Multiple sclerosis**
IV
Adults, Elderly. 12 mg/m^2/dose q3mo.

OFF-LABEL USES
Treatment of breast or hepatic carcinoma, non-Hodgkin's lymphoma

CONTRAINDICATIONS
Baseline left ventricular ejection fraction less than 50%, cumulative lifetime mitoxantrone dose of 140 mg/m^2 or more, multiple sclerosis with hepatic impairment

INTERACTIONS
Drug
Antigout medications: May decrease the effects of these drugs.
Bone marrow depressants: May increase myelosuppression.
Live-virus vaccines: May potentiate virus replication, increase vaccine side effects, and decrease the patient's antibody response to the vaccine.
Herbal
None known.

Food
None known.

DIAGNOSTIC TEST EFFECTS
May increase serum bilirubin and uric acid, AST (SGOT), and ALT (SGPT) levels.

▨ IV INCOMPATIBILITIES
Heparin, paclitaxel (Taxol), piperacillin and tazobactam (Zosyn)

▨ IV Compatibilities
Allopurinol (Aloprim), etoposide (VePesid), gemcitabine (Gemzar), granisetron (Kytril), ondansetron (Zofran), potassium chloride

SIDE EFFECTS
Frequent (greater than 10%)
Nausea, vomiting, diarrhea, cough, headache, stomatitis, abdominal discomfort, fever, alopecia
Occasional (9%-4%)
Ecchymosis, fungal infection, conjunctivitis, UTI
Rare (3%)
Arrhythmias

SERIOUS REACTIONS
• Myelosuppression may be severe, resulting in GI bleeding, hematologic toxicity, sepsis, and pneumonia.
• Renal failure, seizures, jaundice, and CHF may occur.

PRECAUTIONS & CONSIDERATIONS
Caution is warranted with impaired hepatobiliary function and preexisting myelosuppression and in those who have previously been treated with cardiotoxic medications. Mitoxantrone use should be avoided during pregnancy, especially during the first trimester, because it can cause fetal harm. Contraceptive measures should be used during mitoxantrone therapy. Breast-feeding also is not recommended. The safety and efficacy of mitoxantrone have not been established in children. No age-related precautions have been noted in the elderly. Vaccinations and coming in contact with crowds and people with known infections should be avoided.

Urine will appear blue or green and sclera may have a blue tint for 24 hours after mitoxantrone administration. Notify the physician if fever, signs of local infection, unusual bleeding from any site, blush skin, burning or erythema of oral mucosa, difficulty swallowing, oral ulcerations, and sore throat occurs. Adequate hydration should be maintained to protect against renal impairment. Hematologic status and liver, renal, and pulmonary function test.

Storage
Store vials at room temperature.
Administration
! Because mitoxantrone may be carcinogenic, mutagenic, or teratogenic, handle the drug with extreme care during preparation and administration. Dilute the drug before administration, and administer it by IV injection or infusion.

Dilute with at least 50 ml D_5W or 0.9% NaCl. Do not administer by subcutaneous, IM, intrathecal, or intra-arterial injection. Do not give IV push over less than 3 minutes. Give IV bolus over at least 3 minutes or intermittent IV infusion over 15 to 60 minutes. Administer continuous IV infusion of 0.02 to 0.5 mg/ml in D_5W or 0.9% NaCl.

Modafinil
mode-ah-feen′awl
(Alertec [CAN], Provigil)

CATEGORY AND SCHEDULE
Pregnancy Risk Category: C

CLASSIFICATION
Analeptics, stimulants, central nervous system

MECHANISM OF ACTION
An alpha$_1$-agonist that may bind to dopamine reuptake carrier sites, increasing alpha activity and decreasing delta, theta, and beta brain wave activity. *Therapeutic Effect:* Reduces the number of sleep episodes and total daytime sleep.

PHARMACOKINETICS
Well absorbed. Protein binding: 60%. Widely distributed. Metabolized in the liver. Excreted by the kidneys. Unknown if removed by hemodialysis. **Half-life:** 8-10 hr.

AVAILABILITY
Tablets: 100 mg, 200 mg.

INDICATIONS AND DOSAGES
▸ **Narcolepsy, other sleep disorders**
PO
Adults, Elderly. 200-400 mg/day.

OFF-LABEL USES
Treatment of depression

CONTRAINDICATIONS
None known.

INTERACTIONS
Drug
Cyclosporine, oral contraceptives, theophylline: May decrease plasma concentrations of these drugs.

Diazepam, phenytoin, propranolol, tricyclic antidepressants, warfarin: May increase plasma concentrations of these drugs.
Other CNS stimulants: May increase CNS stimulation.
Herbal
None known.
Food
None known.

DIAGNOSTIC TEST EFFECTS
None known.

SIDE EFFECTS
Frequent
Anxiety, insomnia, nausea, nervousness
Occasional
Anorexia, diarrhea, dizziness, dry mouth or skin, muscle stiffness, polydipsia, rhinitis, paraesthesia, tremor, headache, vomiting

SERIOUS REACTIONS
• Agitation, excitation, hypertension, and insomnia may occur.

PRECAUTIONS & CONSIDERATIONS
Caution is warranted with hepatic impairment or a history of clinically significant mitral valve prolapse, left ventricular hypertrophy, and seizures. Nonhormonal contraceptive methods should be used during modafinil therapy and 1 month afterward because modafinil decreases the effectiveness of hormonal contraceptives. It is unknown if modafinil is excreted in breast milk. Use caution when giving modafinil to pregnant women. The safety and efficacy of this drug have not been established in children younger than 16 years. Age-related hepatic or renal impairment may require decreased dosage in the elderly.

Dizziness may occur, so tasks that require mental alertness and motor

M

skills should be avoided until response to the drug is established. Sleep pattern should be assessed throughout therapy. Should only be used in patients with a diagnosis of narcolepsy, OSAHS, or SWSD.

Administration

Take modafinil without regard to food.

Moexipril
moe-ex′a-prile
(Univasc)

CATEGORY AND SCHEDULE
Pregnancy Risk Category: C (D if used in second or third trimesters)

CLASSIFICATION
Angiotensin converting enzyme inhibitors

MECHANISM OF ACTION
An ACE inhibitor that suppresses the renin-angiotensin-aldosterone system and prevents conversion of angiotensin I to angiotensin II, a potent vasoconstrictor; may also inhibit angiotensin II at local vascular and renal sites. *Therapeutic Effect:* Reduces peripheral arterial resistance and lowers B/P.

PHARMACOKINETICS

Route	Onset	Peak	Duration
PO	1 hr	3-6 hr	24 hr

Incompletely absorbed from the GI tract. Food decreases drug absorption. Rapidly converted to active metabolite. Protein binding: 50%. Primarily recovered in feces, partially excreted in urine. Unknown if removed by dialysis. **Half-life:** 1 hr, metabolite 2-9 hr.

AVAILABILITY
Tablets: 7.5 mg, 15 mg.

INDICATIONS AND DOSAGES
▶ **Hypertension**
PO
Adults, Elderly. For patients not receiving diuretics, initial dose is 7.5 mg once a day 1 hr before meals. Adjust according to B/P effect. Maintenance: 7.5-30 mg a day in 1-2 divided doses 1 hr before meals.
▶ **Hypertension in patients with impaired renal function**
PO
Adults, Elderly. 3.75 mg once a day in patients with creatinine clearance of 40 ml/min. Maximum: May titrate up to 15 mg/day.

CONTRAINDICATIONS
History of angioedema from previous treatment with ACE inhibitors

INTERACTIONS
Drug
Alcohol, antihypertensives, diuretics: May increase the effects of moexipril.
Lithium: May increase lithium blood concentration and risk of lithium toxicity.
NSAIDs: May decrease the effects of moexipril.
Potassium-sparing diuretics, potassium supplements: May cause hyperkalemia.
Herbal
None known.
Food
None known.

DIAGNOSTIC TEST EFFECTS
May increase BUN, serum alkaline phosphatase, serum bilirubin, serum creatinine, serum potassium,

AST (SGOT), and ALT (SGPT) levels. May decrease serum sodium levels. May cause positive serum antinuclear antibody titer.

SIDE EFFECTS
Occasional
Cough, headache (6%); dizziness (4%); fatigue (3%)
Rare
Flushing, rash, myalgia, nausea, vomiting

SERIOUS REACTIONS
• Excessive hypotension (first-dose syncope) may occur in patients with CHF and in those who are severely salt or volume depleted.
• Angioedema (swelling of face and lips) and hyperkalemia occur rarely.
• Agranulocytosis and neutropenia may be noted in those with collagen vascular disease, including scleroderma and systemic lupus erythematosus, and impaired renal function.
• Nephrotic syndrome may be noted in those with history of renal disease.

PRECAUTIONS & CONSIDERATIONS
Caution is warranted with angina, aortic stenosis, cerebrovascular disease, cerebrovascular and coronary insufficiency, hypovolemia, ischemic heart disease, renal impairment, severe CHF, sodium depletion, and those on dialysis and/or receiving diuretics. Moexipril crosses the placenta and it is unknown if it is distributed in breast milk. Moexipril has caused fetal or neonatal morbidity or mortality. Safety and efficacy of moexipril have not been established in children. In the elderly, age-related renal impairment may require cautious use of moexipril.

Dizziness may occur. Notify the physician if chest pain, cough, difficulty breathing, fever, sore throat, or swelling of the eyes, face, feet, hands, lips, or tongue occurs. B/P should be obtained immediately before giving each moexipril dose, in addition to regular monitoring. Be alert to fluctuations in B/P. If an excessive reduction in B/P occurs, place the person in the supine position with legs elevated. CBC and blood chemistry should be obtained before beginning moexipril therapy, then every 2 weeks for the next 3 months, and periodically thereafter in patients with autoimmune disease, or renal impairment, and in those who are taking drugs that affect immune response or leukocyte count. BUN, serum creatinine, serum potassium, renal function, and white blood cell count (WBC) should also be monitored. Lungs should be auscultated for rales. Heart rate for irregularities should be assessed.

Administration
! To reduce the risk of hypotension in patients receiving concurrent diuretic therapy, expect to discontinue the diuretic 2 to 3 days before beginning moexipril therapy. However, if the B/P is not controlled, resume diuretic therapy. If diuretics can't be discontinued, administer an initial moexipril dose of 3.75 mg.
! To reduce the risk of hypotension, expect to discontinue diuretics 2 to 3 days before initiating moexipril therapy. If B/P is not controlled, resume diuretic as ordered. If diuretic cannot be discontinued, prepare to give an initial dose of 3.75 mg moexipril.

Take moexipril 1 hour before meals. Crush tablets if necessary.

M

Molindone
moe-lin'done
(Moban)
Do not confuse with Mobic.

CATEGORY AND SCHEDULE
Pregnancy Risk Category: C

CLASSIFICATION
Antipsychotics

MECHANISM OF ACTION
An indole derivative of dihydroin-dole compounds that reduces sponta-neous locomotion and aggressiveness. *Therapeutic Effect:* Suppresses behavioral response in psychosis.

PHARMACOKINETICS
Rapidly absorbed from the gastrointestinal (GI) tract. Metabolized in liver. Excreted feces, and a small amount excreted via lungs as carbon dioxide. Not removed by dialysis. **Half-life:** unknown.

AVAILABILITY
Oral Solutions: 20 mg/ml (Moban).
Tablets: 5 mg, 10 mg, 25 mg, 50 mg, 100 mg (Moban).

INDICATIONS AND DOSAGES
▶ **Schizophrenia**
PO
Adults, Children 12 yr and older.
Initially, 50-75 mg/day, increased to 100 mg/day in 3-4 days.
Maintenance: 5-15 mg 3-4 times/day (mild psychosis). Maintenance: 10-25 mg 3-4 times/day (moderate psychosis). Maintenance: 225 mg/day maximum in divided doses (severe psychosis).
Elderly. Start at a lower dose.

CONTRAINDICATIONS
Severe central nervous system (CNS) depression, hypersensitivity to molindone or any component of the formulation

INTERACTIONS
Drug
Alcohol, CNS depressants: May increase CNS and respiratory depression of molindone.
Lithium: May decrease the absorp-tion of molindone and produce adverse neurologic effects.
Vitex: May decrease effectiveness of molindone.
Herbal
Betel nut: May increase extrapyramidal side effects of molindone.
Kava kava: May add to dopamine antagonist effects.
Food
None known.

DIAGNOSTIC TEST EFFECTS
None known.

▓ IV INCOMPATIBILITIES
None known.
▓ **IV Compatibilities**
None known.

SIDE EFFECTS
Frequent
Blurred vision, constipation, drowsi-ness, headache, extrapyramidal symptoms
Occasional
Mental depression
Rare
Skin rash, hot and dry skin, inability to sweat, muscle weakness, confu-sion, jaundice, convulsions

SERIOUS REACTIONS
• Neuroleptic malignant syndrome or tardive dyskinesia has been reported.

PRECAUTIONS & CONSIDERATIONS

Caution should be used in persons allergic to sulfites (oral concentrate contains sodium metabisulfite), have a history of breast cancer, brain tumor or intestinal obstruction, BPH, urinary retention, glaucoma, and liver impairment. Be aware that neuroleptic agents should not be reintroduced to persons with a history of neuroleptic malignant syndrome; however, in some cases neuroleptic agents have been reintroduced safely, without recurrence of this syndrome. It is unknown if molindone crosses the placenta or is distributed in breast milk. Safety and efficacy of molindone has not been established in children younger than 12 years old. There are no age-related precautions noted in the elderly.

If high fever, muscle stiffness, fast or irregular heartbeat, unexplained weakness or tiredness, muscle spasms, twitching, or uncontrolled tongue occurs, notify the physician. Avoid alcohol or other CNS depressants during molindone therapy.

Storage
Store at room temperature.
Administration and Handling
Take with or without food.

Mometasone
mo-met′a-sone
(Allermax Aqueous [AUS],
Elocon Cream [AUS], Elocon
Ointment [AUS], Nasonex,
Nasonex Nasal Spray [AUS],
Novasone Cream [AUS],
Novasone Lotion [AUS],
Novasone Ointment [AUS])

CATEGORY AND SCHEDULE
Pregnancy Risk Category: C

CLASSIFICATION
Corticosteroids, inhalation, topical, dermatologics

MECHANISM OF ACTION
An adrenocorticosteroid that inhibits the release of inflammatory cells into nasal tissue, preventing early activation of the allergic reaction. *Therapeutic Effect:* Decreases response to seasonal and perennial rhinitis.

PHARMACOKINETICS
Undetectable in plasma. Protein binding: 98%-99%. The swallowed portion undergoes extensive metabolism. Excreted primarily through bile and, to a lesser extent, urine.

AVAILABILITY
Nasal Spray: 50 mcg/spray.

INDICATIONS AND DOSAGES
▸ **Allergic rhinitis**
Nasal spray
Adults, Elderly, Children 12 yr and older. 2 sprays in each nostril once a day.
Children 2-11 yr. 1 spray in each nostril once a day.

CONTRAINDICATIONS
Hypersensitivity to any corticosteroid, persistently positive sputum cultures for *Candida albicans*, systemic fungal infections, untreated localized infection involving nasal mucosa.

INTERACTIONS
Drug
None known.
Herbal
None known.
Food
None known.

DIAGNOSTIC TEST EFFECTS
None known.

SIDE EFFECTS
Occasional
Nasal irritation, stinging
Rare
Nasal or pharyngeal candidiasis

SERIOUS REACTIONS
• An acute hypersensitivity reaction, including urticaria, angioedema, and severe bronchospasm, occurs rarely.
• Transfer from systemic to local steroid therapy may unmask previously suppressed bronchial asthma condition.

PRECAUTIONS & CONSIDERATIONS
Caution is warranted with adrenal insufficiency, cirrhosis, glaucoma, hypothyroidism, osteoporosis, tuberculosis, and untreated infection. It is unknown if mometasone crosses the placenta or is distributed in breast milk. In children, prolonged treatment and high dosages may decrease cortisol secretion and short-term growth rate. No age-related precautions have been noted in the elderly.

Pulse rate and quality, ABG levels, and respiratory rate, depth, rhythm and type should be monitored. Symptoms should start to improve within 2 days of the first dose but the drug's maximum benefit may take up to 2 weeks to appear. Notify the physician of nasal irritation or if symptoms, such as sneezing, fail to improve.
Administration
For inhalation, first shake the container well. Exhale completely and place the mouthpiece between the lips. Inhale and hold breath for as long as possible before exhaling. Allow 1 minute between inhalations to promote deeper bronchial penetration. Rinse mouth with water immediately after inhalation to prevent mouth and throat dryness and oral candidiasis.

Clear the nasal passages before using mometasone. May need to use a topical nasal decongestant 5 to 15 minutes before using mometasone. Tilt head slightly forward. Insert spray tip up into the nostril, pointing toward the inflamed nasal turbinates, away from nasal septum. Spray the drug into the nostril while holding the other nostril closed, and at the same time inhale through the nose.

Monobenzone
mon-oh-benz-one
(Benoquin)

CATEGORY AND SCHEDULE
Pregnancy Risk Category: C

CLASSIFICATION
Dermatologics

MECHANISM OF ACTION
The mechanism of action is not fully understood. Monobenzone may be converted to hydroquinone, which

inhibits the enzymatic oxidation of tyrosine to DOPA; it may have a direct action on tyrosinase; or, it may act as an anti-oxidant to prevent SH-group oxidation so that more SH groups are available to inhibit tyrosinase. *Therapeutic Effect:* Depigmentation in extensive vitiligo.

PHARMACOKINETICS
Not fully understood. Initial response occurs in 1-4 months.

AVAILABILITY
Cream: 20% (Benoquin).

INDICATIONS AND DOSAGES
▸ **Vitiligo**
TOPICAL
Adults, Elderly. Apply 2-3 times/day to affected area.

CONTRAINDICATIONS
History of hypersensitivity to monobenzone or any of its components.

INTERACTIONS
Drug
None known.
Herbal
None known.
Food
None known.

DIAGNOSTIC TEST EFFECTS
None known.

SIDE EFFECTS
Occasional
Irritation, burning sensation, dermatitis

SERIOUS REACTIONS
• None known.

PRECAUTIONS & CONSIDERATIONS
Caution should be used with hyperpigmentation due to

photosensitization. It is unknown if monobenzone is excreted in breast milk. Safety and efficacy of monobenzone have not been established in children. There are no age-related precautions noted in elderly. Sunlight should be avoided. If exposure cannot be avoided, wear clothing that covers the skin.

Monobenzone is a potent dipigmenting agent, not a mild cosmetic bleach. Irritation or burning should be reported.

Administration
Monobenzone is for external use only. Depigmentation is usually observed after 1-4 months of therapy. Treatment should be discontinued if satisfactory results have not been obtained within four months. Apply and rub gently into the pigmented area.

M

Montelukast
mon-te'loo-kast
(Singulair)

CATEGORY AND SCHEDULE
Pregnancy Risk Category: B

CLASSIFICATION
Leukotriene antagonists/ inhibitors

MECHANISM OF ACTION
An antiasthmatic that binds to cysteinyl leukotriene receptors, inhibiting the effects of leukotrienes on bronchial smooth muscle. *Therapeutic Effect:* Decreases bronchoconstriction, vascular permeability, mucosal edema, and mucus production.

PHARMACOKINETICS

Route	Onset	Peak	Duration
PO	N/A	N/A	24 hr
PO (chewable)	N/A	N/A	24 hr

Rapidly absorbed from the GI tract. Protein binding: 99%. Extensively metabolized in the liver. Excreted almost exclusively in feces. **Half-life:** 2.7-5.5 hr (slightly longer in the elderly).

AVAILABILITY

Oral Granules: 4 mg.
Tablets: 10 mg.
Tablets (Chewable): 4 mg, 5 mg.

INDICATIONS AND DOSAGES

▸ **Bronchial asthma**
PO
Adults, Elderly, Adolescents older than 14 yr. One 10-mg tablet a day, taken in the evening.
Children 6-14 yr. One 5-mg chewable tablet a day, taken in the evening.
Children 1-5 yr. One 4-mg chewable tablet a day, taken in the evening.

CONTRAINDICATIONS

None known.

INTERACTIONS

Drug
Phenobarbital, rifampin: May decrease montelukast's duration of action.
Herbal
None known.
Food
None known.

DIAGNOSTIC TEST EFFECTS

May increase AST (SGOT) and ALT (SGPT) levels.

SIDE EFFECTS

Adults, adolescents older than 14 years

Frequent (18%)
Headache
Occasional (4%)
Influenza
Rare (3%-2%)
Abdominal pain, cough, dyspepsia, dizziness, fatigue, dental pain
Children 6-14 years
Rare (less than 2%)
Diarrhea, laryngitis, pharyngitis, nausea, otitis media, sinusitis, viral infection

SERIOUS REACTIONS

• None known.

PRECAUTIONS & CONSIDERATIONS

Caution is warranted with hepatic impairment and those who are tapering systemic corticosteroid dosage during montelukast therapy. Use montelukast during pregnancy only if necessary. It is unknown if montelukast is excreted in breast milk. No age-related precautions have been noted in children older than 6 years or the elderly. Parents of children with phenylketonuria should be informed that montelukast chewable tablets contain phenylalanine, a component of aspartame. Be aware montelukast is not intended to treat acute asthma attacks. Drink plenty of fluids to decrease the thickness of lung secretions. Avoid aspirin and NSAIDs while taking montelukast.

Pulse rate and quality as well as respiratory depth, rate, rhythm, and type should be monitored. Fingernails and lips should also be assessed for a blue or dusky color in light-skinned patients and a gray color in dark-skinned patients, which may be signs of hypoxemia.

Administration
Take montelukast in the evening without regard to food. Don't abruptly substitute montelukast for inhaled or

oral corticosteroids. Take montelukast as prescribed, even during symptom-free periods and exacerbations. Do not alter the dosage or abruptly discontinue other asthma medications.

Moricizine
mor-iss'i-zeen
(Ethmozine)

CATEGORY AND SCHEDULE
Pregnancy Risk Category: B

CLASSIFICATION
Antiarrhythmics, class IA

MECHANISM OF ACTION
An antiarrhythmic that prevents sodium current across myocardial cell membranes. Has potent local anesthetic activity and membrane stabilizing effects. Slows AV and His-Purkinje conduction and decreases action potential duration and effective refractory period. *Therapeutic Effect:* Suppresses ventricular arrhythmias.

AVAILABILITY
Tablets: 200 mg, 250 mg, 300 mg.

INDICATIONS AND DOSAGES
▸ **Arrhythmias**
PO
Adults, Elderly. 200-300 mg q8hr. May increase by 150 mg/day at no less than 3-day intervals.

OFF-LABEL USES
Atrial arrhythmias, complete and non-sustained ventricular arrhythmias, premature ventricular contractions (PVCs)

CONTRAINDICATIONS
Cardiogenic shock, pre-existing second- or third-degree AV block or right bundle-branch block without pacemaker

INTERACTIONS
Drug
Cimetidine: May increase blood concentration of moricizine.
Theophylline: May decrease blood concentrations of theophylline.
Herbal
None known.
Food
None known.

DIAGNOSTIC TEST EFFECTS
May cause EKG changes, such as prolonged PR and QT intervals.

SIDE EFFECTS
Frequent (15%-6%)
Dizziness, nausea, headache, fatigue, dyspnea
Occasional (5%-2%)
Nervousness, paresthesia, sleep disturbances, dyspepsia, vomiting, diarrhea

SERIOUS REACTIONS
• Moricizine may worsen existing arrhythmias or produce new ones.
• Jaundice with hepatitis occurs rarely.
• Overdosage produces vomiting, lethargy, syncope, hypotension, conduction disturbances, exacerbation of CHF, MI, and sinus arrest.

PRECAUTIONS & CONSIDERATIONS
Caution is warranted with CHF, electrolyte imbalance, impaired hepatic or renal function, and sick sinus syndrome.
    Dizziness, GI upset, headache, and nausea may occur. Notify the physician if chest pain or irregular heartbeat occurs. EKG for changes,

especially increase in PR and QRS intervals, should be monitored before and during therapy. Pulse rate, electrolyte levels, intake and output, and liver and renal function should also be assessed.

Administration

Moricizine may be taken without regard to food but give with food if GI upset occurs. Taking the drug 30 minutes after a meal decreases absorption and serum level.

Morphine

mor'feen

(Anamorph [AUS], Astramorph, Avinza, DepoDur, Duramorph, Infumorph, Kadian, Kapanol [AUS], M-Eslon, Morphine Mixtures [AUS], MS Contin, MSIR, MS Mono [AUS], Oramorph SR, RMS, Roxanol, Statex [CAN])

Do not confuse morphine with hydromorphone, or Roxanol with Roxicet.

CATEGORY AND SCHEDULE

Pregnancy Risk Category: C (D if used for prolonged periods or at high dosages at term)
Controlled Substance Schedule: II

CLASSIFICATION

Analgesics, narcotic

MECHANISM OF ACTION

An opioid agonist that binds with opioid receptors in the CNS. *Therapeutic Effect:* Alters the perception of and emotional response to pain; produces generalized CNS depression.

PHARMACOKINETICS

Route	Onset	Peak	Duration
Oral Solution	N/A	1 hr	3-5 hr
Tablets	N/A	1 hr	3-5 hr
Tablets (ER)	N/A	3-4 hr	8-12 hr
IV	Rapid	0.3 hr	3-5 hr
IM	5-30 min	0.5-1 hr	3-5 hr
Epidural	N/A	1 hr	12-20 hr
Subcutaneous	N/A	1.1-5 hr	3-5 hr
Rectal	N/A	0.5-1 hr	3-7 hr

Variably absorbed from the GI tract. Readily absorbed after IM or subcutaneous administration. Protein binding: 20%-35%. Widely distributed. Metabolized in the liver. Primarily excreted in urine. Removed by hemodialysis. **Half-life:** 2-3 hr. (increased in patients with hepatic disease).

AVAILABILITY

Capsules (Extended-Release [Kadian]): 20 mg, 30 mg, 50 mg, 60 mg, 100 mg.
Capsules (Extended-Release [Avinza]): 30 mg, 60 mg, 90 mg, 120 mg.
Solution for Injection: 0.5 mg/ml, 1 mg/ml, 2 mg/ml, 4 mg/ml, 5 mg/ml, 8 mg/ml, 10 mg/ml, 15 mg/ml, 25 mg/ml, 50 mg/ml.
Solution for Injection (Preservative-Free): 0.5 mg/ml, 1 mg/ml, 10 mg/ml, 25 mg/ml, 50 mg/ml.
Epidural and Intrathecal via Infusion Device (Infumorph): 10 mg/ml, 25 mg/ml.
Epidural, Intrathecal, IV Infusion (Astramorph, Duramorph): 0.5 mg/ml, 1 mg/ml, 4 mg/ml.
IV Infusion (via patient-controlled analgesia [PCA]): 1 mg/ml, 5 mg/ml.
Oral Solution (Roxanol): 10 mg/5 ml, 20 mg/5 ml, 20 mg/ml, 100 mg/5 mg.
Suppository (RMS): 5 mg, 10 mg, 20 mg, 30 mg.

Tablets (MSIR): 15 mg/30 mg.
Tablets (Extended-Release [MS Contin, Oramorph SR]): 15 mg, 30 mg, 60 mg, 100 mg, 200 mg.
Liposomal Injection (DepoDur): 10 mg/ml, 15 mg/1.5 ml, 20 mg/2 ml.

INDICATIONS AND DOSAGES
! Dosage should be titrated to desired effect.
▸ **Analgesia**
PO (PROMPT-RELEASE)
Adults, Elderly. 10-30 mg q3-4hr as needed.
Children. 0.15-0.3 mg/kg q3-4hr as needed.
! For the Kadian dosage information below, be aware that this drug is to be administered q12hr or once a day only.
! Be aware that pediatric dosages of extended-release preparations Kadian and Avinza have not been established.
! For the MSContin and Oramorph SR dosage information below, be aware that the daily dosage is divided and given q8hr or q12hr.
PO (EXTENDED-RELEASE [AVINZA])
Adults, Elderly. Dosage requirement should be established using prompt-release formulations and is based on total daily dose (one-half the dose is given q12hr or one-third the dose is given q8hr).
PO (EXTENDED-RELEASE [KADIAN])
Adults, Elderly. Dosage requirement should be established using prompt-release formulations and is based on total daily dose. Dose is given once a day or divided and given q12hr.
PO (EXTENDED-RELEASE [MSCONTIN, ORAMORPH SR]
Adults, Elderly. Dosage requirement should be established using prompt-release formulations and is based on total daily dose. Daily dose is divided and given q8hr or q12hr.

Children. 0.3-0.6 mg/kg/dose q12hr.
IM
Adults, Elderly. 5-10 mg q3-4hr as needed.
Children. 0.1 mg/kg q3-4hr as needed.
IV
Adults, Elderly. 2.5-5 mg q3-4hr as needed. Note: Repeated doses (e.g., 1-2 mg) may be given more frequently (e.g., every hour) if needed.
Children. 0.05-0.1 mg/kg q3-4hr as needed.
IV CONTINUOUS INFUSION
Adults, Elderly. 0.8-10 mg/hr. Range: Up to 80 mg/hr.
Children. 10-30 mcg/kg/hr.
EPIDURAL
Adults, Elderly. Initially, 1-6 mg bolus, infusion rate: 0.1-1 mg/hr. Maximum: 10 mg/24 hr.
INTRATHECAL
Adults, Elderly. One-tenth of the epidural dose: 0.2-1 mg/dose.
▸ **PCA**
IV
Adults, Elderly. Loading dose: 5-10 mg. Intermittent bolus: 0.5-3 mg. Lockout interval: 5-12 min. Continuous infusion: 1-10 mg/hr. 4-hr limit: 20-30 mg.

CONTRAINDICATIONS
Acute or severe asthma, GI obstruction, severe hepatic or renal impairment, severe respiratory depression, asthma, severe liver or renal impairment

INTERACTIONS
Drug
Alcohol, other CNS depressants: May increase CNS or respiratory depression and hypotension.
MAOIs: May produce a severe, sometimes fatal reaction; expect to administer one-quarter of usual morphine dose.

M

Herbal
None known.
Food
None known.

DIAGNOSTIC TEST EFFECTS
May increase serum amylase and lipase levels.

▨ IV INCOMPATIBILITIES
Amphotericin B complex (Abelcet, AmBisome, Amphotec), cefepime (Maxipime), doxorubicin liposomal (Doxil), thiopental

▨ IV Compatibilities
Amiodarone (Cordarone), bumetanide (Bumex), bupivacaine (Marcaine, Sensorcaine), diltiazem (Cardizem), dobutamine (Dobutrex), dopamine (Intropin), heparin, lidocaine, lorazepam (Ativan), magnesium, midazolam (Versed), milrinone (Primacor), nitroglycerin, potassium, propofol (Diprivan)

SIDE EFFECTS
Frequent
Sedation, decreased B/P (including orthostatic hypotension), diaphoresis, facial flushing, constipation, dizziness, somnolence, nausea, vomiting
Occasional
Allergic reaction (rash, pruritus), dyspnea, confusion, palpitations, tremors, urine retention, abdominal cramps, vision changes, dry mouth, headache, decreased appetite, pain or burning at injection site
Rare
Paralytic ileus

SERIOUS REACTIONS
• Overdose results in respiratory depression, skeletal muscle flaccidity, cold or clammy skin, cyanosis, and extreme somnolence progressing to seizures, stupor, and coma.
• The patient who uses morphine repeatedly may develop a tolerance

to the drug's analgesic effect and physical dependence.
• The drug may have a prolonged duration of action and cumulative effect in those with hepatic and renal impairment.

PRECAUTIONS & CONSIDERATIONS
Extreme caution should be used with COPD, cor pulmonale, head injury, hypoxia, hypercapnia, increased intracranial pressure, preexisting respiratory depression, and severe hypotension. Caution is also warranted with Addison's disease, alcoholism, biliary tract disease, CNS depression, hypothyroidism, pancreatitis, benign prostatic hyperplasia, seizure disorders, toxic psychosis, urethral stricture, and in the elderly and debilitated. Morphine crosses the placenta and is distributed in breast milk. Regular use of opioids during pregnancy may produce withdrawal symptoms in the neonate, such as diarrhea, excessive crying, fever, hyperactive reflexes, irritability, seizures, sneezing, tremors, vomiting, and yawning. Morphine may prolong labor if administered in the latent phase of the first stage of labor or before the cervix is dilated 4 to 5 cm. The neonate may develop respiratory depression if the mother receives morphine during labor. Children and the elderly are more prone to experience paradoxical excitement. Children younger than 2 years and the elderly are more susceptible to the drug's respiratory depressant effects. Age-related renal impairment may increase the risk of urine retention in the elderly.

Dizziness and drowsiness may occur, so change positions slowly and avoid alcohol, CNS depressants, and tasks that require mental alertness or motor skills until response to the drug is established. Pattern of daily bowel activity and clinical improvement should be monitored. Vital signs should be monitored for 5 to 10 minutes after IV administration and 15 to 30 minutes after IM or subcutaneous injection. Be alert for bradycardia and hypotension. The drug should be held and the physician should be notified if the respiratory rate is 12 breaths/minute or less in an adult or 20 breaths/minute or less in a child.

Storage
Store vials at room temperature.

Administration
! Expect to reduce morphine dosage for debilitated and elderly patients and those using CNS depressants concurrently. Titrate dosage to desired effect, as prescribed. Morphine's side effects are dependent on the dosage and route of administration. Ambulatory patients and those not in severe pain are more prone to experience dizziness, nausea, and vomiting than those in the supine position and those in severe pain.

For oral use, mix the liquid form with fruit juice to improve the taste. Don't crush, open, or break extended-release capsules. Kadian (extended-release capsules) may be mixed with applesauce just before administration.

Morphine may be given undiluted as IV push. For IV injection, 2.5 to 15 mg morphine may be diluted in 4 to 5 ml sterile water for injection. For continuous IV infusion, dilute to a concentration of 0.1 to 1 mg/ml in D_5W and administer through a controlled infusion device. Place the patient in the recumbent position before giving parenteral morphine. Always administer IV morphine very slowly because rapid IV administration increases the risk of a severe anaphylactic reaction, marked by apnea, cardiac arrest, and circulatory collapse.

For IM and subcutaneous, inject the drug slowly; rotate injection sites. Know that patients with circulatory impairment are at increased risk for overdose because of delayed absorption of repeated injections.

For rectal use, if the suppository is too soft, refrigerate it for 30 minutes or run cold water over the foil wrapper. Moisten the suppository with cold water before inserting it well into the rectum.

Moxifloxacin
moks-i-floks′a-sin
(Avelox, Avelox IV, Vigamox)
Do not confuse with Avonex.

CATEGORY AND SCHEDULE
Pregnancy Risk Category: C

CLASSIFICATION
Anti-infectives, ophthalmics, antibiotics, quinolones

MECHANISM OF ACTION
A fluoroquinolone that inhibits two enzymes, topoisomerase II and IV, in susceptible microorganisms. *Therapeutic Effect:* Interferes with bacterial DNA replication. Prevents or delays emergence of resistant organisms. Bactericidal.

PHARMACOKINETICS
Well absorbed from the gastrointestinal (GI) tract after PO administration. Protein binding: 50%. Widely distributed throughout body with tissue concentration often exceeding plasma concentration. Metabolized in liver. Primarily excreted in urine with a lesser amount in feces. **Half-life:** 10.7-13.3 hr.

AVAILABILITY
Tablets (Avelox): 400 mg.
Injection (Avelox IV): 400 mg.
Ophthalmic Solution (Vigamox):
0.5%.

INDICATIONS AND DOSAGES
▶ **Acute bacterial sinusitis,
community-acquired pneumonia**
IV/PO
Adults, Elderly. 400 mg q24hr for
10 days.
▶ **Acute bacterial exacerbation of
chronic bronchitis**
IV/PO
Adults, Elderly. 400 mg q24hr for
5 days.
▶ **Skin and skin-structure infection**
IV/PO
Adults, Elderly. 400 mg once a day
for 7 days.
▶ **Topical treatment of bacterial
conjunctivitis due to susceptible
strains of bacteria**
OPHTHALMIC
*Adults, Elderly, Children older than
1 yr.* 1 drop 3 times/day for 7 days.

CONTRAINDICATIONS
Hypersensitivity to quinolones

INTERACTIONS
Drug
**Antacids, didanosine chewable,
buffered tablets or pediatric
powder for oral solution, iron
preparations, sucralfate:** May
decrease moxifloxacin absorption.
Herbal
None known.
Food
None known.

DIAGNOSTIC TEST EFFECTS
None known.

▓ IV INCOMPATIBILITIES
Do not add or infuse other drugs
simultaneously through the same IV
line. Flush line before and after use
if same IV line is used with other
medications.

SIDE EFFECTS
Frequent (8%-6%)
Nausea, diarrhea
Occasional (3%-2%)
Dizziness, headache, abdominal
pain, vomiting
Ophthalmic (6%-1%): conjunctival
irritation, reduced visual acuity, dry
eye, keratitis, eye pain, ocular itching, swelling of tissue around cornea,
eye discharge, fever, cough, pharyngitis, rash, rhinitis
Rare (1%)
Change in sense of taste, dyspepsia
(heartburn, indigestion), photosensitivity

SERIOUS REACTIONS
• Pseudomembranous colitis as
evidenced by fever, severe abdominal
cramps or pain, and severe watery
diarrhea may occur.
• Superinfection manifested as anal
or genital pruritus, moderate to
severe diarrhea, and stomatitis may
occur.

PRECAUTIONS & CONSIDERATIONS
Caution is warranted with cerebral
arthrosclerosis, central nervous
system (CNS) disorders, liver or
renal impairment; seizures, those
with a prolonged QT interval, uncorrected hypokalemia, and those
receiving amiodarone, procainamide,
quinidine, and sotalol. Be aware that
moxifloxacin may be distributed in
breast milk and may produce teratogenic effects. Be aware that the
safety and efficacy of moxifloxacin
have not been established in children. There are no age-related
precautions noted in the elderly.
    Avoid exposure to sunlight and
ultraviolet light and wear sunscreen

and protective clothing if photosensitivity develops.

Abdominal pain, altered sense of taste, dyspepsia (heartburn, indigestion), headache, vomiting, and signs and symptoms of infections should be assessed. Pattern of daily bowel activity, stool consistency, and WBC count should be monitored. History of hypersensitivity to moxifloxacin and other quinolones should be determined before therapy.

Storage

Store at room temperature. Do not refrigerate.

Administration

Take oral moxifloxacin without regard to meals. Take 4 hours before or 8 hours after antacids, didanosine chewable, buffered tablets or pediatric powder for oral solution, iron preparations, multivitamins, or sucralfate. Take full course of therapy.

For ophthalmic use, tilt the head back and look up. With a gloved finger, gently pull the lower eyelid down until a pocket is formed. Hold the dropper above the pocket and, without touching the eyelid or conjunctival sac, place drops into the center of the pocket. Close the eye gently and apply gentle finger pressure to the lacrimal sac at the inner canthus. Remove excess solution around the eye with a tissue.

! Infuse IV over 60 minutes or more. IV formulation is available in ready-to-use containers. Give by IV infusion only. Avoid rapid or bolus IV infusion.

Mupirocin

mew-peer′oh-sin
(Bactroban)
Do not confuse with Bactrim or Bacitracin

CATEGORY AND SCHEDULE

Pregnancy Risk Category: B

CLASSIFICATION

Anti-infectives, topical, dermatologics

MECHANISM OF ACTION

An antibacterial agent that inhibits bacterial protein, RNA synthesis. Less effective on DNA synthesis. Nasal: Eradicates nasal colonization of MRSA. *Therapeutic Effect:* Prevents bacterial growth and replication. Bacteriostatic.

PHARMACOKINETICS

Metabolized in skin to inactive metabolite. Transported to skin surface; removed by normal skin desquamation.

AVAILABILITY

Ointment: 2% (Bactroban).
Nasal ointment: 2% (Bactroban).

INDICATIONS AND DOSAGES

▸ **Impetigo, infected traumatic skin lesions**

TOPICAL

Adults, Elderly, Children. Apply 3 times/day (may cover w/gauze).
Nasal colonization of resistant *Staphylococcus aureus*

INTRANASAL

Adults, Elderly, Children 12 yr and older. Apply 2 times/day for 5 days.

OFF-LABEL USES
Treatment of infected eczema, folliculitis, minor bacterial skin infections.

CONTRAINDICATIONS
Hypersensitivity to mupirocin or any component of the formulation

INTERACTIONS
Drug
None known.
Herbal
None known.
Food
None known.

DIAGNOSTIC TEST EFFECTS
None known.

⬚ IV INCOMPATIBILITIES
None known.
⬚ IV Compatibilities
None known.

SIDE EFFECTS
Frequent
Nasal: Headache, rhinitis, upper respiratory congestion, pharyngitis, altered taste
Occasional
Nasal: Burning, stinging, cough
Topical: Pain, burning, stinging, itching
Rare
Nasal: Pruritis, diarrhea, dry mouth, epistaxis, nausea, rash
Topical: Rash, nausea, dry skin, contact dermatitis

SERIOUS REACTIONS
• Superinfection may result in bacterial or fungal infections, especially with prolonged or repeated therapy.

PRECAUTIONS & CONSIDERATIONS
Caution should be used with impaired renal function. It is unknown if mupirocin crosses the placenta or is distributed in breast milk.

Temporarily discontinue nursing while using mupirocin. Safety and efficacy of nasal preparation have not been established in children less than 12 years old. There are no age-related precautions noted in children or the elderly. Neonates or persons with poor hygiene should be kept isolated.
Storage
Store at room temperature.
Administration and Handling
Gown and gloves are to be worn until 24 hours after therapy is effective. Disease is spread by direct contact with moist discharges. Apply small amount to affected areas. Cover affected areas with gauze dressing if desired.

Muromonab-CD3
mur-oo-mon'ab
(Orthoclone, OKT3)

CATEGORY AND SCHEDULE
Pregnancy Risk Category: C

CLASSIFICATION
Immunosuppressives, monoclonal antibodies, recombinant DNA Origin

MECHANISM OF ACTION
A monoclonal antibody derived from purified IgG_2 that reacts with a T-3 (CD3) antigen of human T-cell membranes, blocking the production and function of T cells, which play a major role in acute organ rejection. *Therapeutic Effect:* Reverses organ rejection.

AVAILABILITY
Injection: 1 mg/ml.

INDICATIONS AND DOSAGES
▸ **Treatment of acute renal allograft rejection**
IV
Adults, Elderly, Children 12 yr and older. 5 mg/day for 10-14 days, beginning as soon as acute renal rejection is diagnosed.
Children younger than 12 yr. 0.1 mg/kg/day for 10-14 days, beginning as soon as acute renal rejection is diagnosed.

CONTRAINDICATIONS
History of hypersensitivity to muromonab-CD3 or any murine-derived product, fluid overload (as evidenced by chest X-ray or weight gain of more than 3%) in the week before initial treatment

INTERACTIONS
Drug
Live-virus vaccines: May potentiate virus replication, increase the vaccine's side effects, and decrease the patient's response to the vaccine.
Other immunosuppressants: May increase the risk of infection or lymphoproliferative disorders.
Herbal
Echinacea: May decrease the effects of muromonab.
Food
None known.

DIAGNOSTIC TEST EFFECTS
None known.

▨ IV INCOMPATIBILITIES
Do not mix muromonab with any other medications.

SIDE EFFECTS
Frequent
Fever, chills, dyspnea, malaise (first-dose reaction occurring 30 min-6 hr after first dose reaction that diminishes after the 2nd day of treatment)

Occasional
Chest pain, nausea, vomiting, diarrhea, tremor

SERIOUS REACTIONS
• Symptoms of cytokine release syndrome, a common reaction, may range from mild flu-like symptoms to a life-threatening, shock-like reaction.
• Infection due to immunosuppression generally occurs within 45 days after initial treatment. Cytomegalovirus occurs in 19% of patients, and herpes simplex occurs in 27% of patients. A severe, life-threatening infection occurs in fewer than 5% of patients.
• Severe pulmonary edema occurs in fewer than 2% of patients.
• Fatal hypersensitivity reactions occur occasionally.

PRECAUTIONS & CONSIDERATIONS
Caution is warranted with impaired cardiac, hepatic, or renal function. Avoid receiving immunizations and coming in contact with crowds and people with known infections during muromonab therapy.

A chest X-ray should be obtained within 24 hours of beginning muromonab therapy to ensure that the lungs are free of fluid. Fluid overload should be checked before beginning muromonab treatment to decrease the risk of pulmonary edema. Immunologic test results (including plasma drug levels and quantitative T-lymphocyte surface phenotyping), liver and renal function test results, intake and output, pattern of daily bowel activity and stool consistency, and WBC count should be obtained before and during therapy.
Storage
Refrigerate ampoules. Don't use the drug if it has been left out of the refrigerator for longer than 4 hours.

Administration

Don't shake the ampoule before using. The solution may develop fine translucent particles, which won't affect potency. Draw the solution into the syringe through a 0.22 micron filter. Discard the filter; use a needle for IV administration. Administer by IV push over less than 1 minute. Give 1 mg/kg methylprednisolone 1-4 hours before and 100 mg hydrocortisone 30 minutes after the first dose of muromonab, as prescribed, to decrease the risk and severity of cytokine release syndrome. Expect a first-dose reaction, including chest tightness, chills, fever, diarrhea, nausea, vomiting, and wheezing.

Mycophenolate
my-co-fen'o-late
(CellCept)

CATEGORY AND SCHEDULE
Pregnancy Risk Category: C

CLASSIFICATION
Immunosuppressives

MECHANISM OF ACTION

An immunologic agent that suppresses the immunologically mediated inflammatory response by inhibiting inosine monophosphate dehydrogenase, an enzyme that deprives lymphocytes of nucleotides necessary for DNA and RNA synthesis, thus inhibiting the proliferation of T and B lymphocytes. *Therapeutic Effect:* Prevents transplant rejection.

PHARMACOKINETICS

Rapidly and extensively absorbed after PO administration (food decreases drug plasma concentration but doesn't affect absorption). Protein binding: 97%. Completely hydrolyzed to active metabolite mycophenolic acid. Primarily excreted in urine. Not removed by hemodialysis. **Half-life:** 17.9 hr.

AVAILABILITY

Capsules: 250 mg.
Oral Suspension: 200 mg/ml.
Tablets: 500 mg.
Injection: 500 mg.

INDICATIONS AND DOSAGES
▸ **Prevention of renal transplant rejection**
PO, IV
Adults, Elderly. 1 g twice a day.
▸ **Prevention of heart transplant rejection**
PO, IV
Adults, Elderly. 1.5 g twice a day.
▸ **Prevention of liver transplant rejection**
IV, PO
Adults, Elderly. 1.5 g twice a day.
Adults, Elderly. 1 g twice a day.
▸ **Usual pediatric dosage**
PO
Children. 600 mg/m^2/dose twice a day. Maximum: 2 g/dose.

OFF-LABEL USES

Treatment of liver transplantation rejection, mild heart transplant rejection, moderate to severe psoriasis

CONTRAINDICATIONS

Hypersensitivity to mycophenolic acid

INTERACTIONS
Drug
Acyclovir, ganciclovir: May increase plasma concentrations of both drugs in patients with renal impairment.

Antacids (aluminum and magnesium-containing), cholestyramine: May decrease the absorption of mycophenolate.

Live-virus vaccines: May potentiate virus replication, increase vaccine side effects, and decrease the patient's antibody response to the vaccine.

Other immunosuppressants: May increase the risk of infection or lymphomas.

Probenecid: May increase mycophenolate plasma concentration.

Herbal

Echinacea: May decrease the effects of mycophenolate.

Food

All foods: May decrease mycophenolate plasma concentration.

DIAGNOSTIC TEST EFFECTS

May increase serum cholesterol, alkaline phosphatase, creatinine, AST (SGOT), and ALT (SGPT) levels. May increase or decrease blood glucose as well as serum lipid, calcium, potassium, phosphate, and uric acid levels.

⚙ IV INCOMPATIBILITIES

Mycophenolate is compatible only with D_5W. Do not infuse it concurrently with other drugs or IV solutions.

SIDE EFFECTS

Frequent (37%-20%)

UTI, hypertension, peripheral edema, diarrhea, constipation, fever, headache, nausea

Occasional (18%-10%)

Dyspepsia; dyspnea; cough; hematuria; asthenia; vomiting; edema; tremors; abdominal, chest, or back pain; oral candidiasis; acne

Rare (9%-6%)

Insomnia, respiratory tract infection, rash, dizziness

SERIOUS REACTIONS

• Significant anemia, leukopenia, thrombocytopenia, neutropenia, and leukocytosis may occur, particularly in those undergoing renal transplant rejection.

• Sepsis and infection occur occasionally.

• GI tract hemorrhage occurs rarely.

• Patients receiving mycophenolate have an increased risk of developing neoplasms.

PRECAUTIONS & CONSIDERATIONS

Caution is warranted with active serious digestive disease, neutropenia, renal impairment, and in females of childbearing potential. Females (unless she has had a hysterectomy) should use effective contraception before, during, and for 6 weeks after discontinuing mycophenolate therapy, even if she has had a history of infertility. Two forms of contraception should be used concurrently unless she will remain abstinent. It is unknown if mycophenolate crosses the placenta or is distributed in breast milk. Females taking this drug should avoid breast-feeding. The safety and efficacy of mycophenolate have not been established in children. Age-related renal impairment may require a dosage adjustment in the elderly.

Notify the physician of abdominal pain, fever, sore throat, or unusual bleeding or bruising. A pregnancy test should be performed before therapy. CBC should be obtained weekly during the first month of therapy, twice monthly during the second and third months, then monthly for the rest of the first year. The dosage should be reduced or discontinue if a rapid fall in WBC count occurs.

Storage

Store the reconstituted suspension in the refrigerator or at room

M

temperature. It remains stable for 60 days after reconstitution. Store vials at room temperature.

Administration

Give oral mycophenolate on an empty stomach. Do not open or crush capsules. Avoid inhaling the powder in capsules and keep the powder away from skin and mucous membranes. If contact occurs, wash thoroughly with soap and water, and rinse the eyes profusely with plain water. The suspension can be administered orally or by nasogastric tube (minimum size: 8 French).

For IV use, reconstitute each 500-mg vial with 14 ml D_5W. Gently agitate the vial. For a 1-g dose, further dilute with 140 ml D_5W; for a 1.5-g dose, further dilute with 210 ml D_5W to provide a concentration of 6 mg/ml. Infuse the drug over at least 2 hours.

Nabumetone
na-byu'me-tone
(Apo-Nabumetone, Relafen)

CATEGORY AND SCHEDULE
Pregnancy Risk Category: C (D if used in third trimester or near delivery)

CLASSIFICATION
Analgesics, non-narcotic, nonsteroidal anti-inflammatory drugs

MECHANISM OF ACTION
An NSAID that produces analgesic and anti-inflammatory effects by inhibiting prostaglandin synthesis. *Therapeutic Effect:* Reduces the inflammatory response and intensity of pain.

PHARMACOKINETICS
Readily absorbed from the GI tract. Protein binding: 99%. Widely distributed. Metabolized in the liver to active metabolite. Primarily excreted in urine. Not removed by hemodialysis. **Half-life:** 22-30 hr.

AVAILABILITY
Tablets: 500 mg, 750 mg.

INDICATIONS AND DOSAGES
▸ **Acute or chronic rheumatoid arthritis and osteoarthritis**
PO
Adults, Elderly. Initially, 1000 mg as a single dose or in 2 divided doses. May increase up to 2000 mg/day as a single or in 2 divided doses.

CONTRAINDICATIONS
Active peptic ulcer disease, chronic inflammation of GI tract, GI bleeding or ulceration, history of hypersensitivity to aspirin or NSAIDs, history of significant renal impairment

INTERACTIONS
Drug
Antihypertensives, diuretics: May decrease the effects of these drugs.
Aspirin, other salicylates: May increase the risk of GI side effects such as bleeding.
Bone marrow depressants: May increase the risk of hematologic reactions.
Heparin, oral anticoagulants, thrombolytics: May increase the effects of these drugs.
Lithium: May increase the blood concentration and risk of toxicity of lithium.
Methotrexate: May increase the risk of methotrexate toxicity.
Probenecid: May increase the nabumetone blood concentration.
Herbal
Feverfew: May decrease the effects of feverfew.
Ginkgo biloba: May increase the risk of bleeding.
Food
None known.

DIAGNOSTIC TEST EFFECTS
May increase BUN level; urine protein levels; and serum LDH, alkaline phosphatase, creatinine, potassium, AST (SGOT), and ALT (SGPT) levels. May decrease serum uric acid level.

SIDE EFFECTS
Frequent (14%-12%)
Diarrhea, abdominal cramps or pain, dyspepsia
Occasional (9%-4%)
Nausea, constipation, flatulence, dizziness, headache
Rare (3%-1%)
Vomiting, stomatitis, confusion

N

SERIOUS REACTIONS

- Overdose may result in acute hypotension and tachycardia.
- Rare reactions with long-term use include peptic ulcer disease, GI bleeding, gastritis, nephrotoxicity (dysuria, cystitis, hematuria, proteinuria, nephrotic syndrome), severe hepatic reactions (cholestasis, jaundice), and severe hypersensitivity reactions (bronchospasm, angioedema).

PRECAUTIONS & CONSIDERATIONS

Caution is warranted with CHF, hypertension, hepatic or renal impairment, and in those using anticoagulants concurrently. Nabumetone is distributed in low concentrations in breast milk. Nabumetone should not be used during the last trimester of pregnancy because it may cause adverse effects in the fetus, such as premature closing of the ductus arteriosus. The safety and efficacy of this drug have not been established in children. In the elderly, GI bleeding or ulceration is more likely to cause serious complications and age-related renal impairment may increase the risk of hepatotoxicity or renal toxicity; a reduced drug dosage is recommended. Avoid alcohol and aspirin during therapy because these substances increase the risk of GI bleeding. Tasks that require mental alertness or motor skills should also be avoided.

Blood chemistry studies, renal and liver function studies, and pattern of daily bowel activity and stool consistency should be assessed before and during therapy. Therapeutic response, such as decreased pain, stiffness, swelling, and tenderness, improved grip strength, and increased joint mobility, should be evaluated.

Administration

Swallow tablets whole.
Take nabumetone with food, milk, or antacids if GI distress occurs.

Nadolol
nay-doe'lole
(Apo-Nadol [CAN], Corgard, Novo-Nadolol [CAN])

CATEGORY AND SCHEDULE
Pregnancy Risk Category: C (D if used in second or third trimester)

CLASSIFICATION
Antiadrenergics, beta blocking

MECHANISM OF ACTION
A nonselective beta-blocker that blocks $beta_1$- and $beta_2$-adrenergic receptors. Large doses increase airway resistance. *Therapeutic Effect:* Slows sinus heart rate, decreases cardiac output and B/P. Decreases myocardial ischemia severity by decreasing oxygen requirements.

AVAILABILITY
Tablets: 20 mg, 40 mg, 80 mg, 120 mg, 160 mg.

INDICATIONS AND DOSAGES
▸ **Mild to moderate hypertension, angina**
PO
Adults. Initially, 40 mg/day. May increase by 40-80 mg at 3-7 day intervals. Maximum: 240-360 mg/day.
Elderly. Initially, 20 mg/day. May increase gradually. Range: 20-240 mg/day.

▶ **Dosage in renal impairment**
Dosage is modified based on creatinine clearance.

Creatinine Clearance	% Usual Dosage
10-50 ml/min	50
Less than 10 ml/min	25

OFF-LABEL USES
Treatment of arrhythmias, hypertrophic cardiomyopathy, MI, mitral valve prolapse syndrome, neuroleptic-induced akathisia, pheochromocytoma, tremors, thyrotoxicosis, vascular headaches

CONTRAINDICATIONS
Bronchial asthma, cardiogenic shock, CHF secondary to tachyarrhythmias, COPD, patients receiving MAOI therapy, second- or third-degree heart block, sinus bradycardia, uncontrolled cardiac failure

INTERACTIONS
Drug
Cimetidine: May increase nadolol blood concentration.
Diuretics, other antihypertensives: May increase hypotensive effect.
Insulin, oral hypoglycemics: May mask symptoms of hypoglycemia and prolong the hypoglycemic effect of insulin and oral hypoglycemics.
NSAIDs: May decrease antihypertensive effect.
Sympathomimetics, xanthines: May mutually inhibit effects.
Herbal
None known.
Food
None known.

DIAGNOSTIC TEST EFFECTS
May increase serum antinuclear antibody titer and BUN, serum LDH, serum lipoprotein, serum alkaline phosphatase, serum bilirubin, serum creatinine, serum potassium, serum uric acid, AST (SGOT), ALT (SGPT), and serum triglyceride levels.

SIDE EFFECTS
Nadolol is generally well tolerated, with transient and mild side effects.
Frequent
Diminished sexual ability, drowsiness, unusual fatigue or weakness
Occasional
Bradycardia, difficulty breathing, depression, cold hands or feet, diarrhea, constipation, anxiety, nasal congestion, nausea, vomiting
Rare
Altered taste, dry eyes, itching

SERIOUS REACTIONS
• Overdose may produce profound bradycardia and hypotension.
• Abrupt withdrawal of nadolol may result in diaphoresis, palpitations, headache, tremulousness, exacerbation of angina, MI, and ventricular arrhythmias.
• Nadolol administration may precipitate CHF and MI in patients with cardiac disease; thyroid storm in those with thyrotoxicosis; and peripheral ischemia in those with existing peripheral vascular disease.
• Hypoglycemia may occur in patients with previously controlled diabetes.

N

PRECAUTIONS & CONSIDERATIONS
Caution is warranted with diabetes mellitus, hyperthyroidism, impaired hepatic and renal function, and inadequate cardiac function. Be aware that salt and alcohol intake should be restricted. Nasal decongestants or OTC cold preparations (stimulants) should not be used without physician approval. Tasks that require mental alertness or motor skills should be avoided.

Notify the physician of confusion, depression, difficulty breathing, dizziness, fever, night cough, rash, slow pulse, sore throat, swelling of arms and legs, or unusual bleeding or bruising. B/P for hypotension, respiratory status for shortness of breath, pattern of daily bowel activity and stool consistency, EKG for arrhythmias, and pulse for quality, rate and rhythm should be monitored during treatment. If pulse rate is 60 beats/minute or lower or systolic B/P is less than 90 mm Hg, withhold the medication and contact the physician. In those receiving nadolol for treatment of angina, the onset, type (sharp, dull, squeezing), radiation, location, intensity, and duration of anginal pain and its precipitating factors, including exertion and emotional stress should be recorded. Signs and symptoms of CHF, such as decreased urine output, distended neck veins, dyspnea (particularly on exertion or lying down), night cough, peripheral edema, and weight gain should also be assessed.

Storage
Store at room temperature.

Administration
Take nadolol without regard to meals. Tablets may be crushed.

Nafarelin
naf-ah-rell-in
(Synarel)

CATEGORY AND SCHEDULE
Pregnancy Risk Category: X

CLASSIFICATION
Gonadotropin-releasing hormone analogs, hormones/hormone modifiers

MECHANISM OF ACTION
A gonadotropin inhibitor that initially stimulates the release of the pituitary gonadotropins, luteinizing hormone and follicle-stimulating hormone, then decreases secretion of gonadal steroids. *Therapeutic Effect:* Temporarily increases ovarian steroidogenesis, abolishes the stimulatory effect on the pituitary gland, decreases secretion of gonadal steroids.

PHARMACOKINETICS
Rapidly absorbed after nasal administration. Protein binding: 78%-84%, binds primarily to albumin. Metabolism: unknown. Excreted in urine. **Half-life:** 3 hr.

AVAILABILITY
Nasal Spray: 2 mg/ml (Synarel).

INDICATIONS AND DOSAGES
▸ **Endometriosis**
INTRANASAL
Adults. 400 mcg/day: 200 mcg (1 spray) into 1 nostril in morning, 1 spray into other nostril in evening. For patients with persistent regular menstruation after months of treatment, increase dose to 800 mcg/day (1 spray into each nostril in morning and evening).

▶ **Central precocious puberty**
INTRANASAL
Children. 1600 mcg/day: 400 mcg
(2 sprays into each nostril in morning
and evening; total 8 sprays).

CONTRAINDICATIONS
Pregnancy, other agonist analogues,
undiagnosed abnormal vaginal
bleeding, hypersensitivity to
nafarelin or any component of the
formulation

INTERACTIONS
Drug
None known.
Herbal
None known.
Food
None known.

DIAGNOSTIC TEST EFFECTS
None known.

SIDE EFFECTS
Frequent
Hot flashes, muscle pain, decreased
breast size, myalgia
Occasional
Nasal irritation, decreased libido,
vaginal dryness, headache,
emotional lability, acne
Rare
Insomnia, edema, weight gain,
seborrhea, depression.

SERIOUS REACTIONS
• None reported.

PRECAUTIONS & CONSIDERATIONS
Caution is warranted with history
of osteoporosis, chronic alcohol or
tobacco use, and intercurrent rhinitis. Be aware that nafarelin is
contraindicated in pregnancy and is
distributed in breast milk. Be aware
that safety and efficacy have not
been established in children younger
than 18 years of age. There are no

age-related precautions noted in the
elderly.
Nonhormonal contraception
should be used during nafarelin
therapy. Do not take nafarelin if
pregnancy is suspected (risk to
fetus).
Storage
Store at room temperature.
Administration
Nafarelin is for nasal use only.
Be aware to initiate treatment
between days 2 and 4 of menstrual
cycle. Duration of therapy is
6 months.

Nafcillin
naph-sil'in
(Nafcil, Nallpen, Unipen)

CATEGORY AND SCHEDULE
Pregnancy Risk Category: B

CLASSIFICATION
Antibiotics, penicillins

N

MECHANISM OF ACTION
A penicillin that acts as a bactericidal in susceptible microorganisms.
Therapeutic Effect: Inhibits bacterial
cell wall synthesis. Bactericidal.

PHARMACOKINETICS
Poorly absorbed from gastrointestinal (GI) tract. Protein binding:
87%-90%. Metabolized in liver.
Primarily excreted in urine. Not
removed by hemodialysis. **Half-life:**
10.5-1 hr (half-life increased with
impaired renal function, neonates).

AVAILABILITY
Tablets: 500 mg (Unipen).
Capsules: 250 mg (Unipen).
Powder for Injection: 1 g, 2 g, 10 g
(Nafcil, Nallpen, Unipen).

INDICATIONS AND DOSAGES
▸ **Staphylococcal infections**
IV
Adults, Elderly. 3-6 g/24 hr in divided doses.
Children. 25 mg/kg 2 times/day.
Neonates 7 days and older. 75 mg/kg/day in 4 divided doses.
Neonates less than 7 days old. 50 mg/kg/day in 2-3 divided doses
IM
Adults, Elderly. 500 mg q4-6hr.
Children. 25 mg/kg 2 times/day.
Neonates 7 days and older. 75 mg/kg/day in 4 divided doses.
Neonates less than 7 days old. 50 mg/kg/day in 2-3 divided doses.
PO
Adults, Elderly. 250 mg to 1 g q4-6hr.
Children. 25-50 mg/kg/day in 4 divided doses.

OFF-LABEL USES
Surgical prophylaxis

CONTRAINDICATIONS
Hypersensitivity to any penicillin

INTERACTIONS
Drug
Probenecid: May increase nafcillin blood concentration and risk for nafcillin toxicity.
Herbal
None known.
Food
None known.

DIAGNOSTIC TEST EFFECTS
May cause positive Coombs' test.

▨ IV INCOMPATIBILITIES
Ditiazem (Cardizem), droperidol (Inapsine), fentanyl, insulin, labetalol (Normodyne, Trandate), midazolam (Versed), nalbuphine (Nubain), vancomycin (Vancocin), verapamil (Isoptin)

▨ IV Compatibilities
None known.

SIDE EFFECTS
Frequent
Mild hypersensitivity reaction (fever, rash, pruritus), GI effects (nausea, vomiting, diarrhea) more frequent w/oral administration
Occasional
Hypokalemia with high IV doses, phlebitis, thrombophlebitis (more common in elderly)
Rare
Extravasation with IV administration

SERIOUS REACTIONS
• Superinfections, potentially fatal antibiotic-associated colitis may result from altered bacterial balance.
• Hematologic effects (especially involving platelets, WBCs), severe hypersensitivity reactions, and anaphylaxis occur rarely.

PRECAUTIONS & CONSIDERATIONS
Caution should be used with antibiotic-associated colitis or a history of allergies, especially to cephalosporins. Be aware that amoxicillin crosses the placenta and is distributed in breast milk in low concentrations. There are no age-related precautions noted in the children. Delayed excretion may occur in neonates or infants. Age-related renal impairment may require dosage adjustment in the elderly.
Storage
After oral solution is reconstituted, it is stable for 7 days if refrigerated.
Reconstituted parenteral solution is stable for 3 days at room temperature and 7 days when refrigerated or 12 weeks when frozen. For IV infusion in 0.9% NaCl or D_5W, solution is stable for 24 hours at room temperature and 96 hours when refrigerated.

Administration
Be aware to space doses evenly around the clock.

Take oral formulation 1 hour before or 2 hours after food/beverages.

Limit IV therapy to less than 48 hours, if possible. Stop infusion if person complains of pain. Because of potential for hypersensitivity/anaphylaxis, start initial dose at a few drops per minute, increase slowly to ordered rate; stay with the person first 10-15 minutes, then check every 10 minutes.

For IV push, reconstitute as above, then further dilute each vial with 15-30 ml sterile water for injection or 0.9% NaCl. Administer over 5-10 minutes.

For intermittent IV infusion (piggyback), further dilute with 50-100 ml D_5W, $D_{10}W$, 0.9% NaCl, 0.45% NaCl, 0.2% NaCl, Ringer's, lactated Ringer's or any combination thereof. Infuse over 30-60 minutes.

For IM administration, reconstitute each 500 mg with 1.7 ml sterile water for injection or 0.9% NaCl to provide concentration of 250 mg/ml. Inject into large muscle mass.

Naftifine
naf-ti-feen
(Naftin)
Do not confuse with nafcillin or nafarelin.

CATEGORY AND SCHEDULE
Pregnancy Risk Category: B

CLASSIFICATION
Antifungals, topical, dermatologics

MECHANISM OF ACTION
An antifungal that selectively inhibits the enzyme squalene epoxidase in a dose-dependent manner, which results in the primary sterol, ergosterol, within the fungal membrane not being synthesized. *Therapeutic Effect:* Results in fungal cell death. Fungistatic and fungicidal.

PHARMACOKINETICS
Minimal systemic absorption. Metabolized in the liver. Excreted in the urine as well as the feces and bile. **Half-life:** 48-72 hr.

AVAILABILITY
Gel: 1% (Naftin).
Cream: 1% (Naftin).

INDICATIONS AND DOSAGES
▶ **Tinea pedis, t. cruris, t. corporis**
TOPICAL
Adults, Elderly, Children 12 yr and older. Apply cream 1 time a day for 4 weeks or until signs and symptoms significantly improve. Apply gel 2 times a day for 4 weeks or until signs and symptoms significantly improve.

OFF-LABEL USES
Trichomycosis

CONTRAINDICATIONS
Hypersensitivity to naftifine or any of its components

INTERACTIONS
Drug
None known.
Herbal
None known.
Food
None known.

DIAGNOSTIC TEST EFFECTS
None known.

SIDE EFFECTS
Frequent
Burning, stinging
Occasional
Erythema, itching, dryness,
irritation

SERIOUS REACTIONS
• Excessive irritation may indicate
hypersensitivity reaction.

PRECAUTIONS & CONSIDERATIONS
Occlusive dressings should be
avoided. It is unknown if naftifine is
distributed in breast milk. Safety and
efficacy of naftifine have not been
established in children. There are no
age-related precautions noted in the
elderly.
Administration
Naftifine is for external use only.
Topical therapy should not exceed
4 weeks. Avoid getting topical form
in contact with eyes, mouth, nose, or
other mucous membranes. Wash
hands after application.

Nalbuphine
nal'byoo-feen
(Nubain)
**Do not confuse Nubain with
Navane.**

CATEGORY AND SCHEDULE
Pregnancy Risk Category: B
(D if used for prolonged periods
or at high dosages at term)

CLASSIFICATION
Analgesics, narcotic agonist-
antagonist

MECHANISM OF ACTION
A narcotic agonist-antagonist that
binds with opioid receptors in

the CNS. May displace opioid
agonists and competitively inhibit
their action; may precipitate withdrawal symptoms. *Therapeutic
Effect:* Alters the perception of and
emotional response to pain.

PHARMACOKINETICS

Route	Onset	Peak	Duration
IV	2-3 min	30 min	3-6 hr
IM	Less than 15 min	60 min	3-6 hr
Subcuta-neous	Less than 15 min	N/A	3-6 hr

Well absorbed after IM or subcutaneous administration. Protein binding: 50%. Metabolized in the liver.
Primarily eliminated in feces by
biliary secretion. **Half-life:** 3.5-5 hr.

AVAILABILITY
Injection: 10 mg/ml, 20 mg/ml.

INDICATIONS AND DOSAGES
▸ **Analgesia**
IV, IM, SUBCUTANEOUS
Adults, Elderly. 10 mg q3-6hr as
needed. Don't exceed maximum
single dose of 20 mg or daily dose
of 160 mg. For patients receiving
long-term narcotic analgesics of
similar duration of action, give 25%
of usual dose.
Children. 0.1-0.15 mg/kg q3-6hr as
needed.
▸ **Supplement to anesthesia**
IV
Adults, Elderly. Induction:
0.3-3 mg/kg over 10-15 min.
Maintenance: 0.25-0.5 mg/kg as
needed.

CONTRAINDICATIONS
Respiratory rate less than 12 breaths/
minute

INTERACTIONS
Drug
Alcohol, other CNS depressants: May increase CNS or respiratory depression and hypotension.
Buprenorphine: May decrease the effects of nalbuphine.
MAOIs: May produce a severe, possibly fatal reaction; plan to administer 25% of the usual nalbuphine dose.
Herbal
None known.
Food
None known.

DIAGNOSTIC TEST EFFECTS
May increase serum amylase and lipase levels.

🔲 IV INCOMPATIBILITIES
Amphotericin B complex (Abelcet, AmBisome, Amphotec), cefepime (Maxipime), docetaxel (Doxil), methotrexate, nafcillin (Nafcil), piperacillin and tazobactam (Zosyn), sargramostim (Leukine, Prokine), sodium bicarbonate
💉 IV Compatibilities
Diphenhydramine (Benadryl), droperidol (Inapsine), glycopyrrolate (Robinul), hydroxyzine (Vistaril), ketorolac (Toradol), lidocaine, midazolam (Versed), propofol (Diprivan)

SIDE EFFECTS
Frequent (35%)
Sedation
Occasional (9%-3%)
Diaphoresis, cold and clammy skin, nausea, vomiting, dizziness, vertigo, dry mouth, headache
Rare (less than 1%)
Restlessness, emotional lability, paresthesia, flushing, paradoxical reaction

SERIOUS REACTIONS
• Abrupt withdrawal after prolonged use may produce symptoms of narcotic withdrawal, such as abdominal cramping, rhinorrhea, lacrimation, anxiety, fever, and piloerection (goose bumps).
• Overdose results in severe respiratory depression, skeletal muscle flaccidity, cyanosis, and extreme somnolence progressing to seizures, stupor, and coma.
• Repeated use may result in drug tolerance and physical dependence.

PRECAUTIONS & CONSIDERATIONS
Caution is warranted with pregnancy, opioid-dependent, head trauma, increased intracranial pressure, hepatic or renal impairment, recent MI, respiratory depression, and those about to undergo biliary tract surgery. Nalbuphine readily crosses the placenta and is distributed in breast milk. Breast-feeding is not recommended. Children may experience paradoxical excitement. Children younger than 2 years and the elderly are more likely to develop respiratory depression. In the elderly, age-related renal impairment may increase the risk of urine retention.

Dizziness and drowsiness may occur, so change positions slowly and avoid alcohol, CNS depressants, and tasks that require mental alertness or motor skills until response to the drug is established. B/P, pulse rate and quality, respirations, pattern of daily bowel activity and stool consistency, and clinical improvement of pain should be monitored.
Storage
Store at room temperature.
Administration
! Keep in mind that nalbuphine dosage is based on the person's physical condition, the severity of pain, and concurrent use of other drugs.

N

For IV use, nalbuphine may be given undiluted. For IV push, administer each 10 mg over 3 to 5 minutes.

For IM use, rotate IM injection sites.

Nalmefene
nal'meh-feen
(Revex)

CATEGORY AND SCHEDULE
Pregnancy Risk Category: B

CLASSIFICATION
Antagonists, narcotic, antidotes

MECHANISM OF ACTION
A narcotic antagonist that binds to opioid receptors. *Therapeutic Effect:* Prevents and reverses effects of opioids (respiratory depression, sedation, hypotenstion).

PHARMACOKINETICS
Well absorbed. Protein binding: 45%. Metabolized primarily via glucuronidation. Excreted in urine and feces. **Half-life:** 8.5-10.8 hr.

AVAILABILITY
Solution for Injection: 100 mcg/ml ([blue label] Revex), 1000 mcg/ml ([green label] Revex)

INDICATIONS AND DOSAGES
▸ **Solution for Injection: 100 mcg/ml ([blue label] Revex), 1000 mcg/ml ([green label] Revex)**
IV/IM/SUBCUTANEOUS
Adults. Initially, 0.25 mcg/kg followed by additional 0.25 mcg doses at 2 to 5 min intervals until desired response. Cumulative doses >1 mcg/kg do not provide additional therapeutic effect.

Known or suspected opioid overdose
IV/IM/SUBCUTANEOUS
Adults. Initially, 0.5 mg/70 kg. May give 1 mg/70 kg in 2-5 min. If physical opioid dependence suspected, initial dose is 0.1 mg/70 kg.

CONTRAINDICATIONS
Hypersensitivity to nalmefene

INTERACTIONS
Drug
None known.
Herbal
None known.
Food
None known.

DIAGNOSTIC TEST EFFECTS
None known.

▓ IV INCOMPATIBILITIES
None known.
🍷 **IV Compatibilities**
None known.

SIDE EFFECTS
Frequent
Nausea, headache, hypertension
Occasional
Postop pain, fever, dizziness, headache, chills, hypotension, vasodilation

SERIOUS REACTIONS
• Signs and symptoms of opioid withdrawal include stuffy or runny nose, tearing, yawning, sweating, tremor, vomiting, piloerection, feeling of temperature change, joint, bone or muscle pain, abdominal cramps, and feeling of skin crawling.

PRECAUTIONS & CONSIDERATIONS
Caution should be used with active liver disease, cardiovascular disease or who have received potentially cardiotoxic drugs, and physical dependence on narcotic or

narcotic-like agents. Be aware that nalmefene should not be used as primary treatment for ventilatory failure. Be aware that nalmefene may not completely reverse buprenorphine-induced respiratory depression. Be aware that nalmefene, particularly in higher doses (1 or 2 mg), may produce long-lasting antianalgesia effects when used to reverse opioid effects in postoperative patients or outpatients undergoing surgical procedures. It is unknown if nalmefene crosses the placenta or is distributed in breast milk. Be aware that nalmefene should be avoided in newborns. There are no age-related precautions noted in children or the elderly.

If a person administers heroin or other opiates, these drugs will have no effect during nalmefene therapy. Any attempt to overcome nalmefene's prolonged 24 to 72 hour blockade of opioid effects by taking large amount of opioids is very dangerous and may result in coma, serious injury, or fatal overdose. Notify the physician of abdominal pain that lasts longer than 3 days, dark-colored urine, white bowel movements, or yellow of the whites of the eyes occurs.

Storage
Store at room temperature.

Administration
Be aware that nalmefene is supplied in 2 concentrations. Labeling is color-coded. Postoperative reversal — blue. Overdose management — green. Be aware that if recurrence of respiratory depression occurs, dose may again be titrated to clinical effect using incremental doses.

Administer IV push. Dilute drug 1:1 with diluent and use smaller doses in persons known to be at increased cardiovascular risk. May be given IM or subcutaneous if venous access is not available.

Single dose is usually effective 5-15 min after IM/subcutaneous doses of 1 mg.

Naloxone
nal-oks'one
(Narcan)
Do not confuse naltrexone, Narcan with Norcuron.

CATEGORY AND SCHEDULE
Pregnancy Risk Category: B

CLASSIFICATION
Antagonists, narcotic, antidotes

MECHANISM OF ACTION

A narcotic antagonist that displaces opioids at opioid-occupied receptor sites in the CNS. *Therapeutic Effect:* Reverses opioid-induced sleep or sedation, increases respiratory rate, raises B/P to normal range.

PHARMACOKINETICS

Route	Onset	Peak	Duration
IV	1-2 min	N/A	20-60 min
IM	2-5 min	N/A	20-60 min
Subcuta-neous	2-5 min	N/A	20-60 min

Well absorbed after IM or subcutaneous administration. Metabolized in the liver. Primarily excreted in urine. **Half-life:** 60-100 min.

AVAILABILITY
Injection: 0.02 mg/ml, 0.4 mg/ml, 1 mg/ml.

INDICATIONS AND DOSAGES
▸ **Opioid toxicity**
IV, IM, SUBCUTANEOUS
Adults, Elderly. 0.4-2 mg q2-3min

as needed. May repeat q20-60min.
Children 5 yr and older and weighing 22 kg or more. 2 mg/dose; if no response, may repeat q2-3min. May need to repeat q20-60min.
Children younger than 5 yr and weighing less than 22 kg.
0.1 mg/kg; if no response, repeat q2-3min. May need to repeat q20-60min.
▸ **Postanesthesia narcotic reversal**
IV
Children. 0.01 mg/kg; may repeat q2-3min.
▸ **Neonatal opioid-induced depression**
IV
Neonates. May repeat q2-3min as needed. May need to repeat q1-2hr.

OFF-LABEL USES
Treatment of PCP, ethanol ingestion

CONTRAINDICATIONS
Respiratory depression due to non-opioid drugs

INTERACTIONS
Drug
Butorphanol, nalbuphine, opioid agonist analgesics, pentazocine:
Reverses the analgesic and adverse effects of these drugs and may precipitate withdrawal symptoms.
Herbal
None known.
Food
None known.

DIAGNOSTIC TEST EFFECTS
None known.

▨ IV INCOMPATIBILITIES
Amphotericin B complex (Abelcet, AmBisome, Amphotec)
▨ IV Compatibilities
Heparin, ondansetron (Zofran), propofol (Diprivan)

SIDE EFFECTS
None known; little or no pharmacologic effect in absence of narcotics.

SERIOUS REACTIONS
• Too-rapid reversal of narcotic-induced respiratory depression may result in nausea, vomiting, tremors, increased B/P, and tachycardia.
• Excessive dosage in postoperative patients may produce significant excitement, tremors, and reversal of analgesia.
• Patients with cardiovascular disease may experience hypotension or hypertension, ventricular tachycardia and fibrillation, and pulmonary edema.

PRECAUTIONS & CONSIDERATIONS
Caution is warranted with chronic cardiovascular or pulmonary disease, postoperative (to avoid cardiovascular complications), and suspect of opioid dependence. It is unknown if naloxone crosses the placenta or is distributed in breast milk. No age-related precautions have been noted in children or the elderly. Notify the physician of pain or increased sedation. Vital signs, especially respiratory rate and rhythm, should be monitored.
Storage
Store the parenteral form at room temperature, and protect it from light. The reconstituted solution remains stable in D_5W or 0.9% NaCl at 4 mcg/ml for 24 hours; discard any unused solution.
Administration
! The American Academy of Pediatrics recommends an initial dose of 0.1 mg/kg for infants and children younger than 5 years and weighing less than 20 kg, and an initial dose of 2 mg for children 5 years and older and weighing more than 20 kg. Obtain body weight of children to calculate the drug dosage.

For IV injection, dilute 1 mg/ml with 50 ml sterile water for injection to provide a concentration of 0.02 mg/ml. For continuous IV infusion, dilute each 2 mg of naloxone with 500 ml D_5W or 0.9% NaCl to provide a concentration of 0.004 mg/ml. Naloxone may also be administered undiluted. Give each 0.4 mg as IV push over 15 seconds. Use the 0.4-mg/ml and 1-mg/ml vials for adults and the 0.02-mg/ml concentration for neonates.

For IM use, inject naloxone in a large muscle mass.

Naltrexone
nal-trex′one
(Revia)

CATEGORY AND SCHEDULE
Pregnancy Risk Category: C

CLASSIFICATION
Antagonists, narcotic, antidotes

MECHANISM OF ACTION
A narcotic antagonist that displaces opioids at opioid-occupied receptor sites in the CNS. *Therapeutic Effect:* Blocks physical effects of opioid analgesics; decreases craving for alcohol and relapse rate in alcoholism.

AVAILABILITY
Tablets: 50 mg.

INDICATIONS AND DOSAGES
▶ **Naloxone challenge test to determine if patient is opioid dependent**
! Expect to perform the naloxone challenge test if there is any question

that the patient is opioid dependent. Don't administer naltrexone until the naloxone challenge test is negative.
IV
Adults, Elderly. Draw 2 ml (0.8 mg) of naloxone into syringe. Inject 0.5 ml (0.2 mg); while needle is still in vein, observe patient for 30 sec for withdrawal signs or symptoms. If no evidence of withdrawal, inject remaining 1.5 ml (0.6 mg); observe patient for additional 20 min for withdrawal signs or symptoms.
SUBCUTANEOUS
Adults, Elderly. Inject 2 ml (0.8 mg) of naloxone; observe patient for 45 min for withdrawal signs or symptoms.
▶ **Treatment of opioid dependence in patients who have been opioid free for at least 7-10 days**
PO
Adults, Elderly. Initially, 25 mg. Observe patient for 1 hr. If no withdrawal signs or symptoms appear, give another 25 mg. May be given as 100 mg every other day or 150 mg every 3 days.
▶ **Adjunctive treatment of alcohol dependence**
PO
Adults, Elderly. 50 mg once a day.

OFF-LABEL USES
Treatment of eating disorders, post-concussional syndrome unresponsive to other treatments

CONTRAINDICATIONS
Acute hepatitis, acute opioid withdrawal, failed naloxone challenge test, hepatic failure, history of hypersensitivity to naltrexone, opioid dependence, positive urine screen for opioids

N

INTERACTIONS
Drug
**Opioid-containing products
(including analgesics, antidiar-
rheals, and antitussives):** Blocks
the therapeutic effects of these
drugs.
Thioridazine: May produce
lethargy and somnolence.
Herbal
None known.
Food
None known.

DIAGNOSTIC TEST EFFECTS
May increase AST (SGOT) and ALT
(SGPT) levels.

SIDE EFFECTS
Frequent
Alcoholism (10%-7%): Nausea,
headache, depression
Narcotic addiction (10%-5%):
Insomnia, anxiety, nervousness,
headache, low energy, abdominal
cramps, nausea, vomiting, arthralgia,
myalgia
Occasional
Alcoholism (4%-2%): Dizziness,
nervousness, fatigue, insomnia,
vomiting, anxiety, suicidal ideation
Narcotic addiction (5%-2%):
Irritability, increased energy, dizziness, anorexia, diarrhea or constipation, rash, chills, increased thirst

SERIOUS REACTIONS
• Signs and symptoms of opioid
withdrawal include stuffy or runny
nose, tearing, yawning, diaphoresis,
tremor, vomiting, piloerection, feeling of temperature change, bone
pain, arthralgia, myalgia, abdominal
cramps, and feeling of skin crawling.
• Accidental naltrexone overdose
produces withdrawal symptoms
within 5 minutes of ingestion that
may last for up to 48 hours.
Symptoms include confusion, visual

hallucinations, somnolence, and
significant vomiting and diarrhea.
• Hepatocellular injury may occur
with large doses.

PRECAUTIONS & CONSIDERATIONS
Caution is warranted with active
hepatic disease. Before treatment,
baseline laboratory tests, including
creatinine clearance, serum bilirubin,
AST (SGOT), and ALT (SGPT)
levels, should be obtained. Liver
function should be monitored
throughout therapy.
    Be aware that opioid-containing
drugs used during naltrexone therapy
will have no effect. Any attempt to
overcome naltrexone's prolonged
24-72-hour blockade of opioid
effects by taking large amounts of
opioids may result in coma, serious
injury, or death. Notify the physician
if abdominal pain lasts longer than
3 days, dark urine, white stools, or
yellowing of the whites of the eyes,
occurs.
Storage
Store the parenteral form at room
temperature, and protect it from
light. The reconstituted solution
remains stable in D_5W or 0.9% NaCl
at 4 mcg/ml for 24 hours; discard
any unused solution.
Administration
Take naltrexone with antacids, after
meals, or with food to avoid adverse
GI effects.

Nandrolone
nan'droe-lone
(Deca-Durabolin,
Durabolin [CAN])
**Do not confuse with
testolactone.**

CATEGORY AND SCHEDULE
Pregnancy Risk Category: X
Controlled Substance:
Schedule III

CLASSIFICATION
Anabolic steroids,
hormones/hormone modifiers

MECHANISM OF ACTION
An anabolic steroid that promotes
tissue-building processes, increases
production of erythropoietin, causes
protein anabolism, and increases
hemoglobin and red blood cell
volume. *Therapeutic Effect:* Controls
metastatic breast cancer and
helps manage anemia of renal
insufficiency.

PHARMACOKINETICS
Well absorbed after IM administration (about 77%). Metabolized in
liver. Primarily excreted in urine.
Half-life: 6-8 days.

AVAILABILITY
*Injection, as decanoate (in sesame
oil):* 100 mg/ml, 200 mg/ml (Deca-
Durabolin).

INDICATIONS AND DOSAGES
▶ **Breast cancer**
IM
Adults, Elderly. 50-100 mg/week.
Anemia of renal insufficiency
IM
Adults, Elderly (male).
100-200 mg/week.

Adults, Elderly (female).
50-100 mg/week.
Children, 2-13 yr. 25-50 mg every
3-4 weeks.

OFF-LABEL USES
Hyperlipidemia, lung cancer, male
contraception, malnutrition, postmenopausal osteoporosis, rheumatoid arthritis, Sjogren's syndrome,
trauma/surgery

CONTRAINDICATIONS
Nephrosis, pregnancy, carcinoma of
breast or prostate, not for use in
infants, hypersensitivity to nandrolone
or any component of the formulation
such as sesame oil

INTERACTIONS
Drug
Adrenal steroids: May increase the
effects of adrenal steroids.
Insulin, oral hypoglycemic agents:
May increase the effects of insulin
and hypoglycemic agents.
Oral anticoagulants: May increase
the effects of oral anticoagulants.
Herbal
Chaparral: May increase liver
enzymes.
Comfrey: May increase liver
enzymes.
Eucalyptus: May increase risk of
heptotoxicity.
Germander: May increase liver
enzymes.
Jin bu huan: May increase liver
enzymes.
Kava kava: May increase risk of
liver damage.
Pennyroyal: May increase liver
enzymes.
Skullcap: May increase the risk of
liver damage.
Valerian: May increase the risk of
heptotoxicity.
Food
None known.

DIAGNOSTIC TEST EFFECTS
None known.

▦ IV INCOMPATIBILITIES
None known.
⬚ IV Compatibilities
None known.

SIDE EFFECTS
Frequent
Male, postpubertal: Gynecomastia, acne, bladder irritability, priapism
Male, prepubertal: Acne, virilism
Females: Virilism
Occasional
Male, postpubertal/prepubertal: Insomnia, chills, decreased libido, hepatic dysfunction, nausea, diarrhea, prostatic hyperplasia (elderly), iron-deficiency anemia, suppression of clotting factors
Male, prepubertal: Chills, insomnia, hyperpigmentation, diarrhea, nausea, iron deficiency anemia, suppression of clotting factors
Female: Chills, insomnia, hypercalcemia, nausea, diarrhea, iron deficiency anemia, suppression of clotting factors, hepatic dysfunction
Rare
Hepatic necrosis, heptocellular carcinoma

SERIOUS REACTIONS
• Peliosis hepatitis of liver, spleen replaced with blood-filled cysts, hepatic neoplasms and hepatocellular carcinoma have been associated with prolonged high-dosage, anaphylactic reactions.

PRECAUTIONS & CONSIDERATIONS
Caution is warranted with diabetes, epilepsy, and liver or renal impairment. Nandrolone use is contraindicated during lactation. Safety and efficacy of nandrolone have not been established in children, so use with caution. Nandrolone use in the elderly may increase the risk of hyperplasia or stimulate growth of occult prostate carcinoma. Adequate calories and protein should be consumed.

Acne, nausea, pedal edema, or vomiting may occur. Women should report deepening of voice, hoarseness, and menstrual irregularities. Men should report difficulty urinating, frequent erections, and gynecomastia. Weight should be obtained each day. Weekly weight gains of more than 5 pounds should be reported.
Administration
Give IM injection deep in gluteal muscle. Do not give as IV injection.

Naphazoline
naf-az′oh-leen
(AK-Con, Albalon Liquifilm [AUS], Clear Eyes [AUS], Naphcon, Privine, Vasocon)

CATEGORY AND SCHEDULE
Pregnancy Risk Category: C

CLASSIFICATION
Decongestants, nasal, ophthalmic

MECHANISM OF ACTION
A sympathomimetic that directly acts on alpha-adrenergic receptors in conjunctival arterioles and nasal blood vessels.
Therapeutic Effect: Causes vasoconstriction, resulting in decreased congestion.

AVAILABILITY
Ophthalmic Solution: 0.012%, 0.1%.
Nasal Drops: 0.05%.
Nasal Spray: 0.05%.

INDICATIONS AND DOSAGES

‣ **Nasal congestion due to acute or chronic rhinitis, common cold, hay fever, or other allergies**
INTRANASAL
Adults, Elderly, Children older than 12 yr. 1-2 drops or sprays in each nostril q3-6hr.
Children 6-12 yr. 1 spray or drop in each nostril q6hr as needed.
‣ **Control of hyperemia in patients with superficial corneal vascularity; relief of congestion and inflammation; for use during ocular diagnostic procedures**
OPHTHALMIC
Adults, Elderly, Children older than 6 yr. 1-2 drops in affected eye q3-4hr for 3-4 days.

CONTRAINDICATIONS

Angle-closure glaucoma, before peripheral iridectomy, patients with a narrow angle who do not have glaucoma

INTERACTIONS

Drug
Maprotiline, tricyclic antidepressants: May increase the effects of naphazoline.
Herbal
None known.
Food
None known.

DIAGNOSTIC TEST EFFECTS

None known.

SIDE EFFECTS

Occasional
Nasal: Burning, stinging, or drying of nasal mucosa; sneezing; rebound congestion
Ophthalmic: Blurred vision, dilated pupils, increased eye irritation

SERIOUS REACTIONS

• If naphazoline is systemically absorbed, the patient may experience tachycardia, palpitations, headache, insomnia, lightheadedness, nausea, nervousness, and tremor.
• Large doses may produce tachycardia, palpitations, lightheadedness, nausea, and vomiting.
• Overdose in patients older than 60 years may produce hallucinations, CNS depression, and seizures.

PRECAUTIONS & CONSIDERATIONS

Caution is warranted with cerebral arteriosclerosis, diabetes, heart disease (including coronary artery disease), hypertension, hypertensive cardiovascular disease, hyperthyroidism, and long-standing bronchial asthma. Avoid performing tasks that require visual acuity in those using ophthalmic naphazoline. B/P should be monitored for increases. Tell the physician if taking tricyclic antidpressants.
Storage
Store nasal and ophthalmic drugs in a tightly closed container. Do not freeze.
Administration
Whenever possible, place oneself in the upright position to instill nasal spray. To minimize the risk of systemic absorption, tilt head slightly downward and avoid directing the spray towards the nasopharynx. Do not use naphazoline for more than 72 hours without consulting a physician because too-frequent use may cause rebound congestion. Discontinue the drug and contact the physician if acute eye redness or eye pain, floating spots, vision changes, headache, dizziness, insomnia, irregular heartbeat, tremor, or weakness occurs.

N

Naproxen

na-prox′en
(Crysanal [AUS], EC-Naprosyn,
Inza [AUS], Naprelan, Naprosyn)
(Aleve, Anaprox, Anaprox DS,
Apo-Naprosyn [CAN],
Naprogesic [AUS], Novo-Naprox
[CAN], Nu-Naprox [CAN],
Pamprin)
**Do not confuse with Allese,
Anaspaz.**

CATEGORY AND SCHEDULE
Pregnancy Risk Category: B
(D if used in third trimester or
near delivery)
OTC (220-mg gelcaps, 220-mg
tablets)

CLASSIFICATION
Analgesics, non-narcotic,
nonsteroidal anti-inflammatory
drugs

MECHANISM OF ACTION
An NSAID that produces
analgesic and anti-inflammatory
effects by inhibiting prostaglandin
synthesis. *Therapeutic Effect:*
Reduces the inflammatory
response and intensity of
pain.

PHARMACOKINETICS

Route	Onset	Peak	Duration
PO (anal-gesic)	Less than 1 hr	N/A	7 hr or less
PO (anti-rheumatic)	Less than 14 days	2-4 wk	N/A

Completely absorbed from the (GI)
tract. Protein binding: 99%. Metabolized in the liver. Primarily excreted
in urine. Not removed by hemodialysis. Half-life: 13 hr.

AVAILABILITY
Gelcaps (Aleve): 220 mg naproxen
sodium (equivalent to 200 mg
naproxen) (OTC).
Oral Suspension (Naprosyn):
125 mg/5 ml naproxen.
Tablets (Aleve): 220 mg naproxen
(OTC).
Tablets (Anaprox): 275 mg naproxen
sodium (equivalent to 250 mg
naproxen).
Tablets (Anaprox DS): 550 mg
naproxen sodium (equivalent to
500 mg naproxen).
*Tablets (Controlled-Release
[EC-Naprosyn]):* 375 mg naproxen,
500 mg naproxen.
*Tablets (Controlled-Release
[Naprelan]):* 421 mg naproxen,
550 mg naproxen sodium
(equivalent to 500 mg
naproxen).

INDICATIONS AND DOSAGES
▶ **Rheumatoid arthritis,
osteoarthritis, ankylosing
spondylitis**
PO
Adults, Elderly. 250-500 mg
naproxen (275-550 mg naproxen
sodium) twice a day or 250 mg
naproxen (275 mg naproxen sodium)
in morning and 500 mg naproxen
(550 mg naproxen sodium) in
evening. Naprelan: 750-1000 mg
once a day.
▶ **Acute gouty arthritis**
PO
Adults, Elderly. Initially, 750 mg
naproxen (825 mg naproxen
sodium), then 250 mg naproxen
(275 mg naproxen sodium)
q8hr until attack subsides. Naprelan:
Initially, 1000-1500 mg, then
1000 mg once a day until attack
subsides.

▸ **Mild to moderate pain, dysmenor-rhea, bursitis, tendinitis**
PO
Adults, Elderly. Initially, 500 mg naproxen (550 mg naproxen sodium), then 250 mg naparoxen (275 mg naproxen sodium) q6-8hr as needed. Maximum: 1.25 g/day naproxen (1.375 g/day naproxen sodium). Naprelan: 1000 mg once a day.
▸ **Juvenile rheumatoid arthritis**
PO (NAPROXEN ONLY)
Children. 10-15 mg/kg/day in 2 divided doses. Maximum: 1000 mg/day.

OFF-LABEL USES
Treatment of vascular headaches

CONTRAINDICATIONS
Hypersensitivity to aspirin, naproxen, or other NSAIDs

INTERACTIONS
Drug
Antihypertensives, diuretics: May decrease the effects of these drugs.
Aspirin, other salicylates: May increase the risk of GI side effects such as bleeding.
Bone marrow depressants: May increase the risk of hematologic reactions.
Heparin, oral anticoagulants, thrombolytics: May increase the effects of these drugs.
Lithium: May increase the blood concentration and risk of toxicity of lithium.
Methotrexate: May increase the risk of methotrexate toxicity.
Probenecid: May increase the naproxen blood concentration.
Herbal
Feverfew: May decrease the effects of feverfew.
Ginkgo biloba: May increase the risk of bleeding.

Food
None known.

DIAGNOSTIC TEST EFFECTS
May prolong bleeding time and alter blood glucose level. May increase serum hepatic function test results. May decrease serum sodium and uric acid levels.

SIDE EFFECTS
Frequent (9%-4%)
Nausea, constipation, abdominal cramps or pain, heartburn, dizziness, headache, somnolence
Occasional (3%-1%)
Stomatitis, diarrhea, indigestion
Rare (less than 1%)
Vomiting, confusion

SERIOUS REACTIONS
• Rare reactions with long-term use include peptic ulcer disease, GI bleeding, gastritis, severe hepatic reactions (cholestasis, jaundice), nephrotoxicity (dysuria, hematuria, proteinuria, nephrotic syndrome), and a severe hypersensitivity reaction (fever, chills, bronchospasm).

PRECAUTIONS & CONSIDERATIONS
Caution is warranted with cardiac disease, GI disease, impaired hepatic or renal function and those using anticoagulants concurrently. Naproxen crosses the placenta and is distributed in breast milk. Naproxen should not be used during the third trimester of pregnancy because it may cause adverse effects in the fetus, such as premature closing of the ductus arteriosus. The safety and efficacy of naproxen have not been established in children younger than 2 years. Children older than 2 years are at an increased risk for developing a rash during naproxen therapy. In the elderly, GI bleeding or ulceration is more likely to cause serious

complications and age-related renal impairment may increase the risk of hepatotoxicity and renal toxicity; a reduced dosage is recommended. Avoid alcohol and aspirin during therapy because these substances increase the risk of GI bleeding. Tasks that require mental alertness or motor skills should also be avoided.

Notify the physician if black or tarry stools, persistent headache, rash, visual disturbances, or weight gain occur. CBC (particularly Hgb, Hct, and platelet count), BUN level, serum alkaline phosphatase, bilirubin, creatinine, AST (SGOT), ALT (SGPT) levels to assess hepatic and renal function, and pattern of daily bowel activity and stool consistency should be assessed during therapy. Therapeutic response, such as decreased pain, stiffness, swelling, and tenderness, improved grip strength, and increased joint mobility, should be evaluated.

Administration
! Be aware that each 275- or 550-mg tablet of naproxen sodium equals 250 or 500 mg of naproxen, respectively.

Swallow enteric-coated tablets whole; scored tablets may be broken or crushed. Take naproxen with food, milk, or antacids if GI distress occurs.

Naratriptan
nare-a-trip'tan
(Amerge, Naramig [AUS])
Do not confuse Amerge with Amaryl.

CATEGORY AND SCHEDULE
Pregnancy Risk Category: C

CLASSIFICATION
Serotonin receptor agonists

MECHANISM OF ACTION
A serotonin receptor agonist that binds selectively to vascular receptors producing a vasoconstrictive effect on cranial blood vessels. *Therapeutic Effect:* Relieves migraine headache.

PHARMACOKINETICS
Well absorbed after PO administration. Protein binding: 28%-31%. Metabolized by the liver to inactive metabolite. Eliminated primarily in urine and, to a lesser extent, in feces. **Half-life:** 6 hr (increased in hepatic or renal impairment).

AVAILABILITY
Tablets: 1 mg, 2.5 mg.

INDICATIONS AND DOSAGES
▸ **Acute migraine attack**
PO
Adults. 1 mg or 2.5 mg. If headache improves but then returns, dose may be repeated after 4 hr. Maximum: 5 mg/24 hr.
▸ **Dosage in mild to moderate hepatic or renal impairment**
A lower starting dose is recommended. Don't exceed 2.5 mg/24 hr.

CONTRAINDICATIONS

Basilar or hemiplegic migraine, cerebrovascular or peripheral vascular disease, coronary artery disease, ischemic heart disease (including angina pectoris, history of MI, silent ischemia, and Prinzmetal's angina), severe hepatic impairment—(Child-Pugh grade C), severe renal impairment (serum creatinine less than 15 ml/min), uncontrolled hypertension, use within 24 hours of ergotamine-containing preparations or another serotonin receptor agonist, use within 14 days of MAOIs

INTERACTIONS
Drug
Ergotamine-containing medications: May produce a vasospastic reaction.
Fluoxetine, fluvoxamine, paroxetine, sertraline: May produce hyperreflexia, incoordination, and weakness.
Oral contraceptives: Decrease naratriptan clearance and volume of distribution.
Herbal
None known.
Food
None known.

DIAGNOSTIC TEST EFFECTS
None known.

SIDE EFFECTS
Occasional (5%)
Nausea
Rare (2%)
Paresthesia; dizziness; fatigue; somnolence; jaw, neck, or throat pressure

SERIOUS REACTIONS
• Corneal opacities and other ocular defects may occur.
• Cardiac reactions (including ischemia, coronary artery vasospasm, and MI) and noncardiac vasospasm-related reactions (such as hemorrhage and CVA), occur rarely, particularly in patients with hypertension, diabetes, or a strong family history of coronary artery disease; obese patients; smokers; males older than 40 years; and postmenopausal women.

PRECAUTIONS & CONSIDERATIONS
Caution is warranted with mild to moderate hepatic or renal impairment and cardiovascular risk factors. It is unknown if naratriptan is excreted in breast milk. The safety and efficacy of naratriptan have not been established in children. Naratriptan is not recommended for the elderly. Tasks that require mental alertness or motor skills should be avoided.

Notify the physician immediately if anxiety, chest pain, palpitations, or tightness in the throat occurs. Migraines and associated symptoms, including nausea and vomiting, photophobia, and phonophobia (sound sensitivity) should be assessed before and during treatment.
Administration
Take naratriptan without regard to food. Swallow tablets whole; don't crush them. Take another dose of naratriptan, if needed, 4 hours after the first dose for a maximum of 5 mg/24 hours.

Natalizumab
nat-ah-lih′zoo-mab
(Tysabri)

CATEGORY AND SCHEDULE
Pregnancy Risk Category: C

CLASSIFICATION
Immunologic agents

MECHANISM OF ACTION
A monoclonal antibody that binds to the surface of leukocytes, inhibiting their adhesion to the vascular endothelial cells of the GI tract and preventing them from migrating across the endothelium into inflamed parenchymal tissue. *Therapeutic Effect:* Decreases clinical exacerbations of multiple sclerosis.

PHARMACOKINETICS
Half-life: 11 days.

AVAILABILITY
Injection Solution: 300 mg/15 ml concentrate.

INDICATIONS AND DOSAGES
▸ **Relapses of multiple sclerosis**
IV
Adults 18 yr and older, Elderly.
300 mg every 4 wk.

CONTRAINDICATIONS
None known.

INTERACTIONS
Drug
None known.
Herbal
None known.
Food
None known.

DIAGNOSTIC TEST EFFECTS
Increases basophil, eosinophil, lymphocyte, monocyte, and RBC counts (increases are reversible, usually within 16 wk after last natalizumab dose). May alter liver function test results.

▨ IV INCOMPATIBILITIES
Don't mix natalizumab with any other medication or with any diluent other than 0.9% NaCl.

SIDE EFFECTS
Frequent (35%-15%)
Headache, fatigue, depression, arthralgia
Occasional (10%-5%)
Abdominal discomfort, rash, urinary frequency or urgency, menstrual irregularities, dysmenorrhea, dermatitis
Rare (4%-2%)
Pruritus, chest discomfort, local bleeding, rigors, tremor, syncope

SERIOUS REACTIONS
• UTI, lower respiratory tract infection, gastroenteritis, vaginitis, allergic reaction, and tonsillitis occur occasionally.

PRECAUTIONS & CONSIDERATIONS
Caution is warranted with chronic progressive multiple sclerosis and in children younger than 18 years. It is unknown if natalizumab crosses the placenta or is distributed in breast milk. The safety and efficacy of natalizumab have not been established in children younger than 18 years. No age-related precautions have been noted for the elderly.

Notify the physician of arthralgia, rash, depression, menstrual irregularities, or urinary changes. CBC and liver function test results should be monitored.
Storage
Protect natalizumab vials from light. Don't freeze them. After reconstitution, the solution is stable for 8 hours if refrigerated.

Administration

To reconstitute, withdraw 15 ml natalizumab from the vial and inject it into 100 ml 0.9% NaCl. Invert the vial to mix the solution completely. Do not shake it. Inspect the solution for particles. Discard it if it contains particles or becomes discolored. Infuse natalizumab over 1 hour. Following the infusion, flush the IV line with 0.9% NaCl.

Natamycin
na ta-myc′sin
(Natacyn)
Do not confuse with naproxen.

CATEGORY AND SCHEDULE
Pregnancy Risk Category: C

CLASSIFICATION
Antifungals, ophthalmics

MECHANISM OF ACTION

A polyene antifungal agent that increases cell membrane permeability in susceptible fungi. *Therapeutic Effect:* Fungicidal.

PHARMACOKINETICS

Minimal systemic absorption. Adheres to cornea and retained in conjunctival fornices.

AVAILABILITY

Ophthalmic Suspension:
5% (Natacyn).

INDICATIONS AND DOSAGES
▶ Fungal keratitis, ophthalmic fungal infections
OPHTHALMIC
Adults, Elderly. Instill 1 drop in conjunctival sac every 1-2 hours. After 3-4 days, reduce to 1 drop

6-8 times daily. Usual course of therapy is 2-3 weeks.

OFF-LABEL USES

Oral and vaginal candidiasis, onychomycosis, pulmonary aspergillosis

CONTRAINDICATIONS

Hypersensitivity to natamycin or any component of the formulation

INTERACTIONS
Drug
Topical corticosteroids: May increase risk of toxicity. Concomitant use is contraindicated.
Herbal
None known.
Food
None known.

DIAGNOSTIC TEST EFFECTS

None known.

▓ IV INCOMPATIBILITIES

None known.
💉 **IV Compatibilities**
None known.

SIDE EFFECTS
Occasional (10%-3%)
Blurred vision, eye irritation, eye pain, photophobia

SERIOUS REACTIONS

• Vomiting and diarrhea have occurred with large doses in the treatment of systemic mycoses.

PRECAUTIONS & CONSIDERATIONS

If symptoms do not improve within 7 to 10 days, or become worse, notify the physician. It is unknown if natamycin is excreted in breast milk. Safety and efficacy of natamycin have not been established in children. There are no age-related precautions in the elderly.

N

Administration
Shake ophthalmic suspension before using. Do not touch dropper to eye.

Nateglinide
na-teg′lin-ide
(Starlix)

CATEGORY AND SCHEDULE
Pregnancy Risk Category: C

CLASSIFICATION
Antidiabetic agents, meglitinides

MECHANISM OF ACTION
An antihyperglycemic that stimulates release of insulin from beta cells of the pancreas by depolarizing beta cells, leading to an opening of calcium channels. Resulting calcium influx induces insulin secretion. *Therapeutic Effect*: Lowers blood glucose concentration.

AVAILABILITY
Tablets: 60 mg, 120 mg.

INDICATIONS AND DOSAGES
▶ **Diabetes mellitus**
PO
Adult, Elderly. 120 mg 3 times a day before meals. Initially, 60 mg may be given.

CONTRAINDICATIONS
Diabetic ketoacidosis, type 1 diabetes mellitus

INTERACTIONS
Drug
Beta blockers, MAOIs, NSAIDs, salicylates: May increase hypoglycemic effect of nateglinide.

Corticosteroids, thiazide diuretics, thyroid medication, sympathomimetics: May decrease hypoglycemic effect of nateglinide.
Herbal
None known.
Food
Liquid meal: Peak plasma levels may be significantly reduced if administered 10 minutes before a liquid meal.

DIAGNOSTIC TEST EFFECTS
None known.

SIDE EFFECTS
Frequent (10%)
Upper respiratory tract infection
Occasional (4%-3%)
Back pain, flu symptoms, dizziness, arthropathy, diarrhea
Rare (2%)
Bronchitis, cough

SERIOUS REACTIONS
• Hypoglycemia occurs in less than 2% of patients.

PRECAUTIONS & CONSIDERATIONS
Caution is warranted with hepatic or renal impairment. Food intake and blood glucose should be monitored before and during therapy. Be aware of signs and symptoms of hypoglycemia (anxiety, cool wet skin, diplopia, dizziness, headache, hunger, numbness in mouth, tachycardia, tremors), or hyperglycemia (deep rapid breathing, dim vision, fatigue, nausea, polydipsia, polyphagia, polyuria, vomiting); carry candy, sugar packets, or other sugar supplements for immediate response to hypoglycemia. Consult the physician when glucose demands are altered (such as with fever, heavy physical activity, infection, stress, trauma). Exercise, good personal hygiene (including foot care), not smoking,

and weight control are essential parts of therapy.

Administration
Ideally, take within 15 minutes of a meal; however, may take immediately to as long as 30 minutes before a meal. Allow at least 1 week to elapse to assess the response to the drug before new dose adjustment is made.

Nedocromil
ned-oh-crow'mil
(Alocril, Mireze [CAN], Tilade)

CATEGORY AND SCHEDULE
Pregnancy Risk Category: B

CLASSIFICATION
Mast cell stabilizers

MECHANISM OF ACTION
A mast cell stabilizer that prevents the activation and release of inflammatory mediators, such as histamine, leukotrienes, mast cells, eosinophils, and monocytes. *Therapeutic Effect:* Prevents both early and late asthmatic responses.

AVAILABILITY
Aerosol for Inhalation (Tilade): 1.75 mg/activation.
Ophthalmic Solution (Alocril): 2%.

INDICATIONS AND DOSAGES
▶ **Mild to moderate asthma**
ORAL INHALATION
Adults, Elderly, Children 6 yr and older. 2 inhalations 4 times a day. May decrease to 3 times a day then twice a day as asthma becomes controlled.
▶ **Allergic conjunctivitis**
OPHTHALMIC
Adults, Elderly, Children 3 yr and older. 1-2 drops in each eye twice a day.

OFF-LABEL USES
Prevention of bronchospasm in patients with reversible obstructive airway disease

CONTRAINDICATIONS
None known.

INTERACTIONS
Drug
None known.
Herbal
None known.
Food
None known.

DIAGNOSTIC TEST EFFECTS
None known.

SIDE EFFECTS
Frequent (10%-6%)
Cough, pharyngitis, bronchospasm, headache, altered taste
Occasional (5%-1%)
Rhinitis, upper respiratory tract infection, abdominal pain, fatigue
Rare (less than 1%)
Diarrhea, dizziness

SERIOUS REACTIONS
• None known.

PRECAUTIONS & CONSIDERATIONS
Nedocromil is not used to reverse acute bronchospasm. Drink plenty of fluids to decrease the thickness of lung secretions. Therapeutic response, such as less frequent or severe asthmatic attacks or reduced dependence on antihistamines, should be monitored. A log of peak flow meter values should be kept.
Storage
Protect the drug from direct exposure to light.

N

Administration

Shake the container well before each use. Administer nedocromil at regular intervals, even when symptom-free, to achieve optimal results. Rinse mouth with water immediately after inhalation to help relieve unpleasant taste.

Nefazodone
neh-faz'oh-doan
(Serzone)
Do not confuse with Seroquel.

CATEGORY AND SCHEDULE
Pregnancy Risk Category: C

CLASSIFICATION
Antidepressants, miscellaneous

MECHANISM OF ACTION

Exact mechanism is unknown. Appears to inhibit neuronal uptake of serotonin and norepinephrine and to antagonize $alpha_1$-adrenergic receptors. *Therapeutic Effect:* Relieves depression.

PHARMACOKINETICS

Rapidly and completely absorbed from the GI tract; food delays absorption. Protein binding: 99%. Widely distributed in body tissues, including CNS. Extensively metabolized to active metabolites. Excreted in urine and eliminated in feces. Unknown if removed by hemodialysis. **Half-life:** 2-4 hr.

AVAILABILITY

Tablets: 50 mg, 100 mg, 150 mg, 200 mg, 250 mg.

INDICATIONS AND DOSAGES
▸ **Depression, prevention of relapse of acute depressive episode**
PO
Adults. Initially, 200 mg/day in 2 divided doses. Gradually increase by 100-200 mg/day at intervals of at least 1 wk. Range: 300-600 mg/day.
Elderly. Initially, 100 mg/day in 2 divided doses. Subsequent dosage titration based on clinical response. Range: 200-400 mg/day.
Children. 300-400 mg/day.

CONTRAINDICATIONS
Use within 14 days of MAOIs

INTERACTIONS
Drug
Alprazolam, triazolam: May increase the blood concentration and risk of toxicity of these drugs.
MAOIs: May produce severe reactions.
Herbal
St. John's wort: May increase the risk of adverse effects.
Food
None known.

DIAGNOSTIC TEST EFFECTS
None known.

SIDE EFFECTS
Frequent
Headache (36%); dry mouth, somnolence (25%); nausea (22%); dizziness (17%); constipation (14%); insomnia, asthenia, lightheadedness (10%).
Occasional
Dyspepsia, blurred vision (9%); diarrhea, infection (8%); confusion, abnormal vision (7%); pharyngitis (6%); increased appetite (5%); orthostatic hypotension, flushing, feeling of warmth (4%); peripheral edema, cough, flu-like symptoms (3%).

SERIOUS REACTIONS

• Serious reactions, such as hyperthermia, rigidity, myoclonus, extreme agitation, delirium, and coma, will occur if the patient takes an MAOI concurrently or fails to let enough time elapse when switching from an MAOI to nefazodone or vice versa.

PRECAUTIONS & CONSIDERATIONS

Caution is warranted with cerebrovascular or cardiovascular disease, recent MI, dehydration, hypovolemia, cirrhosis, a history of hypomania or mania, and a history of seizures. It is unknown if nefazodone crosses the placenta or is distributed in breast milk. The safety and efficacy of this drug have not been established in children. The elderly and debilitated are more susceptible to side effects. Lower dosages are recommended for the elderly, although no age-related precautions have been noted for this age-group.

Drowsiness, dizziness, and lightheadedness may occur, so avoid alcohol and tasks that require mental alertness or motor skills. B/P and pulse rate should be assessed during therapy.

Administration

! Allow at least 14 days to elapse before switching the patient from an MAOI to nefazodone and at least 7 days to elapse before switching the patient from nefazodone to an MAOI.

Take nefazodone without regard to food.

Nelfinavir
nel-fin'eh-veer
(Viracept)

CATEGORY AND SCHEDULE
Pregnancy Risk Category: B

CLASSIFICATION
Antivirals, protease inhibitors

MECHANISM OF ACTION
Inhibits the activity of HIV-1 protease, the enzyme necessary for the formation of infectious HIV. *Therapeutic Effect:* Formation of immature noninfectious viral particles rather than HIV replication.

PHARMACOKINETICS
Well absorbed after PO administration (absorption increased with food). Protein binding: 98%. Metabolized in the liver. Highly bound to plasma proteins. Eliminated primarily in feces. Unknown if removed by hemodialysis. **Half-life:** 3.5-5 hr.

AVAILABILITY
Powder for Oral Suspension: 50 mg/g.
Tablets: 250 mg, 625 mg.

INDICATIONS AND DOSAGES
▸ **HIV infection**
PO
Adults. 750 mg (three 250-mg tablets) 3 times a day or 1250 mg twice a day in combination with nucleoside analogues (enhances antiviral activity).
Children 2-13 yr. 20-30 mg/kg/dose 3 times a day. Maximum: 750 mg q8hr.

CONTRAINDICATIONS

Concurrent administration with midazolam, rifampin, or triazolam

INTERACTIONS

Drug

Alcohol, psychoactive drugs: May produce additive CNS effects.
Anticonvulsants, rifabutin, rifampin: Decrease nelfinavir plasma concentration.
Indinavir, saquinavir: Increases plasma concentration of these drugs.
Oral contraceptives: Decreases the effects of these drugs.
Ritonavir: Increases nelfinavir plasma concentration.
Herbal
St. John's wort: May decrease plasma concentration and effects of nelfinavir.
Food
All foods: Increase nelfinavir plasma concentration.

DIAGNOSTIC TEST EFFECTS

May decrease Hgb values and neutrophil and WBC counts. May increase serum CK, AST (SGOT), and ALT (SGPT) levels.

SIDE EFFECTS

Frequent (20%)
Diarrhea
Occasional (7%-3%)
Nausea, rash
Rare (2%-1%)
Flatulence, asthenia

SERIOUS REACTIONS

• None known.

PRECAUTIONS & CONSIDERATIONS

Caution is warranted with liver function impairment. Be aware that it is unknown if nelfinavir is distributed in breast milk. There are no age-related precautions noted in children over 2 years old. There is no information on the effects of this drug's use in the elderly. Nelfinavir is not a cure for HIV infection nor does it reduce the risk of transmitting HIV to others, and illnesses associated with advanced HIV infection, including opportunistic infections, may occur.

! Monitor the patient for signs and symptoms of opportunistic infections as evidenced by chills, cough, fever, and myalgia. Expect to check hematology and liver function tests to establish an accurate baseline before beginning drug therapy. Assess pattern of daily bowel activity and stool consistency.

Administration

Take with food, a light meal, or snack. Mix oral powder with a small amount of dietary supplement, formula, milk, soy formula, soy milk, or water. The entire contents must be consumed in order to ingest a full dose. Do not mix with acidic food such as apple juice, applesauce, or orange juice, or with water in its original container. Take the medication every day as prescribed and evenly space drug doses around the clock.

Neomycin

nee-oh-mye'sin
(Myciguent, NeoFradin, Neosulf [AUS])

CATEGORY AND SCHEDULE

Pregnancy Risk Category: C
OTC (topical ointment 0.5% only)

CLASSIFICATION

Antibiotics, aminoglycosides

MECHANISM OF ACTION

An aminoglycoside antibiotic that binds to bacterial micro-organisms. *Therapeutic Effect:* Interferes with bacterial protein synthesis.

AVAILABILITY

Tablets: 500 mg.
Ointment: 0.5% (Myciguent).
Oral Solution: 125 mg/5 ml (Neo-Fradin).

INDICATIONS AND DOSAGES

▸ **Preoperative bowel antisepsis**
PO
Adults, Elderly. 1 g/hr for 4 doses; then 1 g q4hr for 5 doses or 1 g at 1 PM, 2 PM, and 10 PM.
(with erythromycin) on day before surgery.
Children. 90 mg/kg/day in divided doses q4hr for 2 days or 25 mg/kg at 1 PM, 2 PM, and 10 PM on day before surgery.
▸ **Hepatic encephalopathy**
PO
Adults, Elderly. 4-12 g/day in divided doses q4-6hr.
Children. 2.5-7 g/m^2/day in divided doses q4-6hr.
▸ **Diarrhea caused by *Escherichia coli***
PO
Adults, Elderly. 3 g/day in divided doses q6hr.
Children. 50 mg/kg/day in divided doses q6hr.
▸ **Minor skin infections**
TOPICAL
Adults, Elderly, Children. Usual dosage, apply to affected area 1-3 times/day.

CONTRAINDICATIONS

Hypersensitivity to neomycin, other aminoglycosides (cross-sensitivity), or their components

INTERACTIONS

Drug
Nephrotoxic medications, other aminoglycosides, ototoxic medications: May increase nephrotoxicity and ototoxicity if significant systemic absorption occurs.
Herbal
None known.
Food
None known.

DIAGNOSTIC TEST EFFECTS

None known.

SIDE EFFECTS

Frequent
Systemic: Nausea, vomiting, diarrhea, irritation of mouth or rectal area
Topical: Itching, redness, swelling, rash
Rare
Systemic: Malabsorption syndrome, neuromuscular blockade (difficulty breathing, drowsiness, weakness)

SERIOUS REACTIONS

• Nephrotoxicity (as evidenced by increased BUN and serum creatinine levels and decreased creatinine clearance) may be reversible if the drug is stopped at the first sign of nephrotoxic symptoms.
• Irreversible ototoxicity (manifested as tinnitus, dizziness, and impaired hearing) and neurotoxicity (as evidenced by headache, dizziness, lethargy, tremor, and visual disturbances) occur occasionally.
• Severe respiratory depression and anaphylaxis occur rarely.
• Superinfections, particularly fungal infections, may occur.

N

PRECAUTIONS & CONSIDERATIONS

Caution is warranted in elderly patients, infants, and other patients with renal insufficiency or immaturity as well as those with neuromuscular disorders, hearing loss, or vertigo.

Expect to correct dehydration before beginning neomycin therapy. Establish the patient's baseline hearing acuity before beginning therapy. Signs and symptoms of hypersensitivity reaction should be monitored. With topical application, symptoms may include a rash, redness, or itching. If dizziness, impaired hearing, or ringing in the ears occurs, notify the physician.

Administration

Continue taking neomycin for the full course of treatment and space doses evenly around the clock.

Clean the affected area gently before applying the topical preparation.

Neostigmine
nee-oh-stig′meen
(Prostigmin)
Do not confuse neostigmine with physostigmine.

CATEGORY AND SCHEDULE
Pregnancy Risk Category: C

CLASSIFICATION
Cholinesterase inhibitors, musculoskeletal agents, stimulants, muscle

MECHANISM OF ACTION
A cholinergic that prevents destruction of acetylcholine by inhibiting the enzyme acetylcholinesterase, thus enhancing impulse transmission across the myoneural junction. *Therapeutic Effect:* Improves intestinal and skeletal muscle tone; stimulates salivary and sweat gland secretions.

AVAILABILITY
Tablets: 15 mg.
Injection: 0.5 mg/ml, 1 mg/ml.

INDICATIONS AND DOSAGES
▸ **Myasthenia gravis**
PO
Adults, Elderly. Initially, 15-30 mg 3-4 times a day. Increase as necessary. Maintenance: 150 mg/day (range of 15-375 mg).
Children. 2 mg/kg/day or 60 mg/m^2/day divided q3-4hr.
IV, IM, SUBCUTANEOUS
Adults. 0.5-2.5 mg as needed.
Children. 0.01-0.04 mg/kg q2-4hr.
▸ **Diagnosis of myasthenia gravis**
IM
Adults, Elderly. 0.022 mg/kg. If cholinergic reaction occurs, discontinue tests and administer 0.4-0.6 mg or more atropine sulfate
IV
Children. 0.025-0.04 mg/kg preceded by atropine sulfate 0.011 mg/kg subcutaneously.
▸ **Prevention of postoperative urinary retention**
IM, SUBCUTANEOUS
Adults, Elderly. 0.25 mg q4-6hr for 2-3 days.
▸ **Postoperative abdomonial distention and urine retention**
IM, SUBCUTANEOUS
Adults, Elderly. 0.5-1 mg. Catheterize patient if voiding does not occur within 1 hr. After voiding, administer 0.5 mg q3hr for 5 injections.
▸ **Reversal of neuromuscular blockade**
IV
Adults, Elderly. 0.5-2.5 mg given slowly.
Children. 0.025-0.08 mg/kg/dose.
Infants. 0.025-0.1 mg/kg/dose.

CONTRAINDICATIONS
GI or GU obstruction, peritonitis

INTERACTIONS
Drug
Anticholinergics: Reverse or prevent the effects of neostigmine.
Cholinesterase inhibitors: May increase the risk of toxicity.
Neuromuscular blockers: Antagonizes the effects of these drugs.
Procainamide, quinidine: May antagonize the action of neostigmine.
Herbal
None known.
Food
None known.

DIAGNOSTIC TEST EFFECTS
None known.

🔳 IV INCOMPATIBILITIES
None known.
🔳 IV Compatibilities
Glycopyrrolate (Robinul), heparin, ondansetron (Zofran), potassium chloride, thiopental (Pentothal)

SIDE EFFECTS
Frequent
Muscarinic effects (diarrhea, diaphoresis, increased salivation, nausea, vomiting, abdominal cramps or pain)
Occasional
Muscarinic effects (urinary urgency or frequency, increased bronchial secretions, miosis, lacrimation)

SERIOUS REACTIONS
• Overdose produces a cholinergic crisis manifested as abdominal discomfort or cramps, nausea, vomiting, diarrhea, flushing, facial warmth, excessive salivation, diaphoresis, lacrimation, pallor, bradycardia or tachycardia, hypotension, bronchospasm, urinary urgency, blurred vision, miosis, and fasciculation (involuntary muscular contractions visible under the skin).

PRECAUTIONS & CONSIDERATIONS
Caution is warranted with arrhythmias, asthma, bradycardia, epilepsy, hyperthyroidism, peptic ulcer disease, and recent coronary occlusion.

Notify the physician of diarrhea, difficulty breathing, increased salivation, irregular heartbeat, muscle weakness, nausea and vomiting, severe abdominal pain, or increased sweating. Vital signs, muscle strength, and fluid intake and output should be monitored. Therapeutic response to the drug, including decreased fatigue, improved chewing and swallowing, and increased muscle strength, should also be assessed.
Administration
! Discontinue all anticholinesterase therapy at least 8 hours before testing, as prescribed. Plan to give 0.011 mg/kg atropine sulfate IV simultaneously with neostigmine or IM 30 minutes before administering neostigmine to prevent adverse effects. Expect to give larger doses when the patient is most tired.

N

Nesiritide
neh-sir′i-tide
(Natrecor)

CATEGORY AND SCHEDULE
Pregnancy Risk Category: C

CLASSIFICATION
Natriuretic peptide, human B-type

MECHANISM OF ACTION
A brain natriuretic peptide that facilitates cardiovascular homeostasis and fluid status through

counterregulation of the renin-angiotensin-aldosterone system, stimulating cyclic guanosine monophosphate, thereby leading to smooth-muscle cell relaxation. *Therapeutic Effect:* Promotes vasodilation, natriuresis, and diuresis, correcting CHF.

PHARMACOKINETICS

Route	Onset	Peak	Duration
IV	15-30 min	1-2 hr	4 hr

Excreted primarily in the heart by the left ventricle. Metabolized by the natriuretic neutral endopeptidase enzymes on the vascular luminal surface. **Half-life:** 18-23 min.

AVAILABILITY

Injection Powder for Reconstitution: 1.5 mg/5-ml vial.

INDICATIONS AND DOSAGES

▸ **Treatment of acutely decompensated CHF in patients with dyspnea at rest or with minimal activity**
IV BOLUS
Adults, Elderly. 2 mcg/kg followed by a continuous IV infusion of 0.01 mcg/kg/min. May be incrementally increased q3hr to a maximum of 0.03 mcg/kg/min.

CONTRAINDICATIONS

Cardiogenic shock, systolic B/P less than 90 mm Hg

INTERACTIONS

Drug
ACE inhibitors, IV nitroglycerin, milrinone, nitroprusside: May increase risk of hypotension.
Herbal
None known.
Food
None known.

DIAGNOSTIC TEST EFFECTS

None known.

▧ IV INCOMPATIBILITIES

Sodium metabisulfite, bumetanide (Bumex), enalapril (Vasotec), ethacrynic acid (Edecrin), furosemide (Lasix), heparin, hydralazine (Apresoline), insulin

SIDE EFFECTS

Frequent (11%)
Hypotension
Occasional (8%-2%)
Headache, nausea, bradycardia
Rare (1% or less)
Confusion, paresthesia, somnolence, tremor

SERIOUS REACTIONS

• Ventricular arrhythmias, including ventricular tachycardia, atrial fibrillation, AV node conduction abnormalities, and angina pectoris occur rarely.

PRECAUTIONS & CONSIDERATIONS

Caution is warranted with atrial conduction defects, constrictive pericarditis, hypotension, hepatic impairment, pericardial tamponade, renal impairment, restrictive or obstructive cardiomyopathy, significant valvular stenosis, suspected low cardiac filling pressures, and ventricular conduction defects. It is unknown if nesiritide crosses the placenta or is distributed in breast milk. The safety and efficacy of nesiritide have not been established in children. No age-related precautions have been noted in the elderly.

B/P should be obtained immediately before each nesiritide dose, in addition to regular monitoring. Be alert to B/P fluctuations. Place the patient in the supine position with legs elevated unless an excessive reduction in B/P occurs. Intake and output records should be maintained. Notify the physician of chest pain, palpitations, cardiac arrhythmias, decreased urine output, or severe decrease in B/P or heart rate.

Storage

Store vial at room temperature. Once reconstituted, store at room temperature or refrigerate; use within 24 hours.

Administration

! Do not mix with other injections or infusions. Do not give IM.

Reconstitute one 1.5-mg vial with 5 ml D$_5$W, 0.9% NaCl, 0.2% NaCl, or any combination thereof. Swirl or rock gently, and add to 250-ml bag D$_5$W, 0.9% NaCl, 0.2% NaCl, or any combination thereof yielding a solution of 6 mcg/ml. Give initially as an IV bolus over approximately 60 seconds, followed by continuous IV infusion.

Nevirapine

neh-veer′a-peen
(Viramune)

CATEGORY AND SCHEDULE

Pregnancy Risk Category: C

CLASSIFICATION

Antivirals, non-nucleoside reverse transcriptase inhibitors

MECHANISM OF ACTION

A nonnucleoside reverse transcriptase inhibitor that binds directly to HIV-1 reverse transcriptase, thus changing the shape of this enzyme and blocking RNA- and DNA-dependent polymerase activity. *Therapeutic Effect:* Interferes with HIV replication, slowing the progression of HIV infection.

PHARMACOKINETICS

Readily absorbed after PO administration. Protein binding: 60%. Widely distributed. Extensively metabolized in the liver. Excreted primarily in urine. **Half-life:** 45 hr (single dose), 25-30 hr (multiple doses).

AVAILABILITY

Tablets: 200 mg.
Oral Suspension: 50 mg/5 ml.

INDICATIONS AND DOSAGES
▸ **HIV infection**
PO
Adults. 200 mg once a day for 14 days (to reduce the risk of rash). Maintenance: 200 mg twice a day in combination with nucleoside analogues.
Children older than 8 yr. 4 mg/kg once a day for 14 days; then 4 mg/kg twice a day. Maximum: 400 mg/day.
Children 2 mo-8 yr. 4 mg/kg once a day for 14 days; then 7 mg/kg twice a day.

OFF-LABEL USES

To reduce the risk of transmitting HIV from infected mother to newborn

CONTRAINDICATIONS

None known.

INTERACTIONS
Drug
Ketoconazole, oral contraceptives, protease inhibitors: May decrease the plasma concentrations of these drugs.
Rifabutin, rifampin: May decrease nevirapine blood concentration.
Herbal
St. John's wort: May decrease blood concentration and effects of nevirapine.

N

Food
None known.

DIAGNOSTIC TEST EFFECTS
May significantly increase serum bilirubin, GGT, AST (SGOT), and ALT (SGPT) levels. May significantly decrease Hgb level and neutrophil and platelet counts.

SIDE EFFECTS
Frequent (8%-3%)
Rash, fever, headache, nausea, granulocytopenia (more common in children)
Occasional (3%-1%)
Stomatitis (burning, erythema, or ulceration of the oral mucosa; dysphagia)
Rare (less than 1%)
Paresthesia, myalgia, abdominal pain

SERIOUS REACTIONS
• Hepatitis and rash may become severe and life-threatening.

PRECAUTIONS & CONSIDERATIONS
Caution is warranted in elderly patients, infants, and other patients with renal insufficiency or immaturity as well as those with neuromuscular disorders, hearing loss, or vertigo. Expect to correct dehydration before beginning neomycin therapy. Establish the patient's baseline hearing acuity before beginning therapy. Signs and symptoms of hypersensitivity reaction should be monitored. With topical application, symptoms may include a rash, redness, or itching. If dizziness, impaired hearing, or ringing in the ears occur, notify the physician.
Administration
Continue taking neomycin for the full course of treatment and space doses evenly around the clock.
Clean the affected area gently before applying the topical preparation.

Niacin (Vitamin B$_3$; Nicotinic Acid)
nye′a-sin
(Niacor, Niaspan, Nicotinex, Slo-Niacin)
Do not confuse niacin, Niacor, or Niaspan with minocin, Nitro-Bid.
OTC

CATEGORY AND SCHEDULE
Pregnancy Risk Category: A (C if used at dosages above the recommended daily allowance)

CLASSIFICATION
Antihyperlipidemics, nicotinic acid derivatives, vitamins/minerals

MECHANISM OF ACTION
An antihyperlipidemic, water-soluble vitamin that is a component of two coenzymes needed for tissue respiration, lipid metabolism, and glycogenolysis. Inhibits synthesis of VLDLs. *Therapeutic Effect:* Reduces total, LDL, and VLDL cholesterol levels and triglyceride levels; increases HDL cholesterol concentration.

PHARMACOKINETICS
Readily absorbed from the GI tract. Widely distributed. Metabolized in the liver. Primarily excreted in urine. **Half-life:** 45 min.

AVAILABILITY
Capsules (Timed-Release): 125 mg, 250 mg, 400 mg, 500 mg.
Tablets (Niacor): 50 mg, 100 mg, 250 mg, 500 mg.
Tablets (Timed-Release [Slo-Niacin]): 250 mg, 500 mg, 750 mg.

Tablets (Timed-Release [Niaspan]):
500 mg, 750 mg, 1000 mg.
Elixir (Nicotinex): 50 mg/5 ml.

INDICATIONS AND DOSAGES
▸ **Hyperlipidemia**
PO (IMMEDIATE-RELEASE)
Adults, Elderly. Initially, 50-100 mg
twice a day for 7 days. Increase
gradually by doubling dose qwk up
to 1-1.5 g/day in 2-3 doses.
Maximum: 3 g/day.
Children. Initially, 100-250 mg/day
(maximum: 10 mg/kg/day) in
3 divided doses. May increase by
100 mg/wk or 250 mg q2-3wk.
Maximum: 2250 mg/day.
PO (TIMED-RELEASE)
Adults, Elderly. Initially, 500 mg/day
in 2 divided doses for 1 wk; then
increase to 500 mg twice a day.
Maintenance: 2 g/day.
▸ **Nutritional supplement**
PO
Adults, Elderly. 10-20 mg/day.
Maximum: 100 mg/day.
▸ **Pellegra**
PO
Adults, Elderly. 50-100 mg
3-4 times a day. Maximum:
500 mg/day.
Children. 50-100 mg 3 times a day.

CONTRAINDICATIONS
Active peptic ulcer disease, arterial
hemorrhaging, hepatic dysfunction,
hypersensitivity to niacin or
tartrazine (frequently seen in patients
sensitive to aspirin), severe hypotension

INTERACTIONS
Drug
**Lovastatin, pravastatin,
simvastatin:** May increase the risk
of acute renal failure and
rhabdomyolysis.
Herbal
None known.

Food
Alcohol: May increase risk of
niacin side effects, such as flushing.

DIAGNOSTIC TEST EFFECTS
May increase serum uric acid level.

SIDE EFFECTS
Frequent
Flushing (especially of the face and
neck) occurring within 20 minutes
of drug administration and lasting
for 30-60 minutes, GI upset,
pruritus
Occasional
Dizziness, hypotension, headache,
blurred vision, burning or tingling of
skin, flatulence, nausea, vomiting,
diarrhea
Rare
Hyperglycemia, glycosuria, rash,
hyperpigmentation, dry skin

SERIOUS REACTIONS
• Arrhythmias occur rarely.

N

PRECAUTIONS & CONSIDERATIONS
Caution is warranted with diabetes
mellitus, gallbladder disease, gout,
and a history of hepatic disease or
jaundice. Niacin is not recommended for use during pregnancy
and lactation. Niacin is distributed in
breast milk and is not recommended
during lactation. No age-related
precautions have been noted in children or the elderly. Niacin use is not
recommended for use in children
younger than 2 years of age.
  Be aware that itching, flushing of
the skin, sensation of warmth, and
tingling may occur. Notify the physician of dark urine, dizziness, loss of
appetite, nausea, vomiting, weakness, yellowing of the skin, blurred
vision, or headache. Pattern of daily
bowel activity and stool consistency
should be assessed. Blood glucose
level, serum cholesterol and

triglyceride levels, and hepatic function test results should be checked at baseline and periodically during treatment.

Administration

Take niacin at bedtime without regard to meals.

Nicardipine

nye-card'i-peen

(Cardene, Cardene IV, Cardene SR)

Do not confuse nicardipine with nifedipine, Cardene with codeine, or Cardene SR with Cardizem SR or codeine.

CATEGORY AND SCHEDULE

Pregnancy Risk Category: C

CLASSIFICATION

Calcium channel blockers

MECHANISM OF ACTION

An antianginal and antihypertensive agent that inhibits calcium ion movement across cell membranes, depressing contraction of cardiac and vascular smooth muscle. *Therapeutic Effect:* Increases heart rate and cardiac output. Decreases systemic vascular resistance and B/P.

PHARMACOKINETICS

Route	Onset	Peak	Duration
PO	N/A	1-2 hr	8 hr

Rapidly, completely absorbed from the GI tract. Protein binding: 95%. Undergoes first-pass metabolism in the liver. Primarily excreted in urine.

Not removed by hemodialysis. **Half-life:** 2-4 hr.

AVAILABILITY

Capsules (Cardene): 20 mg, 30 mg.
Capsules, (Sustained-Release [Cardene SR]): 30 mg, 45 mg, 60 mg.
Injection (Cardene IV): 2.5 mg/ml.

INDICATIONS AND DOSAGES

▶ **Chronic stable (effort-associated) angina**

PO

Adults, Elderly. Initially, 20 mg 3 times a day. Range: 20-40 mg 3 times a day.

▶ **Essential hypertension**

PO

Adults, Elderly. Initially, 20 mg 3 times a day. Range: 20-40 mg 3 times a day.

PO (SUSTAINED-RELEASE)

Adults, Elderly. Initially, 30 mg twice a day. Range: 30-60 mg twice a day.

▶ **Short-term treatment of hypertension when oral therapy is not feasible or desirable (substitute for oral nicardipine)**

IV

Adults, Elderly. 0.5 mg/hr (for patient receiving 20 mg PO q8hr); 1.2 mg/hr (for patient receiving 30 mg PO q8hr); 2.2 mg/hr (for patient receiving 40 mg PO q8hr).

▶ **Patients not already receiving nicardipine**

IV

Adults, Elderly (gradual B/P decrease). Initially, 5 mg/hr. May increase by 2.5 mg/hr q15min. After B/P goal is achieved, decrease rate to 3 mg/hr.

Adults, Elderly (rapid B/P decrease). Initially, 5 mg/hr. May increase by 2.5 mg/hr q5min. Maximum: 15 mg/hr until desired B/P attained. After B/P goal achieved, decrease rate to 3 mg/hr.

▸ **Changing from IV to oral antihypertensive therapy**
Adults, Elderly. Begin antihypertensives other than nicardipine when IV has been discontinued; for nicardipine, give first dose 1 hr before discontinuing IV.
▸ **Dosage in hepatic impairment**
For adults and elderly patients, initially give 20 mg twice a day; then titrate.
▸ **Dosage in renal impairment**
For adults and elderly patients, initially give 20 mg q8hr (30 mg twice a day [sustained-release capsules]); then titrate.

OFF-LABEL USES
Treatment of associated neurologic deficits, Raynaud's phenomenon, subarachnoid hemorrhage, vasospastic angina

CONTRAINDICATIONS
Atrial fibrillation or flutter associated with accessory conduction pathways, cardiogenic shock, CHF, second- or third-degree heart block, severe hypotension, sinus bradycardia, ventricular tachycardia, within several hours of IV beta-blocker therapy

INTERACTIONS
Drug
Beta-blockers: May have additive effect.
Digoxin: May increase nicardipine blood concentration.
Hypokalemia-producing agents (such as furosemide and certain other diuretics): May increase risk of arrhythmias.
Procainamide, quinidine: May increase risk of QT-interval prolongation.
Herbal
None known.
Food
Grapefruit, grapefruit juice: May alter absorption of nicardipine.

DIAGNOSTIC TEST EFFECTS
None known.

IV INCOMPATIBILITIES
Furosemide (Lasix), heparin, thiopental (Pentothal)
IV Compatibilities
Diltiazem (Cardizem), dobutamine (Dobutrex), dopamine (Intropin), epinephrine, hydromorphone (Dilaudid), labetalol (Trandate), lorazepam (Ativan), midazolam (Versed), milrinone (Primacor), morphine, nitroglycerin, norepinephrine (Levophed)

SIDE EFFECTS
Frequent (10%-7%)
Headache, facial flushing, peripheral edema, lightheadedness, dizziness
Occasional (6%-3%)
Asthenia (loss of strength, energy), palpitations, angina, tachycardia
Rare (less than 2%)
Nausea, abdominal cramps, dyspepsia, dry mouth, rash

SERIOUS REACTIONS
• Overdose produces confusion, slurred speech, somnolence, marked hypotension, and bradycardia.

PRECAUTIONS & CONSIDERATIONS
Caution is warranted with cardiomyopathy, edema, hepatic or renal impairment, severe left ventricular dysfunction, sick sinus syndrome and in those concurrently receiving beta blockers or digoxin. It is unclear if nicardipine crosses the placenta. It should only be administered when the benefit to the mother exceeds the risk to the fetus. It is unknown if nicardipine is distributed in breast milk. The safety and efficacy of nicardipine have not been established in children. In the elderly, age-related renal impairment may require cautious use. Alcohol and caffeine

N

should be limited while taking nicardipine.

Notify the physician if anginal pain is not relieved by the medication and if constipation, dizziness, irregular heartbeat, nausea, shortness of breath, or swelling, or symptoms of hypotension such as lightheadedness occurs. B/P for hypotension, skin for dermatitis, facial flushing and rash, liver function test results, EKG and pulse for tachycardia should be assessed. The onset, type (sharp, dull, or squeezing), radiation, location, intensity, and duration of anginal pain and its precipitating factors, such as exertion and emotional stress should be recorded. Be aware that concurrent administration of sublingual nitroglycerin therapy may be used for relief of anginal pain.

Storage
Store at room temperature. Store diluted IV solution for up to 24 hours at room temperature.

Administration
Do not crush, open, or break sustained-release capsules. Take oral nicardipine without regard to food.

For IV use, dilute each 25-mg ampoule with 250 ml D_5W, 0.9% NaCl, 0.45% NaCl, or any combination thereof to provide a concentration of 1 mg/10 ml. Maximum concentration is 4 mg/10 ml. Give by slow IV infusion. Change IV site every 12 hours if drug is administered by a peripheral rather than a central venous catheter line.

Nicotine
nik'o-teen
(Commit, Habitrol [CAN], NicoDerm [CAN], NicoDerm CQ, Nicorette, Nicorette Plus [CAN], Nicotrol, Nicotrol NS, Nicotrol Patch [CAN])
Do not confuse Nicoderm with Nitroderm.

CATEGORY AND SCHEDULE
Pregnancy Risk Category: C (chewing gum), D (transdermal) OTC (Nicoderm transdermal patch, Nicotrol transdermal patch, Nicorette chewing gum)

CLASSIFICATION
Stimulants, central nervous system

MECHANISM OF ACTION
A cholinergic-receptor agonist binds to acetylcholine receptors, producing both stimulating and depressant effects on the peripheral and central nervous systems. *Therapeutic Effect:* Provides a source of nicotine during nicotine withdrawal and reduces withdrawal symptoms.

PHARMACOKINETICS
Absorbed slowly after transdermal administration. Protein binding: 5%. Metabolized in the liver. Excreted primarily in urine. **Half-life:** 4 hr.

AVAILABILITY
Chewing Gum (Nicorette, OTC): 2 mg, 4 mg.
Lozenge (Commit): 2 mg, 4 mg.
Transdermal patch (NicoDerm CQ, Nicotrol): 7 mg, 14 mg, 21 mg.
Nasal Spray (Nicotrol NS): 0.5 mg/spray.
*Inhalation (Nicotrol Inhaler):*10 mg cartridge.

INDICATIONS AND DOSAGES
▸ **Smoking cessation aid to relieve nicotine withdrawal symptoms**
PO (CHEWING GUM)
Adults, Elderly. Usually, 10-12 pieces/day. Maximum: 30 pieces/day.
PO (LOZENGE)
! For those who smoke the first cigarette within 30 min of waking, administer the 4-mg lozenge; otherwise administer the 2-mg lozenge
Adults, Elderly. One 4-mg or 2-mg lozenge q1-2hr for the first 6 wk; one lozenge q2-4hr for wk 7-9; and one lozenge q4-8hr for wk 10-12. Maximum: one lozenge at a time, 5 lozenges/6 hr, 20 lozenges/day.
TRANSDERMAL
Adults, Elderly who smoke 10 cigarettes or more per day. Follow the guidelines below.
Step 1: 21 mg/day for 4-6 wk.
Step 2: 14 mg/day for 2 wk.
Step 3: 7 mg/day for 2 wk.
Adults, Elderly who smoke less than 10 cigarettes per day. Follow the guidelines below.
Step 1: 14 mg/day for 6 wk.
Step 2: 7 mg/day for 2 wk.
Patients weighing less than 100 lb, patients with a history of cardiovascular disease. Initially, 14 mg/day for 4-6 wk, then 7 mg/day for 2-4 wk.
TRANSDERMAL (NICOTROL)
Adults, Elderly. One patch a day for 6 wk.
NASAL
Adults, Elderly. 1-2 doses/hr (1 dose = 2 sprays [1 in each nostril] = 1 mg). Maximum: 5 doses (5 mg)/hr; 40 doses (40 mg)/day.
INHALER (NICOTROL)
Adults, Elderly. Puff on nicotine cartridge mouthpiece for about 20 min as needed.

CONTRAINDICATIONS
Immediate post MI period, life-threatening arrhythmias, severe or worsening angina

INTERACTIONS
Drug
Beta-adrenergic blockers, bronchodilators (such as theophylline), insulin, propoxyphene: May increase the effects of these drugs.
Herbal
None known.
Food
None known.

DIAGNOSTIC TEST EFFECTS
None known.

SIDE EFFECTS
Frequent
All forms: Hiccups, nausea
Gum: Mouth or throat soreness, nausea, hiccups
Transdermal: Erythema, pruritus, or burning at application site
Occasional
All forms: Eructation, GI upset, dry mouth, insomnia, diaphoresis, irritability
Gum: Hiccups, hoarseness
Inhaler: Mouth or throat irri cough
Rare
All forms: Dizines arthralgia

SERIOUS RE mias,
fusion,
• Overdo, rapid or
palpita ea,
seizu is 40-60 mg.
dia espiratory

N

PRECAUTIONS & CONSIDERATIONS

Caution is warranted with eczematous dermatitis, esophagitis, hyperthyroidism, insulin dependent diabetes mellitus, oral or pharyngeal inflammation, peptic ulcer disease, pheochromocytoma and severe renal impairment. Nicotine passes freely into breast milk and smoking or nicotine gum are associated with a decrease in fetal breathing movements. The use of nicotine is not recommended for breast-feeding women. Nicotine use is not recommended for children. In the elderly, an age-related decrease in cardiac function may require cautious use.

Notify the physician of itching or a persistent rash during treatment with the transdermal patch. Vital signs, including B/P and pulse rate, should be obtained before and during treatment. A baseline EKG should be performed.

Administration

! Expect to individualize nicotine dosage and to administer the drug when the person plans to stop moking.

Chew 1 piece of gum slowly and rmittently for 30 minutes when is an urge to smoke. Chew the distinctive, peppery nicotine slight tingling in mouth When the tingling is almost approximately 1 minute, ewing procedure to slow buccal absorp- too rapidly cause excessive of or resulting in and th r to those the gu s nausea ! For t not swallow dosage,

ase the sons

taking more than 600 mg cimetidine (Tagamet) daily.

Apply the patch as soon as it has been removed from the protective pouch. This wrapping prevents evaporation and loss of nicotine. Use only an intact pouch. Do not cut the patch. Apply the patch only once daily to a hairless, clean, dry area on the upper body or outer arm. Rotate application sites; don't use the same site for 7 days or the same patch for longer than 24 hours. Wash hands with water alone after applying the patch because soap may increase nicotine absorption. To discard a used patch, fold it in half with the sticky sides together, place it in the pouch of the new patch, and discard it in a receptacle that is not accessible to children or pets. Do not smoke while wearing the patch.

To use the inhaler, insert the cartridge into mouthpiece and puff vigorously for 20 minutes.

Nifedipine

nye-fed′i-peen

(Adalat 5 [AUS], Adalat 10 [AUS], Adalat 20 [AUS], Adalat CC, Adalat Oros [AUS], Apo-Nifed [CAN], Nifecard [AUS], Nifedicol XL, Nifehexal [AUS], Novo-Nifedin [CAN], Nyefax [AUS], Procardia, Procardia XL)

Do not confuse nifedipine with nicardipine or nimodipine.

CATEGORY AND SCHEDULE

Pregnancy Risk Category: C

CLASSIFICATION

Calcium channel blockers

MECHANISM OF ACTION

An antianginal and antihypertensive agent that inhibits calcium ion movement across cell membranes, depressing contraction of cardiac and vascular smooth muscle. *Therapeutic Effect:* Increases heart rate and cardiac output. Decreases systemic vascular resistance and B/P.

PHARMACOKINETICS

Route	Onset	Peak	Duration
Sublingual	1-5 min	N/A	N/A
PO	20-30 min	N/A	4-8 hr
PO (extended release)	2 hr	N/A	24 hr

Rapidly, completely absorbed from the GI tract. Protein binding: 92%-98%. Undergoes first-pass metabolism in the liver. Primarily excreted in urine. Not removed by hemodialysis. **Half-life:** 2-5 hr.

AVAILABILITY

Capsules (Procardia): 10 mg.
Tablets (Extended-Release [Adalat CC, Procardia XL]): 30 mg, 60 mg, 90 mg.
Tablets (Extended-Release [Nifedical XL]): 30 mg, 60 mg.

INDICATIONS AND DOSAGES

▶ **Prinzmetal's variant angina, chronic stable (effort-associated) angina**
PO
Adults, Elderly. Initially, 10 mg 3 times a day. Increase at 7- to 14-day intervals. Maintenance: 10 mg 3 times a day up to 30 mg 4 times a day.
PO (Extended-release)
Adults, Elderly. Initially, 30-60 mg/day. Maintenance: Up to 120 mg/day.

▶ **Essential hypertension**
PO (Extended-release)
Adults, Elderly. Initially, 30-60 mg/day. Maintenance: Up to 120 mg/day.

OFF-LABEL USES

Treatment of Raynaud's phenomenon

CONTRAINDICATIONS

Advanced aortic stenosis, severe hypotension

INTERACTIONS

Drug
Beta blockers: May have additive effect.
Digoxin: May increase digoxin blood concentration.
Hypokalemia-producing agents (such as furosemide and certain other diuretics): May increase risk of arrhythmias.
Herbal
None known.
Food
Grapefruit, grapefruit juice: May increase nifedipine plasma concentration.

DIAGNOSTIC TEST EFFECTS

May cause positive ANA and direct Coombs' test.

SIDE EFFECTS

Frequent (30%-11%)
Peripheral edema, headache, flushed skin, dizziness
Occasional (12%-6%)
Nausea, shakiness, muscle cramps and pain, somnolence, palpitations, nasal congestion, cough, dyspnea, wheezing
Rare (5%-3%)
Hypotension, rash, pruritus, urticaria, constipation, abdominal discomfort, flatulence, sexual difficulties

N

SERIOUS REACTIONS

- Nifedipine may precipitate CHF and MI in patients with cardiac disease and peripheral ischemia.
- Overdose produces nausea, somnolence, confusion, and slurred speech.

PRECAUTIONS & CONSIDERATIONS

Caution is warranted with impaired hepatic and renal function. It is unclear if nifedipine crosses the placenta. It should be administered only when the benefit to the mother outweighs the risk to the fetus. An insignificant amount of nifedipine is distributed in breast milk. The safety and efficacy of nifedipine have not been established in children. In the elderly, age-related renal impairment may require cautious use. Grapefruit juice, which may increase nifedipine blood concentration, should be avoided. Alcohol and tasks that require alertness and motor skills should also be avoided.

Dizziness or lightheadedness may occur. Notify the physician if irregular heartbeat, prolonged dizziness, nausea, or shortness of breath occurs. B/P and liver function should be monitored. Skin should be assessed for flushing and peripheral edema, especially behind the medial malleolus and the sacral area. The onset, type (sharp, dull, or squeezing), radiation, location, intensity, and duration of anginal pain and its precipitating factors, such as exertion and emotional stress should be recorded. Be aware that concurrent administration of sublingual nitroglycerin therapy may be used for relief of anginal pain.

Storage

Store at room temperature. Store diluted IV solution for up to 24 hours at room temperature.

Administration

Do not crush or break extended-release tablets. Take oral nifedipine without regard to meals.

! May give 10-20 mg of nifedipine sublingually as needed for acute attack of angina.

Capsules must be punctured with a sterile pin or needle and squeezed to express liquid under the tongue.

Nilutamide
nih-lute′ah-myd
(Anandron [CAN], Nilandron)

CATEGORY AND SCHEDULE
Pregnancy Risk Category: C

CLASSIFICATION
Antineoplastics, antiandrogens, hormones/hormone modifiers

MECHANISM OF ACTION

An antiandrogen hormone and antineoplastic agent that competitively inhibits androgen action by binding to androgen receptors in target tissue. *Therapeutic Effect:* Decreases growth of abnormal prostate tissue.

AVAILABILITY
Tablets: 150 mg.

INDICATIONS AND DOSAGES
▸ **Prostatic carcinoma**
PO
Adults, Elderly. 300 mg once a day for 30 days, then 150 mg once a day. Begin on day of, or day after, surgical castration.

CONTRAINDICATIONS
Severe hepatic impairment, severe respiratory insufficiency

INTERACTIONS
Drug
None known.
Herbal
None known.
Food
None known.

DIAGNOSTIC TEST EFFECTS
May increase serum bilirubin, creatinine, AST (SGOT), and ALT (SGPT) levels.

SIDE EFFECTS
Frequent (greater than 10%)
Hot flashes, delay in recovering vision after bright illumination (such as sun, television, bright lights), decreased libido, diminished sexual function, mild nausea, gynecomastia, alcohol intolerance
Occasional (less than 10%)
Constipation, hypertension, dizziness, dyspnea, UTIs

SERIOUS REACTIONS
• Interstitial pneumonitis occurs rarely.

PRECAUTIONS & CONSIDERATIONS
Caution is warranted with hepatitis and markedly increased serum hepatic function test results. Avoid driving at night. Tinted glasses are recommended to help decrease the visual effect of bright headlights and streetlights.

Notify the physician if signs of hepatotoxicity occur, such as abdominal pain, dark urine, fatigue, and jaundice. A baseline chest X-ray and liver function test results should be obtained before therapy and periodically during long-term therapy.
Administration
Take oral nilutamide with or without food.

Nimodipine
nye-mode′i-peen
(Nimotop)
Do not confuse with nifedipine.

CATEGORY AND SCHEDULE
Pregnancy Risk Category: C

CLASSIFICATION
Calcium channel blockers

MECHANISM OF ACTION
A cerebral vasospasm agent that inhibits movement of calcium ions across vascular smooth-muscle cell membranes. *Therapeutic Effect:* Produces favorable effect on severity of neurologic deficits due to cerebral vasospasm. Exerts greatest effect on cerebral arteries; may prevent cerebral spasm.

PHARMACOKINETICS
Rapidly absorbed from the GI tract. Protein binding: 95%. Metabolized in the liver. Excreted in urine; eliminated in feces. Not removed by hemodialysis. **Half-life:** terminal, 3 hr.

AVAILABILITY
Capsules: 30 mg.

INDICATIONS AND DOSAGES
▶ **Improvement neurologic deficits after subarachnoid hemorrhage from ruptured congenital aneurysms**
PO
Adults, Elderly. 60 mg q4hr for 21 days. Begin within 96 hr of subarachnoid hemorrhage.

OFF-LABEL USES
Treatment of chronic and classic migraine, chronic cluster headaches

CONTRAINDICATIONS
Atrial fibrillation or flutter, cardiogenic shock, CHF, heart block, sinus bradycardia, ventricular tachycardia, within several hours of IV beta-blocker therapy

INTERACTIONS
Drug
Beta-blockers: May prolong SA and AV conduction, which may lead to severe hypotension, bradycardia, and cardiac failure.
Erythromycin, itraconazole, ketoconazole, protease inhibitors: May inhibit the metabolism of nimodipine.
Rifabutin, rifampin: May increase the metabolism of nimodipine.
Herbal
Garlic: May increase antihypertensive effect.
Ginseng, yohimbe: May worsen hypertension.
Food
Grapefruit juice: May increase nimodipine blood concentration and risk of toxicity.

DIAGNOSTIC TEST EFFECTS
None known.

SIDE EFFECTS
Occasional (6% -2%)
Hypotension, peripheral edema, diarrhea, headache
Rare (less than 2%)
Allergic reaction (rash, hives), tachycardia, flushing of skin

SERIOUS REACTIONS
• Overdose produces nausea, weakness, dizziness, somnolence, confusion, and slurred speech.

PRECAUTIONS & CONSIDERATIONS
Caution is warranted with impaired hepatic and renal function. It is unknown if nimodipine crosses the placenta or is distributed in breast milk. The safety and efficacy of nimodipine have not been established in children. In the elderly, age-related renal impairment may require cautious use. The elderly may also experience greater hypotensive response and constipation.

Notify the physician if constipation, dizziness, irregular heartbeat, nausea, shortness of breath, or swelling occurs. Liver function, neurologic response, B/P, and heart rate should be assessed before and during therapy. If the pulse rate is 60 beats/minute or lower or systolic B/P is less than 90 mm Hg, withhold the medication and contact the physician.
Administration
If unable to swallow, place a hole in both ends of a capsule with an 18-gauge needle to extract contents into a syringe. Empty contents of syringe into an NG tube; flush tube with 30 ml normal saline.

Nisoldipine
nye-soul-dih-peen
(Sular)
Do not confuse with nicardipine.

CATEGORY AND SCHEDULE
Pregnancy Risk Category: C

CLASSIFICATION
Calcium channel blockers

MECHANISM OF ACTION
A calcium channel blocker that inhibits calcium ion movement across cell membrane, depressing

contraction of cardiac and vascular smooth muscle. *Therapeutic Effect:* Increases heart rate and cardiac output. Decreases systemic vascular resistance and blood pressure (B/P).

PHARMACOKINETICS
Poor absorption from the gastrointestinal (GI) tract. Food increases bioavailability. Protein binding: more than 99%. Metabolism occurs in the gut wall. Primarily excreted in urine. Not removed by hemodialysis.
Half-life: 7-12 hr.

AVAILABILITY
Tablets (extended-release): 10 mg, 20 mg, 30 mg, 40 mg (Sular).

INDICATIONS AND DOSAGES
▸ **Hypertension**
PO
Adults. Initially, 20 mg once daily, then increase by 10 mg per week, or longer intervals until therapeutic B/P response is attained.
Elderly. Initially, 10 mg once daily. Increase by 10 mg per week to therapeutic response. Maintenance: 20-40 mg once daily. Maximum: 60 mg once daily.

OFF-LABEL USES
Stable angina pectoris, CHF

CONTRAINDICATIONS
Sick-sinus syndrome/second- or third-degree AV block (except in presence of pacemaker), hypersensitivity to nisoldipine or any component of the formulation

INTERACTIONS
Drug
Amiodarone: May increase risk of bradycardia, atrioventricular block and/or sinus arrest.
Beta-blockers: May have additive effect.

Delavirdine, ketoconazole, voriconazole: May increase serum nisoldipine concentrations.
Digoxin: May increase digoxin blood concentration.
Epirubicin: May increase risk of heart failure.
Fentanyl: May increase risk of severe hypotension.
Phenytoin, fosphenytoin: May decrease nisoldipine concentrations.
NSAIDs, oral anticoagulants: May increase risk of gastrointestinal hemorrhage and/or antagonism of hypotensive effect.
Quinidine: May increase risk of quinidine toxicity.
Quinupristin/dalfopristin, saquinavir: May increase risk of nisoldipine toxicity.
Rifampin: May decrease nisoldipine efficacy.
Herbal
Licorice, Ma huang, peppermint oil, yohimbine: May decrease effectiveness of nisoldipine.
St. John's Wort: May decrease bioavailability of nisoldipine.
Food
Grapefruit and grapefruit juice: May increase nisoldipine plasma concentration.

DIAGNOSTIC TEST EFFECTS
None known.

✹ IV INCOMPATIBILITIES
None known.
▧ IV Compatibilities
None known.

SIDE EFFECTS
Frequent
Giddiness, dizziness, lightheadedness, peripheral edema, headache, flushing, weakness, nausea
Occasional
Transient hypotension, heartburn, muscle cramps, nasal congestion,

N

cough, wheezing, sore throat, palpitations, nervousness, mood changes
Rare
Increase in frequency, intensity, duration of anginal attack during initial therapy

SERIOUS REACTIONS
• May precipitate congestive heart failure (CHF) and myocardial infarction (MI) in patients with cardiac disease and peripheral ischemia.
• Overdose produces nausea, drowsiness, confusion, and slurred speech.

PRECAUTIONS & CONSIDERATIONS
Caution is warranted with impaired liver or renal function, aortic stenosis, or cirrhosis. It is unknown if nisoldipine crosses the placenta or is distributed in breast milk. Safety and efficacy of nisoldipine have not been established in children. Age-related renal impairment may require cautious use in the elderly. Avoid high fat meals and grapefruit juice after taking medication because it may alter absorption.

Rise slowly from lying to sitting position and permit legs to dangle from bed momentarily before standing to reduce hypotensive effect. Contact physician if irregular heartbeat, shortness of breath, pronounced dizziness, or nausea occurs.
Storage
Store at room temperature.
Administration
Swallow capsule whole. Do not chew, divide, or crush. Take at the same time each day to ensure minimal fluctuation of serum levels.

Nitazoxanide
nigh-tazz-oks'ah-nide
(Alinia)

CATEGORY AND SCHEDULE
Pregnancy Risk Category: B

CLASSIFICATION
Antiprotozoals

MECHANISM OF ACTION
An antiparasitic that interferes with the body's reaction to pyruvate ferredoxin oxidoreductase, an enzyme essential for anaerobic energy metabolism. *Therapeutic Effect:* Produces antiprotozoal activity, reducing or terminating diarrheal episodes.

PHARMACOKINETICS
Rapidly hydrolyzed to an active metabolite. Protein binding: 99%. Excreted in the urine, bile, and feces. **Half-life:** 2-4 hr.

AVAILABILITY
Powder for Oral Suspension: 100 mg/5 ml.

INDICATIONS AND DOSAGES
▸ **Diarrhea**
PO
Children 12 yr and older. 200 mg q12hr.
Children 4-11 yr. 200 mg (10 ml) q12hr for 3 days.
Children 12-47 mo. 100 mg (5 ml) q12hr for 3 days.

CONTRAINDICATIONS
History of sensitivity to aspirin and salicylates

INTERACTIONS
Drug
None known.

Herbal
None known.
Food
None known.

DIAGNOSTIC TEST EFFECTS
May increase serum creatinine and
ALT (SGPT) levels.

SIDE EFFECTS
Occasional (8%)
Abdominal pain
Rare (2%-1%)
Diarrhea, vomiting, headache

SERIOUS REACTIONS
• None known.

PRECAUTIONS & CONSIDERATIONS
Caution is warranted with biliary or
hepatic disease, GI disorders, and
renal impairment. It is unknown if
nitazoxanide is distributed in breast
milk. The safety and efficacy of nitazoxanide have not been established
in children older than 11 years of
age. Nitazoxanide is not indicated
for use in the elderly. Pattern of daily
bowel activity and stool consistency,
electrolytes, and hydration status
should be monitored.
Storage
Store unreconstituted powder at
room temperature. Reconstituted
solution is stable for 7 days at room
temperature.
Administration
Reconstitute oral suspension with
48 ml water to provide a concentration of 100 mg/5 ml. Shake vigorously to suspend powder. Take with
food. Be aware that the oral suspension of nitazoxanide contains 1.48 g
of sucrose per 5 ml.

Nitrofurantoin
nye-troe-fyoor'an-toyn
(Apo-Nitrofurantoin [CAN],
Furadantin, Macrobid,
Macrodantin, Novo-Furan [CAN],
Ralodantin [AUS])

CATEGORY AND SCHEDULE
Pregnancy Risk Category: B

CLASSIFICATION
Antibiotics, nitrofurans

MECHANISM OF ACTION
An antibacterial UTI agent that
inhibits the synthesis of bacterial
DNA, RNA, proteins, and cell walls
by altering or inactivating ribosomal
proteins. *Therapeutic Effect:*
Bacteriostatic (bactericidal at high
concentrations).

PHARMACOKINETICS
Microcrystalline form rapidly and
completely absorbed; macrocrys-
talline form more slowly absorbed.
Food increases absorption. Protein
binding: 40%. Primarily concentrated
in urine and kidneys. Metabolized in
most body tissues. Primarily excreted
in urine. Removed by hemodialysis.
Half-life: 20-60 min.

AVAILABILITY
*Capsules (Macrobid [macrocrys-
talline]):* 100 mg.
*Capsules (Macrodantin [macrocrys-
talline]):* 25 mg, 50 mg, 100 mg
*Oral Suspension (Furadantin
[microcrystalline]):* 25 mg/5 ml.

INDICATIONS AND DOSAGES
▸ **Urinary tract infections (UTIs)**
PO
Adults, Elderly. (Furadantin,
Macrodantin): 50-100 mg q6hr.

N

(Macrobid): 100 mg 2 times/day.
Maximum: 400 mg/day.
Children. (Furadantin,
Macrodantin): 5-7 mg/kg/day in
divided doses q6hr. Maximum:
400 mg/day.
▶ **Long-term prevention of UTIs**
PO
Adults, Elderly. 50-100 mg at
bedtime.
Children. 1-2 mg/kg/day as a single
dose. Maximum: 100 mg/day.

OFF-LABEL USES
Prevention of bacterial UTIs

CONTRAINDICATIONS
Anuria, oliguria, substantial renal
impairment (creatinine clearance
less than 40 ml/min); infants
younger than 1 mo old because of
the risk of hemolytic anemia

INTERACTIONS
Drug
Hemolytics: May increase the risk
of nitrofurantoin toxicity.
Neurotoxic medications:
May increase the risk of
neurotoxicity.
Probenecid: May increase blood
concentration and toxicity of nitrofu-
rantoin.
Herbal
None known.
Food
None known.

DIAGNOSTIC TEST EFFECTS
None known.

SIDE EFFECTS
Frequent
Anorexia, nausea, vomiting, dark
urine
Occasional
Abdominal pain, diarrhea, rash,
pruritus, urticaria, hypertension,
headache, dizziness, drowsiness

Rare
Photosensitivity, transient alopecia,
asthmatic exacerbation in those with
history of asthma

SERIOUS REACTIONS
• Superinfection, hepatotoxicity,
peripheral neuropathy (may be irreversible), Stevens-Johnson
syndrome, permanent pulmonary
function impairment, and anaphylaxis occur rarely.

PRECAUTIONS & CONSIDERATIONS
Caution is warranted with debilitated
patients (greater risk of peripheral
neuropathy) and in patients with
anemia, diabetes mellitus, electrolyte
imbalance, G6PD deficiency
(greater risk of hemolytic anemia),
renal impairment, or vitamin B deficiency. Nitrofurantoin readily crosses
the placenta and is distributed in
breast milk. Nitrofurantoin use is
contraindicated at term and during
breast-feeding if the infant is
suspected of having glucose-6-
phosphate dehydrogenase (G6PD)
deficiency. No age-related precautions
have been noted in children older
than 1 month. Elderly patients are
more likely to develop acute
pneumonitis and peripheral neuropathy and may require a dosage adjustment because of age-related renal
impairment. Avoid sun and ultraviolet light.
   Urine may turn dark yellow or
brown. Hair loss may occur but is
only temporary. Notify the physician
if chest pain, cough, difficult breathing, fever, or numbness and tingling
occur. Intake and output, renal
function, bowel activity, skin for rash,
and breathing should be monitored.
Administration
Take nitrofurantoin with food or
milk to enhance absorption and
reduce GI upset.

Nitrofurazone
nye-troe-fyoor′a-zone
(Furacin)
**Do not confuse with
nitrofurantoin.**

CATEGORY AND SCHEDULE
Pregnancy Risk Category: C
OTC (ointment)

CLASSIFICATION
Anti-infectives, topical, antibiotics, nitrofurans, dermatologics

MECHANISM OF ACTION
A synthetic nitrofuran that inhibits bacterial enzymes involved in carbohydrate metabolism. *Therapeutic Effect:* Inhibits a variety of enzymes. Bactericidal.

PHARMACOKINETICS
Not known.

AVAILABILITY
Cream: 0.2% (Furacin).
Ointment: 0.2% (Furacin).
Solution: 0.2% (Furacin).

INDICATIONS AND DOSAGES
▸ **Burns, catheter-related urinary tract infection, skin grafts**
TOPICAL
Adults. Apply directly on lesion with spatula or place on a piece of gauze first. Use of a bandage is optional. Preparation should remain on lesion for at least 24 hours. Dressing may be changed several times daily or left on the lesion for a longer period.

OFF-LABEL USES
Fire and ant bites, scabies, urethritis, vaginal malodor, vasectomy, wounds

CONTRAINDICATIONS
Hypersensitivity to nitrofurazone or any of its components

INTERACTIONS
Drug
None known.
Herbal
None known.
Food
None known.

DIAGNOSTIC TEST EFFECTS
None known.

SIDE EFFECTS
Occasional
Itching, rash, swelling

SERIOUS REACTIONS
• Use of nitrofurazone may result in bacterial or fungal overgrowth of nonsusceptible pathogens, which may lead to secondary infection.

PRECAUTIONS & CONSIDERATIONS
Caution should be used with renal impairment and glucose-6-phosphate dehydrogenase deficiency. It is unknown if nitrofurazone is distributed in breast milk. Safety and efficacy of nitrofurazone has not been established in children. Age-related renal impairment may require dosage adjustment in the elderly. Irritation, inflammation, or rash should be reported.
Administration
Apply topical formulation directly on the lesion with a spatula or first place on a piece of gauze. Use of a bandage is optional. The preparation should remain on the lesion for at least 24 hours.

Nitroglycerin
nye-troe-gli'ser-in
(Anginine [AUS], Minitran,
Nitradisc [AUS], Nitrek, Nitro-Bid,
Nitro-Dur, Nitrogard, Nitroject
[CAN], Nitrolingual, Nitrong-SR,
NitroQuick, Nitrostat, Nitro-Tab,
Rectogesic [AUS], Transiderm
Nitro [AUS], Trinipatch [CAN])
**Do not confuse nitroglycerin
with nitroprusside; Nitro-Bid
with Nicobid; Nitro-Dur with
Nicoderm; Nitrostat with
Hyperstat, Nilstat, or Nystatin;
or Nitrong-SR with Nizoral.**

CATEGORY AND SCHEDULE
Pregnancy Risk Category: B

CLASSIFICATION
Vasodilators

MECHANISM OF ACTION
A nitrate that decreases myocardial
oxygen demand. Reduces left
ventricular preload and afterload.
Therapeutic Effect: Dilates
coronary arteries and improves
collateral blood flow to ischemic
areas within myocardium.
IV form produces peripheral
vasodilation.

PHARMACOKINETICS

Route	Onset	Peak	Duration
Sublingual	1-3 min	4-8 min	30-60 min
Translingual spray	2 min	4-10 min	30-60 min
Buccal tablet	2-5 min	4-10 min	2 hr
PO (extended-release)	20-45 min	45-120 min	4-8 hr
Topical	15-60 min	30-120 min	2-12 hr
Transdermal patch	40-60 min	60-180 min	18-24 hr
IV	1-2 min	Immediate	3-5 min

Well absorbed after PO, sublingual,
and topical administration.
Undergoes extensive first-pass
metabolism. Metabolized in the liver
and by enzymes in the bloodstream.
Primarily excreted in urine. Not
removed by hemodialysis. **Half-life:**
1-4 min.

AVAILABILITY
*Capsules (Extended-Release
[NitroBid]):* 2.5 mg, 6.5 mg,
9 mg.
Tablets (Buccal [Nitrogard]): 2 mg,
3 mg.
*Tablets (Sublingual [NitroQuick,
Nitrostat, Nitro-Tab]):* 0.4 mg,
0.6 mg.
Spray (Translingual [Nitrolingual]):
0.4 mg/spray.
Infusion Solution: 0.1 mg/ml,
0.2 mg/ml, 0.4 mg/ml.
*Topical Ointment (Nitro-Bid,
Nitrol):* 2%.
Transdermal Patch (Minitran):
0.1 mg/hr, 0.2 mg/hr, 0.3 mg/hr,
0.4 mg/hr.
Transdermal Patch (NitroDur):
0.1 mg/hr, 0.2 mg/hr, 0.3 mg/hr,
0.4 mg/hr, 0.6 mg/hr, 0.8 mg/hr.
Transdermal Patch (Nitrek):
0.2 mg/hr, 0.4 mg/hr, 0.6 mg/hr.

INDICATIONS AND DOSAGES
▸ **Acute relief of angina
pectoris, acute
prophylaxis**
LINGUAL SPRAY
Adults, Elderly. 1 spray onto or
under tongue q3-5min until relief is
noted (no more than 3 sprays in
15-min period).
SUBLINGUAL
Adults, Elderly. 0.4 mg q5min
until relief is noted (no more than
3 doses in 15-min period). Use
prophylactically 5-10 min before
activities that may cause an acute
attack.

▶ **Long-term prophylaxis of angina**
PO (EXTENDED-RELEASE)
Adults, Elderly. 2.5-9 mg q8-12hr.
TOPICAL
Adults, Elderly. Initially, ½ inch
q8hr. Increase by ½ inch with each
application. Range: 1-2 inches q8hr
up to 4-5 inches q4hr.
TRANSDERMAL PATCH
Adults, Elderly. Initially, 0.2-0.4 mg/hr.
Maintenance: 0.4-0.8 mg/hr. Consider
patch on for 12-14 hr, patch off for
10-12 hr (prevents tolerance).
▶ **CHF associated with acute MI**
IV
Adults, Elderly. Initially, 5 mcg/min
via infusion pump. Increase in 5-
mcg/min increments at 3- to 5-min
intervals until B/P response is noted
or until dosage reaches 20 mcg/min,
then increase as needed by
10 mcg/min. Dosage may be further
titrated according to clinical, therapeutic response up to 200 mcg/min.
Children. Initially, 0.25-0.5 mcg/kg/
min; titrate by 0.5-1 mcg/kg/min up
to 20 mcg/kg/min.

CONTRAINDICATIONS
Allergy to adhesives (transdermal),
closed-angle glaucoma, constrictive
pericarditis (IV), early MI (sublingual), GI hypermotility or malabsorption (extended-release), head
trauma, hypotension (IV), inadequate
cerebral circulation (IV), increased
intracranial pressure, nitrates, orthostatic hypotension, pericardial
tamponade (IV), severe anemia,
uncorrected hypovolemia (IV)

INTERACTIONS
Drug
**Other antihypertensives, vasodila-
tors:** May increase risk of orthosta-
tic hypotension.
Sildenafil, tadalafil, vardenafil:
Concurrent use of these drugs
produces significant hypotension.

Herbal
None known.
Food
Alcohol: May increase risk of
orthostatic hypotension.

DIAGNOSTIC TEST EFFECTS
May increase blood methemoglobin,
urine catecholamine, and urine vanillylmandelic acid concentrations.

▓ IV INCOMPATIBILITIES
Alteplase (Activase)
▓ **IV Compatibilities**
Amiodarone (Cordarone), diltiazem
(Cardizem), dobutamine (Dobutrex),
dopamine (Intropin), epinephrine,
famotidine (Pepcid), fentanyl
(Sublimaze), furosemide (Lasix),
heparin, hydromorphone (Dilaudid),
insulin, labetalol (Trandate), lidocaine, lorazepam (Ativan), midazolam (Versed), milrinone (Primacor),
morphine, nicardipine (Cardene),
nitroprusside (Nipride), norepinephrine (Levophed), propofol (Diprivan)

SIDE EFFECTS
Frequent
Headache (possibly severe; occurs
mostly in early therapy, diminishes
rapidly in intensity, and usually
disappears during continued treatment), transient flushing of face and
neck, dizziness (especially if patient
is standing immobile or is in a warm
environment), weakness, orthostatic
hypotension
Sublingual: Burning, tingling sensation at oral point of dissolution
Ointment: Erythema, pruritus
Occasional
GI upset
Transdermal: Contact dermatitis

SERIOUS REACTIONS
• Nitroglycerin should be discontinued if blurred vision or dry mouth
occur.

N

• Severe orthostatic hypotension may occur, manifested by fainting, pulselessness, cold or clammy skin, and diaphoresis.

• Tolerance may occur with repeated, prolonged therapy; minor tolerance may occur with intermittent use of sublingual tablets.

• High doses of nitroglycerin tend to produce severe headache.

PRECAUTIONS & CONSIDERATIONS

Caution is warranted with acute MI, blood volume depletion from therapy, glaucoma (contraindicated in closed-angle glaucoma), hepatic or renal disease, and systolic B/P less than 90 mm Hg. It is unknown if nitroglycerin crosses the placenta or is distributed in breast milk. The safety and efficacy of nitroglycerin have not been established in children. The elderly are more susceptible to the hypotensive effects of nitroglycerin. In the elderly, age-related renal impairment may require cautious use. Alcohol should be avoided because it intensifies the drug's hypotensive effect. If alcohol is ingested soon after taking nitrates, an acute hypotensive episode marked by pallor, vertigo, and a drop in B/P may occur.

Dizziness, lightheadedness, and headache may occur. Rise slowly from a lying to a sitting position and dangle legs momentarily before standing to avoid the drug's hypotensive effect. Notify the physician of facial or neck flushing. The onset, type (sharp, dull, or squeezing), radiation, location, intensity, and duration of anginal pain and its precipitating factors, such as exertion and emotional stress should be recorded before therapy begins. Apical pulse and B/P should be determined before administration and periodically after the dose has been

given. EKG should be closely monitored during IV administration.

Storage

Keep sublingual tablets in their original container. Store solution for injection at room temperature. Keep away from heat and moisture.

Administration

! The cardioverter or defibrillator must not be discharged through a paddle electrode overlying a nitroglycerin system as this may cause burns to the patient or damage the paddle via arching. Do not give nitrates if the patient has recently taken Cialis, Levitra, or Viagra. Swallow extended-release capsules whole; capsules should not be chewed or crushed. Take nitroglycerin preferably on an empty stomach; take the medication with meals if headache occurs during therapy.

Do not shake aerosol canister before lingual spraying. Use the translingual spray only when lying down. Spray under the tongue and avoid inhaling or swallowing lingual spray.

For sublingual use, dissolve under the tongue and avoid swallowing. Administer while seated. To lessen the burning sensation under the tongue, place the tablet in the buccal pouch. Take sublingual tablets at the first sign of angina. If anginal pain is not relieved within 5 minutes of the first dose, dissolve a second tablet under the tongue. If the second dose does not relive anginal pain within 5 minutes, dissolve a third tablet under the tongue. If anginal pain continues, with no relief from the third tablet, immediately notify the physician or seek emergency medical help.

For topical use, spread a thin layer on clean, dry, hairless skin of the upper arm or body, and not below the knee or elbow, using the applicator or dose-measuring papers. Do not use fingers; do not rub or massage into skin.

! Transdermal patch should be removed before cardioversion or defibrillation because the electrical current may cause arching which can burn the person and damage the paddles.

For transdermal use, apply patch on clean, dry, hairless skin of the upper arm or body and not below the knee or elbow.

The IV form is available in ready-to-use injectable containers. To use, dilute vials in 250 or 500 ml D$_5$W or 0.9% NaCl to a maximum concentration of 250 mg/250 ml. Use microdrop or infusion pump.

Nitroprusside

nye-troe-pruss'ide
(Nipride [CAN], Nitropress)
Do not confuse nitroprusside with nitroglycerin or Nitrostat.

CATEGORY AND SCHEDULE
Pregnancy Risk Category: C

CLASSIFICATION
Vasodilators

MECHANISM OF ACTION
A potent vasodilator used to treat emergent hypertensive conditions; acts directly on arterial and venous smooth muscle. Decreases peripheral vascular resistance, preload and after-load; improves cardiac output.
Therapeutic Effect: Dilates coronary arteries, decreases oxygen consumption, and relieves persistent chest pain.

PHARMACOKINETICS

Route	Onset	Peak	Duration
IV	1-10 min	Dependent on infusion rate	Dissipates rapidly after stopping IV

Reacts with Hgb in erythrocytes, producing cyanmethemoglobin, and cyanide ions. Primarily excreted in urine. **Half-life:** less than 10 min.

AVAILABILITY
Injection: 25 mg/ml.
Powder for Injection: 50 mg.

INDICATIONS AND DOSAGES
▶ **Immediate reduction of B/P in hypertensive crisis; to produce controlled hypotension in surgical procedures to reduce bleeding; treatment of acute CHF**
IV
Adults, Elderly, Children.
Initially, 0.3 mcg/kg/min.
Range: 0.5-10 mcg/kg/min.
Do not exceed 10 mcg/kg/min (risk of precipitous drop in B/P).

OFF-LABEL USES
Control of paroxysmal hypertension before and during surgery for pheochromocytoma, peripheral vasospasm caused by ergot alkaloid overdose, treatment adjunct for MI, valvular regurgitation

CONTRAINDICATIONS
Compensatory hypertension (atrioventricular [AV] shunt or coarctation of aorta), inadequate cerebral circulation, moribund patients

N

INTERACTIONS
Drug
Dobutamine: May increase cardiac output and decrease pulmonary wedge pressure.
Hypotension-producing medications: May increase hypotensive effect.
Herbal
None known.
Food
None known.

DIAGNOSTIC TEST EFFECTS
None known.

IV INCOMPATIBILITIES
Cisatracurium (Nimbex)
IV Compatibilities
Diltiazem (Cardizem), dobutamine (Dobutrex), dopamine (Intropin), enalapril (Vasotec), heparin, insulin, labetalol (Normodyne, Trandate), lidocaine, midazolam (Versed), milrinone (Primacor), nitroglycerin, propofol (Diprivan)

SIDE EFFECTS
Occasional
Flushing of skin, increased intracranial pressure, rash, pain or redness at injection site

SERIOUS REACTIONS
• A too rapid IV infusion rate reduces B/P too quickly.
• Nausea, vomiting, diaphoresis, apprehension, headache, restlessness, muscle twitching, dizziness, palpitations, retrosternal pain, and abdominal pain may occur. Symptoms disappear rapidly if rate of administration is slowed or drug is temporarily discontinued.
• Overdose produces metabolic acidosis and tolerance to therapeutic effect.

PRECAUTIONS & CONSIDERATIONS

Caution is warranted with hyponatremia, hypothyroidism, severe hepatic or renal impairment, and in the elderly. It is unknown if nitroprusside crosses the placenta or is distributed in breast milk. The safety and efficacy of nitroprusside have not been established in children. The elderly are more sensitive to the drug's hypotensive effect. In the elderly, age-related renal impairment may require cautious use. Be aware of signs and symptoms of metabolic acidosis, including disorientation, headache, hyperventilation, nausea, vomiting, and weakness. Alcohol should be avoided because it intensifies the drug's hypotensive effect. If alcohol is ingested soon after taking nitrates, an acute hypotensive episode marked by pallor, vertigo, and a drop in B/P may occur.

Notify the physician of pain, redness or swelling at the IV insertion, dizziness, headache, nausea, palpitations, or other unusual signs or symptoms. Desired B/P levels should be determined with the physician before treatment; it is normally maintained at about 30% to 40% below pretreatment levels. B/P and EKG should be monitored before and during treatment. Acid-base balance, electrolyte levels, intake and output, and laboratory results should also be assessed. Nitroprusside should be discontinued if the therapeutic response is not achieved within 10 minutes after IV infusion at 10 mcg/kg/min is initiated.
Storage
Protect solution from light. Use only freshly prepared solution. Once the solution has been prepared, it must be used within 24 hours; do not keep it for longer than 24 hours. Discard unused portion.

Administration
Inspect IV solution, which normally appears as very faint brown. A color change from brown to blue, green, or dark red indicates drug deterioration. Use only freshly prepared solution. Once the solution has been prepared, it must be used within 24 hours; do not keep it for longer than 24 hours. Discard unused portion. Reconstitute 50-mg vial with 2-3 ml D_5W or sterile water for injection without preservative. Further dilute with 250 to 1000 ml D_5W to provide a concentration of 200 mcg/ml to 50 mcg/ml, respectively, up to a maximum concentration of 200 mg/250 ml. Wrap infusion bottle in aluminum foil immediately after mixing. Give by IV infusion only using infusion rate chart provided by manufacturer or facility protocol. Administer using IV infusion pump and lock in rate. The rate of infusion should be monitored frequently. Be alert for extravasation, which produces severe pain and sloughing.

Nizatidine
ni-za'ti-deen
(Axid, Axid AR, Tazac [AUS])

CATEGORY AND SCHEDULE
Pregnancy Risk Category: B
OTC Capsules: 75 mg

CLASSIFICATION
Antihistamines, H2, gastrointestinals

MECHANISM OF ACTION
An antiulcer agent and gastric acid secretion inhibitor that inhibits histamine action at histamine 2 receptors of parietal cells. *Therapeutic Effect:* Inhibits basal and nocturnal gastric acid secretion.

PHARMACOKINETICS
Rapidly, well absorbed from the GI tract. Protein binding: 35%. Metabolized in the liver. Primarily excreted in urine. Not removed by hemodialysis. **Half-life:** 1-2 hr (increased with impaired renal function).

AVAILABILITY
Capsules: 75 mg (OTC), 150 mg, 300 mg.
Oral Solution.

INDICATIONS AND DOSAGES
▶ **Active duodenal ulcer**
PO
Adults, Elderly. 300 mg at bedtime or 150 mg twice a day.
▶ **Prevention of duodenal ulcer recurrence**
PO
Adults, Elderly. 150 mg at bedtime.
▶ **Gastroesophageal reflux disease**
PO
Adults, Elderly. 150 mg twice a day.
▶ **Active benign gastric ulcer**
PO
Adults, Elderly. 150 mg twice a day or 300 mg at bedtime.
▶ **Dyspepsia**
PO (OTC)
Adults, Elderly. 75 mg 30-60 min before meals; no more than 2 tablets a day.
▶ **Dosage in renal impairment**
Dosage adjustment is based on creatinine clearance.

N

Creatinine Clearance	Active Ulcer	Maintenance Therapy
20-50 ml/min	150 mg at bedtime	150 mg every other day
Less than 20 ml/min	150 mg every other day	150 mg q3 days

OFF-LABEL USES
Gastric hypersecretory conditions, multiple endocrine adenoma, Zollinger-Ellison syndrome, weight gain reduction in patients taking Zyprexa

CONTRAINDICATIONS
None known.

INTERACTIONS
Drug
Antacids: May decrease the absorption of nizatidine.
Ketoconazole: May decrease the absorption of ketoconazole.
Herbal
None known.
Food
None known.

DIAGNOSTIC TEST EFFECTS
Interferes with skin tests using allergen extracts. May increase serum alkaline phosphatase, AST (SGOT), and ALT (SGPT) levels.

SIDE EFFECTS
Occasional (2%)
Somnolence, fatigue
Rare (1%)
Diaphoresis, rash

SERIOUS REACTIONS
• Asymptomatic ventricular tachycardia, hyperuricemia not associated with gout, and nephrolithiasis occur rarely.

PRECAUTIONS & CONSIDERATIONS
Caution is warranted with impaired hepatic or renal function. It is unknown if nizatidine crosses the placenta or is distributed in breast milk. The safety and efficacy of nizatidine have not been established in children younger than 16 years of age. No age-related precautions have been noted in the elderly. Tasks that require mental alertness or motor skills should be avoided until response to the drug has been established. Also, avoid alcohol, aspirin, and coffee, all of which may cause GI distress, during nizatidine therapy.

Notify the physician if acid indigestion, gastric distress, or heartburn occurs after 2 weeks of continuous nizatidine therapy. Blood chemistry laboratory test results, including BUN, serum alkaline phosphatase, bilirubin, creatinine, AST (SGOT), and ALT (SGPT) levels to assess hepatic and renal function, should be obtained before and during therapy.
Administration
Take nizatidine without regard to meals; however, it's best given after meals or at bedtime. Take right before eating for heartburn prevention. Do not administer within 1 hour of magnesium- or aluminum-containing antacids because it can decrease the absorption of nizatidine.

Norepinephrine

nor-ep-i-nef'rin
(Levophed)
**Do not confuse Levophed with
Levid, or norepinephrine with
epinephrine.**

CATEGORY AND SCHEDULE
Pregnancy Risk Category: C

CLASSIFICATION
Adrenergic agonists, inotropes

MECHANISM OF ACTION
A sympathomimetic that stimulates
$beta_1$-adrenergic receptors and
alpha-adrenergic receptors, increasing peripheral resistance. Enhances
contractile myocardial force,
increases cardiac output. Constricts
resistance and capacitance vessels.
Therapeutic Effect: Increases
systemic B/P and coronary blood
flow.

PHARMACOKINETICS

Route	Onset	Peak	Duration
IV	Rapid	1-2 min	N/A

Localized in sympathetic tissue.
Metabolized in the liver. Primarily
excreted in urine.

AVAILABILITY
Injection: 1-mg/ml ampules.

INDICATIONS AND DOSAGES
▸ **Acute hypotension unresponsive to
fluid volume replacement**
IV
Adults, Elderly. Initially, administer
at 0.5-1 mcg/min. Adjust rate of flow
to establish and maintain desired B/P
(40 mm Hg below preexisting systolic
pressure). Average maintenance

dose: 8-12 mcg/min.
Children. Initially, 0.05-
0.1 mcg/kg/min; titrate to desired
effect. Maximum: 1-2 mcg/kg/min.
Range: 0.5-3 mcg/min.

CONTRAINDICATIONS
Hypovolemic states (unless as an
emergency measure), mesenteric or
peripheral vascular thrombosis,
profound hypoxia

INTERACTIONS
Drug
Beta blockers: May have mutually
inhibitory effects.
Digoxin: May increase risk of
arrhythmias.
Ergonovine, oxytocin: May
increase vasoconstriction.
**Maprotiline, tricyclic antidepres-
sants:** May increase cardiovascular
effects.
Methyldopa: May decrease the
effects of methyldopa.
Herbal
None known.
Food
None known.

DIAGNOSTIC TEST EFFECTS
None known.

▓ IV INCOMPATIBILITIES
Regular insulin
▓ **IV Compatibilities**
Amiodarone (Cordarone), calcium
gluconate, diltiazem (Cardizem),
dobutamine (Dobutrex), dopamine
(Intropin), epinephrine, esmolol
(Brevibloc), fentanyl (Sublimaze),
furosemide (Lasix), haloperidol
(Haldol), heparin, hydromorphone
(Dilaudid), labetalol (Trandate),
lorazepam (Ativan), magnesium,
midazolam (Versed), milrinone
(Primacor), morphine, nicardipine
(Cardene), nitroglycerin, potassium
chloride, propofol (Diprivan)

N

SIDE EFFECTS

Norepinephrine produces less pronounced and less frequent side effects than epinephrine.

Occasional (5%-3%)

Anxiety, bradycardia, palpitations

Rare (2%-1%)

Nausea, anginal pain, shortness of breath, fever

SERIOUS REACTIONS

• Extravasation may produce tissue necrosis and sloughing.

• Overdose is manifested as severe hypertension with violent headache (which may be the first clinical sign of overdose), arrhythmias, photophobia, retrosternal or pharyngeal pain, pallor, excessive sweating, and vomiting.

• Prolonged therapy may result in plasma volume depletion. Hypotension may recur if plasma volume is not restored.

PRECAUTIONS & CONSIDERATIONS

Caution is warranted with hypertension, hypothyroidism, severe cardiac disease, and concurrent MAOI therapy. Norepinephrine readily crosses the placenta and may produce fetal anoxia due to constriction of uterine blood vessels and uterine contraction. No age-related precautions have been noted in children or the elderly.

B/P and EKG should be monitored continuously. Be alert to precipitous drops in B/P. Intake and output should be assessed hourly, or as ordered. If urine output is less than 30 ml/hour, the infusion should be stopped unless the systolic B/P falls below 80 mm Hg.

Storage

Store ampoules at room temperature.

Administration

! Expect to restore blood and fluid volume before administering norepinephrine.

Do not use if solution is brown or contains precipitate. Add 4 ml (4 mg) to 1 liter of D_5W for a 4-mcg/ml solution. Maximum concentration: 128 mcg/ml. Administer infusion through a central venous catheter, if available, to avoid extravasation. Closely monitor the infusion flow rate with a microdrip or infusion pump. Monitor the B/P every 2 minutes during the infusion until desired therapeutic response is achieved, then every 5 minutes during the remainder of the infusion. Never leave unattended during the infusion. Be alert to any complaint of headache. Plan to maintain B/P at 80 to 100 mm Hg in previously normotensive patients, and 30 to 40 mm Hg below preexisting B/P in previously hypertensive patients. Reduce the infusion gradually, as prescribed. Avoid abrupt withdrawal. Check the peripherally inserted catheter IV site frequently for signs of extravasation, including blanching, coldness, hardness, and pallor to the extremity. If extravasation occurs, expect to infiltrate the affected area with 10 to 15 ml sterile saline containing 5 to 10 mg phentolamine. Know that phentolamine does not alter the pressor effects of norepinephrine.

Norethindrone

nor-eth'in-drone
(Aygestin, Camila, Errin,
Jolivette, Micronor,
Nora-BE, Nor-QD,
Norlutate [CAN])

CATEGORY AND SCHEDULE
Pregnancy Risk Category: X

CLASSIFICATION
Contraceptives,
hormones/hormone modifiers,
progestins

MECHANISM OF ACTION
A synthetic progestin that is
used as a single agent or in
combination with estrogens for
the treatment of gynecological
disorders. It inhibits secretion of
pituitary gonadotropin (LH) which
prevents follicular maturation and
ovulation. *Therapeutic Effect:*
Transforms endometrium from
proliferative to secretory in an
estrogen-primed endometrium,
promotes mammary gland
development, relaxes uterine
smooth muscle.

PHARMACOKINETICS
Rapidly absorbed from the
gastrointestinal (GI) tract. Widely
distributed. Protein binding:
61%. Metabolized in liver. Excreted
in urine and feces. **Half-life:**
4-13 hr.

AVAILABILITY
Tablets: 0.35 mg (Camila, Errin,
Jolivette, Micronor, Nora-BE,
Nor-QD).
Tablets, as norethindrone acetate:
5 mg (Aygestin).

INDICATIONS AND DOSAGES
▸ **Contraception**
PO
Adults. 1 tablet/day.
▸ **Amenorrhea and abnormal uterine bleeding**
PO
Adults. 5-20 mg/day cyclically
(21 days on; 7 days off or continuously) or for acetate salt formulation, 2.5-10 mg cyclically.
▸ **Endometriosis**
PO
Adults. 10 mg/day for 2 weeks,
increase at increments of 5 mg/day
every 2 weeks until 30 mg/day;
continue for 6-9 months or until
breakthrough bleeding demands
temporary termination. For acetate
salt formulation, 5 mg/day for
14 days, increase at increments
of 2.5 mg/day every 2 weeks
up to 15 mg/day continue for
6-9 months or until breakthrough
bleeding demands temporary
termination.

OFF-LABEL USES
Treatment of corpus luteum
dysfunction

CONTRAINDICATIONS
Acute liver disease, benign or malignant liver tumors, hypersensitivity to
norethindrone and any component of
the formulation, known or suspected
carcinoma of the breast, known or
suspected pregnancy, undiagnosed
abnormal genital bleeding

INTERACTIONS
Drug
**Antibiotics such as the penicillins
and erythromycin:** May decrease
effectiveness of norethindrone.
Aprepitant: May decrease the
effects of both drugs.
Benzodiazepines: May increase
risk of benzodiazepine toxicity.

N

Cyclosporine: May increase risk of cyclosporine toxicity.

CYP3A4 inducers (carbamazepine, phenobarbital, phenytoin, rifampin, rifabutin): May decrease the levels and/or effects of norethindrone.

Atorvastatin, rosuvastatin: May increase concentrations of norethindrone.

Amprenavir, nelfinavir, nevirapine, ritonavir: May decrease norethindrone concentrations.

Corticosteroids: May prolong the effects of cortisones.

Fluconazole: May increase risk of adverse effects of norethindrone.

Griseofulvin, modafinil, primidone: May decrease effectiveness of norethindrone.

Lamotrigine: May increase or decrease plasma lamotrigine concentrations.

Thiazolidinediones: May decrease the effects of norethindrone.

Selegiline: May increase the risk of adverse effects of selegiline.

Theophylline: May increase the risk of theophylline toxicity.

Warfarin: May increase or decrease anticoagulant effects.

Zolmitriptan: May increase risk of adverse effects of zolmitriptan.

Herbal

Licorice: May increase risk of fluid retention and elevated blood pressure.

Red clover: May alter effectiveness of norethindrone or increase side effects.

St. John's wort: May decrease plasma concentrations of norethindrone.

Vitamin C (at high doses, more than 1 g/day): May increase adverse effects of norethindrone.

Food

Caffeine: May increase CNS stimulation.

DIAGNOSTIC TEST EFFECTS

May increase LDL concentrations and serum alkaline phosphatase levels. May decrease glucose tolerance and HDL concentrations. May cause abnormal thyroid, metapyrone, liver, and endocrine function tests.

SIDE EFFECTS

Occasional

Breast tenderness, dizziness, headache, breakthrough bleeding, amenorrhea, menstrual irregularity, nausea, weakness

Rare

Mental depression, fever, insomnia, rash, acne, increased breast tenderness, weight gain/loss, changes in cervical erosion and secretions, cholestatic jaundice

SERIOUS REACTIONS

• Thrombophlebitis, cerebrovascular disorders, retinal thrombosis, cholestatic jaundice, and pulmonary embolism occur rarely.

PRECAUTIONS & CONSIDERATIONS

Caution is warranted with conditions aggravated by fluid retention, delayed follicular atresia or ovarian cysts, asthma, cardiac dysfunction, epilepsy, migraine headache, renal insufficiency, diabetes mellitus, and a history of mental depression. Norethindrone is distributed in breast milk and may be harmful to fetus. If pregnancy is suspected, notify physician immediately. Norethindrone should not be used during breast-feeding. Safety and efficacy of this drug have not been established in children. There are no age-related precautions noted in the elderly. Avoid smoking while taking norethindrone.

Menstrual spotting may occur between periods. Pain, redness, swelling, or warmth in the calf, chest pain, migraine headache, peripheral paresthesia, sudden decrease in vision, and sudden shortness of breath should be reported immediately.

Administration

Take norethindrone at the same time each day. Do not take a break between packs.

Norfloxacin

nor-flox′a-sin

(Apo-Norflox [CAN], Insensye [AUS], Norfloxacine [CAN], Noroxin, Novo-Norfloxacin [CAN], PMS-Norfloxacin [CAN], Roxin [AUS])

CATEGORY AND SCHEDULE

Pregnancy Risk Category: C

CLASSIFICATION

Anti-infectives, ophthalmics, antibiotics, quinolones

MECHANISM OF ACTION

A quinolone that inhibits DNA gyrase in susceptible microorganisms, interfering with bacterial cell replication and repair. *Therapeutic Effect:* Bactericidal.

AVAILABILITY

Tablets: 400 mg.
Ophthalmic Solution (Chibroxin): 0.3%.

INDICATIONS AND DOSAGES

▶ **Bacterial conjunctivitis**

The recommended dose in adults and pediatric patients (1 year and older) is 1 or 2 drops 4 times/day for up to 7 days. First day of therapy may be 1 or 2 drops every 2 hours during the working hours.

▶ **Urinary tract infections (UTIs)**

PO

Adults, Elderly. 400 mg twice a day for 7-21 days.

▶ **Prostatitis**

PO

Adults. 400 mg twice a day for 28 days.

▶ **Uncomplicated gonococcal infections**

PO

Adults. 800 mg as a single dose.

▶ **Dosage in renal impairment**

Dosage and frequency are modified based on creatinine clearance.

Creatinine Clearance	Dosage
30 ml/min or higher	400 mg twice a day
Less than 30 ml/min	400 mg once a day

CONTRAINDICATIONS

Children younger than 18 years because of risk arthropathy; hypersensitivity to norfloxacin, other quinolones, or their components

INTERACTIONS

Drug

Antacids, sucralfate: May decrease norfloxacin absorption.

Oral anticoagulants: May increase effects of oral anticoagulants.

Theophylline: Decreases clearance and may increase blood concentration and risk of toxicity of theophylline.

Herbal

None known.

Food

None known.

DIAGNOSTIC TEST EFFECTS

May increase BUN level and serum alkaline phosphatase, bilirubin, creatinine, LDH, AST (SGOT), and ALT (SGPT) levels.

N

SIDE EFFECTS

Burning or discomfort. Other reactions were conjunctival hypermia, chemosis, corneal deposits, photophobia, and a bitter taste following installations.

Frequent
Nausea, headache, dizziness

Rare
Vomiting, diarrhea, dry mouth, bitter taste, nervousness, drowsiness, insomnia, photosensitivity, tinnitus, crystalluria, rash, fever, seizures

SERIOUS REACTIONS

• Superinfection, anaphylaxis, Stevens-Johnson syndrome, and arthropathy occur rarely.
• Hypersensitivity reactions, including photosensitivity (as evidenced by rash, pruritus, blisters, edema, and burning skin), have occurred in patients receiving fluoroquinolones.

PRECAUTIONS & CONSIDERATIONS

Caution is warranted with impaired renal function and a predisposition to seizures. Dizziness, headache, nausea, signs of infection, and vaginitis should be evaluated. Food tolerance should be assessed.

Administration

Take norfloxacin with 8 oz of water 1 hour before or 2 hours after a meal and consume several glasses of water between meals as well as citrus fruits and cranberry juice to acidify urine. Do not take antacids within 2 hours of norfloxacin.

Norgestrel
nor-jes′trel
(Ovrette)

CATEGORY AND SCHEDULE
Pregnancy Risk Category: X

CLASSIFICATION
Contraceptives, hormones/hormone modifiers, progestins

MECHANISM OF ACTION

A progestin that inhibits secretion of pituitary gonadotropin (LH) which prevents follicular maturation and ovulation. *Therapeutic Effect:* Transforms endometrium from proliferative to secretory in an estrogen-primed endometrium, promotes mammary gland development, relaxes uterine smooth muscle.

PHARMACOKINETICS

Well absorbed from the gastrointestinal (GI) tract. Widely distributed. Protein binding: 97%. Metabolized in liver via reduction and conjugation. Primarily excreted in urine. **Half-life:** 20 hr.

AVAILABILITY

Tablets: 0.075 mg (Ovrette).

INDICATIONS AND DOSAGES
▸ **Contraception, female**
PO
Adults. 0.075 mg/day.

OFF-LABEL USES

Endometrial protection, endometriosis, menorrhagia

CONTRAINDICATIONS

Hypersensitivity to norgestrel or any component of the formulation, hypersensitivity to tartrazine, thromboembolic disorders, severe hepatic disease; breast cancer; undiagnosed vaginal bleeding, pregnancy

INTERACTIONS
Drug
Antibiotics, such as the penicillins: May decrease contraceptive efficacy.
Amprenavir, nevirapine, ritonavir: May decrease contraceptive efficacy.
Bromocriptine: May interfere with the effects of bromocriptine.
Aprepitant: May reduce efficacy of norgestrel.
Caffeine: May increase the effects of caffeine.
Fluconazole: May increase risk of norgestrel adverse effects.
Griseofulvin: May decrease contraceptive effectiveness.
Phenobarbital, phenytoin: May decrease contraceptive effectiveness.
Pioglitazone, troglitazone: May decrease contraceptive effectiveness.
Rifampin: May decrease contraceptive effectiveness.
Rosuvastatin: May increase plasma concentrations of norgestrel.
Warfarin: May decrease or increase anticoagulant effects.
Herbal
St. John's wort: May decrease levels of St. John's wort.
Dong quai, black cohosh: May add estrogen activity.
Saw palmetto, red clover, ginseng: May alter contraceptive effectiveness or increase side effects.
Food
None known.

DIAGNOSTIC TEST EFFECTS
None known.

▨ IV INCOMPATIBILITIES
None known.
▨ IV Compatibilities
None known.

SIDE EFFECTS
Frequent
Breakthrough bleeding or spotting at beginning of therapy, amenorrhea, change in menstrual flow, breast tenderness
Occasional
Edema, weight gain or loss, rash, pruritus, photosensitivity, skin pigmentation
Rare
Pain or swelling at injection site, acne, mental depression, alopecia, hirsutism

SERIOUS REACTIONS
• Thrombophlebitis, cerebrovascular disorders, retinal thrombosis, and pulmonary embolism occur rarely.

PRECAUTIONS & CONSIDERATIONS
Caution is necessary with conditions aggravated by fluid retention, diabetes mellitus, and a history of mental depression. Norgestrel is distributed in breast milk and may be harmful to fetus. Norgestrel should not be used during breastfeeding. Safety and efficacy of this drug have not been established in children. There are no age-related precautions noted in the elderly. Avoid smoking while taking norgestrel.

Menstrual spotting may occur between periods. Pain, redness, swelling, or warmth in the calf, chest pain, migraine headache, peripheral paresthesia, sudden decrease in vision, and sudden shortness of breath should be reported immediately.
Administration
If one dose is missed, take as soon as remembered, then next tablet at regular time; if two doses are missed, take 1 tablet as soon as it is remembered, followed by an additional dose that same day at the usual time. When one or two doses

are missed, additional contraceptive measures should be used until 14 consecutive tablets have been taken. If three doses are missed, discontinue norgestrel and use an additional form of birth control until menses or pregnancy is ruled out.

Nortriptyline
nor-trip'ti-leen
(Allegron [AUS], Aventyl, Norventyl, Pamelor)
Do not confuse nortriptyline with amitriptyline, or Aventyl with Ambenyl or Bentyl.

CATEGORY AND SCHEDULE
Pregnancy Risk Category: D

CLASSIFICATION
Antidepressants, tricyclic

MECHANISM OF ACTION
A tricyclic antidepressant that blocks reuptake of the neurotransmitters norepinephrine and serotonin at neuronal presynaptic membranes, increasing their availability at postsynaptic receptor sites. *Therapeutic Effect:* Relieves depression.

AVAILABILITY
Capsules (Aventyl): 10 mg, 25 mg.
Capsules (Pamelor): 10 mg, 25 mg, 75 mg.
Oral Solution (Aventyl, Pamelor): 10 mg/5 ml.

INDICATIONS AND DOSAGES
▸ **Depression**
PO
Adults. 75-100 mg/day in 1-4 divided doses until therapeutic response is achieved. Reduce dosage gradually to effective maintenance level.

Elderly. Initially, 10-25 mg at bedtime. May increase by 25 mg every 3-7 days. Maximum: 150 mg/day.
Children 12 yr and older. 30-50 mg/day in 3-4 divided doses.
Children 6-11 yr. 10-20 mg/day in 3-4 divided doses.
▸ **Enuresis**
PO
Children 12 yr and older. 25-35 mg/day.
Children 8-11 yr. 10-20 mg/day.
Children 6-7 yr. 10 mg/day.

OFF-LABEL USES
Treatment of neurogenic pain, panic disorder; prevention of migraine headache

CONTRAINDICATIONS
Acute recovery period after MI, use within 14 days of MAOIs

INTERACTIONS
Drug
Alcohol, other CNS depressants: May increase CNS and respiratory depression and the hypotensive effects of nortriptyline.
Antithyroid agents: May increase the risk of agranulocytosis.
Cimetidine: May increase the blood concentration and risk of toxicity of nortriptyline.
Clonidine, guanadrel: May decrease the effects of these drugs.
MAOIs: May increase the risk of neuroleptic malignant syndrome, seizures, hyperpyrexia, and hypertensive crisis.
Phenothiazines: May increase the anticholinergic and sedative effects of nortriptyline.
Sympathomimetics: May increase the risk of cardiac effects.
Herbal
None known.
Food
None known.

DIAGNOSTIC TEST EFFECTS

May alter blood glucose level and EKG readings. The therapeutic peak serum level is 6-10 mcg/ml; the therapeutic trough serum level is 0.5-2 mcg/ml. The toxic peak serum level is greater than 12 mcg/ml; the toxic trough serum level is greater than 2 mcg/ml.

SIDE EFFECTS

Frequent
Somnolence, fatigue, dry mouth, blurred vision, constipation, delayed micturition, orthostatic hypotension, diaphoresis, impaired concentration, increased appetite, urine retention
Occasional
GI disturbances (nausea, GI distress, metallic taste), photosensitivity
Rare
Paradoxical reactions (agitation, restlessness, nightmares, insomnia), extrapyramidal symptoms (particularly fine hand tremor)

SERIOUS REACTIONS

• Overdose may produce seizures; cardiovascular effects, such as severe orthostatic hypotension, dizziness, tachycardia, palpitations, and arrhythmias; and altered temperature regulation, such as hyperpyrexia or hypothermia.
• Abrupt discontinuation after prolonged therapy may produce headache, malaise, nausea, vomiting, and vivid dreams.

PRECAUTIONS & CONSIDERATIONS

Caution is warranted with cardiac disease, diabetes mellitus, glaucoma, hiatal hernia, history of seizures, history of urinary obstruction or urine retention, hyperthyroidism, increased IOP, prostatic hypertrophy, hepatic or renal disease, and schizophrenia. Sunscreens and protective clothing should be worn because the drug may cause photosensitivity to sunlight.

Anticholinergic, sedative, and hypotensive effects may occur but tolerance usually develops. Since dizziness may occur, change positions slowly, avoid alcohol and tasks that require alertness or motor skills. Pattern of daily bowel activity and stool consistency, bladder for urine retention, B/P and pulse rate, and EKG should be assessed during therapy.

Administration
! Make sure at least 14 days elapse between the use of MAOIs and nortriptyline. Be aware nortriptyline's therapeutic peak serum level is 6-10 mcg/ml and therapeutic trough serum level is 0.5-2 mcg/ml; nortriptyline's toxic peak serum level is greater than 12 mcg/ml and toxic trough serum level is greater than 2 mcg/ml.

Take nortriptyline with food or milk if GI distress occurs. Nortriptyline's therapeutic effect may be noted in 2 weeks or longer.

N

Nystatin

nye-stat′in
(Mycostatin, Nilstat [CAN], Nyaderm, Nystop)
Do not confuse with Nitrostat.

CATEGORY AND SCHEDULE

Pregnancy Risk Category: C

CLASSIFICATION

Antifungals, topical, dermatologics

MECHANISM OF ACTION
A fungistatic antifungal that binds to sterols in the fungal cell membrane. *Therapeutic Effect:* Increases fungal cell-membrane permeability, allowing loss of potassium and other cellular components.

PHARMACOKINETICS
PO: Poorly absorbed from the GI tract. Eliminated unchanged in feces. Topical: Not absorbed systemically from intact skin.

AVAILABILITY
Oral Suspension (Mycostatin): 100,000 units/ml.
Tablets (Mycostatin): 500,000 units.
Vaginal Tablets: 100,000 units.
Cream (Mycostatin): 100,000 units/g.
Ointment: 100,000 units/g.
Topical Powder (Mycostatin, Nystop): 100,000 units/g.

INDICATIONS AND DOSAGES
▸ **Intestinal infections**
PO
Adults, Elderly. 500,000-1,000,000 units q8hr.
▸ **Oral candidiasis**
PO
Adults, Elderly, Children. 400,000-600,000 units 4 times/day.
Infants. 200,000 units 4 times/day.
▸ **Vaginal infections**
VAGINAL
Adults, Elderly, Adolescents. 1 tablet/day at hs for 14 days.
▸ **Cutaneous candidal infections**
TOPICAL
Adults, Elderly, Children. Apply 2-4 times/day.

OFF-LABEL USES
Prophylaxis and treatment of oropharyngeal candidiasis, tinea barbae, tinea capitis

CONTRAINDICATIONS
None known.

INTERACTIONS
Drug
None known.
Herbal
None known.
Food
None known.

DIAGNOSTIC TEST EFFECTS
None known.

SIDE EFFECTS
Occasional
PO: None known
Topical: Skin irritation
Vaginal: Vaginal irritation

SERIOUS REACTIONS
• High dosages of oral form may produce nausea, vomiting, diarrhea, and GI distress.

PRECAUTIONS & CONSIDERATIONS
It is unknown if nystatin is distributed in breast milk. During pregnancy, vaginal applicators may be contraindicated, requiring manual insertion of tablets. There are no age-related precautions noted for suspension or topical use in children. Be aware that lozenges are not recommended for use in children 5 years old or younger. There are no age-related precautions noted in the elderly.

Confirm that cultures or histologic tests were done for accurate diagnosis before giving the drug. Assess for increased irritation with topical application or increased vaginal discharge with vaginal application. Separate personal items that come in contact with affected areas. Notify the physician if diarrhea, nausea, stomach pain, or vomiting develops.

Administration

Dissolve lozenges (troches) slowly and completely in the mouth for optimal therapeutic effect. Lozenges should not be chewed or swallowed whole.

Shake suspension well before administration. Place and hold the suspension in the mouth or swish throughout the mouth as long as possible before swallowing.

Use nystatin cream or powder sparingly on erythematous areas. Rub the topical form well into affected areas, keep affected areas clean and dry, and wear light clothing for ventilation. Avoid contact with eyes.

Insert the vaginal form high into the vagina at bedtime. Vaginal use should be continued during menses.

N

Octreotide
ok-tree'oh-tide
(Sandostatin, Sandostatin LAR)
Do not confuse octreotide with OctreoScan, or Sandostatin with Sandimmune or Sandoglobulin.

CATEGORY AND SCHEDULE
Pregnancy Risk Category: B

CLASSIFICATION
Antidiarrheals,
gastrointestinals,
hormones/hormone modifiers

MECHANISM OF ACTION
An antidiarrheal and growth hormone suppressant that suppresses the secretion of serotonin and gastroenteropancreatic peptides and enhances fluid and electrolyte absorption from the GI tract. *Therapeutic Effect:* Prolongs intestinal transit time.

PHARMACOKINETICS

Route	Onset	Peak	Duration
Subcuta-neous	N/A	N/A	Up to 12 hr

Rapidly and completely absorbed from injection site. Excreted in urine. Removed by hemodialysis. **Half-life:** 1.5 hr.

AVAILABILITY
Injection (Sandostatin): 0.05 mg/ml, 0.1 mg/ml, 0.2 mg/ml, 0.5 mg/ml, 1 mg/ml.
Suspension for Injection (Sandostatin LAR): 10-mg, 20-mg, 30-mg vials.

INDICATIONS AND DOSAGES
▶ **Diarrhea**
IV (SANDOSTATIN)
Adults, Elderly. Initially, 50-100 mcg q8hr. May increase by 100 mcg/dose q48hr. Maximum: 500 mcg q8hr.
SUBCUTANEOUS (SANDOSTATIN)
Adults, Elderly. 50 mcg 1-2 times a day.
IV, SUBCUTANEOUS (SANDOSTATIN)
Children. 1-10 mcg/kg q12hr.
▶ **Carcinoid tumors**
IV, SUBCUTANEOUS (SANDOSTATIN)
Adults, Elderly. 100-600 mcg/day in 2-4 divided doses.
IM (SANDOSTATIN LAR)
Adults, Elderly. 20 mg q4wk.
▶ **Vipomas**
IV, SUBCUTANEOUS (SANDOSTATIN)
Adults, Elderly. 200-300 mcg/day in 2-4 divided doses.
IM (SANDOSTATIN LAR)
Adults, Elderly. 20 mg q4wk.
▶ **Esophageal varices**
IV (SANDOSTATIN)
Adults, Elderly. Bolus of 25-50 mcg followed by IV infusion of 25-50 mcg/hr.
▶ **Acromegaly**
IV, SUBCUTANEOUS (SANDOSTATIN)
Adults, Elderly. 50 mcg 3 times a day. Increase as needed. Maximum: 500 mcg 3 times a day.
▶ **Acromegaly**
IM (SANDOSTATIN LAR)
Adults, Elderly. 20 mg q4wk for 3 mo. Maximum: 40 mg q4wk.

OFF-LABEL USES
Treatment of AIDS-associated secretory diarrhea, chemotherapy-induced diarrhea, insulinomas, small-bowel fistulas, control of bleeding esophageal varices

CONTRAINDICATIONS
None known.

INTERACTIONS
Drug
Glucagon, growth hormone, insulin, oral antidiabetics: May alter glucose concentrations.
Herbal
None known.
Food
None known.

DIAGNOSTIC TEST EFFECTS
May decrease serum thyroxine (T_4) concentration.

SIDE EFFECTS
Frequent (10%-6%, 58% 30% in acromegaly patients)
Diarrhea, nausea, abdominal discomfort, headache, injection site pain
Occasional (5%-1%)
Vomiting, flatulence, constipation, alopecia, facial flushing, pruritus, dizziness, fatigue, arrhythmias, ecchymosis, blurred vision
Rare (less than 1%)
Depression, diminished libido, vertigo, palpitations, dyspnea

SERIOUS REACTIONS
• Patients using octreotide may develop cholelithiasis or, with prolonged high dosages, hypothyroidism.
• GI bleeding, hepatitis, and seizures occur rarely.

PRECAUTIONS & CONSIDERATIONS
Caution is warranted with insulin-dependent diabetes and renal failure. It is unknown if octreotide is excreted in breast milk. The children's dosage has not been established. No age-related precautions have been noted in the elderly.

Notify the physician of unusual signs or symptoms, such as palpitations or unusual bleeding. Blood glucose levels, B/P, pulse rate, respiratory rate, weight, growth hormone, pattern of daily bowel activity and stool consistency, fecal fat, fluid and electrolyte balance, and thyroid function test results should be monitored. Be alert for decreased urine output and peripheral edema, especially of the ankles.
Administration
! Sandostatin may be given IV, IM, or subcutaneously. Sandostatin LAR may be given only IM.

Don't use solution if it becomes discolored or contains particulates.

Give the drug immediately after mixing. Inject octreotide deep IM in a large muscle mass at 4-week intervals. Avoid deltoid injections.

May also be administered as a subcutaneous injection. Avoid multiple injections at the same site within a short period.

Ofloxacin
o-flox′a-sin
(Apo-Oflox [CAN], Floxin, Floxin Otic, Ocuflox)
Do not confuse Floxin with Flexeril or Flexon, or Ocuflox with Ocufen.

CATEGORY AND SCHEDULE
Pregnancy Risk Category: C

CLASSIFICATION
Anti-infectives, ophthalmics, antibiotics, quinolones

MECHANISM OF ACTION
A fluoroquinolone antibiotic that inhibits DNA gyrase in susceptible microorganisms, interfering with bacterial cell replication and repair. *Therapeutic Effect:* Bactericidal.

PHARMACOKINETICS

Rapidly and well absorbed from the GI tract. Protein binding: 20%-25%. Widely distributed (including to CSF). Metabolized in the liver. Primarily excreted in urine. Removed by hemodialysis. **Half-life:** 4.7-7 hr (increased in impaired renal function, cirrhosis, and the elderly).

AVAILABILITY

Tablets (Floxin): 200 mg, 300 mg, 400 mg.
Injection Solution (Floxin): 40 mg/ml.
Premixed Infusion Solution (Floxin): 200 mg/50 ml, 400 mg/100 ml.
Ophthalmic Solution (Ocuflox): 0.3%.
Otic Solution (Floxin): 0.3%.

INDICATIONS AND DOSAGES

▸ **UTIs**
PO, IV
Adults. 200 mg q12hr.
▸ **Pelvic inflammatory disease (PID)**
PO
Adults. 400 mg q12hr for 10-14 days.
▸ **Lower respiratory tract, skin and skin-structure infections**
PO, IV
Adults. 400 mg q12hr for 10 days.
▸ **Prostatitis, sexually transmitted diseases (cervicitis, urethritis)**
PO
Adults. 300 mg q12hr.
▸ **Prostatitis**
IV
Adults. 300 mg q12hr.
▸ **Sexually transmitted diseases**
IV
Adults. 400 mg as a single dose.
▸ **Acute, uncomplicated gonorrhea**
PO
Adults. 400 mg 1 time.
▸ **Usual elderly dosage**
PO

Elderly. 200-400 mg q12-24hr for 7 days up to 6 wk.
▸ **Bacterial conjunctivitis**
OPHTHALMIC
Adults, Elderly. 1-2 drops q2-4hr for 2 days, then 4 times a day for 5 days.
▸ **Corneal ulcers**
OPHTHALMIC
Adults. 1-2 drops q30min while awake for 2 days, then q60min while awake for 5-7 days, then 4 times a day.
▸ **Acute otitis media**
OTIC
Children 1-12 yr. 5 drops into the affected ear 2 times/day for 10 days.
▸ **Otitis externa**
OTIC
Adults, Elderly, Children 12 yr and older. 10 drops into the affected ear once a day for 7 days.
Children 6 mo-11 yr. 5 drops into the affected ear once a day for 7 days.
▸ **Dosage in renal impairment**
After a normal initial dose, dosage and frequency are based on creatinine clearance.

Creatinine Clearance	Adjusted Dose	Dosage Interval
Greater than 50 ml/min	None	q12hr
10-50 ml/min	None	q24hr
Less than 10 ml/min	½	q24hr

CONTRAINDICATIONS

Children younger than 18 years, hypersensitivity to any quinolones

INTERACTIONS
Drug

Antacids, sucralfate: May decrease absorption and effects of ofloxacin.
Caffeine: May increase the effects of caffeine.
Theophylline: May increase theophylline blood concentration and risk of toxicity.

Herbal
None known.
Food
None known.

DIAGNOSTIC TEST EFFECTS
None known.

▨ IV INCOMPATIBILITIES
Amphotericin B complex (Abelcet, AmBisome, Amphotec), cefepime (Maxipime), doxorubicin liposomal (Doxil)
⚕ IV Compatibilities
Propofol (Diprivan)

SIDE EFFECTS
Frequent (10%-7%)
Nausea, headache, insomnia
Occasional (5%-3%)
Abdominal pain, diarrhea, vomiting, dry mouth, flatulence, dizziness, fatigue, drowsiness, rash, pruritus, fever
Rare (less than 1%)
Constipation, paraesthesia

SERIOUS REACTIONS
• Antibiotic-associated colitis and other superinfections may occur from altered bacterial balance.
• Hypersensitivity reactions, including photosensitivity (as evidenced by rash, pruritus, blisters, edema, and burning skin), have occurred in patients receiving fluoroquinolones.
• Arthropathy (swelling, pain, and clubbing of fingers and toes, degeneration of stress-bearing portion of a joint) may occur if the drug is given to children.

PRECAUTIONS & CONSIDERATIONS
Caution is warranted with CNS disorders, renal impairment, or seizures and those taking caffeine or theophylline. Caution should also be used regarding syphilis because ofloxacin may mask or delay symptoms of syphilis; serologic test for syphilis should be done at diagnosis and 3 months after treatment. Ofloxacin is distributed in breast milk. If possible, pregnant or breast-feeding women should avoid taking the drug because of the risk of arthropathy in the fetus or infant. The safety and efficacy of ofloxacin have not been established in children (children younger than 1 year for otic form). Age-related renal impairment may require a dosage adjustment for oral and parenteral forms in the elderly. No age-related precautions for the otic form have been noted in the elderly. There are no age-related precautions noted in the elderly. Avoid exposure to sunlight and ultraviolet light and wear sunscreen and protective clothing if photosensitivity develops.

Dizziness, drowsiness, headache, and insomnia may occur while taking ofloxacin. Avoid tasks requiring mental alertness or motor skills until response to ofloxacin is established. Signs and symptoms of infection, mental status, WBC count, skin for rash, pattern of daily bowel activity and stool consistency should be monitored. Be alert for signs of superinfection, such as anal or genital pruritus, fever, stomatitis, and vaginitis.
Storage
Store single-use vials at room temperature.
Administration
Do not take ofloxacin with food. The preferred dosing time is 1 hour before or 2 hours after a meal. Take with 8 oz of water and provide additional liquids between meals. Consume citrus fruits and cranberry juice to acidify urine. Take antacids containing aluminum or magnesium or products containing iron or zinc within 2 hours before or after taking ofloxacin.

For IV use, know that ofloxacin is also available in premixed, ready-to-hang solutions. Dilute each 200-mg vial with 50 ml D_5W or 0.9% NaCl (each 400-mg vial with 100 ml) to provide a concentration of 4 mg/ml. After dilution, the IV solution may be stored for 72 hours at room temperature and 14 days if refrigerated. Give by IV infusion only over at least 60 minutes; avoid rapid or bolus IV administration. Discard unused portions. Don't infuse other medications simultaneously through the same IV line.

For ophthalmic use, tilt the head back and place the solution in the conjunctival sac. Close the eye; then press gently on the lacrimal sac for 1 minute. Don't use ophthalmic solutions for injection. Unless the infection is very superficial, expect to also administer systemic drug therapy.

For otic use, lie down with the head turned so that the affected ear is upright. Instill drops toward the canal wall, not directly on the eardrum. Pull the auricle down and back in children and up and back in adults.

Olanzapine

oh-lan′za-peen
(Zyprexa, Zyprexa Intramuscular, Zyprexa Zydis)
Do not confuse olanzapine with olsalazine, or Zyprexa with Zyrtec.

CATEGORY AND SCHEDULE
Pregnancy Risk Category: C

CLASSIFICATION
Antipsychotics

MECHANISM OF ACTION
A dibenzepin derivative that antagonizes alpha$_1$-adrenergic, dopamine, histamine, muscarinic, and serotonin receptors. Produces anticholinergic, histaminic, and CNS depressant effects. *Therapeutic Effect:* Diminishes manifestations of psychotic symptoms.

PHARMACOKINETICS
Well absorbed after PO administration. Protein binding: 93%. Extensively distributed throughout the body. Undergoes extensive first-pass metabolism in the liver. Excreted primarily in urine and, to a lesser extent, in feces. Not removed by dialysis. **Half-life:** 21-54 hr.

AVAILABILITY
Tablets (Zyprexa): 2.5 mg, 5 mg, 7.5 mg, 10 mg, 15 mg, 20 mg).
Tablets (Orally Disintegrating [Zyprexa Zydis]): 5 mg, 10 mg, 15 mg, 20 mg.
Injection (Zyprexa Intramuscular). 10 mg.

INDICATIONS AND DOSAGES
▸ **Schizophrenia**
PO
Adults. Initially, 5-10 mg once daily. May increase by 10 mg/day at 5-7 day intervals. If further adjustments are indicated, may increase by 5-10 mg/day at 7 day intervals. Range: 10-30 mg/day.
Elderly. Initially, 2.5 mg/day. May increase as indicated. Range: 2.5-10 mg/day.
Children. Initially, 2.5 mg/day. Titrate as necessary up to 20 mg/day.
▸ **Bipolar mania**
PO
Adults. Initially, 10-15 mg/day. May increase by 5 mg/day at intervals of at least 24 hr. Maximum: 20 mg/day.
Children. Initially, 2.5 mg/day. Titrate as necessary up to 20 mg/day.

▶ **Dosage for elderly or debilitated patients and those predisposed to hypotensive reactions**
The initial dosage for these patients is 5 mg/day.

▶ **Control agitation in schizophrenic or bipolar patients**
IM
Adults, Elderly. 2.5-10 mg. May repeat 2h after first dose and 4h after 2nd dose. Maximum: 30 mg/day.

OFF-LABEL USES
Treatment of anorexia, maintenance of long-term treatment response in schizophrenic patients, nausea, vomiting

CONTRAINDICATIONS
None known.

INTERACTIONS
Drug
Alcohol, other CNS depressants: May increase CNS depressant effects.
Antihypertensives: May increase the hypotensive effects of these drugs.
Carbamazepine: Increases olanzapine clearance.
Ciprofloxacin, fluvoxamine: May increase the olanzapine blood concentration.
Dopamine agonists, levodopa: May antagonize the effects of these drugs.
Imipramine, theophylline: May inhibit the metabolism of these drugs.
Herbal
None known.
Food
None known.

DIAGNOSTIC TEST EFFECTS
May significantly increase serum GGT, prolactin, AST (SGOT), and ALT (SGPT) levels.

SIDE EFFECTS
Frequent
Somnolence (26%), agitation (23%), insomnia (20%), headache (17%), nervousness (16%), hostility (15%), dizziness (11%), rhinitis (10%)
Occasional
Anxiety, constipation (9%); nonaggressive atypical behavior (8%); dry mouth (7%); weight gain (6%); orthostatic hypotension, fever, arthralgia, restlessness, cough, pharyngitis, visual changes (dim vision) (5%)
Rare
Tachycardia; back, chest, abdominal, or extremity pain; tremor

SERIOUS REACTIONS
• Rare reactions include seizures and neuroleptic malignant syndrome, a potentially fatal syndrome characterized by hyperpyrexia, muscle rigidity, irregular pulse or B/P, tachycardia, diaphoresis, and cardiac arrhythmias.
• Extrapyramidal symptoms and dysphagia may also occur.
• Overdose (300 mg) produces drowsiness and slurred speech.

O

PRECAUTIONS & CONSIDERATIONS
Caution is warranted with a hypersensitivity to clozapine, hepatic impairment, cerebrovascular disease, cardiovascular disease (such as conduction abnormalities, heart failure, or history of MI or ischemia), history of seizures or conditions that lower the seizure threshold (such as Alzheimer's disease), and conditions predisposing to hypotension (such as dehydration, hypovolemia, and use of antihypertensives). Extreme caution should be used with the elderly who are at risk for aspiration pneumonia, concurrently taking hepatotoxic drugs, and those who should avoid anticholinergics (such as persons with benign prostatic hyperplasia).

It is unknown if olanzapine crosses the placenta or is distributed in breast milk. The safety and efficacy of olanzapine have not been established in children. No age-related precautions have been noted in the elderly.

Drowsiness may occur but generally subsides with continued therapy. Tasks requiring mental alertness or motor skills should be avoided. Dehydration, particularly during exercise, exposure to extreme heat, and concurrent use of medications that cause dry mouth or other drying effects, should also be avoided. A healthy diet and exercise program should be maintained to prevent weight gain. Notify the physician of extrapyramidal symptoms. B/P and therapeutic response should be assessed.

Administration

Caution should be used with each dosage increase. Take olanzapine without regard to food. Take as ordered and do not abruptly discontinue the drug or increase the dosage.

Olmesartan Medoxomil

ohl-me-sar′-tan
(Benicar)

CATEGORY AND SCHEDULE

Pregnancy Risk Category: C (D if used in second or third trimester)

CLASSIFICATION

Angiotensin II receptor antagonists

MECHANISM OF ACTION

An angiotensin II receptor, type AT_1, antagonist that blocks the vasoconstrictor and aldosterone-secreting effects of angiotensin II, inhibiting the binding of angiotensin II to the AT_1 receptors. *Therapeutic Effect:* Causes vasodilation, decreases peripheral resistance, and decreases B/P.

PHARMACOKINETICS

Rapidly and completely absorbed after PO administration. Metabolized in the liver. Recovered primarily in feces and, to a lesser extent, in urine. Not removed by hemodialysis. **Half-life:** 13 hr.

AVAILABILITY

Tablets: 5 mg, 20 mg, 40 mg.

INDICATIONS AND DOSAGES
▸ **Hypertension**
PO
Adults, Elderly, Patients with mildly impaired hepatic or renal function. 20 mg once a day in patients who are not volume depleted. After 2 weeks of therapy, if further reduction in B/P is needed, may increase dosage to 40 mg/day.

CONTRAINDICATIONS

Bilateral renal artery stenosis

INTERACTIONS
Drug
Diuretics: Further reduces B/P.
Herbal
None known.
Food
None known.

DIAGNOSTIC TEST EFFECTS

May increase blood Hgb and Hct levels.

SIDE EFFECTS
Occasional (3%)
Dizziness
Rare (less than 2%)
Headache, diarrhea, upper respiratory tract infection

SERIOUS REACTIONS
* Overdosage may manifest as hypotension and tachycardia. Bradycardia occurs less often.

PRECAUTIONS & CONSIDERATIONS
Caution is warranted with hepatic and renal impairment and renal arterial stenosis. It is unknown if olmesartan is distributed in breast milk. It may cause fetal or neonatal morbidity or mortality. Safety and efficacy of olmesartan have not been established in children. No age-related precautions have been noted in the elderly.

Dizziness may occur. Tasks that require mental alertness or motor skills should be avoided. Apical pulse and B/P should be assessed immediately before each olmesartan dose, and regularly throughout therapy. Be alert to fluctuations in apical pulse and B/P. If an excessive reduction in B/P occurs, place the person in the supine position with feet slightly elevated and notify the physician. Diagnostic tests, such as Hgb and Hct levels and liver function tests, should be assessed. Maintain adequate hydration; exercising outside during hot weather should be avoided in order to decrease the risk of dehydration and hypotension.
Administration
Take olmesartan without regard to meals.

Olsalazine
ohl-sal'ah-zeen
(Dipentum)
Do not confuse with olanzapine.

CATEGORY AND SCHEDULE
Pregnancy Risk Category: C

CLASSIFICATION
Gastrointestinals, salicylates

MECHANISM OF ACTION
A salicylic acid derivative that is converted to mesalamine in the colon by bacterial action. Blocks prostaglandin production in bowel mucosa. *Therapeutic Effect:* Reduces colonic inflammation in inflammatory bowel disease.

AVAILABILITY
Capsules: 250 mg.

INDICATIONS AND DOSAGES
▸ **Maintenance of controlled ulcerative colitis**
PO
Adults, Elderly. 1 g/day in 2 divided doses, preferably q12hr.

OFF-LABEL USES
Treatment of inflammatory bowel disease

CONTRAINDICATIONS
History of hypersensitivity to salicylates

INTERACTIONS
Drug
None known.
Herbal
None known.
Food
None known.

DIAGNOSTIC TEST EFFECTS
May increase AST (SGOT) and ALT (SGPT) levels.

SIDE EFFECTS
Frequent (10%-5%)
Headache, diarrhea, abdominal pain or cramps, nausea
Occasional (5%-1%)
Depression, fatigue, dyspepsia, upper respiratory tract infection, decreased appetite, rash, itching, arthralgia
Rare (1%)
Dizziness, vomiting, stomatitis

SERIOUS REACTIONS
• Sulfite sensitivity may occur in susceptible patients, manifested by cramping, headache, diarrhea, fever, rash, hives, itching, and wheezing. Discontinue drug immediately.
• Excessive diarrhea associated with extreme fatigue is noted rarely.

PRECAUTIONS & CONSIDERATIONS
Caution is warranted with preexisting renal disease. Serum alkaline phosphatase, AST, and ALT levels should be obtained before therapy. Adequate fluid intake should be maintained. Daily bowel activity and stool consistency and skin for rash should be assessed. Notify physician if persistent or increasing cramping, diarrhea, fever, pruritus, or rash occurs; olsalazine should be discontinued.
Administration
Take olsalazine with food in evenly divided doses.

Omalizumab
oh-mah-liz′uw-mab
(Xolair)

CATEGORY AND SCHEDULE
Pregnancy Risk Category: B

CLASSIFICATION
Monoclonal antibodies

MECHANISM OF ACTION
A monoclonal antibody that selectively binds to human immunoglobulin E (IgE) preventing it from binding to the surface of mast cells and basophiles. *Therapeutic Effect:* Prevents or reduces the number of asthmatic attacks.

PHARMACOKINETICS
Absorbed slowly after subcutaneous administration, with peak concentration in 7-8 days. Excreted in the liver, reticuloendothelial system, and endothelial cells. **Half-life:** 26 days.

AVAILABILITY
Powder for Injection:
202.5 mg/1.2 ml or 150 mg/1.2 ml after reconstitution.

INDICATIONS AND DOSAGES
▸ **Moderate to severe persistent asthma in patients who are reactive to a perennial allergen and whose asthma symptoms have been inadequately controlled with inhaled corticosteroids**
SUBCUTANEOUS
Adults, Elderly, Children 12 yr and older. 150-375 mg every 2 or 4 wk; dose and dosing frequency are individualized based on weight and pretreatment immunoglobulin E (IgE) level (as shown below).

▶ **4-week dosing table**

Pretreatment Serum IgE Levels (units/ml)	Weight 30-60 kg	Weight 61-70 kg	Weight 71-90 kg	Weight 91-150 kg
30 to 100	150 mg	150 mg	150 mg	300 mg
101- 200	300 mg	300 mg	300 mg	See next table
201- 300	300 mg	See next table	See next table	See next table

▶ **2-week dosing table**

Pretreatment Serum IgE Levels (units/ml)	Weight 30-60 kg	Weight 61-70 kg	Weight 71-90 kg	Weight 91-150 kg
101-200	See previous table	See preceding table	See preceding table	225 mg
201-300	See previous table	225 mg	225 mg	300 mg
301-400	225 mg	225 mg	300 mg	Do not dose
401-500	300 mg	300 mg	375 mg	Do not dose
501-600	300 mg	375 mg	Do not dose	Do not dose
601-700	375 mg	Do not dose	Do not dose	Do not dose

OFF-LABEL USES
Treatment of seasonal allergic rhinitis

CONTRAINDICATIONS
None known.

INTERACTIONS
Drug
None known.
Herbal
None known.
Food
None known.

DIAGNOSTIC TEST EFFECTS
May increase serum IgE levels.

SIDE EFFECTS
Frequent (45%-11%)
Injection site ecchymosis, redness, warmth, stinging, and urticaria; viral infections; sinusitis; headache; pharyngitis

Occasional (8%-3%)
Arthralgia, leg pain, fatigue, dizziness
Rare (2%)
Arm pain, earache, dermatitis, pruritus

SERIOUS REACTIONS
• Anaphylaxis occurs within 2 hours of the first dose or subsequent doses in 0.1% of patients.
• Malignant neoplasms occur in 0.5% of patients.

PRECAUTIONS & CONSIDERATIONS
Omalizumab is not intended to reverse acute bronchospasm or status asthmaticus. Since IgE is present in breast milk, omalizumab is also believed to be present in breast milk. Use omalizumab only if clearly needed. The safety and efficacy of omalizumab have not been established in children younger than 12 years. No age-related precautions

have been noted in the elderly. Drink plenty of fluids to decrease the thickness of lung secretions.

Serum total IgE levels should be obtained before beginning omalizumab therapy because the drug dosage is based on these pretreatment levels. Pulse rate and quality as well as respiratory depth, rate, rhythm, and type should be monitored. Fingernails and lips should also be assessed for a blue or dusky color in light skinned patients and a gray color in dark-skinned patients, which may be signs of hypoxemia.

Storage

Store omalizumab in the refrigerator. The reconstituted solution is stable for 8 hours if refrigerated or 4 hours if stored at room temperature.

Administration

! Expect to base omalizumab dosage on serum IgE levels obtained before beginning treatment. Don't use serum IgE levels obtained during treatment to determine omalizumab dosage because IgE levels remain elevated for up to 1 year after the drug has been discontinued.

Use only clear or slightly opalescent solution; the solution is slightly viscous. Use only sterile water for injection to prepare for subcutaneous administration. Draw 1.4 ml sterile water for injection into a 3-ml syringe with a 1-inch, 18-gauge needle and inject contents into the vial of powder. Swirl the vial for approximately 1 minute; do not shake it. Then swirl the vial again for 5 to 10 seconds every 5 minutes until no gel-like particles appear in the solution. The drug takes 15 to 20 minutes to dissolve. Don't use the solution if the contents fail to dissolve completely in 40 minutes. Invert the vial for 15 seconds to allow the solution to drain toward the stopper. Using a new 3-ml syringe with a

1-inch, 18-gauge needle, withdraw the required 1.2-ml dose and replace the 18-gauge needle with a 25-gauge needle for subcutaneous administration. Subcutaneous administration may take 5 to 10 seconds because of omalizumab's viscosity.

Omeprazole
om-eh-pray′zole
(Losec [CAN], Maxor [AUS], Prilosec, Prilosec TOC, Probitor [AUS], Rapinex)
Do not confuse Prilosec with prilocaine, Prinivil, or Prozac.

CATEGORY AND SCHEDULE
Pregnancy Risk Category: C

CLASSIFICATION
Gastrointestinals, proton pump inhibitors

MECHANISM OF ACTION
A benzimidazole that is converted to active metabolites that irreversibly bind to and inhibit hydrogen-potassium adenosine triphosphatase, an enzyme on the surface of gastric parietal cells. Inhibits hydrogen ion transport into gastric lumen.
Therapeutic Effect: Increases gastric pH, reduces gastric acid production.

PHARMACOKINETICS

Route	Onset	Peak	Duration
PO	1 hr	2 hr	72 hr

Rapidly absorbed from the GI tract. Protein binding: 99%. Primarily distributed into gastric parietal cells.

Metabolized extensively in the liver. Primarily excreted in urine. Unknown if removed by hemodialysis. **Half-life:** 0.5-1 hr (increased in patients with hepatic impairment).

AVAILABILITY

Capsules (Delayed-Release [Prilosec]): 10 mg, 20 mg, 40 mg.
Oral Suspension (Rapinex): 20 mg.

INDICATIONS AND DOSAGES
▶ **Erosive esophagitis, poorly responsive gastroesophageal reflux disease, active duodenal ulcer, prevention and treatment of NSAID-induced ulcers**
PO
Adults, Elderly. 20 mg/day.
▶ **To maintain healing of erosive esophagitis**
PO
Adults, Elderly. 20 mg/day.
▶ **Pathologic hypersecretory conditions**
PO
Adults, Elderly. Initially, 60 mg/day up to 120 mg 3 times a day.
▶ **Duodenal ulcer caused by** *Helicobacter Pylori*
PO
Adults, Elderly. 20 mg twice a day for 10 days.
▶ **Active benign gastric ulcer**
PO
Adults, Elderly. 40 mg/day for 4-8 wk.
▶ **Usual pediatric dosage**
Children older than 2 yr weighing 20 kg and more. 20 mg/day.
Children older than 2 yr weighing less than 20 kg. 10 mg/day.

OFF-LABEL USES

H. pylori-associated duodenal ulcer (with amoxicillin and clarithromycin), prevention and treatment of NSAID-induced ulcers, treatment of active benign gastric ulcers

CONTRAINDICATIONS
None known.

INTERACTIONS
Drug
Diazepam, oral anticoagulants, phenytoin: May increase the blood concentration of diazepam, oral anticoagulants, and phenytoin.
Herbal
None known.
Food
None known.

DIAGNOSTIC TEST EFFECTS
May increase serum alkaline phosphatase, AST (SGOT), and ALT (SGPT) levels.

SIDE EFFECTS
Frequent (7%)
Headache
Occasional (3%-2%)
Diarrhea, abdominal pain, nausea
Rare (2%)
Dizziness, asthenia or loss of strength, vomiting, constipation, upper respiratory tract infection, back pain, rash, cough

SERIOUS REACTIONS
• None known.

PRECAUTIONS & CONSIDERATIONS
It is unknown if omeprazole crosses the placenta or is distributed in breast milk. Safety and efficacy of omeprazole have not been established in children. No age-related precautions have been noted in the elderly.

Notify the physician if headache, diarrhea, discomfort, or nausea occurs during omeprazole therapy. Serum chemistry laboratory values, particularly serum alkaline phosphatase, AST and ALT levels should be obtained to assess liver function.

Administration
Take omeprazole before meals. Do not crush or open capsules; swallow capsules whole.

Ondansetron
on-dan-seh′tron
(Zofran, Zofran ODT)
Do not confuse Zofran with Zantac or Zosyn.

CATEGORY AND SCHEDULE
Pregnancy Risk Category: B

CLASSIFICATION
Antiemetics/antivertigo, serotonin receptor antagonists

MECHANISM OF ACTION
An antiemetic that blocks serotonin, both peripherally on vagal nerve terminals and centrally in the chemoreceptor trigger zone. *Therapeutic Effect:* Prevents nausea and vomiting.

PHARMACOKINETICS
Readily absorbed from the GI tract. Protein binding: 70%-76%. Metabolized in the liver. Primarily excreted in urine. Unknown if removed by hemodialysis. **Half-life:** 4 hr.

AVAILABILITY
Oral Solution (Zofran): 4 mg/5 ml.
Tablets (Zofran): 4 mg, 8 mg, 24 mg.
Tablets (Orally Disintegrating [Zofran ODT]): 4 mg, 8 mg.
Injection (Zofran): 2 mg/ml.
Injection (Premix): 32 mg/50 ml.

INDICATIONS AND DOSAGES
▸ **Prevention of chemotherapy-induced nausea and vomiting**
PO

Adults, Elderly, Children older than 11 yr. 24 mg as a single dose 30 min before starting chemotherapy. Or 8 mg 30 min before chemotherapy and again 8 hr after first dose, then q12hr for 1-2 days.
Children 4-11 yr. 4 mg 30 min before chemotherapy and again 4 and 8 hr after chemotherapy, then q8hr for 1-2 days.
IV
Adults, Elderly, Children 4-18 yr. 32 mg as a single dose or 0.15 mg/kg/dose 30 min before chemotherapy, then 4 and 8 hr after chemotherapy.
▸ **Prevention of radiation-induced nausea and vomiting**
PO
Adults, Elderly. 8 mg 3 times a day.
▸ **Prevention of postoperative nausea and vomiting**
IV, IM
Adults, Elderly. 4 mg undiluted over 2-5 min.
Children weighing less than 40 kg. 0.1 mg/kg.
Children weighing 10 kg and more. 4 mg.

OFF-LABEL USES
Treatment of postoperative nausea and vomiting

CONTRAINDICATIONS
None known.

INTERACTIONS
Drug
None known.
Herbal
None known.
Food
None known.

DIAGNOSTIC TEST EFFECTS
May transiently increase serum bilirubin, AST (SGOT), and ALT (SGPT) levels.

▨ IV INCOMPATIBILITIES

Acyclovir (Zovirax), allopurinol (Aloprim), aminophylline, amphotericin B (Fungizone), amphotericin B complex (Abelcet, AmBisome, Amphotec), ampicillin (Polycillin), ampicillin and sulbactam (Unasyn), cefepime (Maxipime), cefoperazone (Cefobid), 5-fluorouracil, lorazepam (Ativan), meropenem (Merrem IV), methylprednisolone (Solu-Medrol)

▨ IV Compatibilities

Carboplatin (Paraplatin), cisplatin (Platinol), cyclophosphamide (Cytoxan), cytarabine (Cytosar), dacarbazine (DTIC-Dome), daunorubicin (Cerubidine), dexamethasone (Decadron), diphenhydramine (Benadryl), docetaxel (Taxotere), dopamine (Intropin), etoposide (VePesid), gemcitabine (Gemzar), heparin, hydromorphone (Dilaudid), ifosfamide (Ifex), magnesium, mannitol, mesna (Mesnex), methotrexate, metoclopramide (Reglan), mitomycin (Mutamycin), mitoxantrone (Novantrone), morphine, paclitaxel (Taxol), potassium chloride, teniposide (Vumon), topotecan (Hycamtin), vinblastine (Velban), vincristine (Oncovin), vinorelbine (Navelbine)

SIDE EFFECTS

Frequent (13%-5%)
Anxiety, dizziness, somnolence, headache, fatigue, constipation, diarrhea, hypoxia, urine retention
Occasional (4%-2%)
Abdominal pain, xerostomia, fever, feeling of cold, redness and pain at injection site, paresthesia, asthenia
Rare (1%)
Hypersensitivity reaction (including rash and pruritus), blurred vision

SERIOUS REACTIONS

• Overdose may produce a combination of CNS stimulant and depressant effects.

PRECAUTIONS & CONSIDERATIONS

It is unknown if ondansetron crosses the placenta or is distributed in breast milk. The safety and efficacy of ondansetron have not been established in children. No age-related precautions have been noted in the elderly. Alcohol, barbiturates, and tasks that require mental alertness or motor skills should be avoided.

Dizziness or drowsiness may occur. Pattern of daily bowel activity and stool consistency, hydration status, bilirubin, AST (SGOT), and ALT (SGPT) levels should be monitored.

Storage
Store vials at room temperature. The solution is stable for 48 hours after dilution.

Administration
! Give all oral doses 30 minutes before chemotherapy and repeat at 8-hour intervals, as prescribed.

Take ondansetron without regard to food.

For IV use, ondansetron may be given undiluted as an IV push over 2 to 5 minutes. For IV infusion, dilute with 50 ml D_5W or 0.9% NaCl before administration, and infuse over 15 minutes. May also give IM.

O

Opium Tincture

oh'pee-um

Do not confuse with paregoric, camphorated tincture of opium.

CATEGORY AND SCHEDULE

Pregnancy Risk Category: B, D if used for prolonged periods, high dosages at term
Controlled substance: Schedule II

CLASSIFICATION

Antidiarrheals, gastrointestinals

MECHANISM OF ACTION

An opioid agonist that contains many narcotic alkaloids including morphine. It inhibits gastric motility due to its morphine content. *Therapeutic Effect:* Decreases digestive secretions, increases in gastrointestinal (GI) muscle tone, and reduces GI propulsion.

PHARMACOKINETICS

Duration of action is 4-5 hr. Variably absorbed from the gastrointestinal (GI) tract. Protein binding: unknown. Metabolized in liver. Primarily excreted in urine. Unknown if removed by hemodialysis. **Half-life:** unknown.

AVAILABILITY

Liquid: 10%.

INDICATIONS AND DOSAGES

▸ **Analgesia**
PO
Adults, Elderly. 0.6-1.5 ml q3-4hr. Maximum: 6 ml/day.
Children. 0.01-0.02 ml/kg/dose q3-4hr. Maximum: 6 doses/day.

▸ **Antidiarrheal**
PO
Adults, Elderly. 0.3-1 ml q2-6hr. Maximum: 6 ml/day.
Children. 0.005-0.01 ml/kg/dose q3-4hr. Maximum: 6 doses/day.

OFF-LABEL USES

Narcotic withdrawal symptoms in neonates

CONTRAINDICATIONS

Hypersensitivity to morphine sulfate or any component of the formulation, increased intracranial pressure, severe respiratory depression, severe hepatic or renal insufficiency, pregnancy (prolonged use or high dosages near term)

INTERACTIONS

Drug
Alcohol, central nervous system (CNS) depressants: May increase CNS or respiratory depression, and hypotension.
MAOIs, tricyclic antidepressants: May produce severe, fatal reactions unless dose reduced by one quarter.
Dextroamphetamine: May increase the analgesic effect of opium.
Herbal
None known.
Food
None known.

DIAGNOSTIC TEST EFFECTS

May increase serum SGOT (AST), and SGPT (ALT) levels.

SIDE EFFECTS

Frequent
Constipation, drowsiness, nausea, vomiting
Occasional
Paradoxical excitement, confusion, pounding heartbeat, facial flushing, decreased urination, blurred vision, dizziness, dry mouth, headache,

hypotension, decreased appetite, redness, burning, pain at injection site
Rare
Hallucinations, depression, stomach pain, insomnia

SERIOUS REACTIONS

• Overdosage results in cold or clammy skin, confusion, convulsions, decreased blood pressure (B/P), restlessness, pinpoint pupils, bradycardia, respiratory depression, decreased level of consciousness (LOC), and severe weakness.
• Tolerance to analgesic effect and physical dependence may occur with repeated use.

PRECAUTIONS & CONSIDERATIONS

Extreme caution is warranted with acute alcoholism, anoxia, central nervous system (CNS) depression, hypercapnia, respiratory depression, respiratory dysfunction, seizures, shock, and untreated myxedema. Opium tincture crosses the placenta and is distributed in breast milk. Be aware that respiratory depression may occur in the neonate if the mother received opiates during labor. Regular use of opiates during pregnancy may produce withdrawal symptoms in neonate, such as diarrhea, excessive crying, fever, hyperactive reflexes, irritability, seizures, sneezing, tremors, vomiting, and yawning. Be aware that children may experience paradoxical excitement. Children younger than 3 months of age and the elderly are more susceptible to the respiratory depressant effects of opium tincture. Opium tincture use in the elderly may mask dehydration and electrolyte depletion. Avoid alcohol during therapy.

Drowsiness and dizziness may occur during treatment. Avoid tasks that require mental alertness or motor skills until response to the drug

is established. Change positions slowly to avoid orthostatic hypotension.
Storage
Store away from heat and direct light.
Administration
Be aware that opium tincture is not the same as paregoric. Opium tincture contains 10 mg/ml whereas paregoric has 0.4 mg/ml of morphine—a 25-fold difference. Do not exceed the prescribed dose.

Oprelvekin (Interleukin-2, IL-2)
oh-prel've-kin
(Neumega)
Do not confuse Neumega with Neupogen.

CATEGORY AND SCHEDULE
Pregnancy Risk Category: C

CLASSIFICATION
Hematopoietic agents

MECHANISM OF ACTION
A hematopoietic that stimulates production of blood platelets, essential to the blood-clotting process. *Therapeutic Effect:* Increases platelet production.

AVAILABILITY
Injection: 5 mg.

INDICATIONS AND DOSAGES
▸ **Prevention of thrombocytopenia**
SUBCUTANEOUS
Adults. 50 mcg/kg once a day.
Children. 75-100 mcg/kg once a day. Continue for 14-28 days or until platelet count reaches 50,000 cells/mcl after its nadir.

CONTRAINDICATIONS
None known.

INTERACTIONS
Drug
None known.
Herbal
None known.
Food
None known.

DIAGNOSTIC TEST EFFECTS
May decrease Hgb and Hct, usually within 3-5 days of initiation of therapy; reverses about 1 week after discontinuance of therapy.

SIDE EFFECTS
Frequent
Nausea or vomiting (77%); fluid retention (59%); neutropenic fever (48%); diarrhea (43%); rhinitis (42%); headache (41%); dizziness (38%); fever (36%); insomnia (33%); cough (29%); rash, pharyngitis (25%); tachycardia (20%); vasodilation (19%)

SERIOUS REACTIONS
• Transient atrial fibrillation or flutter occurs in 10% of patients and may be caused by increased plasma volume; oprelvekin is not directly arrhythmogenic. Arrhythmias usually are brief in duration and spontaneously convert to normal sinus rhythm.
• Papilledema may occur in children.

PRECAUTIONS & CONSIDERATIONS
Caution is warranted with or susceptible to developing CHF and in those with a history of atrial arrhythmia or heart failure. An electric razor and soft toothbrush should be used to prevent bleeding until platelet count is within normal range.

Notify the physician of palpitations or dyspnea. Fluid and electrolyte status should be closely monitored, particularly if the person is receiving diuretic therapy. Fluid retention should be assessed as evidenced by dyspnea on exertion and peripheral edema; fluid retention generally occurs during the first week of therapy and continues for the duration of treatment. An EKG should be obtained to assess for an underlying arrhythmia. Platelet count should also be periodically assessed for therapeutic response. CBC should be obtained before chemotherapy and at regular intervals thereafter; discontinue oprelvekin more than 2 days before starting next round of chemotherapy.

Storage
Store in refrigerator. Once reconstituted, use within 3 hours.
Administration
! Begin oprelvekin administration 6 to 24 hours following completion of chemotherapy dose.

For subcutaneous use, add 1 ml sterile water for injection to provide concentration of 5 mg/ml oprelvekin. Inject along inside surface of vial, and swirl contents gently to avoid excessive agitation. Discard unused portion. Give single injection in the abdomen, thigh, hip, or upper arm. Continue drug dosing until postnadir platelet count is greater than 50,000 cells/mcl.

Orlistat
ohr'lih-stat
(Xenical)
Do not confuse with Xeloda.

CATEGORY AND SCHEDULE
Pregnancy Risk Category: B

CLASSIFICATION
Gastrointestinals, lipase
inhibitors

MECHANISM OF ACTION
A gastric and pancreatic lipase
inhibitor that inhibits absorption
of dietary fats by inactivating
gastric and pancreatic enzymes.
Therapeutic Effect: Resulting caloric
deficit may positively affect weight
control.

PHARMACOKINETICS
Minimal absorption after administration. Protein binding: 99%. Primarily
eliminated unchanged in feces.
Unknown if removed by hemodialysis. **Half-life:** 1-2 hr.

AVAILABILITY
Capsules: 120 mg.

INDICATIONS AND DOSAGES
▶ **Weight reduction**
PO
Adults, Elderly, Children 12-16 yr.
120 mg 3 times a day.

CONTRAINDICATIONS
Cholestasis, chronic malabsorption
syndrome

INTERACTIONS
Drug
Pravastatin: May increase the
blood concentration of pravastatin
and risk of rhabdomyolysis.

Herbal
None known.
Food
None known.

DIAGNOSTIC TEST EFFECTS
Decreases blood glucose, total
cholesterol, and serum LDL levels.
Decreases absorption and levels of
vitamins A and E.

SIDE EFFECTS
Frequent (30%-20%)
Headache, abdominal discomfort,
flatulence, fecal urgency, fatty or
oily stool
Occasional (14%-5%)
Back pain, menstrual irregularity,
nausea, fatigue, diarrhea, dizziness
Rare (less than 4%)
Anxiety, rash, myalgia, dry skin,
vomiting

SERIOUS REACTIONS
• None known.

PRECAUTIONS & CONSIDERATIONS
It is unknown if orlistat is excreted
in breast milk. Orlistat use is not
recommended during pregnancy or
in breast-feeding women. Safety and
efficacy of orlistat have not been
established in children. No age-
related precautions have been noted
in the elderly.
   Unpleasant side effects, such as
flatulence and urgency, may occur
but should diminish with time.
Laboratory studies, such as blood
glucose levels and lipid profile,
should be obtained before and
during therapy. Changes in coagulation parameters as well as height and
weight should also be monitored.
Administration
! Orlistat's side effects tend to
be mild and transient in nature,
gradually diminishing during
treatment.

Take orlistat without regard to food. A nutritionally balanced, reduced-calorie diet should be maintained. Carbohydrates, fats, and protein should be distributed over three main meals.

Orphenadrine

or-fen'a-dreen
(Norflex, Orphenace [CAN], Rhoxal-orphenadrine [CAN])

CATEGORY AND SCHEDULE

Pregnancy Risk Category: C

CLASSIFICATION

Musculoskeletal agents, relaxants, skeletal muscle

MECHANISM OF ACTION

A skeletal muscle relaxant that is structurally related to diphenhydramine and may thought to indirectly affect skeletal muscle by central atropine-like effects. *Therapeutic Effect:* Relieves musculoskeletal pain.

PHARMACOKINETICS

Well absorbed after PO and IM absorption. Protein binding: low. Metabolized in liver. Primarily excreted in urine and feces. **Half-life:** 14 hr.

AVAILABILITY

Injection: 30 mg/ml (Norflex). *Tablets, extended-release:* 100 mg (Norflex).

INDICATIONS AND DOSAGES

▸ **Musculoskeletal pain**
IM/IV
Adults, Elderly. 60 mg 2 times/day. Switch to oral form for maintenance.

PO
Adults, Elderly. 100 mg 2 times/day.

OFF-LABEL USES

Drug-induced extrapyramidal reactions

CONTRAINDICATIONS

Angle-closure glaucoma, myasthenia gravis, pyloric or duodenal obstruction, stenosing peptic ulcer, prostatic hypertrophy, obstruction of the bladder neck, achalasia, cardiospasm (megaesophagus), hypersensitivity to orphenadrine or any component of the formulation

INTERACTIONS

Drug
Alcohol, CNS depressants: May increase sedative effects.
Anticholinergics: May increase anticholinergic effects
Cisapride: May decrease effectiveness of cisapride
Levodopa: May decrease effects of orphenadrine.
Herbal
St. John's wort, kava kava, gotu kola: May increase CNS depression.
Food
None known.

DIAGNOSTIC TEST EFFECTS

None known.

🖾 IV INCOMPATIBILITIES

None known.
🍶 **IV Compatibilities**
None known.

SIDE EFFECTS

Frequent
Drowsiness, dizziness, muscular weakness, hypotension, dry mouth, nose, throat, and lips, urinary retention, thickening of bronchial secretions
Elderly

Frequent
Sedation, dizziness, hypotension
Occasional
Flushing, visual or hearing distur-
bances, paresthesia, diaphoresis, chill

SERIOUS REACTIONS
• Hypersensitivity reaction, such as
eczema, pruritus, rash, cardiac
disturbances, and photosensitivity,
may occur.
• Overdosage may vary from CNS
depression, including sedation,
apnea, hypotension, cardiovascular
collapse, or death to severe paradoxical reaction, such as hallucinations,
tremor, and seizures.

PRECAUTIONS & CONSIDERATIONS
Caution is warranted with tachycardia
or urinary retention. It is unknown if
orphenadrine crosses the placenta or
is distributed in breast milk. Safety
and efficacy of orphenadrine have not
been established in children. There are
no age-related precautions noted in
the elderly.
    Drowsiness and dizziness may
occur but usually diminishes with
continued therapy. Avoid alcohol and
tasks that require mental alertness or
motor skills.
Storage
Store oral and injection formulations
at room temperature. Solution for
injection normally appears clear,
colorless; discard if cloudy or
precipitate is present. If bloody or
tarry stools, continued weakness,
diarrhea, fatigue, itching, nausea,
or skin rash occurs, notify the
physician.
Administration
Do not crush extended release product. Take two tablets per day, one in
the morning and one in the evening.
    The usual parenteral dose is 60 mg
IV or IM twice daily. Switch to oral
form for maintenance.

Oseltamivir
ah-suhl-tahm′ah-veer
(Tamiflu)

CATEGORY AND SCHEDULE
Pregnancy Risk Category: C

CLASSIFICATION
Antivirals

MECHANISM OF ACTION
A selective inhibitor of influenza
virus neuraminidase, an enzyme
essential for viral replication. Acts
against both influenza A and B
viruses. *Therapeutic Effect:*
Suppresses the spread of infection
within the respiratory system and
reduces the duration of clinical
symptoms.

PHARMACOKINETICS
Readily absorbed. Protein
binding: 3%. Extensively converted
to active drug in the liver.
Primarily excreted in urine.
Half-life: 6-10 hr.

AVAILABILITY
Capsules: 75 mg.
Oral Suspension: 12 mg/ml.

INDICATIONS AND DOSAGES
▸ **Influenza**
PO
Adults, Elderly. 75 mg 2 times a day
for 5 days.
Children weighing more than 40 kg.
75 mg twice a day.
Children weighing 24-40 kg. 60 mg
twice a day.
Children weighing 15-23 kg. 45 mg
twice a day.
Children weighing less than 15 kg.
30 mg twice a day.

▸ **Prevention of influenza**
PO
Adults, Elderly. 75 mg once a day.
▸ **Dosage in renal impairment**
PO
For adult and elderly patients,
dosage is decreased to 75 mg once a
day for at least 7 days and possibly
up to 6 wk.

CONTRAINDICATIONS
None known.

INTERACTIONS
Drug
None known.
Herbal
None known.
Food
None known.

DIAGNOSTIC TEST EFFECTS
None known.

SIDE EFFECTS
Frequent (5%)
Nausea, vomiting, diarrhea
Occasional (4%-1%)
Abdominal pain, bronchitis, dizzi-
ness, headache, cough, insomnia,
fatigue, vertigo

SERIOUS REACTIONS
• Colitis, pneumonia, and pyrexia
occur rarely.

PRECAUTIONS & CONSIDERATIONS
Caution is warranted with renal
function impairment. Be aware that it
is unknown if oseltamivir is excreted
in breast milk. Be aware that the
safety and efficacy of this drug have
not been established in children
younger than 1 year of age. There
are no age-related precautions noted
in the elderly. Be aware that
oseltamivir is not a substitute for a
flu shot. Blood glucose should be
monitored.

Administration
Give oseltamivir without regard to
food. The drug should be started as
soon as possible at the first appearance of flu symptoms.

Oxacillin
ox-a-sill′in

CATEGORY AND SCHEDULE
Pregnancy Risk Category: B

CLASSIFICATION
Antibiotics, penicillins

MECHANISM OF ACTION
A penicillin that binds to bacterial
membranes. *Therapeutic Effect:*
Bactericidal.

AVAILABILITY
Powder for Injection: 1-g vials,
2-g vials.

INDICATIONS AND DOSAGES
▸ **Upper respiratory tract, skin, and
skin-structure infections**
IV, IM
*Adults, Elderly, Children weighing
40 kg or more.* 250-500 mg q4-6hr.
Children weighing less than 40 kg.
50 mg/kg/day in divided doses q6hr.
Maximum: 12 g/day.
▸ **Lower respiratory tract and other
serious infections**
IV, IM
*Adults, Elderly, Children weighing
40 kg or more.* 1 g q4-6hr.
Maximum: 12 g/day.
Children weighing less than 40 kg.
100 mg/kg/day in divided doses q4-6hr.

CONTRAINDICATIONS
Hypersensitivity to any penicillin

INTERACTIONS
Drug
Probenecid: May increase oxacillin blood concentration and risk of toxicity.
Herbal
None known.
Food
None known.

DIAGNOSTIC TEST EFFECTS
May increase AST (SGOT) levels.
May cause a positive Coombs' test.

SIDE EFFECTS
Frequent
Mild hypersensitivity reaction (fever, rash, pruritus), GI effects (nausea, vomiting, diarrhea)
Occasional
Phlebitis, thrombophlebitis (more common in elderly), hepatotoxicity (with high IV dosage)

SERIOUS REACTIONS
• Antibiotic-associated colitis and other superinfections may result from altered bacterial balance.
• A mild to severe hypersensitivity reaction may occur in those allergic to penicillins.

PRECAUTIONS & CONSIDERATIONS
Caution is warranted with impaired renal function or a history of allergies, especially to cephalosporins. History of allergies, especially to cephalosporins or penicillins, should be determined before giving the drug. Withhold and promptly notify the physician if rash or diarrhea occurs. Severe diarrhea with abdominal pain, blood or mucus in stool, and fever may indicate antibiotic-associated colitis. Signs and symptoms of superinfection, including anal or genital pruritus, black hairy tongue, diarrhea, increased fever, sore throat, ulceration or changes of oral mucosa, and vomiting should be monitored. Intake and output, renal function tests, urinalysis, and the injection sites should be assessed.
Storage
Store vials at room temperature. Once reconstituted, the solution remains stable for 3 days at room temperature or 7 days refrigerated. When further diluted with D_5W or 0.9% NaCl, the solution is stable for 24 hours.
Administration
For IV use, add 10 ml sterile water for injection to each 1-g vial to provide a concentration of 100 mg/ml. For piggyback administration, further dilute with 50 to 100 mg D_5W or 0.9% NaCl. Administer IV push over 10 minutes and IV piggyback over 30 minutes.

For IM use, reconstitute each 1.5-g vial with 3.2 ml or each 3-g vial with 6.4 ml of sterile water for injection to provide a concentration of 250 mg ampicillin/125 mg sulbactam per milliliter. Administer the injection deep into a large muscle mass within 1 hour of preparation.

O

Oxandrolone
ox-an'droe-lone
(Lonavar [AUS], Oxandrin)
Do not confuse with testolactone.

CATEGORY AND SCHEDULE
Pregnancy Risk Category: X
Controlled Substance:
Schedule III

CLASSIFICATION
Anabolic steroids, hormones/hormone modifiers

MECHANISM OF ACTION
A synthetic testosterone derivative that promotes growth and development of male sex organs, maintains secondary sex characteristics in androgen-deficient males. *Therapeutic Effect:* Androgenic and anabolic actions.

PHARMACOKINETICS
Well absorbed from the gastrointestinal (GI) tract. Protein binding: 94%-97%. Metabolized in liver. Primarily excreted in urine. Unknown if removed by hemodialysis. **Half-life:** 5-13 hr.

AVAILABILITY
Tablets: 2.5 mg, 10 mg (Oxandrin).

INDICATIONS AND DOSAGES
▸ **Weight gain**
Adults, Elderly. 2.5-20 mg in divided doses 2-4 times/day usually for 2-4 weeks. Course of therapy is based on individual response. Repeat intermittently as needed.
Children. Total daily dose is 0.1 mg/kg. Repeat intermittently as needed.

OFF-LABEL USES
AIDS wasting syndrome, alcoholic hepatitis, athletic performance enhancement, burns, growth hormone deficiency, hyperlipidemia, Turner syndrome

CONTRAINDICATIONS
Nephrosis, carcinoma of breast or prostate hypercalcemia, pregnancy, hypersensitivity to oxandrolone or any component of the formulation

INTERACTIONS
Drug
ACTH: May increase the risk of edema and acne.
Adrenal steroids: May increase the risk of edema and acne.

Bupropion: May lower seizure threshold.
Oral anticoagulants: May increase the effects of oral anticoagulants.
Herbal
Chaparral: May increase liver enzymes.
Comfrey: May increase liver enzymes.
Eucalyptus: May increase risk of hepatoxicity.
Germander: May increase liver enzymes.
Jin bu huan: May increase liver enzymes.
Kava kava: May increase liver enzymes.
Pennyroyal: May increase liver enzymes.
Skullcap: May increase the risk of liver damage.
Velerian: May increase risk of hepatotoxicity.
Food
None known.

DIAGNOSTIC TEST EFFECTS
May decrease levels of thyroxine-binding globulin, resulting in decreased total T_4 serum levels and increased resin uptake of T_3 and T_4. May increase PBI and radioactive iodine uptake.

SIDE EFFECTS
Frequent
Gynecomastia, acne, amenorrhea, other menstrual irregularities
Females: Hirsutism, deepening of voice, clitoral enlargement that may not be reversible when drug is discontinued
Occasional
Edema, nausea, insomnia, oligospermia, priapism, male pattern of baldness, bladder irritability, hypercalcemia in immobilized patients or those with breast cancer, hypercholesterolemia

Rare
Polycythemia with high dosage

SERIOUS REACTIONS
• Peliosis hepatitis of the liver, spleen replaced with blood-filled cysts, hepatic neoplasms and hepatocellular carcinoma have been associated with prolonged high-dosage, anaphylactic reactions.

PRECAUTIONS & CONSIDERATIONS
Caution is warranted with diabetes, epilepsy, and liver, cardiac, and renal disease. Oxandrolone use is contraindicated during lactation and is excreted in breast milk. Oxandrolone may accelerate bone maturation more rapidly than linear growth in children and the effect may continue for 6 months after the drug has been stopped. Its use in the elderly may increase the risk of hyperplasia or stimulate growth of occult prostate carcinoma. Salt intake should be reduced.

Acne, nausea, pedal edema, or vomiting may occur. Women should report deepening of voice, hoarseness, and menstrual irregularities. Men should report difficulty urinating, frequent erections, and gynecomastia. Weight should be obtained each day. Weekly weight gains of more than 5 pounds should be reported.

Storage
Store oxandrolone at room temperature away from moisture, heat, and direct light.

Administration
Take oxandrolone with or without food. Take with a full glass of water. Duration of therapy will depend on the response of the patient.

Oxaprozin
ox-a-pro'zin
(Daypro)
Do not confuse oxaprozin with oxazepam.

CATEGORY AND SCHEDULE
Pregnancy Risk Category: C (D if used in third trimester or near delivery)

CLASSIFICATION
Analgesics, non-narcotic, nonsteroidal anti-inflammatory drugs

MECHANISM OF ACTION
An NSAID that produces analgesic and anti-inflammatory effects by inhibiting prostaglandin synthesis. *Therapeutic Effect:* Reduces the inflammatory response and intensity of pain.

PHARMACOKINETICS
Well absorbed from the GI tract. Protein binding: 99%. Widely distributed. Metabolized in the liver. Primarily excreted in urine; partially eliminated in feces. Not removed by hemodialysis. **Half-life:** 42-50 hr.

AVAILABILITY
Tablets: 600 mg.

INDICATIONS AND DOSAGES
▸ **Osteoarthritis**
PO
Adults, Elderly. 1200 mg once a day (600 mg in patients with low body weight or mild disease). Maximum: 1800 mg/day.

> **Rheumatoid arthritis**
PO
Adults, Elderly. 1200 mg once a day.
Range: 600-1800 mg/day.
> **Juvenile rheumatoid arthritis**
Children weighing more than 54 kg.
1200 mg/day.
Children weighing 32-54 kg.
900 mg/day.
Children weighing 22-31 kg.
600 mg/day.
> **Dosage in renal impairment**
For adults and elderly patients
with renal impairment, the recom-
mended initial dose is 600 mg/day;
may be increased up to 1200 mg/day.

CONTRAINDICATIONS
Active peptic ulcer disease, chronic
inflammation of GI tract, GI bleeding or ulceration, history of hypersensitivity to aspirin or NSAIDs

INTERACTIONS
Drug

Antihypertensives, diuretics:
May decrease the effects of these
drugs.
Aspirin, other salicylates: May
increase the risk of GI side effects
such as bleeding.
Bone marrow depressants: May
increase the risk of hematologic
reactions.
**Heparin, oral anticoagulants,
thrombolytics:** May increase the
effects of these drugs.
Lithium: May increase the blood
concentration and risk of toxicity of
lithium.
Methotrexate: May increase the
risk of methotrexate toxicity.
Probenecid: May increase the
oxaprozin blood concentration.
Herbal
Feverfew: May decrease the effects
of feverfew.
Ginkgo biloba: May increase the
risk of bleeding.

Food
None known.

DIAGNOSTIC TEST EFFECTS
May increase BUN, serum creatinine,
AST (SGOT), and ALT (SGPT) levels.

SIDE EFFECTS
Occasional (9%-3%)
Nausea, diarrhea, constipation,
dyspepsia, edema
Rare (less than 3%)
Vomiting, abdominal cramps or pain,
flatulence, anorexia, confusion,
tinnitus, insomnia, somnolence

SERIOUS REACTIONS
* Hypertension, acute renal failure,
respiratory depression, GI bleeding,
and coma occur rarely.

PRECAUTIONS & CONSIDERATIONS
Caution is warranted with a history
of GI tract disease, hepatic or renal
impairment, and a predisposition to
fluid retention. It is unknown if
oxaprozin is excreted in breast milk.
Oxaprozin should not be used during
the third trimester of pregnancy
because it may cause adverse effects
in the fetus, such as premature
closure of the ductus arteriosus. The
safety and efficacy of oxaprozin have
not been established in children. In
the elderly, GI bleeding or ulceration
is more likely to cause serious
complications and age-related renal
impairment may increase the risk of
hepatotoxicity or renal toxicity; a
decreased dosage is recommended.
Avoid alcohol and aspirin during
therapy because these substances
increase the risk of GI bleeding.
Tasks that require mental alertness
or motor skills should also be
avoided.
    Notify the physician if bleeding,
ecchymosis, edema, confusion or
weight gain occurs. BUN, serum

alkaline phosphatase, bilirubin, creatinine, AST (SGOT), and ALT (SGPT) levels to assess hepatic and renal function should be assessed during therapy. Therapeutic response, such as decreased pain, stiffness, swelling, and tenderness, improved grip strength, and increased joint mobility, should be evaluated.

Administration

Take oxaprozin with food, milk, or antacids if GI distress occurs.

Oxazepam
ox-a′ze-pam
(Alepam [AUS],
Apo-Oxazepam [CAN],
Murelax [AUS], Serax,
Serepax [AUS])
Do not confuse oxazepam with oxaprozin, or Serax with Eurax or Xerac.

CATEGORY AND SCHEDULE
Pregnancy Risk Category: D
Controlled Substance:
Schedule IV

CLASSIFICATION
Anxiolytics, benzodiazepines

MECHANISM OF ACTION
A benzodiazepine that potentiates the effects of gamma-aminobutyric acid and other inhibitory neurotransmitters by binding to specific receptors in the CNS. *Therapeutic Effect:* Produces anxiolytic effect and skeletal muscle relaxation.

PHARMACOKINETICS
Well absorbed from the GI tract. Protein binding: 97%. Metabolized in the liver. Primarily excreted in urine.

Not removed by hemodialysis.
Half-life: 5-20 hr.

AVAILABILITY
Capsules: 10 mg, 15 mg, 30 mg.
Tablet: 15 mg.

INDICATIONS AND DOSAGES
▸ **Mild to moderate anxiety**
PO
Adults. 10-15 mg 3-4 times a day.
▸ **Severe anxiety**
PO
Adults. 15-30 mg 3-4 times a day.
▸ **Alcohol withdrawal**
PO
Adults. 15-30 mg 3-4 times a day.
Elderly. Initially, 10-20 mg 3 times a day. May gradually increase up to 30-45 mg/day.

CONTRAINDICATIONS
Angle-closure glaucoma; pre-existing CNS depression; severe, uncontrolled pain

INTERACTIONS
Drug
Alcohol, other CNS depressants: May potentiate CNS depression.
Herbal
Kava kava, valerian: May increase CNS depression.
Food
None known.

DIAGNOSTIC TEST EFFECTS
May elevate serum alkaline phosphatase, bilirubin, LDH, AST (SGOT), and ALT (SGPT) levels. May produce abnormal renal function test results. Therapeutic serum drug level is 0.2-1.4 mcg/ml; toxic serum drug level has not been established.

SIDE EFFECTS
Frequent
Mild, transient somnolence at beginning of therapy

Occasional
Dizziness, headache
Rare
Paradoxical CNS reactions, such as
hyperactivity or nervousness in children and excitement or restlessness
in the elderly or debilitated (generally noted during the first 2 weeks of
therapy)

SERIOUS REACTIONS
• Abrupt or too-rapid withdrawal
may result in pronounced restlessness, irritability, insomnia, hand
tremor, abdominal or muscle cramps,
diaphoresis, vomiting, and seizures.
• Overdose results in somnolence,
confusion, diminished reflexes, and
coma.

PRECAUTIONS & CONSIDERATIONS
Caution is warranted with a history
of drug dependence. Females on
long-term therapy should use effective contraception during therapy and
notify the physician if she becomes
or may be pregnant. Alcohol and
other CNS depressants should be
avoided while taking oxazepam.
    Drowsiness and dizziness may
occur. Tasks requiring mental alertness
or motor skills should be avoided.
CBC, blood chemistry, and hepatic
and renal function should be monitored especially during long-term
therapy.
Administration
! Plan to use the smallest effective
dose in the elderly or debilitated and
in those with hepatic disease or a
low serum albumin level. Do not
abruptly discontinue after long-term
use. The therapeutic serum level for
oxazepam is 0.2-1.4 mcg/ml; the
toxic serum level is not established.

Oxcarbazepine
oks-kar-bays'uh-peen
(Trileptal)

CATEGORY AND SCHEDULE
Pregnancy Risk Category: C

CLASSIFICATION
Anticonvulsants

MECHANISM OF ACTION
An anticonvulsant that blocks
sodium channels, resulting in stabi-
lization of hyperexcited neural
membranes, inhibition of repetitive
neuronal firing, and diminishing
synaptic impulses. *Therapeutic
Effect:* Prevents seizures.

PHARMACOKINETICS
Completely absorbed from GI tract
and extensively metabolized in the
liver to active metabolite. Protein
binding: 40%. Primarily excreted in
urine. **Half-life:** 2 hr; metabolite,
6-10 hr.

AVAILABILITY
Oral Suspension: 300 mg/5 ml.
Tablets: 150 mg, 300 mg, 600 mg.

INDICATIONS AND DOSAGES
▸ **Adjunctive treatment of seizures**
PO
Adults, Elderly. Initially, 600 mg/day
in 2 divided doses. May increase by
up to 600 mg/day at weekly intervals.
Maximum: 2400 mg/day.
Children 4-16 yr. 8-10 mg/kg.
Maximum: 600 mg/day. Maintenance
(based on weight): 1800 mg/day for
children weighing more than 39 kg;
1200 mg/day for children weighing
29.1-39 kg; and 900 mg/day for children weighing 20-29 kg.

▶ **Conversion to monotherapy**
PO
Adults, Elderly. 600 mg/day in
2 divided doses (while decreasing
concomitant anticonvulsant over
3-6 wk). May increase by 600 mg/day
at weekly intervals up to
2400 mg/day.
Children. Initially, 8-10 mg/kg/day
in 2 divided doses with simultaneous
initial reduction of dose of concomitant antiepileptic.
▶ **Initiation of monotherapy**
PO
Adults, Elderly. 600 mg/day in
2 divided doses. May increase by
300 mg/day every 3 days up to
1200 mg/day.
Children. Initially, 8-10 mg/kg/day
in 2 divided doses. Increase at 3 day
intervals by 5 mg/kg/day to achieve
maintenance dose by weight;
(70 kg): 1500-2100 mg/day;
(60-69 kg): 1200-2100 mg/day;
(50-59 kg): 1200-1800 mg/day;
(41-49 kg): 1200-1500 mg/day;
(35-40 kg): 900-1500 mg/day;
(25-34 kg): 900-1200 mg/day;
(20-24 kg): 600-900 mg/day.
▶ **Dosage in renal impairment**
For patients with creatinine
clearance less than 30 ml/min,
give 50% of normal starting
dose, then titrate slowly to desired
dose.

OFF-LABEL USES
Atypical panic disorder

CONTRAINDICATIONS
None known.

INTERACTIONS
Drug
**Carbamazepine, phenobarbital,
phenytoin, valproic acid, verapamil:** May decrease the blood
concentration and effects of
oxcarbazepine.

Felodipine, oral contraceptives:
May decrease the effectiveness of
these drugs.
Phenobarbital, phenytoin: May
increase the blood concentration and
risk of toxicity of these drugs.
Herbal
None known.
Food
None known.

DIAGNOSTIC TEST EFFECTS
May increase GGT level and other
hepatic function test results. May
increase or decrease blood glucose
level. May decrease serum calcium,
potassium, and sodium levels.

SIDE EFFECTS
Frequent (22%-13%)
Dizziness, nausea, headache
Occasional (7%-5%)
Vomiting, diarrhea, ataxia, nervous-
ness, heartburn, indigestion, epigas-
tric pain, constipation
Rare (4%)
Tremor, rash, back pain, epistaxis,
sinusitis, diplopia

SERIOUS REACTIONS
• Clinically significant hyponatremia may occur.

PRECAUTIONS & CONSIDERATIONS
Caution is warranted with renal
impairment and a hypersensitivity
to carbamazepine. Oxcarbazepine
crosses the placenta and is distributed in breast milk. No age-related
precautions have been noted in children older than 4 years. In the
elderly, age-related renal impairment
may require dosage adjustment.
  Drowsiness may occur, so alcohol
and tasks requiring mental alertness
or motor skills should be avoided.
Notify the physician if dizziness,
headache, nausea, and rash occur.
Seizure disorder, including the onset,

duration, frequency, intensity, and type of seizures, should be assessed before and during treatment. Serum sodium levels should be monitored; signs and symptoms of hyponatremia include confusion, headache, lethargy, malaise, and nausea.

Administration

! Plan to give all doses in a twice-daily regimen.

Take oxcarbazepine without regard to food.

Oxiconazole
ox-i-con'a-zole
(Oxistat, Oxizole [CAN])
Do not confuse with Nitrostat.

CATEGORY AND SCHEDULE
Pregnancy Risk Category: B

CLASSIFICATION
Antifungals, topical, dermatologics

MECHANISM OF ACTION
An antifungal agent that inhibits ergosterol synthesis. *Therapeutic Effect:* Destroys cytoplasmic membrane integrity of fungi. Fungicidal.

PHARMACOKINETICS
Low systemic absorption. Absorbed and distributed in each layer of the dermis. Excreted in the urine.

AVAILABILITY
Cream: 1% (Oxistat).
Lotion: 1% (Oxistat).

INDICATIONS AND DOSAGES
▸ **Tinea pedis**
TOPICAL
Adults, Elderly, Children 12 yr and older. Apply 1-2 times daily for one

month or until signs and symptoms significantly improve.
▸ **Tinea cruris, Tinea corporis**
TOPICAL
Adults, Elderly, Children 12 yr and older. Apply 1-2 times daily for two weeks or until signs and symptoms significantly improve.

CONTRAINDICATIONS
Not for ophthalmic use, hypersensitivity to oxiconazole or any other azole fungals

INTERACTIONS
Drug
None known.
Herbal
None known.
Food
None known.

DIAGNOSTIC TEST EFFECTS
None known.

SIDE EFFECTS
Occasional
Itching, local irritation, stinging, dryness

SERIOUS REACTIONS
• Hypersensitivity reactions characterized by rash, swelling, pruritus, maceration, and a sensation of warmth may occur.

PRECAUTIONS & CONSIDERATIONS
Caution should be used with known hypersensitivity to other antifungal agents. It is unknown if oxiconazole is distributed in breast milk. Safety and efficacy of oxiconazole have not been established in children younger than 12 years. There are no age-related precautions noted in the elderly.

Signs and symptoms of a local reaction include blistering, burning, irritation, itching, oozing, redness, and swelling. Oxiconazole should be discontinued and the physician should be notified immediately.

Administration

Oxiconazole is for external use only. Shake lotion well before using. Apply and rub gently into the affected and surrounding area. Avoid contact with eyes, mouth, nose, or other mucous membranes. Topical therapy may be used for 2 to 4 weeks. Area should not be covered with an occlusive dressing. Keep area clean and dry and wear light clothing to promote ventilation.

Oxtriphylline

ox-trye′fi-lin
(Apo Oxtriphyllin [CAN]; Brondecon-PD Elixir [AUS], Choledyl [CAN], Choledyl SA)
Do not confuse with amitriptyline.

CATEGORY AND SCHEDULE

Pregnancy Risk Category: C

CLASSIFICATION

Bronchodilators, xanthine derivatives

MECHANISM OF ACTION

A choline salt of theophylline acts as a bronchodilator by directly relaxing smooth muscle of the bronchial airway and pulmonary blood vessels. *Therapeutic Effect:* Relieves bronchospasm, increases vital capacity. Produces cardiac skeletal muscle stimulation.

PHARMACOKINETICS

Absorbed slowly due to extended release formulation. Protein binding: 40%. Distributed rapidly into peripheral non-adipose tissues and body water, including cerebrospinal fluid (CSF). Metabolized in liver. Eliminated in urine. **Half-life:** Adults, 6-12 hr; Children, 1.2-7 hr.

AVAILABILITY

Tablet (extended release): 400 mg, 600 mg (Choledyl SA).

INDICATIONS AND DOSAGES

▸ **Asthma**
PO
Adults, Elderly, Children.
400-600 mg q12hr
Children (younger than 5 yr).
24-36 mg/kg/day given in divided doses.
Children (5-9 yr). 200-400 mg/day given in divided doses.
Children (10-14 yr). 400-800 mg/day given in divided doses.

CONTRAINDICATIONS

Active peptic ulcer disease, seizure disorder (unless receiving appropriate anticonvulsant medication, history of hypersensitivity to xanthines)

INTERACTIONS

Drug
Allopurinol (high dose): May increase serum theophylline levels.
Beta-blockers: May decrease effects of theophylline.
Cimetidine, ciprofloxacin, erythromycin, norfloxacin: May increase theophylline blood concentration and risk of theophylline toxicity.
Lithium: May increase renal excretion of lithium.
Oral Contraceptives: May increase theophylline levels.
Phenytoin: May decrease theophylline and phenytoin serum levels.
Rifampin: May decrease serum theophylline levels.

Smoking: May decrease theophylline blood concentration.
Herbal
None known.
Food
None known.

DIAGNOSTIC TEST EFFECTS
May decrease serum alkaline phosphatase, bilirubin, and LDH levels. May increase serum glucose and uric acid. May increase urine albumin and catecholamines.

SIDE EFFECTS
Frequent
Headache, shakiness, restlessness, tachycardia, trembling
Occasional
Nausea, vomiting, epigastric pain, diarrhea, headache, mild diuresis, insomnia
Rare
Alopecia, hyperglycemia, SIADH, rash

SERIOUS REACTIONS
• Nausea, vomiting, seizures, and coma can result from overdosage.

PRECAUTIONS & CONSIDERATIONS
Caution is warranted with diabetes mellitus, glaucoma, hypertension, hyperthyroidism, impaired cardiac, renal or liver function, peptic ulcer disease, or seizure disorder. It is unknown if oxtriphylline is distributed in breast milk. Children may be more sensitive to the effects of xanthines. There are no age-related precautions noted in the elderly. Caffeine and caffeine derivatives such as chocolate, coffee, cola, cocoa, and tea should be avoided. Smoking, charcoal-broiled food, and a high-protein, low-carbohydrate diet may decrease theophylline level.
Administration
Give with food to avoid gastrointestinal (GI) distress. Do not crush or break extended-release forms. Dosage is based on peak serum theophylline concentrations, clinical condition, and absence of theophylline toxicity. The following mg equivalents assist when changing from one xanthine preparation to another: theophylline anhydrous 100 mg = aminophylline 118 mg = oxtriphylline 156 mg = theophylline sodium glycinate 200 mg.

Oxybutynin
ox-i-byoo′ti-nin
(Ditropan, Ditropan XL, Oxytrol)
Do not confuse oxybutynin with Oxycontin, or Ditropan with diazepam.

CATEGORY AND SCHEDULE
Pregnancy Risk Category: B

CLASSIFICATION
Anticholinergics, relaxants, urinary tract

MECHANISM OF ACTION
An anticholinergic that exerts antispasmodic (papaverine-like) and antimuscarinic (atropine-like) action on the detrusor smooth muscle of the bladder. *Therapeutic Effect:* Increases bladder capacity and delays desire to void.

PHARMACOKINETICS

Route	Onset	Peak	Duration
PO	0.5-1 hr	3-6 hr	6-10 hr

Rapidly absorbed from the GI tract. Metabolized in the liver.

Primarily excreted in urine. Unknown if removed by hemodialysis. **Half-life:** 1-2.3 hr.

AVAILABILITY

Syrup (Ditropan): 5 mg/5 ml.
Tablets (Ditropan): 5 mg.
Tablets (Extended-Release [Ditropan XL]): 5 mg, 10 mg, 15 mg.
Transdermal (Oxytrol): 3.9 mg.

INDICATIONS AND DOSAGES
▸ **Neurogenic bladder**
PO
Adults. 5 mg 2-3 times a day up to 5 mg 4 times a day.
Elderly. 2.5-5 mg twice a day. May increase by 2.5 mg/day every 1-2 days.
Children 5 yr and older. 5 mg twice a day up to 5 mg 4 times a day.
Children 1-4 yr. 0.2 mg/kg/dose 2-4 times a day.
PO (EXTENDED RELEASE)
Adults. 5-10 mg/day up to 30 mg/day.
TRANSDERMAL
Adults. 3.9 mg applied twice a week. Apply every 3-4 days.

CONTRAINDICATIONS
GI or GU obstruction, glaucoma, myasthenia gravis, toxic megacolon, ulcerative colitis

INTERACTIONS
Drug
Medications with anticholinergic effects (such as antihistamines): May increase the anticholinergic effects of oxybutynin.
Herbal
None known.
Food
None known.

DIAGNOSTIC TEST EFFECTS
None known.

SIDE EFFECTS
Frequent
Constipation, dry mouth, somnolence, decreased perspiration
Occasional
Decreased lacrimation or salivation, impotence, urinary hesitancy and retention, suppressed lactation, blurred vision, mydriasis, nausea or vomiting, insomnia

SERIOUS REACTIONS
• Overdose produces CNS excitation (including nervousness, restlessness, hallucinations, and irritability), hypotension or hypertension, confusion, tachycardia, facial flushing, and respiratory depression.

PRECAUTIONS & CONSIDERATIONS
Caution is warranted with cardiovascular disease, hypertension, hyperthyroidism, hepatic or renal impairment, neuropathy, benign prostatic hyperplasia, and reflux esophagitis. It is unknown if oxybutynin crosses the placenta or is distributed in breast milk. No age-related precautions have been noted in children older than 5 years. The elderly may be more sensitive to the drug's anticholinergic effects, such as dry mouth and urine retention. Avoid alcohol and tasks that require mental alertness and motor skills until response to the drug is established.

Drowsiness and dizziness may occur. Intake and output, pattern of daily bowel activity and stool consistency, symptomatic relief should be assessed.
Administration
Take oxybutynin without regard to food.

Oxycodone
ox-ee-koe′done
(Endone [AUS], OxyContin,
Oxydose, OxyFast,
OxyIR, Oxynorm [AUS],
Roxicodone, Roxicodone
Intensol)
**Do not confuse oxycodone with
oxybutynin.**

CATEGORY AND SCHEDULE
Pregnancy Risk Category: B
(D if used for prolonged
periods or at high dosages
at term)
Controlled Substance:
Schedule II

CLASSIFICATION
Analgesics, narcotic

MECHANISM OF ACTION
An opioid analgesic that binds
with opioid receptors in the CNS.
Therapeutic Effect: Alters the perception of and emotional response to
pain.

PHARMACOKINETICS

Route	Onset	Peak	Duration
PO, Immediate-release	N/A	N/A	4-5 hr
PO, Controlled-release	N/A	N/A	12 hr

Moderately absorbed from the GI
tract. Protein binding: 38%-45%.
Widely distributed. Metabolized in
the liver. Excreted in urine.
Unknown if removed by hemodialysis. **Half-life:** 2-3 hr (3.2 hr
controlled-release).

AVAILABILITY
*Capsules (Immediate-Release
[OxyIR]):* 5 mg.
*Oral Concentrate (Oxydose,
OxyFast, Roxicodone Intensol):*
20 mg/ml.
Oral Solution (Roxicodone): 5 mg/5 ml.
Tablets (Roxicodone): 5 mg, 15 mg,
30 mg.
*Tablets (Extended-Release
[OxyContin]):* 10 mg, 20 mg, 40 mg,
80 mg, 160 mg.

INDICATIONS AND DOSAGES
▸ **Analgesia**
PO (CONTROLLED-RELEASE)
Adults, Elderly. Initially, 10 mg
q12hr. May increase every
1-2 days by 25%-50%. Usual:
40 mg/day (100 mg/day for
cancer pain).
PO (IMMEDIATE-RELEASE)
Adults, Elderly. Initially, 5 mg q6hr
as needed. May increase up to 30 mg
q4hr. Usual: 10-30 mg q4hr as
needed.
Children. 0.05-0.15 mg/kg/dose
q4-6hr.

CONTRAINDICATIONS
None known.

INTERACTIONS
Drug
Alcohol, other CNS depressants:
May increase CNS or respiratory
depression and hypotension.
MAOIs: May produce a severe,
sometimes fatal reaction; expect to
administer one-quarter of usual
oxycodone dose.
Herbal
None known.
Food
None known.

DIAGNOSTIC TEST EFFECTS
May increase serum amylase and
lipase levels.

SIDE EFFECTS
Frequent
Somnolence, dizziness, hypotension (including orthostatic hypotension), anorexia
Occasional
Confusion, diaphoresis, facial flushing, urine retention, constipation, dry mouth, nausea, vomiting, headache
Rare
Allergic reaction, depression, paradoxical CNS hyperactivity or nervousness in children, paradoxical excitement and restlessness in elderly or debilitated patients

SERIOUS REACTIONS
• Overdose results in respiratory depression, skeletal muscle flaccidity, cold or clammy skin, cyanosis, and extreme somnolence progressing to seizures, stupor, and coma.
• Hepatotoxicity may occur with overdose of the acetaminophen component of fixed-combination products.
• The patient who uses oxycodone repeatedly may develop a tolerance to the drug's analgesic effect and physical dependence.

PRECAUTIONS & CONSIDERATIONS
Extreme caution should be used with acute alcoholism, anoxia, CNS depression, hypercapnia, respiratory depression or dysfunction, seizures, shock, or untreated myxedema. Caution is also warranted with acute abdominal conditions, Addison's disease, chronic obstructive pulmonary disease (COPD), hypothyroidism, hepatic impairment, increased intracranial pressure, prostatic hypertrophy, and urethral stricture. Oxycodone readily crosses the placenta and is distributed in breast milk. Regular use of opioids during pregnancy may produce withdrawal symptoms in the neonate, including irritability, diarrhea, excessive crying, fever, hyperactive reflexes, irritability, seizures, sneezing, tremors, vomiting, and yawning. The neonate may develop respiratory depression if the mother receives oxycodone during labor. Children are more prone to experience paradoxical excitement. Children younger than 2 years and the elderly are more susceptible to the drug's respiratory depressant effects. Age-related renal impairment may increase the risk of urine retention in the elderly.

Dizziness and drowsiness may occur, so change positions slowly and avoid alcohol, CNS depressants, and tasks that require mental alertness or motor skills until response to the drug is established. B/P, respiratory rate, mental status, pattern of daily bowel activity, and clinical improvement should be monitored. The drug should be withheld and the physician should be notified if the respiratory rate is 12 breaths/minute or less in an adult or 20 breaths/minute or less in a child.

Storage
Store vials at room temperature.

Administration
! Be aware that oxycodone's side effects are dependent on the dosage. Know that ambulatory patients and patients not in severe pain are more likely to experience dizziness, hypotension, nausea, and vomiting than those in the supine position or those in severe pain. Swallow controlled-release tablets (OxyContin) whole because crushing, breaking, or chewing them may lead to the rapid release and absorption of a potentially fatal dose. Be aware that OxyContin has a potential for abuse and accidental overdose may result in death.

Take oral oxycodone without regard to food. Crush immediate-release tablets as needed.

O

Oxymetazoline

ox-ee-met-az'oh-leen
(Afrin, Afrin 12-Hour,
Afrin Children's Strength
Nose Drops, Ocuclear,
Sinex 12-Hour
Long-Acting)

CATEGORY AND SCHEDULE
Pregnancy Risk Category: C
OTC

CLASSIFICATION
Imidazoline derivative,
decongestant

MECHANISM OF ACTION
A direct-acting sympathomimetic
amine that acts on alpha-adrenergic
receptors in arterioles of the nasal
mucosa to produce constriction.
Therapeutic Effect: Causes
vasoconstriction resulting in
decreased blood flow and
decreased nasal congestion.

PHARMACOKINETICS
Onset of action is about 10 min,
and a duration of action is 7 hr or
more. Absorption occurs from the
nasal mucosa and can produce
systemic effects, primarily
following overdose or excessive
use. Excreted mostly in the
urine as well as the feces.
Half-life: 5-8 hr.

AVAILABILITY
Eye Drops: 0.025%
(Ocuclear).
Nasal Drops: 0.025% (Afrin
Children's Strength Nose Drops),
0.05% (Afrin).
Nasal Spray: 0.05% (Afrin, Afrin
12-Hour, Sinex 12-Hour
Long-Acting).

INDICATIONS AND DOSAGES
▸ **Rhinitis**
INTRANASAL
*Adults, Elderly, Children older
than 6 yr.* 2-3 drops/sprays
(0.05% nasal solution) in each
nostril q12hr.
Children (2-5 yr). 2-4 drops/sprays
(0.025% nasal solution) in each
nostril q12hr for up to 3 days.
▸ **Conjunctivitis**
OPHTHALMIC
*Adults, Elderly, Children older
than 6 yr.* 1-2 drops (0.025%
ophthalmic solution) q6hr for
3-4 days.

OFF-LABEL USES
Otitis media surgical procedures

CONTRAINDICATIONS
Narrow-angle glaucoma or hypersensitivity to oxymetazoline or other
adrenergic agents

INTERACTIONS
Drug
Maprotiline, tricyclic antidepres-
sants: May increase the effects of
oxymetazoline.
Herbal
None known.
Food
None known.

DIAGNOSTIC TEST EFFECTS
None known.

SIDE EFFECTS
Occasional
Burning, stinging, drying nasal
mucosa, sneezing, rebound congestion, insomnia, nervousness

SERIOUS REACTIONS
• Large doses may produce tachycardia, hypertension, arrhythmias,
palpitations, lightheadedness,
nausea, and vomiting.

PRECAUTIONS & CONSIDERATIONS

Caution is warranted with cerebral arteriosclerosis, coronary artery disease, diabetes, heart disease, hypertension, hypertensive cardio-vascular disease, concurrent monoamine oxidase inhibitors or tricyclic antidepressants, prostatic enlargement and hyperthyroidism. It is unknown if oxymetazoline crosses the placenta and is distributed in breast milk. Safety and efficacy of oxymetazoline have not been established in children younger than 2 years of age using oxymetazoline intranasally and younger than 6 years of age using the drug ophthamoli-cally. There are no age-related precautions noted in the elderly. Prolonged use of oxymetazoline intranasally should be monitored for rebound nasal congestion or rhinitis medicamentosa.

Be aware that if oxymetazoline is systemically absorbed it may cause fast, irregular and pounding heartbeat, headache, insomnia, lightheadedness, nausea, nervousness, and trembling.

Administration

Be aware that oxymetazoline should be used up to 3 days.

Blow nose gently before using the nasal drops. Tilt head back while standing or sitting and squeeze drop in nostril. Keep head tilted back for few minutes. Rinse the dropper with hot water and dry with a clean tissue.

Blow nose gently before using the nasal spray. Stand upright, and spray the medicine once into nostril, sniffing while squeezing the bottle quickly and firmly. Wait 3 to 5 minutes to allow the drug to work, and then blow nose again. Rinse tip of nasal spray with hot water and dry with a clean tissue.

Wash hands before administering oxymetazoline eye drops. With the middle finger, put pressure to the inside corner of the eye. Tilt the head back and with the index finger of the same hand, pull the lower eyelid away from the eye to form a pouch. Drop the medicine into the pouch and gently close the eyes. Tell the patient not to blink. Keep the eyes closed for 1 or 2 minutes to allow the medicine to be absorbed.

Oxymetholone

ox-ee-meth′oh-lone
(Anadrol, Anapolon [CAN])
Do not confuse with oxycodone.

CATEGORY AND SCHEDULE

Pregnancy Risk Category: X
Controlled Substance: Schedule III

CLASSIFICATION

Anabolic steroids, hormones/hormone modifiers

MECHANISM OF ACTION

An androgenic-anabolic steroid that is a synthetic derivative of testosterone synthesized to accentuate anabolic as opposed to androgenic effects. *Therapeutic Effect:* Improves nitrogen balance in conditions of unfavorable protein metabolism with adequate caloric and protein intake, stimulates erythropoiesis, suppress gonadotropic functions of pituitary and may exert a direct effect upon the testes.

PHARMACOKINETICS

The pharmacokinetics of oxymetholone has been studied. Metabolized in the liver via reduction and oxidation. Unchanged oxymetholone and its metabolites are excreted in urine. **Half-life:** Unknown.

AVAILABILITY

Tablets: 50 mg (Anadrol).

INDICATIONS AND DOSAGES

▸ **Anemia, chronic renal failure, acqured aplastic anemia, chemotherapy-induced myelosuppresion, Fanconi's anemia, red cell aplasia**
PO
Adults, Elderly, Children.
1-5 mg/kg/day. Response is not immediate and a minimum of 3-6 months should be given.

OFF-LABEL USES

Amegakaryocytic thrombocytopenia, familial antithrombin III deficiency, hereditary angioedema, HIV wasting, metastatic breast cancer in women, relief of bone pain associated with osteoporosis, neutropenia, Turner's syndrome, xeroderma pigmentosum

CONTRAINDICATIONS

Cardiac impairment, hypercalcemia, pregnancy/lactation, prostatic or breast cancer in males, metastatic breast cancer in women with active hypercalcemia, nephrosis or nephritic phase nephritis, severe liver disease, hypersensitivity to oxymetholone or any of its components

INTERACTIONS

Drug
Bupropion: May lower seizure threshold.
Liver toxic medications: May increase liver toxicity.

Oral anticoagulants: May increase effects of oral anticoagulants.
Herbal
Chaparral: May increase liver enzymes.
Comfrey: May increase liver enzymes.
Eucalyptus: May increase risk of heptotoxicity.
Germander: May increase liver enzymes.
Jin bu huan: May increase liver enzymes.
Kava kava: May increase risk of liver damage.
Pennyroyal: May increase liver enzymes.
Skullcap: May increase risk of liver damage.
Valerian: May increase risk of heptotoxicity.
Food
None known.

DIAGNOSTIC TEST EFFECTS

May increase blood Hgb and Hct, LDL concentrations, serum alkaline phosphatase, bilirubin, calcium, potassium, SGOT (AST) levels and sodium levels. May decrease HDL concentrations.

SIDE EFFECTS

Frequent
Gynecomastia, acne, amenorrhea, menstrual irregularities
Females: Hirsutism, deepening of voice, clitoral enlargement that may not be reversible when drug is discontinued
Occasional
Edema, nausea, insomnia, oligospermia, priapism, male pattern of baldness, bladder irritability, hypercalcemia in immobilized patients or those with breast cancer, hypercholesterolemia, inflammation and pain at IM injection site

Transdermal: Itching, erythema, skin irritation
Rare
Liver damage, hypersensitivity

SERIOUS REACTIONS

• Cholestatic jaundice, hepatic necrosis, and death occur rarely but have been reported in association with long-term androgenic-anabolic steroid use.

PRECAUTIONS & CONSIDERATIONS

Caution is warranted with diabetes, liver and renal impairment, congestive heart failure, hypertension, coronary artery disease, previous myocardial infarction, lipid-lipoprotein abnormalities, benign prostatic hyperplasia, suppression of clotting factors II, V, VII, and X, and an increase in prothrombin time. Oxymetholone use is contraindicated during lactation and is excreted in breast milk. Safety and efficacy of oxymethalone have not been established in children and elderly. Adequate calories and protein should be consumed.

Acne, nausea, pedal edema, or vomiting may occur. Women should report deepening of voice, hoarseness, and menstrual irregularities. Men should report difficulty urinating, frequent erections, and gynecomastia. Weight should be obtained each day. Weekly weight gains of more than 5 pounds should be reported.
Administration
Dose should be individualized. Response is not often immediate and a minimum trial of 3-6 months should be given.

Oxymorphone
ox-ee-mor′fone
(Numorphan)

CATEGORY AND SCHEDULE
Pregnancy Risk Category B, D if used for prolonged periods or at high dosages at term
Controlled Substance: Schedule II

CLASSIFICATION
Analgesics, narcotic

MECHANISM OF ACTION
An opioid agonist, similar to morphine, that binds at opiate receptor sites in the central nervous system (CNS). *Therapeutic Effect:* Reduces intensity of pain stimuli incoming from sensory nerve endings, altering pain perception and emotional response to pain; suppresses cough reflex.

PHARMACOKINETICS

Route	Onset	Peak	Duration
Subcutaneous	5-10 min	30-90 min	4-6 hr
IM	5-10 min	30-60 min	3-6 hr
IV	5-10 min	15-30 min	3-6 hr
Rectal	15-30 min	N/A	3-6 hr

Well absorbed from the gastrointestinal (GI) tract, after IM administration. Widely distributed. Metabolized in liver via glucuronidation. Excreted in urine. **Half-life:** 1-2 hr.

AVAILABILITY
Injection: 1 mg/ml, 1.5 mg/ml (Numorphan).
Suppository: 5 mg (Numorphan).

INDICATIONS AND DOSAGES
▸ **Analgesic, Anxiety, Preanesthesia**
IV
Adults, Elderly, Children 12 yr and older. Initially 0.5 mg.
SC/IM
Adults, Elderly, Children 12 yr and older. 1-1.5 mg IM or SC q4-6hr as needed
RECTAL
Adults, Elderly, Children 12 yr and older. 0.5-1 mg q4-6hr.
▸ **Obstetrical analgesic**
IM
Adults, Elderly, Children 12 yr and older. 0.5-1 mg IM during labor.

OFF-LABEL USES
Cancer pain, intractable pain in narcotic-tolerant patients

CONTRAINDICATIONS
Paralytic ileus, acute asthma attack, pulmonary edema secondary to chemical respiratory irritant, severe respiratory depression, upper airway obstruction

INTERACTIONS
Drug
Alcohol, CNS depressants, tricyclic antidepressants: May increase CNS or respiratory depression, hypotension.
MAOIs: May produce severe, fatal reaction; plan to reduce dose to one quarter usual dose.
Phenothiazines: May decrease effect of oxymorphone.
Herbal
Ginseng: May decrease opioid analgesic effectiveness.
Gotu kola, kava kava, valerian: May increase CNS or respiratory depression.
St. John's Wort: May increase sedation.
Food
None known.

DIAGNOSTIC TEST EFFECTS
May increase serum amylase levels and plasma lipase concentrations.

🏵IV INCOMPATIBILITIES
None known.
💉IV Compatibilities
Glycopyrrolate (Robinul), hydroxyzine (Vistaril), ranitidine (Zantac)

SIDE EFFECTS
Frequent
Drowsiness, dizziness, hypotension, decreased appetite, tolerance, or dependence
Occasional
Confusion, diaphoresis, facial flushing, urinary retention, constipation, dry mouth, nausea, vomiting, headache, pain at injection site, abdominal cramps
Rare
Allergic reaction, depression

SERIOUS REACTIONS
• Hypotension, paralytic ileus, respiratory depression, and toxic megacolon rarely occur.
• Overdosage results in respiratory depression, skeletal muscle flaccidity, cold or clammy skin, cyanosis, extreme somnolence progressing to seizures, stupor and coma.
• Tolerance to analgesic effect and physical dependence may occur with repeated use.
• Prolonged duration of action and cumulative effect may occur in patients with impaired liver or renal function.

PRECAUTIONS & CONSIDERATIONS
Caution is warranted with acute alcoholism, anoxia, CNS depression, hypercapnia, respiratory depression or dysfunction, seizures, shock, untreated myxedema, acute abdominal conditions, Addison's disease, chronic obstructive pulmonary

disease (COPD), hypothyroidism, impaired liver function, increased intracranial pressure, and urethral stricture. Oxymorphone readily crosses the placenta and it is unknown if oxymorphone is distributed in breast milk. Its use may prolong labor if administered in the latent phase of the first stage of labor or before cervical dilation of 4 to 5 cm has occurred. Respiratory depression may occur in neonate if mother receives opiates during labor. Regular use of opiates during pregnancy may produce withdrawal symptoms in the neonate, including diarrhea, excessive crying, fever, hyperactive reflexes, irritability, seizures, sneezing, tremors, vomiting, and yawning. Safety and efficacy of oxymorphone have not been established in children younger than 12 years. The elderly may be more susceptible to respiratory depression and the drug may cause paradoxical excitement. Age-related prostatic hypertrophy or obstruction and renal impairment may increase the risk of urinary retention, and dosage adjustment is recommended in the elderly. Alcohol and tasks that require mental alertness and motor skills should be avoided during therapy. Drug dependence and tolerance may occur with prolonged use at high dosages.

Dizziness, hypotension, nausea, and vomiting may be experienced more frequently than those in supine position or having severe pain.

Storage

Store injection formulation at room temperature and protect from light.

Keep rectal suppositories refrigerated.

Administration

Oxymorphone's side effects depend on the dosage amount and route of administration but occur infrequently with oral antitussives. A high concentration injection should be used only in patients currently receiving high doses of another opiate agonist for severe, chronic pain caused by cancer or tolerance to opiate agonists. Slight yellow discoloration of parenteral form does not indicate loss of potency. May give undiluted as IV push.

Unwrap rectal suppository before inserting. Moisten suppository with cold water before inserting well up into rectum.

Oxytetracycline

ox'ee-tet-tra-sye'kleen
(Terramycin [CAN], Terramycin IM)

CATEGORY AND SCHEDULE

Pregnancy Risk Category: D (B with topical)

CLASSIFICATION

Antibiotics, tetracyclines

MECHANISM OF ACTION

A tetracycline antibiotic that inhibits bacterial protein synthesis by binding to ribosomes. Cell wall synthesis is not affected. *Therapeutic Effect:* Prevents bacterial cell growth. Bacteriostatic.

PHARMACOKINETICS

Poorly absorbed after IM administration. Protein binding: 27%-35%. Metabolized in liver. Excreted in urine. Eliminated in feces via biliary system. Not removed by hemodialysis. **Half-life:** 8.5-9.6 hr (half-life is increased with impaired renal function).

AVAILABILITY

Injection, solution: 5% (Terramycin IM).

INDICATIONS AND DOSAGES

▶ **Treatment of inflammatory acne, anthrax, gonorrhea, skin infections, urinary tract infection (UTI)**

IM
Adults, Elderly. 250 mg/day or 300 mg/day divided q8-12hr
Children 8 yr and older. 15-25 mg/kg/day in divided doses q8-12hr. Maximum: 250 mg/dose.

▶ **Dosage in renal impairment**

Creatinine Clearance	Dosage Interval
Less than 10 ml/min	q24hr

OFF-LABEL USES

Chlamydia, non-specific urethritis, peptic ulcer

CONTRAINDICATIONS

Hypersensitivity to tetracyclines or any component of the formulation, children 8 years and younger

INTERACTIONS

Drug

Carbamazepine, phenytoin: May decrease oxytetracycline blood concentration.
Cholestyramine, colestipol: May decrease oxytetracycline absorption.
Oral contraceptives: May decrease the effects of these drugs.

Herbal

St. John's wort: May increase risk of photosensitivity.

Food

Dairy products: Inhibit oxytetracycline absorption.

DIAGNOSTIC TEST EFFECTS

May increase BUN, serum alkaline phosphatase, serum amylase, serum bilirubin, SGOT (AST), and SGPT (ALT) levels.

▓ IV INCOMPATIBILITIES

Acetylcysteine (Mucomyst), amphotericin B, ampicillin, carbenicillin (Geocillin), cefazolin (Ancef), cephalothin (Ceporacin), cephapirin (Cefadyl), cloxacillin (Cloxapen), erythromycin, iron, methohexital (Brevital), nafcillin (Unipen), oxacillin, penicillin G (Pfizerpen), pentobarbital (Nembutal), phenobarbital (Luminal), phenytoin, prochlorperazine, riboflavin, sodium bicarbonate

▓ IV Compatibilities

Aminophylline, calcium gluconate, colistin, isoproterenol (Isuprel), lidocaine (Xylocaine), methyldopa (Aldomet), norepinephrine (Levophed), polymyxin B, potassium, vancomycin (Vancocin)

SIDE EFFECTS

Frequent
Dizziness, lightheadedness, diarrhea, nausea, vomiting, stomach cramps, increased sensitivity of skin to sunlight
Occasional
Pigmentation of skin, mucous membranes, itching in rectal or genital area, sore mouth or tongue, increased BUN, irritation at injection site

SERIOUS REACTIONS

• Superinfection (especially fungal), anaphylaxis, and increased intracranial pressure may occur.
• Bulging fontanelles occur rarely in infants.

PRECAUTIONS & CONSIDERATIONS

Caution should be used in those who cannot avoid sun or ultraviolet light exposure because this may produce a severe photosensitivity reaction as well as those who have liver disease. Be aware that the patient's history of allergies, especially to tetracyclines before beginning drug therapy should be determined before therapy. Oxytetracycline readily crosses the placenta and is distributed in breast milk. Avoid oxytetracycline use in women during the last half of pregnancy. Be aware that oxytetracycline use may produce permanent tooth discoloration or enamel hypoplasia and inhibit fetal skeletal growth in children 8 years of age or younger. Be aware that oxytetracycline use is not recommended in children 8 years of age and younger. There are no age-related precautions noted in the elderly. Skin should be protected from sun exposure and overexposure to sun or ultraviolet light should be avoided to prevent photosensitivity reactions.

Be alert for signs and symptoms of superinfection as evidenced by anal or genital pruritus, diarrhea, and ulceration or changes of the oral mucosa.

Administration
Injection is for intramuscular use only. Give without regard to meals. Continue the antibiotic for the full length of treatment and evenly space drug doses around the clock.

Oxytocin
ox-ee-toe′sin
(Pitocin, Syntocinon INJ [AUS])
Do not confuse Pitocin with Pitressin.

CATEGORY AND SCHEDULE
Pregnancy Risk Category: X

CLASSIFICATION
Hormones/hormone modifiers, oxytocics, stimulants, uterine

MECHANISM OF ACTION
An oxytocic that affect uterine myofibril activity and stimulates mammary smooth muscle.
Therapeutic Effect: Contracts uterine smooth muscle. Enhances lactation.

PHARMACOKINETICS

Route	Onset	Peak	Duration
IV	Immediate	N/A	1 hr
IM	3-5 min	N/A	2 3 hr

Rapidly absorbed through nasal mucous membranes. Protein binding: 30%. Distributed in extracellular fluid. Metabolized in the liver and kidney. Primarily excreted in urine. **Half-life:** 1-6 min.

AVAILABILITY
Injection: 10 units/ml.
Nasal Spray: 40 units/ml

INDICATIONS AND DOSAGES
▸ **Induction or stimulation of labor**
IV
Adults. 0.5-1 milliunit/min. May gradually increase in increments of 1-2 milliunit/min. Rates of 9-10 milliunit/min are rarely required.

▸ **Abortion**
IV
Adults. 10-20 milliunit/min.
Maximum: 30 unit/12h dose.
▸ **Control of postpartum bleeding**
IV INFUSION
Adults. 10-40 units in 1 liter IV
fluid at a rate sufficient to control
uterine atony.
IM
Adults. 10 units (total dose) after
delivery.

CONTRAINDICATIONS

Adequate uterine activity that fails to
progress, cephalopelvic disproportion, fetal distress without imminent
delivery, grand multiparity, hyperactive or hypertonic uterus, obstetric
emergencies that favor surgical intervention, prematurity, unengaged fetal
head, unfavorable fetal position or
presentation, when vaginal delivery
is contraindicated, such as active
genital herpes infection, placenta
previa, or cord presentation

INTERACTIONS
Drug
**Caudal block anesthetics, vasopres-
sors:** May increase pressor effects.
Other oxytocics: May cause cervi-
cal lacerations, uterine hypertonus,
or uterine rupture.
Herbal
None known.
Food
None known.

DIAGNOSTIC TEST EFFECTS
None known.

▓ IV INCOMPATIBILITIES
No known incompatibilities via
Y-site administration.
▓ IV Compatibilities
Heparin, insulin, multivitamins,
potassium chloride

SIDE EFFECTS
Occasional
Tachycardia, premature ventricular
contractions, hypotension, nausea,
vomiting
Rare
Nasal: Lacrimation or tearing, nasal
irritation, rhinorrhea, unexpected
uterine bleeding or contractions

SERIOUS REACTIONS
• Hypertonicity may occur with
tearing of the uterus, increased
bleeding, abruptio placentae, and
cervical and vaginal lacerations.
• In the fetus, bradycardia, CNS or
brain damage, trauma due to rapid
propulsion, low Apgar score at
5 minutes, and retinal hemorrhage
occur rarely.
• Prolonged IV infusion of oxytocin
with excessive fluid volume has
caused severe water intoxication
with seizures, coma, and death.

PRECAUTIONS & CONSIDERATIONS
Induction of labor should be for
medical, not elective, reasons.
Oxytocin should be used as indicated,
and is not known to cause fetal
abnormalities. Oxytocin is present in
small amounts in breast milk. Nasal
oxytocin is used only for initial
breast milk propulsion and ejection
during the first postpartal week, and
is not meant for continued use.
Oxytocin is not recommended for
use in pregnant women because it
may precipitate contractions and
abortions. Oxytocin is not used in
children or the elderly.
     B/P, pulse, respiration rates, intake
and output, uterine contractions,
including duration, frequency and
strength, and fetal heart rate should
be monitored every 15 minutes. If
uterine contractions last longer than
1 minute, occur more frequently than

every 2 minutes, or stop, notify the physician. Be alert to potential water intoxication and for unexpected or increased blood loss.

Storage
Store at room temperature.

Administration
Dilute 10 to 40 units (1 to 4 ml) in 1000 ml of 0.9% NaCl, lactated Ringer's solution, or D_5W to provide a concentration of 10 to 40 mUnits/ml solution. Give by IV infusion and use an infusion device to carefully control prescribed rate of flow.

O

Palifermin
pal-ih-fur′min
(Kepivance)

CATEGORY AND SCHEDULE
Pregnancy Risk Category: C

CLASSIFICATION
Growth factor, epithelial cell

MECHANISM OF ACTION
An antineoplastic adjunct that binds to the keratinocyte growth factor receptor, present on epithelial cells of the buccal mucosa and tongue, resulting in the proliferation, differentiation, and migration of epithelial cells. *Therapeutic Effect:* Reduces incidence and duration of severe oral mucositis.

AVAILABILITY
Injection: 6.25-mg vials.

INDICATIONS AND DOSAGES
▸ **Mucositis (premyelotoxic therapy)**
IV
Adults, Elderly. 60 mcg/kg/day for 3 consecutive days, with the 3rd dose 24-48 hr before chemotherapy.
▸ **Mucositis (post-myelotoxic therapy)**
IV
Adults, Elderly. The last 3 doses should be administered after myelotoxic therapy; the first of these doses should be administered after, but on the same day of, hematopoietic stem cell infusion and at least 4 days after the most recent administration of palfermin.

CONTRAINDICATIONS
Patients allergic to *Escherichia coli*-derived proteins

INTERACTIONS
Drug
Heparin: Palfermin binds to heparin.

Myelotoxic chemotherapy:
Administration of palfermin during or within 24 hours before or after myelotoxic chemotherapy results in increased severity and duration of oral mucositis.
Herbal
None known.
Food
None known.

DIAGNOSTIC TEST EFFECTS
May elevate serum lipase and amylase levels.

SIDE EFFECTS
Frequent (62%-28%)
Rash, fever, pruritus, erythema, edema
Occasional (17%-10%)
Mouth and tongue thickness or discoloration, altered taste, dysesthesia (hyperesthesia, hypoesthesia, paresthesia), arthralgia

SERIOUS REACTIONS
• Transient hypertension occurs occasionally.

PRECAUTIONS & CONSIDERATIONS
Use palfermin cautiously in women who are pregnant or breast-feeding.
Storage
If not used immediately, the reconstituted solution may be stored in the refrigerator for 24 hours. Protect it from light. The reconstituted solution may be warmed to room temperature for up to 1 hour before administration. Discard the solution if it's left at room temperature for more than 1 hour or if it becomes discolored or contains particles.
Administration
Reconstitute palfermin using aseptic technique. Slowly inject 1.2 ml sterile water for injection to yield a final concentration of 5 mg/ml. Swirl gently to dissolve. Don't shake or

agitate the solution. Dissolution takes less than 3 minutes. Administer by IV bolus injection. If heparin is being used to maintain an IV line, use 0.9% NaCl to rinse the IV line before and after palifermin administration.

Palonosetron
pal-oh-noe'seh-tron
(Aloxi)

CATEGORY AND SCHEDULE
Pregnancy Risk Category: B

CLASSIFICATION
Antiemetics/antivertigo, serotonin receptor antagonists

MECHANISM OF ACTION
A 5-HT$_3$ receptor antagonist that acts centrally in the chemoreceptor trigger zone and peripherally at the vagal nerve terminals.
Therapeutic Effect: Prevents nausea and vomiting associated with chemotherapy.

PHARMACOKINETICS
Protein binding: 52%. Eliminated in urine. **Half-life:** 40 hr.

AVAILABILITY
Injection: 0.25 mg/5 ml.

INDICATIONS AND DOSAGES
▸ **Chemotherapy-induced nausea and vomiting**
IV
Adults, Elderly. 0.25 mg as a single dose 30 min before starting chemotherapy.

CONTRAINDICATIONS
None known.

INTERACTIONS
Drug
None known.
Herbal
None known.
Food
None known.

DIAGNOSTIC TEST EFFECTS
May transiently increase serum bilirubin, AST (SGOT), and ALT (SGPT) levels.

▨ IV INCOMPATIBILITIES
Don't mix palonosetron with any other drugs.

SIDE EFFECTS
Occasional (9%-5%)
Headache, constipation
Rare (less than 1%)
Diarrhea, dizziness, fatigue, abdominal pain, insomnia

SERIOUS REACTIONS
• Overdose may produce a combination of CNS stimulant and depressant effects.

PRECAUTIONS & CONSIDERATIONS   P
Caution is warranted with history of cardiovascular disease. It is unknown if palonosetron is excreted in breast milk. The safety and efficacy of palonosetron have not been established in children. No age-related precautions have been noted in the elderly.

Alcohol, barbiturates, and tasks that require mental alertness or motor skills should be avoided.

Dizziness or drowsiness may occur. Pattern of daily bowel activity and stool consistency and hydration status should be monitored.
Storage
Store vials at room temperature. The solution normally appears clear and colorless. Discard it if it appears cloudy or contains precipitate.

Administration
Give the drug undiluted as an IV push over 30 seconds. Flush the IV line with 0.9% NaCl before and after administration.

Pamidronate
pam-id'drow-nate
(Aredia)
Do not confuse with Adriamycin.

CATEGORY AND SCHEDULE
Pregnancy Risk Category: D

CLASSIFICATION
Bisphosphonates

MECHANISM OF ACTION
A bisphosphate that binds to bone and inhibits osteoclast-mediated calcium resorption. *Therapeutic Effect:* Lowers serum calcium concentrations.

PHARMACOKINETICS

Route	Onset	Peak	Duration
IV	24-48 hr	5-7 days	N/A

After IV administration, rapidly absorbed by bone. Slowly excreted unchanged in urine. Unknown if removed by hemodialysis. Half-life: bone, 300 days; unmetabolized, 2.5 hr.

AVAILABILITY
Powder for Injection: 30 mg, 90 mg.
Injection Solution: 3 mg/ml, 6 mg/ml, 9 mg/ml.

INDICATIONS AND DOSAGES
▸ **Hypercalcemia**
IV infusion
Adults, Elderly. Moderate hypercalcemia (corrected serum calcium level 12-13.5 mg/dl): 60-90 mg. Severe hypercalcemia (corrected serum calcium level greater than 13.5 mg/dl): 90 mg.
▸ **Paget's disease**
IV infusion
Adults, Elderly. 30 mg/day for 3 days.
▸ **Osteolytic bone lesion**
IV infusion
Adults, Elderly. 90 mg over 2-4 hr once a month.

CONTRAINDICATIONS
Hypersensitivity to other bisphosphonates, such as etidronate, tiludronate, risedronate, and alendronate

INTERACTIONS
Drug
Calcium-containing medications, vitamin D: May antagonize effects of pamidronate in treatment of hypercalcemia.
Herbal
None known.
Food
None known.

DIAGNOSTIC TEST EFFECTS
May decrease serum phosphate, magnesium, calcium, and potassium levels.

▨ IV INCOMPATIBILITIES
Calcium-containing IV fluids

SIDE EFFECTS
Frequent (greater than 10%)
Temperature elevation (at least 1° C) 24-48 hr after administration (27%); redness, swelling, induration, pain at catheter site in patients receiving 90 mg (18%); anorexia, nausea, fatigue
Occasional (10%-1%)
Constipation, rhinitis

SERIOUS REACTIONS

• Hypophosphatemia, hypokalemia, hypomagnesemia, and hypocalcemia occur more frequently with higher dosages.
• Anemia, hypertension, tachycardia, atrial fibrillation, and somnolence occur more frequently with 90-mg doses.
• GI hemorrhage occurs rarely.

PRECAUTIONS & CONSIDERATIONS

Caution is warranted with cardiac failure and renal impairment. Because there are no adequate and well-controlled studies in pregnant women, it is unknown if pamidronate causes fetal harm or is excreted in breast milk. Safety and efficacy of pamidronate have not been established in children. The elderly may become overhydrated and require careful monitoring of fluid and electrolytes. Dilute the drug in a smaller volume for the elderly. Avoid drugs containing calcium and vitamin D, such as antacids, because they might antagonize the effects of pamidronate. Hct, Hgb, BUN, creatinine levels, and serum electrolyte levels, including serum calcium and creatinine levels, should be established. Pattern of daily bowel activity and stool consistency, B/P, pulse, and temperature should also be monitored.

Storage

Store parenteral form at room temperature. The reconstituted vial is stable for 24 hours when refrigerated; the IV solution is stable for 24 hours after dilution.

Administration

Reconstitute each 30-mg vial with 10 ml sterile water for injection to provide concentration of 3 mg/ml. Allow the drug to dissolve before withdrawing. Further dilute with 1000 ml sterile 0.45% or 0.9% NaCl or D_5W. Administer as IV infusion over 2 to 24 hours for treatment of hypercalcemia and over 2 to 4 hours for other indications. Adequate hydration is essential during pamidronate administration. Avoid overhydration in those with the potential for heart failure. Be alert for potential GI hemorrhage in those receiving a 90-mg dose.

Pancrelipase
pan-kre-li′pase
(Ku-Zyme,
Pancreatin)(Cotazym-S [AUS],
Cotazym-S Forte [AUS], Creon,
Pancrease [CAN], Pancrease MT,
Ultrase, Viokase)

CATEGORY AND SCHEDULE
Pregnancy Risk Category: C

CLASSIFICATION
Enzymes, gastrointestinal,
gastrointestinals

MECHANISM OF ACTION
Digestive enzymes that replace endogenous pancreatic enzymes. *Therapeutic Effect:* Assist in digestion of protein, starch, and fats.

AVAILABILITY
Capsules.
Tablets.

INDICATIONS AND DOSAGES
▸ **Pancreatic enzyme replacement or supplement when enzymes are absent or deficient, such as with chronic pancreatitis, cystic fibrosis, or ductal obstruction from cancer of the pancreas or common bile duct; to reduce malabsorption; treatment of steatorrhea associated with**

bowel resection or postgastrectomy syndrome
PO
Adults, Elderly. 1-3 capsules or tablets before or with meals or snacks. May increase to 8 tablets/dose.
Children. 1-2 tablets with meals or snacks.

CONTRAINDICATIONS
Acute pancreatitis, exacerbation of chronic pancreatitis, hypersensitivity to pork protein

INTERACTIONS
Drug
Antacids: May decrease the effects of pancreatin and pancrelipase.
Iron supplements: May decrease the absorption of iron supplements.
Herbal
None known.
Food
None known.

DIAGNOSTIC TEST EFFECTS
May increase serum uric acid level.

SIDE EFFECTS
Rare
Allergic reaction, mouth irritation, shortness of breath, wheezing

SERIOUS REACTIONS
• Excessive dosage may produce nausea, cramping, and diarrhea.
• Hyperuricosuria and hyper-uricemia have occurred with extremely high dosages.

PRECAUTIONS & CONSIDERATIONS
Pancreatin and pancrelipase should be used cautiously because inhala-tion of the powder form may precipi-tate an asthma attack. It is unknown if pancreatin or pancrelipase cross the placenta or are distributed in breast milk. Information is not avail-able on pancreatin or pancrelipase

use in children. No age-related precautions have been noted in the elderly. Tell the physician if allergic to pork because hypersensitivity to pancreatin and pancrelipase may exist. Brands should not be changed without first consulting the physician.
Administration
Take pancreatin or pancrelipase before or with meals or snacks. Do not crush enteric-coated form. Do not chew capsules or tablets, to minimize irritation to the mouth, lips, and tongue. If unable to swal-low capsules, open capsules and spread contents over applesauce, mashed fruit, or rice cereal. Spilling Viokase powder on the hands may irritate skin. Inhaling powder may irritate mucous membranes and produce bronchospasm.

Pantoprazole
pan-toe-pra′zole
(Protonix, Pantoloc, Somac [AUS])
Do not confuse Protonix with Lotronex.

CATEGORY AND SCHEDULE
Pregnancy Risk Category: B

CLASSIFICATION
Gastrointestinals, proton pump inhibitors

MECHANISM OF ACTION
A benzimidazole that is converted to active metabolites that irreversibly bind to and inhibit hydrogen-potassium adenosine triphosphate, an enzyme on the surface of gastric parietal cells. Inhibits hydrogen ion transport into gastric lumen.
Therapeutic Effect: Increases gastric

pH and reduces gastric acid production.

PHARMACOKINETICS

Route	Onset	Peak	Duration
PO	N/A	N/A	24 hr

Rapidly absorbed from the GI tract. Protein binding: 98%. Primarily distributed into gastric parietal cells. Metabolized extensively in the liver. Primarily excreted in urine. Not removed by hemodialysis. **Half-life:** 1 hr.

AVAILABILITY

Tablets (Delayed-Release): 20 mg, 40 mg.
Powder for Injection: 40 mg.

INDICATIONS AND DOSAGES
▸ **Erosive esophagitis**
PO
Adults, Elderly. 40 mg/day for up to 8 wk. If not healed after 8 wk, may continue an additional 8 wk.
IV
Adults, Elderly. 40 mg/day for 7-10 days.
▸ **Hypersecretory conditions**
PO
Adults, Elderly. Initially, 40 mg twice a day. May increase to 240 mg/day.
IV
Adults, Elderly. 80 mg twice a day. May increase to 80 mg q8hr.

CONTRAINDICATIONS
None known.

INTERACTIONS
Drug
None known.
Herbal
None known.
Food
None known.

DIAGNOSTIC TEST EFFECTS
May increase serum creatinine, cholesterol, and uric acid levels.

▦ IV INCOMPATIBILITIES
Do not mix with other medications. Flush IV with D_5W, 0.9% NaCl, or lactated Ringer's solution before and after administration.

SIDE EFFECTS
Rare (less than 2%)
Diarrhea, headache, dizziness, pruritus, rash

SERIOUS REACTIONS
• None known.

PRECAUTIONS & CONSIDERATIONS
Caution is warranted with a chronic or current hepatic disease. It is unknown if pantoprazole crosses the placenta or is distributed in breast milk. Safety and efficacy of pantoprazole have not been established in children. No age-related precautions have been noted in the elderly. Serum chemistry laboratory values, including serum creatinine and cholesterol levels, should be obtained before therapy.
Storage
Refrigerate vials and protect from light; do not freeze reconstituted vials. Once diluted, the drug is stable for 2 hours at room temperature.
Administration
Take oral pantoprazole without regard to meals. Do not crush or split tablet; swallow tablet whole. For IV use, mix 40-mg vial with 10 ml 0.9% NaCl injection. Infuse over 2 minutes or 15 minutes.

P

Paregoric

par-e-gor′ik

Do not confuse with opium tincture.

CATEGORY AND SCHEDULE

Pregnancy Risk Category: B, D if used for prolonged periods, high dosages at term
Controlled Substance: Schedule III

CLASSIFICATION

Analgesics, narcotic, antidiarrheals, gastrointestinals

MECHANISM OF ACTION

An opioid agonist that contains many narcotic alkaloids including morphine. It inhibits gastric motility due to its morphine content. *Therapeutic Effect:* Decreases digestive secretions, increases in gastrointestinal (GI) muscle tone, and reduces GI propulsion.

PHARMACOKINETICS

Variably absorbed from the gastrointestinal (GI) tract. Protein binding: low. Metabolized in liver. Primarily excreted in urine primarily as morphine glucuronide conjugates and unchanged drug—morphine, codeine, papaverine, etc. Unknown if removed by hemodialysis. **Half-life:** 2-3 hr.

AVAILABILITY

Tincture: 2 mg/5 ml (Paregoric).

INDICATIONS AND DOSAGES

▶ **Antidiarrheal**
PO
Adults, Elderly. 5-10 ml 1-4 times/day.
Children. 0.25-0.5 ml/kg/dose 1-4 times/day.

OFF-LABEL USES

Narcotic withdrawal symptoms in neonates

CONTRAINDICATIONS

Diarrhea caused by poisoning until the toxic material is removed, hypersensitivity to morphine sulfate or any component of the formulation, pregnancy (prolonged use or high dosages near term)

INTERACTIONS

Drug
Alcohol, central nervous system (CNS) depressants: May increase CNS or respiratory depression, and hypotension.
MAOIs, tricyclic antidepressants: May produce severe, fatal reaction unless dosage reduced by one quarter.
Herbal
None known.
Food
None known.

DIAGNOSTIC TEST EFFECTS

None known.

SIDE EFFECTS

Frequent
Constipation, drowsiness, nausea, vomiting
Occasional
Paradoxical excitement, confusion, pounding heartbeat, facial flushing, decreased urination, blurred vision, dizziness, dry mouth, headache, hypotension, decreased appetite, redness, burning, pain at injection site
Rare
Hallucinations, depression, stomach pain, insomnia

SERIOUS REACTIONS

• Overdosage results in cold or clammy skin, confusion, convulsions, decreased blood pressure (B/P), restlessness, pinpoint pupils, bradycardia, respiratory depression, decreased level of consciousness (LOC), and severe weakness.

• Tolerance to analgesic effect and physical dependence may occur with repeated use.

PRECAUTIONS & CONSIDERATIONS

Extreme caution is warranted with acute alcoholism, central nervous system (CNS) depression, respiratory depression, hepatic, renal or respiratory dysfunction, severe prostatic hyperplasia, history of narcotic abuse, and seizures. Paregoric crosses the placenta and is distributed in breast milk. Be aware that respiratory depression may occur in the neonate if the mother received opiates during labor. Regular use of opiates during pregnancy may produce withdrawal symptoms in neonate, such as diarrhea, excessive crying, fever, hyperactive reflexes, irritability, seizures, sneezing, tremors, vomiting, and yawning. Children may experience paradoxical excitement. Be aware that children younger than 3 months of age and the elderly are more susceptible to the respiratory depressant effects of paregoric. Paregoric use in the elderly may mask dehydration and electrolyte depletion.

Drowsiness and dizziness may occur during treatment. Avoid tasks that require mental alertness or motor skills until response to the drug is established. Change positions slowly to avoid orthostatic hypotension.

Storage
Store away from heat and direct light.

Administration
Be aware that paregoric, or camphorated tincture of opium, is not the same as opium tincture. Paregoric has just 0.4 mg/ml of morphine, whereas opium tincture contains 10 mg/ml—a 25-fold difference.

Paricalcitol
pare-i-cal'sih-tal
(Zemplar)

CATEGORY AND SCHEDULE
Pregnancy Risk Category: C

CLASSIFICATION
Vitamins/minerals

MECHANISM OF ACTION
A fat-soluble vitamin that is essential for absorption, utilization of calcium phosphate, and normal calcification of bone. *Therapeutic Effect:* Stimulates calcium and phosphate absorption from small intestine, promotes secretion of calcium from bone to blood, promotes renal tubule phosphate resorption, acts on bone cells to stimulate skeletal growth and on parathyroid gland to suppress hormone synthesis and secretion.

PHARMACOKINETICS
Protein binding: more than 99%. Metabolized in liver. Primarily eliminated in feces; minimal excretion in urine. Not removed by hemodialysis. **Half-life:** 14-15 hr.

AVAILABILITY
Injection: 5 mcg/ml (Zemplar).

INDICATIONS AND DOSAGES
▸ **Hypoparathyroidism**
IV
Adults, Elderly, Children. 0.04-0.1 mcg/kg (2.8-7 mcg) given as a bolus dose no more frequently than every other day at any time during dialysis; dose as high as 0.24 mcg/kg (16.8 mcg) have been administered safely. Usually start with 0.04 mcg/kg

3 times/week as a bolus, increased by 0.04 mcg/kg every 2 weeks. Dose adjust based on serum PTH levels:
Same or increasing serum PTH level: Increase dose
Serum PTH level decreased by <30%: Increase dose
Serum PTH level decreased by >30% and <60%: Maintain dose
Serum PTH level decrease by >60%: Decrease dose
Serum PTH level 1.5-3 times upper limit of normal: Maintain dose

CONTRAINDICATIONS
Hypercalcemia, malabsorption syndrome, vitamin D toxicity, hypersensitivity to other vitamin D products or analogs

INTERACTIONS
Drug
Aluminum-containing antacid (long-term use): May increase aluminum concentration and aluminum bone toxicity.
Calcium-containing preparations, thiazide diuretics: May increase the risk of hypercalcemia.
Digoxin: May increase the risk of digitalis toxicity.
Magnesium-containing antacids: May increase magnesium concentration.
Herbal
None known.
Food
None known.

DIAGNOSTIC TEST EFFECTS
May decrease serum alkaline phosphatase.

SIDE EFFECTS
Occasional
Edema, nausea, vomiting, headache, dizziness

Rare
Palpitations

SERIOUS REACTIONS
• Early signs of overdosage are manifested as weakness, headache, somnolence, nausea, vomiting, dry mouth, constipation, muscle and bone pain, and metallic taste sensation.
• Later signs of overdosage are evidenced by polyuria, polydipsia, anorexia, weight loss, nocturia, photophobia, rhinorrhea, pruritus, disorientation, hallucinations, hyperthermia, hypertension, and cardiac arrhythmias.
• Hypercalcemia occur rarely.

PRECAUTIONS & CONSIDERATIONS
Caution is necessary with contrary artery disease, kidney stones, renal impairment, and concomitant use of digoxin. Mineral oil should be avoided during paricalcitol use. It is unknown if paricalcitol crosses the placenta or is distributed in breast milk. Safety and efficacy have not been established in children. There are no age-related precautions noted in the elderly. Consume foods rich in vitamin D including eggs, leafy vegetables, margarine, meats, milk, vegetable oils, and vegetable shortening.

Serum alkaline phosphatase, BUN, serum calcium, serum creatinine, serum magnesium, serum phosphate, and urinary calcium levels should be monitored. The therapeutic serum calcium level is 9 to 10 mg/dl.
Storage
Store at room temperature.
Administration
Administer as a bolus. Discard any unused portion.

Paromomycin
par-oh-moe-mye′sin
(Humatin)
Do not confuse with Humira.

CATEGORY AND SCHEDULE
Pregnancy Risk Category: C

CLASSIFICATION
Antibiotics, aminoglycosides, antiprotozoals

MECHANISM OF ACTION
An antibacterial agent that acts directly on amoebas and against normal and pathogenic organisms in the GI tract. Interferes with bacterial protein synthesis by binding to 30S ribosomal subunits. *Therapeutic Effect:* Produces amoebicidal effects.

PHARMACOKINETICS
Poorly absorbed from the gastrointestinal (GI) tract and most of the dose is eliminated unchanged in feces.

AVAILABILITY
Capsules: 250 mg (Humantin).

INDICATIONS AND DOSAGES
▸ **Intestinal amebiasis**
PO
Adults, Elderly, Children. 25-35 mg/kg/day q8hr for 5-10 days.
▸ **Hepatic coma**
PO
Adults, Elderly. 4 g/day q6-12hr for 5-6 days.

OFF-LABEL USES
Cryptosporidiosis, giardiasis, leishmaniasis, microsporidiosis, mycobacterial infections, tapeworm infestation, trichomoniasis, typhoid carriers.

CONTRAINDICATIONS
Intestinal obstruction, renal failure, hypersensitivity to paromomycin or any of its components

INTERACTIONS
Drug
Digoxin: May decrease digoxin serum concentrations and efficacy.
Herbal
None known.
Food
Xylose, sucrose, fats: May cause decreased absorption of xylose, sucrose, and fats.

DIAGNOSTIC TEST EFFECTS
May increase LDH concentrations, SGOT (AST) and SGPT (ALT) levels.

SIDE EFFECTS
Occasional
Diarrhea, abdominal cramps, nausea, vomiting, heartburn
Rare
Rash, pruritus, vertigo

SERIOUS REACTIONS
• Overdosage may result in nausea, vomiting, and diarrhea.

PRECAUTIONS & CONSIDERATIONS
Caution should be used with proven ulcerative bowel disease. Be aware that paromomycin is contraindicated in renal failure. Liver and renal function tests should be performed before administering paromomycin. It is unknown if paromomycin crosses the placenta and is distributed in breast milk. There are no precautions noted in children or the elderly. Impaired hearing should be reported immediately.
Administration
Give with or without food. Take full course of therapy and do not skip doses.

Paroxetine

par-ox'e-teen
(Paxeva, Paxil, Paxil CR)
Do not confuse paroxetine with pyridoxine, or Paxil with Doxil or Taxol.

CATEGORY AND SCHEDULE
Pregnancy Risk Category: C

CLASSIFICATION
Antidepressants, serotonin specific reuptake inhibitors

MECHANISM OF ACTION
An antidepressant, anxiolytic, and antiobsessional agent that selectively blocks uptake of the neurotransmitter serotonin at neuronal presynaptic membranes, thereby increasing its availability at postsynaptic receptor sites. *Therapeutic Effect:* Relieves depression, reduces obsessive-compulsive behavior, decreases anxiety.

PHARMACOKINETICS
Well absorbed from the GI tract. Protein binding: 95%. Widely distributed. Metabolized in the liver. Excreted in urine. Not removed by hemodialysis.
Half-life: 24 hr.

AVAILABILITY
Oral Suspension (Paxil): 10 mg/5 ml.
Tablets (Paxil, Pexeva): 10 mg, 20 mg, 30 mg, 40 mg.
Tablets (Controlled-Release [Paxil CR]): 12.5 mg, 25 mg, 37.5 mg.

INDICATIONS AND DOSAGES
▸ **Depression**
PO
Adults. Initially, 20 mg/day. May increase by 10 mg/day at intervals of more than 1 wk. Maximum: 50 mg/day.
PO (Controlled-Release)
Adults. Initially, 25 mg/day. May increase by 12.5 mg/day at intervals of more than 1 wk. Maximum: 62.5 mg/day.
▸ **Generalized anxiety disorder**
PO
Adults. Initially, 20 mg/day. May increase by 10 mg/day at intervals of more than 1 wk. Range: 20-50 mg/day.
▸ **Obsessive compulsive disorder**
PO
Adults. Initially, 20 mg/day. May increase by 10 mg/day at intervals of more than 1 wk. Range: 20-60 mg/day.
▸ **Panic disorder**
PO
Adults. Initially, 10-20 mg/day. May increase by 10 mg/day at intervals of more than 1 wk. Range: 10-60 mg/day.
▸ **Social anxiety disorder**
PO
Adults. Initially 20 mg/day. Range: 20-60 mg/day.
▸ **Post traumatic stress disorder**
PO
Adults. Initially, 20 mg/day. May increase by 10 mg/day at intervals of more than 1 wk. Range: 20-50 mg/day.
▸ **Premenstrual dysphoric disorder**
PO
Adults. (Paxil CR) Initially, 12.5 mg/day. May increase by 12.5 mg at weekly intervals to a maximum of 25 mg/day.
▸ **Usual elderly dosage**
PO: Initially, 10 mg/day. May increase by 10 mg/day at intervals of more than 1 wk. Maximum: 40 mg/day.
PO (Controlled-Release): Initially, 12.5 mg/day. May increase by 12.5 mg/day at intervals of more than 1 wk. Maximum: 50 mg/day.

CONTRAINDICATIONS
Use within 14 days of MAOIs

INTERACTIONS
Drug
Cimetidine: May increase paroxetine blood concentration.
MAOIs: May cause serotonin syndrome, marked by excitement, diaphoresis, rigidity, hyperthermia, autonomic hyperactivity, coma, and neuroleptic malignant syndrome.
Phenytoin: May decrease paroxetine blood concentration.
Risperidone: May increase risperidone blood concentration and cause extrapyramidal symptoms.
Herbal
St. John's wort: May increase paroxetine's pharmacologic effects and risk of toxicity.
Food
None known.

DIAGNOSTIC TEST EFFECTS
May increase serum hepatic enzyme levels. May decrease blood Hgb level, Hct, and WBC count.

SIDE EFFECTS
Frequent
Nausea (26%); somnolence (23%); headache, dry mouth (18%); asthenia (15%); constipation (15%); dizziness, insomnia (13%); diarrhea (12%); diaphoresis (11%); tremor (8%)
Occasional
Decreased appetite, respiratory disturbance (such as increased cough) (6%); anxiety, nervousness (5%); flatulence, paresthesia, yawning (4%); decreased libido, sexual dysfunction, abdominal discomfort (3%)
Rare
Palpitations, vomiting, blurred vision, altered taste, confusion

SERIOUS REACTIONS
- None known.

PRECAUTIONS & CONSIDERATIONS
Caution is warranted with suicidal tendency, cardiac disease, a history of seizures, impaired platelet aggregation, mania, hepatic and renal impairment, in those with volume-depleted, and in those using diuretics. Paroxetine use may impair reproductive function; it is not distributed in breast milk. The safety and efficacy of this drug have not been established in children. In the elderly, age-related renal impairment may require dosage adjustment. Be aware St. John's wort should be avoided while taking paroxetine.

Alcohol and tasks that require mental alertness or motor skills should be avoided. CBC and liver and renal function tests should be performed before and periodically during therapy, especially with long-term use.

Administration
! Make sure at least 14 days elapse between the use of MAOIs and paroxetine. Expect to reduce paroxetine dosage in the elderly and patients with severe hepatic or renal impairment. Keep in mind that dosage changes should occur at intervals of 1 week or longer.

Take paroxetine as a single morning dose. Give it with food or milk if GI distress occurs. Scored tablets may be crushed or broken.

P

Pegaspargase
peg-as´par-jase
(Oncaspar)

CATEGORY AND SCHEDULE
Pregnancy Risk Category: C

CLASSIFICATION
Antineoplastics, enzymes

MECHANISM OF ACTION
An enzyme that breaks down extra-cellular supplies of the amino acid asparagine, which is necessary for the survival of leukemic cells. Binding to polyethylene glycol decreases the antigenicity of pegaspargase, making it less likely to cause a hypersensitivity reaction. Cell cycle–phase specific for G1 phase of cell division. *Therapeutic Effect:* Interferes with DNA, RNA, and protein synthesis in leukemic cells.

AVAILABILITY
Injection: 7500 international units/ml.

INDICATIONS AND DOSAGES
▶ **Acute lymphocytic leukemia**
IV, IM
Adults, Elderly, Children with a body surface area of 0.6 m² or more. 2500 international units/m² every 14 days.
Children with a body surface area of less than 0.6 m². 82.5 international units/kg every 14 days.

CONTRAINDICATIONS
Previous anaphylactic reaction or significant hemorrhagic event associated with pegaspargase therapy, pancreatitis (current or previous)

INTERACTIONS
Drug
Antigout medications: May decrease the effects of these drugs.
Live-virus vaccine: May potentiate virus replication, increase vaccine side effects, and decrease the patient's antibody response to the vaccine.
Methotrexate: May block the effects of methotrexate.
Steroids, vincristine: May increase hyperglycemia, risk of neuropathy, and disturbances of erythropoiesis.
Herbal
None known.
Food
None known.

DIAGNOSTIC TEST EFFECTS
May increase BUN, blood ammonia, and blood glucose levels; serum alkaline phosphatase, bilirubin, uric acid, AST (SGOT), and ALT (SGPT) levels; PT; and aPTT. May decrease blood clotting factors (including plasma fibrinogen, antithrombin, and plasminogen) as well as serum albumin, calcium, and cholesterol levels.

SIDE EFFECTS
Frequent
Allergic reaction (including rash, urticaria, arthralgia, facial edema, hypotension, and respiratory distress)
Occasional
CNS effects (including confusion, drowsiness, depression, nervousness, and fatigue), stomatitis, hypoalbuminemia, uric acid nephropathy (manifested as edema of the feet or lower legs), hyperglycemia
Rare
Hyperthermia (fever or chills)

SERIOUS REACTIONS
• The patient may have a hypersensitivity reaction, including anaphylaxis, during therapy.

• Pancreatitis, as evidenced by severe abdominal pain with nausea and vomiting, is a common reaction.

• Hepatotoxicity, as evidenced by jaundice and abnormal hepatic enzyme test results, may occur, especially in patients with pre-existing hepatic impairment.

• An increased risk of hematologic toxicity and coagulation disorders occurs occasionally.

• Seizures occur rarely.

PRECAUTIONS & CONSIDERATIONS

Caution is warranted in those concurrently taking aspirin, NSAIDs, and anticoagulants. Vaccinations and coming in contact with crowds and people with known infections should be avoided.

Nausea may occur but will decrease during therapy. Notify the physician if fever, signs of local infection, unusual bleeding from any site occurs. Antihistamines, epinephrine, and corticosteroids should be kept readily available before and during pegaspargase administration to ensure an adequate airway and treat any allergic reaction.

Adequate hydration should be maintained to protect against renal impairment. CBC, bone marrow tests, fibrinogen level, PT, aPTT, liver, pancreatic and renal function test results should be monitored before beginning therapy and whenever a week or more has elapsed between drug doses.

Storage

Refrigerate—do not freeze—vials. Discard the solution if it's cloudy or contains a precipitate. Also discard it if it has been stored at room temperature for longer than 48 hours or if the vial has been previously frozen because freezing destroys the drug's potency.

Administration

! Handle pegaspargase with care because the drug is a contact irritant. Wear gloves, avoid inhaling vapors, and avoid contact with skin or mucous membranes. In case of contact, wash with a copious amount of water for at least 15 minutes. Avoid excessive agitation of the vial (do not shake). The IM administration route is preferred because it poses less risk of coagulopathy, hepatotoxicity, and GI or renal disorders than the IV route. Use one dose per vial; do not re-enter the vial. Discard any unused portion.

Administer no more than 2 ml at any one IM site. Use multiple injection sites if more than 2 ml is being administered.

Add 100 ml 0.9% NaCl or D_5W, and administer the drug through IV infusion that is already running. Infuse over 1 to 2 hours.

Pegfilgrastim
pehg-phil-gras′tim
(Neulasta)
Do not confuse Neulasta with Neumega.

CATEGORY AND SCHEDULE
Pregnancy Risk Category: C

CLASSIFICATION
Hematopoietic agents

MECHANISM OF ACTION
A colony-stimulating factor that regulates production of neutrophils within bone marrow. Also a glycoprotein that primarily affects neutrophil progenitor proliferation, differentiation, and selected end-cell

functional activation. *Therapeutic Effect:* Increases phagocytic ability and antibody-dependent destruction; decreases incidence of infection.

PHARMACOKINETICS
Readily absorbed after subcutaneous administration. **Half-life:** 15-80 hr.

AVAILABILITY
Solution for Injection: 10 mg/ml.

INDICATIONS AND DOSAGES
▸ **Myelosuppression**
SUBCUTANEOUS
Adults, Elderly. Give as a single 6-mg injection once per chemotherapy cycle.

CONTRAINDICATIONS
Hypersensitivity to *Escherichia coli*–derived proteins, within 14 days before and 24 hours after cytotoxic chemotherapy

INTERACTIONS
Drug
Lithium: May potentiate the release of neutrophils.
Herbal
None known.
Food
None known.

DIAGNOSTIC TEST EFFECTS
May increase LDH concentrations, leukocyte alkaline phosphatase scores, and serum alkaline phosphatase and uric acid levels.

SIDE EFFECTS
Frequent (72%-15%)
Bone pain, nausea, fatigue, alopecia, diarrhea, vomiting, constipation, anorexia, abdominal pain, arthralgia, generalized weakness, peripheral edema, dizziness, stomatitis, mucositis, neutropenic fever

SERIOUS REACTIONS
• Allergic reactions, such as anaphylaxis, rash, and urticaria, occur rarely.
• Cytopenia resulting from an antibody response to growth factors occurs rarely.
• Splenomegaly occurs rarely; assess for left upper abdominal or shoulder pain.
• Adult respiratory distress syndrome (ARDS) may occur in patients with sepsis.

PRECAUTIONS & CONSIDERATIONS
Caution is warranted with concurrent use of medications with mycelioid properties and in those with sickle cell disease. It is unknown if pegfilgrastim crosses the placenta or is distributed in breast milk. Safety and efficacy of pegfilgrastim have not been established in children. Its use should be avoided in infants, children, and adolescents weighing less than 45 kg. No age-related precautions have been noted in the elderly.

CBC and platelet count should be obtained before initiation of pegfilgrastim therapy and routinely thereafter. Pattern of daily bowel activity and stool consistency should be assessed. Be aware of signs of peripheral edema, particularly behind the medial malleolus, which is usually the first area to show peripheral edema, and for evidence of mucositis (such as red mucous membranes, white patches, and extreme mouth soreness) and stomatitis.
Storage
Store in refrigerator, but may warm to room temperature up to 48 hours before use. Discard if left at room temperature for longer than 48 hours. Protect from light. Avoid freezing, but if accidentally frozen, may allow to thaw in refrigerator

before administration. Discard if freezing takes place a second time. Discard if discoloration or precipitate is present.

Administration

! Do not administer from 14 days before to 24 hours after cytotoxic chemotherapy, as prescribed. Do not use pegfilgrastim in infants, children, and adolescents weighing less than 45 kg.

Pegfilgrastim should be injected subcutaneously. Compliance with pegfilgrastim regimen is important.

Peginterferon Alfa-2a

peg-inn-ter-fear'on
(Pegasys)

CATEGORY AND SCHEDULE
Pregnancy Risk Category: C

CLASSIFICATION
Antivirals, immunomodulators

MECHANISM OF ACTION
An immunomodulator that binds to specific membrane receptors on the cell surface, inhibiting viral replication in virus-infected cells, suppressing cell proliferation, and producing reversible decreases in leukocyte and platelet counts. *Therapeutic Effect:* Inhibits hepatitis C virus.

PHARMACOKINETICS
Readily absorbed after subcutaneous administration. Excreted by the kidneys. **Half-life:** 80 hr.

AVAILABILITY
Injection: 180 mcg/ml.

INDICATIONS AND DOSAGES
▶ **Hepatitis C**
SUBCUTANEOUS
Adults 18 yr and older, Elderly.
180 mcg (1 ml) injected in abdomen or thigh once weekly for 48 wk.
▶ **Dosage in renal impairment**
For patients who require hemodialysis, dosage is 135 mg injected in abdomen or thigh once weekly for 48 wk.
▶ **Dosage in hepatic impairment**
For patients with progressive ALT (SGPT) increases above baseline values, dosage is 90 mcg injected in abdomen or thigh once weekly for 48 wk.

CONTRAINDICATIONS
Autoimmune hepatitis, decompensated hepatic disease, infants, neonates

INTERACTIONS
Drug
Bone marrow depressants: May increase myelosuppression.
Theophylline: May increase the serum level of theophylline.
Herbal
None known.
Food
None known.

DIAGNOSTIC TEST EFFECTS
May increase ALT (SGPT) level. May decrease the absolute neutrophil, platelet, and WBC counts. May cause a slight decrease in blood Hgb level and Hct.

SIDE EFFECTS
Frequent (54%)
Headache
Occasional (23%-13%)
Alopecia, nausea, insomnia, anorexia, dizziness, diarrhea, abdominal pain, flu-like symptoms, psychiatric reactions (depression, irritability, anxiety), injection site reaction

P

Rare (8%-5%)
Impaired concentration, diaphoresis, dry mouth, nausea, vomiting

SERIOUS REACTIONS
* Serious, acute hypersensitivity reactions, such as urticaria, angioedema, bronchoconstriction, and anaphylaxis, may occur. Other rare reactions include pancreatitis, colitis, hyperthyroidism or hypothyroidism, ophthalmologic disorders, and pulmonary disorders.

PRECAUTIONS & CONSIDERATIONS
Caution is warranted with autoimmune, cardiac, endocrine (diabetes mellitus, hyperthyroidism, hypothyroidism), pulmonary or ophthalmic disorders, colitis, compromised CNS function, myelosuppression, history of neuropsychiatric disorders, and renal impairment (creatinine clearance less than 50 ml/minute). Peginterferon alfa-2a may cause spontaneous abortion. It is unknown if peginterferon alfa-2a is distributed in breast milk. The safety and efficacy of peginterferon alfa-2a have not been established in children younger than 18 years. Cardiac, CNS, and systemic effects may be more severe in the elderly, particularly in those with renal impairment. Avoid performing tasks requiring mental alertness or motor skills until response to the drug has been established.

Flu-like symptoms may occur but usually diminish with continued therapy. Notify the physician of depression or suicidal thoughts. CBC, EKG, urinalysis, BUN level, and serum alkaline phosphatase, creatinine, AST (SGOT), and ALT (SGPT) levels should be obtained before and routinely during therapy. Chest X-ray should be assessed for pulmonary infiltrates.

Storage
Refrigerate vials.
Administration
! For moderate to severe adverse reactions, expect to decrease the dose to 135 mcg (0.75 ml) or 90 mcg (0.5 ml), as prescribed. For patients with an absolute neutrophil count less than 750 cells/mm^3, reduce dose to 135 mcg (0.75 ml). For those with an absolute neutrophil count less than 500 cells/mm^3, discontinue treatment until the count returns to 1000 cells/mm^3. For those with a platelet count less than 50,000 cells/mm^3, reduce dose to 90 mcg.

Vials are for single use only; discard unused portions. Inject the drug subcutaneously in the abdomen or thigh. The drug's therapeutic effect should appear in 1 to 3 months.

Peginterferon Alfa-2b
peg-in-ter-feer'on
(PEG-Intron)

CATEGORY AND SCHEDULE
Pregnancy Risk Category: C

CLASSIFICATION
Antivirals, immunomodulators

MECHANISM OF ACTION
An immunomodulator that inhibits viral replication in virus-infected cells, suppresses cell proliferation, increases phagocytic action of macrophages, and augments specific cytotoxicity of lymphocytes for target cells. *Therapeutic Effect:* Inhibits hepatitis C virus.

AVAILABILITY
Injection Powder for Reconstitution:
50 mcg, 80 mcg, 120 mcg, 150 mcg.

INDICATIONS AND DOSAGES
▸ **Chronic hepatitis C, monotherapy**
SUBCUTANEOUS
Adults 18 yr and older, Elderly.
Administer appropriate dosage
(see chart below) once weekly for
1 yr on the same day each wk.

Vial Strength	Weight (kg)	mcg*	ml*
100 mcg/ml	37-45	40	0.4
	46-56	50	0.5
160 mcg/ml	57-72	64	0.4
	73-88	80	0.5
240 mcg/ml	89-106	96	0.4
	107-136	120	0.5
300 mcg/ml	137-160	150	0.5

*Of peginterferon alpha-2b to administer

▸ **Chronic hepatitis C**
SUBCUTANEOUS
*Combination therapy with ribavirin
(400 mg twice a day).* Initially,
1.5 mcg/kg/wk.

CONTRAINDICATIONS
Autoimmune hepatitis, decompensated hepatic disease, history of psychiatric disorders

INTERACTIONS
Drug
Bone marrow depressants: May
increase myelosuppression.
Herbal
None known.
Food
None known.

DIAGNOSTIC TEST EFFECTS
May increase blood glucose and
ALT (SGPT) levels. May decrease
blood neutrophil and platelet
counts.

SIDE EFFECTS
Frequent (50%-47%)
Flu-like symptoms; inflammation,
bruising, pruritus, and irritation at
injection site
Occasional (29%-18%)
Psychiatric reactions (depression,
anxiety, emotional lability, irritability),
insomnia, alopecia, diarrhea
Rare
Rash, diaphoresis, dry skin, dizziness, flushing, vomiting, dyspepsia

SERIOUS REACTIONS
• Serious, acute hypersensitivity
reactions (such as urticaria,
angioedema, bronchoconstriction,
and anaphylaxis), pulmonary disorders, hypothyroidism, hyperthyroidism, and pancreatitis occur rarely.
• Ulcerative colitis may occur within
12 weeks of starting treatment.

PRECAUTIONS & CONSIDERATIONS
Caution is warranted with autoimmune, cardiac, endocrine (diabetes
mellitus, hyperthyroidism, hypothyroidism), pulmonary or ophthalmic
disorders, colitis, compromised
CNS function, myelosuppression,
renal impairment (creatinine clearance less than 50 ml/minute), and in
the elderly. Peginterferon alfa-2b
may cause spontaneous abortion. It
is unknown if peginterferon alfa-2b
is distributed in breast milk. The
safety and efficacy of peginterferon
alfa-2b have not been established in
children younger than 18 years.
Cardiac, CNS, and systemic effects
may be more severe in the elderly,
particularly in patients with renal
impairment.

Flu-like symptoms may occur but
usually diminish with continued
therapy. Notify the physician of bloody
diarrhea, fever, persistent abdominal
pain, depression, signs of infection,
or unusual bruising or bleeding.

P

CBC, EKG, urinalysis, BUN level, and serum alkaline phosphatase, creatinine, AST (SGOT), and ALT (SGPT) levels should be obtained before and routinely during therapy. Chest X-ray should be assessed for pulmonary infiltrates.

Storage

Store vials at room temperature. Use it immediately or after reconstitution or, if necessary, refrigerate it for up to 24 hours.

Administration

! If severe adverse reactions occur, modify the dosage or temporarily discontinue the drug, as prescribed. Know that the dosage is based on weight. Remember that the drug's side effects are dose-related.

Reconstitute the drug by adding 0.7 ml sterile water for injection (the supplied diluent) to the vial. Administer as subcutaneous injection.

Pegvisomant

peg-vis'oh-mant
(Somavert)
Do not confuse Somavert with somatrem or somatropin.

CATEGORY AND SCHEDULE

Pregnancy Risk Category: B

CLASSIFICATION

Hormones/hormone modifiers

MECHANISM OF ACTION

A protein that selectively binds to growth hormone (GH) receptors on cell surfaces, blocking the binding of endogenous growth hormones and interfering with growth hormone signal transduction. *Therapeutic Effect:* Decreases serum concentrations of insulin-like growth factor 1 (IGF-1) and other GH-responsive serum proteins.

PHARMACOKINETICS

Not distributed extensively into tissues after subcutaneous administration. Less than 1% excreted in urine. **Half-life:** 6 days.

AVAILABILITY

Powder for Injection: 10-mg, 15-mg, 20-mg vials.

INDICATIONS AND DOSAGES

▸ **Acromegaly**

SUBCUTANEOUS

Adults, Elderly. Initially, 40 mg, as a loading dose, then 10 mg daily. After 4-6 wk, adjust dosage in 5-mg increments if serum IGF-1 level is still elevated, or in 5-mg decrements if IGF-1 level has decreased below the normal range. Maximum: 30 mg daily.

CONTRAINDICATIONS

Latex allergy (stopper on vial contains latex)

INTERACTIONS

Drug

Insulin, oral antidiabetics: May enhance effects of these drugs, possibly resulting in hypoglycemia. Dosage should be decreased when initiating pegvisomant therapy.

Opioids: Decrease serum pegvisomant level.

Herbal

None known.

Food

None known.

DIAGNOSTIC TEST EFFECTS

Interferes with measurement of serum growth hormone concentration. May increase AST (SGOT), ALT (SGPT), and transaminase levels.

Decreases effect of insulin on carbohydrate metabolism.

SIDE EFFECTS

Frequent (23%)
Infection (cold symptoms, upper
respiratory tract infection, blister, ear
infection)
Occasional (8%-5%)
Back pain, dizziness, injection site
reaction, peripheral edema, sinusitis,
nausea
Rare (less than 4%)
Diarrhea, paresthesia

SERIOUS REACTIONS

• Pegvisomant use may markedly
elevate liver function test results,
including serum transaminase levels.
• Substantial weight gain occurs
rarely.

PRECAUTIONS & CONSIDERATIONS

Caution is warranted with diabetes
mellitus and in the elderly. It is
unknown if pegvisomant is excreted
in breast milk. The safety and efficacy of pegvisomant have not
been established in children. In
the elderly, treatment should begin
at the low end of the dosage
range.

Notify the physician of yellowing
of the skin or sclera of eyes or any
other adverse effects. Serum alkaline
phosphatase, bilirubin, AST (SGOT),
and ALT (SGPT) levels should be
monitored. Serum IGF-1 concentrations should be obtained 4 to 6 weeks
after therapy begins and periodically
thereafter. The drug dosage should
be adjusted based on these results,
not on growth hormone assays.
Progressive tumor growth with
periodic imaging scans of the sella
turcica should be monitored with
tumors that secrete growth hormone.
Diabetics should be assessed for
hypoglycemia.

Storage
Store unreconstituted vials in the
refrigerator. Administer the drug
within 6 hours of reconstitution.

Administration
The solution normally appears clear
after reconstitution. Discard the solution if it appears cloudy or contains
particles. Withdraw 1 ml sterile water
for injection and inject it into the vial
of pegvisomant, aiming the stream
against the glass wall. Hold the vial
between the palms of both hands and
roll it gently to dissolve the powder;
do not shake. Administer only one
dose from each vial subcutaneously.

Pemetrexed
pem-eh-trex′ed
(Alimta)

CATEGORY AND SCHEDULE
Pregnancy Risk Category: D

CLASSIFICATION
Antineoplastics, antimetabolites

P

MECHANISM OF ACTION
An antimetabolite that disrupts
folate-dependent enzymes essential
for cell replication. *Therapeutic
Effect:* Inhibits the growth of
mesothelioma cell lines.

PHARMACOKINETICS
Protein binding: 81%. Drug is not
metabolized; excreted in urine.
Half-life: 3.5 hr.

AVAILABILITY
Powder for Injection: 500 mg.

INDICATIONS AND DOSAGES

! Pre-treatment with dexamethasone
(or equivalent will reduce the risk and

severity of a cutaneous reaction; treatment with folic acid and vitamin B12) beginning 1 week before treatment and continuing for 21 days after the last pemetrexed dose will reduce the risk of side effects.

▸ **Malignant pleural mesothelioma**
IV
Adults, Elderly. 600 mg/m^2
600 mg/m^2 every 3 wk when used as a single agent; 500 mg/m^2 every 3 wk when used in combination with cisplatin 75 mg/m^2.

CONTRAINDICATIONS
None known.

INTERACTIONS
Drug
Nephrotoxic agents, probenecid: May delay pemetrexed clearance.
NSAIDs (particularly ibuprofen): Increase the risk of myelosuppression and GI and renal toxicity.
Herbal
None known.
Food
None known.

DIAGNOSTIC TEST EFFECTS
May decrease platelet, RBC, and WBC counts.

▒ IV INCOMPATIBILITIES
Use only 0.9% NaCl to reconstitute; flush the line before and after the infusion. Don't add any other medications to the IV line.

SIDE EFFECTS
Frequent (12%-10%)
Fatigue, nausea, vomiting, rash or desquamation
Occasional (8%-4%)
Stomatitis, pharyngitis, diarrhea, anorexia, hypertension, chest pain
Rare (less than 3%)
Constipation, depression, dysphagia

SERIOUS REACTIONS
• Myelosuppression, manifested as neutropenia, thrombocytopenia, or anemia, may occur.

PRECAUTIONS & CONSIDERATIONS
Caution is warranted with liver and renal impairment as well as concurrent therapy with aspirin or other NSAIDs (interrupt dosing for at least 5 days prior, the day of, and 2 days after pemetrexed therapy). Pemetrexed may be harmful to a fetus and that it is unknown if pemetrexed is distributed in breast milk. Do not breast-feed once treatment has been initiated. Safety and efficacy of pemetrexed in children younger than 18 years of age have not been established. Be aware that the elderly may have higher incidence of fatigue, leukopenia, neutropenia, and thrombocytopenia.

Fastidious oral hygiene should be maintained. Do not have immunizations without physician's approval (drug lowers body's resistance). Crowds and/or those with infection should be avoided. Contraceptive measures should be used during therapy. Report fever, sore throat, signs of local infection, easy bruising, and unusual bleeding from any site immediately.
Storage
Store undiluted vial at room temperature. Reconstituted solution is stable for up to 24 hours at room temperature or if refrigerated.
Administration
Be aware that pre-treatment with dexamethasone (or equivalent) will reduce risk of incidence and severity of cutaneous reaction; treatment with folic acid and vitamin B$_{12}$ beginning 1 week prior to treatment and for 21 days after the last pemetrexed dose will reduce risk of side effects.

Dilute 500-mg vial with 20 ml 0.9% NaCl to provide a concentration of 25 mg/ml. Gently swirl each vial until powder is completely dissolved. Solution appears clear and ranges in color from colorless to yellow or green-yellow. Further dilute reconstituted solution with 100 ml 0.9% NaCl.

Use only 0.9% NaCl to reconstitute. Flush line prior to and following infusion. Do not add any other medications to IV line. Infuse over 10 minutes.

Pemoline
pem'oh-leen
(Cylert, PemADD, PemADD CT)

CATEGORY AND SCHEDULE
Pregnancy Risk Category: B
Controlled Substance:
Schedule IV

CLASSIFICATION
Stimulants, central nervous system

MECHANISM OF ACTION
A CNS stimulant that blocks the reuptake mechanism present in dopaminergic neurons in the cerebral cortex and subcortical structures. *Therapeutic Effect:* Reduces motor restlessness and fatigue, increases alertness, elevates mood.

AVAILABILITY
Tablets (Cylert, PemADD): 18.75 mg, 37.5 mg, 75 mg.
Tablets (Chewable [PemADD CT]): 37.5 mg.

INDICATIONS AND DOSAGES
▸ ADHD
PO
Children 6 yr and older. Initially, 37.5 mg/day as a single dose in morning. May increase by 18.75 mg at weekly intervals until therapeutic response is achieved. Range: 56.25-75 mg/day. Maximum: 112.5 mg/day.

CONTRAINDICATIONS
Family history of Tourette syndrome, hepatic impairment, motor tics

INTERACTIONS
Drug
Other CNS stimulants: May increase CNS stimulation.
Herbal
None known.
Food
None known.

DIAGNOSTIC TEST EFFECTS
May increase serum LDH, AST (SGOT), and ALT (SGPT) levels.

SIDE EFFECTS
Frequent
Anorexia, insomnia
Occasional
Nausea, abdominal discomfort, diarrhea, headache, dizziness, somnolence

SERIOUS REACTIONS
• Visual disturbances, rash, and dyskinetic movements of the tongue, lips, face, and extremities have occurred.
• Large doses of pemoline may produce extreme nervousness and tachycardia.
• Hepatic effects, such as hepatitis and jaundice, appear to be reversible when the drug is discontinued.
• Prolonged administration to children with ADHD may temporarily delay growth.

PRECAUTIONS & CONSIDERATIONS

Caution is warranted with hypertension, psychosis, renal impairment, seizures, and a history of drug abuse. Hepatic function tests should be performed before and periodically during therapy. Height and weight should be obtained before and during pemoline therapy. Notify the physician if dark urine, GI complaints, loss of appetite, or yellow skin occurs. Tasks that require mental alertness or motor skills, alcohol, and caffeine should be avoided.

Administration

Do not abruptly discontinue the drug.

Penbutolol

pen-beaut-oh-lol
(Levatol)
Do not confuse with pindolol

CATEGORY AND SCHEDULE

Pregnancy Risk Category: C (D if used in the second or third trimester)

CLASSIFICATION

Antiadrenergics, beta blocking

MECHANISM OF ACTION

An antihypertensive that possesses nonselective beta-blocking. Has moderate intrinsic sympathomimetic activity. *Therapeutic Effect:* Reduces cardiac output, decreases blood pressure (B/P), increases airway resistance, and decreases myocardial ischemia severity.

PHARMACOKINETICS

Rapidly and extensively absorbed from the gastrointestinal (GI) tract. Protein binding: 80%-90%. Metabolized in liver. Excreted primarily via urine. **Half-life:** 17-26 hr.

AVAILABILITY

Tablets: 20 mg (Levatol).

INDICATIONS AND DOSAGES

▶ **Hypertension**
PO
Adults. Initially, 20 mg/day as a single dose. May increase to 40-80 mg/day.
Elderly. Initially, 10 mg/day.

CONTRAINDICATIONS

Bronchial asthma or related bronchospastic conditions, cardiogenic shock, pulmonary edema, second- or third-degree atrioventricular (AV) block, severe bradycardia, overt cardiac failure, hypersensitivity to penbutolol or any component of the formulation

INTERACTIONS

Drug

Calcium blockers: Increase risk of conduction disturbances.
Clonidine: May potentiate blood pressure (B/P) effects.
Cimetidine: May increase penbutolol concentrations.
Digoxin: Increases concentrations of this drug.
Diuretics, other hypotensives: May increase hypotensive effect.
Fentanyl: May cause severe hypotension.
Insulin, oral hypoglycemics: May mask symptoms of hypoglycemia and prolong hypoglycemic effect of these drugs.
Lidocaine: May prolong the elimination of lidocaine
NSAIDs: May decrease antihypertensive effect.
Verapamil: May increase risk of hypotension and bradycardia.

Sympathomimetics, xanthines:
May mutually inhibit effects.
Herbal
Dong quai: May decrease blood
pressure.
St. John's Wort, yohimbine: May
decrease effectiveness of penbutolol.
Food
None known.

DIAGNOSTIC TEST EFFECTS
May increase ANA titer, SGOT
(AST), SGPT (ALT), alkaline phosphatase, LDH, bilirubin, BUN, creatinine, potassium, uric acid,
lipoproteins, triglycerides

SIDE EFFECTS
Frequent
Decreased sexual ability, drowsiness,
trouble sleeping, unusual
tiredness/weakness
Occasional
Diarrhea, bradycardia, depression,
cold hands/feet, constipation, anxiety,
nasal congestion, nausea, vomiting
Rare
Altered taste, dry eyes, itching,
numbness of fingers, toes, scalp

SERIOUS REACTIONS
• Abrupt withdrawal may result in
sweating, palpitations, headache, and
tremulousness.
• Hypoglycemia may occur in
patients with previously controlled
diabetes.

PRECAUTIONS & CONSIDERATIONS
Caution is warranted with inadequate
cardiac function, impaired renal/
hepatic function, diabetes mellitus,
and hyperthyroidism. It is unknown
if penbutolol crosses the placenta or
is distributed in breast milk. Safety
and efficacy of penbutolol has not
been established in children. In the
elderly, the incidence of dizziness
may be increased.

Dizziness and drowsiness may be
experienced during treatment.
Avoid alcohol and tasks that require
mental alertness or motor skills. In
addition, avoid nasal decongestants
and over-the-counter (OTC) cold
preparations, especially those
containing stimulants, without
physician approval.
Storage
Store at room temperature.
Administration
Take with food, which slows the rate
of absorption and reduces the risk of
orthostatic hypotension. To assess
the tolerance of the drug, assess a
standing systolic B/P 1 hour after
giving penbutolol. The full antihypertensive effect of penbutolol
should take in 1 to 2 weeks. Do not
abruptly discontinue penbutolol.

Penciclovir
pen-sye'kloe-veer
(Denavir, Vectavir [SOUTH
AFRICA, COSTA RICA, DOMINICAN
REPUBLIC, EL SALVADOR, GERMANY,
GUATEMALA, HONDURAS, ISRAEL,
NICARAGUA, PANAMA])
Do not confuse with acyclovir

CATEGORY AND SCHEDULE
Pregnancy Risk Category: B

CLASSIFICATION
Antivirals

MECHANISM OF ACTION
Penciclovir triphosphate inhibits
HSV polymerase competitively with
deoxyguanosine triphosphate.
Consequently, herpes viral DNA
synthesis and, therefore, replication
are selectively inhibited. *Therapeutic
Effect:* An antiviral compound that

has inhibitory activity against herpes simplex virus types 1 (HSV-1) and 2 (HSV-2).

PHARMACOKINETICS

Measurable penciclovir concentrations were not detected in plasma or urine. The systemic absorption of penciclovir following topical administration has not been evaluated.

AVAILABILITY

Cream: 10 mg/g

INDICATIONS AND DOSAGES
▸ **Herpes labialis (cold sores)**
TOPICAL
Adolescents, Adults. Penciclovir should be applied every 2 hours during waking hours for a period of 4 days. Treatment should be started as early as possible (i.e., during the prodrome or when lesions appear).

OFF-LABEL USES

Varicella-zoster virus

CONTRAINDICATIONS

Hypersensitivity to penciclovir or any of its components.

INTERACTIONS
Drug
None known.
Herbal
None known.
Food
None known.

DIAGNOSTIC TEST EFFECTS

None known.

SIDE EFFECTS
Frequent
Headache
Occasional
Change in sense of taste; decreased sensitivity of skin, particularly to touch; redness of the skin; skin rash

(maculopapular, erythematous) local edema, skin discoloration; pruritis; hypoesthesia; parathesias; parosmia; urticaria; oral/pharyngeal edema
Rare
Mild pain, burning, or stinging

PRECAUTIONS & CONSIDERATIONS

It is unknown if penciclovir crosses the placenta or is distributed into breast milk. Safety and efficacy have not been established in children. There are no age-related precautions noted in the elderly. Headache may occur while taking penciclovir.
Storage
Store at room temperature.
Administration
Penciclovir is for external use only. Apply every 2 hours during waking hours for 4 days. Continue medication for the full time of treatment.

Penicillamine
pen-i-sil-a-meen
(Cuprimine, Depen)
Do not confuse with penicillin.

CATEGORY AND SCHEDULE
Pregnancy Risk Category: D

CLASSIFICATION
Chelators, cystine depleting agents, disease modifying antirheumatic drugs

MECHANISM OF ACTION

A heavy metal antagonist that chelates copper, iron, mercury, lead to form complexes, promoting excretion of copper. Combines with cystine-forming complex, thus reducing concentration of cystine to below levels for formation of cystine stones. Exact mechanism for rheumatoid arthritis is unknown. May decrease cell-mediated immune response. May inhibit collagen formation. *Therapeutic Effect:* Promotes excretion of copper, prevents renal calculi, dissolves existing stones, acts as anti-inflammatory drug

PHARMACOKINETICS
Moderately absorbed from the gastrointestinal (GI) tract. Protein binding: 80% to albumin. Metabolized in small amounts in liver. Excreted unchanged in urine. **Half-life:** 1.7-3.2 hr.

AVAILABILITY
Capsules: 125 mg, 250 mg (Cuprimine).
Tablets: 250 mg (Depen).

INDICATIONS AND DOSAGES
▸ **Wilson's disease**
PO
Adults, Elderly, Children. Initially, 250 mg 4 times/day (some pts may begin at 250 mg/day; gradually increase). Dosages of 750-1500 mg/day that produce initial 24 hr cupruresis >2 mg should be continued for 3 mo. Maintenance: Based on serum-free copper concentration (<10 mcg/dl indicative of adequate maintenance). Maximum: 2 g/day.
▸ **Cystinuria**
PO
Adults, Elderly. Initially, 250 mg/day. Gradually increase dose. Maintenance: 2 g/day. Range: 1-4 g/day.
Children. 30 mg/kg/day.
▸ **Rheumatoid arthritis**
PO
Adults, Elderly. Initially, 125-250 mg/day. May increase by 125-250 mg/day at 1-3 mo intervals. Maintenance: 500-750 mg/day. After 2-3 mo with no improvement or toxicity, may increase by 250 mg/day at 2-3 mo intervals until remission or toxicity. Maximum: 1 g up to 1.5 g/day.

OFF-LABEL USES
Treatment of rheumatoid vasculitis, heavy metal toxicity.

CONTRAINDICATIONS
History of penicillamine-related aplastic anemia or agranulocytosis, rheumatoid arthritis patients with history or evidence of renal insufficiency, pregnancy, breast-feeding

INTERACTIONS
Drug
Iron supplements, antacids: May decrease absorption of penicillamine. **Bone marrow depressants, gold compounds, immunosuppressants:** May increase risk of hematologic and renal adverse effects.
Herbal
None known.
Food
May decrease absorption of penicillamine.

DIAGNOSTIC TEST EFFECTS
None known.

▦ IV INCOMPATIBILITIES
None known.
ᨀ IV Compatibilities
None known.

SIDE EFFECTS
Frequent
Rash (pruritic, erythematous, maculopapular, morbilliform), reduced/altered sense of taste (hypogeusia), GI disturbances (anorexia, epigastric pain, nausea, vomiting, diarrhea), oral ulcers, glossitis
Occasional
Proteinuria, hematuria, hot flashes, drug fever

P

Rare
Alopecia, tinnitus, pemphigoid rash (water blisters)

SERIOUS REACTIONS
• Aplastic anemia, agranulocytosis, thrombocytopenia, leukopenia, myasthenia gravis, bronchiolitis, erythematouslike syndrome, evening hypoglycemia, skin friability at sites of pressure/trauma producing extravasation or white papules at venipuncture, surgical sites reported.
• Iron deficiency (particularly children, menstruating women) may develop.

PRECAUTIONS & CONSIDERATIONS
Caution should be used in the elderly who may have age-related decreased renal function. Caution should also be used with penicillin allergy and impaired renal and hepatic function. Be aware that penicillamine crosses the placenta and is distributed in breast milk. Use only when the drug's benefits outweigh the possible hazard to the fetus. There are no age-related precautions noted in children.

Baseline WBC, differential, hemoglobin, platelet count should be performed before therapy begins, every 2 weeks thereafter for first 6 months, then monthly during therapy. Liver function tests (GGT, SGOT, SGPT, LDH) and x-ray for renal stones should also be ordered. If WBC <3500, neutrophils <2000/mm^3, monocytes >500/mm^3, or platelet counts <100,000, or if a progressive fall in either platelet count or WBC in three successive determinations noted, and inform physician (drug withdrawal necessary).

If missed menstrual periods/other indications of pregnancy, fever, sore throat, chills, bruising, bleeding, difficulty breathing on exertion, unexplained cough or wheezing occurs, notify the physician promptly.

Storage
Store in tight, well-closed containers.

Administration
Take 1 hr before or 2 hr after meals or at least 1 hr from any other drug, food, or milk. May mix contents of capsule with fruit juice or chilled fruit if the person cannot swallow capsules.

A 2-hour interval is necessary between iron and penicillamine therapy.

In event of upcoming surgery, dosage should be reduced to 250 mg/day until wound.

Be aware that for Wilson's disease, base dosage on urinary copper excretion, serum-free copper concentration that produces/maintains negative copper balance. Give with 10-40 mg sulfurated potash at each meal for 6-12 months.

Be aware for cystinuria, give in 4 equal doses; if not feasible, give larger dose at bedtime. Dose based on urinary cystine excretion. Maintain high fluid intake.

Penicillin

pen-i-sil'in
amoxicillin, ampicillin,
bacampicillin, carbenicillin,
cloxacillin, dicloxacillin,
flucloxacillin, methicillin,
mezlocillin, nafcillin, oxacillin,
penicillin G benzathine,
penicillin G potassium,
penicillin V potassium,
piperacillin, pivampicillin,
pivmecillinam, ticarcillin;
Penicillin and beta-lactamase
inhibitors; amoxicillin/
clavulanate potassium,
ampicillin/ sulbactam sodium,
piperacillin sodium/tazobactam
sodium, ticarcillin disodium/
clavulanate potassium

CATEGORY AND SCHEDULE
Pregnancy Risk Category: B

CLASSIFICATION
Penicillin, natural, antibiotic

MECHANISM OF ACTION
Penicillins bind to bacterial cell wall,
inhibiting bacterial cell wall synthesis. *Therapeutic Effect:* Inhibits
bacterial cell wall synthesis.
Beta-lactamase inhibitors: inhibit
the action of bacterial beta-lactamase.
Therapeutic Effect: Protects the
penicillin from enzymatic
degradation.

PHARMACOKINETICS
Penicillins are generally well
absorbed from the gastrointestinal
(GI) tract after oral administration.
Widely distributed to most
tissues and body fluids. Protein
binding: 20%. Partially metabolized
in liver. Primarily excreted in urine.

Half-life: varies (half-life increased
in reduced renal function).

AVAILABILITY
Penicillins are available in tablets,
chewable tablets, capsules, powder
for oral suspension, powder for injection, prefilled syringes for injection,
premixed dextrose solutions for
injection, and solutions for infusion.

INDICATIONS AND DOSAGES
Penicillins may be used to treat
a large number of infections, including pneumonia and other respiratory
diseases, urinary tract infections,
septicemia, meningitis, intra-
abdominal infections, gonorrhea,
syphilis, and bone and joint
infections.
Doses vary depending on the drug
used. In general, penicillins should
be taken on an empty stomach.
Patients with impaired renal function
may require dose adjustment.

OFF-LABEL USES
Some penicillins, such as amoxicillin, have been used in the treatment
of Lyme disease and typhoid
fever.

CONTRAINDICATIONS
Hypersensitivity to any penicillin,
infectious mononucleosis

INTERACTIONS
Drug
Allopurinol: May increase inci-
dence of rash.
Oral contraceptives: May decrease
effects of oral contraceptives.
Probenecid: May increase peni-
cillin blood concentration and risk
for penicillin toxicity.
Herbal
None known.
Food
None known.

P

DIAGNOSTIC TEST EFFECTS
May increase BUN, LDH, serum bilirubin, serum creatinine, SGOT (AST), and SGPT (ALT) levels. May cause positive Coombs' test.

SIDE EFFECTS
Frequent
Gastrointestinal (GI) disturbances (mild diarrhea, nausea, or vomiting), headache, oral or vaginal candidiasis
Occasional
Generalized rash, urticaria

SERIOUS REACTIONS
• Altered bacterial balance may result in potentially fatal superinfections and antibiotic-associated colitis as evidenced by abdominal cramps, watery or severe diarrhea, and fever.
• Severe hypersensitivity reactions, including anaphylaxis and acute interstitial nephritis occur rarely.

PRECAUTIONS & CONSIDERATIONS
Caution is warranted with antibiotic-associated colitis or a history of allergies, especially to cephalosporins. Be aware that penicillins cross the placenta and are distributed in breast milk in low concentrations. Be aware that penicillin administration may lead to allergic sensitization, candidiasis, diarrhea, and skin rash in infants. Many penicillins are used in children and are generally well tolerated. Be aware that immature renal function in neonates and young infants may delay renal excretion of penicillins. In the elderly, age-related renal impairment may require dosage adjustment.

Notify the physician of signs and symptoms of superinfection, including anal or genital pruritus, black hairy tongue, diarrhea, increased fever, sore throat, ulceration or changes of oral mucosa, and vomiting.

Storage
Store capsules or tablets at room temperature.

In general, after reconstitution, oral solutions are stable for 14 days whether at room temperature or refrigerated.

Store solutions for injection according to manufacturer's instructions.
Administration
Take oral formulations without regard to meals. If GI upset occurs, take with food. Chew or crush chewable tablets thoroughly before swallowing. Take full length of treatment and space doses evenly around the clock.

For IM use, reconstitution and stability vary with each penicillin for injection. Reconstitute and store based on manufacturer's instructions. Give injection deeply in a large muscle mass.

For IV use, reconstitution, rate of infusion, and stability vary with each penicillin for injection. Reconstitute, administer, and store based on manufacturer's instructions.

Penicillin G Benzathine
pen-i-sill'in G ben'za-theen
(Bicillin LA, Permapen)
Do not confuse with penicillin G potassium, penicillin G procaine.

CATEGORY AND SCHEDULE
Pregnancy Risk Category: B

CLASSIFICATION
Antibiotics, penicillins

MECHANISM OF ACTION
A penicillin that inhibits bacterial cell wall synthesis by binding to one

or more of the penicillin-binding proteins of bacteria. *Therapeutic Effect:* Bactericidal.

AVAILABILITY
Injection (Prefilled Syringe [Bicillin LA, Permapen]): 600,000 units/ml.

INDICATIONS AND DOSAGES
▶ **Group A streptococcal infections**
IM
Adults, Elderly. 1.2 million units as a single dose.
Children. 25,000-50,000 units/kg as a single dose.
▶ **Prevention of rheumatic fever**
IM
Adults, Elderly. 1.2 million units every 3-4 wk or 600,000 units twice monthly.
Children. 25,000-50,000 units/kg every 3-4 wk.
▶ **Early syphilis**
IM
Adults, Elderly. 2.4 million units divided and administered in two separate injection sites.
▶ **Congenital syphilis**
IM
Children. 50,000 units/kg weekly for 3 wk.
▶ **Syphilis of more than 1 year's duration**
IM
Adults, Elderly. 2.4 million units divided and administered in two separate injection sites weekly for 3 wk.
Children. 50,000 units/kg weekly for 3 wk.

CONTRAINDICATIONS
Hypersensitivity to any penicillin

INTERACTIONS
Drug
Erythromycin: May antagonize effects of penicillin.
Probenecid: Increases serum concentration of penicillin.

Herbal
None known.
Food
None known.

DIAGNOSTIC TEST EFFECTS
May cause a positive Coombs' test.

SIDE EFFECTS
Occasional
Lethargy, fever, dizziness, rash, pain at injection site
Rare
Seizures, interstitial nephritis

SERIOUS REACTIONS
• Hypersensitivity reactions, ranging from chills, fever, and rash to anaphylaxis, may occur.

PRECAUTIONS & CONSIDERATIONS
Caution is warranted with a hypersensitivity to cephalosporins, impaired cardiac or renal function, or seizure disorders. History of allergies, especially to cephalosporins or penicillins, should be determined before giving the drug. Signs and symptoms of superinfection, including anal or genital pruritus, black hairy tongue, diarrhea, increased fever, sore throat, ulceration or changes of oral mucosa, and vomiting should be monitored. CBC, renal function test results, and urinalysis should be assessed.
Storage
Store prefilled syringes in the refrigerator. Do not freeze them.
Administration
Administer the drug undiluted by deep IM injection.
! Do not administer penicillin G benzathine IV, intra-arterially, or subcutaneously because doing so may cause heart attack, severe neurovascular damage, thrombosis, and death.

Penicillin G Potassium

pen-i-sill'in G

(Megacillin [CAN], Novepen-G [CAN], Pfizerpen)

Do not confuse with penicillin G benzathine, penicillin G procaine.

CATEGORY AND SCHEDULE

Pregnancy Risk Category: B

CLASSIFICATION

Antibiotics, penicillins

MECHANISM OF ACTION

A penicillin that inhibits bacterial cell wall synthesis by binding to one or more of the penicillin-binding proteins of bacteria. *Therapeutic Effect:* Bactericidal.

AVAILABILITY

Injection: 5 million units.
Premixed Dextrose Solution: 1 million units, 2 million units, 3 million units.

INDICATIONS AND DOSAGES

▶ **Sepsis, meningitis, pericarditis, endocarditis, pneumonia due to susceptible gram-positive organisms (not Staphylococcus aureus) and some gram-negative organisms**
IV, IM
Adults, Elderly. 2-24 million units/day in divided doses q4-6hr.
Children. 100,000-400,000 units/ kg/day in divided doses q4-6hr.
▶ **Dosage in renal impairment**
Dosage interval is modified based on creatinine clearance.

Creatinine Clearance	Dosage Interval
10-30 ml/min	Usual dose q8-12hr
Less than 10 ml/min	Usual dose q12-18hr

CONTRAINDICATIONS

Hypersensitivity to any penicillin

INTERACTIONS

Drug
Erythromycin: May antagonize effects of penicillin.
Probenecid: Increases serum concentration of penicillin.
Herbal
None known.
Food
Food, milk: Decrease penicillin absorption.

DIAGNOSTIC TEST EFFECTS

May cause a positive Coombs' test.

▦ IV INCOMPATIBILITIES

Amikacin (Amikin), aminophylline, amphotericin B, dopamine (Intropin)
◗ **IV Compatibilities**
Amiodarone (Cordarone), calcium gluconate, diltiazem (Cardizem), diphenhydramine (Benadryl), furosemide (Lasix), heparin, hydromorphone (Dilaudid), lidocaine, magnesium sulfate, methylprednisolone (Solu-Medrol), morphine, potassium chloride

SIDE EFFECTS

Occasional
Lethargy, fever, dizziness, rash, electrolyte imbalance, diarrhea, thrombophlebitis
Rare
Seizures, interstitial nephritis

SERIOUS REACTIONS

• Hypersensitivity reactions ranging from rash, fever, and chills to anaphylaxis occur.

PRECAUTIONS & CONSIDERATIONS

Caution is warranted with a hypersensitivity to cephalosporins, impaired hepatic or renal function, or seizure disorders. CBC, electrolyte levels, renal function test results, and urinalysis results should be monitored.

Storage
The reconstituted solution is stable for 7 days if refrigerated.

Administration
For IV use, follow the manufacturer's guidelines for dilution. After reconstitution, further dilute with 50 to 100 ml D$_5$W or 0.9% NaCl to yield a final concentration of 100,000 to 500,000 units/ml (50,000 units/ml for infants and neonates). Infuse the solution over 15 to 60 minutes.

Penicillin V Potassium
pen-i-sill'in V
(Abbocillin VK [AUS], Apo-Pen-VK [CAN], Cilicaine VK [AUS], L.P.V. [AUS], Novo-Pen-VK [CAN], Veetids)

CATEGORY AND SCHEDULE
Pregnancy Risk Category: B

CLASSIFICATION
Antibiotics, penicillins

MECHANISM OF ACTION
A penicillin that inhibits cell wall synthesis by binding to bacterial cell membranes. *Therapeutic Effect:* Bactericidal.

PHARMACOKINETICS
Moderately absorbed from the GI tract. Protein binding: 80%. Widely distributed. Metabolized in the liver. Primarily excreted in urine. **Half-life:** 1 hr (increased in impaired renal function).

AVAILABILITY
Tablets: 250 mg, 500 mg.

Powder for Oral Solution:
125 mg/5 ml, 250 mg/5 ml.

INDICATIONS AND DOSAGES
▸ **Mild to moderate respiratory tract or skin or skin-structure infections, otitis media, necrotizing ulcerative gingivitis**
PO
Adults, Elderly, Children 12 yr and older. 125-500 mg q6-8hr.
Children younger than 12 yr.
25-50 mg/kg/day in divided doses q6-8hr. Maximum: 3 g/day.
▸ **Primary prevention of rheumatic fever**
PO
Adults, Elderly. 500 mg 2-3 times/day for 10 days.
Children. 250 mg 2-3 times/day for 10 days.
▸ **Primary prevention of rheumatic fever**
PO
Adults, Elderly, Children. 250 mg twice a day.

CONTRAINDICATIONS
Hypersensitivity to any penicillin

INTERACTIONS
Drug
Probenecid: May increase penicillin blood concentration and risk of toxicity.
Herbal
None known.
Food
None known.

DIAGNOSTIC TEST EFFECTS
May cause a positive Coombs' test.

SIDE EFFECTS
Frequent
Mild hypersensitivity reaction (chills, fever, rash), nausea, vomiting, diarrhea

P

Rare
Bleeding, allergic reaction

SERIOUS REACTIONS
• Severe hypersensitivity reactions, including anaphylaxis, may occur.
• Nephrotoxicity, antibiotic-associated colitis, and other superinfections may result from high dosages or prolonged therapy.

PRECAUTIONS & CONSIDERATIONS
Caution is warranted with renal impairment, a history of seizures, or a history of allergies, particularly to cephalosporins. Penicillin V readily crosses the placenta, appears in cord blood and amniotic fluid, and is distributed in breast milk in low concentrations. Penicillin V may lead to allergic sensitization, candidiasis, diarrhea, and skin rash in infants. Use caution when giving penicillin V to neonates and young infants because their immature renal function may delay renal excretion of the drug. Age-related renal impairment may require dosage adjustment in the elderly.

History of allergies, especially to cephalosporins or penicillins, should be determined before giving the drug. Withhold and promptly notify the physician if rash or diarrhea occur. Severe diarrhea with abdominal pain, blood or mucus in stool, and fever may indicate antibiotic-associated colitis. Signs of bleeding, including ecchymosis, overt bleeding, and swelling, should be assessed. Signs and symptoms of superinfection, including anal or genital pruritus, black hairy tongue, diarrhea, increased fever, sore throat, ulceration or changes of oral mucosa, and vomiting should also be monitored. Intake and output, renal function tests, Hgb levels, and urinalysis should be obtained and reviewed.

Storage
Store tablets at room temperature. After reconstitution, the oral solution is stable for 14 days if refrigerated.
Administration
Take the drug without regard to food. Space drug doses evenly around the clock.

Pentamidine
pen-tam′i-deen
(NebuPent, Pentacarinat [CAN], Pentam-300)

CATEGORY AND SCHEDULE
Pregnancy Risk Category: C

CLASSIFICATION
Antiprotozoals

MECHANISM OF ACTION
An anti-infective, that interferes with nuclear metabolism and incorporation of nucleotides, inhibiting DNA, RNA, phospholipid, and protein synthesis. *Therapeutic Effect:* Produces antibacterial and antiprotozoal effects.

PHARMACOKINETICS
Well absorbed after IM administration; minimally absorbed after inhalation. Widely distributed. Primarily excreted in urine. Minimally removed by hemodialysis. **Half-life:** 6.5 hr (increased in impaired renal function).

AVAILABILITY
Injection (Pentam-300): 300 mg.
Powder for Nebulization (Nebupent): 300 mg.

INDICATIONS AND DOSAGES
▶ *Pneumocystis carinii* **pneumonia (PCP)**
IV, IM
Adults, Elderly. 4 mg/kg/day once a day for 14-21 days.
Children. 4 mg/kg/day once a day for 10-14 days.
▶ **Prevention of PCP**
INHALATION
Adults, Elderly. 300 mg once q4wk.
Children 5 yr and older. 300 mg q3-4wk.
Children younger than 5 yr.
8 mg/kg/dose once q3-4wk.

OFF-LABEL USES
Treatment of African trypanosomiasis, cutaneous or visceral leishmaniasis

CONTRAINDICATIONS
Concurrent use with didanosine

INTERACTIONS
Drug
Blood dyscrasia-producing medications, bone marrow depressants: May increase the abnormal hematologic effects of pentamidine.
Didanosine: May increase the risk of pancreatitis.
Foscarnet: May increase the risk of hypocalcemia, hypomagnesemia, and nephrotoxicity of pentamidine.
Nephrotoxic medications: May increase the risk of nephrotoxicity.
Herbal
None known.
Food
None known.

DIAGNOSTIC TEST EFFECTS
May increase BUN and serum alkaline phosphatase, bilirubin, creatinine, AST (SGOT), and ALT (SGPT) levels. May decrease serum calcium and magnesium levels. May alter blood glucose levels.

▒ IV INCOMPATIBILITIES
Cefazolin (Ancef), cefotaxime (Claforan), ceftazidime (Fortaz), ceftriaxone (Rocephin), fluconazole (Diflucan), foscarnet (Foscavir), interleukin (Proleukin)
▯ IV Compatibilities
Diltiazem (Cardizem), zidovudine (Retrovir)

SIDE EFFECTS
Frequent
Injection (greater than 10%):
Abscess, pain at injection site
Inhalation (greater than 5%):
Fatigue, metallic taste, shortness of breath, decreased appetite, dizziness, rash, cough, nausea, vomiting, chills
Occasional
Injection (10%-1%): Nausea, decreased appetite, hypotension, fever, rash, altered taste, confusion
Inhalation (5%-1%): Diarrhea, headache, anemia, muscle pain
Rare
Injection (less than 1%): Neuralgia, thrombocytopenia, phlebitis, dizziness

SERIOUS REACTIONS
- Rare reactions include life-threatening or fatal hypotension, arrhythmias, hypoglycemia, leukopenia, nephrotoxicity or renal failure, anaphylactic shock, Stevens-Johnson syndrome, and toxic epidural necrolysis.
- Hyperglycemia and insulin-dependent diabetes mellitus (often permanent) may occur even months after therapy has stopped.

PRECAUTIONS & CONSIDERATIONS
Caution is warranted with diabetes mellitus, hypertension, hypotension, or renal or hepatic impairment. It is unknown if pentamidine crosses the placenta or is distributed in breast milk. No age-related precautions

P

have been noted in children. No information is available regarding pentamidine use in the elderly. Avoid alcohol.

Report any lightheadedness, palpitations, shakiness, or sweating, shortness of breath, cough, or fever. Drowsiness, decreased appetite, and increased thirst and urination may develop in the months following therapy. Adequate hydration should be maintained.

IV and IM sites should be evaluated. Skin should be examined for rash. Hematology, liver, and renal function tests should be performed. Be alert for respiratory difficulty when administering pentamidine by inhalation.

Storage
Store vials at room temperature. After reconstitution, the IV solution is stable at room temperature for 48 hours. Store the aerosol at room temperature for 48 hours.

Administration
! Make sure the person is in the supine position during administration and has frequent B/P checks until stable because of the risk of a life-threatening hypotensive reaction. Have resuscitative equipment readily available.

For intermittent IV infusion (piggyback), reconstitute each vial with 3 to 5 ml D_5W or sterile water for injection. Withdraw the desired dose and further dilute with 50 to 250 ml D_5W. Infuse the drug over 60 minutes. Discard any unused portion. Don't give the drug by IV injection or rapid IV infusion because this increases the risk of severe hypotension.

For IM use, reconstitute each 300-mg vial with 3 ml sterile water for injection to provide a concentration of 100 mg/ml.

For aerosol (nebulizer) use, reconstitute each 300-mg vial with 6 ml

sterile water for injection. Avoid using 0.9% NaCl because it may cause a precipitate to form. Don't mix pentamidine with other medications in the nebulizer reservoir.

Pentazocine
pen-tah-zoe-seen
(Talwin)
Combination Products
With naloxone, a narcotic antagonist (oral) (Talwin NX); with aspirin (oral) (Talwin Compound); with acetaminophen (oral) (Talacen)

CATEGORY AND SCHEDULE
With naloxone, a narcotic antagonist (oral) (Talwin NX); with aspirin (oral) (Talwin Compound); with acetaminophen (oral) (Talacen)

CLASSIFICATION
Analgesics, narcotic agonist-antagonist

MECHANISM OF ACTION
An opioid antagonist that binds with opioid receptors within CNS.
Therapeutic Effect: Alters processes affecting pain perception, emotional response to pain.

PHARMACOKINETICS
Well absorbed after administration. Widely distributed including CSF. Metabolized in liver via oxidative and glucuronide conjugation pathways, extensive first-pass effect. Excreted in small amounts as unchanged drug. **Half-life:** 2-3 hr, prolonged with hepatic impairment.

AVAILABILITY
Tablets: 12.5 mg and 325 mg aspirin (Talwin Compound), 25 mg and 650 mg acetaminophen (Talacen), 50 mg pentazocine and 0.5 mg naloxone (Talwin NX), 50 mg (Talwin).
Injection: 30 mg (Talwin).

INDICATIONS AND DOSAGES
▸ **Analgesia**
PO
Adults. 50 mg q3-4hr. May increase to 100 mg q3-4hr, if needed. Maximum: 600 mg/day.
Elderly. 50 mg q4hr.
SUBCUTANEOUS/IM/IV
Adults. 30 mg q3-4hr. Do not exceed 30 mg IV or 60 mg subcutaneous/IM per dose. Maximum: 360 mg/day.
IM
Elderly. 25 mg q4hr.
▸ **Obstetric labor**
IM
Adults. 30 mg as a single dose.
IV
Adults. 20 mg when contractions are regular. May repeat 2-3 times q2-3hr.

CONTRAINDICATIONS
Hypersensitivity to pentazocine or any component of the formulation

INTERACTIONS
Drug
Alcohol, CNS depressants: May increase CNS or respiratory depression and hypotension.
Fluoxetine: May cause hypertension, diaphoresis, ataxia, flushing, nausea, dizziness, and anxiety.
MAOIs: May produce severe, fatal reaction.
Opioid analgesics: May increase withdrawal symptoms.
Sibutramine: May increase risk of serotonin syndrome.
Herbal
None known.

Food
None known.

DIAGNOSTIC TEST EFFECTS
May increase amylase and lipase.

SIDE EFFECTS
Frequent
Drowsiness, euphoria, nausea, vomiting
Occasional
Allergic reaction, histamine reaction (decreased B/P, increased sweating, flushing, wheezing), decreased urination, altered vision, constipation, dizziness, dry mouth, headache, hypotension, pain/burning at injection site

SERIOUS REACTIONS
• Overdosage results in severe respiratory depression, skeletal muscle flaccidity, cyanosis, extreme somnolence progressing to convulsions, stupor, and coma.
• Abrupt withdrawal after prolonged use may produce symptoms of narcotic withdrawal (abdominal cramps, rhinorrhea, lacrimation, nausea, vomiting, restlessness, anxiety, increased temperature, piloerection).

P

PRECAUTIONS & CONSIDERATIONS
Caution is warranted with head injury, respiratory disease, prior to biliary tract surgery (produces spasm of sphincter of Oddi), acute myocardial infarction, opioid dependence or abuse, and impaired hepatic and renal function. It is unknown if pentazocine crosses the placenta or is distributed in breast milk. Safety and efficacy have not been established in children. Age-related renal or liver impairment may require decreased dosage. Caution should be used in the elderly and debilitated.
Pentazocine may cause withdrawal in patients currently dependent

on narcotics. It may cause drowsiness and impaired judgment or coordination. Alcohol should be avoided.

Storage
Store parenteral form for 3 months at room temperature.

Administration
Rotate injection site for IM and subcutaneous use. Avoid intra-arterial injection.

May take oral pentazocine with food if GI upset occurs.

Pentobarbital
pen-toe-bar′bi-tal
(Nembutal, Phenobarbitone [AUS])
Do not confuse with phenobarbital.

CATEGORY AND SCHEDULE
Pregnancy Risk Category: D
Controlled Substance: Schedule II (capsules, injection), Schedule III (suppositories)

CLASSIFICATION
Anticonvulsants, barbiturates, preanesthetics, sedatives/hypnotics

MECHANISM OF ACTION
A barbiturate that binds at the GABA receptor complex, enhancing GABA activity. *Therapeutic Effect:* Depresses central nervous system (CNS) activity and reticular activating system.

PHARMACOKINETICS
Well absorbed after PO, parenteral administration. Protein binding: 35%-55%. Rapidly, widely distributed. Metabolized in liver. Primarily excreted in urine. Removed by hemodialysis. **Half-life:** 15-48 hr.

AVAILABILITY
Capsules: 50 mg, 100 mg.
Injection: 50 mg/ml.
Suppositories: 30 mg, 120 mg, 200 mg.

INDICATIONS AND DOSAGES
▸ **Preanesthetic**
PO
Adults, Elderly. 100 mg.
Children. 2-6 mg/kg. Maximum: 100 mg/dose.
IM
Adults, Elderly. 150-200 mg.
Children. 2-6 mg/kg. Maximum: 100 mg/dose.
RECTAL
Children 12-14 yr. 60 or 120 mg.
Children 5-12 yr. 60 mg.
Children 1-4 yr. 30-60 mg.
Children 1 yr-2 mo. 30 mg.
▸ **Hypnotic**
PO
Adults, Elderly. 100 mg at bedtime.
IM
Adults, Elderly. 150-200 mg at bedtime.
Children. 2-6 mg/kg. Maximum: 100 mg/dose at bedtime.
IV
Adults, Elderly. 100 mg initially then, after 1 minute, may give additional small doses at 1 minute intervals, up to 500 mg total.
Children. 50 mg initially then, after 1 minute, may give additional small doses at 1 minute intervals, up to desired effect.
RECTAL
Adults, Elderly. 120-200 mg at bedtime.
Children 12-14 yr. 60 or 120 mg at bedtime.
Children 5-12 yr. 60 mg at bedtime.

Children 1-4 yr. 30-60 mg at bedtime.
Children 2 mo-1 yr. 30 mg at bedtime.
▶ **Anticonvulsant**
IV
Adults, Elderly. 2-15 mg/kg loading dose given slowly over 1-2 hours. Maintenance infusion: 0.5-5 mg/kg/hr.
Children. 5-15 mg/kg loading dose given slowly over 1-2 hours. Maintenance infusion: 0.5-3 mg/kg/hr.

OFF-LABEL USES
Intracranial hypertension, psychiatric interviews, sedative withdrawal, drug abuse withdrawal

CONTRAINDICATIONS
Porphyria, hypersensitivity to barbiturates

INTERACTIONS
Drug
Alcohol, CNS depressants: May increase the effects of pentobarbital.
Alprenolol, metoprolol: May decrease alprenolol and metoprolol effectiveness.
Barbituates: May increase the risk of respiratory depression.
Chloral hydrate: May increase the risk of respiratory depression.
Dicumarol: May decrease the anticoagulant effectiveness.
Opioid analgesics: May increase the risk of respiratory depression.
Prednisolone, prednisone: May decrease therapeutic effect of prednisolone and prednisone.
Procarbazine: May increase the risk of CNS depression.
Quetiapine: May decrease serum quetiapine concentrations.
Theophylline: May decrease theophylline effectiveness.
Herbal
Catnip oil: May increase risk of CNS depression.

Eucalyptol: May decrease effectiveness of barbiturates.
Kava kava: May increase CNS depression.
St. John's Wort: May decrease CNS depressive effect of barbiturates.
Valerian: May increase CNS depression.
Food
None known.

DIAGNOSTIC TEST EFFECTS
None known.

🖳 IV INCOMPATIBILITIES
Anileridine, atracurium (Tacrium), benzquinamide, butorphanol, cefazolin (Ancef), chlordiazepoxide (Librium), chlorpheniramine, clindamycin (Cleocin), codeine, cyclizine, diphenhydramine (Benadryl), droperidol (Inapsine), fenoldopam (Corlopam), fentanyl, glycopyrrolate (Robinul), hydrocortisone (Solu-Cortef), insulin, kanamycin (Kantrex), levorphanol (Levo-Dromoran), meperidine (Demerol), metaraminol (Aramin), methadone, methyldopa (Aldomet), metocurine (Metubine), midazolam (Versed), nalbuphine (Nubain), opium alkaloids, oxytetracycline, pancuronium (Pavulon), penicillin G (Pfizerpen), pentazocine (Talwin), perphenazine (Trilafon), phytonadione (Aqua-Mephyton), prochlorperazine (Compazine), promazine (Sparine), protein hydrolysate (Nembutal), sodium bicarbonate, streptomycin, thiamine, triflupromazine (Stelazine), tripelennamine (PBZ), vancomycin (Vancocin)

🖳 IV Compatibilities
Acyclovir (Zovirax), amikacin (Amikin), aminophylline, calcium chloride, cephapirin (Cefadyl), chloramphenicol, hyaluronidase (Wydase), hydromorphone

P

(Dilaudid), lidocaine, neostigmine
(Prostigmin), propofol (Diprivan),
ranitidine (Zantac), scopolamine,
sodium iodide, thiopental
(Pentothal), verapamil

SIDE EFFECTS
Occasional
Agitation, confusion, dizziness,
somnolence
Rare
Confusion, paradoxical CNS hyper-
activity or nervousness in children,
excitement or restlessness in elderly

SERIOUS REACTIONS
• Agranulocytosis, megaloblastic
anemia, apnea, hypoventilation,
bradycardia, hypotension, syncope,
hepatic damage, and Stevens-Johnson
syndrome occur rarely.
• Abrupt withdrawal after prolonged
therapy may produce effects ranging
from markedly increased dreaming,
nightmares or insomnia, tremor,
sweating and vomiting, to hallucinations, delirium, seizures, and status
epilepticus.
• Skin eruptions appear as hypersensitivity reactions.
• Overdosage produces cold or
clammy skin, hypothermia, severe
CNS depression, cyanosis, and rapid
pulse.

PRECAUTIONS & CONSIDERATIONS
Caution is warranted with liver or
renal impairment, the elderly or
debilitated, suicidal tendencies, and
history of drug or alcohol abuse.
Pentobarbital readily crosses the
placenta and is distributed in breast
milk. Withdrawal symptoms may
appear in neonates born to women
receiving barbiturates during last
trimester of pregnancy. Its use may
cause paradoxical excitement in children. The elderly taking pentobarbital
may exhibit confusion, excitement,

and mental depression. Alcohol
consumption and caffeine should be
avoided while taking pentobarbital.
Tasks that require mental alertness
or motor skills should be avoided
because pentobarbital may cause
dizziness and drowsiness.

Storage
Store vials at room temperature.
Refrigerate suppositories.

Administration
Be aware that dosage must be individualized based on patient's age,
weight, and condition.
Give oral pentobarbital without
regard to meals.
Do not inject more than 5 ml in
any one IM injection site because it
produces tissue irritation. Inject IM
deeply into gluteus maximus or
lateral aspect of thigh.
May give IV injection undiluted,
or may dilute with NaCl, D_5W,
lactated Ringer's.
Expect to adequately hydrate
before and immediately after infusion to decrease the risk of adverse
renal effects. Parenteral routes
should only be pursued when oral
administration is impossible or
impractical. Beware that inadvertent
intra-arterial injection may result in
arterial spasm with severe pain and
tissue necrosis. Also know that
extravasation in subcutaneous tissue
may produce redness, tenderness,
and tissue necrosis. If either occurs,
treat with 0.5% procaine solution
injected into affected area and apply
moist heat.
Unwrap rectal suppository before
insertion. Moisten suppository with
cold water before inserting well up
into rectum.

Pentosan Polysulfate

pen-toe-san
(Elmiron)
**Do not confuse with
pentostatin.**

CATEGORY AND SCHEDULE
Pregnancy Risk Category: B

CLASSIFICATION
Anticoagulants

MECHANISM OF ACTION
A negatively-charged synthetic
sulfated polysaccharide with
heparin-like properties that appears
to adhere to bladder wall mucosal
membrane, may act as a buffering
agent to control cell permeability
preventing irritating solutes in the
urine. Has anticoagulant/ fibrinolytic
effects. *Therapeutic Effect:* Relieves
bladder pain.

PHARMACOKINETICS
Poorly and erratically absorbed from
the gastrointestinal tract. Distributed
in uroepithelium of GU tract with
lesser amount found in the liver,
spleen, lung, skin, periosteum and
bone marrow. Metabolized in liver
and kidney (secondary). Eliminated
in the urine. **Half-life:** 4.8 hr.

AVAILABILITY
Capsules: 100 mg (Elmiron).

INDICATIONS AND DOSAGES
▶ **Interstitial cystitis**
PO
Adults, Elderly. 100 mg 3 times/day.

OFF-LABEL USES
Urolithiasis

CONTRAINDICATIONS
Hypersensitivity to pentosan polysulfate sodium or structurally related
compounds

INTERACTIONS
Drug
Anticoagulants: May increase risk
of bleeding.
Herbal
Chondroitin, ginseng: May increase
INR serum values and increase anticoagulant effects.
Alfalfa, coenzyme Q, green tea:
May decrease anticoagulant effectiveness.
**Arnica, bilberry, black currant,
bromelain, cat's claw, chamomile,
clove oil, curcumin, dong quai,
primrose oil, fenugreek, garlic,
ginger, kava kava, licorice, red
clover, skullcap, tan-shen,
vitamin A:** May increase risk of
bleeding.
Food
Avocado: May decrease anticoagulant effectiveness.
Rhubarb: May increase risk of
bleeding.

DIAGNOSTIC TEST EFFECTS
May increase transaminase, alkaline
phosphatase, PTT, PT. May decrease
WBC count, thrombocytes.

▓ IV INCOMPATIBILITIES
None known.
⬛ **IV Compatibilities**
None known.

SIDE EFFECTS
Frequent
Alopecia areata (a single area on
the scalp), diarrhea, nausea,
headache, rash, abdominal pain,
dyspepsia.
Occasional
Dizziness, depression, increased
liver function tests.

P

SERIOUS REACTIONS
- Ecchymosis, epistaxis, gum hemorrhage have been reported (drug produces weak anticoagulant effect).
- Overdose may produce liver function abnormalities.

PRECAUTIONS & CONSIDERATIONS

Caution is warranted with gastrointestinal (GI) ulcerations, polyps, diverticula, history of heparin-induced thrombocytopenia, hepatic or splenic function impairment, concurrent anticoagulant, thrombolytic or antiplatelet therapy, and recent intracranial, intraspinal, or ophthalmological surgery. It is unknown if pentosan polysulfate sodium is distributed in breast milk. Safety and efficacy of pentosan polysulfate sodium have not been established in children less than 16 years of age. There are no age-related precautions noted in the elderly.

The physician should be notified if any bleeding from gums or nose, bloody or black bowel movements, coughing up blood, bloody vomit or vomit that looks like coffee grounds, or severe stomach pain or diarrhea that does not stop occurs.

Administration
Take with water at least 1 hr before or 2 hr after meals.

Pentoxifylline
pen-tox-if′ih-lin
(Albert [CAN], Apo-Pentoxifylline SR [CAN], Pentoxifylline [CAN], Pentoxyl, Trental)
Do not confuse Trental with Tegretol, Trandate.

CATEGORY AND SCHEDULE
Pregnancy Risk Category: C

CLASSIFICATION
Hemorrheologic agents, xanthine derivatives

MECHANISM OF ACTION
A blood viscosity-reducing agent that alters the flexibility of RBCs; inhibits production of tumor necrosis factor, neutrophil activation, and platelet aggregation. *Therapeutic Effect:* Reduces blood viscosity and improves blood flow.

PHARMACOKINETICS
Well absorbed after oral administration. Undergoes first-pass metabolism in the liver. Primarily excreted in urine. Unknown if removed by hemodialysis. **Half-life:** 24-48 min; metabolite, 60-90 min.

AVAILABILITY
Tablets (Controlled-Release [Pentoxil, Trental]): 400 mg.

INDICATIONS AND DOSAGES
▸ **Intermittent claudication**
PO
Adults, Elderly. 400 mg 3 times a day. Decrease to 400 mg twice a day if GI or CNS adverse effects occur. Continue for at least 8 wk.

CONTRAINDICATIONS
History of intolerance to xanthine derivatives, such as caffeine, theophylline, or theobromine; recent cerebral or retinal hemorrhage

INTERACTIONS
Drug
Antihypertensives: May increase the effects of antihypertensives.
Herbal
None known.
Food
None known.

DIAGNOSTIC TEST EFFECTS
None known.

SIDE EFFECTS
Occasional (5%-2%)
Dizziness, nausea, altered taste, dyspepsia, marked by heartburn, epigastric pain, and indigestion
Rare (less than 2%)
Rash, pruritus, anorexia, constipation, dry mouth, blurred vision, edema, nasal congestion, anxiety

SERIOUS REACTIONS
• Angina and chest pain occur rarely and may be accompanied by palpitations, tachycardia, and arrhythmias.
• Signs and symptoms of overdose, such as flushing, hypotension, nervousness, agitation, hand tremor, fever, and somnolence, appear 4-5 hours after ingestion and last for 12 hours.

PRECAUTIONS & CONSIDERATIONS
Caution is warranted with chronic occlusive arterial disease, insulin-treated diabetes, hepatic or renal impairment, peptic ulcer disease, and recent surgery. It is unknown if pentoxifylline crosses the placenta and is distributed in breast milk. Safety and efficacy of pentoxifylline have not been established in children. In the elderly, age-related renal impairment may require cautious use. Caffeine should be limited and smoking should be avoided; smoking causes constriction and occlusion of peripheral blood vessels.

Dizziness may occur. Avoid tasks requiring mental alertness or motor skills until response to the drug has been established. Notify the physician of hand tremor. Notify the physician of red or dark urine, muscular pain or weakness, abdominal or back pain, gingival bleeding, black or red stool, coffee-ground vomitus, or blood-tinged mucus from cough. B/P, heart rate and rhythm, and pulse rate, serum creatinine kinase and AST (SGOT) levels should be monitored. Relief of signs and symptoms of intermittent claudication should be monitored; symptoms generally occur while walking or exercising or with weight bearing in the absence of walking or exercising.
Administration
Do not crush or break film-coated tablets. Take with meals to avoid GI upset. Therapeutic effect is generally noted in 2 to 4 weeks.

P

Pergolide
per´go-lide
(Permax)
Do not confuse Permax with Pentrax or Pernox.

CATEGORY AND SCHEDULE
Pregnancy Risk Category: B

CLASSIFICATION
Antiparkinson agents, dermatologics, ergot alkaloids and derivatives

MECHANISM OF ACTION

A centrally active dopamine agonist that directly stimulates dopamine receptors. *Therapeutic Effect:* Decreases signs and symptoms of Parkinson's disease.

PHARMACOKINETICS

Well absorbed from the GI tract. Protein binding: 90%. Undergoes extensive first-pass metabolism in the liver. Primarily excreted in urine. Unknown if removed by hemodialysis.

AVAILABILITY

Tablets: 0.05 mg, 0.25 mg, 1 mg.

INDICATIONS AND DOSAGES

▶ **Parkinsonism**
PO
Adults, Elderly. Initially, 0.05 mg/day for 2 days. May increase by 0.1-0.15 mg/day every 3 days over the next 12 days; afterward may increase by 0.25 mg/day every 3 days. Range: 2-3 mg/day in 3 divided doses. Maximum: 5 mg/day.

CONTRAINDICATIONS

Hypersensitivity to pergolide or other ergot derivatives

INTERACTIONS

Drug
Haloperidol, loxapine, methyldopa, metoclopramide, phenothiazines: May decrease the effectiveness of pergolide.
Hypotension-producing medications: May increase the hypotensive effect.
Herbal
None known.
Food
None known.

DIAGNOSTIC TEST EFFECTS

May increase the serum growth hormone level.

SIDE EFFECTS

Frequent (24%-10%)
Nausea, dizziness, hallucinations, constipation, rhinitis, dystonia, confusion, somnolence
Occasional (9%-3%)
Orthostatic hypotension, insomnia, dry mouth, peripheral edema, anxiety, diarrhea, dyspepsia, abdominal pain, headache, abnormal vision, anorexia, tremor, depression, rash
Rare (less than 2%)
Urinary frequency, vivid dreams, neck pain, hypotension, vomiting

SERIOUS REACTIONS

• Symptoms of overdose may vary from CNS depression, characterized by sedation, apnea, cardiovascular collapse, and death, to severe paradoxical reactions, such as hallucinations, tremor, and seizures.

PRECAUTIONS & CONSIDERATIONS

Caution is warranted with pre-existing cardiac arrhythmias, confusion, and hallucinations. It is unknown if pergolide crosses the placenta or is distributed in breast milk. However, pergolide may interfere with lactation. The safety and efficacy of this drug have not been established in children. No age-related precautions have been noted in the elderly.

Dizziness, drowsiness, and dry mouth may occur. Alcohol and tasks that require mental alertness or motor skills should be avoided. Notify the physician if agitation, headache, lethargy, or confusion occurs. A baseline EKG should be performed in those with a history of cardiac disease. B/P and pulse rate should be monitored to detect hypotension and irregularities that could indicate an arrhythmia. Also, ABG and serum electrolyte levels should be monitored. Relief of parkinsonian symptoms, such as improvement of masklike facial expression, muscular rigidity, shuffling gait, and resting tremors of the hands and head, should be assessed.

Administration

! Pergolide is usually given in 3 divided doses daily.

Crush scored tablets as needed. Take pergolide without regard to food.

Perindopril
per-in′doh-pril
(Aceon)

CATEGORY AND SCHEDULE
Pregnancy Risk Category: C (D if used in second or third trimester)

CLASSIFICATION
Angiotensin converting enzyme inhibitors

MECHANISM OF ACTION
An ACE inhibitor that suppresses the renin-angiotensin-aldosterone system and prevents conversion of angiotensin I to angiotensin II, a potent vasoconstrictor; may also inhibit angiotensin II at local vascular and renal sites. *Therapeutic Effect:* Reduces peripheral arterial resistance and B/P.

AVAILABILITY
Tablets: 2 mg, 4 mg, 8 mg.

INDICATIONS AND DOSAGES
▶ **Hypertension**
PO
Adults, Elderly. 2-8 mg/day as single dose or in 2 divided doses. Maximum: 16 mg/day.

OFF-LABEL USES
Management of heart failure

CONTRAINDICATIONS
History of angioedema from previous treatment with ACE inhibitors

INTERACTIONS
Drug
Alcohol, antihypertensives, diuretics: May increase the effects of perindopril.
Lithium: May increase lithium blood concentration and risk of lithium toxicity.
NSAIDs: May decrease the effects of benazepril.
Potassium-sparing diuretics, potassium supplements: May cause hyperkalemia.
Herbal
None known.
Food
None known.

DIAGNOSTIC TEST EFFECTS
May increase BUN, serum alkaline phosphatase, serum bilirubin, serum creatinine, serum potassium, AST (SGOT), and ALT (SGPT) levels. May decrease serum sodium levels. May cause positive antinuclear antibody titer.

SIDE EFFECTS
Occasional (5%-1%)
Cough, back pain, sinusitis, upper extremity pain, dyspepsia, fever, palpitations, hypotension, dizziness, fatigue, syncope

SERIOUS REACTIONS
• Excessive hypotension (first-dose syncope) may occur in patients with CHF and in those who are severely salt or volume depleted.
• Angioedema (swelling of face and lips) and hyperkalemia occur rarely.

P

• Agranulocytosis and neutropenia may be noted in those with collagen vascular disease, including scleroderma and systemic lupus erythematosus, and impaired renal function.
• Nephrotic syndrome may be noted in those with history of renal disease.

PRECAUTIONS & CONSIDERATIONS

Caution is warranted with cerebrovascular insufficiency, coronary insufficiency, hypovolemia, renal impairment, and sodium depletion, and those on dialysis and/or receiving diuretics. Perindopril crosses the placenta and it is unknown if it is distributed in breast milk. Perindopril has caused fetal or neonatal morbidity or mortality. Safety and efficacy of perindopril have not been established in children. In the elderly, age-related renal impairment may require cautious use of perindopril.

Dizziness may occur. Be alert to fluctuations in B/P. If an excessive reduction in B/P occurs, place the person in the supine position with legs elevated. CBC and blood chemistry should be obtained before beginning perindopril therapy, then every 2 weeks for the next 3 months, and periodically thereafter in patients with autoimmune disease, or renal impairment, and in those who are taking drugs that affect immune response or leukocyte count. BUN, serum creatinine, serum potassium, AST (SGOT) and ALT (SGPT) levels should also be monitored. Pattern of daily bowel activity and stool consistency should be assessed.

Administration

Take perindopril 1 hour before meals. Do not skip doses or voluntarily discontinue the drug to avoid severe, rebound hypertension.

Permethrin
per-meth'ren
(A200 Lice, Acticin, Elimite, Kwellada-P [CAN], Nix, RID Spray)

CATEGORY AND SCHEDULE
Pregnancy Risk Category: B

CLASSIFICATION
Anti-infectives, topical, dermatologics, scabicides/pediculicides

MECHANISM OF ACTION
An antiparasitic agent that inhibits sodium influx through nerve cell membrane channels. *Therapeutic Effect:* Results in delayed repolarization, paralysis, and death of parasites.

PHARMACOKINETICS
Less than 2% absorption after topical application. Detected in residual amounts on hair for at least 10 days following treatment. Metabolized by liver to inactive metabolites. Excreted in urine.

AVAILABILITY
Cream: 5% (Acticin).
Liquid, topical: 1% (Nix).
Shampoo: 0.33% (A200 Lice).
Solution: 0.25% (Nix), 0.5% (A200 Lice, RID).

INDICATIONS AND DOSAGES
▸ **Head lice**
SHAMPOO
Adults, Elderly, Children 2 mo and older. Shampoo hair, towel dry, apply to scalp, leave on for 10 minutes and rinse. Remove nits with nit comb. Repeat application if live lice present 7 days after initial treatment.

▸ **Scabies**
TOPICAL
Adults, Elderly, Children 2 mo and older. Apply from head to feet, leave on for 8-14 hr. Wash with soap and water. Repeat application if living mites present 14 days after initial treatment.

OFF-LABEL USES
Demodicidosis, insect bite prophylaxis, leishmaniasis prophylaxis, malaria prophylaxis

CONTRAINDICATIONS
Infants less than 2 months of age, hypersensitivity to pyrethyroid, pyrethrin, chrysanthemums or any component of the formulation

INTERACTIONS
Drug
None known.
Herbal
None known.
Food
None known.

DIAGNOSTIC TEST EFFECTS
None known.

SIDE EFFECTS
Occasional
Burning, pruritus, stinging, erythema, rash, swelling

SERIOUS REACTIONS
• Shortness of breath and difficulty breathing have been reported.

PRECAUTIONS & CONSIDERATIONS
Caution should be used during pregnancy and with asthma, pruritus, edema, and erythema. It is unknown if permethrin is distributed in breast milk. There are no age-related precautions noted for suspension or topical use in children. Permethrin is not recommended for use in children

2 months or younger. There are no age-related precautions noted in the elderly.
Administration
Because scabies and lice are contagious, use caution to avoid spreading or infecting oneself. Use gloves when applying.

Shampoo hair, towel dry, apply rinse to scalp, leave on for 10 minutes then rinse. Remove nits with nit comb. Repeat application if live lice present 7 days after initial treatment. If live lice are detected 14 days after the initial application of permethrin, retreatment is indicated. Also, in epidemic settings, a second application is recommended 2 weeks after the first.

When using the topical formulation, apply and rub gently into the affected and surrounding area. Apply from head to feet and leave on for 8-14 hr. Wash with soap and water. Repeat application if living mites present 14 days after initial treatment.

P

Perphenazine
per-fen-ah-zeen
(Trilafon)
Do not confuse with promazine.

CATEGORY AND SCHEDULE
Pregnancy Risk Category: C

CLASSIFICATION
Antiemetics/antivertigo, antipsychotics, phenothiazines

MECHANISM OF ACTION
An antipsychotic agent and antiemetic that blocks postsynaptic

dopamine receptor sites in the brain.
Therapeutic Effect: Suppresses behavioral response in psychosis, and relieves nausea and vomiting.

AVAILABILITY
Oral Concentrate: 15 mg/5 ml.
Tablets: 2 mg, 4 mg, 8 mg, 16 mg.

INDICATIONS AND DOSAGES
▸ **Severe schizophrenia**
PO
Adults. 4-16 mg 2-4 times/day.
Maximum: 64 mg/day.
Elderly. Initially, 2-4 mg/day. May increase at 4-7 day intervals by 2-4 mg/day up to 32 mg/day.
▸ **Severe nausea and vomiting**
PO
Adults. 8-16 mg/day in divided doses up to 24 mg/day.

CONTRAINDICATIONS
Coma, myelosuppression, severe cardiovascular disease, severe CNS depression, subcortical brain damage

INTERACTIONS
Drug
Alcohol, other CNS depressants:
May increase hypotensive effects and CNS and respiratory depression.
Antihypotensives: May increase the risk of hypotension.
Antithyroid agents: May increase the risk of agranulocytosis.
Extrapyramidal symptom–producing medications: May increase the severity and frequency of extrapyramidal symptoms.
Levodopa: May decrease the effects of this drug.
Lithium: May decrease perphenazine absorption and produce adverse neurologic effects.
MAOIs, tricyclic antidepressants:
May increase anticholinergic and sedative effects.

Herbal
None known.
Food
Apple juice, caffeine- or tannic-containing beverages (such as tea):
Don't mix oral concentrate with these beverages.

DIAGNOSTIC TEST EFFECTS
May produce false-positive pregnancy and phenylketonuria test results. May produce EKG changes, including prolonged QT and QTc intervals and T-wave depression or inversion.

▦ IV INCOMPATIBILITIES
Aminophylline, cefoperazone (Cefobid), midazolam (Versed), opium alkaloids, oxytocin, pentobarbital (Nembutal), secobarbital (Seconal), thiopental (Pentothal)
▯ IV Compatibilities
Atropine, chlorpromazine (Librium), dimenhydrinate (Dramamine), diphenhydramine (Benadryl), droperidol (Inapsine), fentanyl (Sublimaze), hydroxyzine (Vistaril), meperidine (Demerol), morphine, pentazocine (Talwin), prochlorperazine (Compazine), promethazine (Phenergan), ranitidine (Zantac), scopolamine (Transderm)

SIDE EFFECTS
Occasional
Marked photosensitivity, somnolence, dry mouth, blurred vision, lethargy, constipation or diarrhea, nasal congestion, peripheral edema, urine retention
Rare
Ocular changes, altered skin pigmentation, hypotension, dizziness, syncope

SERIOUS REACTIONS
• Extrapyramidal symptoms appear to be dose-related and are divided into 3 categories: akathisia (characterized

by inability to sit still, tapping of feet), parkinsonian symptoms (including masklike face, tremors, shuffling gait, hypersalivation), and acute dystonias (such as torticollis, opisthotonos, and oculogyric crisis).

• Tardive dyskinesia occurs rarely.

• Abrupt withdrawal after long-term therapy may precipitate nausea, vomiting, gastritis, dizziness, and tremors.

PRECAUTIONS & CONSIDERATIONS

Caution is warranted with impaired respiratory, hepatic, renal or cardiac function, alcohol withdrawal, history of seizures, urinary retention, glaucoma, prostatic hypertrophy, and hypocalcemia (increases susceptibility to dystonias). Be aware that perphenazine crosses the placenta and is distributed in breast milk. Be aware that children may develop extrapyramidal symptoms (EPS), or neuromuscular symptoms, especially dystonias. The elderly are more prone to anticholinergic effects, such as dry mouth, EPS, orthostatic hypotension, and sedation symptoms.

Urine may darken and drowsiness may occur. Alcohol and tasks that require mental alertness or motor skills should be avoided. Exposure to artificial light and sunlight should also be avoided during therapy. EPS, tardive dyskinesia, and potentially fatal, rare neuroleptic malignant syndrome, such as altered mental status, fever, irregular pulse or B/P, and muscle rigidity should be monitored. Hydration status should also be assessed.

Administration

Skin should not come in contact with solutions (contact dermatitis). Therapeutic effect may take up to 6 weeks to appear. Do not abruptly discontinue perphenazine.

Phenazopyridine

fen-az′o-peer′i-deen
(Azo-Gesic, Azo-Standard, Phenazo [CAN], Prodium, Pyridium, Uristat)
Do not confuse phenazopyridine with pyridoxine, or Prodium with Perdiem.

CATEGORY AND SCHEDULE

Pregnancy Risk Category: B

CLASSIFICATION

Analgesics, non-narcotic

MECHANISM OF ACTION

An interstitial cystitis agent that exerts topical analgesic effect on urinary tract mucosa. *Therapeutic Effect:* Relieves urinary pain, burning, urgency, and frequency.

PHARMACOKINETICS

Well absorbed from the GI tract. Partially metabolized in the liver. Primarily excreted in urine.

AVAILABILITY

Tablets (Azo-Gesic, Azo-Standard, Prodium, Uristat): 100 mg, 200 mg.
Tablets (Pyridium): 95 mg.

INDICATIONS AND DOSAGES

▶ **Urinary analgesic**
PO
Adults. 100-200 mg 3-4 times a day.
Children 6 yr and older.
12 mg/kg/day in 3 divided doses for 2 days.

▶ **Dosage in renal impairment**
Dosage interval is modified based on creatinine clearance.

Creatinine Clearance	Interval
50-80 ml/min	Usual dose q8-16hr
Less than 50 ml/min	Avoid use

CONTRAINDICATIONS
Hepatic or renal insufficiency

INTERACTIONS
Drug
None known.
Herbal
None known.
Food
None known.

DIAGNOSTIC TEST EFFECTS
May interfere with urinalysis tests based on color reactions, such as urinary glucose, ketones, protein, and 17-ketosteroids.

SIDE EFFECTS
Occasional
Headache, GI disturbance, rash, pruritus

SERIOUS REACTIONS
• Overdose may lead to hemolytic anemia, nephrotoxicity, or hepatotoxicity. Patients with renal impairment or severe hypersensitivity to the drug may also develop these reactions.
• A massive and acute overdose may result in methemoglobinemia.

PRECAUTIONS & CONSIDERATIONS
Notify the physician and expect to discontinue the drug if skin or sclera turns yellow because this signifies impaired renal excretion. It is unknown if phenazopyridine crosses the placenta or is distributed in breast milk. No age-related precautions have been noted in children older than 6 years. Age-related renal impairment

may increase the risk of toxicity in the elderly.
    Urine may turn a reddish orange color. Therapeutic response, including relief of urinary frequency, pain, and burning, should be assessed.
Administration
Take phenazopyridine with food. Expect to discontinue the drug after 2 days because there's no evidence that it's effective after this time period.

Phendimetrazine
fen-dye-me′tra-zeen
(Adipost, Bontril PDM, Bontril Slow-Release, Melfiat, Obezine, Phendiet, Phendiet-105, Plegine, Prelu-2)

CATEGORY AND SCHEDULE
Pregnancy Risk Category: C

CLASSIFICATION
Anorexiants, stimulants, central nervous system

MECHANISM OF ACTION
A phenylalkylamine sympathomimetic with activity similar to amphetamines that stimulates the central nervous system (CNS) and elevates blood pressure (B/P) most likely mediated via norepinephrine and dopamine metabolism. Causes stimulation of the hypothalamus.
Therapeutic Effect: Decreases appetite.

PHARMACOKINETICS
The pharmacokinetics of phendimetrazine tartrate has not been well established. Metabolized to active metabolite, phendimetrazine. Excreted in urine. **Half-life:** 2-4 hr.

AVAILABILITY
Tablets: 35 mg (Bontril PDM, Obezine, Phendiet, Plegine)
Capsules (extended-release): 105 mg (Adipost, Bontril Slow-Release, Melfiat, Phendiet-105, Prelu-2).

INDICATIONS AND DOSAGES
▶ **Obesity**
PO
Adults, Elderly. 105 mg/day in the morning or before the morning meal (sustained-release); 35 mg 2-3 times/day (immediate-release). Maximum: 70 mg 3 times/day.

CONTRAINDICATIONS
Advanced arteriosclerosis, agitated states, glaucoma, history of drug abuse, history of hypersensitivity to sympathomimetic amines, hyperthyroidism, moderate to severe hypertension, symptomatic cardiovascular disease, use within 14 days of discontinuation MAOI, hypersensitivity to phendimetrazine or sympathomimetics

INTERACTIONS
Drug
Guanethidine: May decrease hypotensive effect of guanethidine.
MAOIs: May increase risk of hypertensive crisis.
Sibutramine: May increase risk of hypertension and tachycardia.
Tricyclic antidepressants: May increase cardiovascular effects.
Herbal
None known.
Food
None known.

DIAGNOSTIC TEST EFFECTS
None known.

SIDE EFFECTS
Occasional
Constipation, nausea, diarrhea, dry mouth, dysuria, libido changes, flushing, hypertension, insomnia, nervousness, headache, dizziness, irritability, agitation, restlessness, palpitations, increased heart rate, sweating, tremor, urticaria

SERIOUS REACTIONS
• Multivalvular heart disease, primary pulmonary hypertension and arrhythmias occur rarely.
• Overdose may produce flushing, arrhythmias, and psychosis.
• Abrupt withdrawal following prolonged administration of high doses may produce extreme fatigue and depression.

PRECAUTIONS & CONSIDERATIONS
Caution is warranted with diabetes mellitus and mild hypertension as well as with guanethidine because phendimetrazine may decrease the hypotensive effect of guanethidine. Caution should be used with pregnancy. It is unknown if phendimetrazine is excreted in breast milk. Be aware that safety and efficacy of this drug have not been established in children. There are no age-related precautions noted in the elderly. Tasks that require mental alertness or motor skills should be avoided. Palpitations, dizziness, dry mouth, and pronounced nervousness should be reported.
Administration
Take one hour before a meal, usually the first meal of the day. Tell the patient to swallow capsules whole.

P

Phenelzine
fen'el-zeen
(Nardil)

CATEGORY AND SCHEDULE
Pregnancy Risk Category: C

CLASSIFICATION
Antidepressants, monoamine oxidase inhibitors

MECHANISM OF ACTION
An MAOI that inhibits the activity of the enzyme monoamine oxidase at CNS storage sites, leading to increased levels of the neurotransmitters epinephrine, norepinephrine, serotonin, and dopamine at neuronal receptor sites. *Therapeutic Effect:* Relieves depression.

AVAILABILITY
Tablets: 15 mg.

INDICATIONS AND DOSAGES
▶ **Depression refractory to other antidepressants or electroconvulsive therapy**
PO
Adults. 15 mg 3 times a day. May increase to 60-90 mg/day.
Elderly. Initially, 7.5 mg/day. May increase by 7.5-15 mg/day q3-4wk up to 60 mg/day in divided doses.

OFF-LABEL USES
Treatment of panic disorder, vascular or tension headaches

CONTRAINDICATIONS
Cardiovascular or cerebrovascular disease, hepatic or renal impairment, pheochromocytoma

INTERACTIONS
Drug
Alcohol, other CNS depressants: May increase CNS depression.
Buspirone: May increase B/P.
Caffeine-containing medications: May increase the risk of cardiac arrhythmias and hypertension.
Carbamazepine, cyclobenzaprine, maprotiline, other MAOIs: May precipitate hypertensive crisis.
Dopamine, tryptophan: May cause sudden, severe hypertension.
Fluoxetine, trazodone, tricyclic antidepressants: May cause serotonin syndrome.
Insulin, oral antidiabetics: May increase the effects of these drugs.
Meperidine, other opioid analgesics: May produce diaphoresis, immediate excitation, rigidity, and severe hypertension or hypotension, sometimes leading to severe respiratory distress, vascular collapse, seizures, coma, and death.
Methylphenidate: May increase the CNS stimulant effects of methylphenidate.
Sympathomimetics: May increase the cardiac stimulant and vasopressor effects of phenelzine.
Herbal
None known.
Food
Caffeine, chocolate, tyramine-containing foods (such as aged cheese): May cause sudden, severe hypertension.

DIAGNOSTIC TEST EFFECTS
None known.

SIDE EFFECTS
Frequent
Orthostatic hypotension, restlessness, GI upset, insomnia, dizziness, headache, lethargy, asthenia, dry mouth, peripheral edema

Occasional
Flushing, diaphoresis, rash, urinary frequency, increased appetite, transient impotence
Rare
Visual disturbances

SERIOUS REACTIONS
• Hypertensive crisis occurs rarely and is marked by severe hypertension, occipital headache radiating frontally, neck stiffness or soreness, nausea, vomiting, diaphoresis, fever or chilliness, clammy skin, dilated pupils, palpitations, tachycardia or bradycardia, and constricting chest pain.

PRECAUTIONS & CONSIDERATIONS
Caution is warranted with cardiac arrhythmias, frequent or severe headaches, hypertension, suicidal tendencies, and within several hours of ingestion of a contraindicated substance, such as tyramine-containing foods. Foods that require bacteria or molds for their preparation or preservation (such as yogurt and aged cheese), foods containing tyramine (including avocados, bananas, broad beans, figs, papayas, raisins, sour cream, soy sauce, beer, wine, yeast extracts, meat tenderizers, and smoked or pickled meats), and excessive amounts of caffeine-containing foods or beverages (such as chocolate, coffee, and tea) should be avoided during therapy.

Alcohol and tasks that require mental alertness or motor skills should be avoided. Notify the physician if headache or neck soreness or stiffness occurs. If hypertensive crisis occurs, phentolamine 5-10 mg IV should be administered. Liver function tests should be performed before and periodically during therapy, especially with long-term use.

Storage
Store phenelzine tablets at room temperature. Don't freeze.
Administration
Take the drug with food or milk to alleviate GI symptoms. Crush them and give with food or fluids. Depression may start to lift during the first week of therapy but phenelzine's full therapeutic effect may require 2 to 6 weeks of therapy.

Phenobarbital
fee-noe-bar'bi-tal
(Luminal, Phenobarbitone [AUS])
Do not confuse Phenobarbital with pentobarbital, or Luminal with Tuinal.

CATEGORY AND SCHEDULE
Pregnancy Risk Category: D
Controlled Substance: Schedule IV

CLASSIFICATION
Anticonvulsants, barbiturates, preanesthetics, sedatives/hypnotics

MECHANISM OF ACTION
A barbiturate that enhances the activity of gamma-aminobutyric acid (GABA) by binding to the GABA receptor complex. *Therapeutic Effect:* Depresses CNS activity.

PHARMACOKINETICS

Route	Onset	Peak	Duration
PO	20-60 min	N/A	6-10 hr
IV	5 min	30 min	4-10 hr

Well absorbed after PO or parenteral administration. Protein binding: 35%-50%. Rapidly and widely distributed.

Metabolized in the liver. Primarily excreted in urine. Removed by hemodialysis. **Half-life:** 53-118 hr.

AVAILABILITY
Elixir: 20 mg/5 ml.
Tablets: 30 mg, 100 mg.
Injection: 60 mg/ml, 130 mg/ml.

INDICATIONS AND DOSAGES
▸ **Status epilepticus**
IV
Adults, Elderly, Children, Neonates.
Loading dose of 15-20 mg/kg as a single dose or in divided doses.
▸ **Seizure control**
PO, IV
Adults, Elderly, Children 12 yr and older. 1-3 mg/kg/day.
Children 6-12 yr. 4-6 mg/kg/day.
Children 1-5 yr. 6-8 mg/kg/day.
Children younger than 1 yr.
5-6 mg/kg/day.
Neonates. 3-4 mg/kg/day.
▸ **Sedation**
PO, IM
Adults, Elderly. 30-120 mg/day in 2-3 divided doses.
Children. 2 mg/kg 3 times a day.
▸ **Hypnotic**
PO, IV, IM, Subcutaneous
Adults, Elderly. 100-320 mg at bedtime.
Children. 3-5 mg/kg at bedtime.

OFF-LABEL USES
Prevention and treatment of hyper-bilirubinemia

CONTRAINDICATIONS
Porphyria, pre-existing CNS depression, severe pain, severe respiratory disease

INTERACTIONS
Drug
Alcohol, other CNS depressants: May increase the effects of pheno-barbital.

Carbamazepine: May increase the metabolism of carbamazepine.
Digoxin, glucocorticoids, metronida-zole, oral anticoagulants, quinidine, tricyclic antidepressants: May decrease the effects of these drugs.
Valproic acid: Increases the blood concentration and risk of toxicity of phenobarbital.
Herbal
None known.
Food
None known.

DIAGNOSTIC TEST EFFECTS
May decrease serum bilirubin level. Therapeutic serum level is 10-40 mcg/ml; toxic serum level is greater than 40 mcg/ml.

▨ IV INCOMPATIBILITIES
Amphotericin B complex (Abelcet, AmBisome, Amphotec), hydrocorti-sone (Solu-Cortef), hydromorphone (Dilaudid), insulin
▨ **IV Compatibilities**
Calcium gluconate, enalapril (Vasotec), fentanyl (Sublimaze), fosphenytoin (Cerebyx), morphine, propofol (Diprivan)

SIDE EFFECTS
Occasional (3%-1%)
Somnolence
Rare (less than 1%)
Confusion; paradoxical CNS reactions, such as hyperactivity or nervousness in children and excite-ment or restlessness in the elderly (generally noted during first 2 weeks of therapy, particularly in presence of uncontrolled pain)

SERIOUS REACTIONS
• Abrupt withdrawal after prolonged therapy may produce increased dreaming, nightmares, insomnia, tremor, diaphoresis, and vomiting,

hallucinations, delirium, seizures, and status epilepticus.
- Skin eruptions may be a sign of a hypersensitivity reaction.
- Blood dyscrasias, hepatic disease, and hypocalcemia occur rarely.
- Overdose produces cold or clammy skin, hypothermia, severe CNS depression, cyanosis, tachycardia, and Cheyne-Stokes respirations.
- Toxicity may result in severe renal impairment.

PRECAUTIONS & CONSIDERATIONS
Caution is warranted with hepatic and renal impairment. Phenobarbital readily crosses the placenta and is distributed in breast milk. Phenobarbital use lowers serum bilirubin concentrations in neonates, produces respiratory depression in neonates during labor, and may increase the risk of maternal bleeding and neonatal hemorrhage during delivery. Neonates born to women who use barbiturates during the last trimester of pregnancy may experience withdrawal symptoms. Phenobarbital use may cause paradoxical excitement in children. The elderly taking phenobarbital may exhibit confusion, excitement, and mental depression.

Drowsiness and dizziness may occur, so alcohol and tasks requiring mental alertness or motor skills should be avoided. Notify the physician if headache, nausea, and rash occur. B/P, heart rate, respiratory rate, CNS status, renal and hepatic function, and seizure activity should be monitored.

Storage
Store vials at room temperature.

Administration
Take oral phenobarbital without regard to food. Crush tablets as needed. The elixir may be mixed with fruit juice, milk, or water.

! Expect to administer the maintenance dose 12 hours after the loading dose. Therapeutic serum drug level is 10-40 mcg/ml; the toxic serum drug level is greater than 40 mcg/ml.

Phenobarbital may be given undiluted or may be diluted with NaCl, D_5W, or lactated Ringer's solution. Expect to adequately hydrate the patient before and immediately after infusion to decrease the risk of adverse renal effects. Don't exceed an injection rate of 30 mg/minute for children and 60 mg/minute for adults. Injecting too rapidly may produce marked respiratory depression and severe hypotension. Be aware that inadvertent intra-arterial injection may result in arterial spasm with severe pain and tissue necrosis and that extravasation in subcutaneous tissue may produce redness, tenderness, and tissue necrosis. If either occurs, inject 0.5% procaine solution into the affected area and apply moist heat, as ordered.

For IM use, don't inject more than 5 ml in any one injection site because doing so may cause tissue irritation. Inject the drug deep intramuscularly.

P

Phenoxybenzamine
fen-ox-ee-ben'za-meen
(Dibenzyline)

CATEGORY AND SCHEDULE
Pregnancy Risk Category: C

CLASSIFICATION
Antiadrenergics, alpha blocking

MECHANISM OF ACTION

An antihypertensive that produces long-lasting noncompetitive alpha-adrenergic blockade of postganglionic synapses in exocrine glands and smooth muscles. Relaxes urethra and increases opening of the bladder. *Therapeutic Effect:* Controls hypertension.

PHARMACOKINETICS

Well absorbed from the gastrointestinal (GI) tract. Distributed into fatty tissue. Metabolized in liver. Eliminated in urine and feces. Not removed by hemodialysis. **Half-life:** 24 hr.

AVAILABILITY

Tablets: 10 mg (Dibenzyline).

INDICATIONS AND DOSAGES
▸ **Pheochromocytoma**
PO
Adults. Initially, 10 mg twice daily. May increase dose every other day to 20-40 mg 2-3 times/day
Children. 1-2 mg/kg/day in divided doses.

OFF-LABEL USES

Bladder instability, complex regional pain syndrome (CRPS), contraception, prostatic obstruction, Raynaud's disease

CONTRAINDICATIONS

Any condition compromised by hypotension, hypersensitivity to phenoxybenzamine or any component of the formulation

INTERACTIONS
Drug
Beta-blockers (used concurrently): May increase risk of toxicity (hypotension, tachycardia).

Hypotensive-producing medications: May increase the effects of phenoxybenzamine.
Alpha-adrenergic agonists: May decrease the effects of phenoxybenzamine.
Herbal
Licorice, Ma huang, yohimbine: May decrease the effects of phenoxybenzamine.
Food
None known.

DIAGNOSTIC TEST EFFECTS

None known.

SIDE EFFECTS
Frequent
Headache, lethargy, confusion, fatigue
Occasional
Nausea, postural hypotension, syncope, dry mouth
Rare
Palpitations, diarrhea, constipation, inhibition of ejaculation, weakness, altered vision, dizziness

SERIOUS REACTIONS
• Overdosage produces severe hypotension, irritability, lethargy, tachycardia, dizziness, and shock.

PRECAUTIONS & CONSIDERATIONS

Caution is warranted with congestive heart failure, coronary artery disease, and renal function impairment. It is unknown if phenoxybenzamine crosses the placenta or is distributed into breast milk. Safety and efficacy have not been established in children. The elderly may be more sensitive to hypotensive effects and may be at risk of developing phenoxybenzamine-induced hypothermia.

Miosis, nasal congestion, dizziness, lightheadedness, and fast heartbeat may occur. Caution when driving and change positions slowly. Alcohol should be avoided.

Administration
Dosage increments should not be made more frequently than every 4 days. If GI irritation occurs, take with meals or milk.

Phentermine

(Adipex-P, Fastin, Ionamin, Oby-Cap, Phentercot, Pro-Fast HS, Pro-Fast SA, Pro-Fast SR, T-Diet, Teramine, Zantryl)

CATEGORY AND SCHEDULE
Pregnancy Risk Category: B
Controlled Substance:
Schedule IV

CLASSIFICATION
Anorexiants, stimulants, central nervous system

MECHANISM OF ACTION
A sympathomimetic amine structurally similar to dextroamphetamine and is most likely mediated via norephinephrine and dopamine metabolism. Causes stimulation of the hypothalamus. *Therapeutic Effect:* Decreased appetite.

PHARMACOKINETICS
Well absorbed from the gastrointestinal (GI) tract; resin absorbed slower. Excreted unchanged in urine. **Half-life:** 20 hrs.

AVAILABILITY
Capsules (as hydrochloride): 15 mg, 18.75 mg, 30 mg (Fastin), 37.5 mg (Adipex-P).
Capsules (as resin complex): 15 mg (Ionamin), 30 mg (Ionamin).

Tablets (as hydrochloride): 8 mg, 37.5 mg (Adipex-P).

INDICATIONS AND DOSAGES
▶ **Obesity**
PO
Adults, Children older than 16 yr.
Adipex-P: 37.5 mg as a single daily dose or in divided doses.
Ionamin: 15-37.5 mg/day before breakfast or 1-2 hr. after breakfast.
Fastin: 30 mg/day taken in the morning

CONTRAINDICATIONS
Advanced arteriosclerosis, agitated states, cardiovascular disease, concurrent use or within 14 days of discontinuation of MAOI therapy, glaucoma, history of drug abuse, hypertension (moderate-to-severe), hyperthyroidism, hypersensitivity to phentermine or sympathomimetic amines

INTERACTIONS
Drug
Fenfluramine: May increase risk of pulmonary hypertension and valvular heart disease.
MAOIs: May increase risk of hypertensive crisis (headache, hyperpyrexia, hypertension).
Sibutramine: May increase risk of hypertension and tachycardia.
Herbal
None known.
Food
None known.

DIAGNOSTIC TEST EFFECTS
May interfere and give false positive amphetamine EMIT assay result.

SIDE EFFECTS
Occasional
Restlessness, insomnia, tremor, palpitations, tachycardia, elevation in blood pressure, headache, dizziness,

dry mouth, unpleasant taste, diarrhea or constipation, changes in libido

SERIOUS REACTIONS
• Primary pulmonary hypertension (PPH), psychotic episodes, and valvular heart disease rarely occur.
• Anorectic agents have been associated with regurgitant multivalvular heart disease involving mitral, aortic, and/or tricuspid valves.
• Prolonged use may cause physical or psychological dependence.

PRECAUTIONS & CONSIDERATIONS
Caution is warranted with cardiovascular disease, psychosis, diabetes, insomnia, porphyria, mild hypertension, Tourette's syndrome, seizure disorders, and history of substance abuse. It is unknown if phentermine is excreted in breast milk. Be aware that the safety and efficacy of this drug have not been established in children younger than 16 years of age. Age-related liver or renal impairment may require decreased dosage in the elderly. Phentermine may be habit-forming, and it should not be abruptly discontinued.

Fast, pounding, or irregular heartbeat, chest pain, severe headache, trouble breathing, skin rash, blurred vision, confusion, or unexplained sore throat should be reported immediately.

Administration
Do not take phentermine in afternoon or evening because it can cause insomnia. May take before breakfast or 1-2 hours after breakfast.

Phentolamine
fen-tole'a-meen
(Regitine)

CATEGORY AND SCHEDULE
Pregnancy Risk Category: C

CLASSIFICATION
Antiadrenergics, alpha blocking

MECHANISM OF ACTION
An alpha-adrenergic blocking agent which produces peripheral vasodilation and cardiac stimulation.
Therapeutic Effect: Decreases blood pressure (B/P).

PHARMACOKINETICS
Poorly absorbed from the gastrointestinal (GI) tract. Protein binding: 72%. Metabolized in liver. Eliminated in urine and feces. Not removed by hemodialysis.
Half-life: 19 min.

AVAILABILITY
Injection: 5 mg/ml (Regitine).

INDICATIONS AND DOSAGES
▸ **Extravasation—norepinephrine**
SC
Adults, Elderly. Infiltrate area with a small amount (1 ml) of solution (made by diluting 5-10 mg in 10 ml of NS) within 12 hours of extravasation. Do not exceed 0.1-0.2 mg/kg or 5 mg total. If dose is effective, normal skin color should return to the blanched area within 1 hour.
Children. Infiltrate area with a small amount (1 ml) of solution (made by diluting 5-10 mg in 10 ml of NS) within 12 hours of extravasation.

Do not exceed 0.1-0.2 mg/kg or 5 mg total.

▶ **Diagnosis of pheochromocytoma**
IM/IV
Adults, Elderly. 5 mg as a single dose. *Children.* 0.05-0.1 mg/kg/dose. Maximum single dose: 5 mg.

▶ **Surgery for pheochromocytoma: Hypertension**
IM/IV
Adults, Elderly. 5 mg given 1-2 hours before procedure and repeated as needed every 2-4 hours.
Children. 0.05-0.1 mg/kg/dose given 1-2 hours before procedure. Repeat as needed every 2-4 hours until hypertension is controlled. Maximum single dose: 5 mg.

▶ **Hypertensive crisis**
IV
Adults, Elderly. 5-20 mg as a single dose.

OFF-LABEL USES

Treatment of pralidoxime-induced hypertension, arrhythmias, asthma, bladder instability, cardiac diseases, diabetes mellitus, erectile dysfunction, extravasation-dopamine, epinephrine, hyperhidrosis, myocardial infarction, Raynaud's phenomenon, surgery, sympathetic maintained pain

CONTRAINDICATIONS

Renal impairment, coronary or cerebral arteriosclerosis, concurrent use with phosphodiesterase-5 (PDE-5) inhibitors including sildenafil (>25 mg), tadalafil, or vardenafil, hypersensitivity to phentolamine or related compounds.

INTERACTIONS
Drug
Alcohol: May increase the risk of disulfiram-type reactions.
Beta-blockers: May exaggerate hypotensive effects.

Epinephrine, ephedrine: May decrease the effects of phentolamine
Sildenafil, tadalafil, vardenafil: May increase blood pressure-lowering effects.
Herbal
None known.
Food
None known.

DIAGNOSTIC TEST EFFECTS

May increase liver function tests.

▒ IV INCOMPATIBILITIES
Iron
▒ **IV Compatibilities**
Amiodarone (Cordarone), dobutamine (Dobutrex), norepinephrine (Levophed), papaverine (Papacon), verapamil

SIDE EFFECTS
Occasional
Hypotension, tachycardia, arrhythmia, flushing, orthostatic hypotension, weakness, dizziness, nausea, vomiting, diarrhea, nasal congestion, pulmonary hypertension

SERIOUS REACTIONS

• Symptoms of overdosage include tachycardia, shock, vomiting, and dizziness.
• Mixed agents, such as epinephrine, may cause more hypotension.

PRECAUTIONS & CONSIDERATIONS

Caution is warranted with arrhythmias, cerebral vascular spasm or occlusion, hypotension, and tachycardia. Be aware that it is unknown if phentolamine crosses the placenta or is distributed into breast milk. There are no age-related precautions in children or the elderly.

Nasal congestion, increased heartbeat, palpitations, dizziness, headache, and hypotension are

P

common side effects of phentolamine. Blood pressure should be monitored during its use.

Storage

Store at room temperature.

Administration

Phentolamine mesylate for injection is reconstituted for parenteral use by adding 1 ml of sterile water for injection to the vial, producing a solution containing 5 mg of phentolamine mesylate per ml. Discard any unused portion.

Persons undergoing diagnostic testing for pheochromocytoma should be maintained in the supine position during phentolamine administration.

Phenylephrine (Systemic)

(Af-Taf [ISRAEL]; AK-Dilate; Albalon Relief [NEW ZEALAND]; Despec-SF; Drosin [INDIA]; Efrin-10 [ISRAEL]; Efrisel [INDONESIA]; Isopto Frin [BELGIUM, CZECH REPUBLIC, ECUADOR, MALAYSIA]; Metaoxedrin [DEN, NOR, SWE]; Minims Phenylephrine HCL 10% [SOUTH AFRICA]; Minims Phenylephrine Hydrochloride [ENG]; Mydfrin; Nefrin-Ofteno [COSTA RICA, DOMINICAN REPUBLIC, EL SALVADOR, GUATEMALA, HONDURAS, NICARAGUA, PANAMA]; Neofrin; Neosynephrine [BELGIUM, SWE]; Neosynephrine 10% Chibret [FRA]; Neosynephrine Faure 10% [FRA]; Neo-Synephrine Ophthalmic Viscous 10% [AUS]; Neo-Synephrine Ophthalmic; Neosynephrin-POS [KOR]; Ocu-Phrin; Oftan-Metaoksedrin [FIN]; Optistin [ITL]; Phenoptic; Phenylephrine [NETHERLANDS]; Prefrin [AUSTRIA, ECUADOR, GREECE, HONG KONG, INDONESIA, NEW ZEALAND, SOUTH AFRICA, THAILAND]; Pupiletto Forte [INDIA]; Rectasol; Vistafrin [SPA]; Vistosan [GER])

Do not confuse with pseudoephedrine, epinephrine

CATEGORY AND SCHEDULE

Pregnancy Risk Category: C

MECHANISM OF ACTION

Phenylephrine is a powerful postsynaptic alpha-receptor stimulant with

little effect on the beta receptors of the heart, lacking chronotropic and inotropic actions on the heart.
Therapeutic Effect: Vasoconstriction, decreases heart rate, increases stroke output, increases blood pressure

PHARMACOKINETICS

Phenylephrine is irregularly absorbed from and readily metabolized in the GI tract. After IV administration, a pressor effect occurs almost immediately and persists for 15-20 minutes. After IM administration, a pressor effect occurs within 10-15 minutes and persists for 50 minutes to 1 hour. After oral inhalation of phenylephrine in combination with isoproterenol, pulmonary effects occur within a few minutes and persist for about 3 hours. The pharmacologic effects of phenylephrine are terminated at least partially by the uptake of the drug into the tissues. Phenylephrine is metabolized in the liver and intestine by the enzyme monoamine oxidase (MAO). The metabolites and their route and rate of excretion have not been identified.

AVAILABILITY

Solution (ophthalmic): 2.5%, 10%
Solution (nasal): 0.125%, 0.16%, 0.25%, 0.5%
Solution (injection): 10 mg/ml
Solution (oral): 5 mg/ml
Suppository (rectal): 0.25%

INDICATIONS AND DOSAGES
▸ **Paroxysmal supraventricular tachycardia (PSVT)**
Adults. The initial dose, given by rapid IV injection, should not exceed 0.5 mg. Subsequent doses may be increased in increments of 0.1 to 0.2 mg. Maximum single dose is 1 mg IV.
Children. 5 to 10 mcg/kg IV over 20-30 seconds.

▸ **Mild to Moderate Hypotension**
SC/IM
Adults. 2-5 mg IM or SC (range 1-10 mg), repeated no more than every 10-15 minutes. Maximum initial IM or SC dose is 5 mg.
Children. 0.1 mg/kg IM or SC every 1-2 hours as needed. Maximum dose is 5 mg.
IV
Adults. 0.2 mg IV (range 0.1 to 0.5 mg), given no more frequently than every 10-15 minutes. Maximum initial IV dose is 0.5 mg.
▸ **Severe Hypotension or Shock**
IV
Adults. Initially, 100-180 mcg/min IV infusion, with dose titration to the desired MAP and SVR. A maintenance infusion rate of 40-60 mcg/min IV is usually adequate after blood pressure stabilizes. If necessary to produce the desired pressor response, additional phenylephrine in increments of 10 mg or more may be added to the infusion solution and the rate of flow adjusted according to the response of the patient.
Children. 5-20 mcg/kg IV bolus, followed by an initial IV infusion of 0.1 to 0.5 mcg/kg/min, titrated to desired effect. Doses up to 3-5 mcg/kg/min IV may be required.
▸ **Hypotensive emergencies during spinal anesthesia**
IV
Adults. Initially, 0.2 mg IV.
Subsequent doses should not exceed the previous dose by more than 0.1 to 0.2 mg. Maximum of 0.5 mg per dose.
▸ **Hypotension during spinal anesthesia in children**
IM/SC
Children. A dose of 0.044 to 0.088 mg/kg IM or SC is recommended by the manufacturer.

P

▸ **Hypotension prophylaxis during spinal anesthesia**
IM/SC
Adults. 2 to 3 mg SC or IM, 3 or 4 minutes before anesthesia. A dose of 2 mg SC or IM is usually adequate with low spinal anesthesia, 3 mg IM or SC may be necessary with high spinal anesthesia.

▸ **Vasoconstriction in regional anesthesia**
IV
Adults. The manufacturer states that the optimum concentration of phenylephrine HCl is 0.05 mg/ml (1:20,000). Solutions may be prepared for regional anesthesia by adding 1 mg of phenylephrine HCl to each 20 ml of local anesthesia solution. Some pressor response can be expected when at least 2 mg is injected.

▸ **Prolongation of spinal anesthesia.**
IV
Adults. The addition of 2-5 mg added to the anesthetic solution increases the duration of motor block by as much as 50% without an increase in the incidence of complications such as nausea, vomiting, or blood pressure disturbances.

▸ **Hypotension during special anesthesia in children.**
IM/SC
Children. A dose of 0.5 mg to 1 mg per 25 pounds body weight, administered subcutaneously or IM, is recommended.

CONTRAINDICATIONS
Phenylephrine HCl injection should not be used with patients with severe hypertension, ventricular tachycardia or fibrillation, acute myocardial infarction (MI), atrial flutter or fibrillation, cardiac arrhythmias, cardiac disease, cardiomyopathy, closed-angle glaucoma, coronary artery disease, women who are in labor, during obstetric delivery, or in patients who have a known hypersensitivity to phenylephrine, sulfitres, or to any one of its components.

INTERACTIONS
Drug
MAO Inhibitors: The pressor effect of sympathomimetic pressor amines and adrenergic agents is markedly potentiated in patients receiving MAO inhibitors.
Halothane: Vasopressors may cause serious cardiac arrhythmias during halothane anesthesia and therefore should be used only with great caution or not at all.
Oxytocics: The pressure effect of sympathomimetic pressor amines is potentiated.
Herbal
None known.
Food
None known.

DIAGNOSTIC TEST EFFECTS
None known.

SIDE EFFECTS
Occasional
Headache, reflex bradycardia, excitability, restlessness, and rarely arrhythmias.

SERIOUS REACTIONS
• Overdose may induce ventricular extrasystoles and short paroxysms of ventricular tachycardia, a sensation of fullness in the head and tingling of the extremities. Should an excessive elevation of blood pressure occur, it may be immediately relieved by an α-adrenergic blocking agent, e.g., phentolamine. The oral LD_{50} in the rat is 350 mg/kg, in the mouse 120 mg/kg.

PRECAUTIONS & CONSIDERATIONS

Caution is warranted with metabolic acidosis, hypercapnia, hypoxia, atrial fibrillation, narrow angle glaucoma, pulmonary hypertension, hypovolemia, mechanical obstruction such as severe valvular aortic stenosis, myocardial infarction, arterial embolism, atherosclerosis, Buerger's disease, cold injury such as frostbite, diabetic endarteritis, Raynaud's syndrome, and sensitivity to other sympathomimetics. It is unknown if phenylephrine (systemic) crosses the placenta or is distributed into breast milk. Phenylephrine (systemic) should be used cautiously in children and the elderly.

Storage

Store at room temperature.

Administration

To prepare a solution of phenylephrine for direct intravenous injection, 10 mg (1 ml) of phenylephrine hydrochloride injection should be diluted with 9 ml of sterile water for injection to provide a solution containing 1 mg of phenylephrine per ml.

Phenylephrine (Topical)

(Af-Taf [ISRAEL]; AK-Dilate; Albalon Relief [NEW ZEALAND]; Despec-SF; Drosin [INDIA]; Efrin-10 [ISRAEL]; Efrisel [INDONESIA]; Isopto Frin [BELGIUM, CZECH REPUBLIC, ECUADOR, MALAYSIA]; Metaoxedrin [AEN, NOR, SWE]; Minims Phenylephrine HCL 10% [SOUTH AFRICA]; Minims Phenylephrine Hydrochloride [ENG]; Mydfrin; Nefrin-Ofteno [COSTA RICA, DOMINICAN REPUBLIC, EL SALVADOR, GUATEMALA, HONDURAS, NICARAGUA, PANAMA]; Neofrin; Neosynephrine [BELGIUM, SWE]; Neosynephrine 10% Chibret [FRA]; Neosynephrine Faure 10% [FRA]; Neo-Synephrine Ophthalmic Viscous 10% [AUS]; Neo-Synephrine Ophthalmic; Neosynephrin-POS [KOR]; Ocu-Phrin; Oftan-Metaoksedrin [FIN]; Optistin [ITL]; Phenoptic; Phenylephrine [NETHERLANDS]; Prefrin [AUSTRIA, ECUADOR, GREECE, HONG KONG, INDONESIA, NEW ZEALAND, SOUTH AFRICA, THAILAND]; Pupiletto Forte [INDIA]; Rectasol; Vistafrin [SPA]; Vistosan [GER])

Do not confuse with pseudoephedrine, epinephrine

CATEGORY AND SCHEDULE

Pregnancy Risk Category: C

CLASSIFICATION

Substituted phenylethylamine, decongestant, mydriatic

P

MECHANISM OF ACTION

Phenylephrine HCl is an alpha receptor sympathetic agonist used in local ocular disorders because of its vasoconstrictor and mydriatic action. It exhibits rapid and moderately prolonged action, and it produces little rebound vasodilatation. Systemic side effects are uncommon. *Therapeutic effect:* Vasoconstriction and pupil dilation.

PHARMACOKINETICS

Some absorption occurs systemically. The duration of action of intranasal administration ranges from 30 minutes to 4 hours. The duration of the mydriatic effect is roughly 3 hours after administration of the 2.5% solution but may be as long as 7 hours after the 10% solution.

AVAILABILITY

Solution (ophthalmic): 2.5%, 10%
Solution (nasal): 0.125%, 0.16%, 0.25%, 0.5%
Solution (injection): 10 mg/ml
Solution (oral): 5 mg/ml
Suppository (rectal): 0.25%

INDICATIONS AND DOSAGES
▸ **Mydriasis induction (ophthalmic)**
TOPICAL
Adults, Adolescents, Elderly. Instill 1 or 2 drops of a 2.5% or 10% solution in eye before procedure. May be repeated in 10-60 minutes if needed. In general, the 2.5% solution is preferred in the elderly to avoid cardiac reactions.
Children. Instill 1 or 2 drops of a 2.5% solution in the eye before procedure. May be repeated in 10-60 minutes if needed.
Infants <1 yr. 1 drop of 2.5% solution 15-30 minutes before procedure.

▸ **Uveitis (Posterior Synechia)**
TOPICAL
Adults, Elderly. Instill 1 drop of 10% solution in eye 3 or more times daily with atropine sulfate. In general, the 2.5% solution is preferred in elderly to avoid adverse cardiac reactions.
Adults and children over age 12 (intranasal). Apply 2-3 drops or 1-2 sprays of a 0.25% to 0.5% solution instilled in each nostril or a small quantity of 0.5% nasal jelly applied into each nostril. Apply every 4 hours as needed. The 1% solution may be used in adults with severe congestion.
Children 6-12 yr (intranasal). 2-3 drops of the 0.25% solution in each nostril every 4 hours as needed.
Children <6 yr (intranasal). Apply 2-3 drops or sprays of a 0.125% or 0.16% solution in each nostril every 4 hours as needed.
Infants >6 mo (intranasal). 1 to 2 drops of the 0.16% solution in each nostril every 3 hours.

▸ **Conjunctival Congestion**
TOPICAL
Adults, Elderly. 1 to 2 drops of a 0.12% to 0.25% solution applied to the conjunctiva every 3 to 4 hours as needed. In general, the 2.5% solution is preferred in elderly to avoid cardiac reactions.

▸ **Postoperative Malignant Glaucoma**
TOPICAL
Adults, Elderly. Instill 1 drop of a 10% solution with 1 drop of a 1% to 4% solution 3 or more times per day. In general, the 2.5% solution is preferred in elderly to avoid cardiac reactions.

▸ **Vasoconstriction and Pupil Dilatation**
TOPICAL
Adults. A drop of a suitable topical anesthetic may be applied, followed

in a few minutes by 1 drop on the upper limbus.

▸ **Surgery**

TOPICAL

Adults. When a short-acting mydriatic is needed for wide dilatation of the pupil before intraocular surgery, phenylephrine HCl 2.5% (or the 10%) may be applied topically from 30 to 60 minutes before the operation.

▸ **Cycloplegia**

TOPICAL

Adults. One drop of the preferred cycloplegic is placed in each eye, followed in 5 minutes by one drop of phenylephrine HCl 2.5%.

Children. For a "one application method," phenylephrine HCl 2.5% may be combined with one of the preferred rapid acting cycloplegics to produce adequate cycloplegia.

▸ **Ophthalmoscopic Examination**

TOPICAL

Adults. One drop of phenylephrine HCl 2.5% is placed in each eye.

▸ **Blanching Test**

TOPICAL

Adults. One or two drops of phenylephrine HCl 2.5% should be applied to the injected eye.

▸ **Glaucoma**

TOPICAL

Adults. In certain patients with glaucoma, temporary reduction of intraocular tension may be attained by producing vasoconstriction of the intraocular vessels; this may be accompanied by placing 1 drop of the 10% solution on the upper surface of the cornea. This treatment may be repeated as often as necessary.

▸ **Nasal Congestion**

INTRANASAL

Adults, Children 12 and older. Use 2 or 3 drops or sprays of a 0.25% to 0.5% solution in the nose every 4 hours as needed

Children 6 to 12 yr. Use 2 or 3 drops or sprays of a 0.25% solution in the nose every 4 hours as needed. *Children 2 to 6 yr.* Use 2 or 3 drops of a 0.125% to 0.16% solution in the nose every 4 hours as needed.

CONTRAINDICATIONS

Ophthalmic solutions, (both strengths), of phenylephrine HCl are contraindicated in patients with anatomically narrow angles or narrow angle glaucoma, some low birth weight infants and some elderly adults with severe arteriosclerotic cardiovascular or cerebrovascular disease, use during intraocular operative procedures when the corneal epithelial barrier has been disturbed, and in persons with a known sensitivity to phenylephrine, sulfites, or any of its components including preservatives. The 10% solution is contraindicated in infants and in patients with aneurysms.

INTERACTIONS

Drug

Adrenergic drugs, MAO inhibitors: May increase adrenergic effects.

Tricyclic Antidepressants: May increase the pressor response of adrenergic agents.

Beta-blockers: This drug may potentiate the cardiovascular depressant effects of potent inhalation anesthetic agents.

Herbal

None known.

Food

None known.

DIAGNOSTIC TEST EFFECTS

None known.

SIDE EFFECTS

Frequent

Burning or stinging of eyes, headache or browache, sensitivity to light,

watering of the eyes, increase in runny or stuffy nose, burning, stinging, dryness of inside the nose
Occasional
Rare
Irritation, dizziness, fast and/or irregular and/or pounding heartbeat, increased sweating, increase in blood pressure, paleness, trembling, headache, nervousness, trouble sleeping

SERIOUS REACTIONS
• There have been reports associating the use of phenylephrine HCl 10% ophthalmic solutions with the development of serious cardiovascular reactions, including ventricular arrhythmias and myocardial infarctions. These episodes, some ending fatally, have usually occurred in elderly patients with preexisting cardiovascular diseases.

PRECAUTIONS & CONSIDERATIONS
Caution is necessary with advanced arteriosclerotic changes, cardiac disease, diabetes mellitus, angle-closure glaucoma, hypertension, idiopathic orthostatic hypotension, and sensitivity to sulfites. It is unknown if phenylephrine (topical) crosses the placenta or is distributed into breast milk. Children may be more sensitive to the effects of phenylephrine. The 10% strength is not recommended in infants. Repeated use may increase the chance of adverse effects such as miosis and reduced mydriatic effects in the elderly.
    Burning or stinging of the eyes, headache, browache, sensitivity of eyes to light, and watering of eyes may occur.
Storage
Store at room temperature. Prolonged exposure to strong light may cause oxidation and discoloration. Do not

use if solution is brown or precipitate is present.
Administration
Apply digital pressure to the lacrimal sac during and for 2 or 3 minutes following instillation. The recommended dose should not be exceeded.

Phenylephrine Hydrochloride
fen-ill-ef´rin
(AK-Dilate, AD-Nephrin, Isopto Frin [AUS], Mydfrin, Neo-Synephrine, Prefrin)

CATEGORY AND SCHEDULE
Pregnancy Risk Category: C
OTC (nasal solution, nasal spray, ophthalmic solution)

CLASSIFICATION
Adrenergic agonists, decongestants, ophthalmics

MECHANISM OF ACTION
A sympathomimetic, alpha receptor stimulant that acts on the alpha-adrenergic receptors of vascular smooth muscle. Causes vasoconstriction of arterioles of nasal mucosa or conjunctiva, activates dilator muscle of the pupil to cause contraction, produces systemic arterial vasoconstriction. *Therapeutic Effect:* Decreases mucosal blood flow and relieves congestion and increases systolic B/P.

PHARMACOKINETICS

Route	Onset	Peak	Duration
IV	Immediate	N/A	15-20 min
IM	10-15 min	N/A	0.5-2 hr
subcuta-neous	10-15 min	N/A	1 hr

Minimal absorption after intranasal and ophthalmic administration. Metabolized in the liver and GI tract. Primarily excreted in urine. **Half-life:** 2.5 hr.

AVAILABILITY
Injection: 1% (10 mg/ml).
Nasal Solution Drops (Neosynephrine): 0.5%, 1%.
Nasal Spray (Neosynephrine): 0.25%, 0.5%, 1%.
Ophthalmic Solution (Ak-Nephrin): 0.12%.
Ophthalmic Solution (AK-Dilate): 2.5%, 10%.
Ophthalmic Solution (Mydfrin, Neosynephrine): 2.5%.

INDICATIONS AND DOSAGES
▶ **Nasal decongestant**
Nasal Spray, Nasal Solution
Adults, Elderly, Children 12 yr and older. 2-3 drops or 1-2 sprays of 0.25%-0.5% solution into each nostril.
Children 6-11 yr. 2-3 drops or 1-2 sprays of 0.25% solution into each nostril.
Children younger than 6 yr. 2-3 drops of 0.125% solution (dilute 0.5% solution with 0.9% NaCl to achieve 0.125%) in each nostril. Repeat q4hr as needed. Do not use for more than 3 days.
▶ **Conjunctival congestion, itching, and minor irritation; whitening of sclera**
OPHTHALMIC
Adults, Elderly, Children 12 yr and older. 1-2 drops of 0.12% solution q3-4hr.
▶ **Hypotension, shock**
IM, SUBCUTANEOUS
Adults, Elderly. 2-5 mg/dose q1-2hr.
Children. 0.1 mg/kg/dose q1-2hr.
IV bolus
Adults, Elderly. 0.1-0.5 mg/dose q10-15min as needed.

Children. 5-20 mcg/kg/dose q10-15min.
IV INFUSION
Adults, Elderly. 100-180 mcg/min.
Children. 0.1-0.5 mcg/kg/min. Titrate to desired effect.

CONTRAINDICATIONS
Acute pancreatitis, heart disease, hepatitis, narrow-angle glaucoma, pheochromocytoma, severe hypertension, thrombosis, ventricular tachycardia

INTERACTIONS
Drug
Beta blockers: May have mutually inhibitory effects.
Digoxin: May increase risk of arrhythmias.
Ergonovine, oxytocin: May increase vasoconstriction.
MAOIs: May increase vasopressor effects.
Maprotiline, tricyclic antidepressants: May increase cardiovascular effects.
Methyldopa: May decrease effects of methyldopa.
Herbal
None known.
Food
None known.

DIAGNOSTIC TEST EFFECTS
None known.

▨ IV INCOMPATIBILITIES
Thiopentothal (Pentothal)
▨ IV Compatibilities
Amiodarone (Cordarone), dobutamine (Dobutrex), lidocaine, potassium chloride, propofol (Diprivan)

SIDE EFFECTS
Frequent
Nasal: Rebound nasal congestion due to overuse, especially when used longer than 3 days

P

Occasional
Mild CNS stimulation (restlessness, nervousness, tremors, headache, insomnia, particularly in those hypersensitive to sympathomimetics, such as elderly patients)
Nasal: Stinging, burning, drying of nasal mucosa
Ophthalmic: Transient burning or stinging, brow ache, blurred vision

SERIOUS REACTIONS

• Large doses may produce tachycardia and palpitations (particularly in those with cardiac disease), lightheadedness, nausea, and vomiting.
• Overdose in those older than 60 years may result in hallucinations, CNS depression, and seizures.
• Prolonged nasal use may produce chronic swelling of nasal mucosa and rhinitis.

PRECAUTIONS & CONSIDERATIONS

Caution is warranted with bradycardia, heart block, hyperthyroidism, and severe arteriosclerosis. If phenylephrine 10% ophthalmic is instilled into denuded or damaged corneal epithelium, corneal clouding may result. Phenylephrine crosses the placenta and is distributed in breast milk. Children may exhibit increased absorption and toxicity with nasal preparation. No age-related precautions have been noted with systemic use in children. The elderly are more likely to experience adverse effects. The drug should be immediately discontinued if dizziness, feeling of irregular heartbeat, insomnia, tremor, or weakness occurs. B/P and heart rate should be monitored before and during therapy.

Storage
Store vials at room temperature.

Administration
For nasal administration, blow nose before giving the medication. Tilt head back and instill the drops in one nostril, as prescribed. Remain in the same position; wait 5 minutes before applying drops in other nostril. Administer nasal spray into each nostril with the head erect. Sniff briskly while squeezing container; then wait 3 to 5 minutes before blowing nose gently. Rinse tip of spray bottle. Do not use for longer than 5 days because of the risk of rebound nasal congestion.

For ophthalmic use, tilt head backward and look up. With a gloved finger, gently pull the lower eyelid down to form a pouch; instill medication into the pouch. Do not touch tip of applicator to eyelids or any surface. When lower eyelid is released, keep eye open without blinking for at least 30 seconds. Apply gentle finger pressure to lacrimal sac, which is located at the bridge of the nose at inside corner of the eye, for 1 to 2 minutes. Remove excess solution around eye with tissue. Wash hands immediately to remove medication on hands. Notify the physician if swelling of eyelids or itching occurs.

For IV push, dilute 1 ml of 10 mg/ml solution with 9 ml sterile water for injection to provide a concentration of 1 mg/ml. Give over 20 to 30 seconds. For IV infusion, dilute 10-mg vial with 500 ml D_5W or 0.9% NaCl to provide a concentration of 2 mcg/ml. Maximum concentration: 500 mg/250 ml. Titrate as prescribed.

Tablets (Chewable [Dilantin]): 50 mg.
Injection: 50 mg/ml.

INDICATIONS AND DOSAGES
▶ **Status epilepticus**
IV
Adults, Elderly, Children. 15-
18 mg/kg. Maintenance dose:
300 mg/day in 2-3 divided doses for
adults and elderly; 6-7 mg/kg/day for
children 10-16 yr; 7-8 mg/kg/day
for children 7-9 yr; 7.5-9 mg/kg/
day for children 4-6 yr; 8-10 mg/kg/
day for children 6 mo-3 yr.
Neonates. Loading dose:
15-20 mg/kg. Maintenance dose:
5-8 mg/kg/day.
▶ **Seizure control**
PO
Adults, Elderly, Children. Loading
dose: 15-20 mg/kg in 3 divided
doses 2-4 hr apart. Maintenance
dose: Same as for status epilepticus.
▶ **Arrhythmias**
IV
Adults, Elderly, Children. Loading
dose: 1.25 mg/kg q5min. May repeat
up to total dose of 15 mg/kg.
Children. Maintenance dose:
5-10 mg/kg/day in 2-3 divided doses.
PO
Adults, Elderly. Loading dose:
250 mg 4 times a day for 1 day, then
250 mg twice a day for 2 days.
Maintenance dose: 300-400 mg/day
1-4 times a day.
Children. Maintenance dose:
5-10 mg/kg/day in 2-3 divided doses.

OFF-LABEL USES
Adjunctive treatment of tricyclic
antidepressant toxicity; treatment of
muscle hyperirritability, digoxin-
induced arrhythmias, and trigeminal
neuralgia

CONTRAINDICATIONS
Hypersensitivity to hydantoins,
seizures due to hypoglycemia

Phenytoin
fen′-i-toyn
(Dilantin, Epamin,
Phenytek)(Dilantin)
**Do not confuse phenytoin with
mephenytoin, or Dilantin with
Dilaudid.**

CATEGORY AND SCHEDULE
Pregnancy Risk Category: D

CLASSIFICATION
Anticonvulsants, hydantoins

MECHANISM OF ACTION
A hydantoin anticonvulsant that
stabilizes neuronal membranes in the
motor cortex by decreasing sodium
and calcium ion influx into the
neurons. Also acts as an antiarrhythmic agent by decreasing abnormal
ventricular automaticity and shortening the refractory period, QT interval,
and action potential duration.
Therapeutic Effect: Limits the spread
of seizure activity. Restores normal
cardiac rhythm.

PHARMACOKINETICS
Slowly and variably absorbed after PO
administration; slowly but completely
absorbed after IM administration.
Protein binding: 90%-95%. Widely
distributed. Metabolized in the liver.
Primarily excreted in urine. Not
removed by hemodialysis. **Half-life:**
22 hr.

AVAILABILITY
Capsules (Prompt-Release): 100 mg.
*Capsules (Extended-Release
[Dilantin]):* 30 mg.
*Capsules (Extended-Release
[Phenytek]):* 200 mg, 300 mg.
Oral Suspension (Dilantin):
125 mg/5 ml.

IV: Adam-Stokes syndrome, second-
and third-degree AV block, sinoatrial
block, sinus bradycardia

INTERACTIONS
Drug
Alcohol, other CNS depressants:
May increase CNS depression.
**Amiodarone, anticoagulants,
cimetidine, disulfiram, fluoxetine,
isoniazid, sulfonamides:** May
increase phenytoin blood concentration, effects, and risk of toxicity.
Antacids: May decrease phenytoin
absorption.
**Fluconazole, ketoconazole,
miconazole:** May increase pheny-
toin blood concentration.
Glucocorticoids: May decrease the
effects of glucocorticoids.
Lidocaine, propranolol: May
increase cardiac depressant
effects.
Valproic acid: May decrease the
metabolism and increase the blood
concentration of phenytoin.
Xanthine: May increase the metabolism of these drugs.
Herbal
None known.
Food
None known.

DIAGNOSTIC TEST EFFECTS
May increase blood glucose level
and serum GGT and alkaline phosphatase levels. Therapeutic serum
level is 10-20 mcg/ml; toxic
serum level is greater than
20 mcg/ml.

▒ IV INCOMPATIBILITIES
Diltiazem (Cardizem), dobutamine
(Dobutrex), enalapril (Vasotec),
heparin, hydromorphone (Dilaudid),
insulin, lidocaine, morphine, nitroglycerin, norepinephrine (Levophed),
potassium chloride, propofol
(Diprivan)

SIDE EFFECTS
Frequent
Drowsiness, lethargy, confusion,
slurred speech, irritability, gingival
hyperplasia, hypersensitivity reaction
(including fever, rash, and
lymphadenopathy), constipation,
dizziness, nausea
Occasional
Headache, hirsutism, coarsening of
facial features, insomnia, muscle
twitching

SERIOUS REACTIONS
• Abrupt withdrawal may precipitate status epilepticus.
• Blood dyscrasias, lymphadenopathy, and osteomalacia (caused by
impaired vitamin D metabolism)
may occur.
• Toxic phenytoin blood concentration (25 mcg/ml or more) may
produce ataxia, nystagmus, or
diplopia. As the level increases,
extreme lethargy may lead to coma.

PRECAUTIONS & CONSIDERATIONS
Extreme caution should be used
with CHF, myocardial damage,
MI, and respiratory depression.
Caution is also warranted with
hyperglycemia, hypotension, hepatic
and renal impairment, and severe
myocardial insufficiency. Phenytoin
crosses the placenta and is distributed in small amounts in breast milk.
Fetal hydantoin syndrome, marked
by craniofacial abnormalities, digital
or nail hypoplasia, and prenatal
growth deficiency, have been
reported. Pregnant women may
experience more frequent seizures
because of altered drug absorption
and metabolism. Phenytoin use may
increase the risk of neonatal hemorrhage and maternal bleeding during
delivery. Children are more susceptible to coarsening of facial hair,
hirsutism, and gingival hyperplasia.

Lower dosages are recommended for the elderly, although no age-related precautions have been noted for this age-group.

Drowsiness, dizziness, and lethargy may occur, so alcohol and tasks that require mental alertness or motor skills should be avoided. Notify the physician if fever, swollen glands, sore throat, a skin reaction, or signs of hematologic toxicity (such as a bleeding tendency, bruising, fatigue, or fever) occurs. History of the seizure disorder, including the duration, frequency, and intensity of seizures should be assessed. CBC and blood chemistry tests should be performed to assess hepatic function before and periodically during phenytoin therapy. Repeat the CBC 2 weeks after beginning phenytoin therapy and 2 weeks after the phenytoin maintenance dose is established. CBC should be performed every month for 1 year after the maintenance dose is established and every 3 months thereafter. Therapeutic serum drug level is 10-20 mcg/ml; the toxic serum drug level is greater than 20 mcg/ml.

Storage

If refrigerated, the solution may form a precipitate that dissolves at room temperature.

Administration

Take oral phenytoin with food if GI distress occurs. Don't chew, open, or break capsules. Tablets may be chewed. Shake the oral suspension well before using.

! Give phenytoin by IV push. Remember that the maintenance dose is usually given 12 hours after the loading dose.

Don't use the solution if it's not clear. A slight yellow discoloration of the solution won't affect its potency. Phenytoin may be given undiluted or may be diluted with 0.9% NaCl.

Don't exceed an injection rate of 50 mg/minute for adults to avoid cardiovascular collapse and severe hypotension. For elderly patients, administer 50 mg over 2 to 3 minutes. For neonates, don't exceed 1-3 mg/kg/minute. To minimize pain from chemical irritation of the vein, flush the catheter with sterile saline solution after each bolus dose of phenytoin.

Phosphates
(Fleet Enema, Fleet Phospho Soda, K-Phos ME, K-Phos Neutral, Neutra-Phos, Uro-KP-Neutral)

CATEGORY AND SCHEDULE
Pregnancy Risk Category: C

CLASSIFICATION
Electrolyte, mineral

MECHANISM OF ACTION
Electrolytes that participate in bone deposition, calcium metabolism, and utilization of B complex vitamins and act as a buffer in maintaining acid-base balance. Also exert an osmotic effect in small intestine, producing distention and promoting peristalsis. *Therapeutic Effect:* Correct hypophosphatemia, acidify urine in UTIs, help prevent calcium deposits in urinary tract, and promote evacuation of the bowel.

PHARMACOKINETICS
Poorly absorbed after PO administration. PO form excreted in feces; IV form excreted in urine.

AVAILABILITY
Oral Solution (Fleet Phospha-Soda): 4 mmol phosphate per ml.

Powder (Neutra-Phos, Neutra-Phos K): 250 mg (8 mmol) phosphate.
Tablets (K-Phos ME): 125 mg (4 mmol) phosphate.
Tablets (K-Phos Neutral, Uro-KP-Neutral): 250 mg (8 mmol) phosphate.
Enema (Fleet Enema): 2.25 oz, 4.5 oz.
Injection (potassium phosphate): 3 mmol phosphate and 4.4 mEq potassium per ml.
Injection (sodium phosphate): 3 mmol phosphate and 4 mEq sodium per ml.

INDICATIONS AND DOSAGES
▸ **Hypophosphatemia**
PO (Neutra-Phos, Neutra-Phos K, K-Phos ME, K-Phos-Neutral, Uro-KP-Neutral)
Adults, Elderly. 50-150 mmol/day.
Children. 2-3 mmol/kg/day.
IV
Adults, Elderly. 50-70 mmol/day.
Children. 0.5-1.5 mmol/kg/day.
▸ **Laxative**
PO (Neutra-Phos, Neutra-Phos K, Uro-KP-Neutral)
Adults, Elderly, Children 4 yr and older. 1-2 capsules/packets 4 times a day.
Children younger than 4 yr. 1 capsule/packet 4 times a day.
RECTAL
Adults, Elderly, Children 12 yr and older. 4.5-oz enema as single dose. May repeat.
Children younger than 12 yr. 2.25-oz enema as single dose. May repeat.
▸ **Urine acidification**
PO
Adults, Elderly. 8 mmol 4 times a day.

OFF-LABEL USES
Prevention of calcium renal calculi

CONTRAINDICATIONS
Abdominal pain or fecal impaction (from rectal dosage form), CHF, hyperkalemia, hypernatremia, hyperphosphatemia, hypocalcemia, hypomagnesemia, phosphate renal calculi, severe renal impairment

INTERACTIONS
Drug
ACE inhibitors, NSAIDs, potassium-containing medications, potassium-sparing diuretics, salt substitutes containing potassium phosphate: May increase potassium blood concentration.
Antacids: May decrease the absorption of phosphates.
Calcium-containing medications: May increase the risk of calcium deposition in soft tissues and decrease phosphate absorption.
Digoxin: May increase the risk of heart block caused by hyperkalemia when given with potassium phosphates.
Glucocorticoids: May cause edema when given with sodium phosphate.
Phosphate-containing medications: May increase the risk of hyperphosphatemia.
Sodium-containing medications: May increase the risk of edema when given with sodium phosphate.
Herbal
None known.
Food
None known.

DIAGNOSTIC TEST EFFECTS
None known.

▨ IV INCOMPATIBILITIES
Dobutamine (Dobutrex)
▨ IV Compatibilities
Diltiazem (Cardizem), enalapril (Vasotec), famotidine (Pepcid), magnesium sulfate, metoclopramide (Reglan)

SIDE EFFECTS
Frequent
Mild laxative effect (in first few days of therapy)
Occasional
Diarrhea, nausea, abdominal pain, vomiting
Rare
Headache; dizziness; confusion; heaviness of lower extremities; fatigue; muscle cramps; paraesthesia; peripheral edema; arrhythmias, weight gain; thirst

SERIOUS REACTIONS
• Hyperphosphatemia may produce extra-skeletal calcification.

PRECAUTIONS & CONSIDERATIONS
Caution is warranted with adrenal insufficiency, cirrhosis, renal impairment, and concurrent use of potassium- sparing drugs. It is unknown if phosphates cross the placenta or are distributed in breast milk. No age-related precautions have been noted in children or the elderly.

Notify the physician of abdominal pain. Baseline phosphate levels and urinary pH should be obtained. Serum alkaline phosphatase, bilirubin, calcium, phosphorus, potassium, sodium, AST (SGOT), and ALT (SGPT) levels should be monitored throughout therapy. Pattern of daily bowel activity and stool consistency should also be assessed.
Storage
Store vials at room temperature.
Administration
For oral use, dissolve tablets in water. Give phosphates after meals or with food to decrease GI upset. Maintain high fluid intake to prevent renal calculi.

For IV use, dilute the drug before using. Infuse at a maximum rate of 0.06 mmol phosphate/kg/hour, as prescribed.

Phosphorated Carbohydrate Solution
(Emetrol)

CATEGORY AND SCHEDULE
Pregnancy Risk Category: NR
OTC

CLASSIFICATION
Hyperosmolar carbohydrate with phosphoric acid, antiemetic

MECHANISM OF ACTION
An antiemetic whose mechanism of action has not been determined. Phosphorated carbohydrate solution consists of fructose, dextrose, and phosphoric acid, and may directly act on the wall of the gastrointestinal (GI) tract and reduce smooth muscle contraction and delays gastric emptying time through high osmotic pressure exerted by the solution of simple sugars.
Therapeutic Effect: Relieves nausea and vomiting.

PHARMACOKINETICS
Fructose is slowly absorbed from the gastrointestinal (GI) tract. Metabolized in liver by phosphorylation and partly converted to liver glycogen and glucose. Excreted in urine.
Dextrose is rapidly absorbed from GI tract. Distributed and stored throughout tissues. Metabolized in liver to carbon dioxide and water.

AVAILABILITY
Solution: 1.87 g fructose/1.87 g dextrose/21.5 mg phosphoric acid/5 ml (Emetrol).

P

INDICATIONS AND DOSAGES
▸ **Antiemetic**
PO
Adults, Elderly. 15-30 ml initially.
May repeat dose every 15 minutes
until distress subsides. Maximum:
5 doses in a 1-hr period
Children 3 yr and older. 5-15 ml
initially. May repeat dose every
15 minutes until distress subsides.
Maximum: 5 doses in a 1-hour
period

CONTRAINDICATIONS
Symptoms of appendicitis or
inflamed bowel, hereditary
fructose intolerance, hypersensitivity to any component of the
formulation

INTERACTIONS
Drug
None known.
Herbal
None known.
Food
None known.

DIAGNOSTIC TEST EFFECTS
May increase blood glucose concentrations.

SIDE EFFECTS
Frequent
Diarrhea, abdominal pain

SERIOUS REACTIONS
• Fructose intolerance includes
symptoms of fainting, swelling of
face, arms and legs, unusual bleeding, vomiting, weight loss, and
yellow eyes and skin.

PRECAUTIONS & CONSIDERATIONS
Caution is warranted with diabetes
mellitus because condition may be
aggravated due to solution's high
carbohydrate content as well as with
children and elderly due to risk

of fluid and electrolyte loss due
to vomiting. It is unknown if
phosphorated carbohydrate
solution crosses the placenta or is
distributed in breast milk. Safety
and efficacy of phosphorated carbohydrate solution have not been
established in children younger
than 3 years of age. Be aware of
the risk of fluid and electrolyte
loss in the elderly.
Administration
Take 1 or 2 tablespoonfuls until
nausea stops. May repeat dose after
15 minutes if distress does not
subside. Do not dilute phosphorated
carbohydrate solution. Do not
exceed more than 5 doses in 1-hour
period.

Physostigmine
fi-zoe-stig′meen
(Antilirium)
**Do not confuse physostigmine
with Prostigmin or
pyridostigmine.**

CATEGORY AND SCHEDULE
Pregnancy Risk Category: C

CLASSIFICATION
Antidotes, cholinesterase
inhibitors

MECHANISM OF ACTION
A cholinergic that inhibits destruction of acetylcholine by enzyme
acetylcholinesterase, thus enhancing
impulse transmission across the
myoneural junction. *Therapeutic
Effect:* Improves skeletal muscle
tone, stimulates salivary and sweat
gland secretions.

AVAILABILITY
Injection: 1 mg/ml.

INDICATIONS AND DOSAGES
▸ **To reverse CNS effects of anti-cholinergic drugs and tricyclic antidepressants**
IV, IM
Adults, Elderly. Initially, 0.5-2 mg. If no response, repeat q20min until response or adverse cholinergic effects occur. If initial response occurs, may give additional doses of 1-4 mg q30-60min as life-threatening signs, such as arrhythmias, seizures, and deep coma, recur.
Children. 0.01-0.03 mg/kg. May give additional doses q5-10min until response or adverse cholinergic effects occur or total dose of 2 mg is given.

OFF-LABEL USES
Treatment of hereditary ataxia

CONTRAINDICATIONS
Active uveal inflammation, angle-closure glaucoma before iridectomy, asthma, cardiovascular disease, concurrent use of ganglionic-blocking agents, diabetes, gangrene, glaucoma associated with iridocyclitis, hypersensitivity to cholinesterase inhibitors or their components, mechanical obstruction of intestinal or urogenital tract, vagotonic state

INTERACTIONS
Drug
Cholinesterase agents, including bethanechol and carbachol: May increase the effects of these drugs.
Succinylcholine: May prolong the action of succinylcholine.
Herbal
None known.
Food
None known.

DIAGNOSTIC TEST EFFECTS
None known.

SIDE EFFECTS
Expected
Miosis, increased GI and skeletal muscle tone, bradycardia
Occasional
Marked drop in B/P (hypertensive patients)
Rare
Allergic reaction

SERIOUS REACTIONS
• Parenteral overdose produces a cholinergic crisis manifested as abdominal discomfort or cramps, nausea, vomiting, diarrhea, flushing, facial warmth, excessive salivation, diaphoresis, urinary urgency, and blurred vision. If overdose occurs, stop all anticholinergic drugs and immediately administer 0.6-1.2 mg atropine sulfate IM or IV for adults, or 0.01 mg/kg for infants and children younger than 12 years.

PRECAUTIONS & CONSIDERATIONS
Caution is warranted with bradycardia, bronchial asthma, epilepsy, GI disturbances, hypotension, parkinsonism, peptic ulcer disease, and disorders that may be adversely affected by drug's vagotonic effects and in those who have recently had an MI. Avoid driving at night and activities requiring visual acuity in dim light during physostigmine therapy.

Adverse effects usually subside after the first few days of therapy. Vital signs should be assessed immediately before and every 15 to 30 minutes after physostigmine administration. Cholinergic reactions, such as abdominal pain, dyspnea, hypotension, arrhythmias, muscle weakness, and diaphoresis, after drug administration should be assessed.

Administration
For adults, administer at a rate not
exceeding 1 mg/minute. For children, administer no more than
0.02 mg/kg over at least 1 minute.

**Pilocarpine
Hydrochloride**
pye-loe-kar′peen
(Salagen)

CATEGORY AND SCHEDULE
Pregnancy Risk Category: C

CLASSIFICATION
Cholinergics, miotics, ophthalmics

MECHANISM OF ACTION
A cholinergic that increases exocrine
gland secretions by stimulating
cholinergic receptors. *Therapeutic
Effect:* Improves symptoms of dry
mouth in patients with salivary gland
hypofunction.

PHARMACOKINETICS

Route	Onset	Peak	Duration
PO	20 min	1 hr	3-5 hr

Absorption decreased if taken
with a high-fat meal. Inactivation of
pilocarpine thought to occur at
neuronal synapses and probably in
plasma. Excreted in urine. **Half-life:**
4-12 hr.

AVAILABILITY
Tablets: 5 mg.

INDICATIONS AND DOSAGES
▸ **Dry mouth associated with radiation
treatment for head and neck cancer**
PO
Adults, Elderly. 5 mg three times
a day. Range: 15-30 mg/day.
Maximum: 2 tablets/dose.
▸ **Dry mouth associated with
Sjögren's syndrome**
PO
Adults, Elderly. 5 mg four times a
day. Range: 20-40 mg/day.
▸ **Dosage in hepatic impairment**
Dosage decreased to 5 mg twice a
day for adults and elderly with
hepatic impairment.

CONTRAINDICATIONS
Conditions in which miosis is
undesirable, such as acute iritis and
angle-closure glaucoma;
uncontrolled asthma

INTERACTIONS
Drug
Anticholinergics: May
antagonize the effects of anticholin-
ergics.
Beta blockers: May produce
conduction disturbances.
Herbal
None known.
Food
High-fat meals: May decrease
the absorption rate of
pilocarpine.

DIAGNOSTIC TEST EFFECTS
None known.

SIDE EFFECTS
Frequent (29%)
Diaphoresis
Occasional (11%-5%)
Headache, dizziness, urinary
frequency, flushing, dyspepsia,
nausea, asthenia, lacrimation, visual
disturbances
Rare (less than 4%)
Diarrhea, abdominal pain, peripheral
edema, chills

SERIOUS REACTIONS
• Patients with diaphoresis who don't drink enough fluids may develop dehydration.

PRECAUTIONS & CONSIDERATIONS
Caution is warranted with hepatic impairment, pulmonary disease, and significant cardiovascular disease. Pilocarpine use may impair reproductive function. The safety and efficacy of pilocarpine have not been established in children. The elderly have an increased incidence of diarrhea, dizziness, and urinary frequency. Adequate hydration should be maintained. Avoid tasks that require mental alertness or motor skills until response to the drug has been established.

Visual changes may occur, especially at night. Pattern of daily bowel activity and stool consistency and urinary frequency should be assessed.
Administration
Take pilocarpine without regard to food.

Pimecrolimus
pim-eh-crow-leh-mus
(Elidel)

CATEGORY AND SCHEDULE
Pregnancy Risk Category: C

CLASSIFICATION
Dermatologics, immunosuppressives

MECHANISM OF ACTION
An immunomodulator that inhibits release of cytokine, an enzyme that produces an inflammatory reaction. *Therapeutic Effect:* Produces anti-inflammatory activity.

PHARMACOKINETICS
Minimal systemic absorption with topical application. Metabolized in liver. Excreted in feces.

AVAILABILITY
Cream: 1% (Elidel).

INDICATIONS AND DOSAGES
▸ **Atopic dermatitis (eczema)**
TOPICAL
Adults, Elderly, Children 2-17 yr.
Apply to affected area twice daily for up to 3 weeks (up to 6 weeks in adolescents, children 2-17 yr). Rub in gently and completely.

OFF-LABEL USES
Allergic contact dermatitis, irritant contact dermatitis, psoriasis

CONTRAINDICATIONS
Hypersensitivity to pimecrolimus or any component of the formulation, Netherton's Syndrome (potential for increased systemic absorption), application to active cutaneous viral infections.

INTERACTIONS
Drug
None known.
Herbal
None known.
Food
None known.

DIAGNOSTIC TEST EFFECTS
None known.

IV INCOMPATIBILITIES
None known.
IV Compatibilities
None known.

SIDE EFFECTS
Rare
Transient application-site sensation of burning or feeling of heat

SERIOUS REACTIONS
• Lymphadenopathy and phototoxicity occur rarely.

PRECAUTIONS & CONSIDERATIONS
Caution should be used with those who are immunocompromised and those who are at an increased risk of varicella zoster virus infection, herpes simplex virus infection, or eczema herpeticum. Be aware that clinical infection at treatment sites should be cleared before commencing treatment. Consider discontinuing therapy if lymphadenopathy or in presence of acute infectious mononucleosis develops. It is unknown if pimecrolimus is distributed in breast milk. Safety and efficacy of pimecrolimus has not been established in children younger than 2 years of age. There are no age-related precautions noted in the elderly.

Pimecrolimus may cause a mild to moderate feeling of warmth and/or sensation of burning at the site of application. Artificial sunlight or tanning beds should be avoided.

Administration
Gently cleanse area prior to application. Use occlusive dressings only as ordered. Apply sparingly and rub into area thoroughly. Do not use topical pimecrolimus on broken skin or in areas of infection and do not apply to the face, inguinal areas, or wet skin.

Pimozide
pi′moe-zide
(Orap)

CATEGORY AND SCHEDULE
Pregnancy Risk Category: C

CLASSIFICATION
Antipsychotics

MECHANISM OF ACTION
A diphenylbutylpiperidine that blocks dopamine at postsynaptic receptor sites in the brain. *Therapeutic Effect:* Suppresses behavioral response in psychosis.

AVAILABILITY
Tablets: 1 mg, 2 mg (Orap).

INDICATIONS AND DOSAGES
▶ **Tourette's disorder**
PO
Adults, Elderly. 1-2 mg/day in divided doses 3 times/day. Maximum: 10 mg/day.
Children older than 12 yr. Initially, 0.5 mg/kg/day. Maximum: 10 mg/day.

CONTRAINDICATIONS
Aggressive schizophrenics when sedation is required, concurrent administration of pemoline, methylphenidate or amphetamines, concurrent administration with dofetilide, sotalol, quinidine, other Class IA and III anti-arrhythmics, mesoridazine, thioridazine, chlorpromazine, droperidol, sparfloxacin, gatifloxacin, moxifloxacin, halofantrine, mefloquine, pentamidine, arsenic trioxide, levomethadyl acetate, dolasetron mesylate, probucol, tacrolimus,

ziprasidone, sertraline, macrolide antibiotics, drugs that cause QT prolongation, and less potent inhibitors of CYP3A, congenital or drug-induced long QT syndrome, doses greater than 10 mg daily, history of cardiac arrhythmias, Parkinson's disease, patients with known hypokalemia or hypomagnesemia, severe central nervous system depression, simple tics or tics not associated with Tourette's syndrome, hypersensitivity to pimozide or any of its components

INTERACTIONS
Drug
Alcohol, CNS depressants: May increase CNS and respiratory depression.
Aprepitant: May increase pimozide plasma concentrations.
Drugs that prolong QT interval: May increase risk for QT prolongation and cardiotoxicity.
Belladonna alkaloids: May increase anticholinergic effects.
Lithium: May increase extrapyramidal symptoms.
Phenylalanine: May increase incidence of tardive dyskinesia.
Sertraline: May increase plasma pimozide levels.
Tramadol: May increase risk of seizures.
Vitex: May decrease effectiveness of dopamine antagonists.
Herbal
Betel nut: May increase extrapyramidal side effects of pimozide
Kava kava: May increase dopamine antagonist effects.
Food
Grapefruit juice: May inhibit metabolism of pimozide.

DIAGNOSTIC TEST EFFECTS
None known.

SIDE EFFECTS
Occasional
Akathisia, dystonic extrapyramidal effects, parkinsonian extrapyramidal effects, tardive dyskinesia, blurred vision, ocular changes, constipation, decreased sweating, dry mouth, nasal congestion, dizziness, drowsiness, orthostatic hypotension, urinary retention, somnolence
Rare
Rash, cholestatic jaundice, priapism

SERIOUS REACTIONS
• Serious reactions such as blood dyscrasias, agranulocytosis, leukocytopenia, thrombocytopenia, cholestatic jaundice, neuroleptic malignant syndrome (NMS), constipation or paralytic ileus, priapism, QT prolongation and torsades de pointes, seizure, systemic lupus erythematosus-like syndrome, and temperature regulation dysfunction (heatstroke or hypothermia) occur rarely.
• Abrupt withdrawal following long-term therapy may precipitate nausea, vomiting, gastritis, dizziness, and tremors.

PRECAUTIONS & CONSIDERATIONS
Caution is necessary with history of neuroleptic malignant syndrome, tardive dyskinesia, and impaired liver or kidney function. Caution is warranted with concomitant administration with inhibitors of cytochrome P450 1A2 and 3A4 enzymes as well as CNS depressants and fluoxetine. Safety and effectiveness have not been established in children under the age of 12. The elderly and debilitated may require a lower initial dose. Avoid grapefruit juice and alcohol consumption.

Akathisia, dystonic extrapyramidal effects, parkinsonian extrapyramidal effects, tardive dyskinesia, tardive dystonia, urinary retention, blurred vision, ocular changes, epithelial keratopathy, pigmentary retinopathy, constipation, decreased sweating, dry mouth, nasal congestion, dizziness, drowsiness, hypotension, and orthostatic hypotension may occur.

Administration

The suppression of tics by pimozide requires a slow and gradual introduction of the drug. The dose should be carefully adjusted to a point where the suppression of tics and the relief afforded is balanced against the unpleasant side effects.

Pindolol
pin'doe-loll
(Apo-Pindol [CAN], Visken)

CATEGORY AND SCHEDULE
Pregnancy Risk Category: B
(D if used in second or third trimester)

CLASSIFICATION
Antiadrenergics, beta blocking

MECHANISM OF ACTION
A nonselective beta blocker that blocks beta$_1$- and beta$_2$-adrenergic receptors. *Therapeutic Effect:* Slows heart rate, decreases cardiac output, decreases blood pressure (B/P), and exhibits antiarrhythmic activity. Decreases myocardial ischemia severity by decreasing oxygen requirements.

PHARMACOKINETICS
Completely absorbed from GI tract. Metabolized in liver. Primarily excreted in urine. **Half-life:** 3-4 hr (half-life increased with impaired renal function, elderly).

AVAILABILITY
Capsules: 5 mg, 10 mg (Visken).

INDICATIONS AND DOSAGES
▸ **Mild to moderate hypertension**
PO
Adults. Initially, 5 mg 2 times/day. Gradually increase dose by 10 mg/day at 2-4 week intervals. Maintenance: 10-30 mg/day in 2-3 divided doses. Maximum: 60 mg/day.
Usual elderly dosage:
PO
Initially, 5 mg/day. May increase by 5 mg q3-4 wk.

OFF-LABEL USES
Treatment of chronic angina pectoris, hypertrophic cardiomyopathy, tremors, and mitral valve prolapse syndrome. Increases antidepressant effect with fluoxetine and other SSRIs.

CONTRAINDICATIONS
Bronchial asthma, COPD, uncontrolled cardiac failure, sinus bradycardia, heart block greater than first degree, cardiogenic shock, CHF, unless secondary to tachyarrhythmias

INTERACTIONS
Drug
Diuretics, other hypotensives: May increase hypotensive effect of pindolol.
Sympathomimetics, xanthines: May mutually inhibit effects of pindolol.
Insulin and oral hypoglycemics: May mask symptoms of hypoglycemia and/or prolong hypoglycemic effect.
Herbal
None known.
Food
None known.

DIAGNOSTIC TEST EFFECTS

May increase ANA titer, SGOT (AST), SGPT (ALT), alkaline phosphatase, LDH, bilirubin, BUN, creatinine, potassium, uric acid, lipoproteins, and triglycerides.

SIDE EFFECTS

Frequent

Decreased sexual ability, drowsiness, trouble sleeping, unusual tiredness/weakness

Occasional

Bradycardia, depression, cold hands/feet, diarrhea, constipation, anxiety, nasal congestion, nausea, vomiting

Rare

Altered taste, dry eyes, itching, numbness of fingers, toes, and scalp

SERIOUS REACTIONS

- Overdosage may produce profound bradycardia and hypotension.
- Abrupt withdrawal may result in sweating, palpitations, headache, and tremulousness.
- May precipitate congestive heart failure (CHF) or myocardial infarction (MI) in patients with heart disease; thyroid storm in those with thyrotoxicosis; or peripheral ischemia in those with existing peripheral vascular disease.
- Hypoglycemia may occur in previously controlled diabetics.
- Signs of thrombocytopenia, such as unusual bleeding or bruising, occur rarely.

PRECAUTIONS & CONSIDERATIONS

Caution is warranted with bronchospastic disease, diabetes, hyperthyroidism, impaired renal or liver function, inadequate cardiac function, or peripheral vascular disease. Pindolol readily crosses the placenta and is distributed in breast milk.

During delivery, pindolol may produce apnea, bradycardia, hypoglycemia, and hypothermia as well as low-birth-weight infants. Safety and efficacy have not been established in children. Caution should be used in the elderly who may have age-related peripheral vascular disease. Nasal decongestants or over-the-counter (OTC) cold preparations (stimulants) should be avoided without physician approval. Excess salt and alcohol consumption should be limited.

Excessive fatigue, headache, prolonged dizziness, shortness of breath, or weight gain should be reported.

Administration

May be given with or without regard to meals. Tablets may be crushed. Do not abruptly discontinue the drug.

Pioglitazone

pye-oh-gli′ta-zonc

(Actos)

P

CATEGORY AND SCHEDULE

Pregnancy Risk Category: C

CLASSIFICATION

Antidiabetic agents, thiazolidinediones

MECHANISM OF ACTION

An antidiabetic that improves target-cell response to insulin without increasing pancreatic insulin secretion. Decreases hepatic glucose output and increases insulin-dependent glucose utilization in skeletal muscle. *Therapeutic Effect:* Lowers blood glucose concentration.

PHARMACOKINETICS
Rapidly absorbed. Highly protein bound (99%), primarily to albumin. Metabolized in the liver. Excreted in urine. Unknown if removed by hemodialysis. **Half-life:** 16-24 hr.

AVAILABILITY
Tablets: 15 mg, 30 mg, 45 mg.

INDICATIONS AND DOSAGES
▶ **Diabetes mellitus, combination therapy**
PO
Adult, Elderly. With insulin: Initially, 15-30 mg once a day. Initially continue current insulin dosage; then decrease insulin dosage by 10% to 25% if hypoglycemia occurs or plasma glucose level decreases to less than 100 mg/dl. Maximum: 45 mg/day. With sulfonylureas: Initially, 15-30 mg/day. Decrease sulfonylurea dosage if hypoglycemia occurs. With metformin: Initially, 15-30 mg/day. As monotherapy: Monotherapy is not to be used if patient is well controlled with diet and exercise alone. Initially, 15-30 mg/day. May increase dosage in increments until 45 mg/day is reached.

CONTRAINDICATIONS
Active hepatic disease; diabetic ketoacidosis; increased serum transaminase levels, including ALT (SGPT) greater than 2.5 times normal serum level; type 1 diabetes mellitus

INTERACTIONS
Drug
Gemfibrizol: May increase the effect and toxicity of pioglitazone.
Ketoconazole: May significantly inhibit metabolism of pioglitazone.

Oral contraceptives: May alter the effects of oral contraceptives.
Food
None known.
Herbal
None known.

DIAGNOSTIC TEST EFFECTS
May increase creatine kinase (CK) level. May decrease Hgb levels by 2% to 4% and serum alkaline phosphatase, bilirubin, and ALT (SGOT) levels. Less than 1% of patients experience ALT values 3 times the normal level.

SIDE EFFECTS
Frequent (13%-9%)
Headache, upper respiratory tract infection
Occasional (6%-5%)
Sinusitis, myalgia, pharyngitis, aggravated diabetes mellitus

SERIOUS REACTIONS
• None known.

PRECAUTIONS & CONSIDERATIONS
Caution is warranted with CHF, edema, and hepatic impairment. It is unknown if pioglitazone crosses the placenta or is distributed in breast milk. Pioglitazone use is not recommended in pregnant or breast-feeding women. Safety and efficacy of pioglitazone have not been established in children. No age-related precautions have been noted in the elderly. Avoid alcohol.

Food intake, blood glucose, and Hgb should be monitored before and during therapy. Hepatic enzyme levels should also be obtained before beginning pioglitazone therapy and periodically thereafter. Notify the physician of abdominal or chest pain, dark urine or light stool, hypoglycemic reactions, fever, nausea, palpitations, rash, vomiting, or yellowing of the eyes or skin. Be aware of signs and symptoms of hypoglycemia (anxiety, cool wet skin, diplopia, dizziness, headache, hunger, numbness in mouth, tachycardia, tremors), or hyperglycemia (deep rapid breathing, dim vision, fatigue, nausea, polydipsia, polyphagia, polyuria, vomiting); carry candy, sugar packets, or other sugar supplements for immediate response to hypoglycemia. Consult the physician when glucose demands are altered (such as with fever, heavy physical activity, infection, stress, trauma). Exercise, good personal hygiene (including foot care), not smoking, and weight control are essential parts of therapy.

Administration
Take pioglitazone without regard to meals.

Piperacillin; Piperacillin/ Tazobactam

(Tazocin [CAN], Zosyn)
Do not confuse Zosyn with Zofran or Zyvox.

CATEGORY AND SCHEDULE
Pregnancy Risk Category: B

MECHANISM OF ACTION
Piperacillin inhibits cell wall synthesis by binding to bacterial cell membranes. Tazobactam inactivates bacterial beta-lactamase. *Therapeutic Effect:* Piperacillin is bactericidal in susceptible organisms. Tazobactam protects piperacillin from enzymatic degradation, extends its spectrum of activity, and prevents bacterial overgrowth.

PHARMACOKINETICS
Protein binding: 16%-30%. Widely distributed. Primarily excreted unchanged in urine. Removed by hemodialysis. **Half-life:** 0.7-1.2 hr (increased in hepatic cirrhosis and impaired renal function).

AVAILABILITY
! Piperacillin/tozobactam is a combination product in a ratio of piperacillin to tazobactam.
Powder for Injection: 2.25 g, 3.375 g, 4.5 g.
Premix Ready to Use: 2.25 g, 3.375 g, 4.5 g.

INDICATIONS AND DOSAGES
▸ **Severe infections**
IV
Adults, Elderly, Children 12 yr and older. 4 g/0.5 g q8hr or 3 g/0.375 g q6hr. Maximum: 18 g/2.25 g daily.
▸ **Moderate infections**
IV
Adults, Elderly, Children 12 yr and older. 2 g/0.225g q6-8hr.
▸ **Dosage in renal impairment**
Dosage and frequency are modified based on creatinine clearance.

Creatinine Clearance	Dosage
20-40 ml/min	8 g/1 g/day (2.25 g q6hr)
Less than 20 ml/min	6 g/0.75 g/day (2.25 g q8hr)

▸ **Dosage in hemodialysis patients**
IV
Adults, Elderly. 2.25 g q8hr with additional dose of 0.75 g after each dialysis session.

CONTRAINDICATIONS
Hypersensitivity to any penicillin

INTERACTIONS
Drug
Hepatotoxic medications: May increase the risk of hepatotoxicity.
Probenecid: May increase piperacillin blood concentration and risk of toxicity.
Herbal
None known.
Food
None known.

DIAGNOSTIC TEST EFFECTS
May increase serum sodium, alkaline phosphatase, bilirubin, LDH, AST (SGOT), and ALT (SGPT) levels. May decrease serum potassium level. May cause a positive Coombs' test.

▓ IV INCOMPATIBILITIES
Amphotericin B (Fungizone), amphotericin B complex (Abelcet, AmBisome, Amphotec), chlorpromazine (Thorazine), dacarbazine (DTIC), daunorubicin (Cerubidine), dobutamine (Dobutrex), doxorubicin (Adriamycin), doxorubicin liposomal (Doxil), droperidol (Inapsine), famotidine (Pepcid), haloperidol (Haldol), hydroxyzine (Vistaril), idarubicin (Idamycin), minocycline (Minocin), nalbuphine (Nubain), prochlorperazine (Compazine), promethazine (Phenergan), vancomycin (Vancocin)
▓ IV Compatibilities
Aminophylline, bumetanide (Bumex), calcium gluconate, diphenhydramine (Benadryl), dopamine (Intropin), enalapril (Vasotec), furosemide (Lasix), granisetron (Kytril), heparin, hydrocortisone (Solu-Cortef), hydromorphone (Dilaudid), lorazepam (Ativan), magnesium sulfate, methylprednisolone (Solu-Medrol), metoclopramide (Reglan), morphine, ondansetron (Zofran), potassium chloride

SIDE EFFECTS
Frequent
Diarrhea, headache, constipation, nausea, insomnia, rash
Occasional
Vomiting, dyspepsia, pruritus, fever, agitation, candidiasis, dizziness, abdominal pain, edema, anxiety, dyspnea, rhinitis

SERIOUS REACTIONS
• Antibiotic-associated colitis and other superinfections may result from altered bacterial balance.
• Seizures and other neurologic reactions are more likely to occur in patients with renal impairment and those who have received an overdose.
• Severe hypersensitivity reactions, including anaphylaxis, occur rarely.

PRECAUTIONS & CONSIDERATIONS
Caution is warranted with a history of allergies, especially to cephalosporins, a pre-existing seizure disorder, and renal impairment. Piperacillin readily crosses the placenta, appears in cord blood and amniotic fluid, and is distributed in breast milk in low concentrations. Piperacillin may lead to allergic sensitization, candidiasis, diarrhea, and skin rash in infants. The safety and efficacy of piperacillin have not been established in children younger than 12 years. Age-related renal impairment may require dosage adjustment in the elderly.

History of allergies, especially to cephalosporins or penicillins, should be determined before giving the drug. Withhold and promptly notify the physician if rash or diarrhea occurs. Severe diarrhea with abdominal pain, blood or mucus in stool, and fever may indicate antibiotic-associated colitis. Signs and symptoms of superinfection, including anal or genital pruritus, black hairy tongue, diarrhea, increased fever, sore throat, ulceration or changes of oral mucosa, and vomiting should be monitored. Electrolytes (especially potassium), intake and output, renal function tests, urinalysis, and the injection sites should be assessed.

Storage

The reconstituted vial is stable for 24 hours at room temperature and 48 hours if refrigerated.

Administration

Reconstitute each 1-g vial with 5 ml D₅W or 0.9% NaCl. Shake vigorously to dissolve. Further dilute with at least 50 ml D₅W, 0.9% NaCl, dextrose 5% in 0.9% NaCl, or lactated Ringer's solution. After further dilution, the solution is stable for 24 hours at room temperature and 7 days if refrigerated. Infuse the drug over 30 minutes.

Pirbuterol

peer-beut-er-all
(Maxair, Maxair Autohaler)

CATEGORY AND SCHEDULE

Pregnancy Risk Category: C

CLASSIFICATION

Adrenergic agonists, bronchodilators

MECHANISM OF ACTION

A sympathomimetic, adrenergic agonist, that stimulates β2-adrenergic receptors in the lungs, resulting in relaxation of bronchial smooth muscle. *Therapeutic Effect:* Relieves bronchospasm, reduces airway resistance.

PHARMACOKINETICS

Absorbed from bronchi following inhalation. Metabolized in liver. Primarily excreted in urine. Unknown if removed by hemodialysis. **Half-life:** 2-3 hr.

AVAILABILITY

Oral Inhalation: 0.2 mg/actuation (Autohaler).

INDICATIONS AND DOSAGES

▸ **Prevention of bronchospasm**
INHALATION
Adults, Elderly, Children 12 yr and older. 2 inhalations q4-6hr. Maximum: 12 inhalations daily.

▸ **Treatment of bronchospasm**
INHALATION
Adults, Elderly, Children 12 yr and older. 2 inhalations separated by at least 1-3 minutes, followed by a third inhalation. Maximum: 12 inhalations daily.

CONTRAINDICATIONS

History of hypersensitivity to pirbuterol, albuterol or any of its components

INTERACTIONS

Drug
Beta-adrenergic blocking agents: Antagonizes effects of pirbuterol.
MAOIs, tricyclic antidepressants: May potentiate cardiovascular effects.
Herbal
None known.
Food
None known.

DIAGNOSTIC TEST EFFECTS

May decrease serum potassium levels.

SIDE EFFECTS

Occasional (7%-1%)
Nervousness, tremor, headache, palpitations, nausea, dizziness, tachycardia, cough

P

SERIOUS REACTIONS

• Excessive sympathomimetic stimulation may produce palpitations, extrasystoles, tachycardia, chest pain, slight increases in B/P followed by a substantial decrease, chills, sweating and blanching of skin.

• Too frequent or excessive use may lead to loss of bronchodilating effectiveness and severe, paradoxical bronchoconstriction.

PRECAUTIONS & CONSIDERATIONS

Caution is necessary with cardiovascular disease, diabetes mellitus, hypertension, or hyperthyroidism. Pirbuterol appears to cross the placenta but it is unknown if it is distributed in breast milk. Safety and efficacy have not been established in children less than 12 years of age. The elderly may be more likely to develop tremors or tachycardia because of the age-related increased sympathetic sensitivity. Increase fluid intake to decrease the viscosity pulmonary secretions. Excessive use of caffeine derivatives, such as chocolate, cocoa, coffee, cola, and tea should be avoided.

Administration

Shake container for inhalation well and exhale completely through the mouth. Place the mouthpiece into the mouth and close the lips while holding the inhaler upright. Inhale deeply through the mouth while fully depressing the top of the canister and hold breath as long as possible before exhaling slowly. Wait 2 minutes before inhaling second dose to allow for deeper bronchial penetration. Rinse mouth with water immediately after inhalation to prevent mouth and throat dryness.

Piroxicam

peer-ox′i-kam

(Apo-Piroxicam [CAN], Candyl-D [AUS], Feldene, Fexicam [CAN], Mobilis [AUS], Novopirocam [CAN], Pirohexal-D [AUS], Rosig [AUS], Rosig-D [AUS])

Do not confuse with Seldane.

CATEGORY AND SCHEDULE

Pregnancy Risk Category: C (D if used in third trimester or near delivery)

CLASSIFICATION

Analgesics, non-narcotic, nonsteroidal anti-inflammatory drugs

MECHANISM OF ACTION

An NSAID that produces analgesic and anti-inflammatory effects by inhibiting prostaglandin synthesis. *Therapeutic Effect:* Reduces inflammatory response and intensity of pain.

AVAILABILITY

Capsules: 10 mg, 20 mg.

INDICATIONS AND DOSAGES

▸ **Acute or chronic rheumatoid arthritis and osteoarthritis**
PO
Adults, Elderly. Initially, 10-20 mg/day as a single dose or in divided doses. Some patients may require up to 30-40 mg/day.
Children. 0.2-0.3 mg/kg/day. Maximum: 15 mg/day.

OFF-LABEL USES

Treatment of acute gouty arthritis, ankylosing spondylitis, dysmenorrhea

CONTRAINDICATIONS
Active peptic ulcer disease, chronic inflammation of the GI tract, GI bleeding or ulceration, history of hypersensitivity to aspirin or NSAIDs

INTERACTIONS
Drug
Antihypertensives, diuretics: May decrease the effects of these drugs.
Aspirin, other salicylates: May increase the risk of GI side effects such as bleeding.
Bone marrow depressants: May increase the risk of hematologic reactions.
Heparin, oral anticoagulants, thrombolytics: May increase the effects of these drugs.
Lithium: May increase the blood concentration and risk of toxicity of lithium.
Methotrexate: May increase the risk of methotrexate toxicity.
Probenecid: May increase the piroxicam blood concentration.
Herbal
Feverfew: May decrease the effects of feverfew.
Ginkgo biloba: May increase the risk of bleeding.
St. John's wort: May increase the risk of phototoxicity.
Food
None known.

DIAGNOSTIC TEST EFFECTS
May increase AST (SGOT) and ALT (SGPT) levels. May decrease serum uric acid levels.

SIDE EFFECTS
Frequent (9%-4%)
Dyspepsia, nausea, dizziness
Occasional (3%-1%)
Diarrhea, constipation, abdominal cramps or pain, flatulence, stomatitis

Rare (less than 1%)
Hypertension, urticaria, dysuria, ecchymosis, blurred vision, insomnia, phototoxicity

SERIOUS REACTIONS
• Rare reactions with long-term use include peptic ulcer disease, GI bleeding, gastritis, severe hepatic reaction (cholestasis, jaundice), nephrotoxicity (dysuria, hematuria, proteinuria, nephrotic syndrome), hematologic sensitivity (anemia, leukopenia, eosinophilia, thrombocytopenia), and a severe hypersensitivity reaction (fever, chills, bronchospasm).

PRECAUTIONS & CONSIDERATIONS
Caution is warranted with GI disease, hypertension, impaired cardiac or hepatic function and concurrent anticoagulant use. Notify the physician of pregnancy. Avoid alcohol and aspirin during therapy because these substances increase the risk of GI bleeding. Tasks that require mental alertness or motor skills should also be avoided.

CBC, hepatic and renal function test results, and pattern of daily bowel activity and stool consistency should be assessed before and during therapy. Therapeutic response, such as decreased pain, stiffness, swelling, and tenderness, improved grip strength, and increased joint mobility, should be evaluated.
Administration
Don't crush or break capsules. Take piroxicam with food, milk, or antacids if GI distress occurs.

Podofilox
po-doe-fil'ox
(Condyline [CAN], Condyline
Paint [AUS], Condylox)

CATEGORY AND SCHEDULE
Pregnancy Risk Category: C

CLASSIFICATION
Dermatologics, destructive
agents

MECHANISM OF ACTION
An active component of podophyllin
resin that binds to tubulin to prevent
formation of microtubules resulting
in mitotic arrest. Exercises many
biological effects such as damages
endothelium of small blood vessels,
attenuates nucleoside transport,
suppresses immune responses, inhibits
macrophage metabolism, induces
interleukin-1 and interleukin-2,
decreases lymphocytes response to
mitogens and enhances macrophage
growth. *Therapeutic Effect:* Removes
genital warts.

PHARMACOKINETICS
Time to peak occurs in 1 to 2 hours.
Some degree of absorption. **Half-
life:** 1-4.5 hr.

AVAILABILITY
Gel: 0.5% (Condylox).
Solution: 0.5% (Condylox).

INDICATIONS AND DOSAGES
▸ **Anogenital warts**
TOPICAL
Adults. Apply 0.5% gel for 3 days,
then withhold for 4 days. Repeat
cycle up to 4 times.
▸ **Genital warts (condylomata
acuminate)**

TOPICAL
Adults. Apply 0.5% solution or gel
q12hr in the morning and evening
for 3 days, then withhold for 4 days.
Repeat cycle up to 4 times.

OFF-LABEL USES
Systemic: Treatment of fungal pneumonia, prostate cancer, septicemia

CONTRAINDICATIONS
Bleeding warts, moles, birthmarks or
unusual warts with hair, diabetes,
poor blood circulation, pregnancy,
steroid use, hypersensitivity to
podofilox or any component of its
formulation

INTERACTIONS
Drug
None known.
Herbal
None known.
Food
None known.

DIAGNOSTIC TEST EFFECTS
None known.

SIDE EFFECTS
Occasional
Erosion, inflammation, itching, pain,
burning
Rare
Nausea, vomiting

SERIOUS REACTIONS
• Nausea and vomiting occur rarely
and usually after cumulative doses.

PRECAUTIONS & CONSIDERATIONS
Caution is necessary with mucous
membrane warts. It is unknown if
podofilox is distributed in breast
milk. Safety and efficacy of podofilox
have not been established in children
or elderly. Nausea, vomiting, blood in
urine, or dizziness should be reported
immediately.

Administration
Apply on warts with supplied cotton-tip applicator. Allow to dry completely before putting legs together. Use no more than 10 cm²/day and no more than 0.5 g/day of topical gel. Use no more than 10 cm²/day and no more than 0.5 ml/day of topical solution.

Podophyllum
po-dof-fil-um
(Podocon-25, Pododerm)

CATEGORY AND SCHEDULE
Pregnancy Risk Category: X

CLASSIFICATION
Dermatologics, destructive agents

MECHANISM OF ACTION
A cytotoxic agent that directly affects epithelial cell metabolism by arresting mitosis through binding to a protein subunit of spindle microtubules. *Therapeutic Effect:* Removes soft genital warts.

PHARMACOKINETICS
Topical podophyllum is systemically absorbed. Absorption may be increased if applied to bleeding, friable, or recently biopsied warts.

AVAILABILITY
Liquid: 25% (Podocon-25, Pododerm).

INDICATIONS AND DOSAGES
▶ **Genital warts (condylomata acuminate)**
TOPICAL
Adults, Elderly, Children. Apply 10%-25% solution in compound benzoin tincture to dry surface. Use 1 drop at a time allowing drying between drops until area is covered. Total volume should be limited to less than 0.5 ml per treatment session.

OFF-LABEL USES
Epitheliomatosis, laryngeal papilloma

CONTRAINDICATIONS
Diabetes mellitus, concomitant steroid therapy, circulation disorders, bleeding warts, moles, birthmarks or unusual warts with hair growing from them, pregnancy, hypersensitivity to podophyllum resin preparations

INTERACTIONS
Drug
None known.
Herbal
None known.
Food
None known.

DIAGNOSTIC TEST EFFECTS
May increase BUN, serum alkaline phosphatase, serum creatinine, SGOT (AST), and SGPT (ALT) levels.

P

▦ IV INCOMPATIBILITIES
None known.
🗍 **IV Compatibilities**
None known.

SIDE EFFECTS
Occasional (10%-1%)
Pruritus, nausea, vomiting, abdominal pain, diarrhea

SERIOUS REACTIONS
• Paresthesia, polyneuritis, paralytic ileus, pyrexia, leukopenia, thrombocytopenia, coma and death have been reported with podophyllum resin use.

PRECAUTIONS & CONSIDERATIONS

Caution should be used on skin that appears irritated as well as area surrounding the eyes. Contact should be avoided with the eyes because podophyllum resin can cause corneal damage. Podophyllum resin use should be avoided during pregnancy. It is unknown if podophyllum is distributed in breast milk. There are no age-related precautions noted in children or the elderly.

Painful urination, dizziness, light-headedness, increased heart rate, constipation, or tingling in hands or feet should be reported.

Administration

Podophyllum resin is to be applied only by a physician. It may not be dispensed to the patient. Apply only to intact lesion (no bleeding). Large areas or numerous warts should not be treated at once. Use concentration of 5%-10% for very large lesions (greater than 10-20 cm) in order to minimize the risk of toxicity.

Thoroughly cleanse affected area before use. The first application of podophyllum resin is recommended to be left on contact for only a short time (30-40 minutes) to determine sensitivity. Use supplied applicator to apply podophyllum resin sparingly to lesion. Avoid contact with healthy tissue. Allow to dry thoroughly. After treatment time has elapsed, remove dried podophyllum resin thoroughly with alcohol or soap and water.

Poly-L-Lactic Acid
(Sculptra)

CATEGORY AND SCHEDULE
Pregnancy Risk Category: Not established

CLASSIFICATION
Physical adjunct, lipoatrophy agent

MECHANISM OF ACTION
A lipoatrophy agent containing microparticles of a synthetic polymer that is used as an injectable implant. *Therapeutic Effect:* Restores facial fat.

PHARMACOKINETICS
Biodegradable, biocompatible synthetic polymer.

AVAILABILITY
Powder for Injection (freeze-dried).

INDICATIONS AND DOSAGES
▸ **Facial lipoatrophy**
SUBCUTANEOUS
Adults, Elderly. For severe facial fat loss, one vial usually injected into multiple points of each cheek during each injection session. Volume of drug for each injection and number of injection sessions depend on severity of condition. Typically, 3-6 injection sessions, separated by intervals of at least 2 weeks, are required.

CONTRAINDICATIONS
None known.

INTERACTIONS
Drug
None known.
Herbal
None known.

Food
None known.

DIAGNOSTIC TEST EFFECTS
None known.

SIDE EFFECTS
Frequent
Ecchymosis
Occasional
Discomfort, edema
Rare
Erythema

SERIOUS REACTIONS
• Subcutaneous papules at injection sites and hematoma occur occasionally.

PRECAUTIONS & CONSIDERATIONS
Be aware of the tendency of keloid formation. It is unknown whether poly-L-lactic acid is excreted in breast milk. Safety and efficacy of poly-L-lactic acid have not been established in children younger than 18 years. Age-related liver impairment may require decreased dosage in the elderly.

Redness, swelling or bruising that typically resolves in hours to 1 week. Avoid excessive sunlight or UV lamp exposure until initial swelling and redness has resolved.
Storage
Reconstituted product is stable for up to 72 hours at room temperature.
Administration and Handling
For IV infusion, reconstitute by drawing 3 to 5 ml sterile water for injection. Using an 18-gauge sterile needle, slowly add all sterile water for injection into the vial. Let vial stand for at least 2 hours. Do not shake during this period. After 2 hours, agitate vial until a uniform translucent suspension is obtained.

Withdraw amount of the suspension (usually 1 ml) into a syringe using a new, 18-gauge needle and replace with a 26-gauge needle before injecting the product into the deep dermis or subcutaneous layer.

Polycarbophil
polly-car'bow-fill
(Fibercon, Replens [CAN])

CATEGORY AND SCHEDULE
Pregnancy Risk Category: C
OTC

MECHANISM OF ACTION
A bulk-forming laxative and antidiarrheal. As a laxative, retains water in the intestine and opposes dehydrating forces of the bowel. *Therapeutic Effect:* Promotes well-formed stools. As an antidiarrheal, absorbs fecal-free water, restores normal moisture level, and provides bulk. *Therapeutic Effect:* Forms gel and produces formed stool.

PHARMACOKINETICS

Route	Onset	Peak	Duration
PO	12-72 hr	N/A	N/A

Acts in small and large intestines.

AVAILABILITY
Tablets: 500 mg, 625 mg.
Tablets (Chewable): 500 mg.

INDICATIONS AND DOSAGES
▸ **Constipation, diarrhea**
PO
Adults, Elderly, Children 12 yr and older. 1 g 1-4 times a day, or as needed. Maximum: 4 g/24 hr.

Children 6-11 yr. 500 mg 1-4 times a day, or as needed. Maximum: 2 g/24 hr.
Children younger than 6 yr. Consult product labeling.

CONTRAINDICATIONS

Abdominal pain, dysphagia, nausea, partial bowel obstruction, symptoms of appendicitis, vomiting

INTERACTIONS
Drug
Digoxin, oral anticoagulants, salicylates, tetracyclines: May decrease the effects of digoxin, salicylates, and tetracyclines.
Potassium-sparing diuretics, potassium supplements: May interfere with the effects of potassium-sparing diuretics and potassium supplements.
Herbal
None known.
Food
None known.

DIAGNOSTIC TEST EFFECTS

May increase blood glucose level. May decrease serum potassium levels.

SIDE EFFECTS
Rare
Some degree of abdominal discomfort, nausea, mild cramps, griping, syncope/near syncope

SERIOUS REACTIONS

• Esophageal or bowel obstruction may occur if administered with less than 250 ml or 1 full glass of liquid.

PRECAUTIONS & CONSIDERATIONS

This drug may be used safely in pregnancy. Polycarbophil use is not recommended in children younger than 6 years of age. No age-related precautions have been noted in the elderly.

Pattern of daily bowel activity and stool consistency and serum electrolyte levels should be monitored. Adequate fluid intake should be maintained.
Administration
! For severe diarrhea, give every half hour up to maximum daily dosage; for constipation, give with 8 oz liquid, as prescribed.
  Drink 6 to 8 glasses of water a day to aid in stool softening. To promote defecation, increase fluid intake, exercise, and eat a high-fiber diet.

Polyethylene Glycol-Electrolyte Solution
pol-ee-eth'-ill-een
(CoLyte, GoLYTELY, Klean-Prep [CAN], MiraLax, NuLytely, Peglyte [CAN], Pro-Lax [CAN], TriLyte)

CATEGORY AND SCHEDULE
Pregnancy Risk Category: C

CLASSIFICATION
Bowel evacuants, laxatives

MECHANISM OF ACTION

A laxative that has an osmotic effect. *Therapeutic Effect:* Induces diarrhea and cleanses bowel without depleting electrolytes.

PHARMACOKINETICS

Route	Onset	Peak	Duration
PO (bowel cleansing)	1-2 hr	N/A	N/A
PO (constipation)	2-4 days	N/A	N/A

AVAILABILITY
Powder for Oral Solution.
Oral Solution.

INDICATIONS AND DOSAGES
▸ **Bowel cleansing**
PO
Adults, Elderly. Before GI examination: 240 ml (8 oz) q10min until
4 liters consumed or rectal effluent clear. NG tube: 20-30 ml/min until
4 liters given.
Children. 25-40 ml/kg/hr until rectal effluent clear.
▸ **Constipation**
PO (MiraLax)
Adults. 17 g or 1 heaping tbsp a day.

CONTRAINDICATIONS
Bowel perforation, gastric retention, GI obstruction, megacolon, toxic colitis, toxic ileus

INTERACTIONS
Drug
Oral medications: May decrease the absorption of oral medications if given within 1 hour because they may be flushed from GI tract.
Herbal
None known.
Food
None known.

DIAGNOSTIC TEST EFFECTS
None known.

SIDE EFFECTS
Frequent (50%)
Some degree of abdominal fullness, nausea, bloating
Occasional (10%-1%)
Abdominal cramping, vomiting, anal irritation
Rare (less than 1%)
Urticaria, rhinorrhea, dermatitis

SERIOUS REACTIONS
• None known.

PRECAUTIONS & CONSIDERATIONS
Caution is warranted with ulcerative colitis. It is unknown if polyethylene crosses the placenta or is distributed in breast milk. No age-related precautions have been noted in children or the elderly.
   Notify the physician if severe abdominal pain or bloating occurs. Blood glucose, BUN, serum electrolyte levels, urine osmolality, and pattern of daily bowel activity and stool consistency should be monitored.
Storage
Refrigerate reconstituted solutions; use within 48 hours.
Administration
May use tap water to prepare solution. Shake vigorously for several minutes to ensure complete dissolution of powder. Take nothing by mouth 3 hours or more before ingestion of solution. Give only clear liquids after administration. May give via NG tube. Rapid drinking preferred. Chilled solution is more palatable.

P

Polymyxin B
polly-mix-in
(Aerosporin)

CATEGORY AND SCHEDULE
Pregnancy Risk Category: NR

CLASSIFICATION
Antibiotics, polymyxins

MECHANISM OF ACTION
An antibiotic that alters cell membrane permeability in susceptible microorganisms. *Therapeutic Effect:* Bactericidal activity.

PHARMACOKINETICS

Negligible absorption. Protein binding: low. Excreted in urine. Poor removal in hemodialysis. **Half-life:** 6 hr.

AVAILABILITY

Powder: 500,000 (Aerosporin).

INDICATIONS AND DOSAGES

▸ **Mild to moderate infections**
IV
Adults, Elderly, Children 2 yr and older. 15,000-25,000 units/kg/day in divided doses q12hr.
Infants. Up to 40,000 units/kg/day.
IM
Adults, Elderly, Children 2 yr and older. 25,000-30,000 units/kg/day in divided doses q4-6hr.
Infants. Up to 40,000 units/kg/day.
▸ **Usual irrigation dosage**
Continuous Bladder Irrigation
Adults, Elderly. 1 ml urogenital concentrate (contains 200,000 units polymyxin B, 57 mg neomycin) added to 1000 ml 0.9% NaCl. Give each 1000 ml >24 hr for up to 10 days (may increase to 2000 ml/day when urine output >2 L/day).
▸ **Usual ophthalmic dosage**
OPHTHALMIC
Adults, Elderly, Children. 1 drop q3-4hr.

CONTRAINDICATIONS

Hypersensitivity to polymyxin B or any component of the formulation

INTERACTIONS

Drug
Neuromuscular blocking agents or anesthetics: May produce muscle paralysis and prolonged or increased skeletal muscle relaxation.
Aminoglycosides, other nephrotoxic drugs: may increase nephrotoxicity.

SIDE EFFECTS

Frequent
Severe pain, irritation at IM injection sites, phlebitis, thrombophlebitis with IV administration
Occasional
Fever, urticaria

SERIOUS REACTIONS

• Nephrotoxicity, especially with concurrent/sequential use of other nephrotoxic drugs, renal impairment, concurrent/sequential use of muscle relaxants.
• Superinfection, especially with fungi, may occur.

PRECAUTIONS & CONSIDERATIONS

Caution should be used with impaired renal function. Safety and efficacy of polymyxin B have not been established in pregnant women or children younger than 2 years old. There are no age-related precautions noted in the elderly.

Renal function should be carefully monitored. Serum concentrations of more than 5 mcg/ml are toxic in adults. Neurotoxic reactions may be manifested by drowsiness, irritability, blurred vision, weakness, ataxia, and numbness of the extremities.

Storage
Store at room temperature prior to reconstitution and protect from light. After reconstitution, store under refrigeration. Discard any unused solution after 72 hours.

Administration
For IV use, dissolve 500,000 units in 300-500 ml D_5W for continuous IV drip. Administer every 12 hours. For IM injection, dissolve 500,000 units in 2 ml water for injection, 0.9% NaCl, or 1% procaine solution. IM injection is not routinely recommended because of severe pain at the injection sites.

For intrathecal administration, dissolve 500,000 units in 10 ml physiologic solution. Administer once daily for 3-4 days, then every other day for at least 2 weeks after CSF cultures are negative.

For ophthalmic use, 500,000 units in 20-50 ml sterile water for injection or 0.9% NaCl. Instill drops and close the eye gently for 1 to 2 minutes and roll eyeball to increase contact area of drug to eye. Remove excess solution around the eye with a tissue.

Polythiazide
poly-thi'a-zide
(Renese)

CATEGORY AND SCHEDULE
Pregnancy Risk Category: D

CLASSIFICATION
Diuretics, thiazide and derivatives

MECHANISM OF ACTION
A sulfonamide derivative that acts as a thiazide diuretic and antihypertensive. As a diuretic blocks reabsorption of water, sodium and potassium at cortical diluting segment of distal tubule. As an antihypertensive it reduces plasma and extracellular fluid volume and decreases peripheral vascular resistance (PVR) by direct effect on blood vessels. *Therapeutic Effect:* Promotes diuresis, reduces blood pressure (B/P).

PHARMACOKINETICS
Rapidly absorbed from the gastrointestinal (GI) tract. Primarily excreted unchanged in urine. Not removed by hemodialysis. **Half-life:** 25.7 hr.

AVAILABILITY
Tablets: 1 mg, 2 mg, 4 mg (Renese).

INDICATIONS AND DOSAGES
▶ **Edema**
PO
Adults. 1- 4 mg/day.
▶ **Hypertension**
PO
Adults. 2- 4 mg/day.

OFF-LABEL USES
Prevention of calcium-containing renal stones

CONTRAINDICATIONS
Anuria, history of hypersensitivity to sulfonamides or thiazide diuretics, renal decompensation

INTERACTIONS
Drug
Ace inhibitors: May increase the risk of postural hypotension.
Beta blockers: May increase hyperglycemic effects in patients with Type 2 diabetes mellitus.
Cylcosporine, other thiazides: May increase the risk of gout or renal toxicity.
Cholestyramine, colestipol: May decrease the absorption and effects of polythiazide.
Digoxin: May increase the risk of toxicity of digoxin caused by hypokalcmia.
Lithium: May increase the risk of toxicity of lithium.
Neuromuscular blocking agents: May prolong neuromuscular blockade.
NSAIDs: May decrease the effects of polythiazide.
Herbal
Dong quai, St. John's wort: May cause photosensitization.
Garlic: May increase antihypertensive effect.
Ginkgo biloba: May increase blood pressure.

P

Gossypol: May increase the risk of hypokalemia.
Licorice: May increase the risk of hypokalemia and/or reduce effectiveness of polythiazide.
Ma Huang: May decrease hypotensive effect of polythiazide.
Ephedra, ginseng, yohimbine: May decrease the effects of polythiazide.
Food
None known.

DIAGNOSTIC TEST EFFECTS

May increase blood glucose levels, serum cholesterol, LDL, bilirubin, calcium, creatinine, uric acid, and triglyceride levels. May decrease urinary calcium, and serum magnesium, potassium, and sodium levels.

SIDE EFFECTS

Expected
Increase in urine frequency and volume
Frequent
Potassium depletion
Occasional
Postural hypotension, headache, gastrointestinal (GI) disturbances, photosensitivity reaction

SERIOUS REACTIONS

• Vigorous diuresis may lead to profound water loss and electrolyte depletion, resulting in hypokalemia, hyponatremia, and dehydration.
• Acute hypotensive episodes may occur.
• Hyperglycemia may be noted during prolonged therapy.
• GI upset, pancreatitis, dizziness, paresthesias, headache, blood dyscrasias, pulmonary edema, allergic pneumonitis, and dermatologic reactions occur rarely.
• Overdosage can lead to lethargy and coma without changes in electrolytes or hydration.

PRECAUTIONS & CONSIDERATIONS

Caution should be used with diabetes mellitus, electrolyte imbalance, hyperuricemia or gout, hypotension, systemic lupus erythematosus, impaired liver function and severe renal disease. Polythiazide crosses the placenta and a small amount is distributed in breast milk. Breast-feeding is not recommended in this patient population. Safety and efficacy of polythiazide have not been established in children. Be aware that the elderly may be more sensitive to the drug's electrolyte and hypotensive effects. Age-related renal impairment may require caution in the elderly.

Frequency and volume of urination is expected to increase. Be aware that polythiazide may aggravate digitalis toxicity. Be aware that sensitivity reactions may occur with or without history of allergy or asthma. Skin should be protected from sunlight.

Hypokalemia may result in change in mental status, muscle cramps, nausea, tachycardia, tremor, vomiting, and weakness. Hyponatremia may result in clammy and cold skin, confusion, and thirst. Be especially alert for potassium depletion in persons taking digoxin, such as cardiac arrhythmias. Foods high in potassium such as apricots, bananas, legumes, meat, orange juice, white and sweet potatoes, raisins, and whole grains, such as cereals should be eaten during treatment.

Administration
Take polythiazide with food or milk if GI upset occurs, preferably with breakfast to help prevent nocturia.

Poractant Alfa
poor-ak'tant
(Curosurf)

CATEGORY AND SCHEDULE
Pregnancy Risk Category: This drug is not indicated for use in pregnant women.

CLASSIFICATION
Surfactants, lung

MECHANISM OF ACTION
A pulmonary surfactant that reduces alveolar surface tension during ventilation and stabilizes the alveoli against collapse that may occur at resting transpulmonary pressures. *Therapeutic Effect:* Improves lung compliance and respiratory gas exchange.

AVAILABILITY
Intratracheal Suspension: 1.5 ml (120 mg), 3 ml (240 mg).

INDICATIONS AND DOSAGES
▸ **Respiratory distress syndrome (RDS)**
INTRATRACHEAL
Infants. Initially, 2.5 ml/kg of birth weight. May give up to 2 subsequent doses of 1.25 ml/kg of birth weight at 12-hr intervals. Maximum: 5 ml/kg (total dose).

OFF-LABEL USES
Adult RDS due to viral pneumonia or near-drowning, *Pneumocystis carinii* pneumonia in HIV-infected patients, prevention of RDS

CONTRAINDICATIONS
None known.

INTERACTIONS
Drug
None known.
Herbal
None known.
Food
None known.

DIAGNOSTIC TEST EFFECTS
None known.

SIDE EFFECTS
Frequent
Transient bradycardia, oxygen (O_2) desaturation, increased carbon dioxide (CO_2) retention
Occasional
Endotracheal tube reflux
Rare
Apnea, endotracheal tube blockage, hypotension or hypertension, pallor, vasoconstriction

SERIOUS REACTIONS
• None known.

PRECAUTIONS & CONSIDERATIONS
Caution should be used with persons at risk for circulatory overload. This drug is for use only in neonates. No age-related precautions have been noted.

The infant's oxygenation and ventilation should be monitored using arterial or transcutaneous measurement of systemic oxygen (O_2) and carbon dioxide (CO_2). Heart rate and breath sounds should also be assessed. Visitors should be limited during treatment. Hand washing and other infection control measures should be enforced to minimize the risk of nosocomial infections.
Storage
Refrigerate vials. Unopened, unused vials may be returned to the refrigerator only once after having been warmed to room temperature.

Administration

Warm the vial by letting it stand at room temperature for 20 minutes or warming it in your hand for 8 minutes. Turn the vial upside down and gently swirl it, if needed, to obtain a uniform suspension. Do not shake the vial.

Withdraw the entire contents of the vial into a 3- or 5-ml plastic syringe through a large-gauge needle (20 gauge or larger). Attach the syringe to a catheter that's inserted into the infant's endotracheal tube, and instill the solution through the catheter. Monitor the infant for bradycardia and decreased SaO_2 during administration. Stop the procedure if the infant experiences these effects, and take appropriate measures before reinstituting therapy.

Potassium Iodide
(Pima, SSKI, Thyro-Block [CAN])

CATEGORY AND SCHEDULE
Pregnancy Risk Category: D
OTC (tablets)

CLASSIFICATION
Antithyroid agents, hormones/hormone modifiers

MECHANISM OF ACTION
An agent that reduces viscosity of mucus by increasing respiratory tract secretions. Inhibits secretion of thyroid hormone, fosters colloid accumulation in thyroid follicles. *Therapeutic Effect:* Blocks thyroid radioiodine uptake.

PHARMACOKINETICS
Oral onset 24-48 hr, peak 10-15 days, duration 6 weeks. Primarily excreted in the urine.

AVAILABILITY
Solution: 1 mg/ml (SSKI), 100 mg/ml (Lugol's solution).
Syrup: 325/5 ml (Pima).
Tablets: 130 mg (Iosat).

INDICATIONS AND DOSAGES
▸ **Expectorant**
PO
Adults, Elderly, Children 3 yr and older. 325-650 mg q8hr (Pima); 300-600 mg 3-4 times/day (SSKI).
Children less than 3 yr. 162 mg q8hr.
▸ **Preoperative thyroidectomy**
PO
Adults, Elderly, Children. 0.1-0.3 ml (3-5 drops of Lugol's solution) q8hr or 50-250 mg (1-5 drops of SSKI) q8hr. Administer 10 days before surgery.
▸ **Radiation protectant to radioactive isotopes of iodine**
PO
Adults, Elderly. 195 mg/day (Pima) for 10 days. Start 24 hours prior to exposure.
Children more than 1 yr. 130 mg/day for 10 days. Start 24 hours prior to exposure.
Children less than 1 yr. 65 mg/day for 10 days. Start 24 hours prior to exposure.
▸ **Reduce risk of thyroid cancer following nuclear accident**
PO
Adults, Elderly, Children more than 68 kg. 130 mg/day
Children 3-18 yr. 65 mg/day.
Children 1 mo - 3 yr. 32 mg/day.
Children 1 mo and younger. 16 mg/day.

▶ **Sporotrichosis**
PO
Adults, Elderly. Initally, 5 drops
(SSKI) q8hr and increase to
40-50 drops q8hr as tolerated for
3-6 months.
▶ **Thyrotoxic crisis**
PO
Adults, Elderly. 300-500 mg
(6-19 drops SSKI) q8hr or 1 ml
(Lugol's solution) q8hr.

CONTRAINDICATIONS
Hypersensitivity to potassium, iodine
compounds, or any of its
components, pulmonary edema,
hyperkalemia, impaired renal function, hyperthyroidism, iodine-
induced goiter, pregnancy

INTERACTIONS
Drug
ACE inhibitors: May increase risk
of hyperkalemia, cardiac arrhyth-
mias, or cardiac arrest.
Diuretics, potassium-sparing: May
increase risk of hyperkalemia, cardiac
arrhythmias, or cardiac arrest.
Lithium: May increase the
hypothyroid effects.
**Potassium (and potassium-
containing products):** May increase
risk of hyperkalemia, cardiac arrhyth-
mias, or cardiac arrest.
Herbal
None known.
Food
None known.

DIAGNOSTIC TEST EFFECTS
May alter thyroid function tests.

SIDE EFFECTS
Occasional
Irregular heart beat, confusion,
drowsiness, fever, rash, diarrhea, GI
bleeding, metallic taste, nausea,
stomach pain, vomiting, numbness,
tingling, weakness

Rare
Goiter, salivary gland swelling and
tenderness, thyroid adenoma,
swelling of the throat and neck,
myxedema, lymph node swelling.

SERIOUS REACTIONS
• Hypersensitivity symptoms
include angioedema, muscle weakness, paralysis, peaked T-waves, flattened P-waves, prolongation of QRS
complex, ventricular arrhythmias.

PRECAUTIONS & CONSIDERATIONS
Caution is warranted with CHF,
hypertension, and pulmonary edema.
Be aware citrate use may increase
the risk of urolithiasis.
   CBC (particularly blood Hct and
Hgb level), serum acid-base balance,
and serum creatinine should be
monitored. EKG and urinary pH
should be assessed in those with
cardiac disease.
Administration
Take citrates after meals and at
bedtime. Mix citrates in water or
juice and drink additional liquids
after taking the drug.

P

Potassium Salts
(K-Lyte, Klor-Con EF, Effer K, K-Lyte DS) (Apo-K [CAN], Kaochlor, K-Dur, K-Lor, K-Lor-Con M 15, Kaon-Cl, KSR [AUS], KSR-600 [AUS], Micro-K, Slow-K [AUS], Span-K [AUS]) (Kaon)
Do not confuse K-dur with Cardura.

CATEGORY AND SCHEDULE
Pregnancy Risk Category: C
(A for potassium chloride)

CLASSIFICATION
Electrolytes, minerals

MECHANISM OF ACTION
An electrolyte that is necessary for multiple cellular metabolic processes. Primary action is intracellular. *Therapeutic Effect:* Is necessary for nerve impulse conduction and contraction of cardiac, skeletal, and smooth muscle; maintains normal renal function and acid-base balance.

PHARMACOKINETICS
Well absorbed from the GI tract. Enters cells by active transport from extracellular fluid. Primarily excreted in urine.

AVAILABILITY
Potassium Acetate
Injection: 2 mEq/ml.
Potassium Bicarbonate and Potassium Citrate
Tablet for Solution (Klor-Con EF, Effer-K, K-Lyte): 25 mEq.
Tablet for Solution (K-Lyte DS): 50 mEq.
Potassium Chloride
Capsules (Controlled-Release [Micro-K]): 8 mEq, 10 mEq.

Liquid (Kaochlor): 20 mEq/15 ml.
Liquid (Kaon-Cl): 40 mEq/15 ml.
Powder for Oral Solution (K-Lor): 20 mEq.
Injection: 2 mEq/ml.
Tablets (Extended-Release [Klor-Con, Micro-K]): 8 mEq, 10 mEq.
Tablets (Extended-Release [Kaon-Cl, K-Tab]): 10 mEq.
Tablets (Extended-Release [K-Dur]): 10 mEq, 20 mEq.
Potassium Gluconate
Elixir (Kaon): 20 mEq/15 ml.

INDICATIONS AND DOSAGES
▶ **Prevention of hypokalemia (in patients on diuretic therapy)**
PO
Adults, Elderly. 20-40 mEq/day in 1-2 divided doses.
Children. 1-2 mEq/kg/day in 1-2 divided doses.
▶ **Treatment of hypokalemia**
PO
Adults, Elderly. 40-80 mEq/day; further doses based on laboratory values.
Children. 2-5 mEq/day; further doses based on laboratory values.
IV
Adults, Elderly. 5-10 mEq/hr.
Maximum: 400 mEq/day.
Children. 1 mEq/kg over 1-2 hr.

CONTRAINDICATIONS
Concurrent use of potassium-sparing diuretics, digitalis toxicity, heat cramps, hyperkalemia, postoperative oliguria, severe burns, severe renal impairment, shock with dehydration or hemolytic reaction, untreated Addison's disease

INTERACTIONS
Drug
ACE inhibitors, beta-adrenergic blockers, heparin, NSAIDs,

potassium-containing medications, potassium-sparing diuretics, salt substitutes: May increase potassium blood concentration.
Anticholinergics: May increase the risk of GI lesions.
Herbal
None known.
Food
None known.

DIAGNOSTIC TEST EFFECTS
None known.

IV INCOMPATIBILITIES
Amphotericin B complex (Abelcet, AmBisome, Amphotec), methylprednisolone (Solu-Medrol), phenytoin (Dilantin)

IV Compatibilities
Aminophylline, amiodarone (Cordarone), atropine, aztreonam (Azactam), calcium gluconate, cefepime (Maxipime), ciprofloxacin (Cipro), clindamycin (Cleocin), dexamethasone (Decadron), digoxin (Lanoxin), diltiazem (Cardizem), diphenhydramine (Benadryl), dobutamine (Dobutrex), dopamine (Intropin), enalapril (Vasotec), famotidine (Pepcid), fluconazole (Diflucan), furosemide (Lasix), granisetron (Kytril), heparin, hydrocortisone (Solu-Cortef), insulin, lidocaine, lorazepam (Ativan), magnesium sulfate, methylprednisolone (Solu-Medrol), metoclopramide (Reglan), midazolam (Versed), milrinone (Primacor), morphine, norepinephrine (Levophed), ondansetron (Zofran), oxytocin (Pitocin), piperacillin and tazobactam (Zosyn), procainamide (Pronestyl), propofol (Diprivan), propranolol (Inderal)

SIDE EFFECTS
Occasional
Nausea, vomiting, diarrhea, flatulence, abdominal discomfort with distention, phlebitis with IV administration (particularly when potassium concentration of greater than 40 mEq/L is infused)
Rare
Rash

SERIOUS REACTIONS
• Hyperkalemia (more common in elderly patients and those with impaired renal function) may be manifested as paresthesia, feeling of heaviness in the lower extremities, cold skin, grayish pallor, hypotension, confusion, irritability, flaccid paralysis, and cardiac arrhythmias.

PRECAUTIONS & CONSIDERATIONS
Caution is warranted with cardiac disease and tartrazine sensitivity (most common in those with aspirin hypersensitivity). It is unknown if potassium crosses the placenta or is distributed in breast milk. No age-related precautions have been noted in children. The elderly may be at increased risk for hyperkalemia because of an impaired ability to excrete potassium. Consuming potassium-rich foods, including apricots, avocados, bananas, beans, beef, broccoli, brussel sprouts, cantaloupe, chicken, dates, fish, ham, lentils, milk, molasses, potatoes, prunes, raisins, spinach, turkey, watermelon, veal, and yams, is encouraged.
    Notify the physician of a feeling of heaviness in the lower extremities and paraesthesia. Serum potassium levels should be obtained before and throughout therapy. Intake and output, pattern of daily bowel activity and stool consistency should also be monitored. Be alert for signs and symptoms of hyperkalemia, including cold skin, feeling of heaviness in lower extremities, paraesthesia, and skin pallor.

P

Storage
Store vials at room temperature.
Administration
! Potassium dosage must be individualized.

Give oral potassium with or after meals and with full glass of water to decrease GI upset. Mix effervescent tablets, liquids, and powder with juice or water and let them dissolve before administering. Swallow the tablets whole and do not chew or crush them.

Dilute the drug to a concentration of no more than 40 mEq/L and mix it well before IV infusion. Avoid adding potassium to a hanging IV line. Infuse the drug slowly at a rate not exceeding 20 mEq/hr. Check the IV site closely during the infusion for evidence of phlebitis (hardness of vein; heat, pain, and red streaking of skin over vein) and extravasation (cool skin, little or no blood return, pain, and swelling).

Pralidoxime
pra-li-doks-eem
(Protopam Chloride)

CATEGORY AND SCHEDULE
Pregnancy Risk Category: C

CLASSIFICATION
Antidotes

MECHANISM OF ACTION
Reactivates cholinesterase activity by 2-formyl-1-methylpyridinium ion. *Therapeutic Effect:* Restores cholinesterase activity following organophosphate anticholinesterase poisoning.

PHARMACOKINETICS
Onset of activity is 1 hour and duration of action is short, which may require readministration. Not protein bound. Excreted in urine. **Half-life:** 1.2-2.6 hr.

AVAILABILITY
Injection, powder for reconstitution: 1 g (Protopam Chloride).

INDICATIONS AND DOSAGES
▸ **Anticholinesterase overdosage**
IV
Adults, Elderly. 1-2 g initially, followed by increments of 250 mg q5min until response is observed.
▸ **Organophosphate poisoning**
IV
Adults, Elderly. 1-2 g initially in 100 ml 0.9% NaCl infused over 15-30 minutes or 5% solution in sterile water for injection over not less than 5 minutes. Repeat 1-2 g in 1 hour if muscle weakness persists.
Children. 25-50 mg/kg/dose. Repeat in 1-2 hours if muscle weakness has not been relieved, then at 8-12 hour intervals if cholinergic signs recur.

CONTRAINDICATIONS
Use of aminophylline, morphine, theophylline and succinylcholine, hypersensitivity to pralidoxime or any of its components

INTERACTIONS
Drug
Barbiturates: May increase effect of pralidoxime.
Aminophylline, caffeine, theophylline: May exacerbate effects of organophosphate poisoning.
Succinylcholine: May prolong respiratory paralysis.

Reserpine, phenothiazines: May exacerbate effects of organophosphate poisoning.
Atropine: May decrease effects of pralidoxime.
Thiamine: May delay excretion of pralidoxime due to competition at renal excretory site.
Herbal
None known.
Food
None known.

DIAGNOSTIC TEST EFFECTS
May increase SGOT (AST) and creatine kinase levels.

SIDE EFFECTS
Occasional
Blurred vision, dizziness, headache, laryngospasm, hyperventilation, nausea, tachycardia, hypertension, pain at injection site
Rare
Rash, muscle rigidity, decreased renal function

SERIOUS REACTIONS
* Excessive doses may cause blurred vision, nausea, tachycardia and dizziness.

PRECAUTIONS & CONSIDERATIONS
Caution is warranted with myasthenia gravis and renal impairment as well as in the elderly. It is unknown if pralidoxime crosses the placenta and is distributed in breast milk. Safety and efficacy of pralidoxime have not been established in children. Age-related renal impairment may require dosage adjustment in the elderly. Avoid consuming an excessive amount of caffeine derivatives such as chocolate, cocoa, coffee, cola, or tea.

Resolution of clinical symptoms (muscle weakness, respiratory difficulty, muscarinic effects such as salivation, lacrimation, urination, and defecation) should be assessed.
Storage
Store vials for injection at room temperature.
Administration
Initiation of therapy must not be delayed until results of tests are available. Dilute 1 g with 20 ml of sterile water for injection. Solution may be further diluted and administered as 1-2 g in 100 ml 0.9% NaCl. Slow IV infusion prevents tachycardia, laryngospasm, and muscle rigidity. Do not use if solution appears discolored or contains a precipitate.

Pramipexole
pram-eh-pex′ol
(Mirapex)
Do not confuse Mirapex with Mifeprex or MiraLax.

CATEGORY AND SCHEDULE
Pregnancy Risk Category: C

CLASSIFICATION
Antiparkinson agents, dopaminergics

MECHANISM OF ACTION
An antiparkinson agent that stimulates dopamine receptors in the striatum. *Therapeutic Effect:* Relieves signs and symptoms of Parkinson's disease.

PHARMACOKINETICS
Rapidly and extensively absorbed after PO administration. Protein binding: 15%. Widely distributed. Steady-state concentrations achieved within 2 days. Primarily eliminated

in urine. Not removed by hemodialysis. **Half-life:** 8 hr (12 hr in patients older than 65 yr).

AVAILABILITY
Tablets: 0.125 mg, 0.25 mg, 0.5 mg, 1 mg, 1.5 mg.

INDICATIONS AND DOSAGES
▸ **Parkinson's disease**
PO
Adults, Elderly. Initially, 0.375 mg/day in 3 divided doses. Don't increase dosage more frequently than every 5-7 days. Maintenance: 1.5-4.5 mg/day in 3 equally divided doses.
▸ **Dosage in renal impairment**
Dosage and frequency are modified based on creatinine clearance.

Creatinine Clearance	Initial Dose	Maximum Dose
Greater than 60 ml/min	0.125 mg 3 times a day	1.5 mg 3 times a day
35-59 ml/min	0.125 mg twice a day	1.5 mg twice a day
15-34 ml/min	0.125 mg once a day	1.5 mg once a day

CONTRAINDICATIONS
History of hypersensitivity to pramipexole

INTERACTIONS
Drug
Carbidopa and levodopa, levodopa: May increase plasma level of levodopa.
Cimetidine: Increases pramipexole plasma concentration and half-life.
Cimetidine, diltiazem, quinidine, quinine, ranitidine, triamterene, verapamil: May decrease pramipexole clearance.
Herbal
None known.

Food
All foods: Delay peak drug plasma levels by 1 hour but don't affect drug absorption.

DIAGNOSTIC TEST EFFECTS
None known.

SIDE EFFECTS
Frequent
Early Parkinson's disease (28%-10%): Nausea, asthenia, dizziness, somnolence, insomnia, constipation
Advanced Parkinson's disease (53%-17%): Orthostatic hypotension, extrapyramidal reactions, insomnia, dizziness, hallucinations
Occasional
Early Parkinson's disease (5%-2%): Edema, malaise, confusion, amnesia, akathisia, anorexia, dysphagia, peripheral edema, vision changes, impotence
Advanced Parkinson's disease (10%-7%): Asthenia, somnolence, confusion, constipation, abnormal gait, dry mouth
Rare
Advanced Parkinson's disease (6%-2%): General edema, malaise, chest pain, amnesia, tremor, urinary frequency or incontinence, dyspnea, rhinitis, vision changes

SERIOUS REACTIONS
• None known.

PRECAUTIONS & CONSIDERATIONS
Caution is warranted with hallucinations, syncope, renal impairment, history of orthostatic hypotension and in those using CNS depressants concurrently. It is unknown if pramipexole is distributed in breast milk. The safety and efficacy of pramipexole have not been established in children. The elderly are at increased risk for hallucinations.

Dizziness, drowsiness, lightheadedness, and constipation may occur. Alcohol and tasks that require mental alertness or motor skills should be avoided. Change positions slowly to prevent orthostatic hypotension. Baseline vital signs and renal function should be assessed at baseline. Relief of symptoms, such as improvement of masklike facial expression, muscular rigidity, shuffling gait, and resting tremors of the hands and head should be assessed during treatment.

Administration
Take pramipexole without regard to food. Take with food if nausea is a problem. Do not abruptly discontinue pramipexole.

Pramoxine
pra-mox′een
(Analpram-HC, Anusol, Enzone, Epifoam, Pramosome, Pramox HC [CAN], Prasone [TAIWAN], Prax, Proctofoam [US, ENG, GERMANY], Proctocream, Rectocort, Tronolane, Zone-A)
Do not confuse with pralidoxime, Apisol, Aquasol, Tronothane

CATEGORY AND SCHEDULE
Pregnancy Risk Category: C

CLASSIFICATION
Morpholine derivative, anesthetic, topical

MECHANISM OF ACTION
A surface or local anesthetic which is not chemically related to the "caine" types of local anesthetics. Decreases the neuronal membranes permeability to sodium ions, blocking both initiation and conduction of nerve impulses, therefore inhibiting depolarization of the neuron. *Therapeutic Effect:* Temporarily relieves pain and itching associated with anogenital pruritus or irritation.

PHARMACOKINETICS
Onset of action occurs within a few minutes of application. Peak effect is reached in 3-5 minutes. Duration is several days.

AVAILABILITY
Foam: 1% (Proctofoam NS)
Cream: 1% (Tranolane)
Gel: 1% (Itch-X)
Lotion: 1% (Prax)
Ointment: 1% (Anusol)
Solution: 1% (Itch-X)
Suppository: 1% (Tronolane)

INDICATIONS AND DOSAGES
▶ **Anogenital pruritus or irritation, dermatosis, minor burns, hemorrhoids**
TOPICAL
Adults, Elderly. Apply to affected area 3 or 4 times daily.

CONTRAINDICATIONS
Hypersensitivity to any component of the product.

INTERACTIONS
Drug
None known.
Herbal
None known.
Food
None known.

DIAGNOSTIC TEST EFFECTS
None known.

SIDE EFFECTS
Occassional
Angioedema, contact dermatitis, burning, itching, irritation, stinging

P

Rare
Dryness, folliculitis, hypopigmenta-tion, perioral dermatitis, maceration of the skin, secondary infection, skin atrophy, striae, miliaria.

SERIOUS REACTIONS
• None known.

PRECAUTIONS & CONSIDERATIONS
Caution is warranted with children and the elderly. It is unknown if pramoxine crosses the placenta and is distributed in the breast milk.

Redness, irritation, swelling, burn-ing, stinging, pain, and dryness may occur. If bleeding at affected area, hoarseness, hives, rash, severe itching, difficulty breathing or swallowing, or swelling of the face, throat, lips, eyes, hands, feet, or ankles occurs, notify physician immediately.
Storage
Store at room temperature.
Administration
To use pramoxine cream, gel, spray, or lotion, wash hands first. Clean the affected area with mild soap and warm water. Rinse thoroughly. Pat affected area dry with a clean, soft cloth or tissue. Apply small amount of pramoxine to affected area. Wash hands thoroughly.

To use pramoxine pledgets, wash hands first. Clean affected rectal area with mild soap and warm water. Rinse thoroughly. Gently dry by patting or blotting with a clean, soft cloth or tissue. Open sealed pouch and remove pledget. Apply medica-tion from pledget to affected rectal area by patting. If needed, fold pled-get and leave in place for up to 15 minutes. Remove pledget, and throw away. Wash hands thoroughly.

To use pramoxine hemorrhoidal foam, wash hands first. Clean affected area with mild soap and warm water. Rinse thoroughly. Gently dry by patting or blotting with a clean, soft cloth or tissue. Shake the foam container. Squirt a small amount of foam onto a clean tissue and apply to affected rectal area. Wash hands thoroughly.

Pravastatin
prav-i-sta′tin
(Pravachol)
Do not confuse pravastatin with Prevacid, or Pravachol with propranolol.

CATEGORY AND SCHEDULE
Pregnancy Risk Category: X

CLASSIFICATION
Antihyperlipidemics, HMG CoA reductase inhibitors

MECHANISM OF ACTION
An HMG-CoA reductase inhibitor that interferes with cholesterol biosynthesis by preventing the conversion of HMG-CoA reductase to mevalonate, a precursor to choles-terol. *Therapeutic Effect:* Lowers serum LDL and VLDL cholesterol and plasma triglyceride levels; increases serum HDL concentration.

PHARMACOKINETICS
Poorly absorbed from the GI tract. Protein binding: 50%. Metabolized in the liver (minimal active metabo-lites). Primarily excreted in feces via the biliary system. Not removed by hemodialysis. **Half-life:** 2.7 hr.

AVAILABILITY
Tablets: 10 mg, 20 mg, 40 mg, 80 mg.

INDICATIONS AND DOSAGES
▶ **Hyperlipidemia, primary and secondary prevention of cardiovascular events in patient with elevated cholesterol levels**
PO
Adults, Elderly. Initially, 40 mg/day. Titrate to desired response. Range: 10-80 mg/day.
Children 14-18 yr. 40 mg/day.
Children 8-13 yr. 20 mg/day.
▶ **Dosage in hepatic and renal impairment**
For adults, give 10 mg/day initially. Titrate to desired response.

CONTRAINDICATIONS
Active hepatic disease or unexplained, persistent elevations of liver function test results

INTERACTIONS
Drug
Cyclosporine, erythromycin, gemfibrozil, immunosuppressants, niacin: Increases the risk of acute renal failure and rhabdomyolysis.
Herbal
None known.
Food
None known.

DIAGNOSTIC TEST EFFECTS
May increase serum CK and transaminase concentrations.

SIDE EFFECTS
Pravastatin is generally well tolerated. Side effects are usually mild and transient.
Occasional (7%-4%)
Nausea, vomiting, diarrhea, constipation, abdominal pain, headache, rhinitis, rash, pruritus
Rare (3%-2%)
Heartburn, myalgia, dizziness, cough, fatigue, flu-like symptoms

SERIOUS REACTIONS
• Malignancy and cataracts may occur.
• Hypersensitivity occurs rarely.

PRECAUTIONS & CONSIDERATIONS
Caution is warranted with history of hepatic disease, severe electrolyte, endocrine, and metabolic disorders and in those who consume a substantial amount of alcohol. Withholding or discontinuing pravastatin may be necessary when the person is at risk for renal failure secondary to rhabdomyolysis. It is unknown if pravastatin is distributed in breast milk; because there is risk of serious adverse reactions in breast-feeding infants, pravastatin is contraindicated during lactation. Safety and efficacy of pravastatin have not been established in children. No age-related precautions have been noted in the elderly.

Dizziness and headache may occur. Tasks that require mental alertness or motor skills should be avoided until response to the drug is established. Notify the physician of muscle weakness, myalgia, severe gastric upset, or rash. Pattern of daily bowel activity and stool consistency should be assessed. Serum lipid cholesterol and triglyceride levels and hepatic function should be checked at baseline and periodically during treatment.
Administration
! Before the patient begins pravastatin therapy, he or she should be on a standard cholesterol-lowering diet for a minimum of 3 to 6 months. The patient should continue the diet throughout pravastatin therapy.

Take pravastatin without regard to meals and administer in the evening.

P

Praziquantel
pray-zih-kwon-tel
(Biltricide)

CATEGORY AND SCHEDULE
Pregnancy Risk Category: B

CLASSIFICATION
Antihelmintics

MECHANISM OF ACTION
An antihelmintic that increases cell permeability in susceptible helminths resulting in loss of intracellular calcium, massive contractions and paralysis of their musculature, followed by attachment of phagocytes to the parasites. *Therapeutic Effect:* Vermicidal. Dislodges the dead and dying worms.

PHARMACOKINETICS
Well absorbed from gastrointestinal (GI) tract. Protein binding: 80%. Widely distributed including CSF. Metabolized in liver. Primarily excreted in urine. Not removed by hemodialysis. **Half-life:** 4-5 hr.

AVAILABILITY
Tablets: 600 mg (Biltricide).

INDICATIONS AND DOSAGES
▸ **Schistosomiasis**
PO
Adults, Elderly. 3 doses of 20 mg/kg as 1 day treatment. Do not give doses less than 4 hours or more than 6 hours apart.
▸ **Clonorchiasis/opisthorchiasis**
PO
Adults, Elderly. 3 doses of 25 mg/kg as 1 day treatment.

CONTRAINDICATIONS
Ocular cysticercosis, hypersensitivity to praziquantel or any component of the formulation

INTERACTIONS
Drug
Albendazole: May increase risk of albendazole adverse effects.
Carbamazepine: May decrease praziquantel effectiveness.
Cimetidine: May increase praziquantel concentrations.
Phenytoin, fosphenytoin: May decrease praziquantel effectiveness.
Herbal
None known.
Food
None known.

DIAGNOSTIC TEST EFFECTS
None known.

▧ IV INCOMPATIBILITIES
None known.
▧ **IV Compatibilities**
None known.

SIDE EFFECTS
Frequent
Headache, dizziness, malaise, abdominal pain
Occasional
Anorexia, vomiting, diarrhea, severe cramping abdominal pain may occur within 1 hour of administration w/fever, sweating, bloody stools
Rare
Giddiness, urticaria

SERIOUS REACTIONS
• Overdose should be treated with fast-acting laxative.

PRECAUTIONS & CONSIDERATIONS
Caution should be used with severe liver impairment and cardiac irregularities. It is unknown if praziquantel is distributed in breast milk.

Safety and efficacy have not been established in children. There are no age-related precautions noted in the elderly.

Storage

Store at room temperature.

Administration

Doses should not be spaced not less than four and not more than 6 hours apart. Tablets are scored and may be broken for dosage adjustment. If iron supplements are ordered, continue as directed which may be up to 6 months post therapy.

Prazosin

pra'zoe-sin

(Minipress, Prasig [AUS], Pratisol [AUS], Pressin [AUS])

CATEGORY AND SCHEDULE

Pregnancy Risk Category: C

CLASSIFICATION

Antiadrenergics, alpha blocking, peripheral

MECHANISM OF ACTION

An antidote, antihypertensive, and vasodilator that selectively blocks alpha$_1$-adrenergic receptors, decreasing peripheral vascular resistance. *Therapeutic Effect:* Produces vasodilation of veins and arterioles, decreases total peripheral resistance, and relaxes smooth muscle in bladder neck and prostate.

AVAILABILITY

Capsules: 1 mg, 2 mg, 5 mg.

INDICATIONS AND DOSAGES

▸ **Mild to moderate hypertension**

PO

Adults, Elderly. Initially, 1 mg 2-3 times a day. Maintenance: 3-15 mg/day in divided doses. Maximum: 20 mg/day.

Children. 5 mcg/kg/dose q6hr. Gradually increase up to 25 mcg/kg/dose.

OFF-LABEL USES

Treatment of benign prostate hyperplasia, CHF, ergot alkaloid toxicity, pheochromocytoma, Raynaud's phenomenon

CONTRAINDICATIONS

None known.

INTERACTIONS

Drug

Estrogen, NSAIDs, other sympathomimetics: May decrease the effects of prazosin.

Hypotension-producing medications, such as antihypertensives and diuretics: May increase the effects of prazosin.

Herbal

Licorice: Causes sodium and water retention and potassium loss.

Food

None known.

DIAGNOSTIC TEST EFFECTS

None known.

SIDE EFFECTS

Frequent (10%-7%)

Dizziness, somnolence, headache, asthenia (loss of strength, energy)

Occasional (5%-4%)

Palpitations, nausea, dry mouth, nervousness

Rare (less than 1%)

Angina, urinary urgency

SERIOUS REACTIONS

• First-dose syncope (hypotension with sudden loss of consciousness)

P

may occur 30 to 90 minutes following initial dose of more than 2 mg, a too rapid increase in dosage, or addition of another antihypertensive agent to therapy. First-dose syncope may be preceded by tachycardia (pulse rate of 120-160 beats/minute).

PRECAUTIONS & CONSIDERATIONS

Caution is warranted with chronic renal failure and impaired hepatic function. Caution should be used when driving or operating machinery. Tasks that require mental alertness or motor skills should be avoided until response to the drug is established. Dizziness, lightheadedness, and fainting may occur. Rise slowly from a lying to a sitting position and permit legs to dangle momentarily before standing to avoid the hypotensive effect. Notify the physician if dizziness or palpitations become bothersome. B/P and pulse should be obtained immediately before each dose, and every 15 to 30 minutes thereafter until B/P is stabilized. Be alert for fluctuations in B/P. Pattern of daily bowel activity and stool consistency should also be assessed.

Administration

Take prazosin without regard to food. Take the first dose at bedtime to minimize the risk of fainting from first-dose syncope.

Prednisolone
pred-niss′oh-lone
(AK-Pred, AK-Tate [CAN], Inflamase Forte, Inflamase Mild, Minims-Prednisolone [CAN], Novo-Prednisolone [CAN], Orapred, Pediapred, Pred Forte, Pred Mild, Prelone, Solone [AUS])
Do not confuse prednisolone with prednisone or Primidone.

CATEGORY AND SCHEDULE
Pregnancy Risk Category: C (D if used in first trimester)

CLASSIFICATION
Corticosteroids

MECHANISM OF ACTION
An adrenocortical steroid that inhibits accumulation of inflammatory cells at inflammation sites, phagocytosis, lysosomal enzyme release and synthesis, and release of mediators of inflammation. *Therapeutic Effect:* Prevents or suppresses cell-mediated immune reactions. Decreases or prevents tissue response to inflammatory process.

AVAILABILITY
Oral Solution (Pediapred): 6.7 mg/5 ml.
Oral Solution (Orapred): 20 mg/5 ml.
Tablets: 5 mg.
Syrup (Prelone): 5 mg/5 ml.
Ophthalmic Solution (Inflamase Mild): 0.125%.
Ophthalmic Solution (AK-Pred, Inflamase Forte): 1%.
Ophthalmic Suspension (Pred Mild): 0.12%.

Ophthalmic Suspension (Pred Forte): 1%.

INDICATIONS AND DOSAGES
▶ **Substitution therapy for deficiency states: acute or chronic adrenal insufficiency, congenital adrenal hyperplasia, and adrenal insufficiency secondary to pituitary insufficiency; nonendocrine disorders: arthritis; rheumatic carditis; allergic, collagen, intestinal tract, liver, ocular, renal, skin diseases; bronchial asthma; cerebral edema; malignancies**
PO
Adults, Elderly. 5-60 mg/day in divided doses.
Children. 0.1-2 mg/kg/day in 1-4 divided doses.
▶ **Treatment of conjuctivitis and corneal injury**
OPHTHALMIC
Adults, Elderly. 1-2 drops every hr during day and q2hr during night. After response, decrease dosage to 1 drop q4hr, then 1 drop 3-4 times a day.

CONTRAINDICATIONS
Acute superficial herpes simplex keratitis, systemic fungal infections, varicella

INTERACTIONS
Drug
Amphotericin: May increase hypokalemia.
Digoxin: May increase the risk of digoxin toxicity caused by hypokalemia
Diuretics, insulin, oral hypoglycemics, potassium supplements: May decrease the effects of these drugs.
Hepatic enzyme inducers: May decrease the effects of prednisolone.
Live virus vaccines: May decrease the patient's antibody response to vaccine, increase vaccine side effects, and potentiate virus replication.
Herbal
None known.
Food
None known.

DIAGNOSTIC TEST EFFECTS
May increase blood glucose and serum lipid, amylase, and sodium levels. May decrease serum calcium, potassium, and thyroxine levels.

SIDE EFFECTS
Frequent
Insomnia, heartburn, nervousness, abdominal distention, increased sweating, acne, mood swings, increased appetite, facial flushing, delayed wound healing, increased susceptibility to infection, diarrhea or constipation
Occasional
Headache, edema, change in skin color, frequent urination
Rare
Tachycardia, allergic reaction (such as rash and hives), psychological changes, hallucinations, depression Ophthalmic: stinging or burning, posterior subcapsular cataracts

SERIOUS REACTIONS
• Long-term therapy may cause hypocalcemia, hypokalemia, muscle wasting (especially in the arms and legs), osteoporosis, spontaneous fractures, amenorrhea, cataracts, glaucoma, peptic ulcer disease, and CHF.
• Abruptly withdrawing the drug after long-term therapy may cause anorexia, nausea, fever, headache, severe or sudden joint pain, rebound inflammation, fatigue, weakness, lethargy, dizziness, and orthostatic hypotension.
• Suddenly discontinuing prednisolone may be fatal.

P

PRECAUTIONS & CONSIDERATIONS

Caution is warranted with cirrhosis, CHF, diabetes mellitus, hypertension, hypothyroidism, myasthenia gravis, ocular herpes simplex, osteoporosis, peptic ulcer disease, thromboembolic disorders, and ulcerative colitis. Monitor growth and development of children receiving long-term steroid therapy. Avoid alcohol and limit caffeine intake during therapy.

Mood swings, ranging from euphoria to depression, may occur. Notify the physician of fever, muscle aches, sore throat, and sudden weight gain or swelling. The mouth should be assessed daily for signs and symptoms of candidal infection, such as white patches and painful mucous membranes and tongue. Blood glucose level, intake and output, B/P, serum electrolyte levels, pattern of daily bowel activity, height, and weight should be monitored before and during therapy. Be alert to signs and symptoms of infection caused by reduced immune response, including fever, sore throat, and vague symptoms.

Administration

Shake ophthalmic preparation well before using. Instill drops into conjunctival sac, as prescribed. Avoid touching the applicator tip to the conjunctiva to avoid contamination. Do not abruptly discontinue the drug without physician approval.

Prednisone

pred'ni-sone
(Apo-Prednisone [CAN], Deltasone, Panafcort [AUS], Prednisone Intensol, Sone [AUS], Sterapred, Sterapred DS, Winpred [CAN])

Do not confuse prednisone with prednisolone or Primidone.

CATEGORY AND SCHEDULE

Pregnancy Risk Category: C, D if used in first trimester

CLASSIFICATION

Corticosteroids

MECHANISM OF ACTION

An adrenocortical steroid that inhibits accumulation of inflammatory cells at inflammation sites, phagocytosis, lysosomal enzyme release and synthesis, and release of mediators of inflammation. *Therapeutic Effect:* Prevents or suppresses cell-mediated immune reactions. Decreases or prevents tissue response to inflammatory process.

PHARMACOKINETICS

Well absorbed from the GI tract. Protein binding: 70%-90%. Widely distributed. Metabolized in the liver and converted to prednisolone. Primarily excreted in urine. Not removed by hemodialysis. **Half-life:** 3.4-3.8 hr.

AVAILABILITY

*Oral Concentrate (Prednisone Intensol):*5 mg/ml.
Oral Solution: 5 mg/5 ml.
Tablets (Deltasone): 2.5 mg, 5 mg, 10 mg, 20 mg, 50 mg.
Tablets (Sterapred): 5 mg, 10 mg.

INDICATIONS AND DOSAGES
▶ **Substitution therapy in deficiency states: acute or chronic adrenal insufficiency, congenital adrenal hyperplasia, and adrenal insufficiency secondary to pituitary insufficiency; nonendocrine disorders: arthritis; rheumatic carditis; allergic, collagen, intestinal tract, liver, ocular, renal, skin diseases; bronchial asthma; cerebral edema; malignancies**
PO
Adults, Elderly. 5-60 mg/day in divided doses.
Children. 0.05-2 mg/kg/day in 1-4 divided doses.

CONTRAINDICATIONS
Acute superficial herpes simplex keratitis, systemic fungal infections, varicella

INTERACTIONS
Drug
Amphotericin: May increase hypokalemia.
Digoxin: May increase the risk of digoxin toxicity caused by hypokalemia
Diuretics, insulin, oral hypoglycemics, potassium supplements: May decrease the effects of these drugs.
Hepatic enzyme inducers: May decrease the effects of prednisone.
Live virus vaccines: May decrease the patient's antibody response to vaccine, increase vaccine side effects, and potentiate virus replication.
Herbal
None known.
Food
None known.

DIAGNOSTIC TEST EFFECTS
May increase blood glucose and serum lipid, amylase, and sodium levels.
May decrease serum calcium, potassium, and thyroxine levels.

SIDE EFFECTS
Frequent
Insomnia, heartburn, nervousness, abdominal distention, increased sweating, acne, mood swings, increased appetite, facial flushing, delayed wound healing, increased susceptibility to infection, diarrhea or constipation
Occasional
Headache, edema, change in skin color, frequent urination
Rare
Tachycardia, allergic reaction (including rash and hives), psychological changes, hallucinations, depression

SERIOUS REACTIONS
• Long-term therapy may cause muscle wasting in the arms and legs, osteoporosis, spontaneous fractures, amenorrhea, cataracts, glaucoma, peptic ulcer disease, and CHF.
• Abruptly withdrawing the drug following long-term therapy may cause anorexia, nausea, fever, headache, sudden or severe joint pain, rebound inflammation, fatigue, weakness, lethargy, dizziness, and orthostatic hypotension.
• Suddenly discontinuing prednisone may be fatal.

PRECAUTIONS & CONSIDERATIONS
Caution is warranted with CHF, cirrhosis, hypertension, hyperthyroidism, myasthenia gravis, ocular herpes simplex. Prednisone crosses the placenta and is distributed in breast milk. Prolonged prednisone use in the first trimester of pregnancy causes cleft palate in the neonate. Prolonged treatment or high dosages may decrease the cortisol secretion and short-term growth rate in children. The elderly may be more susceptible to developing hypertension

or osteoporosis. Never give prednisone with live virus vaccines, such as smallpox vaccine; avoid exposure to chickenpox or measles. Dentist or other physician should be informed of prednisone therapy if taken within the past 12 months.

Mood swings, ranging from euphoria to depression, may occur. Notify the physician of fever, muscle aches, sore throat, and sudden weight gain or swelling. Initially, tuberculosis skin test, X-rays, and EKG, should be checked. Blood glucose level, intake and output, B/P, serum electrolyte levels, height, and weight should be monitored before and during therapy. Be alert to signs and symptoms of infection caused by reduced immune response, including fever, sore throat, and vague symptoms. The mouth should be assessed daily for signs and symptoms of candidal infection, such as white patches and painful mucous membranes and tongue.

Administration

Take prednisone without regard to meals; give with food if GI upset occurs. Take single doses before 9 AM; give multiple doses at evenly spaced intervals. Do not abruptly discontinue prednisone without physician approval.

Primaquine
prim-a-kween
(Primacin [AUS])
Do not confuse with primidone.

CATEGORY AND SCHEDULE
Pregnancy Risk Category: C

CLASSIFICATION
Antiprotozoals

MECHANISM OF ACTION
An antimalarial and antirheumatic that eliminates tissue exoerythrocytic forms of Plasmodium falciparum. Disrupts mitochondria and binds to DNA. *Therapeutic Effect:* Inhibits parasite growth.

PHARMACOKINETICS
Well absorbed. Metabolized in the liver to the active metabolite, carboxyprimaquine. Excreted in the urine in small amounts as unchanged drug. **Half-life:** 4-6 hr

AVAILABILITY
Tablets: 26.3 mg (Primaquine phosphate).

INDICATIONS AND DOSAGES
▶ **Treatment of malaria**
PO
Adults, Elderly. 15 mg base daily for 14 days.
Children. 0.3 mg base/kg/wk once daily for 14 days.
Malaria prophylaxis
Adults, Elderly. 30 mg base daily. Begin 1 day before departure and continue for 7 days after leaving malarious area.

CONTRAINDICATIONS
Concomitant medications which cause bone marrow suppression, rheumatoid arthritis, lupus erythematosus, glucose-6-phosphate dehydrogenase (G-6-PD) deficiency, pregnancy, hypersensitivity to primaquine or any of its components

INTERACTIONS
Drug
Aurothioglucose: May increase risk of blood dyscrasias.
Levomethadyl: May increase risk of cardiotoxicity (QT prolongation, torsades de pointes, cardiac arrest).

Herbal
None known.
Food
None known.

DIAGNOSTIC TEST EFFECTS
None known.

SIDE EFFECTS
Frequent
Abdominal pain, nausea, vomiting
Rare
Leukopenia, hemolytic anemia, methemoglobinemia

SERIOUS REACTIONS
• Leukopenia, hemolytic anemia, methemoglobinemia occur rarely.
• Overdosage include symptoms of abdominal cramps, vomiting, burning epigastric distress, central nervous system and cardiovascular disturbances, cyanosis, methemoglobinemia, moderate leukocytosis or leukopenia, and anemia.
• Acute hemolysis occurs, but patients recover completely if the dosage is discontinued.

PRECAUTIONS & CONSIDERATIONS
Caution is warranted with erythrocytic G6PD deficiency or nicotinamide adenine dinucleotide (NADH) methemoglobin reductase deficiency, a family personal history of favism, and a previous idiosyncrasy to primaquine phosphate (as manifested by hemolytic anemia, methemoglobinemia, or leukopenia). Primaquine crosses the placenta but it is unknown if it is distributed in breast milk. Children are especially susceptible to primaquine's fatal effects. Signs suggestive of hemolytic anemia such as darkening of urine, marked fall of hemoglobin or erythrocytic count should be reported and primaquine should be discontinued promptly.

Administration
26.3 mg primaquine = 15 mg base. The dose of 1 tablet (15 mg base) daily for 14 days should not be exceeded. Take dose with food.

Primidone
pri'mi-done
(Apo-Primidone [CAN], Mysoline)
Do not confuse primidone with prednisone.

CATEGORY AND SCHEDULE
Pregnancy Risk Category: D

CLASSIFICATION
Anticonvulsants

MECHANISM OF ACTION
A barbiturate that decreases motor activity from electrical and chemical stimulation and stabilizes the seizure threshold against hyperexcitability. *Therapeutic Effect:* Reduces seizure activity.

AVAILABILITY
Tablets: 50 mg, 250 mg.

INDICATIONS AND DOSAGES
▶ **Seizure control**
PO
Adults, Elderly, Children 8 yr and older. 125-150 mg/day at bedtime. May increase by 125-250 mg/day every 3-7 days. Maximum: 2 g/day.
Children younger than 8 yr. Initially, 50-125 mg/day at bedtime. May increase by 50-125 mg/day every 3-7 days. Usual dose: 10-25 mg/kg/day in divided doses.
Neonates. 12-20 mg/kg/day in divided doses.

OFF-LABEL USES
Treatment of essential tremor

CONTRAINDICATIONS
History of bronchopneumonia, porphyria

INTERACTIONS
Drug
Alcohol, other CNS depressants: May increase the effects of primidone.
Carbamazepine: May increase the metabolism of carbamazepine.
Digoxin, glucocorticoids, metronidazole, oral anticoagulants, quinidine, tricyclic antidepressants: May decrease the effects of these drugs.
Valproic acid: Increases the blood concentration and risk of toxicity of primidone.
Herbal
None known.
Food
None known.

DIAGNOSTIC TEST EFFECTS
May decrease serum bilirubin level. Therapeutic serum level is 4-12 mcg/ml; toxic serum level is greater than 12 mcg/ml.

SIDE EFFECTS
Frequent
Ataxia, dizziness
Occasional
Anorexia, drowsiness, mental changes, nausea, vomiting, paradoxical excitement
Rare
Rash

SERIOUS REACTIONS
• Abrupt withdrawal after prolonged therapy may produce effects ranging from increased dreaming, nightmares, insomnia, tremor, diaphoresis, and vomiting to hallucinations, delirium, seizures, and status epilepticus.

• Skin eruptions may be a sign of a hypersensitivity reaction.
• Blood dyscrasias, hepatic disease, and hypocalcemia occur rarely.
• Overdose produces cold or clammy skin, hypothermia, and severe CNS depression, followed by high fever and coma.

PRECAUTIONS & CONSIDERATIONS
Caution is warranted with hepatic and renal impairment. Dizziness may occur, so change positions slowly—from recumbent to sitting position before standing, and alcohol and tasks requiring mental alertness or motor skills should be avoided. CBC, neurologic status (including duration, frequency, and severity of seizures) and serum concentrations of primidone should be assessed before and during treatment.
Administration
Administer primidone at the same time each day. Do not abruptly discontinue primidone after long-term use because this may precipitate seizures. Strict maintenance of drug therapy is essential for seizure control. Be aware that the therapeutic serum drug level is 4-12 mcg/ml; the toxic serum drug level is greater than 12 mcg/ml.

Probenecid

proe-ben'e-sid
(Benuryl [CAN], Pro-cid [AUS])
**Do not confuse probenecid
with procainamide.**

CATEGORY AND SCHEDULE
Pregnancy Risk Category: C

CLASSIFICATION
Antigout agents, uricosurics

MECHANISM OF ACTION
A uricosuric that competitively
inhibits reabsorption of uric acid
at the proximal convoluted tubule.
Also, inhibits renal tubular secretion
of weak organic acids, such as
penicillins. *Therapeutic Effect:*
Promotes uric acid excretion,
reduces serum uric acid level, and
increases plasma levels of penicillins
and cephalosporins.

AVAILABILITY
Tablets: 500 mg.

INDICATIONS AND DOSAGES
▶ **Gout**
PO
Adults, Elderly. Initially, 250 mg
twice a day for 1 wk; then 500 mg
twice a day. May increase by 500 mg
q4wk. Maximum: 2-3 g/day.
Maintenance: Dosage that maintains
normal uric acid level.
▶ **As adjunct to penicillin or
cephalosporin therapy to prolong
antibiotic plasma levels**
PO
Adults, Elderly. 2 g/day in divided
doses.
Children weighing more than 50 kg.
Receive adult dosage.

Children 2-14 yr. Initially,
25 mg/kg. Maintenance:
40 mg/kg/day in 4 divided doses.
▶ **Gonorrhea**
PO
Adults, Elderly. 1 g 30 min before
penicillin, ampicillin, or amoxicillin.

CONTRAINDICATIONS
Blood dyscrasias, children younger
than 2 years, concurrent high-dose
aspirin therapy, severe renal impairment, uric acid calculi

INTERACTIONS
Drug
Alcohol: May increase serum urate
level.
Antineoplastics: May increase the
risk of uric acid nephropathy.
**Cephalosporins, methotrexate,
nitrofurantoin, NSAIDs, peni-
cillins, zidovudine:** May increase
blood concentrations of these
drugs.
Heparin: May increase and prolong
the effects of heparin.
Salicylates: May decrease uricosuric
effect.
Herbal
None known.
Food
None known.

DIAGNOSTIC TEST EFFECTS
May inhibit renal excretion of serum
PSP (phenolsulfonphthalein),
17-ketosteroids, and BSP (sulfobro-
mophthalein).

SIDE EFFECTS
Frequent (10%-6%)
Headache, anorexia, nausea,
vomiting
Occasional (5%-1%)
Lower back or side pain, rash,
hives, itching, dizziness, flushed
face, frequent urge to urinate,
gingivitis

P

SERIOUS REACTIONS

• Severe hypersensitivity reactions, including anaphylaxis, occur rarely and usually within a few hours after administration following previous use. If severe hypersensitivity reactions develop, discontinue the drug immediately and contact the physician.

• Pruritic maculopapular rash, possibly accompanied by malaise, fever, chills, arthralgia, nausea, vomiting, leukopenia, and aplastic anemias should be considered a toxic reaction.

PRECAUTIONS & CONSIDERATIONS

Caution is warranted with hematuria, peptic ulcer disease, and renal colic. Avoid alcohol and large doses of aspirin or other salicylates. Limit intake of high purine foods, such as fish and organ meats.

High fluid intake (3000 ml/day) should be encouraged; intake and output should be monitored; output should be at least 2000 ml/day. CBC, serum uric acid level, and urine for cloudiness, odor, and unusual color should also be monitored. Signs and symptoms of a therapeutic response, including improved joint range of motion and reduced joint tenderness, redness, and swelling, should be evaluated.

Storage

Store at room temperature.

Administration

! Do not start giving probenecid until acute gouty attack has subsided; continue drug if acute attack occurs during therapy. Probenecid should not be used in those with renal impairment.

Give probenecid orally with or immediately after meals or milk. Drink at least 6 to 8 eight-ounce glasses of fluid each day to prevent renal calculi. It may take more than 1 week for the full therapeutic effect of the drug to be evident.

Procainamide

proe-kane′a-mide
(Apo-Primidone [CAN], Mysoline)
Do not confuse primidone with prednisone.

CATEGORY AND SCHEDULE

Pregnancy Risk Category: D

CLASSIFICATION

Antiarrhythmics, class IA

MECHANISM OF ACTION

A barbiturate that decreases motor activity from electrical and chemical stimulation and stabilizes the seizure threshold against hyperexcitability. *Therapeutic Effect:* Reduces seizure activity.

AVAILABILITY

Tablets: 50 mg, 250 mg.

INDICATIONS AND DOSAGES

▸ **Seizure control**

PO

Adults, Elderly, Children 8 yr and older. 125-150 mg/day at bedtime. May increase by 125-250 mg/day every 3-7 days. Maximum: 2 g/day.

Children younger than 8 yr. Initially, 50-125 mg/day at bedtime. May increase by 50-125 mg/day every 3-7 days. Usual dose: 10-25 mg/kg/day in divided doses.

Neonates. 12-20 mg/kg/day in divided doses.

OFF-LABEL USES

Treatment of essential tremor

CONTRAINDICATIONS

History of bronchopneumonia, porphyria

INTERACTIONS
Drug
Alcohol, other CNS depressants:
May increase the effects of primidone.
Carbamazepine: May increase the
metabolism of carbamazepine.
**Digoxin, glucocorticoids, metron-
idazole, oral anticoagulants, quini-
dine, tricyclic antidepressants:**
May decrease the effects of these
drugs.
Valproic acid: Increases the blood
concentration and risk of toxicity of
primidone.
Herbal
None known.
Food
None known.

DIAGNOSTIC TEST EFFECTS
May decrease serum bilirubin
level. Therapeutic serum level is
4-12 mcg/ml; toxic serum level is
greater than 12 mcg/ml.

SIDE EFFECTS
Frequent
Ataxia, dizziness
Occasional
Anorexia, drowsiness, mental
changes, nausea, vomiting, paradoxi-
cal excitement
Rare
Rash

SERIOUS REACTIONS
• Abrupt withdrawal after
prolonged therapy may produce
effects ranging from increased
dreaming, nightmares, insomnia,
tremor, diaphoresis, and vomiting to
hallucinations, delirium, seizures,
and status epilepticus.
• Skin eruptions may be a sign of a
hypersensitivity reaction.
• Blood dyscrasias, hepatic disease,
and hypocalcemia occur rarely.
• Overdose produces cold or
clammy skin, hypothermia, and
severe CNS depression, followed by
high fever and coma.

PRECAUTIONS & CONSIDERATIONS
Caution is warranted with bundle-
branch block, congestive heart failure
(CHF), liver and renal impairment,
marked AV-conduction disturbances,
severe digoxin toxicity, and supraventricular tachyarrhythmias. Be aware
that procainamide crosses the placenta
and it is unknown if procainamide is
distributed in breast milk. There are
no age-related precautions noted in
children. The elderly are more susceptible to the drug's hypotensive effect.
In the elderly, age-related renal
impairment may require dosage
adjustment. Be aware that cardiotoxic
effects occur most commonly with
IV administration, observed as
conduction changes (50% widening
of QRS complex, frequent ventricular
premature contractions, ventricular
tachycardia, complete atrioventricular [AV] block); prolonged PR and
QT intervals, flattened T waves occur
less frequently. Nasal decongestants
or over-the-counter (OTC) cold preparations, especially those containing
stimulants, should be avoided without
consulting the physician for approval.
Alcohol and salt consumption should
be restricted while taking
procainamide.
  GI upset, headache, dizziness, and
joint pain may occur. Notify the
physician if fever, joint pain or stiffness, and signs of upper respiratory
infection occur. EKG for cardiac
changes, particularly widening of
QRS and prolongation of PR and QT
intervals, should be monitored. Pulse,
pattern of daily bowel activity and
stool consistency, skin for hypertensive reaction, intake and output, serum
electrolyte levels, including chloride,
potassium, and sodium, and B/P
should be assessed during therapy.

P

Storage
When diluted with D$_5$W, solution is stable for up to 24 hours at room temperature or for 7 days if refrigerated.

Administration
! Know that procainamide dosage and the interval of administration are individualized based on age, clinical response, renal function, and underlying myocardial disease. Also be aware that extended-release tablets are used for maintenance therapy.

Do not crush or break sustained-release tablets.

! May give procainamide by IM injection, IV push, or IV infusion. Therapeutic serum level is 4 to 8 mcg/ml and a toxic serum level is greater than 10 mcg/ml.

Solution normally appears clear, colorless to light yellow. Discard if solution darkens or appears discolored or if precipitate forms. For IV push, dilute with 5 to 10 ml D$_5$W. For initial loading IV infusion, add 1 g to 50 ml D$_5$W to provide a concentration of 20 mg/ml. For IV infusion, add 1 g to 250-500 ml D$_5$W to provide concentration of 2 to 4 mg/ml. Know that the maximum concentration is 4 g/250 ml. For IV push, with patient in the supine position, administer at a rate not exceeding 25 to 50 mg/min. For initial loading infusion, infuse 1 ml/min for up to 25 to 30 minutes. For IV infusion, infuse at 1 to 3 ml/min. Check B/P every 5 to 10 minutes during infusion. If a fall in B/P exceeds 15 mm Hg, discontinue drug and contact physician. Monitor EKG for cardiac changes, particularly widening of QRS and prolongation of PR and QT intervals. Notify physician of any significant interval changes. Continuously monitor B/P and EKG during IV administration.

Continuously adjust the rate of infusion to eliminate arrhythmias.

Procaine
proe′kane
(Novocain, Mericaine)

CATEGORY AND SCHEDULE
Pregnancy Risk Category: C

CLASSIFICATION
Anesthetics, local

MECHANISM OF ACTION
Procaine causes a reversible blockade of nerve conduction by decreasing nerve membrane permeability to sodium. *Therapeutic Effect:* Local anesthesia.

PHARMACOKINETICS
Highly plasma protein-bound and distributed to all body tissues. Excreted in the urine (80%). **Half-life:** 40 ± 9 seconds in adults, 84 ± 30 seconds in neonates.

AVAILABILITY
Solution: 0.25%, 0.5%, 10% (Novocaine)

INDICATIONS AND DOSAGES
▸ **Spinal anesthesia**
INTRATHECAL
Adults. 0.5-1 ml of a 10% solution (50-100 mg) mixed with an equal volume of diluent injected into the third or fourth lumber interspace (perineum and lower extremities). 2 ml of a 10% solution (200 mg) mixed with 1 ml of diluent injected into the second, third, or fourth interspace.

▸ **Infiltration anesthesia, dental anesthesia, control of severe pain (post-herpatic neuralgia, cancer pain, or burns)**

TOPICAL

Adults. A single dose of 350-600 mg using a 0.25% or 0.5% solution. Use 0.9% sodium chloride for dilution.

Children. 15 mg/kg of a 0.5% solution is the maximum recommended dose.

▸ **Peripheral or sympathetic nerve block (regional anesthesia)**

TOPICAL

Adults. Up to 200 ml of a 0.5% solution (1 g), 100 ml of a 1% solution (1 g), or 50 ml of a 2% solution (1 g). The 2% solution should only be used when a small volume of anesthetic is required.

OFF-LABEL USES
Severe pain

CONTRAINDICATIONS
Hypersensitivity to ester local anesthetics, sulfites, PABA, patients on anticoagulant therapy, and in patients with coagulopathy, infection, thrombocytopenia. Should not be given intraarterial, intrathecal, or intravenous.

INTERACTIONS
Drug

Local anesthetics: May cause a toxic additive effect.

Medications that cause QT prolongation: May cause additive cardiotoxic effects.

Cholinesterase inhibitors: Procaine may antagonize the effect of these medications.

Antihypertensives, nitrates: May experience additive hypotensive effects.

MAOIs: Increased risk of hypotension.

CNS depressants: May cause additive suppression.

Herbal
None known.

Food
None known.

DIAGNOSTIC TEST EFFECTS
None known.

SIDE EFFECTS
Frequent

Numbness or tingling of the face or mouth, pain at the injection site, dizziness, drowsiness, lightheadedness, nausea, vomiting, back pain, headache

Rare

Anxiety, restlessness, difficulty breathing, shortness of breath, seizures (convulsions), skin rash, itching (hives), slow irregular heartbeat (palpitations), swelling of the face or mouth, tremors, QT prolongation, PR prolongation, atrial fibrillation, sinus bradycardia, hypotension, angina, cardiovascular collapse, fecal or urinary incontinence, loss of perineal sensation and sexual function, persistent motor, sensory, and/or autonomic (sphincter control) deficit

SERIOUS REACTIONS
• Procaine-induced CNS toxicity usually presents with symptoms of stimulation such as anxiety, apprehension, restlessness, nervousness, disorientation, confusion, dizziness, blurred vision, tremor, nausea/vomiting, shivering, or seizures. Subsequently, depressive symptoms can occur including drowsiness, unconsciousness, and respiratory arrest.

• If higher concentrations are introduced into the blood stream, depression of cardiac excitability and contractility may cause AV block, ventricular arrhythmias, or cardiac arrest. CNS toxicity including

P

dizziness, tongue numbness, visual impairment and disturbances, and muscular twitching appear to occur before cardiotoxic effects.

! Procaine should be used with caution in patients that have asthma since there is the increased risk of anaphylactoid reactions including bronchospasm and status asthmaticus.

! Local anesthetics can cause varying degrees of maternal, fetal, and neonatal toxicities during labor and obstetric delivery. Fetal heart rate should be monitored as well as the presence of symptoms indicating fetal bradycardia, fetal acidosis, and maternal hypotension. Epidural procaine may cause decreased uterine contractility or maternal expulsion efforts and alter the forces of parturition.

! Unintentional fetal intracranial injection of procaine occurring during pudenal or paracervical block has been shown to lead to neonatal depression at birth and can lead to seizures within 6 hours as a result of high serum concentrations.

PRECAUTIONS & CONSIDERATIONS
Caution is warranted with cardiac disease, hyperthyroidism, or other endocrine disease. It is unknown if procaine crosses the placenta or is distributed in the breast milk. There are no age-related precautions noted in the elderly. A burning sensation may occur at the site of injection.
Administration
Dosage varies based on procedure, desired depth, and duration of anesthesia, desired muscle relaxation, vascularity of tissues, physical condition, and age of patient. Prior to instillation of anesthetic agent, withdraw plunger to ensure needle is not in artery or vein. Resuscitative

equipment should be available when local anesthetic is administered.

Procarbazine Hydrochloride
pro-kar′ba-zeen
(Matulane, Natulan [CAN])
Do not confuse procarbazine with dacarbazine.

CATEGORY AND SCHEDULE
Pregnancy Risk Category: D

CLASSIFICATION
Antineoplastics, miscellaneous

MECHANISM OF ACTION
A methylhydrazine derivative that inhibits DNA, RNA, and protein synthesis. May also directly damage DNA. Cell cycle-phase specific for S phase of cell division. *Therapeutic Effect:* Causes cell death.

AVAILABILITY
Capsules: 50 mg.

INDICATIONS AND DOSAGES
▸ **Advanced Hodgkin's disease**
PO
Adults, Elderly. Initially, 2-4 mg/kg/day as a single dose or in divided doses for 1 wk, then 4-6 mg/kg/day. Maintenance: 1-2 mg/kg/day.
Children. 50-100 mg/m²/day for 10-14 days of a 28-day cycle. Continue until maximum response occurs, leukocyte count falls below 4000/mm³, or platelet count falls below 100,000/mm³. Maintenance: 50 mg/m²/day.

OFF-LABEL USES
Treatment of lung carcinoma, malignant melanoma, multiple myeloma,

non-Hodgkin's lymphoma, polycythemia vera, primary brain tumors

CONTRAINDICATIONS
Myelosuppression

INTERACTIONS
Drug
Alcohol: May cause a disulfiram-
like reaction.
Anticholinergics, antihistamines:
May increase the anticholinergic
effects of these drugs.
Bone marrow depressants: May
increase myelosuppression.
**Buspirone, caffeine-containing
medications:** May increase B/P.
**Carbamazepine, cyclobenzaprine,
MAOIs, maprotiline:** May cause
hyperpyretic crisis, seizures, or
death.
CNS depressants: May increase
CNS depression.
Insulin, oral antidiabetics: May
increase the effects of these drugs.
Meperidine: May produce coma,
seizures, immediate excitation, rigidity, severe hypertension or hypotension, severe respiratory distress,
diaphoresis, and vascular collapse.
Sympathomimetics: May increase
cardiac stimulant and vasopressor
effects.
Tricyclic antidepressants: May
increase anticholinergic effects; may
cause seizures and hyperpyretic crisis.
Herbal
None known.
Food
Caffeine-containing beverages: May
increase B/P.

DIAGNOSTIC TEST EFFECTS
None known.

SIDE EFFECTS
Frequent
Severe nausea, vomiting, respiratory
disorders (cough, effusion), myalgia,

arthralgia, drowsiness, nervousness,
insomnia, nightmares, diaphoresis,
hallucinations, seizures
Occasional
Hoarseness, tachycardia, nystagmus,
retinal hemorrhage, photophobia,
photosensitivity, urinary frequency,
nocturia, hypotension, diarrhea, stomatitis, paraesthesia, unsteadiness,
confusion, decreased reflexes, foot
drop
Rare
Hypersensitivity reaction (dermatitis,
pruritus, rash, urticaria), hyperpigmentation, alopecia

SERIOUS REACTIONS
• Procarbazine's major toxic effects
are myelosuppression manifested as
hematologic toxicity (mainly
leukopenia, thrombocytopenia, and
anemia) and hepatotoxicity manifested as jaundice and ascites.
• UTIs may occur secondary to
leukopenia.

PRECAUTIONS & CONSIDERATIONS
Caution is warranted with hepatic and
renal impairment. Alcohol should be
avoided because it may cause nausea
and vomiting, sedation, severe
headache, and visual disturbances.
 Notify the physician if bleeding,
easy bruising, fever, or sore throat
occurs. WBC count with differential,
platelet count, and reticulocyte count,
bone marrow test results, urinalysis
results, BUN level, blood Hct and
Hgb levels, serum alkaline phosphatase, AST (SGOT), and ALT
(SGPT) levels should be monitored
before and periodically during
procarbazine therapy. Procarbazine
should be discontinued if stomatitis,
diarrhea, paraesthesia, neuropathy,
confusion, or a hypersensitivity reaction occurs, WBC count falls below
4000/mm^3, or if the platelet count
falls below 100,000/mm^3.

P

Administration
Administer procarbazine with food or fluids if the patient has severe GI side effects or difficulty swallowing.

Prochlorperazine

proe-klor-per'a-zeen
(Compazine, Stemetil [CAN], Stemzine [AUS])
Do not confuse prochlorper-azine with chlorpromazine, or Compazine with Copaxone.

CATEGORY AND SCHEDULE
Pregnancy Risk Category: C

CLASSIFICATION
Antiemetics/antivertigo, antipsy-chotics, phenothiazines

MECHANISM OF ACTION
A phenothiazine that acts centrally to inhibit or block dopamine receptors in the chemoreceptor trigger zone and peripherally to block the vagus nerve in the GI tract.
Therapeutic Effect: Relieves nausea and vomiting and improves psychotic conditions.

PHARMACOKINETICS

Route	Onset*	Peak	Duration
Tablets, oral solution	30-40 min	N/A	3-4 hr
Capsules (extended-release)	30-40 min	N/A	10-12 hr
Rectal	60 min	N/A	3-4 hr

*As an antiemetic

Variably absorbed after PO administration. Widely distributed.

Metabolized in the liver and GI mucosa. Primarily excreted in urine. Unknown if removed by hemodialysis. **Half-life:** 23 hr.

AVAILABILITY
Capsules (Extended-Release): 10 mg, 15 mg.
Oral solution: 5 mg/5 ml.
Tablets: 5 mg, 10 mg.
Suppositories: 2.5 mg, 5 mg, 25 mg.
Injection (Compazine): 5 mg/ml.

INDICATIONS AND DOSAGES
▶ **Nausea and vomiting**
PO
Adults, Elderly. 5-10 mg 3-4 times a day.
Children. 0.4 mg/kg/day in 3-4 divided doses.
PO (Extended-Release)
Adults, Elderly. 10 mg twice a day or 15 mg once a day.
IV
Adults, Elderly. 2.5-10 mg. May repeat q3-4hr.
Children. 0.1-0.15 mg/kg/dose q8-12hr. Maximum: 40 mg/day.
IM
Adults, Elderly. 5-10 mg q3-4hr.
Children. 0.1-0.15 mg/kg/dose q8-12hr. Maximum: 40 mg/day.
RECTAL
Adults, Elderly. 25 mg twice a day.
Children. 0.4 mg/kg/day in 3-4 divided doses.
▶ **Psychosis**
PO
Adults, Elderly. 5-10 mg 3-4 times a day. Maximum: 150 mg/day.
Children. 2.5 mg 2-3 times a day. Maximum: 25 mg for children 6-12 yr; 20 mg for children 2-5 yr.
IM
Adults, Elderly. 10-20 mg q4hr.
Children. 0.13 mg/kg/dose.

CONTRAINDICATIONS

Angle-closure glaucoma, CNS depression, coma, myelosuppression, severe cardiac or hepatic impairment, severe hypotension or hypertension

INTERACTIONS
Drug

Alcohol, other CNS depressants: May increase CNS and respiratory depression and the hypotensive effects of prochlorperazine.
Antihypertensives: May increase hypotension.
Antithyroid agents: May increase the risk of agranulocytosis.
Extrapyramidal symptom-producing medications: May increase extrapyramidal symptoms.
Levodopa: May decrease the effects of levodopa.
Lithium: May decrease the absorption of prochlorperazine and produce adverse neurologic effects.
MAOIs, tricyclic antidepressants: May increase the anticholinergic and sedative effects of prochlorperazine.
Herbal
None known.
Food
None known.

DIAGNOSTIC TEST EFFECTS
None known.

▓ IV INCOMPATIBILITIES
Atropine, furosemide (Lasix), midazolam (Versed)
▓ IV Compatibilities
Calcium gluconate, diphenhydramine (Benadryl), fentanyl, glycopyrrolate (Robinul), heparin, hydromorphone (Dilaudid), morphine, metoclopramide (Reglan), nalbuphine (Nubain), potassium chloride, promethazine (Phenergan), propofol (Diprivan)

SIDE EFFECTS
Frequent
Somnolence, hypotension, dizziness, fainting (commonly occurring after first dose, occasionally after subsequent doses, and rarely with oral form)
Occasional
Dry mouth, blurred vision, lethargy, constipation, diarrhea, myalgia, nasal congestion, peripheral edema, urine retention

SERIOUS REACTIONS

* Extrapyramidal symptoms appear to be dose-related and are divided into three categories: akathisia (marked by inability to sit still, tapping of feet), parkinsonian symptoms (including masklike face, tremors, shuffling gait, hypersalivation), and acute dystonias (such as torticollis, opisthotonos, and oculogyric crisis. A dystonic reaction may also produce diaphoresis or pallor.
* Tardive dyskinesia, manifested as tongue protrusion, puffing of the cheeks, and puckering of the mouth, is a rare reaction that may be irreversible.
* Abrupt withdrawal after long-term therapy may precipitate nausea, vomiting, gastritis, dizziness, and tremors.
* Blood dyscrasias, particularly agranulocytosis and mild leukopenia, may occur.
* Prochlorperazine use may lower the seizure threshold.

P

PRECAUTIONS & CONSIDERATIONS
Caution is warranted with Parkinson's disease, seizures, and in children younger than 2 years.

Prochlorperazine crosses the placenta and is distributed in breast milk. The safety and efficacy of this drug have not been established in children younger than 2 years or weighing less than 9 kg. A decreased prochlorperazine dosage is recommended for the elderly, who are more susceptible to the drug's sedative, anticholinergic, extrapyramidal, and hypotensive effects. Alcohol, barbiturates, and tasks that require mental alertness or motor skills should be avoided and limit caffeine consumption.

B/P, CBC for blood dyscrasias, and hydration status should be monitored. Be alert for extrapyramidal symptoms such as rapid tongue movement.

Storage
Store prochlorperazine at room temperature and protect from light. Solution should be clear or slightly yellow.

Administration
Take oral prochlorperazine without regard to food. Avoid skin contact with prochlorperazine oral solution because it may cause contact dermatitis.

For IV use, keep the person recumbent—head low and legs raised—for 30 to 60 minutes after drug administration, to minimize the drug's hypotensive effect. May give by IV push slowly over 5 to 10 minutes. May give by IV infusion over 30 minutes.

For rectal use, moisten the suppository with cold water before inserting it well into the rectum.

Procyclidine
proe-sye-kli-deen
(Kemadrin)

CATEGORY AND SCHEDULE
Pregnancy Risk Category: C

CLASSIFICATION
Anticholinergics, antiparkinson agents

MECHANISM OF ACTION
An anticholinergic agent that exerts an atropine-like action and produces an antispasmodic effect on smooth muscle, is a potent mydriatic, and inhibits salivation. *Therapeutic Effect:* Relieves symptoms of Parkinson's disease and drug-induced extrapyramidal symptoms.

PHARMACOKINETICS
Well absorbed from the gastrointestinal (GI) tract. Protein binding: extensive. Metabolized in liver—undergoes extensive first-pass effect. Primarily excreted in urine. Unknown if removed by hemodialysis. **Half-life:** 7.7-16.1 hr.

AVAILABILITY
Tablets: 5 mg (Kemadrin).

INDICATIONS AND DOSAGES
▸ **Drug-induced extrapyramidal reactions**
PO
Adults, Elderly. Initially, 2.5 mg 3 times/day. May increase by 2.5 mg daily as needed. Maintenance: 10-20 mg/day in divided doses 3 times/day.
▸ **Parkinson's disease**
PO
Adults, Elderly. Initially, 2.5 mg 3 times/day after meals. Maintenance: 2.5-5 mg/day in divided doses 3 times/day after meals.
▸ **Hepatic function impairment**
PO
Adults, Elderly. 2.5-5 mg/day in divided doses twice a day after meals

CONTRAINDICATIONS
Angle-closure glaucoma

INTERACTIONS
Drug
Alcohol: May increase sedation.

Amantadine, narcotic analgesics, phenothiazines, tricyclic antidepressants, quinidine, antihistamines: May increase anticholinergic effects.
Levodopa: May increase gastric degradation of levodopa and decrease the amount of levodopa absorbed by gastric emptying.
Paroxetine: May increase anticholinergic effects.
Herbal
Betel nut: May decrease anticholinergic effect of procyclidine.
Food
None known.

DIAGNOSTIC TEST EFFECTS
None known.

IV INCOMPATIBILITIES
None known.
IV Compatibilities
None known.

SIDE EFFECTS
Frequent
Blurred vision, mydriasis, disorientation, lightheadedness, nausea, vomiting, dry mouth, nose, throat, and lips

SERIOUS REACTIONS
• Overdosage may vary from severe anticholinergic effects, such as unsteadiness, severe drowsiness, severe dryness of mouth, nose, or throat, tachycardia, shortness of breath, and skin flushing.
• Also produces severe paradoxical reaction, marked by hallucinations, tremor, seizures, and toxic psychosis.

PRECAUTIONS & CONSIDERATIONS
Caution is necessary with hypotension, mental disorders, prostatic hypertrophy, tachycardia, and urinary retention. It is unknown if procyclidine is distributed in breast milk. Procyclidine is not indicated for

pediatric use. The elderly may exhibit increased sensitivity to procyclidine's anticholinergic effects. Tasks that require mental alertness or motor skills should be avoided. Alcoholic beverages should be avoided during procyclidine therapy.

Dizziness, drowsiness, and dry mouth are expected responses to the drug. These symptoms tend to diminish or disappear with continued therapy.
Administration
Take procyclidine after meals to minimize GI upset.

Progesterone
proe-jess'ter-one
(Crinone, Prochieve, Prometrium)

CATEGORY AND SCHEDULE
Pregnancy Risk Category: D

CLASSIFICATION
Contraceptives, hormones/hormone modifiers, progestins

P

MECHANISM OF ACTION
A natural steroid hormone that promotes mammary gland development and relaxes uterine smooth muscle. *Therapeutic Effect:* Decreases abnormal uterine bleeding; transforms endometrium from proliferative to secretory in an estrogen-primed endometrium.

AVAILABILITY
Capsules (Prometrium): 100 mg, 200 mg.
Injection: 50 mg/ml.
Vaginal Gel (Crinone, Prochieve): 4% (45 mg), 8% (90 mg).

INDICATIONS AND DOSAGES
▸ **Amenorrhea**
PO
Adults. 400 mg daily in evening for 10 days.
IM
Adults. 5-10 mg for 6-8 days. Withdrawal bleeding expected in 48-72 hr if ovarian activity produced proliferative endometrium.
VAGINAL
Adults. Apply 45 mg (4% gel) every other day for 6 or fewer doses.
▸ **Abnormal uterine bleeding**
IM
Adults. 5-10 mg for 6 days. When estrogen given concomitantly, begin progesterone after 2 wk of estrogen therapy; discontinue when menstrual flow begins.
▸ **Prevention of endometrial hyperplasia**
PO
Adults. 200 mg in evening for 12 days per 28-day cycle in combination with daily conjugated estrogen.
▸ **Infertility**
VAGINAL
Adults. 90 mg (8% gel) once a day (2 twice a day in women with partial or complete ovarian failure).

OFF-LABEL USES
Treatment of corpus luteum dysfunction

CONTRAINDICATIONS
Breast cancer; history of active cerebral apoplexy; thromboembolic disorders or thrombophlebitis; missed abortion; severe hepatic dysfunction; undiagnosed vaginal bleeding; use as a pregnancy test

INTERACTIONS
Drug
Bromocriptine: May interfere with the effects of bromocriptine.

Herbal
None known.
Food
None known.

DIAGNOSTIC TEST EFFECTS
May increase serum LDL and serum alkaline phosphatase levels. May decrease glucose tolerance and HDL concentrations. May cause abnormal serum thyroid, metapyrone, hepatic, and endocrine function test results.

SIDE EFFECTS
Frequent
Breakthrough bleeding or spotting at beginning of therapy, amenorrhea, change in menstrual flow, breast tenderness
Gel: drowsiness
Occasional
Edema, weight gain or loss, rash, pruritus, photosensitivity, skin pigmentation
Rare
Pain or swelling at injection site, acne, depression, alopecia, hirsutism

SERIOUS REACTIONS
• Thrombophlebitis, cerebrovascular disorders, retinal thrombosis, and pulmonary embolism occur rarely.

PRECAUTIONS & CONSIDERATIONS
Caution is warranted with conditions aggravated by fluid retention, diabetes mellitus, and history of depression. Progesterone use should be avoided during pregnancy. Progesterone is distributed in breast milk. Safety and efficacy of progesterone have not been established in children. No age-related precautions have been noted in the elderly. Females using progesterone vaginal gel form should avoid performing tasks that require mental alertness or motor skills until response to the drug has been established.

Use sunscreen and wear protective clothing until tolerance to sunlight and ultraviolet light has been determined. Avoid smoking because of the increased risk of blood clot formation and MI.

Notify the physician of chest pain, migraine headache, peripheral paresthesia, sudden decrease in vision, sudden shortness of breath, pain, redness, swelling, warmth in the calf, abnormal vaginal bleeding, or other symptoms. B/P and weight should be monitored.

Storage

Store progesterone at room temperature.

Administration

Take the daily dose of oral progesterone in the evening to minimize the effects of dizziness and drowsiness. If the dose is taken in the morning, take it 2 hours after breakfast.

Shake vial well before withdrawing dose. Administer deep IM injection only in the upper arm or upper outer quadrant aspect of the buttock. Rarely, a residual lump, change in skin color, or sterile abscess occurs at the injection site. Rotate injection sites.

Promethazine
proe-meth′a-zeen
(Insomn-Eze [AUS], Phenadoz, Phenergan)
Do not confuse promethazine with promazine.

CATEGORY AND SCHEDULE
Pregnancy Risk Category: C

CLASSIFICATION
Antiemetics/antivertigo, antihistamines, H1, phenothiazines

MECHANISM OF ACTION
A phenothiazine that acts as an antihistamine, antiemetic, and sedative-hypnotic. As an antihistamine, inhibits histamine at histamine receptor sites. As an antiemetic, diminishes vestibular stimulation, depresses labyrinthine function, and acts on the chemoreceptor trigger zone. As a sedative-hypnotic, produces CNS depression by decreasing stimulation to the brain stem reticular formation. *Therapeutic Effect:* Prevents allergic responses mediated by histamine, such as rhinitis, urticaria, and pruritus. Prevents and relieves nausea and vomiting.

PHARMACOKINETICS

Route	Onset	Peak	Duration
PO	20 min	N/A	2-8 hr
IV	3-5 min	N/A	2-8 hr
IM	20 min	N/A	2-8 hr
Rectal	20 min	N/A	2-8 hr

Well absorbed from the GI tract after IM administration. Widely distributed. Metabolized in the liver. Primarily

P

excreted in urine. Not removed by hemodialysis. **Half-life:** 16-19 hr.

AVAILABILITY
Syrup (Phenergan): 6.25 mg/ml.
Tablets (Phenergan): 12.5 mg,
25 mg, 50 mg.
Injection (Phenergan): 25 mg/ml,
50 mg/ml.
Suppositories (Phenergan): 12.5 mg,
25 mg, 50 mg.
Suppositories (Phenadoz): 25 mg.

INDICATIONS AND DOSAGES
▶ **Allergic symptoms**
PO
Adults, Elderly. 6.25-12.5 mg
3 times a day plus 25 mg at bedtime.
Children. 0.1 mg/kg/dose (maximum:
12.5 mg) 3 times a day plus
0.5 mg/kg/dose (maximum: 25 mg)
at bedtime.
IV, IM
Adults, Elderly. 25 mg. May repeat
in 2 hr.
▶ **Motion sickness**
PO
Adults, Elderly. 25 mg 30-60 min
before departure; may repeat in
8-12 hr, then every morning on rising
and before evening meal.
Children. 0.5 mg/kg 30-60 min before
departure; may repeat in 8-12 hr,
then every morning on rising and
before evening meal.
▶ **Prevention of nausea, and
vomiting**
PO, IV, IM, RECTAL
Adults, Elderly. 12.5-25 mg q4-6hr
as needed.
Children. 0.25-1 mg/kg q4-6hr as
needed.
▶ **Preoperative and postoperative
sedation; adjunct to analgesics**
IV, IM
Adults, Elderly. 25-50 mg.
Children. 12.5-25 mg.
▶ **Sedative**
PO, IV, IM, RECTAL

Adults, Elderly. 25-50 mg/dose. May
repeat q4-6hr as needed.
Children. 0.5-1 mg/kg/dose q6hr as
needed. Maximum: 50 mg/dose.

CONTRAINDICATIONS
Angle-closure glaucoma, GI or GU
obstruction, severe CNS depression
or coma

INTERACTIONS
Drug
Alcohol, other CNS depressants:
May increase CNS depressant effects.
Anticholinergics: May increase
anticholinergic effects.
MAOIs: May intensify and prolong
the anticholinergic and CNS depres-
sant effects of promethazine.
Herbal
None known.
Food
None known.

DIAGNOSTIC TEST EFFECTS
May suppress wheal and flare reactions to antigen skin testing unless
the drug is discontinued 4 days before
testing.

▓ IV INCOMPATIBILITIES
Allopurinol (Aloprim), amphotericin
B complex (Abelcet, AmBisome,
Amphotec), heparin, ketorolac
(Toradol), nalbuphine (Nubain),
piperacillin and tazobactam (Zosyn)
▓ IV Compatibilities
Atropine, diphenhydramine
(Benadryl), glycopyrrolate (Robinul),
hydromorphone (Dilaudid), hydroxy-
zine (Vistaril), meperidine
(Demerol), midazolam (Versed),
morphine, nalbuphine (Nubain),
prochlorperazine (Compazine)

SIDE EFFECTS
Expected
Somnolence, disorientation; in elderly,
hypotension, confusion, syncope

Frequent
Dry mouth, nose, or throat; urine retention; thickening of bronchial secretions
Occasional
Epigastric distress, flushing, visual disturbances, hearing disturbances, wheezing, paresthesia, diaphoresis, chills
Rare
Dizziness, urticaria, photosensitivity, nightmares

SERIOUS REACTIONS
• Children may experience paradoxical reactions, such as excitation, nervousness, tremor, hyperactive reflexes, and seizures.
• Infants and young children have experienced CNS depression manifested as respiratory depression, sleep apnea, and sudden infant death syndrome.
• Long-term therapy may produce extrapyramidal symptoms, such as dystonia (abnormal movements), pronounced motor restlessness (most frequently in children), and parkinsonian (most frequently in elderly patients).
• Blood dyscrasias, particularly agranulocytosis, occur rarely.

PRECAUTIONS & CONSIDERATIONS
Caution is warranted with asthma, history of seizures, cardiovascular disease, hepatic impairment, peptic ulcer disease, sleep apnea, and possible Reye's syndrome. Promethazine readily crosses the placenta and may produce extrapyramidal symptoms and jaundice in neonates if taken during pregnancy. It is unknown whether the drug is excreted in breast milk. Children are more likely to experience paradoxical reactions, such as increased excitement, nervousness, and tremor. Promethazine is not recommended for children younger than 2 years. The elderly are more sensitive to the drug's anticholinergic effects, such as dry mouth, confusion, dizziness, hypotension, syncope, and sedation. Avoid CNS depressants, drinking alcoholic beverages and tasks that require alertness or motor skills until response to the drug is established.

Drowsiness and dry mouth may occur. Pulse rate, electrolytes, B/P, and therapeutic response should be monitored.
Storage
Store vials at room temperature. Refrigerate rectal suppositories.
Administration
Take promethazine without regard to food. Crush scored tablets as needed.

For IV use, promethazine may be given undiluted or diluted with 0.9% NaCl; final dilution should not exceed 25 mg/ml. Inject the drug at a rate of 25 mg/minute through the tubing of an infusing IV solution, as prescribed. Injecting the drug too-rapidly may cause a transient drop in B/P, resulting in orthostatic hypotension and reflex tachycardia.
! Avoid giving subcutaneously because significant tissue necrosis may occur. Inject the drug carefully because inadvertent intra-arterial injection may produce severe arteriospasm, possibly resulting in gangrene.

For IM use, inject deep into a large muscle mass.

For rectal use, moisten the suppository with cold water before inserting it well into the rectum.

Propafenone
proe-pa-fen'one
(Rythmol, Rythmol SR)

CATEGORY AND SCHEDULE
Pregnancy Risk Category: C

CLASSIFICATION
Antiarrhythmics, class IC

MECHANISM OF ACTION
An antiarrhythmic that decreases the fast sodium current in Purkinje or myocardial cells. Decreases excitability and automaticity; prolongs conduction velocity and the refractory period. *Therapeutic Effect:* Suppresses arrhythmias.

AVAILABILITY
Tablets (Rythmol): 150 mg, 225 mg, 300 mg).
Capsules (Extended-Release [Rythmol SR]): 225 mg, 325 mg, 425 mg.

INDICATIONS AND DOSAGES
▸ **Documented, life-threatening ventricular arrhythmias, such as sustained ventricular tachycardia**
PO, PROMPT-RELEASE
Adults, Elderly. Initially, 150 mg q8hr; may increase at 3- to 4-day intervals to 225 mg q8hr, then to 300 mg q8hr. Maximum: 900 mg/day.
PO, EXTENDED-RELEASE
Adults, Elderly. Initially, 225 mg q12hr. May increase at 5-day intervals. Maximum: 425 mg q12hr.

OFF-LABEL USES
Treatment of supraventricular arrhythmia

CONTRAINDICATIONS
Bradycardia; bronchospastic disorders; cardiogenic shock; electrolyte imbalance; sinoatrial, AV, and intraventricular impulse generation or conduction disorders, such as sick sinus syndrome or AV block, without the presence of a pacemaker; uncontrolled CHF

INTERACTIONS
Drug
Digoxin, propranolol: May increase concentrations of these drugs.
Warfarin: May increase warfarin effects.
Herbal
None known.
Food
None known.

DIAGNOSTIC TEST EFFECTS
May cause EKG changes, such as QRS widening and PR interval prolongation, and positive ANA titers.

SIDE EFFECTS
Frequent (13%-7%)
Dizziness, nausea, vomiting, altered taste, constipation
Occasional (6%-3%)
Headache, dyspnea, blurred vision, dyspepsia (heartburn, indigestion, epigastric pain)
Rare (less than 2%)
Rash, weakness, dry mouth, diarrhea, edema, hot flashes

SERIOUS REACTIONS
• Propafenone may produce or worsen existing arrhythmias.
• Overdose may produce hypotension, somnolence, bradycardia, and atrioventricular conduction disturbances.

PRECAUTIONS & CONSIDERATIONS
Caution is warranted with CHF, conduction disturbances, impaired

hepatic or renal function, and recent MI.

Altered taste sensation may occur while taking propafenone. Notify the physician if blurred vision, GI upset, dizziness, or headache occurs. Tasks that require mental alertness or motor skills should be avoided until response to the drug has been established. Electrolyte imbalances should be corrected before beginning propafenone therapy. Pulse rate for quality and irregularity, pattern of daily bowel activity and stool consistency, serum electrolyte levels, and hepatic enzymes should be assessed.

Administration

Take without regard to meals. Do not skip doses. Therapeutic serum level is 0.06 to 1 mcg/ml.

Propantheline
proe-pan-the-leen
(Pro-Banthine, Propanthl [CAN])

CATEGORY AND SCHEDULE
Pregnancy Risk Category: C

CLASSIFICATION
Anticholinergics, gastrointestinals

MECHANISM OF ACTION
A quaternary ammonium compound which has anticholinergic properties and that inhibits action of acetylcholine at postganglionic parasympathetic sites. *Therapeutic Effect:* Reduces gastric secretions and urinary frequency, urgency and urge incontinence.

PHARMACOKINETICS
Onset occurs within 90 min but less than 50% is absorbed from gastrointestinal (GI) tract. Extensive hepatic metabolism. Excreted in the urine and feces. **Half-life:** 2.9 hr.

AVAILABILITY
Tablets: 7.5 mg, 15 mg (Pro-Banthine).

INDICATIONS AND DOSAGES
▸ **Peptic ulcer**
PO
Adults, Elderly. 15 mg 3 times/day 30 min before meals and 30 mg at bedtime.
Children. 1-2 mg/kg/day, divided q4-6hr and at bedtime.

CONTRAINDICATIONS
GI or genitourinary (GU) obstruction, myasthenia gravis, narrow-angle glaucoma, toxic megacolon, severe ulcerative colitis, unstable cardiovascular adjustment in acute hemorrhage, hypersensitivity to propantheline or other anticholinergics

INTERACTIONS
Drug
Digoxin: May increase serum digoxin levels by increasing absorption due to decreased gastrointestinal motility.
Herbal
None known.
Food
None known.

SIDE EFFECTS
Frequent
Dry mouth, decreased sweating, constipation
Occasional
Blurred vision, intolerance to light, urinary hesitancy, drowsiness, agitation, excitement

Rare
Confusion, increased intraocular pressure, orthostatic hypotension, tachycardia

SERIOUS REACTIONS
• Overdosage may produce temporary paralysis of ciliary muscle, pupillary dilation, tachycardia, palpitations, hot, dry, or flushed skin, absence of bowel sounds, hyperthermia, increased respiratory rate, EKG abnormalities, nausea, vomiting, rash over face or upper trunk, CNS stimulation, and psychosis, marked by agitation, restlessness, rambling speech, visual hallucinations, paranoid behavior, and delusions, followed by depression.

PRECAUTIONS & CONSIDERATIONS
Caution is warranted with chronic obstructive pulmonary disease (COPD), congestive heart failure (CHF), coronary artery disease, esophageal reflux or hiatal hernia associated with reflux esophagitis, gastric ulcer, hyperthyroidism, hypertension, liver or renal disease, tachyarrhythmias, autonomic neuropathy, diarrhea, known or suspected GI infections, and mild to moderate ulcerative colitis. It is unknown if propantheline crosses the placenta or is distributed in breast milk. Infants and young children are more susceptible to the drug's toxic effects. Propantheline use in the elderly may cause agitation, confusion, drowsiness, or excitement. Hot baths and saunas should be avoided.

Tasks that require mental alertness or motor skills should be avoided.

Dry mouth may be experienced during therapy. Good oral hygiene should be practiced.

Administration
Give propantheline 30 minutes before meals and at bedtime.

Propofol
pro-poe-fall
(Diprivan)

CATEGORY AND SCHEDULE
Pregnancy Risk Category: B

CLASSIFICATION
Anesthetics, general

MECHANISM OF ACTION
A rapidly acting general anesthetic that inhibits sympathetic vasoconstrictor nerve activity and decreases vascular resistance. *Therapeutic Effect:* Produces hypnosis rapidly.

PHARMACOKINETICS

Route	Onset	Peak	Duration
IV	40 sec	N/A	3-10 min

Rapidly and extensively distributed. Protein binding: 97%-99%. Metabolized in the liver. Primarily excreted in urine. Unknown if removed by hemodialysis. **Half-life:** 3-12 hr.

AVAILABILITY
Injection: 10 mg/ml.

INDICATIONS AND DOSAGES
▸ **Intensive care unit sedation**
IV
Adults, Elderly. Initially, 0.3 mg/kg/hr. May increase by 0.3-0.6 mg/kg/hr q5-10 min until

desired effect is obtained.
Maintenance: 0.3-3 mg/kg/hr.

▶ **Anesthesia**
IV
Adults, American Society of Anesthesiologists (ASA) I and II patients. 2-2.5 mg/kg (about 40 mg q10sec until onset of anesthesia). Maintenance: 0.1-0.2 mg/kg/min.
Elderly, Debilitated, Hypovolemic, ASA III or IV patients. 1-1.5 mg/kg (about 20 mg q10sec until onset of anesthesia). Maintenance: 0.05-0.1 mg/kg/min.
Children 3 yr and older, ASA I or II patients. 2.5-3.5 mg/kg (lower dosage for ASA III or IV patients).
Children 2 mo-16 yr. Maintenance dose: 0.125-0.15 mg/kg/min.

CONTRAINDICATIONS
Impaired cerebral circulation, increased ICP

INTERACTIONS
Drug
Alcohol, other CNS depressants: May increase hypotensive and CNS and respiratory depressant effects of propofol.
Herbal
None known.
Food
None known.

DIAGNOSTIC TEST EFFECTS
None known.

▒ IV INCOMPATIBILITIES
Amikacin (Amikin), amphotericin B complex (Abelcet, AmBisome, Amphotec), bretylium (Bretylol), calcium chloride, ciprofloxacin (Cipro), diazepam (Valium), digoxin (Lanoxin), doxorubicin (Adriamycin), gentamicin (Garamycin), methylprednisolone (Solu-Medrol), minocycline (Minocin), phenytoin (Dilantin),

tobramycin (Nebcin), verapamil (Isoptin)

▒ IV Compatibilities
Acyclovir (Zovirax), bumetanide (Bumex), calcium gluconate, ceftazidime (Fortaz), dobutamine (Dobutrex), dopamine (Intropin), enalapril (Vasotec), fentanyl, heparin, insulin, labetalol (Normodyne, Trandate), lidocaine, lorazepam (Ativan), magnesium, milrinone (Primacor), nitroglycerin, norepinephrine (Levophed), potassium chloride, vancomycin (Vancocin)

SIDE EFFECTS
Frequent
Involuntary muscle movements, apnea (common during induction; lasts longer than 60 seconds), hypotension, nausea, vomiting, IV site burning or stinging
Occasional
Twitching, bucking, jerking, thrashing, headache, dizziness, bradycardia, hypertension, fever, abdominal cramps, paresthesia, coldness, cough, hiccups, facial flushing, greenish-colored urine
Rare
Rash, dry mouth, agitation, confusion, myalgia, thrombophlebitis

SERIOUS REACTIONS
• A continuous infusion or repeated intermittent infusions of propofol may result in extreme somnolence, respiratory depression, and circulatory depression.
• Too-rapid IV administration may produce severe hypotension, respiratory depression, and involuntary muscle movements.
• The patient may experience an acute allergic reaction, characterized by abdominal pain, anxiety, restlessness, dyspnea, erythema, hypotension, pruritus, rhinitis, and urticaria.

P

PRECAUTIONS & CONSIDERATIONS

Caution is warranted with circulatory, hepatic, lipid metabolism, renal, or respiratory disorder, history of epilepsy, and in the debilitated. Propofol crosses the placenta and is not recommended for obstetric use. Propofol is distributed in breast milk and is not recommended for breast-feeding women. The safety and efficacy of propofol have not been established in children. However, the Food and Drug Administration has approved the drug for use in children older than 3 years of age. Lower propofol dosages are recommended for the elderly.

Be aware that urine may turn green. Vital signs should be obtained before propofol administration. ABG levels, B/P, heart and respiratory rates, oxygen saturation, depth of sedation, and lipid and triglyceride levels should be monitored if propofol is given for longer than 24 hours.

Storage
Store propofol at room temperature. Don't use propofol if the emulsion separates.

Administration
! Don't give propofol through the same IV line as blood or plasma.

Shake well before using. Propofol may be given undiluted, or it may be diluted only with D₅W to a concentration of no less than 2 mg/ml (4 ml D₅W to 1 ml propofol yields 2 mg/ml). Discard any unused portions of the drug. Too-rapid IV administration of propofol may produce irregular muscle movements, respiratory depression, and severe hypotension. Observe for signs of inadvertent intra-arterial injection, such as delayed onset of drug action, pain or discolored skin near the injection site, or blue or white discoloration of the hand if a hand or arm IV site is used.

Propoxyphene
(Darvon, Doloxene [AUS])
(Darvon-N [CAN])
Do not confuse with Diovan.

CATEGORY AND SCHEDULE
Pregnancy Risk Category: C (D if used for prolonged periods) Controlled Substance: Schedule IV

CLASSIFICATION
Analgesics, narcotic

MECHANISM OF ACTION
An opioid agonist that binds with opioid receptors in the CNS. *Therapeutic Effect:* Alters the perception of and emotional response to pain.

PHARMACOKINETICS

Route	Onset	Peak	Duration
PO	15-60 min	N/A	4-6 hr

Well absorbed from the GI tract. Protein binding: High. Widely distributed. Metabolized in the liver. Primarily excreted in urine. Not removed by hemodialysis. **Half-life:** 6-12 hr; metabolite: 30-36 hr.

AVAILABILITY
Capsules (Hydrochloride): 65 mg.
Tablets (Napsylate): 100 mg.

INDICATIONS AND DOSAGES
▸ **Mild to moderate pain**
PO (propoxyphene hydrochloride)
Adults, Elderly. 65 mg q4hr as needed. Maximum: 390 mg/day.
PO (propoxyphene napsylate)
Adults, Elderly. 100 mg q4hr as needed. Maximum: 600 mg/day.

CONTRAINDICATIONS
None known.

INTERACTIONS
Drug
Alcohol, other CNS depressants:
May increase CNS or respiratory depression and risk of hypotension.
Buprenorphine: May decrease the effects of propoxyphene.
Carbamazepine: May increase the blood concentration and risk of toxicity of carbamazepine.
MAOIs: May produce a severe, sometimes fatal reaction; plan to administer 25% of usual propoxyphene dose.
Herbal
None known.
Food
None known.

DIAGNOSTIC TEST EFFECTS
May increase serum alkaline phosphatase, lipase, amylase, bilirubin, LDH, AST (SGOT), and ALT (SGPT) levels. Therapeutic serum drug level is 100-400 ng/ml; toxic serum drug level is greater than 500 ng/ml.

SIDE EFFECTS
Frequent
Dizziness, somnolence, dry mouth, euphoria, hypotension (including orthostatic hypotension), nausea, vomiting, fatigue
Occasional
Allergic reaction (including decreased B/P, diaphoresis, flushing, and wheezing), trembling, urine retention, vision changes, constipation, headache
Rare
Confusion, increased B/P, depression, abdominal cramps, anorexia

SERIOUS REACTIONS
• Overdose results in respiratory depression, skeletal muscle flaccidity, cold or clammy skin, cyanosis, and extreme somnolence progressing to seizures, stupor, and coma.
• Hepatotoxicity may occur with overdose of the acetaminophen component of fixed-combination products.
• The patient who uses propoxyphene repeatedly may develop a tolerance to the drug's analgesic effect and physical dependence.

PRECAUTIONS & CONSIDERATIONS
Caution is warranted with hepatic or renal impairment and those who are narcotic-dependent. Propoxyphene crosses the placenta and a minimal amount of the drug is distributed in breast milk. Be aware that regular use of opioids during pregnancy may produce withdrawal symptoms in the neonate, including diarrhea, excessive crying, fever, hyperactive reflexes, irritability, seizures, sneezing, tremors, vomiting, and yawning. The neonate may develop respiratory depression if the mother receives propoxyphene during labor. The pediatric dosage of this drug has not been established. Avoid use in the elderly, if possible. They may be more susceptible to propoxyphene's CNS effects and constipation.

Dizziness and drowsiness may occur, so change positions slowly and avoid alcohol, CNS depressants, and tasks that require mental alertness or motor skills until response to the drug is established. Vital signs, pattern of daily bowel activity and clinical improvement should be monitored. The drug should be held and the physician should be notified if the respiratory rate is 12 breaths/minute or less in an adult or 20 breaths/minute or less in a child.
Storage
Store vials at room temperature.

Administration

! Be aware that propoxyphene's side effects are dependent on the dosage. Know that ambulatory patients and patients not in severe pain are more likely to experience dizziness, hypotension, nausea, and vomiting than patients in the supine position and those in severe pain. Expect to reduce the initial dosage with Addison's disease, hypothyroidism, and renal insufficiency, for the debilitated or elderly, and for those concurrently taking CNS depressants. Be aware the therapeutic serum level of propoxyphene is 100 to 400 ng/ml, and the toxic serum level is over 500 ng/ml.

Take oral propoxyphene without regard to food. Empty capsules and mix with food as needed. Do not crush or break film-coated tablets.

Propranolol

proe-pran'oh-lole
(Apo-Propranolol [CAN], Deralin [AUS], Inderal, Inderal LA, InnoPran XL, Nu-Propranolol [CAN], Propranolol Intensol)
Do not confuse Inderal with Adderall or Isordil, or propranolol with Pravachol.

CATEGORY AND SCHEDULE

Pregnancy Risk Category: C (D if used in second or third trimester)

CLASSIFICATION

Antiadrenergics, beta blocking, antiarrhythmics, class II

MECHANISM OF ACTION

An antihypertensive, antianginal, antiarrhythmic, and antimigraine agent that blocks beta$_1$- and beta$_2$-adrenergic receptors. Decreases oxygen requirements. Slows AV conduction and increases refractory period in AV node. Large doses increase airway resistance.
Therapeutic Effect: Slows sinus heart rate; decreases cardiac output, B/P, and myocardial ischemia severity. Exhibits antiarrhythmic activity.

PHARMACOKINETICS

Route	Onset	Peak	Duration
PO	1-2 hr	N/A	6 hr

Well absorbed from the GI tract. Protein binding: 93%. Widely distributed. Metabolized in the liver. Primarily excreted in urine. Not removed by hemodialysis. **Half-life:** 3-5 hr.

AVAILABILITY

Tablets (Inderal): 10 mg, 20 mg, 40 mg, 60 mg, 80 mg.
Capsules (Extended-Release [Inderal LA]): 60 mg, 80 mg, 120 mg, 160 mg.
Capsules (Extended-Release [InnoPran XL]): 80 mg, 120 mg.
Oral Solution (Inderal): 4 mg/ml.
Oral Concentrate (Propranolol Intensol): 80 mg/ml.
Injection (Inderal): 1 mg/ml.

INDICATIONS AND DOSAGES

▶ **Hypertension**
PO
Adults, Elderly. Initially, 40 mg twice a day. May increase dose q3-7 days. Range: Up to 320 mg/day in divided doses. Maximum: 640 mg/day.
Children. Initially, 0.5-1 mg/kg/day in divided doses q6-12hr. May increase at 3- to 5-day intervals.

Usual dose: 1-5 mg/kg/day.
Maximum: 16 mg/kg/day.
▸ **Angina**
PO
Adults, Elderly. 80-320 mg/day in
divided doses. (long acting): Initially,
80 mg/day. Maximum: 320 mg/day.
▸ **Arrhythmias**
IV
Adults, Elderly. 1 mg/dose. May
repeat q5min. Maximum: 5 mg total
dose.
Children. 0.01-0.1 mg/kg.
Maximum: infants, 1 mg; children,
3 mg.
PO
Adults, Elderly. Initially, 10-20 mg
q6-8hr. May gradually increase dose.
Range: 40-320 mg/day.
Children. Initially, 0.5-1 mg/kg/day
in divided doses q6-8hr. May
increase q3-5 days. Usual dosage:
2-4 mg/kg/day. Maximum:
16 mg/kg/day or 60 mg/day.
▸ **Life-threatening arrhythmias**
IV
Adults, Elderly. 0.5-3 mg. Repeat
once in 2 min. Give additional doses
at intervals of at least 4 hr.
Children. 0.01-0.1 mg/kg.
▸ **Hypertrophic subaortic stenosis**
PO
Adults, Elderly. 20-40 mg in 3-4
divided doses. Or 80-160 mg/day as
extended-release capsule.
▸ **Adjunct to alpha-blocking agents
to treat pheochromocytoma**
PO
Adults, Elderly. 60 mg/day in
divided doses with alpha-blocker for
3 days before surgery. Maintenance
(inoperable tumor): 30 mg/day with
alpha-blocker.
▸ **Migraine headache**
PO
Adults, Elderly. 80 mg/day in divided
doses. Or 80 mg once daily as
extended-release capsule. Increase up
to 160-240 mg/day in divided doses.

Children. 0.6-1.5 mg/kg/day in
divided doses q8hr. Maximum:
4 mg/kg/day.
▸ **Reduction of cardiovascular
mortality and reinfarction in patients
with previous MI**
PO
Adults, Elderly. 180-240 mg/day in
divided doses.
▸ **Essential tremor**
PO
Adults, Elderly. Initially, 40 mg
twice a day increased up to
120-320 mg/day in 3 divided doses.

OFF-LABEL USES
Treatment adjunct for anxiety, mitral
valve prolapse syndrome, thyrotoxicosis

CONTRAINDICATIONS
Asthma, bradycardia, cardiogenic
shock, COPD, heart block, Raynaud's
syndrome, uncompensated CHF

INTERACTIONS
Drug
Diuretics, other antihypertensives:
May increase hypotensive effect.
Insulin, oral hypoglycemics: May
mask symptoms of hypoglycemia
and prolong the hypoglycemic effect
of insulin and oral hypoglycemics.
IV phenytoin: May increase cardiac
depressant effect.
NSAIDs: May decrease antihyper-
tensive effect.
Sympathomimetics, xanthines:
May mutually inhibit effects.
Herbal
None known.
Food
None known.

DIAGNOSTIC TEST EFFECTS
May increase serum antinuclear antibody titer and BUN, serum LDH,
serum lipoprotein, serum alkaline
phosphatase, serum bilirubin, serum

creatinine, serum potassium, serum uric acid, AST (SGOT), ALT (SGPT), and serum triglyceride levels.

IV INCOMPATIBILITIES
Amphotericin B complex (Abelcet, AmBisome, Amphotec)
IV Compatibilities
Alteplase (Activase), heparin, milrinone (Primacor), potassium chloride, propofol (Diprivan)

SIDE EFFECTS
Frequent
Diminished sexual ability, drowsiness, difficulty sleeping, unusual fatigue or weakness
Occasional
Bradycardia, depression, sensation of coldness in extremities, diarrhea, constipation, anxiety, nasal congestion, nausea, vomiting
Rare
Altered taste, dry eyes, pruritus, paresthesia

SERIOUS REACTIONS
• Overdose may produce profound bradycardia and hypotension.
• Abrupt withdrawal may result in sweating, palpitations, headache, and tremulousness.
• Propranolol administration may precipitate CHF and MI in patients with cardiac disease; thyroid storm in those with thyrotoxicosis; and peripheral ischemia in those with existing peripheral vascular disease.
• Hypoglycemia may occur in patients with previously controlled diabetes.

PRECAUTIONS & CONSIDERATIONS
Caution should be used in those who are also receiving calcium channel blockers, especially when giving propranolol IV. Caution is also warranted with diabetes and hepatic

and renal impairment. Propranolol crosses the placenta and is distributed in breast milk. Propranolol use should be avoided in pregnant women after the first trimester because it may result in low-birth-weight infants. The drug may also produce apnea, bradycardia, hypoglycemia, hypothermia during childbirth. No age-related precautions have been noted in children. In the elderly, age-related peripheral vascular disease may increase susceptibility to decreased peripheral circulation. Be aware that salt and alcohol intake should be restricted. Nasal decongestants or OTC cold preparations (stimulants) should not be used without physician approval. Tasks that require mental alertness or motor skills should be avoided.

Notify the physician of behavioral changes, fatigue, rash, dizziness, excessively slow pulse rate (less than 60 beats/minute), or peripheral numbness. B/P for hypotension, respiratory status for shortness of breath, pattern of daily bowel activity and stool consistency, EKG for arrhythmias, and pulse for quality, rate and rhythm should be monitored during treatment. If pulse rate is 60 beats/minute or lower or systolic B/P is less than 90 mm Hg, withhold the medication and contact the physician. In those receiving propranolol for treatment of angina, the onset, type (sharp, dull, squeezing), radiation, location, intensity, and duration of anginal pain and its precipitating factors, including exertion and emotional stress should be recorded. Signs and symptoms of CHF, such as decreased urine output, distended neck veins, dyspnea (particularly on exertion or lying down), night cough, peripheral edema, and weight gain should also be assessed.

Storage
Store at room temperature.

Administration
For oral use, crush scored tablets if necessary. Take at same time each day. Do not abruptly discontinue the drug. Compliance with the therapy regimen is essential to control anginal pain, arrhythmias, and hypertension.

For IV use, give undiluted for IV push. For IV infusion, may dilute each 1 mg in 10 ml D_5W. Do not exceed 1 mg/minute injection rate. For IV infusion, give 1 mg over 10 to 15 minutes.

Propylthiouracil
proe-pill-thye-oh-yoor′a-sill
(Propylthiouracil, Propyl-Thyracil
[CAN])

CATEGORY AND SCHEDULE
Pregnancy Risk Category: D

CLASSIFICATION
Antithyroid agents,
hormones/hormone modifiers

MECHANISM OF ACTION
A thiourea derivative that blocks oxidation of iodine in the thyroid gland and blocks synthesis of thyroxine and triiodothyronine.
Therapeutic Effect: Inhibits synthesis of thyroid hormone.

AVAILABILITY
Tablets: 50 mg.

INDICATIONS AND DOSAGES
▸ **Hyperthyroidism**
PO
Adults, Elderly. Initially:
300-450 mg/day in divided doses q8hr.

Maintenance: 100-150 mg/day in divided doses q8-12hr.
Children. Initially: 5-7 mg/kg/day in divided doses q8hr. Maintenance: 33%-66% of initial dose in divided doses q8-12hr.
Neonates. 5-10 mg/kg/day in divided doses q8hr.

CONTRAINDICATIONS
None known.

INTERACTIONS
Drug
Amiodarone, iodinated glycerol, iodine, potassium iodide: May decrease response of propylthiouracil.
Digoxin: May increase digoxin blood concentration as patient becomes euthyroid.
I^{131}: May decrease thyroid uptake of I^{131}.
Oral anticoagulants: May decrease the effects of oral anticoagulants.
Herbal
None known.
Food
None known.

DIAGNOSTIC TEST EFFECTS
May increase LDH, serum alkaline phosphatase, bilirubin, AST (SGOT), and ALT (SGPT) levels and prothrombin time.

SIDE EFFECTS
Frequent
Urticaria, rash, pruritus, nausea, skin pigmentation, hair loss, headache, paraesthesia
Occasional
Somnolence, lymphadenopathy, vertigo
Rare
Drug fever, lupus-like syndrome

SERIOUS REACTIONS
• Agranulocytosis as long as 4 months after therapy,

pancytopenia, and fatal hepatitis have occurred.

PRECAUTIONS & CONSIDERATIONS

Caution is warranted with concurrent use of other agranulocytosis-inducing drugs and in persons older than 40 years of age. Propylthiouracil crosses the placenta and should be avoided during pregnancy. Breastfeeding should be avoided. Use cautiously in children because of the risk of hepatic dysfunction. Restrict the consumption of iodine products and seafood.

Notify the physician of somnolence, jaundice, nausea, vomiting, illness, unusual bleeding or bruising, rash, itching, swollen lymph glands, or a pulse rate less than 60 beats per minute. Weight, pulse, prothrombin time, LDH, serum alkaline phosphatase, bilirubin, AST, and ALT levels should be monitored.

Administration

Space doses evenly around the clock.

Protamine

proe′ta-meen
(Protamine [CAN], Protamine sulfate)
Do not confuse protamine with ProAmatine, Protopam, or Protropin.

CATEGORY AND SCHEDULE

Pregnancy Risk Category: C

CLASSIFICATION

Antidotes, coagulants

MECHANISM OF ACTION

A protein that complexes with heparin to form a stable salt.

Therapeutic Effect: Reduces anticoagulant activity of heparin.

AVAILABILITY

Injection: 10 mg/ml.

INDICATIONS AND DOSAGES
▶ **Heparin overdose (antidote and treatment)**
IV
Adults, Elderly. 1 mg protamine sulfate neutralizes 90-115 units of heparin. Heparin disappears rapidly from circulation, reducing the dosage demand for protamine as time elapses.

OFF-LABEL USES

Treatment of enoxaparin toxicity

CONTRAINDICATIONS

None known.

INTERACTIONS
Drug
None known.
Herbal
None known.
Food
None known.

DIAGNOSTIC TEST EFFECTS

None known.

SIDE EFFECTS
Frequent
Decreased B/P, dyspnea
Occasional
Hypersensitivity reaction (urticaria, angioedema); nausea and vomiting, which generally occur in those sensitive to fish and seafood, vasectomized men, infertile men, those on isophane (NPH) insulin, or those previously on protamine therapy
Rare
Back pain

SERIOUS REACTIONS

• Too rapid IV administration may produce acute hypotension, bradycardia, pulmonary hypertension, dyspnea, transient flushing, and feeling of warmth.

• Heparin rebound may occur several hours after heparin has been neutralized (usually 8-9 hours after protamine administration). Heparin rebound occurs most often after arterial or cardiac surgery.

PRECAUTIONS & CONSIDERATIONS

Caution is warranted with a history of allergy to fish and seafood, in those previously on protamine therapy because of a propensity to hypersensitivity reaction, and in infertile or vasectomized men and those on isophane (NPH) or insulin therapy. An electric razor or soft toothbrush should be used to prevent bleeding until coagulation studies normalize.

Notify the physician of black or red stool, coffee-ground vomitus, dark or red urine, or red-speckled mucus from cough. Activated clotting time, aPTT, B/P, cardiac function, and other coagulation tests should be monitored.

Storage
Store vials at room temperature.
Administration
May give undiluted over 10 minutes. Do not exceed 5 mg/min or 50 mg in any 10-minute period. Make sure the patient is supine while protamine is being administered, to prevent injury from a hypotensive episode or other complication.

Protriptyline
proe-trip′-ti-leen
(Vivactil, Triptil [CAN])

CATEGORY AND SCHEDULE
Pregnancy Risk Category: C

CLASSIFICATION
Antidepressants, tricyclic

MECHANISM OF ACTION
A tricyclic antidepressant that increases synaptic concentration of norepinephrine and/or serotonin by inhibiting their reuptake by presynaptic membranes. *Therapeutic Effect:* Produces antidepressant effect.

PHARMACOKINETICS
Well absorbed from the gastrointestinal (GI) tract. Protein binding: 92%. Widely distributed. Extensively metabolized in liver. Excreted in urine. Not removed by hemodialysis. **Half-life:** 54-92 hr.

AVAILABILITY
Tablets: 5 mg, 10 mg (Vivactil).

INDICATIONS AND DOSAGES
▸ **Depression**
PO
Adults. 15-40 mg/day divided into 3-4 doses/day. Maximum: 600 mg/day.
Elderly. 5 mg 3 times/day. May increase gradually.

OFF-LABEL USES
Narcolepsy, sleep apnea, sleep hypoxemia

CONTRAINDICATIONS
Acute recovery period after myocardial infarction, coadministration with

P

cisapride, use of MAOIs within 14 days, hypersensitivity to protriptyline or any component of the formulation

INTERACTIONS
Drug
Alcohol, central nervous system (CNS) depressants: May increase CNS and respiratory depression and the hypotensive effects of protriptyline.

Antithyroid agents: May increase risk of agranulocytosis.

Cimetidine: May increase protriptyline blood concentration and risk of toxicity.

Clonidine, guanadrel: May decrease the effects of clonidine and guanadrel.

MAOIs: May increase the risk of hyperpyrexia, hypertensive crisis, and seizures.

Phenothiazines: May increase the anticholinergic and sedative effects of protriptyline.

Phenytoin: May decrease protriptyline blood concentration.

Sympathomimetics: May increase the cardiac effects.

Herbal
St. John's wort: May have additive effects.

Food
None known.

DIAGNOSTIC TEST EFFECTS
None known.

🔲 IV INCOMPATIBILITIES
None known.
🔲 IV Compatibilities
None known.

SIDE EFFECTS
Frequent
Drowsiness, weight gain, fatigue, dry mouth, blurred vision, constipation, delayed micturition, postural hypotension, diaphoresis, disturbed concentration, increased appetite, urinary retention
Occasional
Gastrointestinal (GI) disturbances, such as nausea, diarrhea, GI distress, metallic taste sensation
Rare
Paradoxical reaction, marked by agitation, restlessness, nightmares, insomnia, extrapyramidal symptoms, particularly fine hand tremor

SERIOUS REACTIONS
• High dosage may produce confusion, seizures, severe drowsiness, arrhythmias, fever, hallucinations, agitation, shortness of breath, vomiting, and unusual tiredness or weakness.
• Abrupt withdrawal from prolonged therapy may produce severe headache, malaise, nausea, vomiting, and vivid dreams.

PRECAUTIONS & CONSIDERATIONS
Caution is warranted with increased intraocular pressure, overactive or agitated patients, seizure disorder, bipolar disorder, suicidal ideation, cardiovascular disease, hyperthyroidism, urinary retention, and concurrent use of guanethidine or other peripherally-acting antihypertensives. Be aware that protriptyline crosses the placenta and is minimally distributed in breast milk. Safety and efficacy have not been established in children. Expect to use lower dosages in the elderly. Higher dosages are not tolerated well, and increase the risk of toxicity in the elderly.

Protriptyline serum levels should be monitored. The therapeutic serum level for protriptyline is 70 to 250 ng/ml, and the toxic serum level for protriptyline is greater than 500 ng/ml.

Anticholinergic, sedative effects, and postural hypotension usually develop during early therapy. Avoid unnecessary exposure to sunlight.
Storage
Store at room temperature.
Administration
May be taken with food to decrease GI distress. Dose increases should occur during the morning dose.

Pseudoephedrine
soo-doe-e-fed'rin
(Balminil Decongestant [CAN], BioContac Cold 12 Hour Relief Non Drowsy [CAN], Decofed, Dimetapp 12 Hour Non Drowsy Extentabs, Dimetapp Decongestant, Dimetapp sinus liquid caps [AUS], Genaphed, PMS-Pseudoephedrine [CAN], Robidrine [CAN], Sudafed, Sudafed 12hr [AUS], Sudafed 12 Hour, Sudafed 24 Hour)

CATEGORY AND SCHEDULE
Pregnancy Risk Category: C
OTC

CLASSIFICATION
Decongestants, nasal

MECHANISM OF ACTION
A sympathomimetic that directly stimulates alpha-adrenergic and beta-adrenergic receptors. *Therapeutic Effect:* Produces vasoconstriction of respiratory tract mucosa; shrinks nasal mucous membranes; reduces edema, and nasal congestion.

PHARMACOKINETICS

Route	Onset	Peak	Duration
PO (tablets, syrup)	15-30 min	N/A	4-6 hr
PO (extended-release)	N/A	N/A	8-12 hr

Well absorbed from the GI tract. Partially metabolized in the liver. Primarily excreted in urine. Not removed by hemodialysis. **Half-life:** 9-16 hr (children, 3.1 hr).

AVAILABILITY
Gelcaps (Dimetapp Decongestant): 30 mg.
Liquid (Sudafed): 15 mg/5 ml.
Oral Drops (Dimetapp Infant Drops): 7.5 mg/0.8 ml.
Syrup (Biofed, Decofed): 30 mg/5 ml.
Tablets (Genaphed, Sudafed): 30 mg.
Tablets (Chewable [Sudafed]): 15 mg.
Tablets (Extended-Release [Dimetapp 12 Hour Non Drowsy Extentabs, Sudafed 12 Hour]): 120 mg.
Tablets (Extended-Release [Sudafed 24 Hour]): 240 mg.

INDICATIONS AND DOSAGES
▸ **Decongestant**
PO
Adults, Children 12 yr and older. 60 mg q4-6hr. Maximum: 240 mg/day.
Children 6-11 yr. 30 mg q6hr. Maximum: 120 mg/day.
Children 2-5 yr. 15 mg q6hr. Maximum: 60 mg/day.
Children younger than 2 yr. 4 mg/kg/day in divided doses q6hr.
Elderly. 30-60 mg q6hr as needed.
PO (EXTENDED-RELEASE)
Adults, Children 12 yr and older. 120 mg q12hr.

P

CONTRAINDICATIONS

Breast-feeding women, coronary artery disease, severe hypertension, use within 14 days of MAOIs

INTERACTIONS
Drug
Antihypertensive, beta blockers, diuretics: May decrease the effects of these drugs.
MAOIs: May increase cardiac stimulant and vasopressor effects.
Herbal
None known.
Food
None known.

DIAGNOSTIC TEST EFFECTS

None known.

SIDE EFFECTS
Occasional (10%-5%)
Nervousness, restlessness, insomnia, tremor, headache
Rare (4%-1%)
Diaphoresis, weakness

SERIOUS REACTIONS

• Large doses may produce tachycardia, palpitations (particularly in patients with cardiac disease), light-headedness, nausea, and vomiting.
• Overdose in patients older than 60 years may result in hallucinations, CNS depression, and seizures.

PRECAUTIONS & CONSIDERATIONS

Caution is warranted with diabetes, heart disease, hyperthyroidism, benign prostatic hyperplasia, and in the elderly. Pseudoephedrine crosses the placenta and is distributed in breast milk. The safety and efficacy of pseudoephedrine have not been established in children younger than 2 years. Age-related benign prostatic hyperplasia may require a dosage adjustment in the elderly.

B/P should be monitored for increases. Tell the physician if taking antihypertensives, beta blockers, diuretics, or MAOIs before administering pseudoephedrine.
Administration
Don't crush extended-release tablets; swallow them whole. Discontinue therapy and notify the physician if dizziness, insomnia, irregular or rapid heartbeat, tremors, or other side effects occur.

Psyllium
sill'ee-yum
(Fiberall, Hydrocil, Konsyl, Metamucil, Novo-Mucilax [CAN], Perdiem)

CATEGORY AND SCHEDULE
Pregnancy Risk Category: B
OTC

CLASSIFICATION
Psyllium colloid, laxative

MECHANISM OF ACTION
A bulk-forming laxative that dissolves and swells in water providing increased bulk and moisture content in stool. *Therapeutic Effect:* Promotes peristalsis and bowel motility.

PHARMACOKINETICS

Route	Onset	Peak	Duration
PO	12-24 hr	2-3 days	N/A

Acts in small and large intestines.

AVAILABILITY
Powder (Fiberall, Hydrocil, Konsyl, Metamucil).

Wafer(Metamucil): 3.4 g/dose.
Capsules(Metamucil): 0.52 g.
Granules (Perdiem): 4 g/5 ml.

INDICATIONS AND DOSAGES
▸ **Constipation, irritable bowel syndrome**
PO
❗ 3.4 g powder equals 1 rounded tsp, 1 packet pr 1 wafer.
Adults, Elderly. 2-5 capsules/dose 1-3 times a day. 1-2 tsp granules 1-2 times a day. 1 rounded tsp or 1 tbsp of powder 1-3 times a day. 2 wafers 1-3 times a day.
Children 6-11 yr. One half-1 tsp powder in water 1-3 times a day.

CONTRAINDICATIONS
Fecal impaction, GI obstruction

INTERACTIONS
Drug
Digoxin, oral anticoagulants, salicylates: May decrease the effects of digoxin, oral anticoagulants, and salicylates by decreasing absorption.
Potassium-sparing diuretics, potassium supplements: May interfere with the effects of potassium-sparing diuretics and potassium supplements.
Herbal
None known.
Food
None known.

DIAGNOSTIC TEST EFFECTS
May increase blood glucose level. May decrease serum potassium level.

SIDE EFFECTS
Rare
Some degree of abdominal discomfort, nausea, mild abdominal cramps, griping, faintness

SERIOUS REACTIONS
• Esophageal or bowel obstruction may occur if administered less than 250 ml of liquid.

PRECAUTIONS & CONSIDERATIONS
Caution is warranted with esophageal strictures, intestinal adhesions, stenosis, and ulcers. This drug may be used safely in pregnancy. Safety and efficacy of psyllium have not been established in children younger than 6 years of age. No age-related precautions have been noted in the elderly.

Pattern of daily bowel activity and stool consistency and serum electrolyte levels should be monitored. Adequate fluid intake should be maintained.
Administration
Administer at least 2 hours before or after other medication administration. Drink 6 to 8 glasses of water a day to aid in stool softening. Drugs should not be swallowed in dry form but should be mixed with at least 1 full glass (8 oz) of liquid and then followed by 8 ounces of liquid; inadequate amount of fluid may cause GI obstruction. To promote defecation, increase fluid intake, exercise, and eat a high-fiber diet.

P

Pyrantel
pi-ran-tel
(Antiminth, Combantrin [CAN], Pin-Rid, Pin-X, Reese's Pinworm Caplets, Reese's Pinworm Medicine)

CATEGORY AND SCHEDULE
Pregnancy Risk Category: C
OTC (capsules, liquid, suspension)

CLASSIFICATION
Pyrimidine derivative, antihelmintic

MECHANISM OF ACTION
A depolarizing neuromuscular blocking agent that causes the release of acetylcholine and inhibits cholinesterase. *Therapeutic Effect:* Results in a spastic paralysis of the worm and consequent expulsion from the host's intestinal tract.

PHARMACOKINETICS
Poorly absorbed through gastro-intestinal (GI) tract. Time to peak occurs in 1-3 hr. Partially metabo-lized in liver. Primarily excreted in feces; minimal elimination in urine.

AVAILABILITY
Caplets: 180 mg (Reese's Pinworm Caplets).
Capsules: 180 mg (Pin-Rid).
Liquid: 50 mg/ml (Reese's Pinworm Medicine).
Suspension, oral: 50 mg/ml (Antiminth, Pin-X).

INDICATIONS AND DOSAGES
▸ **Enterobiasis vermicularis (pinworm)**
PO
Adults, Elderly, Children older than 2 yr. 11 mg base/kg once.

Repeat in 2 wk. Maximum: 1 g/day.

CONTRAINDICATIONS
Hypersensitivity to pyrantel or any of its components

INTERACTIONS
Drug
Piperazine: May decrease effects of pyrantel.
Herbal
None known.
Food
None known.

DIAGNOSTIC TEST EFFECTS
None known.

SIDE EFFECTS
Occasional
Nausea, vomiting, headache, dizziness, drowsiness, GI distress, weakness

SERIOUS REACTIONS
• Overdosage includes symptoms of anorexia, nausea, abdominal cramps, vomiting, diarrhea, and ataxia.

PRECAUTIONS & CONSIDERATIONS
Caution is necessary in pregnancy and with liver disease. Pyrantel should not be used concurrently with piperazines. It is unknown if pyrantel is distributed in breast milk. There are no age-related precautions noted in children or elderly. The entire family should be treated for pinworms. Wash bedding and clothes in hot soapy water to avoid being re-infected.
Storage
Refrigerate suspension.
Administration
2.9 g pamoate salt = 1 g base.
May be taken with or without food. Shake suspension well before using.

Pyrazinamide
pye-ra-zin′a-mide
(Pyrazinamide, Tebrazid [CAN], Zinamide [AUS])

CATEGORY AND SCHEDULE
Pregnancy Risk Category: C

CLASSIFICATION
Antimycobacterials

MECHANISM OF ACTION
An antitubercular whose exact mechanism of action is unknown. *Therapeutic Effect:* Either bacteriostatic or bactericidal, depending on the drug's concentration at the infection site and the susceptibility of infecting bacteria.

AVAILABILITY
Tablets: 500 mg.

INDICATIONS AND DOSAGES
▶ **Tuberculosis (in combination with other antituberculars)**
PO
Adults. 15-30 mg/kg/day in 1-4 doses. Maximum: 3 g/day.
Children. 20-40 mg/kg/day in 1 or 2 doses. Maximum: 2 g/day.

CONTRAINDICATIONS
Severe hepatic dysfunction

INTERACTIONS
Drug
Allopurinol, colchicine, probenecid, sulfinpyrazone: May decrease the effects of these drugs.
Herbal
None known.
Food
None known.

DIAGNOSTIC TEST EFFECTS
May increase AST (SGOT), ALT (SGPT), and serum uric acid concentrations.

SIDE EFFECTS
Frequent
Arthralgia, myalgia (usually mild and self-limiting)
Rare
Hypersensitivity reaction (rash, pruritus, urticaria), photosensitivity, gouty arthritis

SERIOUS REACTIONS
• Hepatotoxicity, gouty arthritis, thrombocytopenia, and anemia occur rarely.

PRECAUTIONS & CONSIDERATIONS
Caution is warranted with diabetes mellitus, a history of gout, and renal impairment. Caution should be used with possible cross-sensitivity to ethionamide, isoniazid, and niacin. Be aware that the safety and efficacy of pyrazinamide have not been established in children.
Liver function test results should be monitored. Side effects such as anorexia, fever, jaundice, liver tenderness, malaise, nausea, and vomiting may occur. If any liver reactions occur, stop the drug and notify the physician promptly. Serum uric acid levels should be monitored and signs and symptoms of gout, such as hot, painful, swollen joints, especially the ankle, big toe, or knee should be assessed. Blood glucose levels should be evaluated, especially in persons with diabetes mellitus, because pyrazinamide administration may make diabetic management difficult. Skin should be assessed for rash or eruptions.
Administration
Take pyrazinamide with food to reduce GI upset.

Pyridostigmine
peer-id-oh-stig'meen
(Mestinon, Mestinon SR [CAN],
Mestinon Timespan)
**Do not confuse pyridostigmine
with physostigmine or
Mesitonin with Mesantoin or
Metatensin.**

CATEGORY AND SCHEDULE
Pregnancy Risk Category: C

CLASSIFICATION
Cholinesterase inhibitors,
musculoskeletal agents,
stimulants, muscle

MECHANISM OF ACTION
A cholinergic that prevents destruction of acetylcholine by inhibiting the enzyme acetylcholinesterase, thus enhancing impulse transmission across the myoneural junction. *Therapeutic Effect:* Produces miosis; increases tone of intestinal, skeletal muscle tone; stimulates salivary and sweat gland secretions.

AVAILABILITY
Syrup (Mestinon): 60 mg/5 ml.
Tablets (Mestinon): 60 mg.
Tablets (Extended-Release [Mestinon Timespan]): 180 mg.
Injection (Mestinon): 5 mg/ml.

INDICATIONS AND DOSAGES
▸ **Myasthenia gravis**
PO
Adults, Elderly. Initially, 60 mg 3 times a day. Dosage increased at 48-hr intervals. Maintenance: 60 mg-1.5 g a day.
PO (EXTENDED-RELEASE)
Adults, Elderly. 180-540 mg once or twice a day with at least a 6-hr interval between doses.
IV, IM
Adults, Elderly. 2 mg q2-3hr.
Children, Neonates. 0.05-0.15 mg/kg/ dose. Maximum single dose: 10 mg.
▸ **Reversal of nondepolarizing neuromuscular blockade**
IV
Adults, Elderly. 10-20 mg with, or shortly after, 0.6-1.2 mg atropine sulfate or 0.3-0.6 mg glycopyrrolate.
Children. 0.1-0.25 mg/kg/dose preceded by atropine or glycopyrrolate.

CONTRAINDICATIONS
Mechanical GI or urinary tract obstruction

INTERACTIONS
Drug
Anticholinergics: Prevent or reverse the effects of pyridostigmine.
Cholinesterase inhibitors: May increase the risk of toxicity.
Neuromuscular blockers: Antagonizes the effects of these drugs.
Procainamide, quinidine: May antagonize the action of pyridostigmine.
Herbal
None known.
Food
None known.

DIAGNOSTIC TEST EFFECTS
None known.

▒ IV INCOMPATIBILITIES
Don't mix pyridostigmine with any other medications.

SIDE EFFECTS
Frequent
Miosis, increased GI and skeletal muscle tone, bradycardia, constriction of bronchi and ureters, diaphoresis, increased salivation

Occasional

Headache, rash, temporary decrease in diastolic B/P with mild reflex tachycardia, short periods of atrial fibrillation (in hyperthyroid patients), marked drop in B/P (in hypertensive patients)

SERIOUS REACTIONS

• Overdose may produce a cholinergic crisis, manifested as increasingly severe muscle weakness that appears first in muscles involving chewing and swallowing and is followed by muscle weakness of the shoulder girdle and upper extremities, respiratory muscle paralysis, and pelvis girdle and leg muscle paralysis. If overdose occurs, stop all cholinergic drugs and immediately administer 1-4 mg atropine sulfate IV for adults or 0.01 mg/kg for infants and children younger than 12 years.

PRECAUTIONS & CONSIDERATIONS

Caution is warranted with bradycardia, bronchial asthma, cardiac arrhythmias, epilepsy, hyperthyroidism, peptic ulcer disease, recent coronary occlusion, and vagotonia. Keep a log of energy level and muscle strength to help guide drug dosing.

Notify the physician of diarrhea, difficulty breathing, profuse salivation or sweating, irregular heartbeat, muscle weakness, severe abdominal pain, or nausea and vomiting. Therapeutic response to the drug, such as decreased fatigue, improved chewing and swallowing, and increased muscle strength, should be monitored. Respirations should be closely assessed.

Administration

! Drug dosage and frequency of administration are dependent on the daily clinical response, including exacerbations, physical and emotional stress, and remissions.

Crush tablets as needed. Take larger doses at times of increased fatigue, for example 30 to 45 minutes before meals. May break extended-release tablets but do not chew or crush them

For IV and IM use, give large doses concurrently with 0.6 to 1.2 mg atropine sulfate IV, as prescribed, to minimize side effects.

Pyridoxine (Vitamin B₆)

peer-i-dox′een

(Aminoxin, Beesix, Doxine, Nestrex, Pryi, Pyroxin [AUS], Rodex, Vitabee 6)

Do not confuse pyridoxine with paroxetine, pralidoxime, or Pyridium.

CATEGORY AND SCHEDULE

Pregnancy Risk Category: A
OTC

CLASSIFICATION

Vitamins/minerals

MECHANISM OF ACTION

Acts as a coenzyme for various metabolic functions, including metabolism of proteins, carbohydrates, and fats. Aids in the breakdown of glycogen and in the synthesis of gamma-aminobutyric acid in the CNS. *Therapeutic Effect:* Prevents pyridoxine deficiency. Increases the excretion of certain drugs, such as isoniazid, that are pyridoxine antagonists.

PHARMACOKINETICS

Readily absorbed primarily in jejunum. Stored in the liver, muscle, and brain. Metabolized in the liver.

Primarily excreted in urine. Removed by hemodialysis. **Half-life:** 15-20 days.

AVAILABILITY
Capsules: 250 mg.
Tablets: 20 mg, 25 mg, 50 mg, 100 mg, 250 mg, 500 mg.
Injection: 100 mg/ml.

INDICATIONS AND DOSAGES
▸ **Pyridoxine deficiency**
PO
Adults, Elderly. Initially, 2.5-10 mg/day; then 2.5 mg/day when clinical signs are corrected.
Children. Initially, 5-25 mg/day for 3 wk, then 1.5-2.5 mg/day.
▸ **Pyridoxine dependent seizures**
PO, IV, IM
Infants. Initially,10-100 mg/day. Maintenance: PO: 50-100 mg/day.
▸ **Drug-induced neuritis**
PO (treatment)
Adults, Elderly. 100-300 mg/day in divided doses
Children. 10-50 mg/day.
PO (prophylaxis)
Adults, Elderly. 25-100 mg/day.
Children. 1-2 mg/kg/day.

CONTRAINDICATIONS
None known.

INTERACTIONS
Drug
Immunosuppressants, isoniazid, penicillamine: May antagonize pyridoxine, causing anemia or peripheral neuritis.
Levodopa: Reverses the effects of levodopa.
Herbal
None known.
Food
None known.

DIAGNOSTIC TEST EFFECTS
None known.

▨ IV INCOMPATIBILITIES
Don't mix pyridoxine with any other medications.

SIDE EFFECTS
Occasional
Stinging at IM injection site
Rare
Headache, nausea, somnolence; sensory neuropathy (paraesthesia, unstable gait, clumsiness of hands) with high doses

SERIOUS REACTIONS
* Long-term megadoses (2-6 g over more than 2 mo) may produce sensory neuropathy (reduced deep tendon reflexes, profound impairment of sense of position in distal limbs, gradual sensory ataxia). Toxic symptoms subside when drug is discontinued.
* Seizures have occurred after IV megadoses.

PRECAUTIONS & CONSIDERATIONS
Pyridoxine crosses the placenta and is excreted in breast milk. High doses of pyridoxine in pregnancy may produce seizures in neonates. No age-related precautions have been noted in children or the elderly. Foods rich in pyridoxine, including avocados, bananas, bran, carrots, eggs, organ meats, tuna, shrimp, hazelnuts, legumes, soybeans, sunflower seeds, and wheat germ, are encouraged.

Improvement of deficiency symptoms, including CNS abnormalities (anxiety, depression, insomnia, motor difficulty, paraesthesia and tremors) and skin lesions (glossitis, seborrhea-like lesions around eyes, mouth, nose), should be monitored.
Storage
Store vials for parenteral use at room temperature. Use the solution immediately if reconstituted with sterile

water for injection and within 7 days if reconstituted with bacteriostatic water for injection.
Administration
Scored tablets may be crushed.
! Give pyridoxine orally unless malabsorption, nausea, or vomiting occurs.
Avoid IV use in cardiac patients.
Take extended-release capsules and tablets whole without crushing or breaking them. Have the patient avoid chewing the capsule or tablet. For IV use, pyridoxine may be given undiluted or may be added to IV solutions and given as an infusion. IM injections may cause discomfort.

Pyrimethamine
pye-ri-meth'a-meen
(Daraprim, Malocide [FRANCE])
Do not confuse with Dantrium, Daranide.

CATEGORY AND SCHEDULE
Pregnancy Risk Category: C

CLASSIFICATION
Antiprotozoals

MECHANISM OF ACTION
An antiprotozoal with blood and some tissue schizonticidal activity against malaria parasites of humans. Highly selective activity against plasmodia and *Toxoplasma gondii. Therapeutic Effect:* Inhibition of tetrahydrofolic acid synthesis.

PHARMACOKINETICS
Well absorbed, peak levels occurring between 2-6 hours following administration. Protein binding: 87%. Eliminated slowly. **Half-life:** approximately 96 hours.

AVAILABILITY
Tablets: 25 mg (Daraprim)

INDICATIONS AND DOSAGES
▸ **Toxoplasmosis**
PO
Adults. Initially, 50-75 mg daily, with 1-4 g daily of a sulfonamide of the sulfapyrimidine type (e.g., sulfadoxine). Continue for 1-3 weeks, depending on response of patient and tolerance to therapy then reduce dose to one-half that previously given for each drug and continue for additional 4-5 weeks.
Children. 1 mg/kg/day divided into 2 equal daily doses; after 2-4 days reduce to one-half and continue for approximately 1 month. The usual pediatric sulfonamide dosage is used in conjunction with pyrimethamine.
▸ **Acute malaria**
PO
Adults (in combination with sulfonamide). 25 mg daily for 2 days with a sulfonamide
Adults (without concomitant sulfonamide). 50 mg for 2 days
Children 4-10 yr. 25 mg daily for 2 days.
▸ **Chemoprophylaxis of malaria**
PO
Adults and pediatric patients over 10 yr: 25 mg once weekly.
Children 4-10 yr: 12.5 mg once weekly.
Infants and children under 4 yr: 6.25 mg once weekly.

OFF-LABEL USES
Prophylaxis for first episode and recurrence of *Pneumocystis carinii* pneumonia and *Toxoplasma gondii* in HIV-infected patients.

CONTRAINDICATIONS
Hypersensitivity to pyrimethamine, megaloblastic anemia due to folate

P

deficiency, monotherapy for treatment of acute malaria.

INTERACTIONS

Drug

Antifolic drugs: Pyrimethamine may be used with sulfonamides, quinine, and other antimalarials, and with other antibiotics. However, the concomitant use of other antifolic drugs, such as sulfonamides or trimethoprim-sulfamethoxazole combinations, while the patient is receiving pyrimethamine, may increase the risk of bone marrow suppression. If signs of folate deficiency develop, pyrimethamine should be discontinued. Folinic acid (leucovorin) should be administered until normal hematopoiesis is restored.

Benzodiazepines: Mild hepatotoxicity has been reported in some patients when lorazepam and pyrimethamine were administered concomitantly.

Herbal
None known.

Food
None known.

DIAGNOSTIC TEST EFFECTS
None known.

SIDE EFFECTS

Frequent
Anorexia, vomiting

Occasional
Hypersensitivity reactions, Stevens-Johnson syndrome, toxic epidermal necrolysis, erythema multiforme, anaphylaxis, hyperphenylalaninemia, megaloblastic anemia, leukopenia, thrombocytopenia, pancytopenia, atrophic glossitis, hematuria, and disorders of cardiac rhythm

Rare
Pulmonary eosinophilia

SERIOUS REACTIONS
• None known.

PRECAUTIONS & CONSIDERATIONS
Caution is warranted with megaloblastic anemia due to folate deficiency, seizures or epilepsy, kidney disease, and liver disease. It is unknown if pyrimethamine crosses the placenta. It passes through the breast milk and may be harmful to the infant. There are no age-related precautions noted in the elderly.

Storage
Store at room temperature away from heat and moisture.

Administration
Take with food to decrease stomach upset. Take each dose with a full glass of water.

Quazepam
kwaz'ze-pam
(Doral)

CATEGORY AND SCHEDULE
Pregnancy Risk Category: X
Controlled Substance:
Schedule IV

CLASSIFICATION
Benzodiazepines, sedatives/
hypnotics

MECHANISM OF ACTION
A BZ-1 receptor selective benzodiazepine with sedative properties.
Therapeutic Effect: Produces sedative
effect from its central nervous
system (CNS) depressant action.

PHARMACOKINETICS
Rapidly absorbed from gastrointestinal
(GI) tract. Food increases absorption.
Protein binding: 95%. Extensively
metabolized in liver. Excreted in urine
and feces. Unknown if removed by
hemodialysis. **Half-life:** 25-41 hr.

AVAILABILITY
Tablets: 7.5 mg, 15 mg (Doral).

INDICATIONS AND DOSAGES
▶ Insomnia
PO
Adults (older than 18 yr). Initially,
15 mg at bedtime. Adjust dose up or
down from 7.5 mg to 30 mg at
bedtime depending on initial response.
Elderly, debilitated, liver disease.
Initially, 7.5-15 mg at bedtime. Adjust
dose depending on initial response.

CONTRAINDICATIONS
Pregnancy, sleep apnea, hypersensitivity to quazepam or any component
of the formulation

INTERACTIONS
Drug
**Alcohol, central nervous system
(CNS) depressants:** Potentiates
effects of quazepam.
Azole antifungals: May inhibit liver
metabolism and increase quazepam
blood serum concentrations.
Theophylline: May decrease
quazepam effectiveness.
Herbal
**Dong quai, kava kava, magnolia,
passionflower, skullcap, tan-shen,
valerian:** May increase CNS
depressant effect of quazepam
Food
Caffeine: May decrease sedative
and anxiolytic effects of quazepam.

DIAGNOSTIC TEST EFFECTS
None known.

▨ IV INCOMPATIBILITIES
None known.
▨ IV Compatibilities
None known.

SIDE EFFECTS
Frequent
Muscular incoordination (ataxia),
lightheadedness, transient mild drowsiness, slurred speech (particularly in
elderly or debilitated patients)
Occasional
Confusion, depression, blurred vision,
constipation, diarrhea, dry mouth,
headache, nausea
Rare
Behavioral problems such as anger,
impaired memory, paradoxical reactions such as insomnia, nervousness,
or irritability

SERIOUS REACTIONS
• Abrupt or too rapid withdrawal
may result in pronounced restlessness,
irritability, insomnia, hand tremors,
abdominal and muscle cramps, sweating, vomiting, and seizures.

Q

- Overdosage results in somnolence, confusion, diminished reflexes, and coma.
- Blood dyscrasias have been reported rarely.

PRECAUTIONS & CONSIDERATIONS
Caution should be used with impaired renal or liver function. Quazepam crosses the placenta and is distributed in breast milk. Chronic ingestion of quazepam during pregnancy may produce withdrawal symptoms in women and CNS depression in neonates. Safety and efficacy of quazepam have not been established in children. In the elderly, use small initial doses and gradually increase them to avoid excessive sedation or ataxia as evidenced by muscular incoordination.

Drowsiness and dizziness are expected side effects. Avoid tasks that require mental alertness or motor skills as well as alcohol.

Administration
May be taken on an empty stomach. Take quazepam at bedtime. Tablets may be crushed. Do not abruptly stop quazepam.

Quetiapine
kwe-tye′a-peen
(Seroquel)

CATEGORY AND SCHEDULE
Pregnancy Risk Category: C

CLASSIFICATION
Antipsychotics

MECHANISM OF ACTION
A dibenzepin derivative that antagonizes dopamine, serotonin, histamine, and alpha$_1$-adrenergic receptors. *Therapeutic Effect:* Diminishes manifestations of psychotic disorders. Produces moderate sedation, few extrapyramidal effects, and no anticholinergic effects.

PHARMACOKINETICS
Well absorbed after PO administration. Protein binding: 83%. Widely distributed in tissues; CNS concentration exceeds plasma concentration. Undergoes extensive first-pass metabolism in the liver. Primarily excreted in urine. **Half-life:** 6 hr.

AVAILABILITY
Tablets: 25 mg, 100 mg, 200 mg, 300 mg.

INDICATIONS AND DOSAGES
▸ **To manage manifestations of psychotic disorders, Bipolar disorder**
PO
Adults, Elderly. Initially, 25 mg twice a day, then 25-50 mg 2-3 times a day on the second and third days, up to 300-400 mg/day in divided doses 2-3 times a day by the fourth day. Further adjustments of 25-50 mg twice a day may be made at intervals of 2 days or longer. Maintenance: 300-800 mg/day (adults); 50-200 mg/day (elderly).
Dosage in hepatic impairment, elderly or debilitated patients, and those predisposed to hypotensive reactions.
These patients should receive a lower initial dose and lower dosage increases.

CONTRAINDICATIONS
None known.

INTERACTIONS
Drug
Alcohol, other CNS depressants: May increase CNS depression.

Antihypertensives: May increase the hypotensive effects of these drugs.
Hepatic enzyme inducers (such as phenytoin): May increase quetiapine clearance.
Herbal
None known.
Food
None known.

DIAGNOSTIC TEST EFFECTS
May decrease serum total and free thyroxine (T_4) serum levels. May increase serum cholesterol, triglyceride, AST (SGOT), and ALT (SGPT) levels. May produce a false-positive pregnancy test result.

SIDE EFFECTS
Frequent (19%-10%)
Headache, somnolence, dizziness
Occasional (9%-3%)
Constipation, orthostatic hypotension, tachycardia, dry mouth, dyspepsia, rash, asthenia, abdominal pain, rhinitis
Rare (2%)
Back pain, fever, weight gain

SERIOUS REACTIONS
• Overdose may produce heart block hypotension, hypokalemia, and tachycardia.

PRECAUTIONS & CONSIDERATIONS
Caution is warranted with Alzheimer's disease, cardiovascular disease (such as CHF or history of MI), cerebrovascular disease, seizures, hepatic impairment, dehydration, hypothyroidism, hypovolemia, a history of breast cancer, and a history of drug abuse or dependence. It is unknown if quetiapine is distributed in breast milk. However, this drug is not recommended for breast-feeding women. The safety and efficacy of quetiapine have not been established in children. Although no age-related precautions have been noted in the elderly, lower initial and target dosages may be necessary for this age group.

Drowsiness and dizziness may occur but generally subsides with continued therapy. Tasks requiring mental alertness or motor skills should be avoided. Dehydration, particularly during exercise, exposure to extreme heat, and concurrent use of medications that cause dry mouth or other drying effects, should also be avoided. B/P, pulse rate, and pattern of daily bowel activity and stool consistency should be assessed.
Administration
Take quetiapine without regard to food. Know that dosage adjustments should occur at 2-day intervals. When restarting therapy for persons who have been off quetiapine for longer than 1 week, follow the initial titration schedule, as prescribed. When restarting therapy for persons who have been off quetiapine for less than 1 week, titration is not required and the maintenance dose can be reinstituted. Do not abruptly discontinue or increase the dosage.

Q

Quinapril
kwin'na-pril
(Accupril, Asig [AUS])
Do not confuse Accupril with Accolate or Accutane.

CATEGORY AND SCHEDULE
Pregnancy Risk Category: C
(D if used in second or third trimester)

CLASSIFICATION
Angiotensin converting enzyme inhibitors

MECHANISM OF ACTION

An ACE inhibitor that suppresses the renin-angiotensin-aldosterone system and prevents the conversion of angiotensin I to angiotensin II, a potent vasoconstrictor; may also inhibit angiotensin II at local vascular and renal sites. *Therapeutic Effect:* Reduces peripheral arterial resistance, B/P, and pulmonary capillary wedge pressure; improves cardiac output.

PHARMACOKINETICS

Route	Onset	Peak	Duration
PO	1 hr	N/A	24 hr

Readily absorbed from the GI tract. Protein binding: 97%. Metabolized in the liver, GI tract, and extravascular tissue to active metabolite. Primarily excreted in urine. Minimal removal by hemodialysis. **Half-life:** 1-2 hr; metabolite, 3 hr (increased in those with impaired renal function).

AVAILABILITY

Tablets: 5 mg, 10 mg, 20 mg, 40 mg.

INDICATIONS AND DOSAGES

▸ **Hypertension (monotherapy)**
PO
Adults. Initially, 10-20 mg/day. May adjust dosage at intervals of at least 2 wk or longer. Maintenance: 20-80 mg/day as single dose or 2 divided doses. Maximum: 80 mg/day.
Elderly. Initially, 2.5-5 mg/day. May increase by 2.5-5 mg q1-2wk.
▸ **Hypertension (combination therapy)**
PO
Adults. Initially, 5 mg/day titrated to patient's needs.
Elderly. Initially, 2.5-5 mg/day. May increase by 2.5-5 mg q1-2wk.

▸ **Adjunct to manage heart failure**
PO
Adults, Elderly. Initially, 5 mg twice a day. Range: 20-40 mg/day.
▸ **Dosage in renal impairment**
Dosage is titrated to the patient's needs after the following initial doses:

Creatinine Clearance	Initial Dose
More than 60 ml/min	10 mg
30-60 ml/min	5 mg
10-29 ml/min	2.5 mg

OFF-LABEL USES

Treatment of hypertension and renal crisis in scleroderma

CONTRAINDICATIONS

Bilateral renal artery stenosis

INTERACTIONS

Drug
Alcohol, antihypertensives, diuretics: May increase the effects of quinapril.
Lithium: May increase lithium blood concentration and risk of lithium toxicity.
NSAIDs: May decrease the effects of quinapril.
Potassium-sparing diuretics, potassium supplements: May cause hyperkalemia.
Herbal
Garlic: May increase antihypertensive effect.
Ginseng, yohimbe: May worsen hypertension.
Food
None known.

DIAGNOSTIC TEST EFFECTS

May increase BUN, serum alkaline phosphatase, serum bilirubin, serum creatinine, serum potassium,

AST (SGOT), and ALT (SGPT) levels. May decrease serum sodium levels. May cause positive antinuclear antibody titer.

SIDE EFFECTS
Frequent (7%-5%)
Headache, dizziness
Occasional (4%-2%)
Fatigue, vomiting, nausea, hypotension, chest pain, cough, syncope
Rare (less than 2%)
Diarrhea, cough, dyspnea, rash, palpitations, impotence, insomnia, drowsiness, malaise

SERIOUS REACTIONS
• Excessive hypotension (first-dose syncope) may occur in patients with CHF and in those who are severely salt or volume depleted.
• Angioedema and hyperkalemia occur rarely.
• Agranulocytosis and neutropenia may be noted in those with collagen vascular disease, including scleroderma and systemic lupus erythematosus, and impaired renal function.
• Nephrotic syndrome may be noted in those with history of renal disease.

PRECAUTIONS & CONSIDERATIONS
Caution is warranted with CHF, collagen vascular disease, hyperkalemia, hypovolemia, renal impairment, and renal stenosis. Quinapril crosses the placenta and it is unknown if it is distributed in breast milk. Quinapril may cause fetal or neonatal morbidity or mortality. Safety and efficacy of quinapril have not been established in children. The elderly may be more sensitive to the hypotensive effect of quinapril.

Dizziness and headache may occur. Tasks that require mental alertness or motor skills should be avoided. Be alert to fluctuations in B/P. If an

excessive reduction in B/P occurs, place the person in the supine position with legs elevated. CBC and blood chemistry should be obtained before beginning quinapril therapy, then every 2 weeks for the next 3 months, and periodically thereafter in patients with autoimmune disease, or renal impairment, and in those who are taking drugs that affect immune response or leukocyte count. BUN, serum creatinine, and serum potassium levels, and WBC count should also be monitored.

Administration
! Expect to discontinue diuretics 2 to 3 days before beginning quinapril therapy.

Take quinapril without regard to food. Crush tablets as desired.

Quinidine
(Apo-Quin-G [CAN], Apo-Quinidine [CAN], Biquinate [AUS], BioQuin Durules [CAN], Kinidin Durules [AUS], Myoquin [AUS], Quinaglute Dura-Tabs, Quinate [CAN], Quinbisu [AUS], Quinidex Extentabs, Quinoctal [AUS], Quinsul [AUS])
Do not confuse quinidine with clonidine or quinine.

CATEGORY AND SCHEDULE
Pregnancy Risk Category: C

CLASSIFICATION
Antiarrhythmics, class IA, antiprotozoals

Q

MECHANISM OF ACTION
An antiarrhythmic that decreases sodium influx during depolarization,

potassium efflux during repolarization, and reduces calcium transport across the myocardial cell membrane. Decreases myocardial excitability, conduction velocity, and contractility. *Therapeutic Effect:* Suppresses arrhythmias.

AVAILABILITY

Injection: 80 mg/ml.
Tablets: 200 mg, 300 mg.
Tablets (Extended-Release [Quinidex Extentabs]): 300 mg.
Tablets (Extended-Release [Quinaglute Dura-Tabs]): 324 mg.

INDICATIONS AND DOSAGES

▶ **Maintenance of normal sinus rhythm after conversion of atrial fibrillation or flutter; prevention of premature atrial, AV, and ventricular contractions; paroxysmal atrial tachycardia; paroxysmal AV junctional rhythm; atrial fibrillation; atrial flutter; paroxysmal ventricular tachycardia not associated with complete heart block**
PO
Adults, Elderly. 100-600 mg q4-6hr. (Long-acting): 324-972 mg q8-12hr.
Children: 30 mg/kg/day in divided doses q4-6hr.
IV
Adults, Elderly. 200-400 mg.
Children. 2-10 mg/kg.

OFF-LABEL USES

Treatment of malaria (IV only)

CONTRAINDICATIONS

Complete AV block, intraventricular conduction defects (widening of QRS complex)

INTERACTIONS

Drug
Antimyasthenics: May decrease effects of these drugs on skeletal muscle.

Digoxin: May increase digoxin serum concentration.
Other antiarrhythmics, pimozide: May increase cardiac effects.
Neuromuscular blockers, oral anticoagulants: May increase effects of these drugs.
Urinary alkalizers such as antacids: May decrease quinidine renal excretion.
Herbal
None known.
Food
None known.

DIAGNOSTIC TEST EFFECTS

Therapeutic serum level is 2 to 5 mcg/ml; toxic serum level is greater than 5 mcg/ml.

▨ IV INCOMPATIBILITIES

Furosemide (Lasix), heparin
▨ **IV Compatibilities**
Milrinone (Primacor)

SIDE EFFECTS

Frequent
Abdominal pain and cramps, nausea, diarrhea, vomiting (can be immediate, intense)
Occasional
Mild cinchonism (ringing in ears, blurred vision, hearing loss) or severe cinchonism (headache, vertigo, diaphoresis, lightheadedness, photophobia, confusion, delirium)
Rare
Hypotension (particularly with IV administration), hypersensitivity reaction (fever, anaphylaxis, photosensitivity reaction)

SERIOUS REACTIONS

• Cardiotoxic effects occur most commonly with IV administration, particularly at high concentrations, and are observed as conduction changes (50% widening of QRS complex, prolonged QT interval, flattened T waves, and disappearance of P wave), ventricular tachycardia or flutter, frequent premature ventricular contractions (PVCs), or complete AV block.

• Quinidine-induced syncope may occur with the usual dosage.

• Severe hypotension may result from high dosages.

• Patients with atrial flutter and fibrillation may experience a paradoxical, exremely rapid ventricular rate that may be prevented by prior digitalization.

• Hepatotoxicity with jaundice due to drug hypersensitivity may occur.

PRECAUTIONS & CONSIDERATIONS

Caution is warranted with digoxin toxicity, incomplete AV block, hepatic and renal impairment, myasthenia gravis, myocardial depression, and sick sinus syndrome. Direct sunlight and artificial light should be avoided.

B/P and pulse rate should be checked for 1 full minute before giving quinidine unless the person is on a continuous cardiac monitor. Notify the physician if fever, ringing in the ears, or visual disturbances occurs. CBC, BUN, serum alkaline phosphatase, bilirubin, creatinine, AST (SGOT), ALT (SGPT) levels, intake and output, pattern of bowel activity and stool consistency, serum potassium should be monitored in those receiving long-term therapy. EKG for cardiac changes, particularly prolongation of PR or QT interval and widening of the QRS complex should also be assessed; notify the physician of significant EKG changes.

Storage

Solution is stable for 24 hours at room temperature when diluted with D_5W.

Administration

! Quinidine's therapeutic serum level is 2 to 5 mcg/ml and the toxic level is greater than 5 mcg/ml.

Do not crush or chew sustained-release tablets. Take quinidine with food to reduce GI upset.

! Continuously monitor B/P and EKG during IV administration; adjust the rate of the infusion as appropriate and as ordered to minimize arrhythmias and hypotension.

Use only clear, colorless solution. For IV infusion, dilute 800 mg with 40 ml D_5W to provide concentration of 16 mg/ml. Give at rate of 1 ml (16 mg)/min because a rapid rate may markedly decrease arterial pressure. Administer with patient in supine position.

Quinine
kwye'nine
(Quinine)
Do not confuse with quinidine.

CATEGORY AND SCHEDULE
Pregnancy Risk Category: X

CLASSIFICATION
Antiprotozoals

MECHANISM OF ACTION
A cinchone alkaloid that relaxes skeletal muscle by increasing the refractory period, decreasing excitability of motor end plates (curarelike), and affecting distribution of calcium with muscle fiber. Antimalaria: Depresses oxygen uptake, carbohydrate metabolism, elevates pH in intracellular organelles of parasites. *Therapeutic Effect:* Relaxes skeletal muscle; produces parasite death.

PHARMACOKINETICS
Rapidly absorbed mainly from upper small intestine. Protein binding: 70%-95%. Metabolized in liver.

Excreted in feces, saliva, and urine.
Half-life: 8-14 hr (adults), 6-12 hr
(children).

AVAILABILITY
Capsules: 200 mg, 325 mg (Quinine).
Tablets: 260 mg (Quinine).

INDICATIONS AND DOSAGES
▶ **Nocturnal leg cramps**
PO
Adults, Elderly. 260-300 mg at
bedtime as needed.
▶ **Treatment of malaria**
PO
Adults, Elderly. 260-650 mg 3 times
a day for 6-12 days.
Children. 10 mg/kg q8hr for 5-7 days.
Dosage in renal impairment

Creatinine Clearance	Dosage Interval
10-50 ml/min	75% of normal dose or q12hr
Less than 10 ml/min	30%-50% of normal dose or q24hr

CONTRAINDICATIONS
Hypersensitivity to quinine (possible
cross-sensitivity to quinidine), G-6-
PD deficiency, tinnitus, optic neuritis,
history of thrombocytopenia during
previous quinine therapy, blackwater
fever

INTERACTIONS
Drug
**Amiodarone, alkalinizing agents,
cimetidine, verapamil:** May
increase quinine serum concentrations.
Beta blockers: May increase bradycardia.
Digoxin: May increase blood
concentration of digoxin.
Mefloquine: May increase risk of
seizures and EKG abnormalities.

**Phenobarbital, phenytoin,
rifampin:** May decrease quinine
serum concentrations.
Warfarin: May increase anticoagu-
lant effect.
Herbal
St. John's wort: May decrease
quinine levels.
Food
None known.

DIAGNOSTIC TEST EFFECTS
May interfere with 17-OH steroid
determinations. May result in positive
Coombs' test.

SIDE EFFECTS
Frequent
Nausea, headache, tinnitus, slight
visual disturbances (mild cinchonism)
Occasional
Extreme flushing of skin with intense
generalized pruritus is most typical
hypersensitivity reaction; also rash,
wheezing, dyspnea, angioedema.
Prolonged therapy: cardiac conduction
disturbances, decreased hearing

SERIOUS REACTIONS
• Overdosage (severe cinchonism)
may result in cardiovascular effects,
severe headache, intestinal cramps
with vomiting and diarrhea, apprehension, confusion, seizures, blindness, and respiratory depression.
• Hypoprothrombinemia, thrombocytopenic purpura, hemoglobinuria,
asthma, agranulocytosis, hypoglycemia, deafness, and optic atrophy occur rarely.

PRECAUTIONS & CONSIDERATIONS
Caution is warranted with cardiovascular disease, myasthenia gravis, and
asthma. Be aware that quinine is
contraindicated in pregnant women.
Quinine readily crosses the placenta
and is distributed in breast milk. Be
aware that quinine may cause

congenital malformations such as deafness, limb abnormalities, visceral defects, visual changes, stillbirths. Nonhormonal contraception should be used. There are no age-related precautions noted in children. In the elderly, age-related renal impairment may require dosage adjustment.

Fasting blood sugar should be checked and watch for signs of hypoglycemia such as cold sweating, tremors, tachycardia, hunger, anxiety.

Visual/hearing difficulties, shortness of breath, rash, itching, and nausea should be reported. Aluminum-containing antacids should be avoided because of drug absorption problems.

Storage

Store at room temperature.

Administration

Take quinine with food. Do not crush tablets or capsules to avoid bitter taste.

Q

Rabeprazole
rah-bep'rah-zole
(Aciphex, Pariet [CAN])
Do not confuse Aciphex with Accupril or Aricept.

CATEGORY AND SCHEDULE
Pregnancy Risk Category: B

CLASSIFICATION
Gastrointestinals, proton pump inhibitors

MECHANISM OF ACTION
A proton pump inhibitor that converts to active metabolites that irreversibly binds to and inhibit hydrogen-potassium adenosine triphosphate, an enzyme on the surface of gastric parietal cells. Actively secretes hydrogen ions for potassium ions, resulting in an accumulation of hydrogen ions in gastric lumen. *Therapeutic Effect:* Increases gastric pH, reducing gastric acid production.

PHARMACOKINETICS
Rapidly absorbed from the GI tract after passing through the stomach relatively intact. Protein binding: 96%. Metabolized extensively in the liver. Primarily excreted in urine. Unknown if removed by hemodialysis. **Half-life:** 1-2 hr (increased with hepatic impairment).

AVAILABILITY
Tablets (Delayed-Release): 20 mg.

INDICATIONS AND DOSAGES
▸ **Gastroesophageal reflux disease**
PO
Adults, Elderly. 20 mg/day for 4-8 wk. Maintenance: 20 mg/day.

▸ **Duodenal ulcer**
PO
Adults, Elderly. 20 mg/day after morning meal for 4 wk.
▸ **Non-steroidal antiinflammatory disorder (NSAID)-induced ulcer**
PO
Adults, Elderly. 20 mg/day.
▸ **Pathologic hypersecretory conditions**
PO
Adults, Elderly. Initially, 60 mg once a day. May increase to 60 mg twice a day.
▸ *Helicobacter pylori* **infection**
PO
Adults, Elderly. 20 mg 2 times a day for 7 days (given with amoxicillin 1000 mg and clarithromycin 500 mg)

CONTRAINDICATIONS
None known.

INTERACTIONS
Drug
Digoxin: May increase the plasma concentration of digoxin.
Ketoconazole: May decrease the blood concentration of ketoconazole.
Herbal
None known.
Food
None known.

DIAGNOSTIC TEST EFFECTS
May increase serum alkaline phosphatase, AST (SGOT), and ALT (SGPT) levels.

SIDE EFFECTS
Rare (less than 2%)
Headache, nausea, dizziness, rash, diarrhea, malaise

SERIOUS REACTIONS
• Hyperglycemia, hypokalemia, hyponatremia, and hyperlipemia occur rarely.

PRECAUTIONS & CONSIDERATIONS

Caution is warranted with impaired hepatic function. It is unknown if rabeprazole crosses the placenta or is distributed in breast milk. Safety and efficacy of rabeprazole have not been established in children. No age-related precautions have been noted in the elderly.

Notify the physician if diarrhea, GI discomfort, headache, nausea, or skin rash occurs. Laboratory values, especially serum chemistries and liver function test results, should be assessed before therapy.

Administration

Take rabeprazole before meals. Do not crush, chew, or split tablet; swallow it whole.

Raloxifene

ra-lox'i-feen
(Evista)
Do not confuse raloxifene with propoxyphene.

CATEGORY AND SCHEDULE

Pregnancy Risk Category: X

CLASSIFICATION

Estrogen receptor modulators, selective, hormones/hormone modifiers

MECHANISM OF ACTION

A selective estrogen receptor modulator that affects some receptors like estrogen. *Therapeutic Effect:* Like estrogen, prevents bone loss and improves lipid profiles.

PHARMACOKINETICS

Rapidly absorbed after PO administration. Highly bound to plasma proteins (95%) and albumin. Undergoes extensive first-pass metabolism in liver. Excreted mainly in feces and, to a lesser extent, in urine. Unknown if removed by hemodialysis. **Half-life:** 27.7 hr.

AVAILABILITY

Tablets: 60 mg.

INDICATIONS AND DOSAGES

▶ **Prevention or treatment of osteoporosis**
PO
Adults, Elderly. 60 mg a day.

OFF-LABEL USES

Treatment of breast cancer in postmenopausal women, prevention of fractures

CONTRAINDICATIONS

Active or history of venous thromboembolic events, such as deep vein thrombosis, pulmonary embolism, and retinal vein thrombosis; women who are or may become pregnant

INTERACTIONS

Drug
Ampicillin, cholestyramine: Reduce raloxifene absorption.
Hormone replacement therapy, systemic estrogen: Don't use raloxifene concurrently with these drugs.
Warfarin: May decrease PT and the effects of warfarin.
Herbal
None known.
Food
None known.

DIAGNOSTIC TEST EFFECTS

Lowers serum total cholesterol and LDL levels, but does not affect HDL or triglyceride levels. Slightly decreases platelet count and serum inorganic phosphate, albumin, calcium, and protein levels.

SIDE EFFECTS
Frequent (25%-10%)
Hot flashes, flu-like symptoms, arthralgia, sinusitis
Occasional (9%-5%)
Weight gain, nausea, myalgia, pharyngitis, cough, dyspepsia, leg cramps, rash, depression
Rare (4%-3%)
Vaginitis, UTI, peripheral edema, flatulence, vomiting, fever, migraine, diaphoresis

SERIOUS REACTIONS
• Pneumonia, gastroenteritis, chest pain, vaginal bleeding, and breast pain occur rarely.

PRECAUTIONS & CONSIDERATIONS
Caution is warranted with cardiovascular disease, hepatic or renal impairment, and a history of cervical or uterine cancer. It is unknown if raloxifene is distributed in breast milk. However, this drug is not recommended for breast-feeding women. Raloxifene is not used in children. No age-related precautions have been noted in the elderly. Avoid alcohol consumption and cigarette smoking during raloxifene therapy. Also avoid prolonged immobility during travel because limited movement increases the risk of venous thromboembolic events. Exercise is encouraged.

Bone mineral density, platelet count, serum levels of inorganic phosphate, calcium, total and LDL cholesterol, and protein should be monitored.
Administration
Take raloxifene without regard to food at any time of day. Discontinue the drug 72 hours before and during prolonged immobilization, such as postoperative recovery and prolonged bed rest. Resume therapy, as prescribed, only after the patient is fully ambulatory. Take supplemental calcium and vitamin D if daily dietary intake is inadequate.

Ramipril
ram'i-pril
(Altace)
Do not confuse Altace with Alteplase or Artane.

CATEGORY AND SCHEDULE
Pregnancy Risk Category: C (D if used in second or third trimester)

CLASSIFICATION
Angiotensin converting enzyme inhibitors

MECHANISM OF ACTION
An ACE inhibitor that suppresses the renin-angiotensin-aldosterone system. Decreases plasma angiotensin II, increases plasma renin activity, and decreases aldosterone secretion. *Therapeutic Effect:* Reduces peripheral arterial resistance and B/P.

PHARMACOKINETICS
Route	Onset	Peak	Duration
PO	1-2 hr	3-6 hr	24 hr

Well absorbed from the GI tract. Protein binding: 73%. Metabolized in the liver to active metabolite. Primarily excreted in urine. Not removed by hemodialysis. **Half-life:** 5.1 hr.

AVAILABILITY

Capsules: 1.25 mg, 2.5 mg, 5 mg, 10 mg.

INDICATIONS AND DOSAGES

▸ **Hypertension (monotherapy)**
PO
Adults, Elderly. Initially, 2.5 mg/day. Maintenance: 2.5-20 mg/day as single dose or in 2 divided doses.
▸ **Hypertension (in combination with other antihypertensives)**
PO
Adults, Elderly. Initially, 1.25 mg/day titrated to patient's needs.
▸ **CHF**
PO
Adults, Elderly. Initially, 1.25-2.5 mg twice a day. Maximum: 5 mg twice a day.
▸ **Risk reduction for myocardial infarction stroke**
PO
Adults, Elderly. Initially, 2.5 mg/day for 7 days, then 5 mg/day for 21 days, then 10 mg/day as a single dose or in divided doses.
▸ **Dosage in renal impairment**
Creatinine clearance equal to or less than 40 ml/min. 25% of normal dose.
Hypertension. Initially, 1.25 mg/day titrated upward.
CHF. Initially, 1.25 mg/day, titrated up to 2.5 mg twice a day.

OFF-LABEL USES

Treatment of hypertension and renal crisis in scleroderma

CONTRAINDICATIONS

Bilateral renal artery stenosis

INTERACTIONS
Drug
Alcohol, antihypertensives, diuretics: May increase the effects of ramipril.
Lithium: May increase lithium blood concentration and risk of lithium toxicity.
NSAIDs: May decrease the effects of ramipril.
Potassium-sparing diuretics, potassium supplements: May cause hyperkalemia.
Herbal
Garlic: May increase antihypertensive effect.
Ginseng, yohimbe: May worsen hypertension.
Food
None known.

DIAGNOSTIC TEST EFFECTS

May increase BUN, serum alkaline phosphatase, serum bilirubin, serum creatinine, serum potassium, AST (SGOT), and ALT (SGPT) levels. May decrease serum sodium levels. May cause positive antinuclear antibody titer.

SIDE EFFECTS

Frequent (12%-5%)
Cough, headache
Occasional (4%-2%)
Dizziness, fatigue, nausea, asthenia (loss of strength)
Rare (less than 2%)
Palpitations, insomnia, nervousness, malaise, abdominal pain, myalgia

SERIOUS REACTIONS

• Excessive hypotension (first-dose syncope) may occur in patients with CHF and and in those who are severely salt or volume depleted.
• Angioedema and hyperkalemia occur rarely.
• Agranulocytosis and neutropenia may be noted in those with collagen

R

vascular disease, including scleroderma and systemic lupus erythematosus, and impaired renal function.
• Nephrotic syndrome may be noted
in those with history of renal disease.

PRECAUTIONS & CONSIDERATIONS

Caution is warranted with CHF,
collagen vascular disease, hyperkalemia, hypovolemia, renal impairment, and renal stenosis. Ramipril
crosses the placenta, is distributed in
breast milk, and may cause fetal or
neonatal morbidity or mortality.
Safety and efficacy of ramipril have
not been established in children. The
elderly may be more sensitive to the
hypotensive effect of ramipril.

Dizziness and lightheadedness
may occur. Tasks that require mental
alertness or motor skills should be
avoided. Notify the physician if
chest pain, cough, or palpitations
occur. Be alert to fluctuations in B/P.
If an excessive reduction in B/P
occurs, place the person in the
supine position with legs elevated.
CBC and blood chemistry should be
obtained before beginning ramipril
therapy, then every 2 weeks for the
next 3 months, and periodically
thereafter in patients with autoimmune disease, or renal impairment,
and in those who are taking drugs
that affect immune response or
leukocyte count. BUN, serum creatinine, and serum potassium levels, and
WBC count should also be monitored. Crackles and wheezing should
be assessed in persons with CHF.

Administration

❗ Expect to discontinue diuretics 2 to
3 days before beginning ramipril
therapy.

Take ramipril without regard to
food. Swallow the capsules whole
and do not chew or break them. Mix
with apple juice, applesauce, or water
as needed.

Ranitidine
ra-ni'ti-deen
(Apo-Ranitidine [CAN], Ausran
[AUS], Novo-Ranidine [CAN],
Rani-2 [AUS], Ranihexal [AUS],
Zantac, Zantac-75, Zantac
EFFERdose)
**Do not confuse Zantac
with Xanax, Ziac,
or Zyrtec.**

CATEGORY AND SCHEDULE
Pregnancy Risk Category: B
OTC (Tablets, 75 mg)

CLASSIFICATION
Antihistamines, H2,
gastrointestinals

MECHANISM OF ACTION
An antiulcer agent that inhibits histamine action at histamine 2 receptors
of gastric parietal cells. *Therapeutic
Effect:* Inhibits gastric acid secretion
when fasting, at night, or when stimulated by food, caffeine, or insulin.
Reduces volume and hydrogen ion
concentration of gastric juice.

PHARMACOKINETICS
Rapidly absorbed from the GI tract.
Protein binding: 15%. Widely
distributed. Metabolized in the liver.
Primarily excreted in urine. Not
removed by hemodialysis. **Half-life:**
PO, 2.5 hr; IV, 2-2.5 hr (increased
with impaired renal function).

AVAILABILITY
*Tablets (Effervescent [Zantac
EFFERdose]):* 25 mg, 150 mg.
Capsules: 150 mg, 300 mg.
Granules (Zantac EFFERdose):
150 mg.
Syrup (Zantac): 15 mg/ml.
Tablets (Zantac 75): 75 mg (OTC).

Tablets (Zantac): 150 mg, 300 mg.
Injection (Zantac): 25 mg/ml.

INDICATIONS AND DOSAGES
▶ **Duodenal ulcers, gastric ulcers, gastroesophageal reflux disease**
PO
Adults, Elderly. 150 mg twice a day or 300 mg at bedtime. Maintenance: 150 mg at bedtime.
Children. 2-4 mg/kg/day in divided doses twice a day. Maximum: 300 mg/day.
▶ **Erosive esophagitis**
PO
Adults, Elderly. 150 mg 4 times a day. Maintenance: 150 mg 2 times/day or 300 mg at bedtime.
Children. 4-10 mg/kg/day in 2 divided doses. Maximum: 600 mg/day.
▶ **Hypersecretory conditions**
PO
Adults, Elderly. 150 mg twice a day. May increase up to 6 g/day.
▶ **Usual parenteral dosage**
IV, IM
Adults, Elderly. 50 mg/dose q6-8hr. Maximum: 400 mg/day.
Children. 2-4 mg/kg/day in divided doses q6-8hr. Maximum: 200 mg/day.
▶ **Usual neonatal dosage**
PO
Neonates. 2 mg/kg/day in divided doses q12hr.
IV
Neonates. Initially, 1.5 mg/kg/dose; then 1.5-2 mg/kg/day in divided doses q12hr.
▶ **Dosage in renal impairment**
For patients with creatinine clearance less than 50 ml/min, give 150 mg PO q24hr or 50 mg IV or IM q18-24hr.

OFF-LABEL USES
Prevention of aspiration pneumonia

CONTRAINDICATIONS
History of acute porphyria

INTERACTIONS
Drug
Antacids: May decrease the absorption of ranitidine.
Ketoconazole: May decrease the absorption of ketoconazole.
Herbal
None known.
Food
None known.

DIAGNOSTIC TEST EFFECTS
Interferes with skin tests using allergen extracts. May increase hepatic function enzyme, gamma-glutamyl transpeptidase, and serum creatinine levels.

▨ IV INCOMPATIBILITIES
Amphotericin B complex (Abelcet, AmBisome, Amphotec)
▨ **IV Compatibilities**
Diltiazem (Cardizem), dobutamine (Dobutrex), dopamine (Intropin), heparin, hydromorphone (Dilaudid), insulin, lidocaine, lorazepam (Ativan), morphine, norepinephrine (Levophed), potassium chloride, propofol (Diprivan)

SIDE EFFECTS
Occasional (2%)
Diarrhea
Rare (1%)
Constipation, headache (may be severe)

SERIOUS REACTIONS
• Reversible hepatitis and blood dyscrasias occur rarely.

PRECAUTIONS & CONSIDERATIONS
Caution is warranted with impaired hepatic or renal function and in the elderly. It is unknown if ranitidine crosses the placenta or is distributed in breast milk. No age-related precautions have been noted in children. The elderly are more likely to

R

experience confusion, especially those with hepatic or renal impairment. Smoking should be avoided. Also, avoid alcohol, aspirin, and coffee, all of which may cause GI distress, during ranitidine therapy.

Notify the physician if headache occurs. Blood chemistry laboratory test results, including BUN, serum alkaline phosphatase, bilirubin, creatinine, AST (SGOT), and ALT (SGPT) levels to assess hepatic and renal function, should be obtained before and during therapy.

Storage

IV infusion (piggyback) is stable for 48 hours at room temperature. Discard if discolored or precipitate forms.

Administration

Take oral ranitidine without regard to meals; however it's best given after meals or at bedtime. Do not administer within 1 hour of magnesium- or aluminum-containing antacids because they decrease ranitidine absorption by 33%. Give 2 hours after ketoconazole administration.

IV solutions normally appear clear and are colorless to yellow; slight darkening does not affect potency. For IV push, dilute each 50 mg with 20 ml 0.9% NaCl or D_5W. For intermittent IV infusion (piggyback), dilute each 50 mg with 50 ml 0.9% NaCl or D_5W. For IV infusion, dilute with 250 to 1000 ml 0.9% NaCl or D_5W. Administer IV push over minimum of 5 minutes to prevent arrhythmias and hypotension. Infuse IV piggyback over 15 to 20 minutes. Infuse IV infusion over 24 hours.

For IM use, ranitidine may be given undiluted. Give deep IM into large muscle mass, such as the gluteus maximus.

Repaglinide
re-pag′lih-nide
(GlucoNorm [CAN], Prandin)

CATEGORY AND SCHEDULE
Pregnancy Risk Category: C

CLASSIFICATION
Antidiabetic agents, meglitinides

MECHANISM OF ACTION
An antihyperglycemic that stimulates release of insulin from beta cells of the pancreas by depolarizing beta cells, leading to an opening of calcium channels. Resulting calcium influx induces insulin secretion. *Therapeutic Effect:* Lowers blood glucose concentration.

PHARMACOKINETICS
Rapidly, completely absorbed from the GI tract. Protein binding: 98%. Metabolized in the liver to inactive metabolites. Excreted primarily in feces with a lesser amount in urine. Unknown if removed by hemodialysis. **Half-life:** 1 hr.

AVAILABILITY
Tablets: 0.5 mg, 1 mg, 2 mg.

INDICATIONS AND DOSAGES
▸ **Diabetes mellitus**
PO
Adults, Elderly. 0.5-4 mg 2-4 times a day. Maximum: 16 mg/day.

CONTRAINDICATIONS
Diabetic ketoacidosis, type 1 diabetes mellitus

INTERACTIONS
Drug
Beta blockers, chloramphenicol, gemfibrozil, MAOIs, NSAIDs,

probenecid, salicylates, sulfon-
amides, warfarin: May increase the
effects of repaglinide.
Herbal
None known.
Food
Food: Decreases repaglinide plasma
concentration.

DIAGNOSTIC TEST EFFECTS
None known.

SIDE EFFECTS
Frequent (10%-6%)
Upper respiratory tract infection,
headache, rhinitis, bronchitis, back
pain
Occasional (5%-3%)
Diarrhea, dyspepsia, sinusitis,
nausea, arthralgia, urinary tract
infection
Rare (2%)
Constipation, vomiting, paresthesia,
allergy

SERIOUS REACTIONS
• Hypoglycemia occurs in 16% of
patients.
• Chest pain occurs rarely.

PRECAUTIONS & CONSIDERATIONS
Caution is warranted with hepatic or
renal impairment. It is unknown if
repaglinide is distributed in breast
milk. Safety and efficacy of repaglinide have not been established in children. No age-related precautions have
been noted in the elderly, but hypoglycemia may be more difficult to
recognize in this patient population.
Food intake and blood glucose
should be monitored before and
during therapy. Be aware of signs and
symptoms of hypoglycemia (anxiety,
cool wet skin, diplopia, dizziness,
headache, hunger, numbness in
mouth, tachycardia, tremors), or
hyperglycemia (deep rapid breathing,
dim vision, fatigue, nausea, polydipsia,

polyphagia, polyuria, vomiting);
carry candy, sugar packets, or other
sugar supplements for immediate
response to hypoglycemia. Consult
the physician when glucose demands
are altered (such as with fever, heavy
physical activity, infection, stress,
trauma). Exercise, good personal
hygiene (including foot care), not
smoking, and weight control are
essential parts of therapy.
Administration
Ideally, take repaglinide within
15 minutes of a meal; however, it
may be taken immediately or as long
as 30 minutes before a meal. Allow
at least 1 week to elapse to assess
response to the drug before new
dosage adjustment is made.

Reserpine
reh-zer'peen
(Serpalan, Maviserpin [MEX],
Novoreserpine [CAN], Rauserpine
[TAIWAN], Rauverid [PHILIPPINES],
Reserfia [CAN], Serpasil [CAN,
INDONESIA], Serpasol [SPAIN])
**Do not confuse with Risperdal,
risperidone**

CATEGORY AND SCHEDULE
Pregnancy Risk Category: C

CLASSIFICATION
Antiadrenergics, peripheral

MECHANISM OF ACTION
An antihypertensive that depletes
stores of catecholamines and
5-hydroxytryptamine in many organs,
including the brain and adrenal
medulla. Depression of sympathetic
nerve function results in a decreased

heart rate and a lowering of arterial blood pressure. Depletion of cate-cholamines and 5-hydroxytryptamine from the brain is thought to be the mechanism of the sedative and tran-quilizing properties. *Therapeutic Effects:* Decrease blood pressure and heart rate; sedation.

PHARMACOKINETICS

Characterized by slow onset of action and sustained effects. Both cardiovas-cular and central nervous system effects may persist for a period of time following withdrawal of the drug. Mean maximum plasma levels were attained after a median of 3.5 hours. Bioavailability was approx-imately 50% of that of a correspon-ding intravenous dose. Protein binding: 96%. **Half life:** 33 hours.

AVAILABILITY

Tablets: 0.25 mg, 0.1 mg (reserpine)

INDICATIONS AND DOSAGES

▸ **Hypertension**
PO
Adults: Usual initial dosage 0.5 mg daily for 1 or 2 weeks. For mainte-nance, reduce to 0.1 to 0.25 mg daily.
Children: Reserpine is not recom-mended for use in children. If it is to be used in treating a child, the usual recommended starting dose is 20 µg/kg daily. The maximum recom-mended dose is 0.25 mg (total) daily.
▸ **Psychiatric Disorders**
PO
Adults: Initial dosage 0.5 mg daily, may range from 0.1-1.0 mg. Adjust dosage upward or downward accord-ing to response.

OFF-LABEL USES

Cerebral vasospasm, migraines, Raynaud's syndrome, reflex sympathetic dystrophy, refractory

depression, tardive dyskinesia, thyro-toxic crisis.

CONTRAINDICATIONS

Hypersensitivity, mental depression or history of mental depression (espe-cially with suicidal tendencies), active peptic ulcer, ulcerative colitis, patients receiving electroconvulsive therapy.

INTERACTIONS

Drug
MAO inhibitors: May cause hyper-tensive reactions.
Beta-blockers: Reserpine may increase effect.
CNS depressants/ethanol: Reserpine may increase effects.
Levodopa, quinidine, procainamide, digitalis glycosides: Reserpine may increase effects/ toxicity.
Tricyclic antidepressants: May increase antihypertensive effects.
Herbal
Dong quai: Has estrogenic activity
Ephedra/yohimbe: May worsen hypertension
Valerian, St John's wort, kava kava, gotu kola: May increase CNS depression
Garlic: May have increased antihy-pertensive effects
Food
Ethanol: May increase CNS depression.

DIAGNOSTIC TEST EFFECTS

None known.

SIDE EFFECTS

Occasional
Burning in the stomach, nausea, vomiting, diarrhea, dry mouth, nose-bleed, stuffy nose, dizziness, headache, nervousness, nightmares, drowsiness, muscle aches, weight gain, redness of the eyes

Rare
Irregular heart beat, difficulty breathing, heart problems, feeling faint, swelling, gynecomastia, decreased libido

SERIOUS REACTIONS
- None known.

PRECAUTIONS & CONSIDERATIONS

Caution is warranted with kidney disease, gallstones, ulcers, ulcerative colitis, history of depression, electric shock therapy, and allergy to tartrazine. The physician should be aware of other medications being taken especially quinidine, digoxin, and tricyclic antidepressants such as imipramine, amitriptyline, doxepin, and nortriptyline. Be aware that reserpine is excreted in the breast milk. The elderly may be more susceptible to the hypotensive effects of reserpine. A low-salt diet should be followed. Change positions slowly to avoid orthostatic hypotension.

Dizziness, loss of appetite, diarrhea, upset stomach, vomiting, headache, dry mouth, and decreased sexual ability may occur. Notify physician immediately if depression, nightmares, fainting, slow heartbeat, chest pain, or swollen ankles and feet occur.

Storage
Store at room temperature.

Administration
Take with food or milk to avoid GI irritation. Take at the same time each day.

Respiratory Syncytial Immune Globulin
res′purr-ah-tore-ee sin-sish′ee-al ih-mewn′ glah′byew-lin
(RespiGam)

CATEGORY AND SCHEDULE
Pregnancy Risk Category: C

CLASSIFICATION
Immune globulins

MECHANISM OF ACTION
An immune serum with a high concentration of neutralizing and protective antibodies specific for respiratory syncytial virus (RSV).
Therapeutic Effect: Provides protection against RSV infection and decreases the severity of existing infection.

AVAILABILITY
Injection: 2500 mcg RSV immune globulin.

INDICATIONS AND DOSAGES
▸ **Prevention of RSV in children with bronchopulmonary dysplasia and history of premature birth**
IV
Children younger than 24 mo.
750 mg/kg (15 ml/kg) administered at a rate of 1.5 ml/kg/hr for the first 15 min, then 3.6 ml/kg/hr for remainder of infusion. Given once monthly for 5 doses beginning in September or October.

CONTRAINDICATIONS
IgA deficiency

INTERACTIONS
Drug
Live-virus vaccines: May decrease the patient's antibody response to the vaccine.

Herbal
None known.
Food
None known.

DIAGNOSTIC TEST EFFECTS
None known.

SIDE EFFECTS
Occasional (6%-2%)
Fever, vomiting, wheezing
Rare (less than 1%)
Diarrhea, rash, tachycardia, hypertension, hypoxia, injection site inflammation

SERIOUS REACTIONS
* Hypersensitivity reactions, characterized by dizziness, flushing, anxiety, palpitations, pruritus, myalgia, and arthralgia, occur rarely.

PRECAUTIONS & CONSIDERATIONS
Caution is warranted with pulmonary disease. ABG, blood chemistry, serum osmolality electrolyte and total protein levels should be monitored. Cardiopulmonary status and vital signs should be assessed before giving the drug, before each dosage or rate increase, every 30 minutes during the infusion, and 30 minutes after the infusion is completed. Child's body weight should be recorded. Baseline pulmonary assessment, including breath sounds, presence of intercostal retractions, and respiratory rate, should be performed.
Storage
Refrigerate vials. Do not freeze.
Administration
Do not shake the vials. Start the infusion within 6 hours and complete it within 12 hours of opening the vial. Administer the infusion at a rate of 1.5 ml/kg/hr for the first 15 minutes, then 3.6 ml/kg/hr until the end of the infusion.

Reteplase
reh'te-place
(Rapilysin [AUS], Retavase)
Do not confuse reteplase or Retavase with Restasis.

CATEGORY AND SCHEDULE
Pregnancy Risk Category: C

CLASSIFICATION
Thrombolytics

MECHANISM OF ACTION
A tissue plasminogen activator that activates the fibrinolytic system by directly cleaving plasminogen to generate plasmin, an enzyme that degrades the fibrin of the thrombus. *Therapeutic Effect:* Exerts thrombolytic action.

PHARMACOKINETICS
Rapidly cleared from plasma. Eliminated primarily by the liver and kidney. **Half-life:** 13-16 min.

AVAILABILITY
Powder for Injection: 10.4 units (18.1 mg).

INDICATIONS AND DOSAGES
▶ **Acute MI, CHF**
IV bolus
Adults, Elderly. 10 units over 2 min; repeat in 30 min.

CONTRAINDICATIONS
Active internal bleeding, AV malformation or aneurysm, bleeding diathesis, history of cerebrovascular accident, intracranial neoplasm, recent intracranial or intraspinal surgery or trauma, severe uncontrolled hypertension

INTERACTIONS
Drug
Heparin, platelet aggregation antagonists (such as abciximab, aspirin, dipyridamole), warfarin: Increase the risk of bleeding.
Herbal
Ginkgo biloba: May increase the risk of bleeding.
Food
None known.

DIAGNOSTIC TEST EFFECTS
May decrease fibrinogen and serum plasminogen levels.

▒ IV INCOMPATIBILITIES
Do not mix with other medications.

SIDE EFFECTS
Frequent
Bleeding at superficial sites, such as venous injection sites, catheter insertion sites, venous cutdowns, arterial punctures, and sites of recent surgical procedures, gingival bleeding

SERIOUS REACTIONS
• Bleeding at internal sites may occur, including intracranial, retroperitoneal, GI, GU, and respiratory sites.
• Lysis or coronary thrombi may produce atrial or ventricular arrhythmias and stroke.

PRECAUTIONS & CONSIDERATIONS
Caution is warranted with acute pericarditis, bacterial endocarditis, cerebrovascular disease, diabetic retinopathy; hepatic or renal impairment; hypertension, major surgery, including coronary artery bypass graft, obstetric delivery, organ biopsy, mitral stenosis with atrial fibrillation, occluded AV cannula at an infected site, ophthalmic hemorrhage, recent GI or GU bleeding,

septic thrombophlebitis, concurrent use of oral anticoagulants, and in the elderly. It is unknown if reteplase is distributed in breast milk. Safety and efficacy of reteplase have not been established in children. The elderly are more susceptible to bleeding. Use reteplase cautiously in this population. An electric razor and a soft toothbrush should be used to reduce the risk of bleeding.

Notify the physician of black or red stool, coffee-ground vomitus, dark or red urine, red-speckled mucus from cough, chest pain, headache, palpitations, or shortness of breath. Continuous cardiac monitoring should be performed. B/P and pulse and respiration rates should be checked every 15 minutes until stable; then check hourly. Serum creatine kinase (CK), and CK-MB concentrations, 12-lead EKG, electrolyte levels, Hct, platelet count, TT, aPTT, PT, and fibrinogen level should be evaluated before therapy starts.

Storage
Use within 4 hours of reconstitution. Discard any unused portion.

Administration
Reconstitute only with sterile water for injection immediately before use. Reconstituted solution contains 1 unit/ml. Do not shake the vial. Slight foaming may occur; let stand for a few minutes to allow bubbles to dissipate. Give through a dedicated IV line. Give as a 10-unit plus 10-unit double bolus, with each IV bolus administered over 2 minutes. Give the second bolus 30 minutes after the first bolus injection. Do not add other medications to the bolus injection solution. Do not give second IV bolus if serious bleeding occurs after first bolus.

Rho (D) Immune Globulin

(BayRho-D Full Dose, BayRho Minidose, MICRhogam, RhoGAM, Rhophylac,WinRho SDF)

CATEGORY AND SCHEDULE
Pregnancy Risk Category: C

CLASSIFICATION
Immune globulins

MECHANISM OF ACTION

$Rh_o(D)$ immune globulin contains anti-$Rh_o(D)$ antibody to the RBC antigen $Rh_o(D)$. $Rh_o(D)$ immune globulin suppresses the active anti-body response and formation of anti-$Rh_o(D)$ in $Rh_o(D)$-negative women exposed to Rh_o-positive blood from a pregnancy with an $Rh_o(D)$-positive fetus or transfusion with $Rh_o(D)$-positive blood. The anti-$Rh_o(D)$ antibody in $Rh_o(D)$ immune globulin may bind to $Rh_o(D)$ antigen in maternal circulation, preventing stimulation of the primary immune response to $Rh_o(D)$ and subsequent active productiuon of anti-$Rh_o(D)$. Injection of $Rh_o(D)$ immune globulin into an Rh-positive patient with idiopathic thrombocytopenic purpura (ITP) may result in the formation of anti-$Rh_o(D)$-coated RBC complexes; as the RBCs are cleared by the spleen, they saturate the capacity of the spleen to clear antibody-coated cells, sparing antibody-coated platelets. *Therapeutic Effect:* Prevents antibody response and hemolytic disease of the newborn in women who have previously conceived an $Rh_o(D)$-positive fetus. Prevents $Rh_o(D)$ sensitization in patients who have received

$Rh_o(D)$-positive blood. Decreases bleeding in patients with ITP.

AVAILABILITY
Injection, Powder for Reconstitution (WinRho SDF): 120 mcg, 300 mcg.
Injection Solution (BayRho D Full Dose, RhoGAM): 300 mcg.
Injection Solution (BayRho D Mini-Dose, MICRORhoGAM): 50 mcg.
Injection Solution (Rhophylac): 300 mcg/2 ml.

INDICATIONS AND DOSAGES
▸ **ITP**
IV (WinRho SDF)
Adults, Elderly, Children. Initially, 50 mcg/kg as single dose (reduce to 25-40 mcg/kg if Hgb is less than 10 g/dl) Maintenance: 25-60 mcg/kg based on platelet count and Hgb level.
▸ **Suppression of the active antibody response and formation of anti-$Rh_o(D)$ in $Rh_o(D)$-negative women exposed to Rh_o positive blood from a pregnancy with an $Rh_o(D)$-positive fetus**
IM (BayRho-D Full Dose, RhoGAM)
Adults. 300 mcg preferably within 72 hr of delivery.
IV, IM (WinRho SDF)
Adults. 300 mcg at 28 wk gestation. After delivery: 120 mcg preferably within 72 hr.
▸ **Suppression of active antibody response and formation of anti-$Rh_o(D)$ in $Rh_o(D)$-negative women exposed to Rh_o-positive blood from a miscarriage with an $Rh_o(D)$-positive fetus**
IM (BayRho-D Full Dose, RhoGAM)
Adults. 300 mcg as soon as possible.
▸ **Suppresson of the active antibody response and formation of anti-$Rh_o(D)$ in $Rh_o(D)$-negative women exposed to Rh_o-positive blood from an abortion, miscarriage, or**

termination of an ectopic pregnancy
with an $Rh_o(D)$-positive fetus
IM (BayRho-D, RhoGAM)
Adults. 300 mcg if more than 13 wk
gestation, 50 mcg if less than 13 wk
gestation.
IV, IM (WinRho SDF)
Adults. 120 mcg after 34 wk gestation.
▸ **Transfusion incompatibility**
IV
Adults. 3000 units (600 mcg) q8hr
until total dose given.
IM
Adults. 6000 units (1200 mcg)
q12hr until total dose given.

CONTRAINDICATIONS

Hypersensitivity to any component,
IgA deficiency, mothers whose Rh
group or immune status is uncertain,
prior sensitization to $Rh_o(D)$,
$Rh_o(D)$-positive mother or pregnant
woman, transfusion of $Rh_o(D)$-positive
blood in previous 3 months

INTERACTIONS
Drug
Live-virus vaccines: May interfere
with the patient's immune response
to the vaccine.
Herbal
None known.
Food
None known.

DIAGNOSTIC TEST EFFECTS
None known.

SIDE EFFECTS

Hypotension, pallor, vasodilation (IV
formulation), fever, headache, chills,
dizziness, somnolence, lethargy,
rash, pruritus, abdominal pain, diarrhea, discomfort and swelling at
injection site, back pain, myalgia,
arthralgia, asthenia

SERIOUS REACTIONS
• None known.

PRECAUTIONS & CONSIDERATIONS

Caution is warranted with bleeding
disorders, particularly thrombocytopenia, and blood Hgb less than
8 g/dl. Notify the physician of chills,
dizziness, fever, headache, or rash.
CBC (especially Hgb and platelet
count), BUN and serum creatinine
levels, reticulocyte count, and urinalysis results should be monitored.
Storage
Refrigerate vials. Do not freeze. Once
reconstituted, the solution is stable for
12 hours at room temperature.
Administration
For IV use, reconstitute the 120-mcg
and 300-mcg vials with 2.5 ml 0.9%
NaCl (the 1000-mcg vials with
8.5 ml 0.9% NaCl). Gently swirl–do
not shake–the vial. Infuse the solution over 3 to 5 minutes.
    For IM use, reconstitute the
120-mcg and 300-mcg vials with
2.5 ml 0.9% NaCl (the 1000-mg
vials with 8.5 ml 0.9% NaCl). Inject
the IM solution into the deltoid
muscle of the upper arm or the anterolateral aspect of the upper thigh.

Ribavirin

R

rye-ba-vye′rin
(Copegus, Rebetol, Virazole)
**Do not confuse ribavirin with
riboflavin.**

CATEGORY AND SCHEDULE
Pregnancy Risk Category: X

CLASSIFICATION
Antivirals

MECHANISM OF ACTION
A synthetic nucleoside that inhibits
influenza virus RNA polymerase

activity and interferes with expression of messenger RNA. *Therapeutic Effect:* Inhibits viral protein synthesis and replication of viral RNA and DNA.

AVAILABILITY

Capsules (Rebetol): 200 mg.
Tablets (Cepegus): 200 mg.
Powder for Reconstitution (Aerosol [Virazole]): 6 g.
Oral Solution (Rebetol): 40 mg/ml.

INDICATIONS AND DOSAGES
▶ **Chronic hepatitis C**
PO (capsule or oral solution in combination with interferon alfa-2b)
Adults, Elderly. 1000-1200 mg/day in 2 divided doses.
Children weighing 60 kg or more. Use adult dosage. *(51-60 kg):* 400 mg 2 times/day. *(37-50 kg):* 200 mg in morning, 400 mg in evening. *(24-36 kg):* 200 mg 2 times/day.
PO (capsules in combination with peginterferon alfa-2b)
Adults, Elderly. 800 mg/day in 2 divided doses.
PO (tablets in combination with peginterferon alfa-2b)
Adults, Elderly. 800-1200 mg/day in 2 divided doses.
▶ **Severe lower respiratory tract infection caused by respiratory syncytial virus (RSV)**
INHALATION
Children, Infants. Use with Viratek small-particle aerosol generator at a concentration of 20 mg/ml (6 g reconstituted with 300 ml sterile water) over 12-18 hr/day for 3-7 days.

OFF-LABEL USES
Treatment of influenza A or B and west Nile virus

CONTRAINDICATIONS
Pregnancy, women of childbearing age who won't use contraception reliably

INTERACTIONS
Drug
Didanosine: May increase the risk of pancreatitis and peripheral neuropathy and decrease the effects of didanosine.
Nucleoside analogues (including adefovir, didanosine, lamivudine, stavudine, zalcitabine, zidovudine): May increase the risk of lactic acidosis.
Herbal
None known.
Food
None known.

DIAGNOSTIC TEST EFFECTS
None known.

SIDE EFFECTS
Frequent (greater than 10%)
Dizziness, headache, fatigue, fever, insomnia, irritability, depression, emotional lability, impaired concentration, alopecia, rash, pruritus, nausea, anorexia, dyspepsia, vomiting, decreased hemoglobin, hemolysis, arthralgia, musculoskeletal pain, dyspnea, sinusitis, flu-like symptoms
Occasional (10%-1%)
Nervousness, altered taste, weakness

SERIOUS REACTIONS
• Cardiac arrest, apnea and ventilator dependence, bacterial pneumonia, pneumonia, and pneumothorax occur rarely.
• Anemia may occur if ribavirin therapy exceeds 7 days.

PRECAUTIONS & CONSIDERATIONS
Use inhaled ribavirin cautiously with asthma, chronic obstructive pulmonary disease (COPD), and those requiring mechanical ventilation. Caution should be used with oral ribavirin in the elderly and with cardiac or pulmonary disease and a history of psychiatric disorders.

Report any difficulty breathing or itching, redness, or swelling of the eyes. Respiratory tract secretions should be obtained for diagnostic testing before giving the first dose of ribavirin or at least during the first 24 hours of therapy. Complete blood count (CBC) with differential should be obtained and pretreat and test females of childbearing age monthly for pregnancy. Hematology reports should be assessed for anemia due to reticulocytosis when therapy exceeds 7 days. For ventilator-assisted patients, watch for "rainout" in tubing and empty frequently.

Storage
Solution normally appears clear and colorless and is stable for 24 hours at room temperature. Discard solution for nebulization after 24 hours. Discard solution if discolored or cloudy.

Administration
! Ribavirin may be given via nasal or oral inhalation. Add 50 to 100 ml sterile water for injection or inhalation to 6-g vial. Transfer to a flask, serving as reservoir for aerosol generator. Further dilute to final volume of 300 ml, giving a solution concentration of 20 mg/ml. Use only aerosol generator available from manufacturer of drug. Do not give at the same time with other drug solutions for nebulization. Discard reservoir solution when fluid levels are low and at least every 24 hours. Be aware that there is controversy over the safety of administering ribavirin to ventilator-dependent patients; only experienced personnel should administer the drug.

Capsules may be taken without regard to food. Tablets should be given with food.

Rifabutin
rif′a-byoo-ten
(Mycobutin)
Do not confuse rifabutin with rifampin.

CATEGORY AND SCHEDULE
Pregnancy Risk Category: B

CLASSIFICATION
Antimycobacterials

MECHANISM OF ACTION
An antitubercular that inhibits DNA-dependent RNA polymerase, an enzyme in susceptible strains of *Escherichia coli* and *Bacillus subtilis*. Rifabutin has a broad spectrum of antimicrobial activity, including against mycobacteria such as *Mycobacterium avium* complex (MAC). *Therapeutic Effect:* Prevents MAC disease.

PHARMACOKINETICS
Readily absorbed from the GI tract (high-fat meals delay absorption). Protein binding: 85%. Widely distributed. Crosses the blood-brain barrier. Extensive intracellular tissue uptake. Metabolized in the liver to active metabolite. Excreted in urine; eliminated in feces. Unknown if removed by hemodialysis. **Half-life:** 16-69 hr.

AVAILABILITY
Capsules: 150 mg.

INDICATIONS AND DOSAGES
▸ **Prevention of MAC disease (first episode)**
PO
Adults, Elderly. 300 mg as a single dose or in 2 divided doses if gastrointestinal (GI) upset occurs.

▸ **Prevention of recurrent MAC disease**
PO
Adults, Elderly. 300 mg/day (in combination)
▸ **Dosage in renal impairment**
Dosage is modified based on creatinine clearance. If creatinine clearance is less than 30 ml/min, reduce dosage by 50%.

CONTRAINDICATIONS
Active tuberculosis; hypersensitivity to other rifamycins, including rifampin

INTERACTIONS
Drug
Oral contraceptives: May decrease contraceptive effectiveness.
Zidovudine: May decrease blood concentration of zidovudine, but does not affect the drug's inhibition of HIV.
Herbal
None known.
Food
None known.

DIAGNOSTIC TEST EFFECTS
May increase serum alkaline phosphatase, AST (SGOT), and ALT (SGPT) levels.

SIDE EFFECTS
Frequent (30%)
Red-orange or red-brown discoloration of urine, feces, saliva, skin, sputum, sweat, or tears
Occasional (11%-3%)
Rash, nausea, abdominal pain, diarrhea, dyspepsia, belching, headache, altered taste, uveitis, corneal deposits
Rare (less than 2%)
Anorexia, flatulence, fever, myalgia, vomiting, insomnia

SERIOUS REACTIONS
• Hepatitis and thrombocytopenia occur rarely. Anemia and neutropenia may also occur.

PRECAUTIONS & CONSIDERATIONS
Caution should be used with liver or renal impairment. The safety of this drug for use in children is not established. Be aware that it is unknown if rifabutin crosses the placenta or is excreted in breast milk. There are no age-related precautions noted in children or the elderly. Avoid IM injections, taking rectal temperature, and any other trauma that may induce bleeding. Avoid crowds and those with known infection.

Feces, perspiration, saliva, skin, sputum, tears, and urine may be discolored brown-orange during drug therapy. Soft contact lenses may be permanently discolored. Rifabutin may decrease the effectiveness of oral contraceptives. Alternative methods of contraception should be used. Expect to perform a biopsy of suspicious nodes, if present. Also, expect to obtain blood or sputum cultures and a chest x-ray to rule out active tuberculosis. If ordered, obtain baseline complete blood count (CBC) and liver function test results.
Administration
Take without regard to food. Take with food if GI irritation occurs. May mix with applesauce if unable to swallow capsules whole.

Rifampin
rye′fam-pin
(Rifadin, Rimactane, Rimycin
[AUS], Rofact [CAN])
**Do not confuse rifampin with
rifabutin, Rifamate, rifapentine, or Ritalin.**

CATEGORY AND SCHEDULE
Pregnancy Risk Category: C

CLASSIFICATION
Antimycobacterials

MECHANISM OF ACTION
An antitubercular that interferes with
bacterial RNA synthesis by binding
to DNA-dependent RNA polymerase,
thus preventing its attachment to
DNA and blocking RNA transcription. *Therapeutic Effect:* Bactericidal
in susceptible microorganisms.

PHARMACOKINETICS
Well absorbed from the GI tract (food
delays absorption). Protein binding:
80%. Widely distributed.
Metabolized in the liver to active
metabolite. Primarily eliminated by
the biliary system. Not removed by
hemodialysis. **Half-life:** 3-5 hr
(increased in hepatic impairment).

AVAILABILITY
Capsules (Rifadin): 150 mg, 300 mg.
Capsules (Rimactane): 300 mg.
*Injection, Powder for Reconstitution
(Rifadin):* 600 mg.

INDICATIONS AND DOSAGES
▸ **Tuberculosis**
PO, IV
Adults, Elderly. 10 mg/kg/day.
Maximum: 600 mg/day.

Children. 10-20 mg/kg/day in
divided doses q12-24hr.
▸ **Prevention of meningococcal
infections**
PO, IV
Adults, Elderly. 600 mg q12hr for
2 days.
Children 1 month and older.
20 mg/kg/day in divided doses q12-
24hr. Maximum: 600 mg/dose.
Infants younger than 1 mo.
10 mg/kg/day in divided doses q12hr
for 2 days.
▸ **Staphylococcal infections**
PO, IV
Adults, Elderly. 600 mg once a day.
Children. 15 mg/kg/day in divided
doses q12hr.
▸ ***Staphylococcus aureus* infections
(in combination with other
anti-infectives)**
PO
Adults, Elderly. 300-600 mg twice
a day.
Neonates. 5-20 mg/kg/day in
divided doses q12hr.
▸ **Prevention of *Haemophilus
influenzae* infection**
PO
Adults, Elderly. 600 mg/day for
4 days.
Children 1 mo and older. 20 mg/kg/
day in divided doses q12hr for
5-10 days.
Children younger than 1 mo.
10 mg/kg/day in divided doses q12hr
for 2 days.

OFF-LABEL USES
Prophylaxis of *H. influenzae* type b
infection; treatment of atypical mycobacterial infection and serious infections caused by *Staphylococcus* species

CONTRAINDICATIONS
Concomitant therapy with amprenavir, hypersensitivity to rifampin or
any other rifamycins

R

INTERACTIONS
Drug
Alcohol, hepatotoxic medications: May increase the risk of hepato-toxicity.

Aminophylline, theophylline: May increase clearance of these drugs.

Chloramphenicol, digoxin, diso-pyramide, fluconazole, methadone, mexiletine, oral anticoagulants, oral antidiabetics, phenytoin, quinidine, tocainide, verapamil: May decrease the effects of these drugs.

Oral contraceptives: May decrease oral contraceptive effectiveness.
Herbal
None known.
Food
None known.

DIAGNOSTIC TEST EFFECTS
May increase serum alkaline phosphatase, bilirubin, uric acid, AST (SGOT), and ALT (SGPT) levels.

▓ IV INCOMPATIBILITIES
Diltiazem (Cardizem)

SIDE EFFECTS
Expected
Red-orange or red-brown discoloration of urine, feces, saliva, skin, sputum, sweat, or tears
Occasional (5%-2%)
Hypersensitivity reaction (such as flushing, pruritus, or rash)
Rare (2%-1%)
Diarrhea, dyspepsia, nausea, candida as evidenced by sore mouth or tongue

SERIOUS REACTIONS
• Rare reactions include hepatotoxicity (risk is increased when rifampin is taken with isoniazid), hepatitis, blood dyscrasias, Stevens-Johnson syndrome, and antibiotic-associated colitis.

PRECAUTIONS & CONSIDERATIONS
Caution is warranted with active alcoholism, a history of alcohol abuse, or liver dysfunction. Be aware that rifampin crosses the placenta and is distributed in breast milk. There are no age-related precautions noted in children or the elderly. Avoid alcohol and any other medications, including antacids, without consulting with the physician. The reliability of oral contraceptives may be affected by rifampin, so alternative methods of contraception should be used.

Feces, sputum, sweat, tears, or urine may become red-orange colored, and soft contact lenses may be permanently stained. Notify the physician of any new symptoms or if fatigue, fever, flu, nausea, unusual bleeding or bruising, vomiting, weakness, or yellow eyes and skin occurs. CBC results should be evaluated for blood dyscrasias and bleeding, bruising, infection manifested as a fever or sore throat, and unusual tiredness and weakness should be assessed.
Storage
Reconstituted vial is stable for 24 hours. Once the reconstituted vial is further diluted, it is stable for 4 hours in D_5W or 24 hours in 0.9% NaCl.
Administration
Preferably give oral rifampin 1 hour before or 2 hours after meals with 8 oz of water. Rifampin may be given with food to decrease GI upset; but this will delay the drug's absorption. For those unable to swallow capsules, rifampin's contents may be mixed with applesauce or jelly. Give rifampin at least 1 hour before administering antacids, especially antacids containing aluminum.

! Administer rifampin by IV infusion only. Avoid IM and subcutaneous administration. Reconstitute 600-mg vial with 10 ml sterile water for injection to provide a concentration of 60 mg/ml. Withdraw the desired dose and further dilute with 500 ml D$_5$W. Evaluate periodically for extravasation as evidenced by local inflammation and irritation. Infuse over 3 hours (may dilute with 100 ml D$_5$W and infuse over 30 minutes).

Rifapentine
rif-a-pen'teen
(Priftin)
Do not confuse with Rifampin.

CATEGORY AND SCHEDULE
Pregnancy Risk Category: C

CLASSIFICATION
Antimycobacterials

MECHANISM OF ACTION
An antitubercular that inhibits bacterial RNA synthesis by binding to DNA-dependent RNA polymerase in *Mycobacterium tuberculosis*. This action prevents the enzyme from attaching to DNA, thereby blocking RNA transcription. *Therapeutic Effect:* Bactericidal.

AVAILABILITY
Tablets: 150 mg.

INDICATIONS AND DOSAGES
▸ **Tuberculosis**
PO
Adults, Elderly. Intensive phase: 600 mg twice weekly for 2 mo (interval between doses no less than 3 days). Continuation phase: 600 mg weekly for 4 mo.

CONTRAINDICATIONS
None known.

INTERACTIONS
Drug
None known.
Herbal
None known.
Food
None known.

DIAGNOSTIC TEST EFFECTS
May increase serum AST (SGOT), ALT (SGPT), and bilirubin levels.

SIDE EFFECTS
Rare (less than 4%)
Red-orange or red-brown discoloration of urine, feces, saliva, skin, sputum, sweat, or tears; arthralgia, pain, nausea, vomiting, headache, dyspepsia, hypertension, dizziness, diarrhea

SERIOUS REACTIONS
• Hyperuricemia, neutropenia, proteinuria, hematuria, and hepatitis occur rarely.

PRECAUTIONS & CONSIDERATIONS
Caution is warranted with alcoholic and with liver function impairment. Feces, sputum, sweat, tears, and urine may become red-orange or red-brown colored and soft contact lenses may be permanently stained. The reliability of oral contraceptives may be affected by rifapentine, so alternative methods of contraception should be used. Initial complete blood count (CBC) and liver function test results should be evaluated. Evaluate for diarrhea, gastrointestinal (GI) upset, nausea, or vomiting as well as pattern of daily bowel activity and stool consistency.
Administration
❗ Be aware that rifapentine is used only in combination with another antituberculosis agent.

Rifaximin
rye-faks'eh-men
(Xifaxan)

CATEGORY AND SCHEDULE
Pregnancy Risk Category: C

CLASSIFICATION
Antibiotics, miscellaneous

MECHANISM OF ACTION
An anti-infective that inhibits bacterial RNA synthesis by binding to a subunit of bacterial DNA-dependent RNA polymerase. *Therapeutic Effect:* Bactericidal.

PHARMACOKINETICS
Less than 0.4% absorbed after PO administration. **Half-life:** 5.85 hr.

AVAILABILITY
Tablets: 200 mg.

INDICATIONS AND DOSAGES
▶ **Traveler's diarrhea**
PO
Adults, Elderly, Children 12 yr and older. 200 mg 3 times a day for 3 days.
▶ **Hepatic encephalopathy**
PO
Adults, Elderly. 1200 mg/day for 15-21 days.

OFF-LABEL USES
Treatment of hepatic encephalopathy

CONTRAINDICATIONS
Hypersensitivity to rifaximin or other rifamycin antibiotics

INTERACTIONS
Drug
None known.

Herbal
None known.
Food
None known.

DIAGNOSTIC TEST EFFECTS
None known.

SIDE EFFECTS
Occasional (11%-5%)
Flatulence, headache, abdominal discomfort, rectal tenesmus, defecation urgency, nausea
Rare (4%-2%)
Constipation, fever, vomiting

SERIOUS REACTIONS
• Hypersensitivity reactions, including dermatitis, angioneurotic edema, pruritus, rash, and urticaria may occur.
• Superinfection occurs rarely.

PRECAUTIONS & CONSIDERATIONS
Caution should be used with diarrhea complicated by fever and/or blood in the stool, or diarrhea due to pathogens other than Escherichia coli (rifaximin is not considered effective) as well as with diarrhea believed to be caused by Campylobacter jejuni, Shigella spp., or Salmonella spp. It is unknown if rifaximin is distributed in breast milk. Safety and efficacy of rifaximin have not been established in children less than 12 years old. In the elderly with normal renal function, no age-related precautions are noted.

If diarrhea worsens or within 48 hr, if blood in the stool occurs, or if fever develops, notify the physician.
Storage
Store tablets at room temperature.
Administration
Take with or without food. Do not break or crush film-coated tablets.

Riluzole
rye'loo-zole
(Rilutek)

CATEGORY AND SCHEDULE
Pregnancy Risk Category: C

CLASSIFICATION
Neuroprotectives

MECHANISM OF ACTION
An amyotrophic lateral sclerosis (ALS) agent that inhibits presynaptic glutamate release in the CNS and intereferes postsynaptically with the effects of excitatory amino acids. *Therapeutic Effect:* Extends survival of ALS patients.

AVAILABILITY
Tablets: 50 mg.

INDICATIONS AND DOSAGES
▸ ALS
PO
Adults, Elderly. 50 mg q12hr.

CONTRAINDICATIONS
None significant.

INTERACTIONS
Drug
Alcohol: May increase CNS depression.
Amitriptyline, quinolones, theophylline: May increase the effects and risk of toxicity of riluzole.
Omeprazole, rifampin: May decrease the effects of riluzole.
Herbal
None known.
Food
Caffeine: May increase the effects and risk of toxicity of riluzole.
High-fat meals: May decrease the absorption and effects of riluzole.

DIAGNOSTIC TEST EFFECTS
May increase liver function test results.

SIDE EFFECTS
Frequent (greater than 10%)
Nausea, asthenia, reduced respiratory function
Occasional (10%-1%)
Edema, tachycardia, headache, dizziness, somnolence, depression, vertigo, tremor, pruritus, alopecia, abdominal pain, diarrhea, anorexia, dyspepsia, vomiting, stomatitis, increased cough

SERIOUS REACTIONS
• None known.

PRECAUTIONS & CONSIDERATIONS
Caution is warranted with renal or hepatic impairment. Alcohol should be avoided as well as tasks requiring mental alertness or motor skills until response to the medication has been established.
Notify the physician of fever. Blood chemistry tests to evaluate hepatic function should be obtained before and during therapy. The drug should be discontinued if the ALT level exceeds 10 times the upper normal limit.
Administration
Take riluzole at least 1 hour before or 2 hours after a meal at the same time each day.

R

Rimantadine
ri-man′ti-deen
(Flumadine)
**Do not confuse rimantadine
with ranitidine, or Flumadine
with flunisolide or flutamide.**

CATEGORY AND SCHEDULE
Pregnancy Risk Category: C

CLASSIFICATION
Antivirals

MECHANISM OF ACTION
An antiviral that appears to exert an
inhibitory effect early in the viral
replication cycle. May inhibit uncoat-
ing of the virus. *Therapeutic Effect:*
Prevents replication of influenza A
virus.

AVAILABILITY
Syrup: 50 mg/5 ml.
Tablets: 100 mg.

INDICATIONS AND DOSAGES
▸ **Influenza A virus**
PO
Adults, Elderly. 100 mg twice a day
for 7 days.
*Elderly nursing home patients,
patients with severe hepatic or renal
impairment.* 100 mg once a day for
7 days.
▸ **Prevention of influenza A virus**
PO
*Adults, Elderly, Children 10 yr and
older.* 100 mg twice a day for at least
10 days after known exposure (usually
for 6-8 wk).
Children younger than 10 yr.
5 mg/kg once a day. Maximum:
150 mg.
*Elderly nursing home patients,
patients with severe hepatic or renal
impairment.* 100 mg once a day.

CONTRAINDICATIONS
Hypersensitivity to amantadine or
rimantadine

INTERACTIONS
Drug
Acetaminophen, aspirin: May
decrease rimantadine blood concen-
tration.
Anticholinergics, CNS stimulants:
May increase side effects of
rimantadine.
Cimetidine: May increase rimanta-
dine blood concentration.
Herbal
None known.
Food
None known.

DIAGNOSTIC TEST EFFECTS
None known.

SIDE EFFECTS
Occasional (3%-2%)
Insomnia, nausea, nervousness,
impaired concentration, dizziness
Rare (less than 2%)
Vomiting, anorexia, dry mouth,
abdominal pain, asthenia, fatigue

SERIOUS REACTIONS
• None known.

PRECAUTIONS & CONSIDERATIONS
Caution is warranted with a history
of recurrent eczematoid dermatitis,
liver disease, renal impairment,
seizures, uncontrolled psychosis, and
concomitant use of CNS stimulants.
Avoid taking acetaminophen, aspirin,
or compounds containing these
drugs. Avoid contact with those who
are at high risk for developing
influenza A (rimantadine-resistant
virus may be shed during therapy).
　　Dry mouth may occur while taking
rimantadine. Do not drive or perform
tasks that require mental alertness
if decreased concentration or

dizziness occurs. Nervousness, sleep pattern, insomnia, and dizziness should be assessed.
Administration
Give rimantadine without regard to food.

Risedronate
rye-se-droe′nate
(Actonel)

CATEGORY AND SCHEDULE
Pregnancy Risk Category: C

CLASSIFICATION
Bisphosphonates

MECHANISM OF ACTION
A bisphosphonate that binds to bone hydroxyapatite and inhibits osteo-clasts. *Therapeutic Effect:* Reduces bone turnover (the number of sites at which bone is remodeled) and bone resorption.

AVAILABILITY
Tablets: 5 mg, 30 mg, 35 mg.

INDICATIONS AND DOSAGES
▸ **Paget's disease**
PO
Adults, Elderly. 30 mg/day for 2 mo. Retreatment may occur after 2-mo post-treatment observation period.
▸ **Prevention and treatment of post-menopausal osteoporosis**
PO
Adults, Elderly. 5 mg/day or 35 mg once weekly.
▸ **Glucocorticoid-induced osteoporosis**
PO
Adults, Elderly. 5 mg/day.

CONTRAINDICATIONS
Hypersensitivity to other bisphos-phonates, including etidronate, tilu-dronate, risedronate, and alendronate; hypocalcemia; inability to stand or sit upright for at least 20 minutes; renal impairment when serum creati-nine clearance is greater than 5 mg/dl

INTERACTIONS
Drug
Antacids containing aluminum, calcium, magnesium; vitamin D: May decrease the absorption of rise-dronate.
Herbal
None known.
Food
None known.

DIAGNOSTIC TEST EFFECTS
None known.

SIDE EFFECTS
Frequent (30%)
Arthralgia
Occasional (12%-8%)
Rash, flu-like symptoms, peripheral edema
Rare (5%-3%)
Bone pain, sinusitis, asthenia, dry eye, tinnitus

SERIOUS REACTIONS
• Overdose causes hypocalcemia, hypophosphatemia, and significant GI disturbances.

PRECAUTIONS & CONSIDERATIONS
Caution is warranted with cardiac failure or renal impairment. Because there are no adequate and well-controlled studies in pregnant women, it is unknown if risedronate causes fetal harm or is excreted in breast milk. Safety and efficacy of risedronate have not been estab-lished in children. The elderly may become overhydrated and require

R

careful monitoring of fluid and electrolytes. Dilute the drug in a smaller volume for the elderly. Consider beginning weight-bearing exercises and modifying behavioral factors, such as avoiding alcohol consumption and cigarette smoking. Hypocalcemia and vitamin D deficiency, if present, should be corrected before beginning risedronate therapy. BUN, creatinine levels, and serum electrolyte levels, including serum calcium and creatinine levels, should be established before and monitored during therapy.

Administration

Take the drug with a full glass (6-8 ounces) of plain water first thing in the morning and at least 30 minutes before first beverage, food, or medication of the day. Taking risedronate with other beverages, including coffee, mineral water, and orange juice, significantly reduces the absorption of the drug. Lie down for at least 30 minutes after taking risedronate to potentiate delivery to the stomach and reduce the risk of esophageal irritation.

Risperidone

ris-per′i-done
(Risperdal, Risperdal Consta, Risperdol M-Tabs)
Do not confuse risperidone with reserpine.

CATEGORY AND SCHEDULE

Pregnancy Risk Category: C

CLASSIFICATION

Antipsychotics

MECHANISM OF ACTION

A benzisoxazole derivative that may antagonize dopamine and serotonin receptors. *Therapeutic Effect:* Suppresses psychotic behavior.

PHARMACOKINETICS

Well absorbed from the GI tract; unaffected by food. Protein binding: 90%. Extensively metabolized in the liver to active metabolite. Primarily excreted in urine. **Half-life:** 3-20 hr; metabolite: 21-30 hr (increased in elderly).

AVAILABILITY

Oral Solution (Risperdal):
1 mg/ml.
Tablets (Risperdal): 0.25 mg, 0.5 mg, 1 mg, 2 mg, 3 mg, 4 mg.
Tablets (Orally Disintegrating [Risperdal M-Tabs]): 0.5 mg, 1 mg, 2 mg.
Injection (Risperdal Consta): 25 mg, 37.5 mg, 50 mg.

INDICATIONS AND DOSAGES
▸ **Psychotic disorder**
PO
Adults. 0.5-1 mg twice a day. May increase dosage slowly. Range: 2-6 mg/day.
Elderly. Initially, 0.25-2 mg/day in 2 divided doses. May increase dosage slowly. Range: 2-6 mg/day.
IM
Adults, Elderly. 25 mg q2wk. Maximum: 50 mg q2wk.
▸ **Mania**
PO
Adults, Elderly. Initially, 2-3 mg as a single daily dose. May increase at 24-hour intervals of 1 mg/day. Range: 2-6 mg/day.
▸ **Dosage in renal impairment**
Initial dosage for adults and elderly patients is 0.25-0.5 mg twice a day. Dosage is titrated slowly to desired effect.

OFF-LABEL USES

Autism in children, behavioral symptoms associated with dementia, Tourette's disorder

CONTRAINDICATIONS

None known.

INTERACTIONS

Drug

Alcohol, other CNS depressants: May increase CNS depression.
Carbamazepine: May decrease the risperidone blood concentration.
Clozapine: May increase the risperidone blood concentration.
Dopamine agonists, levodopa: May decrease the effects of these drugs.
Paroxetine: May increase the risperidone blood concentration and the risk of extrapyramidal symptoms.
Herbal
None known.
Food
None known.

DIAGNOSTIC TEST EFFECTS

May increase serum prolactin, creatinine, alkaline phosphatase, uric acid, AST (SGOT), ALT (SGPT), and triglyceride levels. May decrease blood glucose and serum potassium, protein, and sodium levels. May cause EKG changes.

SIDE EFFECTS

Frequent (26%-13%)
Agitation, anxiety, insomnia, headache, constipation
Occasional (10%-4%)
Dyspepsia, rhinitis, somnolence, dizziness, nausea, vomiting, rash, abdominal pain, dry skin, tachycardia
Rare (3%-2%)
Visual disturbances, fever, back pain, pharyngitis, cough, arthralgia, angina, aggressive behavior, orthostatic hypotension, breast swelling

SERIOUS REACTIONS

* Rare reactions include tardive dyskinesia (characterized by tongue protrusion, puffing of the cheeks, and chewing or puckering of the mouth) and neuroleptic malignant syndrome (marked by hyperpyrexia, muscle rigidity, change in mental status, irregular pulse or B/P, tachycardia, diaphoresis, cardiac arrhythmias, rhabdomyolysis, and acute renal failure).

PRECAUTIONS & CONSIDERATIONS

Caution is warranted with cardiac disease, breast cancer, hepatic or renal impairment, recent MI, those at risk for aspiration pneumonia, suicidal tendencies, and dementia (may increase risk of CVA). Be aware that risperidone may increase risk of hyperglycemia. It is unknown if risperidone crosses the placenta or is excreted in breast milk. Breast-feeding is not recommended for patients taking this drug. The safety and efficacy of this drug have not been established in children. The elderly are more susceptible to orthostatic hypotension. They may require a dosage adjustment because of age-related renal or hepatic impairment.

Drowsiness and dizziness may occur but generally subsides with continued therapy. Tasks requiring mental alertness or motor skills should be avoided. Notify the physician if altered gait, difficulty breathing, palpitations, pain or swelling in breasts, severe dizziness or fainting, trembling fingers, unusual movements, rash, fever, or visual changes occur. B/P, heart rate, liver function test results, EKG, and weight should be assessed.

Storage

The drug may be given up to 6 hours after reconstitution, but immediate administration is recommended. If 2 minutes pass before the injection, reconstitute the solution by shaking the upright vial vigorously back and forth for as long as it takes to resuspend the microspheres. Store the drug below 77° F (25° C) once it's in suspension.

Administration

Take risperidone without regard to food. Mix the oral solution with water, orange juice, coffee, or low-fat milk, but not with cola or tea.

For IM administration, use only the diluent and needle supplied in the dose pack. You'll require all the components in the dose pack for administration. Don't substitute any components. Prepare the suspension according to the manufacturer's directions. Inject the drug IM into the upper outer quadrant of the gluteus maximus. Do not administer the drug by the IV route.

Ritonavir

ri-tone′a-veer
(Norvir, Norvisec [CAN])
Do not confuse ritonavir with Retrovir.

CATEGORY AND SCHEDULE

Pregnancy Risk Category: B

CLASSIFICATION

Antivirals, protease inhibitors

MECHANISM OF ACTION

Inhibits HIV-1 and HIV-2 proteases, rendering these enzymes incapable of processing the polypeptide precursors; this results in the production of noninfectious, immature HIV particles.

Therapeutic Effect: Impedes HIV replication, slowing the progression of HIV infection.

PHARMACOKINETICS

Well absorbed after PO administration (absorption increased with food). Protein binding: 98%-99%. Extensively metabolized in the liver to active metabolite. Primarily eliminated in feces. Unknown if removed by hemodialysis. **Half-life:** 2.7-5 hr.

AVAILABILITY

Oral Solution: 80 mg/ml.
Soft Gelatin Capsules: 100 mg.

INDICATIONS AND DOSAGES
▶ **HIV infection**
PO
Adults, Children 12 yr and older.
600 mg twice a day. If nausea occurs at this dosage, give 300 mg twice a day for 1 day, 400 mg twice a day for 2 days, 500 mg twice a day for 1 day, then 600 mg twice a day thereafter.
Children younger than 12 yr.
Initially, 250 mg/m^2/dose twice a day. Increase by 50 mg/m^2/dose up to 400 mg/m^2/dose. Maximum: 600 mg/dose twice a day.

CONTRAINDICATIONS

Concurrent use of amiodarone, astemizole, bepridil, bupropion, cisapride, clozapine, encainide, flecainide, meperidine, piroxicam, propafenone, propoxyphene, quinidine, rifabutin, or terfenadine (increased risk of serious or life-threatening drug interactions, such as arrhythmias, hematologic abnormalities, and seizures); concurrent use of alprazolam, clorazepate, diazepam, estazolam, flurazepam, midazolam, triazolam, or zolpidem (may produce extreme sedation and respiratory depression)

INTERACTIONS

Drug

Desipramine, fluoxetine, other antidepressants: May increase the blood concentration of these drugs.

Disulfiram, drugs causing disulfiram-like reaction (such as metronidazole): May produce a disulfiram-like reaction.

Enzyme inducers (including carbamazepine, dexamethasone, nevirapine, phenobarbital, phenytoin, rifabutin, rifampin): May increase the metabolism and decrease the efficacy of ritonavir.

Oral contraceptives, theophylline: May decrease the effectiveness of these drugs.

Herbal

St. John's wort: May decrease the blood concentration and effect of ritonavir.

Food

None known.

DIAGNOSTIC TEST EFFECTS

May alter serum CK, GGT, triglyceride, uric acid, AST (SGOT), and ALT (SGPT) levels as well as creatinine clearance.

SIDE EFFECTS

Frequent

GI disturbances (abdominal pain, anorexia, diarrhea, nausea, vomiting), circumoral and peripheral paresthesias, altered taste, headache, dizziness, fatigue, asthenia

Occasional

Allergic reaction, flu-like symptoms, hypotension

Rare

Diabetes mellitus, hyperglycemia

SERIOUS REACTIONS

• None known.

PRECAUTIONS & CONSIDERATIONS

Caution should be used with impaired hepatic function. Be aware that breast-feeding is not recommended in this population because of the possibility of HIV transmission. There are no age-related precautions noted in children older than 2 years. There are no known effects of this drug's use in the elderly.

When beginning combination therapy with ritonavir and nucleosides, it may promote GI tolerance by first beginning ritonavir alone and then by adding nucleosides before completing 2 weeks of ritonavir monotherapy. Check baseline laboratory test results, if ordered, especially liver function tests and serum triglycerides, before beginning ritonavir therapy and at periodic intervals during therapy. Monitor for signs and symptoms of GI disturbances or neurologic abnormalities, particularly paresthesias.

Storage

Store capsules or solution in the refrigerator. Protect the drug from light. Refrigerate the oral solution unless it is used within 30 days and stored below 77°F.

Administration

May give without regard to meals, but preferably give with food. May improve the taste of the oral solution by mixing it with Advera, chocolate milk, or Ensure within 1 hour of dosing. Continue therapy for the full length of treatment and to evenly space drug doses around the clock.

R

Rituximab

rye-tucks'ih-mab
(monoclonal antibody, antineoplastic)
(Mabthera [AUS], Rituxan)

CATEGORY AND SCHEDULE

Pregnancy Risk Category: C

CLASSIFICATION

Antineoplastics, monoclonal
antibodies

MECHANISM OF AC TION

Binds to CD20, the antigen found
on the surface of B lymphocytes and
B-cell non-Hodgkin's lymphomas.
Therapeutic Effect: Produces cytotoxicity, reducing tumor size.

PHARMACOKINETICS

Rapidly depletes B cells. **Half-life:**
59.8 hr after first infusion and
174 hr after fourth infusion.

AVAILABILITY

Injection: 10 mg/ml.

INDICATIONS AND DOSAGES

▸ **Non-Hodgkin's lymphoma**
IV
Adults. 375 mg/m^2 once weekly for
4-8 wk. May administer a second
4-wk course.

CONTRAINDICATIONS

Hypersensitivity to murine proteins

INTERACTIONS

Drug
None known.
Herbal
None known.
Food
None known.

DIAGNOSTIC TEST EFFECTS

None known.

▓ IV INCOMPATIBILITIES

Don't mix rituximab with any other
medications.

SIDE EFFECTS

Frequent
Fever (49%), chills (32%), asthenia
(16%), headache (14%), angioedema
(13%), hypotension (10%), nausea
(18%), rash or pruritus (10%)
Occasional (less than 10%)
Myalgia, dizziness, abdominal pain,
throat irritation, vomiting, neutropenia, rhinitis, bronchospasm, urticaria

SERIOUS REACTIONS

• A hypersensitivity reaction marked
by hypotension, bronchospasm, and
angioedema may occur.
• Arrhythmias may occur, particularly in those with a history of
pre-existing cardiac conditions.

PRECAUTIONS & CONSIDERATIONS

Caution is warranted with a history
of cardiac disease. Be aware that
rituximab may cause fetal B-cell
depletion. Females with childbearing
potential should use contraceptive
methods during treatment and for up
to 12 months afterward. It is unknown
if rituximab is distributed in breast
milk. The safety and efficacy of
rituximab have not been established
in children. No age-related precautions have been noted in the
elderly.
   Infusion-related reactions,
including chills, fever, hypotension,
and rigors, which usually occur
30 minutes to 2 hours after beginning
the first rituximab infusion should be
monitored; slowing the infusion
resolves these symptoms. CBC
should be obtained before and regularly during therapy.
Storage
Refrigerate unopened vials.
The diluted solution is stable for up
to 24 hours if refrigerated and

up to 36 hours if stored at room temperature.

Administration

! Expect to pretreat the patient with acetaminophen and diphenhydramine before each infusion to help prevent infusion-related reactions. Don't give rituximab by IV push or bolus. Withdraw the needed amount into an infusion bag, and dilute it with 0.9% NaCl or D_5W to a final concentration of 1 to 4 mg/ml. For the initial infusion, infuse the drug at 50 mg/hour. The infusion rate may be increased, as necessary, in increments of 50 mg/hour every 30 minutes to a maximum rate of 400 mg/hour. For subsequent infusions, the drug may be administered initially at 100 mg/hour and increased in increments of 100 mg/hour every 30 minutes to a maximum rate of 400 mg/hr.

Rizatriptan
rize-a-trip′tan
(Maxalt, Maxalt-MLT)

CATEGORY AND SCHEDULE
Pregnancy Risk Category: C

CLASSIFICATION
Serotonin receptor agonists

MECHANISM OF ACTION
A serotonin receptor agonist that binds selectively to vascular receptors, producing a vasoconstrictive effect on cranial blood vessels. *Therapeutic Effect:* Relieves migraine headache.

PHARMACOKINETICS
Well absorbed after PO administration. Protein binding: 14%. Crosses the blood-brain barrier. Metabolized by the liver to inactive metabolite. Eliminated primarily in urine and, to a lesser extent, in feces.

Half-life:
2-3 hr.

AVAILABILITY
Tablets (Maxalt): 5 mg, 10 mg.
Oral Disintegrating Tablets (Maxalt-MLT): 5 mg, 10 mg.

INDICATIONS AND DOSAGES
▸ **Acute migraine attack**
PO
Adults older than 18 yr, Elderly.
5-10 mg. If headache improves, but then returns, dose may be repeated after 2 hr. Maximum: 30 mg/24 hr.

CONTRAINDICATIONS
Basilar or hemiplegic migraine, coronary artery disease, ischemic heart disease (including angina pectoris, history of MI, silent ischemia, and Prinzmetal's angina), uncontrolled hypertension, use within 24 hours of ergotamine-containing preparations or another serotonin receptor agonist, use within 14 days of MAOIs.

INTERACTIONS
Drug
Ergotamine-containing medications: May produce a vasospastic reaction.
Fluoxetine, fluvoxamine, paroxetine, sertraline: May produce hyperreflexia, incoordination, and weakness.
MAOIs, propranolol: May dramatically increase plasma concentration of rizatriptan.
Herbal
None known.
Food
All foods: Delay peak drug concentration by 1 hour.

R

DIAGNOSTIC TEST EFFECTS
None known.

SIDE EFFECTS
Frequent (9%-7%)
Dizziness, somnolence, paraesthesia, fatigue
Occasional (6%-3%)
Nausea, chest pressure, dry mouth
Rare (2%)
Headache; neck, throat, or jaw pressure; photosensitivity

SERIOUS REACTIONS
• Cardiac reactions (such as ischemia, coronary artery vasospasm, and MI) and noncardiac vasospasm-related reactions (including hemorrhage and CVA), occur rarely, particularly in patients with hypertension, diabetes, or a strong family history of coronary artery disease; obese patients; smokers; males older than 40 years; and postmenopausal women.

PRECAUTIONS & CONSIDERATIONS

Caution is warranted with mild to moderate hepatic or renal impairment and cardiovascular risk factors. It is unknown if rizatriptan is excreted in breast milk. The safety and efficacy of rizatriptan have not been established in children. Rizatriptan is not recommended for the elderly. Smoking, exposure to sunlight and ultraviolet rays, and tasks that require mental alertness or motor skills should be avoided.

Dizziness may occur. Notify the physician immediately if anxiety, chest pain, palpitations, or tightness in the throat occurs. BUN level and serum alkaline phosphatase, bilirubin, creatinine AST (SGOT), and ALT (SGPT) levels should be obtained before treatment to assess renal and hepatic function. EKG should also be obtained at baseline.

Migraines and associated symptoms, including nausea and vomiting, photophobia, and phonophobia (sound sensitivity) should be assessed before and during treatment.
Administration
The orally disintegrating tablets come packaged in individual aluminum blister packs. Do not remove the orally disintegrating tablet from the blister pack until just before intending to take it. Open packet with dry hands, and place tablet on the tongue to dissolve. Then swallow it. Don't administer the orally disintegrating tablets with water.

Ropinirole
ro-pin'i-role
(Requip)

CATEGORY AND SCHEDULE
Pregnancy Risk Category: C

CLASSIFICATION
Antiparkinson agents, dopaminergics

MECHANISM OF ACTION
An antiparkinson agent that stimulates dopamine receptors in the striatum. *Therapeutic Effect:* Relieves signs and symptoms of Parkinson's disease.

PHARMACOKINETICS
Rapidly absorbed after PO administration. Protein binding: 40%. Extensively distributed throughout the body. Extensively metabolized. Steady-state concentrations achieved within 2 days. Eliminated in urine.

Unknown if removed by hemodialysis.
Half-life: 6 hr.

AVAILABILITY
Tablets: 0.25 mg, 0.5 mg, 1 mg,
2 mg, 3 mg, 4 mg, 5 mg.

INDICATIONS AND DOSAGES
▸ **Parkinson's disease**
PO
Adults, Elderly. Initially, 0.25 mg
3 times a day. May increase dosage
every 7 days.

CONTRAINDICATIONS
None known.

INTERACTIONS
Drug
**Butyrophenones, metoclopramide,
phenothiazines, thioxanthenes:**
Decrease the effectiveness of
ropinirole.
**Cimetidine, diltiazem, enoxacin,
erythromycin, fluvoxamine,
mexiletine, norfloxacin, tacrine:**
Alter ropinirole blood concentration.
Ciprofloxacin: Increases ropinirole
blood concentration.
CNS depressants: May increase
CNS depressant effects.
Estrogens: Reduce the clearance of
ropinirole.
Levodopa: Increases the blood
concentration of levodopa.
Herbal
None known.
Food
All foods: Delay peak plasma levels
by 1 hour but don't affect drug
absorption.

DIAGNOSTIC TEST EFFECTS
May increase serum alkaline
phosphatase level.

SIDE EFFECTS
Frequent (60%-40%)
Nausea, dizziness, somnolence

Occasional (12%-5%)
Syncope, vomiting, fatigue, viral
infection, dyspepsia, diaphoresis,
asthenia, orthostatic hypotension,
abdominal discomfort, pharyngitis,
abnormal vision, dry mouth, hypertension, hallucinations, confusion
Rare (less than 4%)
Anorexia, peripheral edema,
memory loss, rhinitis, sinusitis,
palpitations, impotence

SERIOUS REACTIONS
• None known.

PRECAUTIONS & CONSIDERATIONS
Caution is warranted with hallucinations (especially the elderly), syncope,
history of orthostatic hypotension,
and those who take CNS depressants
concurrently. Because ropinirole is
distributed in breast milk, it may
cause drug-related effects in the
breast-feeding infant. The safety and
efficacy of ropinirole have not been
established in children. No age-related
precautions have been noted in the
elderly, but they are more likely than
other age-groups to experience
hallucinations.
Dizziness, drowsiness, and orthostatic hypotension are common initial
responses to the drug. Alcohol and
tasks that require mental alertness
or motor skills should be avoided.
Change positions slowly to prevent
orthostatic hypotension. Baseline
vital signs and serum alkaline phosphatase levels should be assessed at
baseline. Relief of symptoms, such
as improvement of masklike facial
expression, muscular rigidity, shuffling gait, and resting tremors of the
hands and head should be assessed
during treatment.
Administration
Expect the dosage schedule to
increase very gradually, as follows:
Week 1, 0.25 mg 3 times a day to total

R

daily dose of 0.75 mg; Week 2, 0.5 mg 3 times a day to total daily dose of 1.5 mg; Week 3, 0.75 mg 3 times a day to total daily dose of 2.25 mg; Week 4, 1 mg 3 times a day to total daily dose of 3 mg, as prescribed. After week 4, dosage may be increased every week, if needed, by 1.5-3 mg/day to a total dose of 24 mg/day.

Plan to discontinue the drug gradually at 7-day intervals, as follows: first decrease the frequency from 3 times a day to twice a day for 4 days; for the remaining 3 days, decrease the frequency to once a day before complete withdrawal, as prescribed.

Rosiglitazone
roz-ih-gli′ta-zone
(Avandia)
Do not confuse with Avalide, Avinza, or Prandin.

CATEGORY AND SCHEDULE
Pregnancy Risk Category: C

CLASSIFICATION
Antidiabetic agents, thiazolidinediones

MECHANISM OF ACTION
An antidiabetic that improves target-cell response to insulin without increasing pancreatic insulin secretion. Decreases hepatic glucose output and increases insulin-dependent glucose utilization in skeletal muscle. *Therapeutic Effect:* Lowers blood glucose concentration.

PHARMACOKINETICS
Rapidly absorbed. Protein binding: 99%. Metabolized in the liver.

Excreted primarily in urine, with a lesser amount in feces. Not removed by hemodialysis. **Half-life:** 3-4 hr.

AVAILABILITY
Tablets: 2 mg, 4 mg, 8 mg.

INDICATIONS AND DOSAGES
▶ **Diabetes mellitus, combination therapy**
PO
Adults, Elderly. Initially, 4 mg as a single daily dose or in divided doses twice a day. May increase to 8 mg/day after 12 wk of therapy if fasting glucose level is not adequately controlled.
▶ **Diabetes mellitus, monotherapy**
Adults, Elderly. Initially, 4 mg as a single daily dose or in divided doses twice a day. May increase to 8 mg/day after 12 wk of therapy.

CONTRAINDICATIONS
Active hepatic disease, diabetic ketoacidosis, increased serum transaminase levels, including ALT (SGPT) greater than 2.5 times the normal serum level, type 1 diabetes mellitus

INTERACTIONS
Drug
None known.
Herbal
None known.
Food
None known.

DIAGNOSTIC TEST EFFECTS
May decrease Hct and Hgb and serum alkaline phosphatase, bilirubin, and AST (SGOT) levels. Less than 1% of patients experience ALT values that are 3 times the normal level.

SIDE EFFECTS
Frequent (9%)
Upper respiratory tract infection

Occasional (4%-2%)
Headache, edema, back pain, fatigue, sinusitis, diarrhea

SERIOUS REACTIONS
- None known.

PRECAUTIONS & CONSIDERATIONS
Caution is warranted with CHF, edema, and hepatic impairment. It is unknown if rosiglitazone crosses the placenta or is distributed in breast milk. Rosiglitazone use is not recommended in pregnant or breast-feeding women. Safety and efficacy of rosiglitazone have not been established in children. No age-related precautions have been noted in the elderly.

Food intake, blood glucose, and Hgb should be monitored before and during therapy. Hepatic enzyme levels should also be obtained before beginning rosiglitazone therapy and periodically thereafter. Notify the physician of abdominal or chest pain, dark urine or light stool, hypoglycemic reactions, fever, nausea, palpitations, rash, vomiting, or yellowing of the eyes or skin. Be aware of signs and symptoms of hypoglycemia (anxiety, cool wet skin, diplopia, dizziness, headache, hunger, numbness in mouth, tachycardia, tremors), or hyperglycemia (deep rapid breathing, dim vision, fatigue, nausea, polydipsia, polyphagia, polyuria, vomiting); carry candy, sugar packets, or other sugar supplements for immediate response to hypoglycemia. Consult the physician when glucose demands are altered (such as with fever, heavy physical activity, infection, stress, trauma). Exercise, good personal hygiene (including foot care), not smoking, and weight control are essential parts of therapy.

Administration
Take rosiglitazone without regard to meals.

Rosuvastatin
ross-uh-vah-stah'tin
(Crestor)

CATEGORY AND SCHEDULE
Pregnancy Risk Category: X

CLASSIFICATION
Antihyperlipidemics, HMG CoA reductase inhibitors

MECHANISM OF ACTION
An antihyperlipidemic that interferes with cholesterol biosynthesis by inhibiting the conversion of the enzyme HMG-CoA to mevalonate, a precursor to cholesterol. *Therapeutic Effect:* Decreases LDL cholesterol, VLDL, and plasma triglyceride levels, increases HDL concentration.

PHARMACOKINETICS
Protein binding: 88%. Minimal hepatic metabolism. Primarily eliminated in the feces. **Half-life:** 19 hr (increased in patients with severe renal dysfunction).

AVAILABILITY
Tablets: 5 mg, 10 mg, 20 mg, 40 mg.

INDICATIONS AND DOSAGES
▸ **Hyperlipidemia, dyslipidemia**
PO
Adults, Elderly. 5 to 40 mg/day. Usual starting dosage is 10 mg/day, with adjustments based on lipid levels; monitor q2-4wk until desired level is achieved.

▶ **Renal impairment (creatinine clearance less than 30 ml/min)**
PO
Adults, Elderly. 5 mg/day; do not exceed 10 mg/day.
▶ **Concurrent cyclosporine use**
PO
Adults, Elderly. 5 mg/day.
▶ **Concurrent lipid-lowering therapy**
PO
Adults, Elderly. 10 mg/day.

CONTRAINDICATIONS
Active hepatic disease, breast-feeding, pregnancy, unexplained, persistent elevations of serum transaminase levels

INTERACTIONS
Drug
Cyclosporine, gemfibrozil, niacin: Increases the risk of myopathy with cyclosporine, gemfibrozil, and niacin.
Erythromycin: Reduces the plasma concentration of erythromycin.
Ethinylestradiol, norgestrel: Increases the plasma concentrations of ethinylestradiol and norgestrel.
Warfarin: Enhances anticoagulant effect.
Herbal
None known.
Food
None known.

DIAGNOSTIC TEST EFFECTS
May increase serum CK and transaminase concentrations. May produce hematuria and proteinuria.

SIDE EFFECTS
Rosuvastatin is generally well tolerated. Side effects are usually mild and transient.
Occasional (9%-3%)
Pharyngitis, headache, diarrhea, dyspepsia, including heartburn and epigastric distress, nausea

Rare (less than 3%)
Myalgia, asthenia or unusual fatigue and weakness, back pain

SERIOUS REACTIONS
• Lens opacities may occur.
• Hypersensitivity reaction and hepatitis occur rarely.

PRECAUTIONS & CONSIDERATIONS
Caution is warranted with history of hepatic disease, hypotension, severe acute infection, severe electrolyte, endocrine, metabolic imbalances or disorders, trauma, and uncontrolled seizures. Caution should also be used in those who consume a substantial amount of alcohol and those who have had recent major surgery. Rosuvastatin use is contraindicated in pregnancy because the suppression of cholesterol biosynthesis may cause fetal toxicity. Rosuvastatin is contraindicated during lactation because it carries the risk of serious adverse reactions in breast-feeding infants. Safety and efficacy of rosuvastatin have not been established in children. No age-related precautions have been noted in the elderly.

Notify the physician of headache, sore throat, muscle weakness and aches, severe gastric upset, or rash. Pattern of daily bowel activity and stool consistency should be assessed. Serum lipid cholesterol and triglyceride levels and hepatic function should be checked at baseline and periodically during treatment. Before beginning rosuvastatin therapy, a standard cholesterol-lowering diet for a minimum of 3 to 6 months should be practiced and then continued throughout rosuvastatin therapy.
Administration
Take rosuvastatin without regard to meals and administer in the evening.

Salicylic Acid

sal-i-sill'ik
(Compound W, Compound W
One Step Wart Remover, DHS
Sal, Dr. Scholl's, Callus
Remover, Dr. Scholl's Clear Away,
DuoFilm, DuoPlant, Freezone,
Fung-O, Gordofilm, Hydrisalic,
Ionil, Ionil Plus, Keralyt,
LupiCare, Dandruff, LupiCare II
Psoriasis, LupiCare Psoriasis,
Mediplast, MG217 Sal-Acid,
Mosco Corn and Callus Remover,
NeoCeuticals Acne Spot
Treatment, Neutrogena Acne
Wash, Neutrogena Body Clear,
Neutrogena Clear Pore,
Neutrogena Clear Pore Shine
Control, Neutrogena Healthy
Scalp, Neutrogena Maximum
Strength T/Sal, Neutrogena On
The Spot Acne Patch, Occlusal
[CAN], Occlusal-HP, Oxy Balance,
Oxy Balance Deep Pore, Palmer's
Skin Success Acne Cleanser,
Pedisilk, Propa pH, SalAc, Sal-
Acid, Salactic, Sal-Plant, Stri-dex,
Stri-dex Body Focus, Stri-dex
Facewipes To Go, Stri-dex
Maximum Strength, Sunspot
Cream [AUS], Tinamed, Tiseb,
Trans-Ver-Sal, Wart-Off
Maximum Strength, Zapzyt Acne
Wash, Zapzyt Pore Treatment,
Salac)

CATEGORY AND SCHEDULE

Pregnancy Risk Category: C
OTC (cream, gel, foam, liquid,
ointment, pads, patch, plaster,
soap, shampoo, solution)

CLASSIFICATION

Antipsoriatics, dermatologics,
keratolytics, salicylates

MECHANISM OF ACTION

A keratolytic agent that produces
desquamation of hyperkeratotic
epithelium by dissolution of intercel-
lular cement and causes the cornified
tissue to swell, soften, macerate, and
desquamate. *Therapeutic Effect:*
Decreases acne, psoriasis, and wart
removal

PHARMACOKINETICS

Absorption differs between formulations. Protein binding: 50%-80%.
Bound to serum albumin.
Metabolized to salicylate glucoro-
nides and salicyluric acid. Excreted
in urine.

AVAILABILITY

Cream: 2% (Neutrogena Acne
Wash), 2.5% (LupiCare Dandruff,
LupiCare Psoriasis, LupiCare II).
Gel: 0.5% (Neutrogena Clean Pore
Shine Control), 2% (NeuCeuticals
Acne Spot Treatment, Neutrogena
Clean Pore, Oxy Balance, Stri-dex
Body Focus, Zapzyt Acne Wash,
Zapzyt Pore Treatment), 6%
(Hydrisalic, Keralyt), 17%
(Compound W, DuoPlant, Sal-Plant).
Foam: 2% (Neutrogena Acne Wash,
Salac).
Liquid: 2% (NeoCeuticals Acne Spot
Treatment, Neutrogena Acne Wash,
Neutrogena Body Clear, Propa pH,
SalAc), 17% (Compound W,
DuoFilm, Freezone, Fung-O,
Gordofilm, Mosco Corn and Callus
Remover, Occlusal-HP, Pedisilk,
Salactic, Tinamed, Wart-Off).
Ointment: 3% (MG217 Sal-Acid).
Pads: 0.5% (Oxy Balance, Oxy
Balance Deep Pore, Stri-dex, Stri-
dex Facewipes To Go), 2%
(Neutrogena Acne Wash, Stri-dex
Maximum Strength).
Patch: 2% (Neutrogena On The Spot
Acne Patch), 15% (Trans-Ver-Sal),
40% (Compound W, Dr. Scholl's

S

Callus Remover, Dr. Scholl's Clear Away, DuoFilm).
Plaster: 40% (Mediplast, Sal-Acid, Tinamed).
Shampoo: 1.8% (Neutrogena Healthy Scalp), 2% (Ionil, Ionil Plus, LupiCare Dandruff, LupiCare Psoriasis, Tiseb), 3% (Neutrogena Maximum Strength T/Sal).
Soap: 2%.
Solution: 17% (Compound W).

INDICATIONS AND DOSAGES
▸ **Acne**
TOPICAL
Adults, Elderly, Children. Apply cream, foam, gel, liquid, pads, patch, or soap 1-3 times/day.
▸ **Callus, corn, wart removal**
TOPICAL
Adults, Elderly, Children. Apply gel, liquid, plaster, or patch to wart 1-2 times/day.
▸ **Dandruff, psoriasis, seborrheic dermatitis**
TOPICAL
Adults, Elderly, Children. Apply cream, ointment, or shampoo 3-4 times/day.

OFF-LABEL USES
Tinea pedis

CONTRAINDICATIONS
Children less than 2 years old, diabetes, impaired circulation, hypersensitivity to salicylic acid or any of its components

INTERACTIONS
Drug
Tolbutamide: May increase risk of hypoglycemia.
Methotrexate: May increase risk of methotrexate toxicity.
Corticosteroids: May decrease plasma salicylate levels.
Ammonium sulfate: May increase plasma salicylate levels.

Heparin: May decrease platelet adhesiveness and interfere with hemostasis in heparin-treated patients.
Pyranzinamide: May inhibit pyrazinamide-induced hyper-uricemia.
Uricosuric agents: May decrease the effects of probenecid, sulfinpyra-zone, and phenylbutazone.
Varicella virus vaccine: May increase risk of developing Reye's syndrome.
Herbal
Tamarind: May increase risk of salicylate toxicity.
Food
None known.

DIAGNOSTIC TEST EFFECTS
May interfere with thyroid function tests (decrease PBI and increase T_3 uptake). May give false negative results with glucose oxidase test and fluorometric test. May give false positive results with clinitest with high-dose salicylate therapy and $FeCl_3$ in Gerhardt reaction. May give false reduced values with 17-OH corticosteroid tests and vanilman-delic acid test. May increase or decrease uric acid levels. May decrease prothrombin levels and slightly increase prothrombin time.

SIDE EFFECTS
Occasional
Burning, erythema, irritation, pruritus, stinging
Rare
Dizziness, nausea, vomiting, diar-rhea, hypoglycemia

SERIOUS REACTIONS
• Symptoms of salicylate toxicity include lethargy, hyperpnea, diarrhea, and psychic disturbances.

PRECAUTIONS & CONSIDERATIONS

Salicylic acid should not be applied to areas that are irritated, infected, reddened, birthmarks, genital or facial warts, or mucous membranes. It is unknown if salicylic acid crosses the placenta or is distributed in breast milk. Salicylic acid is not recommended for use in children younger than 2 years old. There are no age-related precautions noted in the elderly. Use of abrasive soaps and cleansers, alcohol-containing preparations, other topical acne preparations, cosmetic soaps that dry skin, and medicated cosmetics should be avoided.

Administration

Use 2% cream, pads, foam, or liquid cleansers for acne by cleansing the skin 1-2 times/day. Massage gently into skin, work into lather and rinse thoroughly. Pads should be wet with water prior to using and disposed of after use. Do not flush pads.

Use gel (0.5% or 2%) for acne by applying a small amount to clean, dry skin on the face in the morning or evening. If peeling or drying occurs, use every other day. Some products may be used up to 3-4 times/day.

Use pads (0.5% or 2%) for acne to cover clean, dry skin with thin layer 1-3 times/day. Do not leave pad on skin.

Use patches (2%) for acne by washing face and allow skin to dry for at least 5 minutes. Apply patch directly over pimple being treated at bedtime. Remove in the morning.

When using shower/bath gels or soap (2%), use once daily in shower or bath. Massage over skin prone to acne. Rinse well.

Use gel or liquid (17%) for callus, corns, or warts by cleaning and drying the area. Apply to each wart and allow to dry. Repeat 1-2 times/day for up to 12 weeks as needed.

Apply gel (6%) to callus, corns, or warts once daily. Use at night and rinse off in the morning.

Apply plaster or patch (40%) for callus, corns, or warts by cleaning and drying skin. Apply directly over affected area. Leave on for 48 hours. Repeat procedure for up to 12 weeks as needed.

Use patch (15%) for callus, corns, or warts by applying directly over affected area at bedtime. Leave in place overnight and remove in the morning. Repeat daily for up to 12 weeks as needed. May trim patch to fit area.

Use cream (2.5%) for dandruff, psoriasis, or seborrheic dermatitis by cleaning and drying skin. Apply to affected area 3-4 times/day. Apply to clean, dry skin. Some products may remain overnight.

Apply ointment (3%) for dandruff, psoriasis, or seborrheic dermatitis to scales or plaques on skin up to 4 times/day. Do not apply to scalp or face.

Massage shampoo (1.8% to 3%) for dandruff, psoriasis, or seborrheic dermatitis into wet hair. Leave in place for several minutes and rinse thoroughly. Some products may by used 2-3 times/week.

S

Salmeterol

sal-me′te-rol
(Serevent Diskus, Serevent
Inhaler and Disks [AUS])
**Do not confuse Serevent with
Serentil.**

CATEGORY AND SCHEDULE
Pregnancy Risk Category: C

CLASSIFICATION
Adrenergic agonists,
bronchodilators

MECHANISM OF ACTION
An adrenergic agonist that stimulates
beta$_2$-adrenergic receptors in the
lungs, resulting in relaxation of
bronchial smooth muscle.
Therapeutic Effect: Relieves
bronchospasm and reduces airway
resistance.

PHARMACOKINETICS

Route	Onset	Peak	Duration
Inhalation	10-20 min	3 hr	12 hr

Low systemic absorption; acts
primarily in the lungs. Protein
binding: 95%. Metabolized by
hydroxylation. Primarily
eliminated in feces.
Half-life: 3-4 hr.

AVAILABILITY
*Powder for Oral Inhalation (Serevent
Diskus):* 50 mcg.

INDICATIONS AND DOSAGES
▸ **Prevention and maintenance
treatment of asthma**
INHALATION (DISKUS)
*Adults, Elderly, Children 4 yr and
older.* 1 inhalation (50 mcg) q12hr.

▸ **Prevention of exercise-induced
bronchospasm**
INHALATION
*Adults, Elderly, Children 4 yr and
older.* 1 inhalation at least 30 min
before exercise.
▸ **COPD**
INHALATION
Adults, Elderly. 1 inhalation q12hr.

CONTRAINDICATIONS
History of hypersensitivity to
sympathomimetics

INTERACTIONS
Drug
Beta blockers: May decrease the
effects of beta blockers.
Herbal
None known.
Food
None known.

DIAGNOSTIC TEST EFFECTS
May decrease serum potassium level.

SIDE EFFECTS
Frequent (28%)
Headache
Occasional (7%-3%)
Cough, tremor, dizziness, vertigo,
throat dryness or irritation,
pharyngitis
Rare (3%)
Palpitations, tachycardia, tremors,
nausea, heartburn, GI distress,
diarrhea

SERIOUS REACTIONS
• Salmeterol may prolong the QT
interval, which may precipitate
ventricular arrhythmias.
• Hypokalemia and hyperglycemia
may occur.

PRECAUTIONS & CONSIDERATIONS
Caution is warranted with cardiovascular disorders (such as coronary
insufficiency, arrhythmias, and

hypertension), seizure disorders, and thyrotoxicosis. Salmeterol is not for acute asthma symptoms and may cause paradoxical bronchospasm. It is unknown if salmeterol is excreted in breast milk. No age-related precautions have been noted in children older than 4 years. The elderly may require a lower dosage because of increased sensitivity to sympathomimetics and increased susceptibility to tachycardia and tremors. Avoid excessive use of caffeinated products, such as chocolate, cocoa, cola, coffee, and tea.

Notify the physician of chest pain or dizziness. Pulse rate and quality, respiratory rate, depth, rhythm and type, B/P, and serum potassium levels should be monitored. Evidence of cyanosis, a blue or a dusky color in light-skinned patients and a gray color in dark-skinned patients, should also be assessed.

Storage
Keep the drug canister at room temperature because cold decreases the drug's effects.

Administration
Shake the container well. Exhale completely through the mouth. Then place the mouthpiece in the mouth and close lips, holding the inhaler upright. Inhale deeply through the mouth while fully depressing the top of canister. Hold breath for as long as possible before exhaling slowly. Wait 1 minute before inhaling a second dose to allow for deeper bronchial penetration. Rinse mouth with water immediately after inhalation to prevent mouth and throat dryness. Do not abruptly discontinue the drug or exceed the recommended dosage. Keep a log of peak flow measurements.

To prevent exercise-induced bronchospasm, administer the dose at least 30 to 60 minutes before exercising.

Salsalate
sal′sa-late
(Amigesic, Disalcid, Mono-Gesic, Salflex)

CATEGORY AND SCHEDULE
Pregnancy Risk Category: C

CLASSIFICATION
Analgesics, non-narcotic, salicylates

MECHANISM OF ACTION
An NSAID that inhibits prostaglandin synthesis, reducing the inflammatory response and the intensity of pain stimuli reaching the sensory nerve endings. *Therapeutic Effect:* Produces analgesic and anti-inflammatory effects.

AVAILABILITY
Tablets (Amigesic, Disalcid): 500 mg, 750 mg.
Tablets (Mono-Gesic, Slaflex): 750 mg.

INDICATIONS AND DOSAGES
▸ **Rheumatoid arthritis, osteoarthritis pain**
PO
Adults, Elderly. Initially, 3 g/day in 2-3 divided doses. Maintenance: 2-4 g/day.

CONTRAINDICATIONS
Bleeding disorders, hypersensitivity to salicylates or NSAIDs

INTERACTIONS
Drug
Alcohol, NSAIDs: May increase the risk of GI effects, such as ulceration.
Antacids, urinary alkalinizers: Increase the excretion of salsalate.

S

Anticoagulants, heparin, thrombolytics: Increase the risk of bleeding.

Insulin, oral antidiabetics: May increase the effects of these drugs (with large doses of salsalate).

Methotrexate, zidovudine: May increase the toxicity of these drugs.

Ototoxic medications, vancomycin: May increase the risk of ototoxicity.

Platelet aggregation inhibitors, valproic acid: May increase the risk of bleeding.

Probenecid, sulfinpyrazone: May decrease the effects of these drugs.

Herbal
Ginkgo biloba: May increase the risk of bleeding.

Food
None known.

DIAGNOSTIC TEST EFFECTS

May alter serum alkaline phosphatase, uric acid, AST (SGOT), and ALT (SGPT) levels. May prolong PT and bleeding time. May decrease serum cholesterol, potassium, T_3, and T_4 levels.

SIDE EFFECTS

Occasional
Nausea, dyspepsia (including heartburn, indigestion, and epigastric pain)

SERIOUS REACTIONS

- Tinnitus may be the first indication that the serum salicylic acid concentration is reaching or exceeding the upper therapeutic range.
- Salsalate use may also produce vertigo, headache, confusion, drowsiness, diaphoresis, hyperventilation, vomiting, and diarrhea.
- Reye's syndrome may occur in children with chickenpox or the flu.
- Severe overdose may result in electrolyte imbalance, hyperthermia, dehydration, and blood pH imbalance.

- GI bleeding, peptic ulcer, and Reye's syndrome rarely occur.

PRECAUTIONS & CONSIDERATIONS
Caution is warranted with asthma, bleeding disorders, gastritis, history of gastric irritation hepatic or renal impairment peptic ulcer disease, and platelet disorders. Alcohol and NSAIDs should be avoided. Notify the physician if behavioral changes or vomiting occurs because they may be early signs of Reye's syndrome. Baseline liver function and coagulation studies should be obtained. Therapeutic response should be assessed.

Administration
Don't give salsalate to children or teenagers with chickenpox or the flu because this increases their risk of developing Reye's syndrome.

To minimize GI discomfort, take the drug with food.

Saquinavir
sa-kwin'a-veer
(Fortovase, Invirase)
Do not confuse saquinavir with Sinequan.

CATEGORY AND SCHEDULE
Pregnancy Risk Category: B

CLASSIFICATION
Antivirals, protease inhibitors

MECHANISM OF ACTION
Inhibits HIV protease, rendering the enzyme incapable of processing the polyprotein precursors needed to generate functional proteins in HIV-infected cells. *Therapeutic Effect:* Intereferes with HIV replication,

slowing the progression of HIV infection.

PHARMACOKINETICS

Poorly absorbed after PO administration (absorption increased with high-calorie and high-fat meals). Protein binding: 99%. Metabolized in the liver to inactive metabolite. Primarily eliminated in feces. Unknown if removed by hemodialysis. **Half-life:** 13 hr.

AVAILABILITY

Capsules (Invirase): 200 mg.
Capsules, Gelatin (Fortovase): 200 mg.

INDICATIONS AND DOSAGES

▶ **HIV infection in combination with other antiretrovirals**
PO
Adults, Elderly. 1200 mg Fortovase 3 times a day or 600 mg Invirase 3 times a day within 2 hr after a full meal.
Dosage adjustments when given in combination therapy:
Delavirdine: Fortovase 800 mg 3 times/day.
Lopinavir/ritonavir: Fortovase 800 mg 2 times/day.
Nelfinavir: Fortovase 800 mg 3 times/day or 1200 mg 2 times/day.
Ritonavir: Fortovase or Invirase 1000 mg 2 times/day.

CONTRAINDICATIONS

Clinically significant hypersensitivity to saquinavir; concurrent use with ergot medications, lovastatin, midazolam, simvastatin, or triazolam

INTERACTIONS

Drug
Calcium channel blockers, clindamycin, dapsone, quinidine, triazolam: May increase the plasma concentrations of these drugs.

Carbamazepine, dexamethasone, phenobarbital, phenytoin, rifampin: May reduce saquinavir plasma concentration.
Ketoconazole: Increases saquinavir plasma concentration.
Herbal
Garlic, St. John's wort: May decrease the plasma concentration and effect of saquinavir.
Food
Grapefruit juice: May increase saquinavir plasma concentration.

DIAGNOSTIC TEST EFFECTS

May alter serum CK levels, elevate liver function test results, and lower blood glucose levels.

SIDE EFFECTS

Occasional
Diarrhea, abdominal discomfort and pain, nausea, photosensitivity, stomatitis
Rare
Confusion, ataxia, asthenia, headache, rash

SERIOUS REACTIONS

• Ketoacidosis occurs rarely.

PRECAUTIONS & CONSIDERATIONS

Caution is warranted with diabetes mellitus or liver impairment. Breast-feeding is not recommended in this population because of the possibility of HIV transmission. Be aware that the safety and efficacy of saquinavir have not been established in children. There is no information on the effects of this drug's use in the elderly. Avoid exposure to artificial light sources and sunlight and grapefruit products. Saquinavir is not a cure for HIV infection, nor does it reduce the risk of transmission to others; illnesses associated with advanced HIV infection may occur.

S

Check the baseline laboratory and diagnostic test results, especially liver function test results, if ordered, before beginning saquinavir therapy and at periodic intervals during therapy. Closely monitor for signs and symptoms of gastrointestinal (GI) discomfort.

Assess the patient's pattern of daily bowel activity and stool consistency. Inspect the mouth for signs of mucosal ulceration. Notify the physician if nausea, numbness, persistent abdominal pain, tingling, or vomiting occurs.

Administration

Give within 2 hours after a full meal. Keep in mind that if saquinavir is taken on an empty stomach, the drug may not produce antiviral activity. Continue therapy for the full length of treatment and evenly space drug doses around the clock.

Sargramostim (Granulocyte Macrophage Colony-stimulating Factor, GM-CSF)
sar-gram'oh-stim
(Leukine)
Do not confuse Leukine with Leukeran.

CATEGORY AND SCHEDULE
Pregnancy Risk Category: C

CLASSIFICATION
Hematopoietic agents, recombinant DNA Origin

MECHANISM OF ACTION
A colony-stimulating factor that stimulates proliferation and differentiation of hematopoietic cells to activate mature granulocytes and macrophages. *Therapeutic Effect:*
Assists bone marrow in making new WBCs and increases their chemotactic, antifungal, and antiparasitic activity. Increases cytoneoplastic cells and activates neutrophils to inhibit tumor cell growth.

PHARMACOKINETICS

Effect	Onset	Peak	Duration
Increase WBCs	7-14 days	N/A	1 wk

Detected in serum within 5 min after subcutaneous administration. **Half-life:** IV, 1 hr; subcutaneous, 3 hr.

AVAILABILITY
Injection Solution: 500 mcg/ml.
Injection Powder for Reconstitution: 250 mcg.

INDICATIONS AND DOSAGES
▸ **Myeloid recovery following bone marrow transplant (BMT)**
IV INFUSION
Adults, Elderly. Usual parenteral dosage: 250 mcg/m^2/day for 21 days (as 2-hr infusion). Begin 2-4 hr after autologous bone marrow infusion and not less than 24 hr after last dose of chemotherapy or not less than 12 hr after last radiation treatment. Discontinue if blast cells appear or underlying disease progresses.
▸ **Bone marrow transplant failure, engraftment delay**
IV INFUSION
Adults, Elderly. 250 mcg/m^2/day for 14 days. Infuse over 2 hr. May repeat after 7 days off therapy if engraftment has not occurred with 500 mcg/m^2/day for 14 days.
▸ **Stem cell transplant**
IV, SUBCUTANEOUS
Adults. 250 mcg/m^2/day.

OFF-LABEL USES
Treatment of AIDS-related neutropenia; chronic, severe neutropenia;

drug induced neutropenia; myelodys-plastic syndrome

CONTRAINDICATIONS
Twelve hours before or after radiation therapy; 24 hours before or after chemotherapy; excessive leukemic myeloid blasts in bone marrow or peripheral blood (greater than 10%); known hypersensitivity to GM-CSF, yeast-derived products, or components of drug

INTERACTIONS
Drug
Lithium, steroids: May increase the effects of sargramostim.
Herbal
None known.
Food
None known.

DIAGNOSTIC TEST EFFECTS
May increase serum bilirubin, creatinine, and hepatic enzyme levels. May decrease serum albumin level.

▦ IV INCOMPATIBILITIES
Amphotericin B complex (Abelcet, AmBisome, Amphotec), hydromorphone (Dilaudid), lorazepam (Ativan), morphine
🖫 IV Compatibilities
Calcium gluconate, dopamine (Intropin), heparin, magnesium, potassium chloride

SIDE EFFECTS
Frequent
GI disturbances, including nausea, diarrhea, vomiting, stomatitis, anorexia, and abdominal pain; arthralgia or myalgia; headache; malaise; rash; pruritus
Occasional
Peripheral edema, weight gain, dyspnea, asthenia, fever, leukocytosis, capillary leak syndrome (such as fluid retention, irritation at local injection site, and peripheral edema)
Rare
Rapid or irregular heartbeat, thrombophlebitis

SERIOUS REACTIONS
• Pleural or pericardial effusion occurs rarely after infusion.

PRECAUTIONS & CONSIDERATIONS
Caution is warranted with CHF, hypoxia, impaired hepatic or renal function, preexisting cardiac disease, preexisting fluid retention, and pulmonary infiltrates. It is unknown if sargramostim crosses the placenta or is distributed in breast milk. Safety and efficacy of this drug have not been established in children. No age-related precautions have been noted in the elderly. Avoid situations that might place risk for contracting an infectious disease such as influenza.

Notify the physician of chest pain, chills, fever, palpitations, or dyspnea. Follow-up blood tests should be maintained to evaluate the effectiveness of drug therapy. CBC, pulmonary, liver, and kidney function test results, platelet count, vital signs, and weight should be monitored.
Storage
Refrigerate powder, reconstituted solution, and diluted solution for injection. Do not shake. Do not use past expiration date. Reconstituted solution is normally clear and colorless. Use reconstituted solution within 6 hours; discard unused portion. Use one dose/vial; do not reenter vial.
Administration
For IV use, to reconstitute, add 1 ml preservative-free sterile water for

injection to 250-mcg or 500-mcg vial. Direct sterile water for injection to side of vial, and gently swirl contents to avoid foaming. Do not shake or vigorously agitate. After reconstitution, further dilute with 0.9% NaCl. If final concentration is less than 10 mcg/ml, add 1 mg albumin per ml 0.9% NaCl to provide a final albumin concentration of 0.1%.

! Albumin is added before sargramostim to prevent drug adsorption to components of drug delivery system. Give each single dose over 2, 4, or 24 hours, as directed by physician.

Scopolamine
skoe-pol′a-meen
(Trans-Derm Scop, Transderm-V)

CATEGORY AND SCHEDULE
Pregnancy Risk Category: C

CLASSIFICATION
Anticholinergics, antiemetics/antivertigo, cycloplegics, gastrointestinals, mydriatics, ophthalmics, preanesthetics, sedatives/hypnotics

MECHANISM OF ACTION
An anticholinergic that reduces excitability of labyrinthine receptors, depressing conduction in the vestibular cerebellar pathway. *Therapeutic Effect:* Prevents motion-induced nausea and vomiting.

AVAILABILITY
Transdermal System: 1.5 mg.

INDICATIONS AND DOSAGES
▸ **Prevention of motion sickness**
TRANSDERMAL
Adults. 1 system q72hr.
▸ **Post-operative nausea or vomiting**
TRANSDERMAL
Adults, Elderly. 1 system no sooner than 1 hr before surgery and removed 24 hr after surgery.

CONTRAINDICATIONS
Angle-closure glaucoma, GI or GU obstruction, myasthenia gravis, paralytic ileus, tachycardia, thyrotoxicosis

INTERACTIONS
Drug
Antihistamines, tricyclic antidepressants: May increase the anticholinergic effects of scopolamine.
CNS depressants: May increase CNS depression.
Herbal
None known.
Food
None known.

DIAGNOSTIC TEST EFFECTS
May interfere with gastric secretion test.

SIDE EFFECTS
Frequent (greater than 15%)
Dry mouth, somnolence, blurred vision
Rare (5%-1%)
Dizziness, restlessness, hallucinations, confusion, difficulty urinating, rash

SERIOUS REACTIONS
• None known.

PRECAUTIONS & CONSIDERATIONS
Caution is warranted with cardiac disease, renal or hepatic impairment, psychoses, and seizures. Tasks that require mental alertness or motor skills should be avoided.

BUN level, blood chemistry test results, and serum alkaline phosphatase, bilirubin, creatinine, AST (SGOT) and ALT (SGPT) levels to assess hepatic and renal function should be monitored.

Administration

Apply transdermal patch to the hairless area behind one ear. Replace the patch after 72 hours or if it becomes dislodged. Wash hands after applying the patch. Use only one patch at a time and do not cut it.

Secobarbital

see-koe-bar'bi-tal
(Seconal)

CATEGORY AND SCHEDULE
Pregnancy Risk Category: D
Controlled Substance: Schedule II

CLASSIFICATION
Barbiturates, preanesthetics, sedatives/hypnotics

MECHANISM OF ACTION
A barbiturate that depresses the central nervous system (CNS) activity by binding to barbiturate site at the GABA-receptor complex enhancing GABA activity and depressing reticular activity system. *Therapeutic Effect:* Produces hypnotic effect due to central nervous system (CNS) depression.

PHARMACOKINETICS
Well absorbed from the gastrointestinal (GI) tract. Protein binding: 52%-57%. Crosses blood-brain barrier. Widely distributed. Metabolized in liver by microsomal enzyme system to inactive and active metabolites.

Primarily excreted in urine. Not removed by hemodialysis.
Half-life: 15-40 hr.

AVAILABILITY
Capsules: 50 mg (Seconal sodium).

INDICATIONS AND DOSAGES
▸ **Insomnia**
PO
Adults. 100 mg at bedtime.
▸ **Preoperative sedation**
PO
Adults. 100-300 mg 1-2 hr before procedure.
Children. 2-6 mg/kg 1-2 hr before procedure. Maximum: 100 mg/dose.
▸ **Sedation, daytime**
PO
Adults. 30-50 mg 3-4 times/day.
Children. 2 mg/kg 3 times/day.

OFF-LABEL USES
Chemotherapy-induced nausea and vomiting

CONTRAINDICATIONS
History of manifest or latent porphyria, marked liver dysfunction, marked respiratory disease in which dyspnea or obstruction is evident, and hypersensitivity to secobarbital or barbiturates

INTERACTIONS
Drug
Alcohol, CNS depressants: May increase the CNS depressant effects.
Anticoagulants: May decrease anticoagulant activity. Corticosteroids: May increase metabolism of corticosteroids.
Doxycycline: May shorten the half-life of doxycycline.
Griseofulvin: May decrease levels of griseofulvin by interfering with its metabolism.

S

Estradiol, estrone, progesterone, other steroidal hormones: May decrease the effect of these hormones by increasing their metabolism.

MAOIs: May prolong the effects of secobarbital by inhibiting its metabolism.

Phenytoin, sodium valproate, valproic acid: May decreases the metabolism and increase the concentration and risk of toxicity with secobarbital.

Herbal

St. John's wort, kava kava, gotu kola, valerian: May increase CNS depressant effects.

Food

None known.

DIAGNOSTIC TEST EFFECTS

None known.

SIDE EFFECTS

Frequent

Somnolence

Occasional

Agitation, confusion, hyperkinesia, ataxia, CNS depression, nightmares, nervousness, psychiatric disturbance, hallucinations, insomnia, anxiety, dizziness, abnormality in thinking, hypoventilation, apnea, bradycardia, hypotension, syncope, nausea, vomiting, constipation, headache

Rare

Hypersensitivity reactions, fever, liver damage, megaloblastic anemia

SERIOUS REACTIONS

• Agranulocytosis, megaloblastic anemia, apnea, hypoventilation, bradycardia, hypotension, syncope, hepatic damage, and Stevens-Johnson syndrome rarely occur.

• Tolerance and physical dependence may occur with repeated use.

PRECAUTIONS & CONSIDERATIONS

Secobarbital crosses the placenta and is distributed in breast milk. Its use may cause paradoxical excitement in children. The elderly patient taking secobarbital may exhibit confusion, excitement, and mental depression. Alcohol consumption and caffeine intake should be limited while taking secobarbital. Avoid tasks that require mental alertness or motor skills because this drug may cause dizziness and drowsiness.

Administration

Give secobarbital without regard to meals.

Selegiline

seh-leg'ill-ene
(Apo-Selegiline [CAN], Eldepryl, Novo-Selegiline [CAN], Selgene [AUS])
Do not confuse selegiline with Stelazine, or Eldepryl with enalapril.

CATEGORY AND SCHEDULE

Pregnancy Risk Category: C

CLASSIFICATION

Antiparkinson agents, dopaminergics

MECHANISM OF ACTION

An antiparkinson agent that irreversibly inhibits the activity of monoamine oxidase type B, the enzyme that breaks down dopamine, thereby increasing dopaminergic action. *Therapeutic Effect:* Relieves signs and symptoms of Parkinson's disease.

PHARMACOKINETICS
Rapidly absorbed from the GI tract.
Crosses the blood-brain barrier.
Metabolized in the liver to the active
metabolites. Primarily excreted in
urine. **Half-life:** 17 hr (amphetamine),
20 hr (methamphetamine).

AVAILABILITY
Capsules: 5 mg.
Tablets: 5 mg.

INDICATIONS AND DOSAGES
▶ **Adjunctive treatment for parkinsonism**
PO
Adults. 10 mg/day in divided doses,
such as 5 mg at breakfast and lunch,
given concomitantly with each dose
of carbidopa and levodopa.
Elderly. Initially, 5 mg in the morning. May increase up to 10 mg/day.

CONTRAINDICATIONS
None known.

INTERACTIONS
Drug
Fluoxetine: May cause serotonin
syndrome.
Meperidine: May cause a diaphore-
sis, excitation, hypertension or
hypotension, coma, and even death.
Herbal
None known.
Food
Tyramine-rich foods: May produce
a severe hypertensive reaction.

DIAGNOSTIC TEST EFFECTS
None known.

SIDE EFFECTS
Frequent (10%-4%)
Nausea, dizziness, lightheadedness,
syncope, abdominal discomfort
Occasional (3%-2%)
Confusion, hallucinations, dry
mouth, vivid dreams, dyskinesia

Rare (1%)
Headache, myalgia, anxiety, diarrhea,
insomnia

SERIOUS REACTIONS
• Symptoms of overdose may vary
from CNS depression, characterized
by sedation, apnea, cardiovascular
collapse, and death, to severe paradoxical reactions, such as hallucinations, tremor, and seizures.
• Other serious effects may include
involuntary movements, impaired
motor coordination, loss of balance,
blepharospasm, facial grimaces, feeling of heaviness in the lower extremities, depression, nightmares,
delusions, overstimulation, sleep
disturbance, and anger.

PRECAUTIONS & CONSIDERATIONS
Caution is warranted with cardiac
arrhythmias, dementia, history of
peptic ulcer disease, profound tremor,
psychosis, and tardive dyskinesia. It
is unknown if selegiline crosses the
placenta or is distributed in breast
milk. The safety and efficacy of
selegiline have not been established
in children. No age-related precautions have been noted in the elderly.
Be aware tyramine-rich foods, such
as wine and aged cheese, should be
avoided to prevent a hypertensive
reaction.
Dizziness, drowsiness, lightheadedness, and dry mouth are
common side effects of the drug but
will diminish or disappear with
continued treatment. Alcohol and
tasks that require mental alertness or
motor skills should be avoided.
Change positions slowly to prevent
orthostatic hypotension. Notify the
physician if agitation, headache,
lethargy, or confusion occurs. Baseline
vital signs should be assessed at baseline. Relief of symptoms, such as
improvement of masklike facial

expression, muscular rigidity, shuffling gait, and resting tremors of the hands and head should be assessed during treatment.

Administration

! Expect to take selegiline with carbidopa and levodopa therapy. Keep in mind that therapy should begin with the lowest dosage, then increase gradually over 3 to 4 weeks.

Senna

sen'na

(Ex-lax, Senexon, Senna-Glen, Sennatural, Senokot, X-Prep)

CATEGORY AND SCHEDULE

Pregnancy Risk Category: C

OTC

CLASSIFICATION

Anthraquinone derivative, laxative, stimulant

MECHANISM OF ACTION

A GI stimulant that has a direct effect on intestinal smooth musculature by stimulating the intramural nerve plexi. *Therapeutic Effect:* Increases peristalsis and promotes laxative effect.

PHARMACOKINETICS

Route	Onset	Peak	Duration
PO	6-12 hr	N/A	N/A
Rectal	0.5-2 hr	N/A	N/A

Minimal absorption after oral administration. Hydrolyzed to active form by enzymes of colonic flora. Absorbed drug metabolized in the liver. Eliminated in feces via biliary system.

AVAILABILITY

Granules (Senokot): 15 mg/tsp.

Liquid (X-Prep): 8.8 mg/5 ml.
Syrup (Senokot): 8.8 mg/5 ml.
Tablets (Sennatural, Senokot, Senexon, Senna-Gen): 8.6 mg, 15 mg.
Tablets (Ex-Lax).

INDICATIONS AND DOSAGES

▶ **Constipation**

PO (TABLETS)

Adults, Elderly, Children 12 yr and older. 2 tablets at bedtime. Maximum: 4 tablets twice a day.

Children 6-11 yr. 1 tablet at bedtime. Maximum: 2 tablets twice a day.

Children 2-5 yr. ½ tablet at bedtime. Maximum: 1 tablet twice a day.

PO (SYRUP)

Adults, Elderly, Children 12 yr and older. 10-15 ml at bedtime. Maximum: 15 ml twice a day.

Children 6-11 yr. 5-7.5 ml at bedtime. Maximum: 7.5 ml twice a day.

Children 2-5 yr. 2.5-3.75 ml at bedtime. Maximum: 3.75 ml twice a day.

PO (GRANULES)

Adults, Elderly, Children 12 yr and older. 1 tsp at bedtime. Maximum: 2 tsp twice a day.

Children 6-11 yr. One half (½) teaspoon at bedtime up to 1 teaspoon 2 times/day.

Children 2-5 yr. One quarter (¼) teaspoon at bedtime up to one half (½) teaspoon 2 times/day.

▶ **Bowel evacuation**

PO

Adults, Elderly, Children older than 1 yr. 75 ml between 2 PM and 4 PM on day prior to procedure.

CONTRAINDICATIONS

Abdominal pain, appendicitis, intestinal obstruction, nausea, vomiting

INTERACTIONS
Drug
Oral medications: May decrease transit time of concurrently administered oral medications, decreasing absorption of senna.
Herbal
None known.
Food
None known.

DIAGNOSTIC TEST EFFECTS
May increase blood glucose level. May decrease serum potassium level.

SIDE EFFECTS
Frequent
Pink-red, red-violet, red-brown, or yellow-brown discoloration of urine
Occasional
Some degree of abdominal discomfort, nausea, mild cramps, griping, faintness

SERIOUS REACTIONS
• Long-term use may result in laxative dependence, chronic constipation, and loss of normal bowel function.
• Prolonged use or overdose may result in electrolyte and metabolic disturbances (such as hypokalemia, hypocalcemia, and metabolic acidosis or alkalosis), vomiting, muscle weakness, persistent diarrhea, malabsorption, and weight loss.

PRECAUTIONS & CONSIDERATIONS
Senna should be used cautiously for extended periods of time (greater than 1 week). It is unknown if senna is distributed in breast milk. Safety and efficacy of senna have not been established in children younger than 6 years of age. No age-related precautions have been noted in the elderly, but this population should be monitored for signs and symptoms of dehydration and electrolyte loss.

Urine may turn pink-red, red-violet, red-brown, or yellow-brown. Pattern of daily bowel activity and stool consistency and serum electrolyte levels should be monitored. Adequate fluid intake should be maintained.
Administration
Take senna on an empty stomach for faster results. Drink at least 6 to 8 glasses of water a day to aid in stool softening. Avoid giving within 1 hour of other oral medications because drug absorption is decreased. To promote defecation, increase fluid intake, exercise, and eat a high-fiber diet. Oral senna generally produces a laxative effect in 6 to 12 hours but it can take 24 hours.

Sertaconazole
sir-tah-con'ah-zole
(Ertaczo)

CATEGORY AND SCHEDULE
Pregnancy Risk Category: C

CLASSIFICATION
Antifungals, topical, dermatologics

MECHANISM OF ACTION
An imidazole derivative that inhibits synthesis of ergosterol, a vital component of fungal cell formation. *Therapeutic Effect:* Damages the fungal cell membrane, altering its function.

AVAILABILITY
Cream: 2%.

INDICATIONS AND DOSAGES
▸ **Tinea pedis**
TOPICAL
Adults, Elderly, Children 12 yr and older. Apply to affected area twice a day for 4 wk.

S

CONTRAINDICATIONS
None known.

INTERACTIONS
Drug
None known.
Herbal
None known.
Food
None known.

DIAGNOSTIC TEST EFFECTS
None known.

SIDE EFFECTS
Rare (2%)
Burning, tenderness, erythema, dryness, pruritus, hyperpigmentation, and contact dermatitis at application site

SERIOUS REACTIONS
• None known.

PRECAUTIONS & CONSIDERATIONS

It is unknown if sertaconazole is excreted in breast milk. There are no age-related precautions noted in patients younger than 12 years of age or in the elderly. Skin should be assessed for dermatitis, dryness, erythema, hyperpigmentation, burning sensation, or pruritus.
Administration
Rub gently into affected, surrounding areas. Avoid contact with eyes, nose, and mouth. Keep the affected area clean and dry. Continue sertaconazole treatment for the full length of therapy.

Sertraline
sir'trall-een
(Apo-Sertraline [CAN], Novo-Sertraline [CAN], PMS-Sertraline [CAN], Zoloft)
Do not confuse sertraline with Serentil.

CATEGORY AND SCHEDULE
Pregnancy Risk Category: B

CLASSIFICATION
Antidepressants, serotonin specific reuptake inhibitors

MECHANISM OF ACTION
An antidepressant, anxiolytic, and obsessive-compulsive disorder adjunct that blocks the reuptake of the neurotransmitter serotonin at CNS neuronal presynaptic membranes, increasing its availability at postsynaptic receptor sites. *Therapeutic Effect:* Relieves depression, reduces obsessive-compulsive behavior, decreases anxiety.

PHARMACOKINETICS
Incompletely and slowly absorbed from the GI tract; food increases absorption. Protein binding: 98%. Widely distributed. Undergoes extensive first-pass metabolism in the liver to active compound. Excreted in urine and feces. Not removed by hemodialysis.
Half-life: 26 hr.

AVAILABILITY
Oral Concentrate: 20 mg/ml.
Tablets: 25 mg, 50 mg, 100 mg.

INDICATIONS AND DOSAGES
▸ **Depression, obsessive-compulsive disorder**

PO
Adults, Children 13-17 yr. Initially,
50 mg/day with morning or evening
meal. May increase by 50 mg/day at
7-day intervals.
Elderly, Children 6-12 yr. Initially,
25 mg/day. May increase by
25-50 mg/day at 7-day intervals.
Maximum: 200 mg/day.
▸ **Panic disorder, posttraumatic
stress disorder, social anxiety
disorder**
PO
Adults, Elderly. Initially, 25 mg/day.
May increase by 50 mg/day at 7-day
intervals. Range: 50-200 mg/day.
Maximum: 200 mg/day.
▸ **Premenstrual dysphoric disorder**
PO
Adults. Initially, 50 mg/day. May
increase up to 150 mg/day in 50-mg
increments.

CONTRAINDICATIONS
Use within 14 days of MAOIs

INTERACTIONS
Drug
**Highly protein-bound medications
(such as, digoxin and warfarin):**
May increase the blood concentration
and risk of toxicity of these drugs.
MAOIs: May cause neuroleptic
malignant syndrome, hypertensive
crisis, hyperpyrexia, seizures, and
serotonin syndrome (marked by
diaphoresis, diarrhea, fever, mental
changes, restlessness, and shivering).
Herbal
St. John's wort: May increase the
risk of adverse effects.
Food
None known.

DIAGNOSTIC TEST EFFECTS
May increase serum total cholesterol, triglyceride, AST (SGOT), and
ALT (SGPT) levels. May decrease
serum uric acid level.

SIDE EFFECTS
Frequent (26%-12%)
Headache, nausea, diarrhea, insomnia,
somnolence, dizziness, fatigue, rash,
dry mouth
Occasional (6%-4%)
Anxiety, nervousness, agitation,
tremor, dyspepsia, diaphoresis, vomiting, constipation, abnormal ejaculation, visual disturbances, altered taste
Rare (less than 3%)
Flatulence, urinary frequency,
paraesthesia, hot flashes, chills

SERIOUS REACTIONS
• None known.

PRECAUTIONS & CONSIDERATIONS
Caution is warranted with cardiac
disease, hepatic impairment, seizure
disorders, those who have had a recent
MI, and in those with suicidal
tendency. It is unknown if sertraline
crosses the placenta or is distributed
in breast milk. Notify the physician
if pregnancy occurs. No age-related
precautions have been noted in children older than 6 years. Lower initial
sertraline dosages are recommended
for the elderly, although no age-
related precautions have been noted
in this age group.
Dizziness may occur, so alcohol
and tasks that require mental alertness or motor skills should be
avoided. Notify the physician if
fatigue, headache, sexual dysfunction, or tremor occurs. CBC and liver
and renal function tests should be
performed before and periodically
during therapy, especially with long-
term use.
Administration
! Make sure at least 14 days elapse
between the use of MAOIs and
sertraline.
Take sertraline with food or milk
if GI distress occurs.

Sevelamer
seh-vel'a-mer
(Renagel)
**Do not confuse Renagel with
Reglan or Regonol.**

CATEGORY AND SCHEDULE
Pregnancy Risk Category: C

CLASSIFICATION
Metabolics

MECHANISM OF ACTION
An antihyperphosphatemia agent that
binds with dietary phosphorus in the
GI tract, thus allowing phosphorus to
be eliminated through the normal
digestive process and decreasing the
serum phosphorus level. *Therapeutic
Effect:* Decreases incidence of hypercalcemic episodes in patients receiving
calcium acetate treatment.

PHARMACOKINETICS
Not absorbed systemically. Unknown
if removed by hemodialysis.

AVAILABILITY
Capsules: 403 mg.
Tablets: 400 mg, 800 mg.

INDICATIONS AND DOSAGES
▶ **Hyperphosphatemia**
PO
Adults, Elderly. 800-1600 mg with
each meal, depending on severity of
hyperphosphatemia.

CONTRAINDICATIONS
Bowel obstruction, hypophosphatemia

INTERACTIONS
Drug
None known.
Herbal
None known.

Food
None known.

DIAGNOSTIC TEST EFFECTS
None known.

SIDE EFFECTS
Frequent (20%-11%)
Infection, pain, hypotension, diarrhea,
dyspepsia, nausea, vomiting
Occasional (10%-1%)
Headache, constipation, hypertension,
thrombosis, increased cough

SERIOUS REACTIONS
• None known.

PRECAUTIONS & CONSIDERATIONS
Caution is warranted with dysphagia,
severe GI tract motility disorders,
swallowing disorders, and in those
who have undergone major GI tract
surgery. Sevelamer is not distributed
in breast milk. The safety and efficacy
of sevelamer have not been established in children. No age-related
precautions have been noted in the
elderly.
    Serum bicarbonate, chloride,
calcium, and phosphorus levels
should be monitored. Notify the
physician of diarrhea, signs of
hypotension (such as lightheadedness), nausea or vomiting, or a
persistent headache.
Administration
Take sevelamer with food. Don't
break capsules apart because the
contents expand in water. Take other
medications at least 1 hour before or
3 hours after sevelamer.

Sibutramine
sih-byoo′tra-meen
(Meridia)

CATEGORY AND SCHEDULE
Pregnancy Risk Category: C
Controlled Substance:
Schedule IV

CLASSIFICATION
Anorexiants, stimulants, central
nervous system

MECHANISM OF ACTION
A central nervous system (CNS) stimulant inhibits reuptake of serotonin (enhancing satiety) and norepinephrine (raises metabolic rate) centrally. *Therapeutic Effect:* Induces and maintains weight loss.

PHARMACOKINETICS
Rapidly absorbed from the gastrointestinal (GI) tract. Protein binding: 95%-97%. Metabolized in liver, undergoes first-pass metabolism. Primarily excreted in urine, minimal elimination in feces. **Half-life:** 1.1 hr.

AVAILABILITY
Capsules: 5 mg, 10 mg, 15 mg (Meridia).

INDICATIONS AND DOSAGES
▸ **Weight loss**
PO
Adults 16 yr and older. Initially, 10 mg/day. May increase up to 15 mg/day. Maximum: 20 mg/day.

CONTRAINDICATIONS
Anorexia nervosa, concomitant MAOI use, concomitant use of centrally acting appetite suppressants, hypersensitivity to sibutramine or any component of the formulation

INTERACTIONS
Drug
CNS-acting appetite suppressants: May increase risk of hypertension and tachycardia.
Dextromethorphan, dihydroergotamine, ergotamine, fentanyl, lithium, meperidine, MAOIs, pentazocine, SSRIs, serotonin agonists, tryptophan: May increase risk of serotonin syndrome.
Herbal
St. John's wort: May decrease sibutramine levels.
Yohimbine: May increase risk of adverse cardiovascular effects.
Food
None known.

DIAGNOSTIC TEST EFFECTS
None known.

SIDE EFFECTS
Frequent
Headache, dry mouth, anorexia, constipation, insomnia, rhinitis, pharyngitis
Occasional
Back pain, flu syndrome, dizziness, nausea, asthenia (loss of strength, energy), arthralgia, nervousness, dyspepsia, sinusitis, abdominal pain, anxiety, dysmenorrheal
Rare
Depression, rash, cough, sweating, tachycardia, migraine, increased B/P, paresthesia, altered taste

SERIOUS REACTIONS
• Seizures, thrombocytopenia, and deaths have been reported.
• Serotonin syndrome can occur with concomitant use of drugs that increase serotonin.
• Large doses may produce extreme nervousness and tachycardia.

S

PRECAUTIONS & CONSIDERATIONS

Caution is warranted with arrhythmias, congestive heart failure, coronary artery disease, gallstones, hypertension (uncontrolled or poorly controlled), narrow angle glaucoma, seizures, severe liver or renal impairment, and stroke. It is unknown if sibutramine crosses the placenta or is distributed in breast milk. Safety and efficacy have not been established in children younger than 16 years of age. Be aware that sibutramine is not recommended in the elderly. Avoid alcohol. Do not take any over-the-counter medications without consulting with the physician.

Storage

Store at room temperature.

Administration

Take with or without food usually in the morning. Administer sibutramine with a low-calorie diet.

Sibutramine is intended for obese persons with an initial body mass index greater than or equal to 30 kg/m^2 or greater than or equal to 27 kg/m^2 in the presence of other risk factors such as hypertension, diabetes, dyslipidemia. Sibutramine may be habit-forming. Do not abruptly discontinue the medication.

Sildenafil

sill-den′a-fill

(Viagra)

Do not confuse Viagra with Vaniqa.

CATEGORY AND SCHEDULE

Pregnancy Risk Category: B

CLASSIFICATION

Impotence agents, phosphodiesterase inhibitors

MECHANISM OF ACTION

An erectile dysfunction agent that inhibits phosphodiesterase type 5, the enzyme responsible for degrading cyclic guanosine monophosphate in the corpus cavernosum of the penis, resulting in smooth muscle relaxation and increased blood flow. *Therapeutic Effect:* Facilitates an erection.

AVAILABILITY

Tablets: 25 mg, 50 mg, 100 mg.

INDICATIONS AND DOSAGES

▸ **Erectile dysfunction**

PO

Adults. 50 mg (30 min-4 hr before sexual activity). Range: 25-100 mg. Maximum dosing frequency is once daily.

Elderly (over 65 yr). Consider starting dose of 25 mg.

OFF-LABEL USES

Treatment of diabetic gastroparesis, sexual dysfunction associated with the use of selective serotonin reuptake inhibitors

CONTRAINDICATIONS

Concurrent use of sodium nitroprusside or nitrates in any form

INTERACTIONS
Drug
Cimetidine, erythromycin, itracona-zole, ketoconazole: May increase sildenafil plasma concentration.
Nitrates: Potentiates the hypotensive effects of nitrates.
Herbal
None known.
Food
High-fat meals: Delay drug's maximum effectiveness by 1 hour.

DIAGNOSTIC TEST EFFECTS
None known.

SIDE EFFECTS
Frequent
Headache (16%), flushing (10%)
Occasional (7%-3%)
Dyspepsia, nasal congestion, UTI, abnormal vision, diarrhea
Rare (2%)
Dizziness, rash

SERIOUS REACTIONS
• Prolonged erections (lasting over 4 hours) and priapism (painful erections lasting over 6 hours) occur rarely.

PRECAUTIONS & CONSIDERATIONS
Caution is warranted with an anatomic deformity of the penis, cardiac, hepatic or renal impairment, and conditions that increase the risk of priapism, including leukemia, multiple myeloma, and sickle cell anemia. Be aware sildenafil is not effective without sexual stimulation. Avoid using nitrate drugs concurrently with sildenafil. Seek treatment immediately if an erection lasts longer than 4 hours.
Administration
Sildenafil is usually taken 1 hour before sexual activity but may be taken anywhere from 4 hours to 30 minutes beforehand. High-fat meals may affect the drug's absorption rate and effectiveness.

Silver Nitrate

CATEGORY AND SCHEDULE
Pregnancy Risk Category: C

CLASSIFICATION
Anti-infectives, ophthalmics

MECHANISM OF ACTION
Free silver ions precipitate bacterial proteins by combining with chloride in tissue forming silver chloride; coagulates cellular protein to form an eschar or scab. The germicidal action is credited to precipitation of bacterial proteins by free silver ions. *Therapeutic Effect:* Inhibits growth of both gram-positive and gram-negative bacteria.

PHARMACOKINETICS
Minimal gastrointestinal (GI) tract and cutaneous absorption. Minimal excretion in urine.

AVAILABILITY
Applicator sticks: 75% silver nitrate and 25% potassium nitrate.
Ophthalmic solution: 1%.
Topical solution: 10%, 25%, 50%.

INDICATIONS AND DOSAGES
▸ **Exuberant granulations**
APPLICATOR STICKS
Adults, Elderly, Children. Apply to mucous membranes and other moist skin surfaces only on area to be treated 2-3 times/wk for 2-3 wk.
TOPICAL, SOLUTION
Adults, Elderly, Children. Apply a cotton applicator dipped in solution

S

on the affected area 2-3 times/wk for 2-3 wk.

▸ **Gonococcal ophthalmia neonatorum**
OPHTHALMIC
Children. Instill 2 drops in each eye immediately after delivery.

OFF-LABEL USES
Children. Instill 2 drops in each eye immediately after delivery.

CONTRAINDICATIONS
Broken skin, cuts, or wounds, hypersensitivity to silver nitrate or any of its components

INTERACTIONS
Drug
None known.
Herbal
None known.
Food
None known.

DIAGNOSTIC TEST EFFECTS
None known.

SIDE EFFECTS
Occasional
Ophthalmic: Chemical conjunctivitis
Topical: Burning, irritation, staining of the skin
Rare
Hyponatremia, methemoglobinemia

SERIOUS REACTIONS
• Symptoms of overdose include blackening of skin and mucous membranes, pain and burning of the mouth, salivation, vomiting, diarrhea, shock, convulsions, coma, and death.
• Methemoglobinemia is caused by absorbed silver nitrate but occurs rarely.
• Cauterization of the cornea and blindness occur rarely.

PRECAUTIONS & CONSIDERATIONS
Topical preparations should be used cautiously and should not be applied to abraded areas or near the eyes. It is unknown if silver nitrate crosses the placenta and is distributed in breast milk. There are no age-related precautions noted in children or the elderly.

Prolonged use may cause skin discoloration. Repeated applications of silver nitrate ophthalmic solution can cause cauterization of the cornea and blindness.
Storage
Store silver nitrate in a dry place and in a tight, light-resistant container. Exposure to light causes silver to oxidize and turn brown.
Administration
Apply topical preparation by rubbing gently into the affected and surrounding area.

Instill ophthalmic drops of solution in each lower conjunctival sac. Gently massage the closed eyelids to help spread the solution to all areas of the conjunctiva. Gently wipe away excess solution from the eyelids and surrounding skin with sterile cotton.

Silver Sulfadiazine
sul-fa-dye'a-zeen
(Flamazine [CAN], SSD, SSD AF, Silvadene)

CATEGORY AND SCHEDULE
Pregnancy Risk Category: B

CLASSIFICATION
Anti-infectives, topical, dermatologics

MECHANISM OF ACTION

An anti-infective that acts upon cell wall and cell membrane. Releases silver slowly in concentrations selectively toxic to bacteria. *Therapeutic Effect:* Produces bactericidal effect.

PHARMACOKINETICS

Variably absorbed. Significant systemic absorption may occur if applied to extensive burns. Absorbed medication excreted unchanged in urine. **Half-life:** 10 hr (half-life increased with impaired renal function).

AVAILABILITY

Cream: 1% (Silvadene, SSD, SSD AF).

INDICATIONS AND DOSAGES

▶ **Burns**
TOPICAL
Adults, Elderly Children. Apply 1-2 times daily.

OFF-LABEL USES

Treatment of minor bacterial skin infection, dermal ulcer

CONTRAINDICATIONS

Hypersensitivity to silver sulfadiazine or any component of the formulation

INTERACTIONS

Drug
Collagenase, papain, sutilains: May be inactivated.
Herbal
None known.
Food
None known.

DIAGNOSTIC TEST EFFECTS

None known.

SIDE EFFECTS

Side effects characteristic of all sulfonamides may occur when systemically absorbed such as extensive burn areas, anorexia, nausea, vomiting, headache, diarrhea, dizziness, photosensitivity, joint pain
Frequent
Burning feeling at treatment site
Occasional
Brown-gray skin discoloration, rash, itching
Rare
Increased sensitivity or skin to sunlight

SERIOUS REACTIONS

- If significant systemic absorption occurs, less often but serious are hemolytic anemia, hypoglycemia, diuresis, peripheral neuropathy, Stevens-Johnson syndrome, agranulocytosis, disseminated lupus erythematosus, anaphylaxis, hepatitis, and toxic nephrosis.
- Fungal superinfections may occur.
- Interstitial nephritis occurs rarely.

PRECAUTIONS & CONSIDERATIONS

Caution is warranted with impaired renal or hepatic function, G6PD deficiency, premature neonates, and infants less than 2 months. Be aware that silver sulfadiazine is not recommended during pregnancy unless burn area is greater than 20% of body surface. Be aware that it is unknown if silver sulfadiazine is distributed in breast milk. There is a risk of kernicterus in neonates. There are no age-related precautions noted in children or the elderly.

Serum sulfonamide concentrations should be checked. Skin should be assessed for burns, surrounding areas for pain, burning, itching, and rash. Antihistamines may provide relief, silver sulfadiazine therapy should continue unless reactions are severe.
Storage
Store at room temperature. Cream will occasionally darken either in the

S

jar or after application to the skin. This color change results from a light catalyzed reaction which is a common characteristic of all silver salts. The antimicrobial activity of the product is not substantially diminished because of the color change reaction involves such a small amount of the active drug.

Administration

Apply topical preparation to cleansed and debrided burns using sterile glove. Keep burn areas covered with silver sulfadiazine cream at all times. Reapply to areas where removed by activity. Dressings may be ordered on individual basis.

Simethicone
si-meth′i-kone
(Alka-Seltzer Gas Relief, Gas-X, Genasym, Infant Mylicon, Mylanta Gas, Ovol [CAN], Phazyme)

CATEGORY AND SCHEDULE
Pregnancy Risk Category: C
OTC

CLASSIFICATION
Siloxane polymer, antiflatulent

MECHANISM OF ACTION
An antiflatulent that changes surface tension of gas bubbles, allowing easier elimination of gas.
Therapeutic Effect: Drug dispersal, prevents formation of gas pockets in the GI tract.

PHARMACOKINETICS
Does not appear to be absorbed from GI tract. Excreted unchanged in feces.

AVAILABILITY
Oral Drops (Infants Mylicon): 40 mg/0.6 ml.
Softgel (Alka-Seltzer Gas Relief, Gas-Z, Mylanta Gas): 125 mg.
Softgel (Phazyme): 180 mg.
Tablets (Chewable [Gas-X, Mylanta Gas]): 80 mg, 125 mg.

INDICATIONS AND DOSAGES
▶ **Antiflatulent**
PO
Adults, Elderly, Children 12 yr and older. 40-250 mg after meals and at bedtime. Maximum: 500 mg/day.
Children 2-11 yr. 40 mg 4 times a day.
Children younger than 2 yr. 20 mg 4 times a day.

OFF-LABEL USES
Adjunct to bowel radiography and gastroscopy

CONTRAINDICATIONS
None known.

INTERACTIONS
Drug
None known.
Herbal
None known.
Food
None known.

DIAGNOSTIC TEST EFFECTS
None known.

SIDE EFFECTS
None known.

SERIOUS REACTIONS
• None known.

PRECAUTIONS & CONSIDERATIONS
It is unknown if simethicone crosses the placenta or is distributed in breast milk. Simethicone may be used safely in children and the elderly.

Before simethicone administration, the abdomen should be assessed for signs of tenderness, rigidity, and the presence of bowel sounds. Avoid carbonated beverages during simethicone therapy.

Administration

Take simethicone after meals and at bedtime, as needed. Chew tablets thoroughly before swallowing. Shake suspension well before using.

Simvastatin

sim'va-sta-tin

(Apo-Simvastatin [CAN], Lipex [AUS], Zocor)

Do not confuse Zocor with Cozaar.

CATEGORY AND SCHEDULE

Pregnancy Risk Category: X

CLASSIFICATION

Antihyperlipidemics, HMG CoA reductase inhibitors

MECHANISM OF ACTION

An HMG-CoA reductase inhibitor that interferes with cholesterol biosynthesis by inhibiting the conversion of the enzyme HMG-CoA to mevalonate. *Therapeutic Effect:* Decreases serum LDL, cholesterol, VLDL, and plasma triglyceride levels; slightly increases serum HDL concentration.

PHARMACOKINETICS

Route	Onset	Peak	Duration
PO to reduce cholesterol	3 days	14 days	N/A

Well absorbed from the GI tract. Protein binding: 95%. Undergoes extensive first-pass metabolism. Hydrolyzed to active metabolite. Primarily eliminated in feces. Unknown if removed by hemodialysis.

AVAILABILITY

Tablets: 5 mg, 10 mg, 20 mg, 40 mg, 80 mg.

INDICATIONS AND DOSAGES

▸ **To decrease elevated total and LDL cholesterol in hypercholesterolemia (types IIa and IIb), lower triglyceride levels, and increase HDL levels; to reduce risk of death and prevent MI in patients with heart disease and elevated cholesterol level; to reduce risk of revascularization procedures; to decrease risk of stroke or transient ischemic attack; to prevent cardiovascular events.**

PO

Adults. Initially, 10-40 mg/day in evening. Dosage adjusted at 4-wk intervals.

Elderly. Initially, 10 mg/day. May increase by 5-10 mg/day q4wk. Range: 5-80 mg/day. Maximum: 80 mg/day.

CONTRAINDICATIONS

Active hepatic disease or unexplained, persistent elevations of liver function test results, age younger than 18 years, pregnancy

INTERACTIONS

Drug

Cyclosporine, erythromycin, gemfibrozil, immunosuppressants, niacin: Increases the risk of acute renal failure and rhabdomyolysis.

Erythromycin, itraconazole, keto-conazole: May increase simvastatin blood concentration and cause muscle inflammation, myalgia, or weakness.

S

Herbal
None known.
Food
None known.

DIAGNOSTIC TEST EFFECTS
May increase serum CK and serum transaminase concentrations.

SIDE EFFECTS
Simvastatin is generally well tolerated. Side effects are usually mild and transient.
Occasional (3%-2%)
Headache, abdominal pain or cramps, constipation, upper respiratory tract infection
Rare (less than 2%)
Diarrhea, flatulence, asthenia (loss of strength and energy), nausea, or vomiting

SERIOUS REACTIONS
- Lens opacities may occur.
- Hypersensitivity reaction and hepatitis occur rarely.

PRECAUTIONS & CONSIDERATIONS
Caution is warranted with history of hepatic disease, severe electrolyte, endocrine, metabolic disorders and those who consume substantial amounts of alcohol. Withholding or discontinuing simvastatin may be necessary when the person is at risk for renal failure secondary to rhabdomyolysis. Simvastatin use is contraindicated in pregnancy because suppression of cholesterol biosynthesis may cause fetal toxicity. Simvastatin is contraindicated in lactation because there is a risk of serious adverse reactions in breastfeeding infants. Safety and efficacy of simvastatin have not been established in children. No age-related precautions have been noted in the elderly.

Notify the physician of headache or muscle weakness and aches. Pattern of daily bowel activity and stool consistency should be assessed. Serum lipid cholesterol and triglyceride levels and hepatic function should be checked at baseline and periodically during treatment. Before beginning therapy, a standard cholesterol-lowering diet for a minimum of 3 to 6 months should be practiced and then continued throughout simvastatin therapy.
Administration
Take simvastatin without regard to meals and administer in the evening.

Sirolimus
sir-oh-leem'us
(Rapamune)

CATEGORY AND SCHEDULE
Pregnancy Risk Category: C

CLASSIFICATION
Immunosuppressives

MECHANISM OF ACTION
An immunosuppressant that inhibits T-lymphocyte proliferation induced by stimulation of cell surface receptors, mitogens, alloantigens, and lymphokines. Prevents activation of the enzyme target of rapamycin, a key regulatory kinase in cell cycle progression. *Therapeutic Effect:* Inhibits proliferation of T and B cells, essential components of the immune response; prevents organ transplant rejection.

AVAILABILITY
Oral Solution: 1 mg/ml.
Tablets: 1 mg, 2 mg.

INDICATIONS AND DOSAGES
▶ **Prevention of organ transplant rejection**
PO
Adults. Loading dose: 6 mg.
Maintenance: 2 mg/day.
Children 13 yr and older weighing less than 40 kg. Loading dose: 3 mg/m^2. Maintenance: 1 mg/m^2/day.

CONTRAINDICATIONS
Hypersensitivity to sirolimus, malignancy

INTERACTIONS
Drug
Cyclosporine, diltiazem, ketoconazole: May increase the blood concentration and risk of toxicity of sirolimus.
Rifampin: May decrease the blood concentration and effects of sirolimus.
Herbal
None known.
Food
Grapefruit, grapefruit juice: May decrease the metabolism of sirolimus.

DIAGNOSTIC TEST EFFECTS
May decrease blood Hgb level, Hct, and platelet count. May increase serum cholesterol, creatinine, and triglyceride levels.

SIDE EFFECTS
Occasional
Hypercholesterolemia, hyperlipidemia, hypertension, rash; with high doses (5 mg/day): anemia, arthralgia, diarrhea, hypokalemia, and thrombocytopenia

SERIOUS REACTIONS
• None known.

PRECAUTIONS & CONSIDERATIONS
Caution is warranted with chickenpox, herpes zoster, hepatic impairment, and infection. Avoid consuming grapefruit or grapefruit juice during therapy. Also, avoid coming in contact with people with colds or other infections. Liver function tests should be monitored.
Storage
Store vials at room temperature. Use it immediately or after reconstitution or, if necessary, refrigerate it for up to 24 hours.
Administration
Take the drug at the same time each day. Notify the physician if a dose is missed.

Sodium Bicarbonate

CATEGORY AND SCHEDULE
Pregnancy Risk Category: C
OTC

CLASSIFICATION
Alkalinizing agents, electrolyte replacements

MECHANISM OF ACTION
An alkalinizing agent that dissociates to provide bicarbonate ion. *Therapeutic Effect:* Neutralizes hydrogen ion concentration, raises blood and urinary pH.

PHARMACOKINETICS

Route	Onset	Peak	Duration
PO	15 min	N/A	1-3 hr
IV	Immediate	N/A	8-10 min

After administration, sodium bicarbonate dissociates to sodium and bicarbonate ions. With increased hydrogen ion concentrations bicarbonate ions combine with hydrogen ions to form carbonic acid, which then dissociates to CO_2, which is excreted by the lungs.

AVAILABILITY

Tablets: 325 mg, 650 mg.
Injection: 0.5 mEq/ml (4.2%), 0.6 mEq/ml (5%), 0.9 mEq/ml (7.5%), 1 mEq/ml (8.4%).

INDICATIONS AND DOSAGES

▶ **Cardiac arrest**
IV
Adults, Elderly. Initially, 1 mEq/kg (as 7.5%-8.4% solution). May repeat with 0.5 mEq/kg q10min during continued cardiopulmonary arrest. Use in the postresuscitation phase is based on arterial blood pH, partial pressure of carbon dioxide in arterial blood ($PaCO_2$) and base deficit calculation.
Children, Infants. Initially, 1 mEq/kg.

▶ **Metabolic acidosis (not severe)**
IV
Adults, Elderly, Children. 2-5 mEq/kg over 4-8 hr. May repeat based on laboratory values.

▶ **Metabolic acidosis (associated with chronic renal failure)**
PO
Adults, Elderly. Initially, 20-36 mEq/day in divided doses.

▶ **Renal tubular acidosis (distal)**
PO
Adults, Elderly. 0.5-2 mEq/kg/day in 4-6 divided doses.
Children. 2-3 mEq/kg/day in divided doses.

▶ **Renal tubular acidosis (proximal)**
PO
Adults, Elderly, Children. 5-10 mEq/kg/day in divided doses.

▶ **Urine alkalinization**
PO
Adults, Elderly. Initially, 4 g, then 1-2 g q4hr. Maximum: 16 g/day.
Children. 84-840 mg/kg/day in divided doses.

▶ **Antacid**
PO
Adults, Elderly. 300 mg-2 g 1-4 times a day.

▶ **Hyperkalemia**
IV
Adults, Elderly. 1 mEq/kg over 5 minutes.

CONTRAINDICATIONS

Excessive chloride loss due to diarrhea, vomiting, or GI suctioning; hypocalcemia; metabolic or respiratory alkalosis

INTERACTIONS

Drug
Calcium-containing products: May result in milk-alkali syndrome.
Corticosteroids: May cause edema and hypertension.
Lithium, salicylates: May increase the excretion of these drugs.
Methenamine: May decrease the effects of methenamine.
Herbal
None known.
Food
Milk, other dairy products: May result in milk-alkali syndrome.

DIAGNOSTIC TEST EFFECTS

May increase serum and urinary pH.

▧ IV INCOMPATIBILITIES

Ascorbic acid, diltiazem (Cardizem), dobutamine (Dobutrex), dopamine (Intropin), hydromorphone (Dilaudid), magnesium sulfate, midazolam

(Versed), morphine, norepinephrine (Levophed)

IV Compatibilities

Aminophylline, calcium chloride, furosemide (Lasix), heparin, insulin, lidocaine, mannitol, milrinone (Primacor), morphine, phenylephrine (Neo-Synephrine), phenytoin (Dilantin), potassium chloride, propofol (Diprivan), vancomycin (Vancocin)

SIDE EFFECTS

Frequent

Abdominal distention, flatulence, belching

SERIOUS REACTIONS

• Excessive or chronic use may produce metabolic alkalosis (characterized by irritability, twitching, paraesthesias, cyanosis, slow or shallow respirations, headache, thirst, and nausea).

• Fluid overload results in headache, weakness, blurred vision, behavioral changes, incoordination, muscle twitching, elevated B/P, bradycardia, tachypnea, wheezing, coughing, and distended neck veins.

• Extravasation may occur at the IV site, resulting in tissue necrosis and ulceration.

PRECAUTIONS & CONSIDERATIONS

Caution is warranted with CHF, renal insufficiency, edema and concurrent corticosteroid therapy. Sodium bicarbonate use may produce hypernatremia and increased deep tendon reflexes in the neonate or fetus whose mother is administered chronically high doses. Sodium bicarbonate may be distributed in breast milk. No age-related precautions have been noted in children; however sodium bicarbonate should not be used as an antacid in children younger than 6 years. In the elderly, age-related

renal impairment may require cautious use. Check with the physician before taking any OTC drugs because they may contain sodium.

Serum calcium, phosphate and uric acid levels, blood and urinary pH, $PaCO_2$ and CO_2, plasma bicarbonate, and serum electrolyte levels should be monitored. Pattern of daily bowel activity and stool consistency and clinical improvement of metabolic acidosis, including relief from disorientation, hyperventilation, and weakness, should also be assessed.

Storage

Store vials at room temperature.

Administration

! Sodium bicarbonate may be given by IV push, IV infusion, or orally. Dosage is individualized based on age, weight, clinical conditions, and laboratory values and on the severity of acidosis. Metabolic alkalosis may result if the bicarbonate deficit is fully corrected during the first 24 hours.

Take oral sodium bicarbonate 1 to 3 hours after meals. Don't take other oral drugs within 2 hours of sodium bicarbonate administration.

! With acidosis, administer sodium bicarbonate when the plasma bicarbonate level is less than 15 mEq/L. Use a 0.5 mEq/ml concentration for direct IV administration to neonates and infants.

Sodium bicarbonate may be given undiluted. For IV push, give up to 1 mEq/kg over 1 to 3 minutes for cardiac arrest. Don't exceed an infusion rate of 50 mEq/hour. For children younger than 2 years, premature infants, and neonates, administer by slow infusion, up to 8 mEq/minute.

S

Sodium Chloride
(Muro 128, Nasal Mist, Nasal
Moist, Ocean, SalineX, SeaMist,
Slo-Salt)

CATEGORY AND SCHEDULE
Pregnancy Risk Category: C
OTC (Tablets, nasal solution,
ophthalmic solution, ophthalmic
ointment)

CLASSIFICATION
Electrolyte replacements,
vitamins/minerals

MECHANISM OF ACTION
Sodium is a major cation of
extracellular fluid that
controls water distribution,
fluid and electrolyte balance,
and osmotic pressure of body
fluids; it also maintains acid-base
balance.

PHARMACOKINETICS
Well absorbed from the GI tract.
Widely distributed. Primarily excreted
in urine.

AVAILABILITY
Tablets: 1 g
Injection (Concentrate): 23.4%
(4 mEq/ml).
Injection: 0.45%, 0.9%, 3%.
Irrigation: 0.45%, 0.9%.
Nasal Gel (Nasal Moist): 0.65%.
Nasal Solution (OTC [SalineX]):
0.4%.
*Nasal Solution (OTC [Nasal Moist,
SeaMist]):* 0.65%.
*Ophthalmic Solution (OTC [Muro
128]):* 5%.
*Ophthalmic Ointment (OTC [Muro
128]):* 5%.

INDICATIONS AND DOSAGES
▸ **Prevention and treatment of
sodium and chloride deficiencies;
source of hydration**
IV
Adults, Elderly. 1-2 L/day 0.9% or
0.45% or 100 ml 3% or 5% over
1 hr; assess serum electrolyte levels
before giving additional fluid.
▸ **Prevention of heat prostration and
muscle cramps from excessive
perspiration**
PO
Adults, Elderly. 1-2 g 3 times a day.
▸ **Relief of dry and inflamed nasal
membranes**
INTRANASAL
Adults, Elderly. Use as needed.
▸ **Diagnostic aid in ophthalmoscopic
exam, treatment of corneal edema**
OPHTHALMIC SOLUTION
Adults, Elderly. Apply 1-2 drops
q3-4hr.
OPHTHALMIC OINTMENT
Adults, Elderly. Apply once a day or
as directed.

CONTRAINDICATIONS
Fluid retention, hypernatremia

INTERACTIONS
Drug
**Hypertonic saline solution, oxyto-
cics:** May cause uterine hypertonus,
ruptures, or lacerations.
Herbal
None known.
Food
None known.

DIAGNOSTIC TEST EFFECTS
None known.

SIDE EFFECTS
Frequent
Facial flushing
Occasional
Fever; irritation, phlebitis, or extrava-
sation at injection site

Ophthalmic: Temporary burning or irritation

SERIOUS REACTIONS
• Too rapid administration may produce peripheral edema, CHF, and pulmonary edema.
• Excessive dosage may cause hypokalemia, hypervolemia, and hypernatremia.

PRECAUTIONS & CONSIDERATIONS
Caution is warranted with cirrhosis, CHF, hypertension, and renal impairment. Don't administer sodium and chloride preserved with benzyl alcohol to neonates. No age-related precautions have been noted in children or the elderly.

Notify the physician of acute redness of eyes, floating spots, severe eye pain or pain on exposure to light, a rapid change in vision (side and straight ahead), or headache after ophthalmic administration. Fluid balance, weight, acid-base balance, B/P, and serum electrolyte levels should be monitored. Be alert for signs and symptoms of hypernatremia (edema, hypertension, and weight gain) and hyponatremia (dry mucous membranes, muscle cramps, nausea, and vomiting).

Storage
Store vials at room temperature.

Administration
! Dosage is based on acid-base status, age, weight, clinical condition, and fluid and electrolyte status.

Do not crush or break enteric-coated or slow-release tablets. Take tablets with a full glass of water.

For IV use, administer hypertonic solutions (3% or 5%) through a large vein at a rate not exceeding 100 ml/hr. Avoid infiltration. Dilute vials containing 2.5 to 4 mEq/ml (concentrated NaCl) with D_5W or $D_{10}W$ before administration.

For nasal use, inhale slowly just before releasing the drug into nose. Then release air gently through the mouth. Continue this technique for 20 to 30 seconds.

For ophthalmic use, place a finger on the lower eyelid, and pull it out until a pocket is formed between the eye and lower lid. Hold the dropper above the pocket and instill the prescribed number of drops (or apply a thin strip of ointment) in the pocket. Close the eyes gently so that the drug isn't squeezed out of the sac. After administering the solution, apply gentle finger pressure to the lacrimal sac for 1 to 2 minutes to reduce systemic absorption. Release the lower lid, and keep solution in the affected eye open without blinking for at least 30 seconds; close the affected eye with ointment and roll the eyeball to distribute the drug.

Sodium Ferric Gluconate Complex
sew-dee'um fair'ick glue'koe-nate calm'plex
(Ferrlecit)

CATEGORY AND SCHEDULE
Pregnancy Risk Category: B

CLASSIFICATION
Hematinics, vitamins/minerals

MECHANISM OF ACTION
A trace element that repletes total iron content in body. Replaces iron found in Hgb, myoglobin, and specific enzymes; allows oxygen transport via Hgb. *Therapeutic Effect:* Prevents and corrects iron deficiency.

AVAILABILITY
Ampules: 12.5 mg/ml elemental iron.

INDICATIONS AND DOSAGES
▸ **Iron deficiency anemia**
IV INFUSION
Adults, Elderly. 125 mg in 100 ml
0.9% NaCl infused over 1 hr.
Minimum cumulative dose 1 g
elemental iron given over 8 sessions
at sequential dialysis treatments.
May be given during dialysis
session.

CONTRAINDICATIONS
All anemias not associated with iron
deficiency

INTERACTIONS
Drug
None known.
Herbal
None known.
Food
None known.

DIAGNOSTIC TEST EFFECTS
None known.

▨ IV INCOMPATIBILITIES
Do not mix with other medications.

SIDE EFFECTS
Frequent (greater than 3%)
Flushing, hypotension, hypersensitivity reaction
Occasional (3%-1%)
Injection site reaction, headache,
abdominal pain, chills, flu-like
syndrome, dizziness, leg cramps,
dyspnea, nausea, vomiting, diarrhea,
myalgia, pruritus, edema

SERIOUS REACTIONS
• A potentially fatal hypersensitivity
reaction occurs rarely, characterized
by cardiovascular collapse, cardiac
arrest, dyspnea, bronchospasm,
angioedema, and urticaria.

• Rapid administration may cause
hypotension associated with flushing,
lightheadedness, fatigue, weakness,
or severe pain in the chest, back, or
groin.

PRECAUTIONS & CONSIDERATIONS
Caution is warranted with asthma,
iron overload, hepatic impairment,
rheumatoid arthritis, and significant
allergies. It is unknown if sodium
ferric gluconate complex is distributed in breast milk. Safety and efficacy of sodium ferric gluconate
complex have not been established
in children. No age-related precautions have been noted in the elderly.
However, lower initial dosages of
sodium ferric gluconate complex are
recommended in the elderly.
  Stools may become black during
iron therapy, but this effect is harmless unless accompanied by abdominal cramping or pain and red
streaking and sticky consistency of
stool. Notify the physician of
abdominal cramping or pain or red
streaking or sticky consistency of
stool. Laboratory test results, especially CBC, serum iron concentrations, and vital signs, should be
monitored. Test results may not be
meaningful for 3 weeks after beginning sodium ferric gluconate complex
therapy. Patients with rheumatoid
arthritis or iron deficiency anemia
should be assessed for acute exacerbation of joint pain and swelling.
Storage
Store at room temperature.
Administration
! Plan to initially administer a
25-mg test dose that's diluted in
50 ml 0.9% NaCl and given over
60 minutes. May give undiluted as
slow IV injection without test dose.
  Use immediately after dilution.
Remember that the standard recommended dose is 125 mg (10 ml)

diluted with 100 ml 0.9% NaCl. Infuse both test dose and standard dose over 1 hour. Do not give concurrently with oral iron because excessive iron intake may produce excessive iron storage (hemosiderosis). The drug may be administered during dialysis treatments.

Sodium Oxybate
sew-dee′um ox′ee-bate
(Xyrem)

CATEGORY AND SCHEDULE
Pregnancy Risk Category: B
Controlled Substance:
Schedule III

CLASSIFICATION
Depressants, central nervous system

MECHANISM OF ACTION
A naturally occurring inhibitory neurotransmitter that binds to gamma aminobutyric acid (GABA)-B receptors and sodium oxybate specific receptors with its highest concentrations in the basal ganglia, which mediates sleep cycles, temperature regulation, cerebral glucose metabolism and blood flow, memory, and emotion control. *Therapeutic Effect:* Reduces the number of sleep episodes.

PHARMACOKINETICS
Rapidly and incompletely absorbed. Absorption is delayed and decreased by a high fat meal. Protein binding: less than 1%. Widely distributed, including cerebrospinal fluid (CSF). Metabolized in liver. Excretion is less than 5% in the urine and negligible in feces. Unknown if removed by hemodialysis. **Half-life:** 20-53 min.

AVAILABILITY
Oral solution: 500 mg/ml (Xyrem).

INDICATIONS AND DOSAGES
▸ Cataplexy of narcolepsy
PO
Adults, Elderly. 4.5 g/day in 2 equal doses of 2.25 g, the first taken at bedtime while in bed and the second 2.5-4 hr later. Maximum: 9 g/day in two weekly increments of 1.5 g/day.

OFF-LABEL USES
Alcohol withdrawal

CONTRAINDICATIONS
Metabolic/respiratory alkalosis, current treatment with sedative hypnotics, succinic semialdehyde dehydrogenase deficient, hypersensitivity to sodium oxybate or any component of the formulation

INTERACTIONS
Drug
Alcohol, barbiturates, benzodiazepines, centrally-acting muscle relaxants, opioid analgesics: May increase CNS and respiratory depressant effects.
Methamphetamine: May increase risk of unconsciousness and seizure-like tremor.
Herbal
None known.
Food
None known.

DIAGNOSTIC TEST EFFECTS
May increase sodium and glucose level.

SIDE EFFECTS
Frequent
Mild bradycardia
Occasional
Headache, vertigo, dizziness, restless legs, abdominal pain, muscle weakness

S

Rare
Dream-like state of confusion

SERIOUS REACTIONS
• Agitation, excitation, increased blood pressure (B/P), and insomnia may occur upon abrupt discontinuation of sodium oxybate.

PRECAUTIONS & CONSIDERATIONS
Caution is warranted with a history of depression, hypertension, pregnancy, concurrent ingestion of alcohol, other central nervous system depressants and liver impairment. It is unknown if sodium oxybate is excreted in breast milk. Use caution if giving sodium oxybate to pregnant women. Safety and efficacy of this drug have not been established in children. Age-related liver or renal impairment may require decreased dosage in the elderly. High fat meals should be avoided because it will delay absorption of the drug.

Dizziness and lightheadedness may occur. Avoid alcohol and tasks that require mental alertness or motor skills. Notify physician of signs of metabolic alkalosis or irritability, twitching, numbness/tingling of extremities, cyanosis, slow/shallow respiration, headache, thirst, nausea.

Storage
Store at room temperature.

Administration
Be aware that sodium oxybate is available only through restricted distribution. Take sodium oxybate without regard to meals. Mix this medicine with 2 ounces (¼ cup) of water before using. Mix both doses of medicine before going to bed, and store the second dose close to the bed. Take the second dose 2½ to 4 hours of taking the first dose. Set an alarm clock to wake up to take the second dose on time.

Sodium Polystyrene Sulfonate
pol-ee-stye′reen
(Kayexalate, Kionex, PMS-Sodium Polystyrene Sulfonate [CAN], SPS)

CATEGORY AND SCHEDULE
Pregnancy Risk Category: C

CLASSIFICATION
Resins

MECHANISM OF ACTION
An ion exchange resin that releases sodium ions in exchange primarily for potassium ions. *Therapeutic Effect:* Moves potassium from the blood into the intestine so it can be expelled from the body.

AVAILABILITY
Suspension (SPS): 15 g/60 ml.
Powder for Suspension (Kayexalate, Kionex): 454 g.

INDICATIONS AND DOSAGES
▸ **Hyperkalemia**
PO
Adults, Elderly. 60 ml (15 g) 1-4 times a day.
Children. 1 g/kg/dose q6hr.
RECTAL
Adults, Elderly. 30-50 g as needed q6hr.
Children. 1 g/kg/dose q2-6hr.

CONTRAINDICATIONS
Hypernatremia, intestinal obstruction or perforation

INTERACTIONS
Drug
Cation-donating antacids, laxatives (such as magnesium hydroxide): May decrease effect of

sodium polystyrene sulfonate, and cause systemic alkalosis in patients with renal impairment.
Herbal
None known.
Food
None known.

DIAGNOSTIC TEST EFFECTS
May decrease serum calcium and magnesium levels.

SIDE EFFECTS
Frequent
High dosage: Anorexia, nausea, vomiting, constipation
High dosage in elderly: Fecal impaction characterized by severe stomach pain with nausea or vomiting
Occasional
Diarrhea, sodium retention marked by decreased urination, peripheral edema, and increased weight

SERIOUS REACTIONS
• Potassium deficiency may occur. Early signs of hypokalemia include confusion, delayed thought processes, extreme weakness, irritability, and EKG changes (including prolonged QT interval; widening, flattening, or inversion of T wave; and prominent U waves).
• Hypocalcemia, manifested by abdominal or muscle cramps, occurs occasionally.
• Arrhythmias and severe muscle weakness may be noted.

PRECAUTIONS & CONSIDERATIONS
Caution is warranted with edema, hypertension, and severe CHF. It is unknown if sodium polystyrene sulfonate crosses the placenta or is distributed in breast milk. No age-related precautions have been noted in children. The elderly may be at increased risk for fecal impaction.

Foods rich in potassium should be consumed.

Because sodium polystyrene sulfonate does not rapidly correct severe hyperkalemia (it may take hours to days), consider other measures, such as dialysis, IV glucose and insulin, IV calcium, and IV sodium bicarbonate to correct severe hyperkalemia in a medical emergency. Serum potassium levels, calcium and magnesium, and pattern of daily bowel activity and stool consistency should be assessed. Clinical condition and EKG is valuable when determining when treatment should be discontinued.
Administration
Give oral sodium polystyrene sulfonate with 20 to 100 ml sorbitol to aid in potassium removal, facilitate passage of resin through intestinal tract, and prevent constipation. Do not mix this drug with foods or liquids containing potassium. Drink the entire amount of the resin for best results.
  For rectal use, after initial cleansing enema, insert large rubber tube well into sigmoid colon and tape in place. Introduce suspension with 100 ml sorbitol by gravity. Flush with 50 to 100 ml fluid and clamp. Retain for several hours, if possible. Irrigate colon with a non–sodium-containing solution to remove resin.

S

Solifenacin
sohl-e-fen'ah-sin
(VESIcare)

CATEGORY AND SCHEDULE
Pregnancy Risk Category: C

CLASSIFICATION
Anticholinergics, relaxants, urinary tract

MECHANISM OF ACTION
A urinary antispasmodic that acts as a direct antagonist at muscarinic acetylcholine receptors in cholinergically innervated organs. Reduces tonus (elastic tension) of smooth muscle in the bladder and slows parasympathetic contractions. *Therapeutic Effect:* Decreases urinary bladder contractions, increases residual urine volume, and decreases detrusor muscle pressure.

AVAILABILITY
Tablets: 5 mg, 10 mg.

INDICATIONS AND DOSAGES
▸ **Overactive bladder**
PO
Adults, Elderly. 5 mg/day; if tolerated, may increase to 10 mg/day.
▸ **Dosage in renal or hepatic impairment**
For patients with severe renal impairment or moderate hepatic impairment, maximum dosage is 5 mg/day.

CONTRAINDICATIONS
Breast-feeding, GI obstruction, uncontrolled angle-closure glaucoma, urine retention

INTERACTIONS
Drug
Aminoglutethimide, carbamazepine, nafcillin, nevirapine, phenobarbital, phenytoin: May decrease the effects and serum level of solifenacin.
Azole antifungals, ciprofloxacin, clarithromycin, diclofenac, doxycycline, erythromycin, imatinib, isoniazid, nefazodone, nicardipine, propofol, protease inhibitors, quinidine, verapamil: May increase the effects and serum level of solifenacin.
Ketoconazole: May increase the serum level of solifenacin
Herbal
St John's wort: May decrease the effects and serum level of solifenacin.
Food
Grapefruit, grapefruit juice: May increase the effects and serum level of solifenacin.

DIAGNOSTIC TEST EFFECTS
None known.

SIDE EFFECTS
Frequent (11%-5%)
Dry mouth, constipation, blurred vision
Occasional (5%-3%)
UTI, dyspepsia, nausea
Rare (2%-1%)
Dizziness, dry eyes, fatigue, depression, edema, hypertension, upper abdominal pain, vomiting, urine retention

SERIOUS REACTIONS
• Angioneurotic edema and GI obstruction occur rarely.
• Overdose can result in severe central anticholinergic effects.

PRECAUTIONS & CONSIDERATIONS
Caution is warranted with bladder outflow obstruction, congenital or acquired prolonged QT interval,

controlled angle-closure glaucoma, decreased GI motility, GI obstructive disorders, hepatic or renal impairment, and in pregnant women.
Administration
Take solifenacin without regard to food; swallow tablets whole.

Somatrem
soe′-ma-trem
(Protropin)
Do not confuse with Proloprim, Protamine, Protopam, or somatropin.

CATEGORY AND SCHEDULE
Pregnancy Risk Category: C

CLASSIFICATION
Hormones/hormone modifiers, recombinant DNA Origin

MECHANISM OF ACTION
A polypeptide hormone that increases the number, size of muscle cells; increases red blood cell (RBC) mass. Affects carbohydrate metabolism by antagonizing action of insulin, increasing the mobilization of fats, and increasing cellular protein synthesis. *Therapeutic Effect:* Stimulates linear growth.

AVAILABILITY
Powder for Injection: 5 mg, 10 mg.

INDICATIONS AND DOSAGES
▶ **Long-term treatment of children who have growth failure due to endogenous growth hormone deficiency**
IM/SUBCUTANEOUS
Children. Up to 0.1 mg/kg (0.26 IU/kg) 3 times/wk.

CONTRAINDICATIONS
None known.

INTERACTIONS
Drug
Corticosteroids: May inhibit growth response.
Herbal
None known.
Food
None known.

DIAGNOSTIC TEST EFFECTS
May increase serum parathyroid hormone levels, serum alkaline phosphatase, and inorganic phosphorus levels.

SIDE EFFECTS
Frequent (30%)
Persistent antibodies to growth hormone, but generally does not cause failure to respond to somatrem
Occasional
Headache, muscle pain, weakness, mild hyperglycemia, allergic reaction, including rash and itching, pain and swelling at injection site, pain in hip or knee

PRECAUTIONS & CONSIDERATIONS
Caution is warranted with diabetes mellitus, malignancy, and untreated hypothyroidism.
Blood glucose levels, bone age, growth rate, parathyroid, phosphorus, renal function, serum calcium, and thyroid function studies should be monitored.
Administration
May be administered as IM or subcutaneous injection.

Sorbitol
sor'bi-tole

CATEGORY AND SCHEDULE
Pregnancy risk category: C

CLASSIFICATION
Irrigants, genitourinary

MECHANISM OF ACTION
A polyalcoholic sugar with osmotic cathartic actions. Specific mechanism unknown. *Therapeutic effect:* Catharsis, urinary irrigation.

PHARMACOKINETICS
Onset of action within 15-60 minutes. Poorly absorbed by both oral and rectal route. Metabolized in liver to primary metabolite, fructose.

AVAILABILITY
Solution: 3%

INDICATIONS AND DOSAGES
▶ **Hyperosmotic laxative**
PO
Adults, Elderly, Children 12 yr and older: 30-150 mL as a 70% solution
Children 2-11 yr: 2 ml/kg as a 70% solution
RECTAL
Adults, Elderly, Children 12 yr and older: 120 ml as a 25%-30% solution
Children 2-11 yr: 30-60 ml as a 25%-30% solution
▶ **Transurethral surgical procedure**
TOPICAL
Adults, Elderly: 3%-3.3% as transurethral surgical procedure irrigation

CONTRAINDICATIONS
Anuria

INTERACTIONS
Drug
None known.
Herbal
None known.
Food
None known.

DIAGNOSTIC TEST EFFECTS
None known.

SIDE EFFECTS
Acidosis, electrolyte loss, marked diuresis, urinary retention, edema, dryness of mouth and thirst, dehydration, pulmonary congestion, hypotension, tachycardia, angina-like pains, blurred vision, convulsions, nausea, vomiting, diarrhea, rhinitis, chills, vertigo, backache, urticaria.

SERIOUS REACTIONS
• Life-threatening adverse reactions with IV sorbitol infusions have been reported in patients with fructose intolerance.

PRECAUTIONS & CONSIDERATIONS
Caution is warranted with cardiopulmonary dysfunction, diabetes mellitus, fructose intolerance, hyponatremia, and renal dysfunction. Be aware that it is unknown if sorbitol crosses the placenta or is distributed in breast milk. There are no age-related precautions noted in children or the elderly.
Storage
Store at room temperature. Protect from freezing and heat.
Administration
Do not use unless solution is clear.
Do not use oral formulation for more than one week and do not take with additional laxatives or stool softeners. Prolonged use can result in dependence.

Sotalol

soe'ta-lole

(Apo-Sotalol [CAN], Betapace, Betapace AF, Cardol [AUS], Novo-Sotalol [CAN], PMS-Sotalol [CAN], Solavert [AUS], Sorine, Sotab [AUS], Sotacor [AUS], Sotahexal [AUS])

Do not confuse sotalol with Stadol.

CATEGORY AND SCHEDULE

Pregnancy Risk Category: B (D if used in second or third trimester)

CLASSIFICATION

Antiadrenergics, beta blocking, antiarrhythmics, class III

MECHANISM OF ACTION

A beta-adrenergic blocking agent that prolongs action potential, effective refractory period, and QT interval. Decreases heart rate and AV node conduction; increases AV node refractoriness. *Therapeutic Effect:* Produces antiarrhythmic activity.

PHARMACOKINETICS

Well absorbed from the GI tract. Protein binding: None. Widely distributed. Primarily excreted unchanged in urine. Removed by hemodialysis. **Half-life:** 12 hr (increased in the elderly and patients with impaired renal function).

AVAILABILITY

Tablets (Betapace): 80 mg, 120 mg, 160 mg, 240 mg.
Tablets (Betapace AF): 80 mg, 120 mg, 160 mg.
Tablets (Sorine): 80 mg, 120 mg, 160 mg, 240 mg.

INDICATIONS AND DOSAGES

▶ **Documented, life-threatening arrhythmias**
PO
Adults, Elderly. Initially, 80 mg twice a day. May increase gradually at 2- to 3-day intervals. Range: 240-320 mg/day.
▶ **Dosage in renal impairment**
Dosage interval is modified based on creatinine clearance.

Creatinine Clearance	Dosage Interval
30-60 ml/min	24 hr
10-30 ml/min	36-48 hr
Less than 10 ml/min	Individualized

OFF-LABEL USES

Maintenance of normal heart rhythm in chronic or recurring atrial fibrillation or flutter; treatment of anxiety, chronic angina pectoris, hypertension, hypertrophic cardiomyopathy, MI, mitral valve prolapse syndrome, pheochromocytoma, thyrotoxicosis, tremors

CONTRAINDICATIONS

Bronchial asthma, cardiogenic shock, prolonged QT syndrome (unless functioning pacemaker is present), second- and third-degree heart block, sinus bradycardia, uncontrolled cardiac failure

INTERACTIONS

Drug
Antiarrhythmics, phenothiazine, tricyclic antidepressants: May prolong QT interval.
Calcium channel blockers: May increase effect on AV conduction and B/P.
Clonidine: May potentiate rebound hypertension after clonidine is discontinued.

S

Digoxin: May increase risk of proarrhythmias.
Insulin, oral hypoglycemics: May mask signs of hypoglycemia and prolong the effects of insulin and oral hypoglycemics.
Sympathomimetics: May inhibit the effects of sympathomimetics.
Herbal
None known.
Food
None known.

DIAGNOSTIC TEST EFFECTS
May increase blood glucose, serum alkaline phosphatase, serum LDH, serum lipoprotein, AST (SGOT), ALT (SGPT), and serum triglyceride levels.

SIDE EFFECTS
Frequent
Diminished sexual function, drowsiness, insomnia, unusual fatigue or weakness
Occasional
Depression, cold hands or feet, diarrhea, constipation, anxiety, nasal congestion, nausea, vomiting
Rare
Altered taste, dry eyes, itching, numbness of fingers, toes, or scalp

SERIOUS REACTIONS
• Bradycardia, CHF, hypotension, bronchospasm, hypoglycemia, prolonged QT interval, torsades de pointes, ventricular tachycardia, and premature ventricular complexes may occur.

PRECAUTIONS & CONSIDERATIONS
Caution is warranted with cardiomegaly, CHF, diabetes mellitus, excessive QT-interval prolongation, history of ventricular tachycardia, hypokalemia, hypomagnesemia, severe and prolonged diarrhea, sick sinus syndrome, ventricular

fibrillation, and those at risk for developing thyrotoxicosis. Sotalol crosses the placenta and is excreted in breast milk. The safety and efficacy of sotalol have not been established in children. In the elderly, age-related peripheral vascular disease may increase susceptibility to decreased peripheral circulation. Tasks that require mental alertness or motor skills should be avoided.

B/P for hypotension and pulse for bradycardia should be monitored during treatment. If pulse rate is 60 beats/minute or lower or systolic B/P is less than 90 mm Hg, withhold the medication and contact the physician. Continuous cardiac monitoring should be performed when beginning sotalol therapy. If the pulse rate is 60 beats/minute or less, consult the physician before beginning sotalol therapy. Arrhythmias should also be assessed. Signs and symptoms of CHF, such as decreased urine output, distended neck veins, dyspnea (particularly on exertion or lying down), night cough, peripheral edema, and weight gain should also be assessed.
Administration
! Some people may require 480-640 mg/day. Sotalol has a long half-life and administering the drug more than 2 times a day is usually not necessary. Avoid abrupt withdrawal.

Take sotalol without regard to food. Do not abruptly discontinue the drug.

Sparfloxacin
spar-floks′a-sin
(Zagam)

CATEGORY AND SCHEDULE
Pregnancy Risk Category: C

CLASSIFICATION
Antibiotics, quinolones

MECHANISM OF ACTION
A fluoroquinolone that interferes with DNA-gyrase in susceptible microorganisms. *Therapeutic Effect:* Inhibits DNA replication and repair. Bactericidal.

PHARMACOKINETICS
Well absorbed from the gastrointestinal (GI) tract after PO administration. Widely distributed. Metabolized in liver. Primarily excreted in urine with a lesser amount eliminated in the feces. **Half-life:** 16-30 hr.

AVAILABILITY
Tablets: 200 mg (Zagam).

INDICATIONS AND DOSAGES
▸ **Bronchitis, pneumonia**
PO
Adults 18 yr and older, Elderly.
Initially, two 200-mg tablets as a loading dose on first day. Then one 200-mg tablet q24hr for a total of 10 days.
▸ **Dosage in renal impairment (creatinine clearance < 50 ml/min)**
PO
Adults 18 yr and older, Elderly.
Initially, two 200-mg tablets as a loading dose on first day. Then one 200-mg tablet q48hr for a total of 9 days.

CONTRAINDICATIONS
Hypersensitivity to fluoroquinolones, cinoxacin, nalidixic acid

INTERACTIONS
Drug
Antacids, sucralfate, iron preparations: May decrease sparfloxacin plasma concentration and half-life.
Phenothiazines, tricyclic antidepressants, erythromycin: Concurrent use of these drugs may increase the risk of QTc prolongation and life-threatening arrhythmias.
Cyclosporine: Increases the risk of nephrotoxicity.
Herbal
None known.
Food
None known.

DIAGNOSTIC TEST EFFECTS
May increase SGOT (AST), SGOT (ALT), alkaline phosphatase, WBC count.

SIDE EFFECTS
Occasional
Photosensitivity, diarrhea, nausea, headache
Rare
Dyspepsia, dizziness, insomnia, abdominal pain, change in taste

SERIOUS REACTIONS
• Superinfection (particularly enterococcal or fungal overgrowth of nonsusceptible organisms) due to altered bacterial balance may occur (genital-anal pruritus, ulceration or changes in oral mucosa, moderate to severe diarrhea, new or increased fever).
• Hypersensitivity reactions have occurred in those receiving fluoroquinolone therapy.

S

PRECAUTIONS & CONSIDERATIONS

Caution is warranted with liver or renal impairment, prolonged QT interval, and concurrent use of medications known to prolong the QT interval (e.g., erythromycin, tricyclic antidepressants). Determine history of hypersensitivity to sparfloxacin and quinolones before beginning drug therapy. It is unknown if sparfloxacin crosses the placenta or is distributed in breast milk. The safety and efficacy of sparfloxacin have not been established in children. Age-related renal impairment may require dosage adjustment in the elderly.

Be alert for superinfection such as genital/anal pruritus, ulceration or changes in oral mucosa, moderate to severe diarrhea, and new or increased fever. Avoid excessive sunlight/ artificial ultraviolet light (reaction may occur up to several weeks after stopping therapy). Sugarless gum or hard candy may relieve bad taste. Do not take antacids (aluminum, magnesium), sucralfate, iron, and multivitamin preparations with zinc within 2 hours of trovafloxacin administration as these drugs significantly reduce trovafloxacin absorption.

Storage

Store at room temperature.

Administration

Take without regard to meals. Do not crush or break film-coated tablets. Continue medication for full length of treatment.

Spectinomycin
spek-ti-noe-mye′sin
(Trobicin)
Do not confuse with strepto-mycin or tobramycin.

CATEGORY AND SCHEDULE
Pregnancy Risk Category: B

CLASSIFICATION
Antibiotics, miscellaneous

MECHANISM OF ACTION
An anti-infective that inhibits protein synthesis of bacterial cells. *Therapeutic Effect:* Produces bacterial cell death.

PHARMACOKINETICS
Rapid, complete absorption after intramuscular (IM) administration. Protein binding: Unknown. Widely distributed. Excreted unchanged in urine. Partially removed by hemodialysis. **Half-life:** 1.7 hr.

AVAILABILITY
Powder for Reconstitution: 2 g (Trobicin).

INDICATIONS AND DOSAGES
▶ **Treatment of acute gonococcal urethritis, proctitis in males, acute gonococcal cervicitis and proctitis in females**
IM
Adults, Elderly. 2 g once. In areas where antibiotic resistance is known to be prevalent, 4 g (10 ml) divided between 2 injection sites is preferred.

OFF-LABEL USES
Treatment of disseminated gonorrhea

CONTRAINDICATIONS
Hypersensitivity to spectinomycin or any component of the formulation

INTERACTIONS
Drug
None known.
Herbal
None known.
Food
None known.

DIAGNOSTIC TEST EFFECTS
None known.

SIDE EFFECTS
Frequent
Pain at IM injection site
Occasional
Dizziness, insomnia
Rare
Decreased urine output

SERIOUS REACTIONS
• Hypersensitivity reaction characterized as chills, fever, nausea, vomiting, urticaria, and anaphylaxis.

PRECAUTIONS & CONSIDERATIONS
Caution should be used with history of allergies. Be aware that it is unknown if spectinomycin crosses the placenta and/or is distributed in breast milk. Safety and efficacy have not been established in children. There are no age-related precautions noted in the elderly.
Storage
Store at room temperature. After reconstitution, use within 24 hours.
Administration
Shake vial vigorously immediately after adding diluent and before withdrawing dose. Inject deep IM into upper outer quandrant of gluteal muscle.

Spironolactone
speer-on-oh-lak'tone
(Aldactone, Novospiroton [CAN], Spiractin [AUS])
Do not confuse with Aldactazide.

CATEGORY AND SCHEDULE
Pregnancy Risk Category: C
(D if used in pregnancy-induced hypertension)

CLASSIFICATION
Diuretics, potassium sparing

MECHANISM OF ACTION
A potassium-sparing diuretic that interferes with sodium reabsorption by competitively inhibiting the action of aldosterone in the distal tubule, thus promoting sodium and water excretion and increasing potassium retention. *Therapeutic Effect:* Produces diuresis; lowers B/P; diagnostic aid for primary aldosteronism.

PHARMACOKINETICS

Route	Onset	Peak	Duration
PO	24-48 hr	48-72 hr	48-72 hr

Well absorbed from the GI tract (absorption increased with food). Protein binding: 91%-98%. Metabolized in the liver to active metabolite. Primarily excreted in urine. Unknown if removed by hemodialysis.
Half-life: 0-24 hr (metabolite, 13-24 hr).

AVAILABILITY
Tablets: 25 mg, 50 mg, 100 mg.

INDICATIONS AND DOSAGES
▸ **Edema**
PO
Adults, Elderly. 25-200 mg/day as a single dose or in 2 divided doses.
Children. 1.5-3.3 mg/kg/day in divided doses.
Neonates. 1-3 mg/kg/day in 1-2 divided doses.
▸ **Hypertension**
PO
Adults, Elderly. 25-50 mg/day in 1-2 doses/day.
Children. 1.5-3.3 mg/kg/day in divided doses.
▸ **Hypokalemia**
PO
Adults, Elderly. 25-200 mg/day as a single dose or in 2 divided doses.
▸ **Hirsutism**
PO
Adults, Elderly. 50-200 mg/day as a single dose or in 2 divided doses.
▸ **Primary aldosteronism**
PO
Adults, Elderly. 100-400 mg/day as a single dose or in 2 divided doses.
Children. 100-400 mg/m^2/day as a single dose or in 2 divided doses.
▸ **Dosage in renal impairment**
Dosage interval is modified based on creatinine clearance.

Creatinine Clearance	Interval
10-50 ml/min	Usual dose q12-24hr
Less than 10 ml/min	Avoid use

OFF-LABEL USES
Treatment of female hirsutism, polycystic ovary disease

CONTRAINDICATIONS
Acute renal insufficiency, anuria, BUN and serum creatinine levels more than twice normal values, hyperkalemia

INTERACTIONS
Drug
ACE inhibitors (such as captopril), potassium-containing medications, potassium supplements: May increase the risk of hyperkalemia.
Anticoagulants, heparin: May decrease the effects of these drugs.
Digoxin: May increase the half-life of digoxin.
Lithium: May decrease the clearance and increase the risk of toxicity of lithium.
NSAIDs: May decrease the antihypertensive effect of spironolactone.
Herbal
None known.
Food
None known.

DIAGNOSTIC TEST EFFECTS
May increase urinary calcium excretion; BUN and blood glucose levels; serum creatinine, magnesium, potassium, and uric acid levels. May decrease serum sodium level.

SIDE EFFECTS
Frequent
Hyperkalemia (in patients with renal insufficiency and those taking potassium supplements), dehydration, hyponatremia, lethargy
Occasional
Nausea, vomiting, anorexia, abdominal cramps, diarrhea, headache, ataxia, somnolence, confusion, fever
Male: Gynecomastia, impotence, decreased libido
Female: Menstrual irregularities (including amenorrhea and postmenopausal bleeding), breast tenderness
Rare
Rash, urticaria, hirsutism

SERIOUS REACTIONS
• Severe hyperkalemia may produce arrhythmias, bradycardia, and EKG

changes (tented T waves, widening QRS complex and ST segment depression). These may proceed to cardiac standstill or ventricular fibrillation.

• Cirrhosis patients are at risk for hepatic decompensation if dehydration or hyponatremia occurs.

• Patients with primary aldosteronism may experience rapid weight loss and severe fatigue during high-dose therapy.

PRECAUTIONS & CONSIDERATIONS

Caution is warranted with hyponatremia, hepatic or renal impairment, dehydration, and concurrent use of potassium supplements. An active metabolite of spironolactone is excreted in breast milk. Breast-feeding is not recommended for patients taking this drug. No age-related precautions have been noted in children. The elderly may be more susceptible to hyperkalemia. In addition, age-related renal impairment may require cautious use in this age-group. Avoid foods high in potassium such as apricots, bananas, legumes, meat, orange juice, raisins, whole grains, including cereals, and white and sweet potatoes. Also, avoid performing tasks that require mental alertness or motor skills until response to the drug has been established.

An increase in the frequency and volume of urination may occur. Notify the physician of an irregular heartbeat, diarrhea, muscle twitching, cold and clammy skin, confusion, drowsiness, dry mouth, or excessive thirst. Blood pressure (B/P), vital signs, electrolytes, and intake and output should be monitored before and during treatment. Be especially alert for evidence of hyperkalemia, such as arrhythmias, colic, diarrhea, and muscle twitching, followed by paralysis and weakness. Also be aware signs of hyponatremia may result in cold and clammy skin, confusion, and thirst.

Storage

Oral suspension containing crushed tablets in cherry syrup is stable for up to 30 days if refrigerated.

Administration

Take spironolactone with food to enhance its absorption. Crush scored tablets as needed. The drug's therapeutic effect takes several days to begin and can last for several days once the drug is discontinued (unless taking a potassium-losing drug concomitantly).

Stanozolol
stan-oh'zoe-lole
(Winstrol)

CATEGORY AND SCHEDULE
Pregnancy Risk Category: X

CLASSIFICATION
Anabolic steroids, hormones/hormone modifiers

MECHANISM OF ACTION

A synthetic testosterone derivative that increases circulating levels of C1 INH and C4 through an increase in general protein anabolism, and more specifically, through an increase in the synthesis of messenger RNA. *Therapeutic Effect:* Decreases swelling of the face, extremities, genitalia, bowel wall, and upper respiratory tract

PHARMACOKINETICS

Metabolized in liver. Primarily excreted in urine. Unknown if removed by hemodialysis.

S

AVAILABILITY
Tablets: 2 mg (Winstrol).

INDICATIONS AND DOSAGES
▶ **Hereditary angioedema prophylaxis**
PO
Adults. Initially, 2 mg 2 times/day. Decrease at 1-3 month intervals. Maintenance: 2 mg/day.

OFF-LABEL USES
Antithrombin III deficiency, arterial occlusions, hemophilia A, lichen sclerosus et atrophicus, liposclerosis, necrobiosis lipoidica, osteoporosis, protein C deficiency, rheumatoid arthritis, thrombosis, urticaria

CONTRAINDICATIONS
Cardiac impairment, hypercalcemia, pregnancy, prostatic or breast cancer in males, severe liver or renal disease, hypersensitivity to stanozolol or its components

INTERACTIONS
Drug
ACTH: May increase the risk of edema and acne.
Bupropion: May lower seizure threshold. Insulin, oral hypoglycemics: May increase hypoglycemic effects of insulin and oral hypoglycemics.
Oral anticoagulants: May increase the effects of oral anticoagulants.
Herbal
Chaparral: May increase liver enzymes.
Comfrey: May increase liver enzymes.
Eucalyptus: May increase risk of hepatoxicity.
Germander: May increase liver enzymes.
Jin bu huan: May increase liver enzymes.
Kava kava: May increase liver enzymes.

Pennyroyal: May increase liver enzymes.
Skullcap: May increase the risk of liver damage.
Valerian: May increase risk of hepatotoxicity.
Food
None known.

DIAGNOSTIC TEST EFFECTS
May increase blood Hgb and Hct, LDL concentrations, serum alkaline phosphatase, bilirubin, calcium, potassium, SGOT (AST) levels, and sodium levels. May decrease HDL concentrations.

SIDE EFFECTS
Frequent
Gynecomastia, acne
Females: Amenorrhea or other menstrual irregularities, hirsutism deepening of voice, clitoral enlargement that may not be reversible when drug is discontinued
Occasional
Edema, nausea, insomnia, oligospermia, male pattern of baldness, bladder irritability, hypercalcemia in immobilized patients or those with breast cancer, hypercholesterolemia

SERIOUS REACTIONS
• Peliosis hepatitis or liver, spleen replaced with blood-filled cysts, hepatic neoplasms and hepatocellular carcinoma have been associated with prolonged high-dosage.

PRECAUTIONS & CONSIDERATIONS
Caution is warranted with diabetes, epilepsy, and liver or renal impairment. Stanozolol use is contraindicated during lactation. Stanozolol is not recommended for children. Its use in the elderly may increase the risk of hyperplasia or stimulate growth of occult prostate carcinoma.

Acne, nausea, pedal edema, or vomiting may occur. Women should report deepening of voice, hoarseness, and menstrual irregularities. Men should report difficulty urinating, frequent erections, and gynecomastia. Weight should be obtained each day. Weekly weight gains of more than 5 pounds should be reported.

Administration
Take with or without regard to food. Decrease dose to 2 mg/day after 1-3 months. Some people may be maintained on 2 mg every other day.

Stavudine (d4T)
stav'yoo-deen
(Zerit)

CATEGORY AND SCHEDULE
Pregnancy Risk Category: C

CLASSIFICATION
Antivirals, nucleoside reverse transcriptase inhibitors

MECHANISM OF ACTION
Inhibits HIV reverse transcriptase by terminating the viral DNA chain. Also inhibits RNA- and DNA-dependent DNA polymerase, an enzyme necessary for HIV replication. *Therapeutic Effect:* Impedes HIV replication, slowing the progression of HIV infection.

PHARMACOKINETICS
Rapidly, and completely absorbed after PO administration. Undergoes minimal metabolism. Excreted in urine. **Half-life:** 1.5 hr (increased in renal impairment).

AVAILABILITY
Capsules: 15 mg, 20 mg, 30 mg, 40 mg.

Oral Solution: 1 mg/ml.

INDICATIONS AND DOSAGES
▸ **HIV infection (in combination with other antiretrovirals)**
PO
Adults weighing 60 kg or more.
40 mg twice a day.
Adults weighing less than 60 kg.
30 mg twice a day.
Children weighing 30 kg or more.
20 mg twice a day.
Children weighing less than 30 kg.
2 mg/kg/day.
▸ **HIV infection in patients with a recent history and complete resolution of peripheral neuropathy or elevated liver function test results**
Adults weighing 60 kg or more.
20 mg twice a day.
Adults weighing less than 60 kg.
15 mg twice a day.
▸ **Dosage in renal impairment**
Dosage and frequency are modified based on creatinine clearance and patient weight.

Creatinine Clearance	Weight 60 kg or More	Weight Less than 60 kg
Greater than 50 ml/min	40 mg q12hr	30 mg q12hr
26-50 ml/min	20 mg q12hr	15 mg q12hr
10-25 ml/min	20 mg q24hr	15 mg q24hr

CONTRAINDICATIONS
None known.

INTERACTIONS
Drug
Didanosine, ethambutol, isoniazid, lithium, phenytoin, zalcitabine: May increase the risk of peripheral neuropathy development.
Didanosine, hydroxyurea: May increase the risk of hepatotoxicity.
Zidovudine: May have antagonistic antiviral effect.

Herbal
None known.
Food
None known.

DIAGNOSTIC TEST EFFECTS

Commonly increases AST (SGOT) and ALT (SGPT) levels. May decrease neutrophil count.

SIDE EFFECTS

Frequent
Headache (55%), diarrhea (50%), chills and fever (38%), nausea and vomiting, myalgia (35%), rash (33%), asthenia (28%), insomnia, abdominal pain (26%), anxiety (22%), arthralgia (18%), back pain (20%), diaphoresis (19%), malaise (17%), depression (14%)
Occasional
Anorexia, weight loss, nervousness, dizziness, conjunctivitis, dyspepsia, dyspnea
Rare
Constipation, vasodilation, confusion, migraine, urticaria, abnormal vision

SERIOUS REACTIONS

• Peripheral neuropathy, (numbness, tingling, or pain in the hands and feet) occurs in 15% to 21% of patients.
• Ulcerative stomatitis (erythema or ulcers of oral mucosa, glossitis, gingivitis), pneumonia, and benign skin neoplasms occur occasionally.
• Pancreatitis and lactic acidosis occur rarely.

PRECAUTIONS & CONSIDERATIONS

Caution is warranted with a history of peripheral neuropathy or liver or renal impairment. Breast-feeding is not recommended in this population because of the possibility of HIV transmission. There are no age-related precautions noted in children. There is no information on the effects of this drug's use in the elderly. Avoid taking any medications, including over-the-counter (OTC) drugs, without first notifying the physician. Stavudine is not a cure for HIV infection, nor does it reduce risk of transmission to others, and illnesses, including opportunistic infections may develop.

Check baseline laboratory test results, if ordered, especially liver function test results, before beginning stavudine therapy and at periodic intervals during therapy. Monitor for signs and symptoms of peripheral neuropathy, which is characterized by numbness, pain, or tingling in the feet or hands. Be aware that peripheral neuropathy symptoms resolve promptly if stavudine therapy is discontinued. Also, know that symptoms may worsen temporarily after the drug is withdrawn. If symptoms resolve completely, expect to resume drug therapy at a reduced dosage. Assess for dizziness, headache, muscle or joint aches, myalgia, weight loss, conjunctivitis, nausea, and vomiting. Monitor for evidence of a rash and signs of chills or a fever. Determine sleep pattern and pattern of daily bowel activity and stool consistency.
Administration
Take without regard to meals. Continue stavudine therapy for the full length of treatment and evenly space doses around the clock.

Streptokinase

strep-toe-kye'nase
(Streptase)

CATEGORY AND SCHEDULE

Pregnancy Risk Category: C

CLASSIFICATION

Thrombolytics

MECHANISM OF ACTION

An enzyme that activates the fibrinolytic system by converting plasminogen to plasmin, an enzyme that degrades fibrin clots. Acts indirectly by forming a complex with plasminogen, which converts plasminogen to plasmin. Action occurs within the thrombus, on its surface, and in circulating blood. *Therapeutic Effect:* Destroys thrombi.

PHARMACOKINETICS

Rapidly cleared from plasma by antibodies and the reticuloendothelial system. Route of elimination unknown. Duration of action continues for several hours after drug has been discontinued.
Half-life: 23 min.

AVAILABILITY

Powder for Injection: 250,000 units, 750,000 units, 1.5 million units.

INDICATIONS AND DOSAGES

▸ **Acute evolving transmural MI (given as soon as possible after symptoms occur)**
IV INFUSION
Adults, Elderly (1.5 million units diluted to 45 ml). 1.5 million units infused over 60 min.
INTRACORONARY INFUSION
Adults, Elderly (250,000 units diluted to 125 ml). Initially, 20,000-units

(10-ml) bolus; then, 2000 units/min for 60 min. Total dose: 140,000 units.
▸ **Pulmonary embolism, deep vein thrombosis (DVT), arterial thrombosis and embolism (given within 7 days of onset)**
IV INFUSION
Adults, Elderly (1.5 million units diluted to 90 ml). Initially, 250,000 units infused over 30 min; then, 100,000 units/hr for 24-72 hr for arterial thrombosis or embolism, and pulmonary embolism, 72 hr for DVT.
INTRA-ATERIAL INFUSION
Adults, Elderly (1.5 million units diluted to 45 ml). Initially, 250,000 units infused over 30 min; then 100,000 units/hr for maintenance.

CONTRAINDICATIONS

Carcinoma of the brain, cerebrovascular accident, internal bleeding, intracranial surgery, recent streptococcal infection, severe hypertension

INTERACTIONS

Drug
Anticoagulants, heparin: May increase the risk of hemorrhage.
Platelet aggregation inhibitors such as aspirin: May increase the risk of bleeding.
Herbal
None known.
Food
None known.

DIAGNOSTIC TEST EFFECTS

Decreases serum plasminogen and fibrinogen level during infusion, decreasing clotting time and confirming presence of lysis

▧ IV INCOMPATIBILITIES

Do not mix with other medications.
▧ **IV Compatibilities**
Dobutamine (Dobutrex), dopamine (Intropin), heparin, lidocaine, nitroglycerin

S

SIDE EFFECTS

Frequent

Fever, superficial bleeding at puncture sites, decreased B/P

Occasional

Allergic reaction, including rash and wheezing; ecchymosis

SERIOUS REACTIONS

- Severe internal hemorrhage may occur.
- Lysis of coronary thrombi may produce life-threatening arrhythmias.

PRECAUTIONS & CONSIDERATIONS

Caution is warranted with GI bleeding or recent trauma and in those who have had major surgery within past 10 days. Streptokinase should be used during pregnancy only when the benefit to the mother outweighs the risk to the fetus. It is unknown if streptokinase crosses the placenta or is distributed in breast milk. Safety and efficacy of streptokinase have not been established in children. The elderly may have an increased risk of intracranial hemorrhage. Streptokinase should be used cautiously in this population. Females may experience an increase in menstrual flow. An electric razor and a soft toothbrush should be used to reduce the risk of bleeding.

Notify the physician of bruises, back or abdominal pain, black or red stool, coffee-ground vomitus, dark or red urine, red-speckled mucus from cough, chest pain, headache, palpitations, or shortness of breath. Stool should be monitored for occult blood. B/P and pulse and respiration rates should be checked every 15 minutes until stable; then check hourly. Hct and Hgb, platelet count, aPTT, PT, and fibrinogen level should be evaluated before and during therapy.

Storage

Store unopened vials at room temperature. Refrigerate reconstituted solution and use within 24 hours.

Administration

! Streptokinase must be administered within 12 to 14 hours of clot formation. It has little effect on older, organized clots. Do not use within 5 days to 6 months of previous streptokinase treatment if administered for streptococcal infection, such as acute glomerulonephritis secondary to streptococcal infection, pharyngitis, and rheumatic fever.

Reconstitute vial with 5 ml D_5W or 0.9% NaCl (preferred). Add diluent slowly to side of vial; roll and tilt to avoid foaming. Do not shake vial. May dilute further with 50 to 500 ml of D_5W or 0.9% NaCl in 45-ml increments. For peripheral IV administration for coronary artery thrombi, give 1.5 million units over 60 minutes. For direct intracoronary administration of coronary artery thrombi, give bolus dose over 25 to 30 seconds using coronary catheter. Follow with 2000 units/minute for 60 minutes. For treatment of DVT, pulmonary arterial embolism, or arterial thrombi, give single dose over 25 to 30 minutes. Follow with maintenance dose of 100,000 or more units every hour for 24 to 72 hours (72 hours for DVT). Monitor the patient's B/P during infusion. Hypotension, which may be severe, occurs in 1% to 10% of patients. If necessary, decrease the infusion rate, as prescribed. Discontinue the infusion immediately and notify the physician if uncontrolled hemorrhage occurs. Be aware that slowing the rate of infusion instead of discontinuing it may produce worsening hemorrhage. Do not use dextran to control hemorrhage.

Streptomycin
strep-toe-mye′sin

CATEGORY AND SCHEDULE
Pregnancy Risk Category: D

CLASSIFICATION
Antibiotics, aminoglycosides, antimycobacterials

MECHANISM OF ACTION
An aminoglycoside that binds directly to the 30S ribosomal subunits causing a faulty peptide sequence to form in the protein chain. *Therapeutic effect:* Inhibits bacterial protein synthesis.

AVAILABILITY
Injection: 1 g.

INDICATIONS AND DOSAGES
▸ **Tuberculosis**
IM
Adults. 15 mg/kg/day. Maximum: 1 g/day.
Elderly: 10 mg/kg/day. Maximum: 750 mg/day.
Children. 20-40 mg/kg/day. Maximum: 1 g/day.
▸ **Dosage in renal impairment**

Creatinine Clearance	Dosage Interval
10-50 ml/min	q24-72hr
Less than 10 ml/min	q72-96hr

CONTRAINDICATIONS
Pregnancy

INTERACTIONS
Drug
Amphotericin, loop diuretics: May increase the nephrotoxicity of streptomycin.

Neuromuscular blockers: May increase the effects of streptomycin.
Herbal
None known.
Food
None known.

DIAGNOSTIC TEST EFFECTS
None known.

SIDE EFFECTS
Occasional
Hypotension, drowsiness, headache, drug fever, paresthesia, rash, nausea, vomiting, anemia, arthralgia, weakness, tremor

SERIOUS REACTIONS
• Nephrotoxicity (as evidenced by increased BUN and serum creatinine levels and decreased creatinine clearance) may be reversible if the drug is stopped at the first sign of nephrotoxic symptoms.
• Irreversible ototoxicity (manifested as tinnitus, dizziness, ringing or roaring in the ears, and impaired hearing) and neurotoxicity (as evidenced by headache, dizziness, lethargy, tremor, and visual disturbances) occur occasionally.
Symptoms of ototoxicity, nephrotoxicity, and neuromuscular toxicity may occur.

PRECAUTIONS & CONSIDERATIONS
Caution is warranted with tinnitus, vertigo, neuromuscular disorders, and renal impairment. Before giving streptomycin, determine if hypersensitive to aminoglycosides, pregnant, or being treated for other medical conditions such as myasthenia gravis or parkinsonism. Hearing, renal function, and serum concentrations of streptomycin should be monitored. If symptoms of hearing loss, dizziness, or fullness or roaring in the ears occur, notify the physician.

Administration
For IM use, inject streptomycin deep into a large muscle mass. Be aware that for patients who are unable to tolerate IM injections, streptomycin may be given as an IV infusion over 30 to 60 minutes.

Succimer
sux'sim-mer
(Chemet)

CATEGORY AND SCHEDULE
Pregnancy Risk Category: C

CLASSIFICATION
Antidotes, chelators

MECHANISM OF ACTION
An analog of dimercaprol that forms water soluble chelates with heavy metals which are excreted renally. *Therapeutic Effect:* Treats lead intoxication in children.

PHARMACOKINETICS
Rapidly absorbed from the gastrointestinal (GI) tract. Extensively metabolized. Excreted in feces (39%), urine (9%-25%), and lungs (1%). Removed by hemodialysis. **Half-life:** 2 hr-2 days.

AVAILABILITY
Capsules: 100 mg (Chemet).

INDICATIONS AND DOSAGES
▶ **Lead poisoning, in pediatric patients with blood lead levels about 45 mcg/L**
PO
Children 12 mo and older. 10 mg/kg q8hr for 5 days, then 10 mg/kg q12hr for 14 days.

OFF-LABEL USES
Lead poisoning in adults, arsenic intoxication, mercury intoxication

CONTRAINDICATIONS
Hypersensitivity to succimer or any component of its formulation

INTERACTIONS
Drug
None known.
Herbal
None known.
Food
None known.

DIAGNOSTIC TEST EFFECTS
May decrease serum creatine phophokinase and serum uric acid measurements. May cause false-positive results for urinary ketones using nitroprusside reagents such as Ketostix.

SIDE EFFECTS
Occasional
Anorexia, diarrhea, nausea, vomiting, rash, odor to breath and urine, increased liver function tests
Rare
Neutropenia

SERIOUS REACTIONS
• Elevated blood lead levels and symptoms of intoxication may occur after succimer therapy due to redistribution of lead from bone to soft tissues and blood.
• Elevated liver function tests have been reported.

PRECAUTIONS & CONSIDERATIONS
It is unknown if succimer is distributed in breast milk. Safety and efficacy of succimer complex have not been established in children less than 12 months of age. There are no age-related precautions noted in the elderly. Plasma lead levels should

be monitored and kept below
15 mcg/dl.

Sulfurous odor to breath and urine
may occur, but will subside when
succimer is discontinued.

Administration

Keep in mind that succimer is not
a substitute for effective abatement
of lead exposure. Capsules may be
opened and contents sprinkled onto
soft food. Make sure all food is eaten.

Sucralfate

soo-kral′fate
(Apo-Sucralate [CAN], Carafate,
Novo-Sucralate [CAN], Ulcyte
[AUS])
**Do not confuse Carafate with
Cafergot.**

CATEGORY AND SCHEDULE
Pregnancy Risk Category: B

CLASSIFICATION
Cytoprotectives, gastrointestinals

MECHANISM OF ACTION
An antiulcer agent that forms an
ulcer-adherent complex with
proteinaceous exudate, such as
albumin, at ulcer site. Also forms a
viscous, adhesive barrier on the
surface of intact mucosa of the
stomach or duodenum. *Therapeutic
Effect:* Protects damaged mucosa
from further destruction by
absorbing gastric acid, pepsin, and
bile salts.

PHARMACOKINETICS
Minimally absorbed from the GI
tract. Eliminated in feces, with small
amount excreted in urine. Not
removed by hemodialysis.

AVAILABILITY
Oral Suspension: 500 mg/5 ml.
Tablets: 1 g.

INDICATIONS AND DOSAGES
▸ **Active duodenal ulcers**
PO
Adults, Elderly. 1 g 4 times a day
(before meals and at bedtime) for up
to 8 wk.
▸ **Maintenance therapy after healing
of acute duodenal ulcers**
PO
Adults, Elderly. 1 g twice a day.

OFF-LABEL USES
Prevention and treatment of stress-
related mucosal damage, especially
in acutely or critically ill patients;
treatment of gastric ulcer and rheumatoid arthritis; relief of GI symptoms
associated with NSAIDs; treatment
of gastroesophageal reflux disease

CONTRAINDICATIONS
None known.

INTERACTIONS
Drug
Antacids: May interfere with bind-
ing of sucralfate.
**Digoxin, phenytoin, quinolones,
such as ciprofloxacin, theophylline:**
May decrease the absorption of these
drugs.
Herbal
None known.
Food
None known.

DIAGNOSTIC TEST EFFECTS
None known.

SIDE EFFECTS
Frequent (2%)
Constipation
Occasional (less than 2%)
Dry mouth, backache, diarrhea,
dizziness, somnolence, nausea,

indigestion, rash, hives, itching, abdominal discomfort

SERIOUS REACTIONS
• None known.

PRECAUTIONS & CONSIDERATIONS

It is unknown if sucralfate crosses the placenta or is distributed in breast milk. Safety and efficacy of sucralfate have not been established in children. No age-related precautions have been noted in the elderly.

Dry mouth may occur, so take sips of tepid water or suck on sour hard candy to relieve it. Before sucralfate administration, the abdomen should be assessed for signs of tenderness, rigidity, and the presence of bowel sounds. Pattern of daily bowel activity and stool consistency should be monitored throughout therapy.

Administration
! Know that 1 g equals 10 ml suspension.

Take 1 hour before meals, on an empty stomach, and at bedtime. Tablets may be crushed or dissolved in water. Do not take antacids within 30 minutes of sucralfate. Do not take digoxin, phenytoin, quinolones, or theophylline within 2 to 3 hours of sucralfate.

Sulfabenzamide/ Sulfacetamide/ Sulfathiazole
sul-fa-ben'za-mide/sul-fa-see'ta-mide/sul-fa-thye'a-zole
(V.V.S.)

CATEGORY AND SCHEDULE
Pregnancy Risk Category: C

CLASSIFICATION
Anti-infectives, topical, antibiotics, sulfonamides, dermatologics

MECHANISM OF ACTION
Interferes with synthesis of folic acid that bacteria require for growth by inhibition of para-aminobenzoic acid metabolism. *Therapeutic Effect:* Prevents further bacterial growth.

PHARMACOKINETICS
Absorption from vagina is variable and unreliable. Primarily metabolized by acetylation. Excreted in urine. **Half-life:** unknown.

AVAILABILITY
Vaginal Cream: 3.7% sulfabenzamide, 2.86% sulfacetamide, 3.42% sulfathiazole (V.V.S.)

INDICATIONS AND DOSAGES
▸ **Treatment of Haemophilus vaginalis vaginitis**
VAGINAL
Adults, Elderly. Insert one applicatorful into vagina twice daily for 4-6 days. Dosage may then be decreased to ½ to ¼ of an applicatorful twice daily.

CONTRAINDICATIONS
Renal dysfunction, pregnancy (or near term), hypersensitivity to

sulfabenzamide, sulfacetamide, sulfathiazole or any component of preparation

INTERACTIONS
Drug
None known.
Herbal
None known.
Food
None known.

DIAGNOSTIC TEST EFFECTS
None known.

SIDE EFFECTS
Occasional
Local irritation
Rare
Pruritus urticaria, allergic reactions

SERIOUS REACTIONS
• Superinfection and Stevens-Johnson syndrome occur rarely.

PRECAUTIONS & CONSIDERATIONS
Be aware that sulfabenzamide, sulfacetamide, sulfathiazole has been associated with Stevens-Johnson syndrome and therapy should be discontinued if local irritation occurs. It is unknown if sulfabenzamide, sulfacetamide, sulfathiazole crosses the placenta or is distributed in breast milk. Do not use sulfabenzamide, sulfacetamide, sulfathiazole in patients during the third trimester of pregnancy. Safety and efficacy of sulfabenzamide, sulfacetamide, sulfathiazole have not been established in children. There are no age-related precautions noted in the elderly.
Administration
Cream is for intravaginal use only. Complete full course of therapy.

Sulfacetamide
sul-fa-see'ta-mide
(AK-Sulf, Bleph-10, Isopto Cetamide, Diosulf [CAN], Ophthacet, Sodium Sulamyd, Sulfair)

CATEGORY AND SCHEDULE
Pregnancy Risk Category: C

CLASSIFICATION
Anti-infectives, ophthalmics, antibiotics, sulfonamides

MECHANISM OF ACTION
Interferes with synthesis of folic acid that bacteria require for growth. *Therapeutic Effect:* Prevents further bacterial growth. Bacteriostatic.

PHARMACOKINETICS
Small amounts may be absorbed into the cornea. Excreted rapidly in urine. **Half-life:** 7-13 hr.

AVAILABILITY
Lotion: 10% (Carmol, Klaron, Ovace).
Ophthalmic Ointment: 10% (AK-Sulf).
Ophthalmic Solution: 10% (Bleph-10, Ocusulf, Sulf-10).

S

INDICATIONS AND DOSAGES
▸ **Treatment of corneal ulcers, conjunctivitis and other superficial infections of the eye, prophylaxis after injuries to the eye/removal of foreign bodies, adjunctive therapy for trachoma and inclusion conjunctivitis**
OPHTHALMIC
Adults, Elderly. Ointment: Apply small amount in lower conjunctival sac 1-4 times/day and at bedtime.

Solution: 1-3 drops to lower conjunctival sac q2-3hr. Seborrheic dermatitis, seborrheic sicca (dandruff), secondary bacterial skin infections
TOPICAL
Adults, Elderly. Apply 1-4 times/day.

OFF-LABEL USES
Treatment of bacterial blepharitis, blepharoconjunctivitis, bacterial keratitis, keratoconjunctivitis

CONTRAINDICATIONS
Hypersensitivity to sulfonamides or any component of preparation (some products contain sulfite), use in combination with silver-containing products

INTERACTIONS
Drug
Silver-containing preparations: These products are incompatible together.
Herbal
None known.
Food
None known.

DIAGNOSTIC TEST EFFECTS
None known.

SIDE EFFECTS
Frequent
Transient ophthalmic burning, stinging
Occasional
Headache
Rare
Hypersensitivity (erythema, rash, itching, swelling, photosensitivity)

SERIOUS REACTIONS
• Superinfection, drug-induced lupus erythematosus, Stevens-Johnson syndrome occur rarely; nephrotoxicity w/high dermatologic concentrations.

PRECAUTIONS & CONSIDERATIONS
Caution should be used with extremely dry eye. It is unknown if sulfacetamide sodium crosses the placenta or is distributed in breast milk. Do not use sulfacetamide sodium during the third trimester of pregnancy. Safety and efficacy of sulfacetamide have not been established in children. There are no age-related precautions noted in the elderly. Be aware sulfacetamide sodium application of lotion to large infected, denuded, or debrided areas should be avoided.

Eye drops may burn upon instillation. Eye ointment will cause blurred vision.

Sulfacetamide may cause sensitivity to light. Sunglasses should be worn and avoid bright light.
Storage
Store at room temperature and protect from light. Discolored solution should not be used. Discard Sulfacet-R lotion after 4 months.
Administration
For ophthalmic use, tilt the head back. Place solution in conjunctival sac. Close eyes, and then press gently on the lacrimal sac for 1 minute. Wait at least 10 minutes before using another eye preparation.

For topical treatment, cleanse area before application to ensure direct contact with affected area. Apply at bedtime and allow to remain overnight.

Sulfasalazine

sul-fa-sal'a-zeen
(Alti-Sulfasalazine [CAN],
Azulfidine, Azulfidine EN-tabs,
Pyralin EN [AUS], Salazopyrin
[CAN], Salazopyrin EN [AUS],
Salazopyrin EN-Tabs [CAN])
**Do not confuse Azulfidine
with azathioprine, or
sulfasalazine with sulfadiazine,
or sulfisoxazole.**

CATEGORY AND SCHEDULE

Pregnancy Risk Category: B (D
if given near term)

CLASSIFICATION

Disease modifying antirheumatic
drugs, gastrointestinals, salicylates

MECHANISM OF ACTION

A sulfonamide that inhibits
prostaglandin synthesis, acting
locally in the colon. *Therapeutic
Effect:* Decreases inflammatory
response, interferes with GI
secretion.

PHARMACOKINETICS

Poorly absorbed from the GI tract.
Cleaved in colon by intestinal
bacteria, forming sulfapyridine and
mesalamine (5-ASA). Absorbed in
colon. Widely distributed.
Metabolized in the liver.
Primarily excreted in urine.
Half-life: sulfapyridine, 6-14 hr;
5-ASA, 0.6-1.4 hr.

AVAILABILITY

Tablets (Azulfidine): 500 mg.
*Tablets (Delayed-Release [Azulfidine
EN-Tabs]):* 500 mg.

INDICATIONS AND DOSAGES
▶ **Ulcerative colitis**
PO
Adults, Elderly. 1 g 3-4 times a day
in divided doses q4-6hr.
Maintenance: 2 g/day in divided
doses q6-12hr. Maximum: 6 g/day.
Children. 40-75 mg/kg/day in
divided doses q4-6hr. Maintenance:
30-50 mg/kg/day in divided doses
q4-8hr. Maximum: 2 g/day.
Maximum: 6 g/day.
▶ **Rheumatoid arthritis**
PO
Adults, Elderly. Initially, 0.5-1 g/day
for 1 wk. Increase by 0.5 g/wk, up to
3 g/day.
▶ **Juvenile rheumatoid arthritis**
PO
Children. Initially, 10 mg/kg/day.
May increase by 10 mg/kg/day
at weekly intervals. Range:
30-50 mg/kg/day. Maximum: 2 g/day.

OFF-LABEL USES

Treatment of ankylosing spondylitis

CONTRAINDICATIONS

Children younger than 2 years; hypersensitivity to carbonic anhydrase
inhibitors, local anesthetics, salicylates, sulfonamides, sulfonylureas,
sunscreens containing PABA, or
thiazide or loop diuretics; intestinal
or urinary tract obstruction;
porphyria; pregnancy at term; severe
hepatic or renal dysfunction

INTERACTIONS
Drug
**Anticonvulsants, methotrexate,
oral anticoagulants, oral antidiabetics:** May increase the effects of
these drugs.
Hemolytics: May increase the toxicity of sulfasalazine.
Hepatotoxic medications: May
increase the risk of hepatotoxicity.

S

Herbal
None known.
Food
None known.

DIAGNOSTIC TEST EFFECTS
None known.

SIDE EFFECTS
Frequent (33%)
Anorexia, nausea, vomiting, headache, oligospermia (generally reversed by withdrawal of drug)
Occasional (3%)
Hypersensitivity reaction (rash, urticaria, pruritus, fever, anemia)
Rare (less than 1%)
Tinnitus, hypoglycemia, diuresis, photosensitivity

SERIOUS REACTIONS
* Anaphylaxis, Stevens-Johnson syndrome, hematologic toxicity (leukopenia, agranulocytosis), hepatotoxicity, and nephrotoxicity occur rarely.

PRECAUTIONS & CONSIDERATIONS
Caution is warranted with bronchial asthma, G6PD deficiency, impaired hepatic or renal function, or severe allergies. Sulfasalazine may produce infertility and oligospermia in men. Sulfasalazine readily crosses the placenta and is excreted in breast milk. Lactating patients should not breast-feed premature infants or those with hyperbilirubinemia or glucose-6-phosphate dehydrogenase (G6PD) deficiency. If given near term, sulfasalazine may produce hemolytic anemia, jaundice, and kernicterus in the newborn. No age-related precautions have been noted in children older than 2 years or the elderly. Avoid the sun and ultraviolet light; photosensitivity may last for months after the last dose of sulfasalazine.

Adequate hydration should be maintained (minimum output 1500 ml/24 hr) and prevent nephrotoxicity. Skin should be examined for rash; withhold the drug at the first sign of a rash. Pattern of daily bowel activity and stool consistency should be monitored; drug dosage may need to be increased if diarrhea continues or recurs. Report hematologic effects such as bleeding, ecchymosis, fever, jaundice, pallor, purpura, pharyngitis, and weakness.
Administration
Space drug doses evenly at intervals not to exceed 8 hours. Administer sulfasalazine after meals, if possible, to prolong intestinal passage. Swallow delayed-release tablets whole without chewing or crushing them. Take the drug with 8 oz of water.

Sulfinpyrazone
sul-fin-pyr′a-zone
(Anturane, Apo-Sulfinpyrazone [CAN], Nu-Sufinpyrazone [CAN])
Do not confuse with Accutane.

CATEGORY AND SCHEDULE
Pregnancy Risk Category: C/D (near term)

CLASSIFICATION
Uricosurics

MECHANISM OF ACTION
A uricosuric that increases urinary excretion of uric acid, thereby decreasing blood urate levels. *Therapeutic Effect:* Promotes uric acid excretion and reduces serum uric acid levels.

PHARMACOKINETICS

Rapidly and completely absorbed from gastrointestinal (GI) tract. Widely distributed. Metabolized in liver to two active metabolites, p-hydroxy-sulfinpyrazone and a sulfide analogue. Excreted primarily in urine. Not removed by hemodialysis. **Half-life:** 2.7- 6 hr.

AVAILABILITY

Tablets: 100 mg (Anturane).

INDICATIONS AND DOSAGES

▶ **Gout**
PO
Adults, Elderly. 100-200 mg 2 times/day. Maximum: 800 mg/day.

OFF-LABEL USES

Mitral valve replacement, myocardial infarction

CONTRAINDICATIONS

Active peptic ulcer, blood dyscrasias, GI inflammation, pregnancy (near term), hypersensitivity to sulfinpyrazone, phenylbutazone, other pyrazoles, or any of its components

INTERACTIONS

Drug
Acetaminophen: May increase risk of heptotoxicity and decrease effect of sulfinpyrazone.
Aspirin: May decrease uricosuric effect.
Oral anticoagulants: May increase anticoagulant effect.
Oral hypoglycemics: May increase hypoglycemic effect.
Salicylates, niacin: May decrease uricosuric activity.
Theophylline, verapamil: May decrease effects and levels of theophylline and verapamil.
Herbal
Arnica, astragalus, bilberry, black currant, cat's claw, chaparral, chondroitin, clove oil, evening primrose, feverfew, ginger, Ginkgo biloba, hawthorn, kava kava, skullcap, tan-shen: May increase risk of bleeding.
Dong quai, St. John's wort: May increase risk of photosensitization.
Food
Rhubarb: May increase risk of bleeding.

DIAGNOSTIC TEST EFFECTS

May alter serum uric acid levels.

SIDE EFFECTS

Frequent
Nausea, vomiting, stomach pain
Occasional
Flushed face, headache, dizziness, frequent urge to urinate, rash
Rare
Increased bleeding time, hepatic necrosis, nephrotic syndrome, uric acid stones

SERIOUS REACTIONS

• Hematological toxicity including anemia, leukopenia, agranulocytosis, thrombocytopenia, and aplastic anemia occur rarely.
• Overdose causes a drowsiness, dizziness, anorexia, abdominal pain, hemolytic anemia, acidosis, jaundice, fever, and agranulocytosis.

PRECAUTIONS & CONSIDERATIONS

Caution is necessary with urolithiasis. It is unknown if sulfinpyrazone crosses the placenta or is distributed in breast milk. Safety and efficacy of sulfinpyrazone have not been established in children older than 18 years of age. Age-related renal impairment may increase risk of toxicity in the elderly. Avoid citrate containing products as well as use of aspirin or aspirin containing products.

Administration
Do not use in presence of renal impairment. Give sulfinpyrazone with meals or milk to decrease GI irritation. Drink at least 6 to 8 glasses (8 oz) of water each day to prevent renal stone development.

Sulfisoxazole
sul-fi-sox′a-zole
Gantrisin, Novo-Soxazole [CAN], Sulfizole [CAN], Truxazole)
Do not confuse with sulfadiazine, sulfamethoxazole, sulfasalazine, Gastrosed

CATEGORY AND SCHEDULE
Pregnancy risk category: B/D (near term)

CLASSIFICATION
Antibiotics, sulfonamides

MECHANISM OF ACTION
An antibacterial sulphonamide that inhibits bacterial synthesis of dihydrofolic acid by preventing condensation of pteridine with aminobenzoic acid through competitive inhibition of the enzyme dihydropteroate synthetase. *Therapeutic Effect:* Bacteriostatic.

PHARMACOKINETICS
Rapidly and completely absorbed. Small intestine is major site of absorption, but some absorption occurs in the stomach. Exists in the blood as unbound, protein-bound and conjugated forms. Sulfisoxazole is metabolized primarily by acetylation and oxidation in the liver. The free form is considered to be the therapeutically active form. Protein binding: 85%. **Half-life:** 5-8 hr.

AVAILABILITY
Tablet: 500 mg powder: 100%
Suspension: 500 mg/5 mL (Gantrisin)

INDICATIONS AND DOSAGES
▸ **Acute, recurrent or chronic urinary tract infections, meningococcal meningitis, acute otitis media due to Haemophilus influenzae**
PO
Infants over 2 Months of Age, Children: One-half of the 24-hour dose initially then 150 mg/kg daily or 4 g/m^2 daily for maintanence divided q4-6hr. Maximum dose: 6 g daily.
Adults: 2-4 g initially then 4-8 g daily divided q4-6hr.

CONTRAINDICATIONS
Patients with a known hypersensitivity to sulfonamides, children younger than 2 months (except in the treatment of congenital toxoplasmosis as adjunctive therapy with pyrimethamine), pregnant women at term, and mothers nursing infants less than 2 months of age.

INTERACTIONS
Drug
Warfarin: May prolong prothrombin time.
Thiopental: May increase effect of thiopental.
Methotrexate: May increase free methotrexate concentrations.
Sulfonylureas: May increase hypoglycemic effect of sulfonylureas.
Herbal
Dong quai, St. John's wort: May cause photosensitization.
Food
Folate: May decrease folate absorption.

DIAGNOSTIC TEST EFFECTS
May cause false-positive for protein in urine and urine glucose with Clinitest.

SIDE EFFECTS

Anaphylaxis, erythema multiforme
(Stevens-Johnson syndrome), toxic
epidermal necrolysis, exfoliative
dermatitis, angioedema, arteritis and
vasculitis, allergic myocarditis, serum
sickness, rash, urticaria, pruritus,
photosensitivity, conjunctival and
scleral injection, generalized allergic
reactions, generalized skin eruptions,
tachycardia, palpitations, syncope,
cyanosis, goiter, diuresis, hypoglycemia, arthralgia, myalgia, headache,
dizziness, peripheral neuritis, paresthesia, convulsions, tinnitus, vertigo,
ataxia, intracranial hypertension,
cough, shortness of breath,
pulmonary infiltrates

SERIOUS REACTIONS

• Fatalities associated with the
administration of sulfonamides
including Stevens-Johnson syndrome
toxic epidermal necrolysis, fulminant
hepatic necrosis, agranulocytosis,
aplastic anemia and other blood
dyscrasias occur rarely.
• Clinical signs such as rash, sore
throat, fever, arthralgia, pallor,
purpura, or jaundice may be
early indications of serious
reactions.

PRECAUTIONS & CONSIDERATIONS

Caution is necessary with G6PD deficiency and liver or kidney disease.
Avoid prolonged exposure to sunlight.
Sunscreen and protective clothing
should be worn if sunlight is not
avoidable. Be aware that it is unknown
if sulfisoxazole crosses the placenta.
Sulfisoxazole enters the breast milk.
There are no age-related precautions
noted in children or the elderly.
Alcohol should be avoided.

If rash, hives, itching, shortness
of breath, wheezing, cough, or
swelling of face, lips, tongue, and
throat occurs, notify physician.

Administration

Take with or without food and with a
full glass of water. Take with food if
GI upset occurs. Administer around
the clock to promote less variation in
peak and trough levels.

Sulindac
sul-in′dak
(Aclin [AUS], Apo-Sulin [CAN],
Clinoril, Novo Sundac [CAN])
**Do not confuse Clinoril with
Clozaril.**

CATEGORY AND SCHEDULE
Pregnancy Risk Category: B (D
if used in third trimester or near
delivery)

CLASSIFICATION
Analgesics, non-narcotic, nonsteroidal anti-inflammatory drugs

MECHANISM OF ACTION
An NSAID that produces analgesic
and anti-inflammatory effects by
inhibiting prostaglandin synthesis.
Therapeutic Effect: Reduces
inflammatory response and intensity
of pain.

PHARMACOKINETICS

Route	Onset	Peak	Duration
PO (Anti-rheumatic)	7 days	2-3 wk	N/A

Well absorbed from the GI tract.
Metabolized in liver to active
metabolite. Primarily excreted in
urine. Not removed by hemodialysis.
Half-life: 7.8 hr; metabolite:
16.4 hr.

AVAILABILITY
Tablets: 150 mg, 200 mg.

INDICATIONS AND DOSAGES
▸ **Rheumatoid arthritis, osteoarthritis, ankylosing spondylitis**
PO
Adults, Elderly. Initially, 150 mg twice a day; may increase up to 400 mg/day.
▸ **Acute shoulder pain, gouty arthritis, bursitis, tendinitis**
PO
Adults, Elderly. 200 mg twice a day.

CONTRAINDICATIONS
Active peptic ulcer disease, chronic inflammation of GI tract, GI bleeding or ulceration, history of hypersensitivity to aspirin or NSAIDs

INTERACTIONS
Drug
Antacids: May decrease the sulindac blood concentration.
Antihypertensives, diuretics: May decrease the effects of these drugs.
Aspirin, other salicylates: May increase the risk of GI side effects such as bleeding.
Bone marrow depressants: May increase the risk of hematologic reactions.
Heparin, oral anticoagulants, thrombolytics: May increase the effects of these drugs.
Lithium: May increase the blood concentration and risk of toxicity of lithium.
Methotrexate: May increase the risk of methotrexate toxicity.
Probenecid: May increase the sulindac blood concentration.
Herbal
Feverfew: May decrease the effects of feverfew.
Ginkgo biloba: May increase the risk of bleeding.

Food
None known.

DIAGNOSTIC TEST EFFECTS
May increase liver function test results and serum alkaline phosphatase level.

SIDE EFFECTS
Frequent (9%-4%)
Diarrhea or constipation, indigestion, nausea, maculopapular rash, dermatitis, dizziness, headache
Occasional (3%-1%)
Anorexia, abdominal cramps, flatulence

SERIOUS REACTIONS
• Rare reactions with long-term use include peptic ulcer disease, GI bleeding, gastritis, nephrotoxicity (glomerular nephritis, interstitial nephritis, nephrotic syndrome), severe hepatic reactions (cholestasis, jaundice), and severe hypersensitivity reactions (fever, chills, and joint pain).

PRECAUTIONS & CONSIDERATIONS
Caution is warranted with a history of GI tract disease, hepatic or renal impairment, a predisposition to fluid retention, and concurrent use of anticoagulant therapy. It is unknown if sulindac is excreted in breast milk. Sulindac should not be used during the third trimester of pregnancy because it may cause adverse effects in the fetus, such as premature closure of the ductus arteriosus. The safety and efficacy of naproxen have not been established in children. In the elderly, GI bleeding or ulceration is more likely to cause serious complications and age-related renal impairment may increase the risk of hepatotoxicity and renal toxicity; a reduced drug dosage is recommended. Avoid alcohol and aspirin during therapy because these substances increase the risk of GI bleeding.

Tasks that require mental alertness or motor skills should also be avoided.

CBC, especially platelet count, skin for rash, and liver and renal function test results should be assessed before and periodically during therapy. Therapeutic response, such as decreased pain, stiffness, swelling, and tenderness, improved grip strength, and increased joint mobility, should be evaluated.

Administration
Take sulindac orally with food, milk, or antacids if GI distress occurs. Sulindac's therapeutic antiarthritic effect will occur 1 to 3 weeks after therapy begins.

Sumatriptan
soo-ma-trip'tan
(Imigran [AUS], Imitrex, Suvalan [AUS])
Do not confuse sumatriptan with somatropin.

CATEGORY AND SCHEDULE
Pregnancy Risk Category: C

CLASSIFICATION
Serotonin receptor agonists

MECHANISM OF ACTION
A serotonin receptor agonist that binds selectively to vascular receptors, producing a vasoconstrictive effect on cranial blood vessels. *Therapeutic Effect:* Relieves migraine headache.

PHARMACOKINETICS

Route	Onset	Peak	Duration
Nasal	15 min	N/A	24-48 hr
PO	30 min	2 hr	24-48 hr
Sub-cutaneous	10 min	1 hr	24-48 hr

Rapidly absorbed after subcutaneous administration. Absorption after PO administration is incomplete, with significant amounts undergoing hepatic metabolism, resulting in low bioavailability (about 14%). Protein binding: 10%-21%. Widely distributed. Undergoes first-pass metabolism in the liver. Excreted in urine. **Half-life:** 2 hr.

AVAILABILITY
Tablets: 25 mg, 50 mg, 100 mg.
Injection: 6 mg/0.5 ml.
Nasal Spray: 5 mg, 20 mg.

INDICATIONS AND DOSAGES
▸ **Acute migraine attack**
PO
Adults, Elderly. 25-50 mg. Dose may be repeated after at least 2 hr. Maximum: 100 mg/single dose; 200 mg/24 hr.
SUBCUTANEOUS
Adults, Elderly. 6 mg. Maximum: Two 6-mg injections/24 hr (separated by at least 1 hr).
INTRANASAL
Adults, Elderly. 5-20 mg; may repeat in 2 hr. Maximum: 40 mg/24 hr.

CONTRAINDICATIONS
CVA, ischemic heart disease (including angina pectoris, history of MI, silent ischemia, and Prinzmetal's angina), severe hepatic impairment, transient ischemic attack, uncontrolled hypertension, use within 14 days of MAOIs, use within 24 hr of ergotamine preparations

INTERACTIONS
Drug
Ergotamine-containing medications: May produce vasospastic reaction.
MAOIs: May increase sumatriptan blood concentration and half-life.

S

Herbal
None known.
Food
None known.

DIAGNOSTIC TEST EFFECTS
None known.

SIDE EFFECTS
Frequent
Oral (10%-5%): Tingling, nasal discomfort
Subcutaneous (greater than 10%): Injection site reactions, tingling, warm or hot sensation, dizziness, vertigo
Nasal (greater than 10%): Bad or unusual taste, nausea, vomiting
Occasional
Oral (5%-1%): Flushing, asthenia, visual disturbances
Subcutaneous (10%-2%): Burning sensation, numbness, chest discomfort, drowsiness, asthenia
Nasal (5%-1%): Nasopharyngeal discomfort, dizziness
Rare
Oral (less than 1%): Agitation, eye irritation, dysuria
Subcutaneous (less than 2%): Anxiety, fatigue, diaphoresis, muscle cramps, myalgia
Nasal (less than 1%): Burning sensation

SERIOUS REACTIONS
• Excessive dosage may produce tremor, red extremities, reduced respirations, cyanosis, seizures, and paralysis.
• Serious arrhythmias occur rarely, especially in patients with hypertension, diabetes, or a strong family history of coronary artery disease; obese patients; and smokers.

PRECAUTIONS & CONSIDERATIONS
Caution is warranted with epilepsy, a hypersensitivity to sulfonamides, and hepatic or renal impairment. It is unknown if sumatriptan is distributed in breast milk. The safety and efficacy of sumatriptan have not been established in children. No age-related precautions have been noted in the elderly.

Dizziness may occur. Notify the physician immediately if palpitations, a rash, wheezing, pain or tightness in the chest or throat, or facial edema occurs. EKG should be obtained at baseline. Migraines and associated symptoms, including nausea and vomiting, photophobia, and phonophobia (sound sensitivity) should be assessed before and during treatment.

Administration
Swallow oral tablets whole with a full glass of water.

For subcutaneous use, follow the manufacturer's instructions for using the autoinjection device. Inject the drug into an area with adequate subcutaneous tissue because the needle will penetrate the skin and adipose tissue as deeply as 6 mm. Do not administer more than two subcutaneous injections during any 24-hour period and allow at least 1 hour between injections. After injecting the medication, discard the syringe.

For nasal use, each unit contains only one spray, so don't test the spray before use. Blow the nose gently to clear nasal passages. With the head upright, close one of the nostrils with an index finger and breathe gently through the mouth. Insert the nozzle about 1/2 inch into the open nostril. Close mouth, then breathe through the nose while depressing the blue plunger and releasing the spray. Remove the nozzle from the nose, and gently breathe in through the nose and out through the mouth for 10-20 seconds. Do not breathe in deeply.

Tacrine
tack'rin
(Cognex)

CATEGORY AND SCHEDULE
Pregnancy Risk Category: C

CLASSIFICATION
Cholinesterase inhibitors

MECHANISM OF ACTION
A cholinesterase inhibitor that inhibits the enzyme acetylcholinesterase, thus increasing the concentration of acetylcholine at cholinergic synapses and enhancing cholinergic function in the CNS. *Therapeutic Effect:* Slows the progression of Alzheimer's disease.

AVAILABILITY
Capsules: 10 mg, 20 mg, 30 mg, 40 mg.

INDICATIONS AND DOSAGES
▸ **Alzheimer's disease**
PO
Adults, Elderly. Initially, 10 mg 4 times a day for 6 wk, followed by 20 mg 4 times a day for 6 wk, 30 mg 4 times a day for 12 wk, then 40 mg 4 times a day if needed.
▸ **Dosage in hepatic impairment**
For patients with (SGPT) ALT greater than 3-5 times normal, decrease the dose by 40 mg/day and resume the normal dose when (SGPT) ALT returns to normal. For patients with (SGPT) ALT greater than 5 times normal, stop treatment and resume it when (SGPT) ALT returns to normal.

CONTRAINDICATIONS
Active, severe hepatic disease; active and untreated duodenal or gastric ulcers; breast-feeding women; concurrent use of other cholinesterase inhibitors; hypersensitivity to cholinergics; mechanical obstruction of intestine or urinary tract; pregnancy; women with childbearing potential

INTERACTIONS
Drug
Anticholinergics: May decrease the effects of tacrine oranticholinergics.
Cimetidine: May increase the tacrine blood concentration.
NSAIDs: May increase the adverse effects of NSAIDs.
Theophylline: May increase the theophylline blood concentration.
Herbal
None known.
Food
None known.

DIAGNOSTIC TEST EFFECTS
Increases AST (SGOT) and ALT (SGPT) levels. Alters blood Hgb, Hct, and serum electrolyte levels.

SIDE EFFECTS
Frequent (28%-11%)
Headache, nausea, vomiting, diarrhea, dizziness
Occasional (9%-4%)
Fatigue, chest pain, dyspepsia, anorexia, abdominal pain, flatulence, constipation, confusion, agitation, rash, depression, ataxia, insomnia, rhinitis, myalgia
Rare (less than 3%)
Weight loss, anxiety, cough, facial flushing, urinary frequency, back pain, tremor

SERIOUS REACTIONS
• Overdose can cause cholinergic crisis, marked by increased salivation,

T

lacrimation, bradycardia, respiratory depression, hypotension, and increased muscle weakness. Treatment usually consists of supportive measures and an anticholinergic such as atropine.

PRECAUTIONS & CONSIDERATIONS

Caution is warranted with alcohol abuse, asthma, bradycardia, cardiac arrhythmias, COPD, peptic ulcer disease, hyperthyroidism, hepatic dysfunction, and a history of seizures. Be aware that tacrine is not a cure for Alzheimer's disease but may slow the progression of its symptoms. Smoking should be avoided because it reduces the drug's blood level. Liver function tests and EKG and rhythm strips should be periodically monitored.

Administration

! If tacrine therapy is stopped for longer than 14 days, reinstitute therapy as prescribed.

Take tacrine without regard to food. Take tacrine at regular intervals, between meals. Take with food if GI upset occurs. Do not abruptly discontinue or adjust the dosage of tacrine.

Tacrolimus

tak-roe-leem′us

(Prograf, Protopic)

Do not confuse Protopic with Protonix, Protopam, Protopin.

CATEGORY AND SCHEDULE

Pregnancy Risk Category: C

CLASSIFICATION

Dermatologics, immunosuppressives

MECHANISM OF ACTION

An immunologic agent that inhibits T-lymphocyte activation by binding to intracellular proteins, forming a complex, and inhibiting phosphatase activity. *Therapeutic Effect:* Suppresses the immunologically mediated inflammatory response; prevents organ transplant rejection.

PHARMACOKINETICS

Variably absorbed after PO administration (food reduces absorption). Protein binding: 75%-97%. Extensively metabolized in the liver. Excreted in urine. Not removed by hemodialysis. **Half-life:** 11.7 hr.

AVAILABILITY

Capsules (Prograf): 0.5 mg, 1 mg, 5 mg.

Injection (Prograf): 5 mg/ml.

Ointment (Protopic): 0.03%, 0.1%.

INDICATIONS AND DOSAGES

▸ **Prevention of liver transplant rejection**

PO

Adults, Elderly. 0.1-0.15 mg/kg/day in 2 divided doses 12 hr apart.

Children. 0.15-0.2 mg/kg/day in 2 divided doses 12 hr apart.

IV

Adults, Elderly, Children. 0.03-0.05 mg/kg/day as a continuous infusion.

▸ **Prevention of kidney transplant rejection**

PO

Adults, Elderly. 0.2 mg/kg/day in 2 divided doses 12 hr apart

IV

Adults, Elderly. 0.03-0.05 mg/kg/day as continuous infusion.

▸ **Atopic dermatitis**

TOPICAL

Adults, Elderly, Children 2 yr and older. Apply 0.03% ointment to affected area twice a day.

0.1% ointment may be used in adults and the elderly. Continue until 1 wk after symptoms have cleared.

OFF-LABEL USES
Prevention of organ rejection in patients receiving allogeneic bone marrow, heart, pancreas, pancreatic island cell, or small-bowel transplant, treatment of autoimmune disease, severe recalcitrant psoriasis

CONTRAINDICATIONS
Concurrent use with cyclosporine (increases the risk of nephrotoxicity), hypersensitivity to HCO-60 polyoxyl 60 hydrogenated castor oil (used in solution for injection), hypersensitivity to tacrolimus

INTERACTIONS
Drug
Aminoglycosides, amphotericin B, cisplatin: Increase the risk of renal dysfunction.
Antacids: Decrease the absorption of tacrolimus.
Antifungals, bromocriptine, calcium channel blockers, cimetidine, clarithromycin, cyclosporine, danazol, diltiazem, erythromycin, methylprednisolone, metoclopramide: Increase tacrolimus blood concentration.
Carbamazepine, phenobarbital, phenytoin, rifamycin: Decrease tacrolimus blood concentration.
Cyclosporine: Increases the risk of nephrotoxicity.
Live-virus vaccines: May potentiate virus replication, increase vaccine side effects, and decrease the patient's antibody response to the vaccine.
Other immunosuppressants: May increase the risk of infection or lymphomas.
Herbal
Echinacea: May decrease the effects of tacrolimus.

Food
Grapefruit, grapefruit juice: May alter the effects of the drug.

DIAGNOSTIC TEST EFFECTS
May increase blood glucose, BUN, and serum creatinine levels, as well as WBC count. May decrease serum magnesium level and RBC and thrombocyte counts. May alter serum potassium level.

IV INCOMPATIBILITIES
No known drug incompatibilities. Do not mix tacrolimus with other medications if possible.
IV Compatibilities
Calcium gluconate, dexamethasone (Decadron), diphenhydramine (Benadryl), dobutamine (Dobutrex), dopamine (Intropin), furosemide (Lasix), heparin, hydromorphone (Dilaudid), insulin, leucovorin, lorazepam (Ativan), morphine, nitroglycerin, potassium chloride

SIDE EFFECTS
Frequent (greater than 30%)
Headache, tremor, insomnia, paresthesia, diarrhea, nausea, constipation, vomiting, abdominal pain, hypertension
Occasional (29%-10%)
Rash, pruritus, anorexia, asthenia, peripheral edema, photosensitivity

SERIOUS REACTIONS
• Nephrotoxicity (characterized by increased serum creatinine level and decreased urine output), neurotoxicity (including tremor, headache, and mental status changes), and pleural effusion are common adverse reactions.
• Thrombocytopenia, leukocytosis, anemia, atelectasis, sepsis, and infection occur occasionally.

PRECAUTIONS & CONSIDERATIONS

Caution is warranted with immunosuppression and hepatic or renal impairment. Tacrolimus crosses the placenta and is distributed in breast milk. Females taking this drug should not breast-feed. Hyperkalemia and renal dysfunction have been noted in neonates. Children may require a higher dosage because of decreased bioavailability and increased clearance of the drug. Post-transplant lymphoproliferative disorder is more common in children, especially children younger than 3 years. Age-related renal impairment may require a dosage adjustment in the elderly. Avoid crowds and people with infection. Also avoid exposure to sunlight and artificial light because this may cause a photosensitivity reaction.

Notify the physician of change in mental status, chest pain, dizziness, headache, decreased urination, rash, respiratory infection, or unusual bleeding or bruising. CBC should be monitored weekly during the first month of therapy, twice monthly during the second and third months of treatment, then monthly for the rest of the first year. Liver function test results and serum creatinine and potassium levels should also be assessed.

Storage

Store the diluted solution in a glass or polyethylene containers and discard it after 24 hours. Don't store it in a polyvinyl chloride container because the container may absorb the drug or affect its stability.

Administration

! If unable to take capsules, initiate therapy with IV infusion. Give oral dose 8 to 12 hours after discontinuing IV infusion. Titrate dosage based on clinical assessments of rejection and tolerance. With hepatic or renal impairment, give the lowest IV and oral doses, as prescribed. Plan to delay administration for 48 hours or longer with postoperative oliguria.

Take oral tacrolimus on an empty stomach at the same time each day. Notify the physician if a dose is missed. Don't give this drug with grapefruit or grapefruit juice or within 2 hours of antacids.

Keep oxygen and an aqueous solution of epinephrine 1:1000 available at the bedside before beginning the IV infusion. Dilute the drug with 250 to 1000 ml 0.9% NaCl or D_5W, depending on the desired dose, to provide a concentration of 0.004 to 0.02 mg/ml. Administer tacrolimus as a continuous IV infusion. Monitor continuously for the first 30 minutes of the infusion and at frequent intervals thereafter. Stop the infusion immediately at the first sign of a hypersensitivity reaction.

Tacrolimus ointment is for external use only. Rub the ointment gently and completely into clean, dry skin. Don't cover the treated area with an occlusive dressing.

Tadalafil
(Cialis)

CATEGORY AND SCHEDULE

Pregnancy Risk Category: Not applicable

CLASSIFICATION

Impotence agents, phosphodiesterase inhibitors

MECHANISM OF ACTION

An erectile dysfunction agent that inhibits phosphodiesterase type 5, the enzyme responsible for degrading cyclic guanosine monophosphate in the corpus cavernosum of the penis, resulting in smooth muscle relaxation and increased blood flow. *Therapeutic Effect:* Facilitates an erection.

PHARMACOKINETICS

Route	Onset	Peak	Duration
PO	16 min	2 hr	36 hr

Rapidly absorbed after PO administration. Drug has no effect on penile blood flow without sexual stimulation. **Half-life:** 17.5 hr.

AVAILABILITY
Tablets: 5 mg, 10 mg, 20 mg.

INDICATIONS AND DOSAGES
▸ **Erectile dysfunction**
PO
Adults, Elderly. 10 mg 30 min before sexual activity. Dose may be increased to 20 mg or decreased to 5 mg, based on patient tolerance. Maximum dosing frequency is once daily.
▸ **Dosage in renal impairment**
For patients with a creatinine clearance of 31-50 ml/min, the starting dose is 5 mg before sexual activity once a day and the maximum dose is 10 mg no more frequently than once q48hr.
For patients with a creatinine clearance of less than 31 ml/min, the starting dose is 5 mg before sexual activity once a day.
▸ **Dosage in mild or moderate hepatic impairment**
Patients with Child-Pugh class A or B hepatic impairment should take no more than 10 mg once a day.

CONTRAINDICATIONS
Concurrent use of alpha-adrenergic blockers (other than the minimum

dose tamsulosin), concurrent use of sodium nitroprusside or nitrates in any form, severe hepatic impairment

INTERACTIONS
Drug
Alcohol: Increases the risk of orthostatic hypotension.
Alpha-adrenergic blockers, nitrates: Potentiate the hypotensive effects of these drugs.
Doxazosin: May produce additive hypotensive effects.
Erythromycin, indinavir, itraconazole, ketoconazole, ritonavir: May increase tadalafil blood concentration.
Herbal
None known.
Food
None known.

DIAGNOSTIC TEST EFFECTS
None known.

SIDE EFFECTS
Occasional
Headache, dyspepsia, back pain, myalgia, nasal congestion, flushing

SERIOUS REACTIONS
• Prolonged erections (lasting over 4 hours) and priapism (painful erections lasting over 6 hours) occur rarely.

PRECAUTIONS & CONSIDERATIONS
Caution is warranted with an anatomic deformity of the penis, cardiac, hepatic or renal impairment, and conditions that increase the risk of priapism, including leukemia, multiple myeloma, and sickle cell anemia. No age-related precautions have been noted in the elderly. This drug is not indicated for use in women and children. Be aware tadalafil is not effective without sexual stimulation. Avoid using nitrate drugs and alpha-adrenergic blockers concurrently with tadalafil.

Seek treatment immediately if an erection lasts longer than 4 hours.

Administration
Take tadalafil without regard to food. Don't crush or break film-coated tablets.

Talc Powder, Sterile
(Sclerosal)

CATEGORY AND SCHEDULE
Pregnancy Risk Category: B

CLASSIFICATION
Sclerosing agents

MECHANISM OF ACTION
A sclerosing agent that induces inflammatory reaction. *Therapeutic Effect:* Obliterates the pleural space and prevents re-accumulation of pleural fluid.

PHARMACOKINETICS
Systemic absorption after intrapleural administration has not been studied.

AVAILABILITY
Aerosol Spray, intrapleural: 4 g (Sclerosol).

INDICATIONS AND DOSAGES
▸ **Pleural effusions**
AEROSOL
Adults. 8 g as single treatment.

CONTRAINDICATIONS
Sensitivity to talc powder or any component of the formulation

INTERACTIONS
Drug
None known.
Herbal
None known.

Food
None known.

DIAGNOSTIC TEST EFFECTS
None known.

SIDE EFFECTS
Rare
Pain

SERIOUS REACTIONS
• Atrial arrhythmias, hypotension, cardiac arrest, chest pain, tachycardia, hypovolemia, asystolic arrest, myocardial infarction, and respiratory complications have been reported.

PRECAUTIONS & CONSIDERATIONS
Be aware that pulmonary complications can occur with talc use. It is unknown if talc crosses the placenta or is distributed in breast milk. Safety and efficacy have not been established in children. There are no age-related precautions noted in the elderly.

Storage
Store aerosol at room temperature. Protect from direct sunlight.

Administration
Shake canister well, remove protective cap, and securely attach the actuator button with the selected delivery tube (either 15 or 25 cm in length) to the valve stem. The total dose should be administered in several short bursts, given with the delivery tube pointing in different directions. Delivery depends on the extent and duration of manual compression of the actuator button. The canister should be kept in an upright position during administration. The spray valve delivers talc at a rate of approximately 0.4 grams/second, but the medication is not delivered as a metered dose.

Tamoxifen
ta-mox'i-fen
(Apo-Tamox [CAN],
Genox [AUS], Istubol,
Nolvadex, Nolvadex-D [CAN],
Novo-Tamoxifen [CAN],
Tamofen [CAN], Tamosin [AUS])

CATEGORY AND SCHEDULE
Pregnancy Risk Category: D

CLASSIFICATION
Antineoplastics, antiestrogens,
estrogen receptor modulators,
selective, hormones/hormone
modifiers

MECHANISM OF ACTION
A nonsteroidal antiestrogen that
competes with estradiol for estrogen-
receptor binding sites in the breasts,
uterus, and vagina. *Therapeutic
Effect:* Inhibits DNA synthesis and
estrogen response.

PHARMACOKINETICS
Well absorbed from the GI tract.
Metabolized in the liver. Primarily
eliminated in feces by biliary
system. **Half-life:** 7 days.

AVAILABILITY
Tablets: 10 mg, 20 mg.

INDICATIONS AND DOSAGES
▸ **Adjunctive treatment of breast
cancer**
PO
Adults, Elderly. 20-40 mg/day. Give
doses greater than 20 mg/day in
divided doses.
▸ **Prevention of breast cancer in
high-risk women**
PO
Adults, Elderly. 20 mg/day.

OFF-LABEL USES
Induction of ovulation

CONTRAINDICATIONS
None known.

INTERACTIONS
Drug
Estrogens: May decrease the effects
of tamoxifen.
Herbal
None known.
Food
None known.

DIAGNOSTIC TEST EFFECTS
May increase serum cholesterol,
calcium, and triglyceride levels.

SIDE EFFECTS
Frequent
Women (greater than 10%): Hot
flashes, nausea, vomiting
Occasional
Women (9%-1%): Changes in
menstruation, genital itching, vaginal
discharge, endometrial hyperplasia
or polyps
Men: Impotence, decreased libido
Men and women: Headache, nausea,
vomiting, rash, bone pain, confusion,
weakness, somnolence

SERIOUS REACTIONS
• Retinopathy, corneal opacity, and
decreased visual acuity have been
noted in patients receiving extremely
high dosages (240-320 mg/day) for
longer than 17 months.

PRECAUTIONS & CONSIDERATIONS
Caution is warranted with leukopenia
and thrombocytopenia. Tamoxifen
use should be avoided during pregnancy, especially during the first
trimester, because it may cause fetal
harm. Nonhormonal contraception
should be used during treatment. It's
unknown if tamoxifen is distributed in

breast milk; however, breast-feeding is not recommended. Tamoxifen use is safe and effective in girls aged 2 to 10 years with McCune Albright syndrome and precocious puberty. No age-related precautions have been noted in the elderly.

Initially, an increase in bone and tumor pain, may occur which indicates a good tumor response to tamoxifen. Notify the physician if nausea and vomiting, leg cramps, weakness, weight gain, or vaginal bleeding, itching, or discharge, develops. Intake and output, weight, CBC, and serum calcium levels should be monitored before and periodically during tamoxifen therapy. An estrogen receptor assay test should be performed before beginning treatment. Signs and symptoms for hypercalcemia, including constipation, deep bone or flank pain, excessive thirst, hypotonicity of muscles, increased urine output, nausea and vomiting, and renal calculi, should be assessed.

Storage
Store at room temperature.
Administration
Take oral tamoxifen without regard to food.

Tamsulosin
tam-sool′o-sin
(Flomax)
Do not confuse Flomax with Fosamax or Volmax.

CATEGORY AND SCHEDULE
Pregnancy Risk Category: B
(Not indicated for use in women.)

CLASSIFICATION
Antiadrenergics, alpha blocking

MECHANISM OF ACTION
An alpha$_1$ antagonist that targets receptors around bladder neck and prostate capsule. *Therapeutic Effect:* Relaxes smooth muscle and improves urinary flow and symptoms of prostatic hyperplasia.

PHARMACOKINETICS
Well absorbed and widely distributed. Protein binding: 94%-99%. Metabolized in the liver. Primarily excreted in urine. Unknown if removed by hemodialysis. **Half-life:** 9-13 hr.

AVAILABILITY
Capsules: 0.4 mg.

INDICATIONS AND DOSAGES
▸ **Benign prostatic hyperplasia**
PO
Adults. 0.4 mg once a day, approximately 30 min after same meal each day. May increase dosage to 0.8 mg if inadequate response in 2-4 wk.

CONTRAINDICATIONS
History of sensitivity to tamsulosin

INTERACTIONS
Drug
Other alpha-adrenergic blocking agents (such as cimetidine, doxazosin, prazosin, terazosin): May increase the alpha-blockade effects of both drugs.
Warfarin: May alter the effects of warfarin.
Herbal
None known.
Food
None known.

DIAGNOSTIC TEST EFFECTS
None known.

SIDE EFFECTS
Frequent (9%-7%)
Dizziness, somnolence

Occasional (5%-3%)
Headache, anxiety, insomnia, ortho-
static hypotension
Rare (less than 2%)
Nasal congestion, pharyngitis, rhinitis,
nausea, vertigo, impotence

SERIOUS REACTIONS
• First-dose syncope (hypotension
with sudden loss of consciousness)
may occur within 30 to 90 minutes
after administration of initial dose
and may be preceded by tachycardia
(pulse rate of 120-160 beats/minute).

PRECAUTIONS & CONSIDERATIONS
Caution is warranted with renal
impairment. Tamsulosin is not indicated for use in women or children.
No age-related precautions have been
noted in the elderly. Tell the physician if using other alpha-adrenergic
blocking agents or warfarin.
   Dizziness and lightheadedness
may occur. Tasks that require mental
alertness or motor skills should be
avoided until response to the drug is
established. Caution should be used
when getting up from a sitting or
lying position. B/P and renal function
should be monitored.
Administration
Take at the same time each day,
30 minutes after the same meal. Do
not crush or open capsule unless
directed by the physician.

Tazarotene
ta-zare'oh-teen
(Tazorac, Avage)

CATEGORY AND SCHEDULE
Pregnancy Risk Category: X

CLASSIFICATION
Dermatologics, retinoids

MECHANISM OF ACTION
Modulates differentiation and
proliferation of epithelial tissue,
binds, selectively to retinoic acid
receptors. *Therapeutic Effect:*
Restores normal differentiation of
the epidermis and reduction in
epidermal inflammation.

PHARMACOKINETICS
Minimal systemic absorption occurs
through the skin. Binding to plasma
proteins is greater than 99%.
Metabolism is in the skin and liver.
Elimination occurs through the
fecal and renal pathways. **Half-life:**
18 hr.

AVAILABILITY
Gel: 0.05%, 0.1% (Tazorac)
Cream: 0.05%, 0.1% (Tazorac)

INDICATIONS AND DOSAGES
▸ **Psoriasis**
TOPICAL
*Adults, adolescents, children
>12 yr.* Thin film applied once
daily in the evening; only cover the
lesions, and area should be dry
before application
▸ **Acne vulgaris**
TOPICAL
*Adults, adolescents, children
>12 yr.* Thin film applied to
affected areas once daily in the

T

evening, after face is gently cleansed and dried.
Fine facial wrinkles, facial mottled hyperpigmentation (liver spots), hypopigmentation associated with photoaging
TOPICAL
Adults. Thin film applied to affected areas once daily in the evening, after face is gently cleansed and dried.

CONTRAINDICATIONS
Should not be used in pregnant women, patients with hypersensitivity to tazarotene, benzyl alcohol, or any one of its components.

INTERACTIONS
Drug
Ethanol, benzoyl peroxide, resorcinol, salicylic acid, sulfur: Increases the drying effect.
Quinolones, phenothiazines, sulfonamides, sulfonylureas, tetracyclines, thiazide diuretics: Increase the risk of photosensitivity.
Herbal
None known.
Food
None known.

DIAGNOSTIC TEST EFFECTS
None known.

SIDE EFFECTS
Frequent
Desquamation, burning or stinging, dry skin, itching, erythema, worsening of psoriasis, irritation, skin pain, pruritis, xerosis, photosensitivity
Occasional
Irritation, skin pain, fissuring, localized edema, skin discoloration, rash, desquamation, contact dermatitis, skin inflammation, bleeding, dry skin, hypertriglyceridemia, peripheral edema, acne vulgaris, cheilitis

PRECAUTIONS & CONSIDERATIONS
Caution is warranted with other skin conditions such as eczema, sunburn, and undiagnosed skin lesions.
Tazarotene is not recommended during pregnancy. It is unknown if it enters the breast milk. Safety and efficacy have not been established in children or the elderly.
   Burning or stinging after application, dryness, itching, peeling, or redness of the skin may occur during tazarotene therapy. Avoid direct exposure to sunlight.
Storage
Store at room temperature away from heat and direct light.
Administration
Tazarotene is for external use only. Apply only on face, once daily at bedtime, or as directed by physician. Remove any make-up, gently wash face with a mild cleanser, and pat skin dry. Wait at least 20 minutes to make sure face is dry before applying a small, pea-sized amount (about 1/4-inch wide) of medication. Apply in a thin layer over wrinkles and discolored spots. Wash hands after using the medication. In the morning, apply a moisturizing sunscreen with SPF 15 or greater.

Tegaserod
teh-gas′er-od
(Zelnorm)

CATEGORY AND SCHEDULE
Pregnancy Risk Category: B

CLASSIFICATION
Gastrointestinals, serotonin receptor agonists

MECHANISM OF ACTION
An anti-irritable bowel syndrome (IBS) agent that binds to 5-HT$_4$ receptors in the GI tract. *Therapeutic Effect:* Triggers a peristaltic reflex in the gut, increasing bowel motility.

PHARMACOKINETICS
Rapidly absorbed. Widely distributed. Protein binding: 98%. Metabolized by hydrolysis in the stomach and by oxidation and conjugation of the primary metabolite. Primarily excreted in feces. **Half-life:** 11 hr.

AVAILABILITY
Tablets: 2 mg, 6 mg.

INDICATIONS AND DOSAGES
▸ **IBS**
PO
Adults, Elderly women. 6 mg twice a day for 4-6 wk.
▸ **Chronic constipation**
PO
Adults. 6 mg 2 times/day.

CONTRAINDICATIONS
Abdominal adhesions, diarrhea, history of bowel obstruction, moderate to severe hepatic impairment, severe renal impairment, suspected sphincter of Oddi dysfunction, symptomatic gallbladder disease

INTERACTIONS
Drug
None known.
Herbal
None known.
Food
None known.

DIAGNOSTIC TEST EFFECTS
None known.

SIDE EFFECTS
Frequency (greater than 5%)
Headache, abdominal pain, diarrhea, nausea, flatulence
Occasional (5%-2%)
Dizziness, migraine, back pain, extremity pain

SERIOUS REACTIONS
• None known.

PRECAUTIONS & CONSIDERATIONS
It is unknown if tegaserod is distributed in breast milk. Safety and efficacy of tegaserod have not been established in children. No age-related precautions have been noted in the elderly. Avoid tegaserod use if diarrhea is present.

Notify the physician if new or worsening episodes of abdominal pain or severe diarrhea occur. Therapeutic response (relief from abdominal discomfort, bloating, cramping, and urgency) should be assessed.
Administration
Take tegaserod before meals. Crush tablets as needed.

Telithromycin
tell-ith′roe-my-sin
(Ketek)

CATEGORY AND SCHEDULE
Pregnancy Risk Category: C

CLASSIFICATION
Antibiotics, ketolides

MECHANISM OF ACTION
A ketolide that blocks protein synthesis by binding to ribosomal receptor sites on the bacterial cell wall. *Therapeutic Effect:* Bactericidal.

PHARMACOKINETICS

Protein binding: 60%-70%. More of drug is concentrated in WBCs than in plasma, and drug is eliminated more slowly from WBCs than from plasma. Partially metabolized by the liver. Minimally excreted in feces and urine. **Half-life:** 10 hr.

AVAILABILITY

Tablets: 400 mg.

INDICATIONS AND DOSAGES

▶ **Chronic bronchitis, sinusitis**
PO
Adults, Elderly. 800 mg once a day for 5 days.
▶ **Community-acquired pneumonia**
PO
Adults, Elderly. 800 mg once a day for 7-10 days.

CONTRAINDICATIONS

Hypersensitivity to macrolide antibiotics, concurrent use of cisapride or pimozide

INTERACTIONS

Drug
Atorvastatin, digoxin, lovastatin, metoprolol, pimozide, simvastatin, theophylline: May increase the blood concentration and toxicity of these drugs.
Carbamazepine, phenobarbital, phenytoin, rifampin: May decrease the blood concentration of telithromycin.
Cisapride: Increases blood concentration of cisapride, resulting in significantly increased QT interval.
Itraconazole, ketoconazole: May increase the blood concentration of telithromycin.
Sotolol: Decreases the blood concentration of sotalol.
Herbal
None known.

Food
None known.

DIAGNOSTIC TEST EFFECTS

May increase platelet count and AST (SGOT) and ALT (SGPT) levels.

SIDE EFFECTS

Occasional (11%-4%)
Diarrhea, nausea, headache, dizziness
Rare (3%-2%)
Vomiting, loose stools, altered taste, dry mouth, flatulence, visual disturbances

SERIOUS REACTIONS

• Hepatic dysfunction, severe hypersensitivity reaction, and atrial arrhythmias occur rarely.
• Antibiotic-associated colitis and other superinfections may result from altered bacterial balance.

PRECAUTIONS & CONSIDERATIONS

Caution is warranted with uncorrected hypokalemia, hypomagnesemia, bradycardia, concomitant use of class IA or III antiarrhythmics, QTc interval prolongation, myasthenia gravis, and history of hepatitis or jaundice associated with telithromycin use. It is unknown if telithromycin is distributed in breast milk. Safety and efficacy of telithromycin have not been established in children. In those elderly with normal renal function, no age-related precautions are noted. Be aware that there is a potential for visual disturbances. Nausea, vomiting, diarrhea, headache, and dizziness are other possible side effects.
Storage
Store at room temperature.
Administration
Take medication with 8 oz of water at least 1 hour before or 2 hours after consuming any food or beverages. Do not break or crush film-coated tablets.

Telmisartan

tel-meh-sar'tan
(Micardis, Pritor [AUS])

CATEGORY AND SCHEDULE

Pregnancy Risk Category: C
(D if used in second or third
trimester)

CLASSIFICATION

Angiotensin II receptor
antagonists

MECHANISM OF ACTION

An angiotensin II receptor, type AT_1,
antagonist that blocks vasoconstrictor and aldosterone-secreting effects
of angiotensin II, inhibiting the binding of angiotensin II to the AT_1
receptors. *Therapeutic Effect:* Causes
vasodilation, decreases peripheral
resistance, and decreases B/P.

PHARMACOKINETICS

Rapidly and completely absorbed
after PO administration. Protein
binding: 99%. Undergoes metabolism in the liver to inactive metabolite. Excreted in feces. Unknown
if removed by hemodialysis.
Half-life: 24 hr.

AVAILABILITY

Tablets: 20 mg, 40 mg, 80 mg.

INDICATIONS AND DOSAGES

▶ **Hypertension**
PO
Adults, Elderly. 40 mg once a day.
Range: 20-80 mg/day.

OFF-LABEL USES

Treatment of CHF

CONTRAINDICATIONS

None known.

INTERACTIONS

Drug
Digoxin: Increases digoxin plasma
concentration.
Warfarin: Slightly decreases
warfarin plasma concentration.
Herbal
None known.
Food
None known.

DIAGNOSTIC TEST EFFECTS

May increase serum creatinine level.
May decrease blood Hgb and Hct
levels.

SIDE EFFECTS

Occasional (7%-3%)
Upper respiratory tract infection,
sinusitis, back or leg pain, diarrhea
Rare (1%)
Dizziness, headache, fatigue, nausea,
heartburn, myalgia, cough, peripheral
edema

SERIOUS REACTIONS

• Overdosage may manifest as
hypotension and tachycardia.
Bradycardia occurs less often.

PRECAUTIONS & CONSIDERATIONS

Caution is warranted with hepatic
and renal impairment, renal artery
stenosis (bilateral or unilateral), and
volume depletion. It is unknown if
telmisartan is excreted in breast
milk; it may cause fetal harm. Safety
and efficacy of telmisartan have
not been established in children.
No age-related precautions have
been noted in the elderly.

Dizziness may occur. Tasks that
require mental alertness or motor
skills should be avoided. Notify the
physician if fever or sore throat
occurs. Apical pulse and B/P should
be assessed immediately before each
olmesartan dose, and regularly
throughout therapy. Be alert to

T

fluctuations in apical pulse and B/P. If an excessive reduction in B/P occurs, place the person in the supine position with feet slightly elevated and notify the physician. Pulse rate, and BUN, serum creatinine, and serum electrolyte levels should be assessed. Maintain adequate hydration; exercising outside during hot weather should be avoided in order to decrease the risk of dehydration and hypotension.

Administration

! May be given concurrently with other antihypertensives. If B/P is not controlled by telmisartan alone, a diuretic may be added.

Take telmisartan without regard to meals.

Temazepam
te-maz′e-pam
(Apo-Temazepam [CAN], Novo-Temazepam [CAN], PMS-Temazepam [CAN], Restoril)
Do not confuse Restoril with Vistaril or Zestril.

CATEGORY AND SCHEDULE
Pregnancy Risk Category: X
Controlled Substance:
Schedule IV

CLASSIFICATION
Benzodiazepines, sedatives/hypnotics

MECHANISM OF ACTION
A benzodiazepine that enhances the action of the inhibitory neurotransmitter gamma-aminobutyric acid, resulting in CNS depression. *Therapeutic Effect:* Induces sleep.

PHARMACOKINETICS
Well absorbed from the GI tract. Protein binding: 96%. Widely distributed. Crosses the blood-brain barrier. Metabolized in the liver. Primarily excreted in urine. Not removed by hemodialysis. **Half-life:** 4-18 hr.

AVAILABILITY
Capsules: 7.5 mg, 15 mg, 30 mg.

INDICATIONS AND DOSAGES
▸ **Insomnia**
PO
Adults, Children 18 yr and older. 15-30 mg at bedtime.
Elderly, Debilitated. 7.5-15 mg at bedtime.

CONTRAINDICATIONS
Angle-closure glaucoma; CNS depression; pregnancy or breast-feeding; severe, uncontrolled pain; sleep apnea

INTERACTIONS
Drug
Alcohol, other CNS depressants: May increase CNS depression.
Herbal
Kava kava, valerian: May increase CNS depression.
Food
None known.

DIAGNOSTIC TEST EFFECTS
None known.

SIDE EFFECTS
Frequent
Somnolence, sedation, rebound insomnia (may occur for 1-2 nights after drug is discontinued), dizziness, confusion, euphoria
Occasional
Asthenia, anorexia, diarrhea

Rare
Paradoxical CNS excitement or restlessness (particularly in elderly or debilitated patients)

SERIOUS REACTIONS
• Abrupt or too-rapid withdrawal may result in pronounced restlessness, irritability, insomnia, hand tremor, abdominal or muscle cramps, vomiting, diaphoresis, and seizures.
• Overdose results in somnolence, confusion, diminished reflexes, respiratory depression, and coma.

PRECAUTIONS & CONSIDERATIONS
Caution is warranted with mental impairment and the potential for drug dependence. Temazepam crosses the placenta and may be distributed in breast milk. Long-term use of flurazepam during pregnancy may produce withdrawal symptoms and CNS depression in neonates. Keep in mind that the drug is FDA pregnancy risk category X and should not be used during pregnancy. Temazepam use is not recommended for children younger than 18 years. To avoid ataxia or excessive sedation in the elderly, plan to administer small doses initially and to increase dosage gradually.

Drowsiness may occur. Avoid alcohol, CNS depressants, and tasks that require mental alertness and motor skills. B/P, pulse rate, and respiratory rate, rhythm, and depth before should be assessed before administering temazepam. Cardiovascular, mental, and respiratory status should be monitored throughout therapy.

Administration
If desired, open temazepam capsules and mix the contents with food. Take temazepam 30 minutes before bedtime.

Temozolomide
tem-oh-zohl'oh-mide
(Temodal [AUS], Temodar)

CATEGORY AND SCHEDULE
Pregnancy Risk Category: D

CLASSIFICATION
Antineoplastics, alkylating agents

MECHANISM OF ACTION
An imidazotetrazine derivative that acts as a prodrug and is converted to a highly active cytotoxic metabolite. Its cytotoxic effect is associated with methylation of DNA. *Therapeutic Effect:* Inhibits DNA replication, causing cell death.

PHARMACOKINETICS
Rapidly and completely absorbed after PO administration. Protein binding: 15%. Peak plasma concentration occurs in 1 hr. Penetrates the blood-brain barrier. Eliminated primarily in urine and, to a much lesser extent, in feces. **Half-life:** 1.6-1.8 hr.

AVAILABILITY
Capsules: 5 mg, 20 mg, 100 mg, 250 mg.

INDICATIONS AND DOSAGES
▶ **Anaplastic astrocytoma**
PO
Adults, Elderly. Initially, 150 mg/m²/day for 5 consecutive days of a 28-day treatment cycle. Subsequent doses based on platelet count and ANC during previous cycle. ANC greater than 1500 per microliter and platelet: more than 100,000 per microliter. Maintenance: 200 mg/m²/day for 5 days q4wk. Continue until disease progression.

Minimum: 100 mg/m^2/day for 5 days q4wk.

CONTRAINDICATIONS

Hypersensitivity to dacarbazine, pregnancy

INTERACTIONS

Drug

Live-virus vaccines: May potentiate virus replication, increase vaccine side effects, and decrease the patient's antibody response to the vaccine.
Valproic acid: Decreases the clearance of temozolomide.
Herbal
None known.
Food
All foods: Decrease the rate of drug absorption.

DIAGNOSTIC TEST EFFECTS

May decrease blood Hgb levels and neutrophil, platelet, and WBC counts.

SIDE EFFECTS

Frequent (53%-33%)
Nausea, vomiting, headache, fatigue, constipation
Occasional (16%-10%)
Diarrhea, asthenia, fever, dizziness, peripheral edema, incoordination, insomnia
Rare (9%-5%)
Paraesthesia, drowsiness, anorexia, urinary incontinence, anxiety, pharyngitis, cough

SERIOUS REACTIONS

• Elderly patients and women are at increased risk for developing severe myelosuppression, characterized by neutropenia and thrombocytopenia and usually occurring within the first few cycles. Neutrophil and platelet counts reach their nadirs approximately 26-28 days after administration and recover within 14 days of the nadir.

PRECAUTIONS & CONSIDERATIONS

Caution is warranted with severe hepatic or renal impairment. Temozolomide use should be avoided during pregnancy because the drug may cause fetal harm. Although it's unknown if temozolomide is excreted in breast milk, women taking this drug should avoid breast-feeding. The safety and efficacy of temozolomide have not been established in children. The elderly, over 70 years, have a higher risk of developing grade 4 neutropenia and grade 4 thrombocytopenia. Vaccinations and coming in contact with crowds and people with known infections should be avoided.

Notify the physician if he or she experiences easy bruising, fever, signs of local infection, sore throat, or unusual bleeding from any site. Before administration, absolute neutrophil count (ANC) must be greater than 1500/mm^3 and the platelet count must be greater than 100,000/mm^3. To control nausea and vomiting, antiemetics should be administered. A CBC on day 22 (21 days after the first dose) or within 48 hours of that day and then weekly until the ANC is greater than 1500/mm^3 and the platelet count is greater than 100,000/mm^3 should be ordered.

Administration

! Because temozolomide is cytotoxic, avoid touching the contents of an open capsule during preparation and administration.

Administer temozolomide on an empty stomach because food reduces the rate and extent of drug absorption and increases the risk of nausea and vomiting. For best results, take temozolomide at bedtime. Swallow the capsule whole with a glass of water. If the patient can't swallow, open the capsule and mix the contents with applesauce or apple juice.

Tenecteplase
ten'neck-te-place
(Metalyse [AUS], TNKase)

CATEGORY AND SCHEDULE
Pregnancy Risk Category: C

CLASSIFICATION
Thrombolytics

MECHANISM OF ACTION
A tissue plasminogen activator produced by recombinant DNA that binds to fibrin and converts plasminogen to plasmin. Initiates fibrinolysis by degrading fibrin clots, fibrinogen, other plasma proteins. *Therapeutic Effect:* Exerts thrombolytic action.

PHARMACOKINETICS
Extensively distributed to tissues. Completely eliminated by hepatic metabolism. **Half-life:** 11-20 min.

AVAILABILITY
Powder for Injection: 50 mg.

INDICATIONS AND DOSAGES
▸ Acute MI
IV
Adults. Dosage is based on patient's weight. Treatment should be initiated as soon as possible after onset of symptoms.

Weight (kg)	(mg)	(ml)
90 or more	50	10
80 to less than 90	45	9
70 to less than 80	40	8
60 to less than 70	35	7
Less than 60	30	6

CONTRAINDICATIONS
Active internal bleeding, aneurysm, AV malformation, bleeding diathesis, history of cerebrovascular accident, intracranial or intraspinal surgery or trauma within past 2 months, intracranial neoplasm, severe uncontrolled hypertension

INTERACTIONS
Drug
Anticoagulants (such as heparin, warfarin), aspirin, dipyridamole, glycoprotein IIb/IIIa inhibitors: Increase the risk of bleeding.
Herbal
Ginkgo biloba: May increase the risk of bleeding.
Food
None known.

DIAGNOSTIC TEST EFFECTS
Decreases plasminogen and fibrinogen levels during infusion, decreasing clotting time and confirming presence of lysis. Decreases Hct and Hgb.

IV INCOMPATIBILITIES
Do not mix with other medications.

SIDE EFFECTS
Frequent
Bleeding (major, 4.7%; minor, 21.8%)

SERIOUS REACTIONS
• Bleeding at internal sites may occur, including intracranial, retroperitoneal, GI, GU, and respiratory sites.
• Lysis or coronary thrombi may produce atrial or ventricular arrhythmias and stroke.

PRECAUTIONS & CONSIDERATIONS
Caution is warranted with severe hepatic impairment and in those who have previously received tenecteplase. It is unknown if tenecteplase is distributed in breast milk. Safety and

efficacy of tenecteplase have not been established in children. The elderly may have an increased risk of intracranial hemorrhage, major bleeding, and stroke. Tenecteplase should be used cautiously in this population. An electric razor and a soft toothbrush should be used to reduce the risk of bleeding.

Notify the physician of bruises, back or abdominal pain, black or red stool, coffee-ground vomitus, dark or red urine, red-speckled mucus from cough, chest pain, headache, palpitations, or shortness of breath. Continuous cardiac monitoring for arrhythmias, B/P, and pulse and respiration rates every 15 minutes should be performed until the patient is stable, then hourly. Cardiac enzyme concentrations, 12-lead EKG, electrolyte levels, aPTT, Hct, Hgb, fibrinogen level, platelet count, and thrombin time should be evaluated before and during therapy.

Storage

Store at room temperature. If possible, use immediately after reconstitution but may refrigerate for up to 8 hours. Discard after 8 hours.

Administration

❗ Give as a single IV bolus over 5 seconds. Precipitate may occur when given in an IV line containing dextrose. Flush line with saline before and after administration.

Tenecteplase is normally a colorless to pale yellow solution. Do not use if solution is discolored or contains particulates. Add 10 ml sterile water for injection without preservative to vial to provide concentration of 5 mg/ml. Gently swirl until dissolved. Do not shake. If foaming occurs, allow vial to sit undisturbed for several minutes. Administer as IV push over 5 seconds.

Teniposide
ten-i-poe′side
(Vumon)

CATEGORY AND SCHEDULE
Pregnancy Risk Category: D

CLASSIFICATION
Antineoplastics, epipodophyllotoxins

MECHANISM OF ACTION
An epipodophyllotoxin that induces single- and double-strand breaks in DNA, inhibiting or altering DNA synthesis. Acts in the late S and early G_2 phases of cell cycle. *Therapeutic Effect:* Prevents cells from entering mitosis.

AVAILABILITY
Injection: 50 mg.

INDICATIONS AND DOSAGES
▸ **Induction therapy in patients with refractory childhood acute lymphoblastic leukemia (in combination with other antineoplastic agents)**
Children. Dosage is individualized based on the patient's clinical response and tolerance of the drug's adverse effects. When used in combination therapy, consult specific protocols for optimum dosage or sequence of drug administration.

CONTRAINDICATIONS
Absolute neutrophil count less than 500/mm³; hypersensitivity to Cremophor EL (polyoxyethylated castor oil), etoposide, or teniposide; platelet count less than 50,000/mm³

INTERACTIONS
Drug
Bone marrow depressants: May increase myelosuppression.

Live-virus vaccines: May potentiate virus replication, increase vaccine side effects, and decrease the patient's antibody response to the vaccine.
Methotrexate: May increase intracellular accumulation of this drug.
Vincristine: May increase the severity of peripheral neuropathy.
Herbal
None known.
Food
None known.

DIAGNOSTIC TEST EFFECTS
None significant.

SIDE EFFECTS
Frequent (greater than 30%)
Mucositis, nausea, vomiting, diarrhea, anemia
Occasional (5%-3%)
Alopecia, rash
Rare (less than 3%)
Hepatic dysfunction, fever, renal dysfunction, peripheral neurotoxicity

SERIOUS REACTIONS
• Myelosuppression manifested as hematologic toxicity (principally leukopenia, neutropenia, and thrombocytopenia) may be severe and may increase the risk of infection or bleeding.
• Hypersensitivity reaction may include anaphylaxis (marked by chills, fever, tachycardia, bronchospasm, dyspnea, and facial flushing).

PRECAUTIONS & CONSIDERATIONS
Caution is warranted with brain tumors, hepatic dysfunction, Down syndrome, and neuroblastoma (increases the risk of anaphylaxis). Women of childbearing age should be cautioned to avoid pregnancy during teniposide therapy. Contraceptive methods should be practiced. Vaccinations and coming in contact with crowds and people with known infections should be avoided.

Notify the physician if fever, signs of local infection, or unusual bleeding from any site occurs.

Appropriate medication and equipment should be readily available before giving the first dose in case life-threatening anaphylaxis occurs. Hematologic, liver, and renal function test results should be assessed before and frequently during teniposide therapy.
Storage
Refrigerate unopened ampoules, and protect them from light.
Reconstituted solutions are stable for 24 hours at room temperature. They should not be refrigerated.
Administration
! Wear gloves when preparing the solution. If the solution comes in contact with your skin, wash immediately and thoroughly with soap and water.

Dilute with 0.9% NaCl or D_5W to provide a concentration of 0.1 to 1 mg/ml. Prepare and administer the drug in glass containers or polyolefin plastic bags. Do not use polyvinyl chloride containers. Use the 1-mg/ml solution within 4 hours of preparation to reduce the risk of precipitation. Discard the solution if precipitation occurs. Infuse teniposide over at least 30 to 60 minutes. Avoid rapid IV injection.

T

Tenofovir
ten-oh′foh-veer
(Viread)

CATEGORY AND SCHEDULE
Pregnancy Risk Category: B

CLASSIFICATION
Antivirals, nucleotide reverse
transcriptase inhibitors

MECHANISM OF ACTION
A nucleotide analogue that inhibits
HIV reverse transcriptase by being
incorporated into viral DNA, resulting in DNA chain termination.
Therapeutic Effect: Slows HIV replication and reduces HIV RNA levels
(viral load).

AVAILABILITY
Tablets: 300 mg.

INDICATIONS AND DOSAGES
▸ **HIV infection (in combination with
other antiretrovirals)**
PO
*Adults, Elderly, Children 18 yr and
older.* 300 mg once a day.

CONTRAINDICATIONS
None known.

INTERACTIONS
Drug
Didanosine: May increase didano-
sine blood concentration.
**Indinavir, lamivudine, lopinavir,
ritonavir:** May decrease the
blood concentrations of these
drugs.
Herbal
None known.
Food
High-fat food: Increases tenofovir
bioavailability.

DIAGNOSTIC TEST EFFECTS
May elevate liver function test
results. May alter serum CK, GGT,
uric acid, AST (SGOT), ALT
(SGPT), and triglyceride levels as
well as creatinine clearance.

SIDE EFFECTS
Occasional
GI disturbances (diarrhea, flatulence,
nausea, vomiting)

SERIOUS REACTIONS
• Lactic acidosis and hepatomegaly
with steatosis occur rarely, but may
be severe.

PRECAUTIONS & CONSIDERATIONS
Caution should be used with impaired
liver or renal function. Check baseline laboratory test results, if ordered,
especially liver function test results
and serum triglyceride levels before
beginning tenofovir therapy and at
periodic intervals during therapy.
Tenofovir is not a cure for HIV
infection, nor does it reduce risk of
transmission to others; illnesses associated with advanced HIV infection.
Monitor CD4 cell count, complete
blood count (CBC), Hgb levels, HIV
RNA plasma levels, liver function
test results, and reticulocyte count.
Assess pattern of daily bowel activity and stool consistency. Notify the
physician if nausea, persistent
abdominal pain, or vomiting occurs.
Administration
Give with food to increase the drug's
absorption. Continue drug therapy
for the full length of treatment.

Terazosin
ter-a′zoe-sin
(Apo-Terazosin [CAN], Hytrin,
Novo-Terazosin [CAN])

CATEGORY AND SCHEDULE
Pregnancy Risk Category: C

CLASSIFICATION
Antiadrenergics, alpha blocking,
peripheral

MECHANISM OF ACTION
An antihypertensive and benign
prostatic hyperplasia agent that
blocks alpha-adrenergic receptors.
Produces vasodilation, decreases
peripheral resistance, and targets
receptors around bladder neck and
prostate. *Therapeutic Effect:* In
hypertension, decreases B/P. In
benign prostatic hyperplasia, relaxes
smooth muscle and improves urine
flow.

PHARMACOKINETICS

Route	Onset	Peak	Duration
PO	15 min	1-2 hr	12-24 hr

Rapidly, completely absorbed from
the GI tract. Protein binding: 90%-
94%. Metabolized in the liver to
active metabolite. Primarily eliminated in feces via biliary system;
excreted in urine. Not removed by
hemodialysis. **Half-life:** 12 hr.

AVAILABILITY
Capsules: 1 mg, 2 mg, 5 mg, 10 mg.
Tablets: 1 mg, 2 mg, 5 mg, 10 mg.

INDICATIONS AND DOSAGES
▸ **Mild to moderate hypertension**

PO
Adults, Elderly. Initially, 1 mg at
bedtime. Slowly increase dosage to
desired levels. Range: 1-5 mg/day as
single or 2 divided doses. Maximum:
20 mg.
▸ **Benign prostatic hyperplasia**
PO
Adults, Elderly. Initially, 1 mg at
bedtime. May increase up to
10 mg/day. Maximum: 20 mg/day.

CONTRAINDICATIONS
None known.

INTERACTIONS
Drug
**Estrogen, NSAIDs, other sympa-
thomimetics:** May decrease the
effects of terazosin.
**Hypotension-producing medica-
tions, such as antihypertensives
and diuretics:** May increase the
effects of terazosin.
Herbal
**Dong quai, ginseng, garlic,
yohimbe:** May decrease the effects
of terazosin.
Food
None known.

DIAGNOSTIC TEST EFFECTS
May decrease blood Hgb and Hct
levels, serum albumin level, total
serum protein level, and WBC count.

SIDE EFFECTS
Frequent (9%-5%)
Dizziness, headache, unusual
tiredness
Rare (less than 2%)
Peripheral edema, orthostatic
hypotension, myalgia, arthralgia,
blurred vision, nausea, vomiting,
nasal congestion, somnolence

SERIOUS REACTIONS
• First-dose syncope (hypotension
with sudden loss of consciousness)

T

may occur 30 to 90 minutes after initial dose of 2 mg or more, a too rapid increase in dosage, or addition of another antihypertensive agent to therapy. First-dose syncope may be preceded by tachycardia (pulse rate of 120-160 beats/minute).

PRECAUTIONS & CONSIDERATIONS

Caution is warranted with confirmed or suspected coronary artery disease. It is unknown if terazosin crosses the placenta or is distributed in breast milk. The safety and efficacy of terazosin have not been established in children. No age-related precautions have been noted in the elderly, but this age-group may be more sensitive to the drug's hypotensive effects. Caution should be used when driving or operating machinery. Tasks that require mental alertness or motor skills should be avoided until response to the drug is established.

Nasal congestion, dizziness, lightheadedness, and fainting may occur. Rise slowly from a lying to a sitting position and permit legs to dangle momentarily before standing to avoid the hypotensive effect. B/P and pulse should be obtained immediately before each dose, and every 15 to 30 minutes thereafter until B/P is stabilized. Be alert for fluctuations in B/P. GU symptoms and peripheral edema should also be assessed.

Administration

! If terazosin is discontinued for several days, expect to restart therapy with a 1-mg dose at bedtime.

Take terazosin without regard to food. Tablets may be crushed. Administer first dose at bedtime to minimize the risk of fainting due to first-dose.

Terbinafine
ter-been'a-feen
(Apo-Terbinafine [CAN], Lamisil, Lamisil AT, Novo-Terbinafine [CAN])
Do not confuse terbinafine with terbutaline or Lamisil with Lamictal.

CATEGORY AND SCHEDULE
Pregnancy Risk Category: B

CLASSIFICATION
Antifungals, topical, dermatologics

MECHANISM OF ACTION
A fungicidal antifungal that inhibits the enzyme squalene epoxidase, thereby interfering with fungal biosynthesis. *Therapeutic Effect:* Results in death of fungal cells.

AVAILABILITY
Tablets (Lamisil): 250 mg.
Cream (Lamisil AT): 1%.
Topical Solution (Lamisil, Lamisil AT): 1%.

INDICATIONS AND DOSAGES
▸ **Tinea pedis**
TOPICAL
Adults, Elderly, Children 12 yr and older. Apply twice a day until signs and symptoms significantly improve.
▸ **Tinea cruris, tinea corporis**
TOPICAL
Adults, Elderly, Children 12 yr and older. Apply 1-2 times a day until signs and symptoms significantly improve.
▸ **Onychomycosis**
PO
Adults, Elderly, Children 12 yr and older. 250 mg/day for 6 wk (fingernails) or 12 wk (toenails).

▸ **Tinea versicolor**
TOPICAL SOLUTION
Adults, Elderly. Apply to the affected area twice a day for 7 days.
▸ **Systemic mycosis**
PO
Adults, Elderly. 250-500 mg/day for up to 16 mo.

CONTRAINDICATIONS
Oral: Children younger than 12 years, pre-existing hepatic or renal impairment (creatinine clearance of 50 ml/min or less)

INTERACTIONS
Drug
Alcohol, other hepatotoxic medications: May increase the risk of hepatotoxicity.
Hepatic enzyme inducers, including rifampin: May increase terbinafine clearance.
Hepatic enzyme inhibitors, including cimetidine: May decrease terbinafine clearance.
Herbal
None known.
Food
None known.

DIAGNOSTIC TEST EFFECTS
May increase SGOT (AST) and SGPT (ALT) levels.

SIDE EFFECTS
Frequent (13%)
Oral: Headache
Occasional (6%-3%)
Oral: Diarrhea, rash, dyspepsia, pruritus, taste disturbance, nausea
Rare
Oral: Abdominal pain, flatulence, urticaria, visual disturbance
Topical: Irritation, burning, pruritus, dryness

SERIOUS REACTIONS
• Hepatobiliary dysfunction (including cholestatic hepatitis), serious skin reactions, and severe neutropenia occur rarely.
• Ocular lens and retinal changes have been noted.

PRECAUTIONS & CONSIDERATIONS
As appropriate, monitor liver function when receiving treatment for longer than 6 weeks.
! Topical therapy may be used for a minimum of 1 week and is not to exceed 4 weeks. Discontinue the medication and notify the physician if a local reaction occurs. Signs and symptoms of a local reaction include blistering, burning, irritation, itching, oozing, redness, and swelling. Separate personal items that come in contact with affected areas.
Administration
Rub the topical form well into the affected and surrounding area. Keep affected areas clean and dry and wear light clothing to promote ventilation. Avoid contact with eyes, mouth, nose, or other mucous membranes. The treated area should not be covered with an occlusive dressing.

T

Terbutaline

ter-byoo'te-leen
(Brethine, Bricanyl [CAN])
Do not confuse terbutaline with tolbutamide or terbinafine, or Brethine with Brethaire.

CATEGORY AND SCHEDULE
Pregnancy Risk Category: B

CLASSIFICATION
Adrenergic agonists, bronchodilators

MECHANISM OF ACTION
An adrenergic agonist that stimulates beta$_2$-adrenergic receptors, resulting in relaxation of uterine and bronchial smooth muscle. *Therapeutic Effect:* Relieves bronchospasm and reduces airway resistance. Also inhibits uterine contractions.

AVAILABILITY
Tablets: 2.5 mg, 5 mg.
Injection: 1 mg/ml.

INDICATIONS AND DOSAGES
▸ **Bronchospasm**
PO
Adults, Elderly, Children 15 yr and older. Initially, 2.5 mg 3-4 times a day. Maintenance: 2.5-5 mg 3 times a day q6h while awake. Maximum: 15 mg/day.
Children 12-14 yr. 2.5 mg 3 times a day. Maximum: 7.5 mg/day.
Children younger than 12 yr. Initially, 0.05 mg/kg/dose q8hr. May increase up to 0.15 mg/kg/dose. Maximum: 5 mg.

SUBCUTANEOUS
Adults, Children 12 yr and older. Initially, 0.25 mg. Repeat in 15-30 min if substantial improvement does not occur. Maximum: 0.5 mg/4 hr.
Children younger than 12 yr. 0.005-0.01 mg/kg/dose to a maximum of 0.4 mg/dose q15-20 min for 2 doses.
▸ **Preterm labor**
PO
Adults. 2.5-10 mg q4-6hr.
IV
Adults. 2.5-10 mcg/min. May increase gradually q15-20 min up to 17.5-30 mcg/min.

CONTRAINDICATIONS
History of hypersensitivity to sympathomimetics

INTERACTIONS
Drug
Beta blockers: May decrease the effects of beta blockers.
Digoxin, sympathomimetics: May increase the risk of arrhythmias.
MAOIs: May increase the risk of hypertensive crisis.
Tricyclic antidepressants: May increase cardiovascular effects.
Herbal
None known.
Food
None known.

DIAGNOSTIC TEST EFFECTS
May decrease serum potassium level.

SIDE EFFECTS
Frequent (23%-18%)
Tremor, anxiety
Occasional (11%-10%)
Somnolence, headache, nausea, heartburn, dizziness

Rare (3%-1%)
Flushing, asthenia, mouth and throat dryness or irritation (with inhalation therapy)

SERIOUS REACTIONS
• Too-frequent or excessive use may lead to decreased drug effectiveness and severe, paradoxical bronchoconstriction.
• Excessive sympathomimetic stimulation may cause palpitations, extrasystoles, tachycardia, chest pain, a slight increase in B/P followed by a substantial decrease, chills, diaphoresis, and blanching of skin.

PRECAUTIONS & CONSIDERATIONS
Caution is warranted with cardiovascular disorders, hypertension, diabetes mellitus, a history of seizures, and hyperthyroidism. Avoid excessive use of caffeinated products, such as chocolate, cocoa, cola, coffee, and tea.

Anxiety, nervousness, and shakiness may occur. Notify the physician of chest pain, difficulty breathing, dizziness, flushing, headache, muscle tremors, or palpitations. Pulse rate and quality, respiratory rate, depth, rhythm, and type, B/P, ABG levels, and serum potassium levels should be monitored. Fingernails and lips should be assessed for a blue or dusky color in light-skinned patients and a gray color in dark-skinned patients, which are signs of hypoxemia. For women taking terbutaline for preterm labor, maternal B/P and pulse, the duration and frequency of contractions, and the fetal heart rate should be monitored before and during treatment.

Administration
Take terbutaline with food if the patient experiences GI upset. Crush tablets as needed.

For IV use, increase the IV infusion slowly, as prescribed, until contractions stop.

May inject the drug subcutaneously into the lateral deltoid region. Don't use solution if it appears discolored.

Terconazole
ter-kon'a-zole
(Terazol [CAN], Terazol 3, Terazol 7)

CATEGORY AND SCHEDULE
Pregnancy Risk Category: C

CLASSIFICATION
Antifungals, topical, dermatologics

MECHANISM OF ACTION
An antifungal that disrupts fungal cell membrane permeability. *Therapeutic Effect:* Produces antifungal activity.

PHARMACOKINETICS
Extent of systemic absorption after vaginal administration may be dependent on presence of a uterus, 5%-8% in women who had a hysterectomy versus 12%-16% in nonhysterectomy women.

AVAILABILITY
Suppository: 80 mg (Terazol 3).
Cream: 0.4 % (Terazol 7), 0.8% (Terazol 3).

INDICATIONS AND DOSAGES
▸ **Vulvovaginal candidiasis**
INTRAVAGINAL
Adults, Elderly. 1 suppository vaginally at bedtime for 3 days.

Adults, Elderly. One applicatorful at bedtime for 7 days (0.4% cream) or for 3 days (0.8% cream).

CONTRAINDICATIONS
Hypersensitivity to terconazole or any component of the formulation

INTERACTIONS
Drug
None known.
Herbal
None known.
Food
None known.

DIAGNOSTIC TEST EFFECTS
None known.

SIDE EFFECTS
Frequent
Headache, vulvovaginal burning
Occasional
Dysmenorrhea, pain in female fenitalia, abdominal pain, fever, itching
Rare
Chills

SERIOUS REACTIONS
• Flu-like syndrome has been reported.

PRECAUTIONS & CONSIDERATIONS
Caution should be used in the first trimester of pregnancy. It is unknown if terconazole crosses the placenta or is distributed in breast milk. Safety and efficacy of terconazole have not been established in children. There are no age-related precautions noted in the elderly.
Storage
Store at room temperature.
Administration
Insert suppository or administer cream at bedtime. Complete full course of therapy. Contact physician if burning or irritation occurs.

Teriparatide
ter-i-par′a-tide
(Forteo)

CATEGORY AND SCHEDULE
Pregnancy Risk Category: C

CLASSIFICATION
Hormones/hormone modifiers

MECHANISM OF ACTION
A synthetic polypeptide hormone that acts on bone to mobilize calcium; also acts on kidney to reduce calcium clearance, increase phosphate excretion. *Therapeutic Effect:* Promotes an increased rate of release of calcium from bone into blood, stimulates new bone formation.

AVAILABILITY
Injection: 3-ml prefilled pen containing 750 mcg teriparatide (Forteo).

INDICATIONS AND DOSAGES
▸ **Osteoporosis**
SUBCUTANEOUS
Adults, Elderly. 20 mcg once daily into the thigh or abdominal wall.

CONTRAINDICATIONS
Serum calcium above normal level, those at increased risk for osteosarcoma (Paget's disease, unexplained elevations of alkaline phosphatase, open epiphyses, prior radiation therapy that include the skeleton), hypercalcemic disorder (e.g., hyperparathyroidism), hypersensitivity to teriparatide or any of the components of the formulation

INTERACTIONS
Drug
Digoxin: May increase serum digoxin concentration.
Herbal
None known.
Food
None known.

DIAGNOSTIC TEST EFFECTS
May increase serum calcium.

▓ IV INCOMPATIBILITIES
Do not mix with other medications.

SIDE EFFECTS
Occasional
Leg cramps, nausea, dizziness, headache, orthostatic hypotension, increased heart rate

SERIOUS REACTIONS
• None known.

PRECAUTIONS & CONSIDERATIONS
Caution is warranted with bone metastases, cardiovascular disease, history of skeletal malignancies, metabolic bone diseases other than osteoporosis, and concurrent therapy with digoxin. Be aware that teriparatide use for more than 2 years is not recommended. Teriparatide should be used in women who have passed menopause and cannot become pregnant or breast-feed. Teriparatide is not indicated for children.

Teriparatide may cause fast heartbeat, dizziness, lightheadedness, and fainting. Avoid alcohol and tasks that require mental alertness and change positions slowly. Signs of toxicity are rash, nausea, dizziness, and leg cramps.
Storage
Refrigerate and minimize the time out of the refrigerator. Do not freeze. Discard if frozen or if solid particles appear or if the solution is cloudy or colored.
Administration
Administer subcutaneous injection into the thigh or abdominal wall.

Teriparatide Acetate
ter-i-par′a-tide
(Forteo)

CATEGORY AND SCHEDULE
Pregnancy Risk Category: C

CLASSIFICATION
Diagnostics, nonradioactive, hormones/hormone modifiers

MECHANISM OF ACTION
A synthetic hormone that acts on bone to mobilize calcium; also acts on kidney to reduce calcium clearance and increase phosphate excretion. *Therapeutic Effect:* Increases the rate at which calcium is released from bone into blood; stimulates new bone formation.

AVAILABILITY
Injection: 750 mg in 3-ml prefilled pen delivers 20 mcg/dose.

INDICATIONS AND DOSAGES
▶ **Osteoporosis**
SUBCUTANEOUS
Adults, Elderly. 20 mcg once a day into thigh or abdominal wall.

CONTRAINDICATIONS
Conditions that increase the risk of osteosarcoma (including Paget's disease, unexplained elevations of alkaline phosphatase level, open epiphyses, and prior skeletal radiation therapy), hypercalcemia, hypercalcemic disorders (such as hyperparathyroidism)

T

INTERACTIONS
Drug
Digoxin: May increase serum digoxin concentration.
Herbal
None known.
Food
None known.

DIAGNOSTIC TEST EFFECTS
May increase the serum calcium level.

SIDE EFFECTS
Occasional
Leg cramps, nausea, dizziness, headache, orthostatic hypotension, tachycardia

SERIOUS REACTIONS
• None known.

PRECAUTIONS & CONSIDERATIONS
Caution is warranted with bone metastases, history of skeletal malignancies, metabolic bone diseases other than osteoporosis, and concurrent digoxin therapy.

Dizziness or lightheadedness may occur. Notify the physician of hypercalcemia, including loss of energy or strength, lethargy, constipation, nausea, and vomiting.

Bone mineral density, parathyroid hormone level, and urinary and serum calcium levels should be checked. B/P and pulse rate should be monitored for tachycardia.
Storage
Keep teriparatide refrigerated, minimizing the time out of the refrigerator. Don't freeze the drug; discard if it becomes frozen.
Administration
Inject teriparatide into the thigh or abdominal wall.

Testosterone
tess-toss'ter-one
(Andriol [CAN], Androderm, AndroGel, Andropository [CAN], Delatestryl, Depotest [CAN], Depo-Testosterone, Everone [CAN], Striant, Testim, Testoderm, Testoprel, Virilon IM [CAN])
Do not confuse testosterone with testolactone.

CATEGORY AND SCHEDULE
Pregnancy Risk Category: X

CLASSIFICATION
Androgens, hormones/hormone modifiers

MECHANISM OF ACTION
A primary endogenous androgen that promotes growth and development of male sex organs and maintains secondary sex characteristics in androgen-deficient males. *Therapeutic Effect:* Helps relieve androgen deficiency.

PHARMACOKINETICS
Well absorbed after IM administration. Protein binding: 98%. Undergoes first-pass metabolism in the liver. Primarily excreted in urine. Unknown if removed by hemodialysis. **Half-life:** 10-20 min.

AVAILABILITY
Cypionate Injection (Depo-Testosterone): 100 mg/ml, 200 mg/ml.
Ethanate Injection (Delatestryl): 200 mg/ml.
Subcutaneous Pellets (Testopel): 75 mg.
Topical Gel (AndroGel): 25 mg/2.5 g, 50 mg/5 g.
Topical Gel (Testim): 50 mg/5 g.

Transdermal Patch (Androderm):
2.5 mg/day, 5 mg/day.
Transdermal Patch (Testoderm):
4 mg/day, 6 mg/day.
Buccal (Striant): 30 mg.

INDICATIONS AND DOSAGES
▸ **Male hypogonadism**
IM
Adults. 50-400 mg q2-4wk.
Adolescents. Initially 40-50 mg/m^2/
dose monthly until growth rate falls
to prepubertal levels. 100 mg/m^2/dose
until growth ceases. Maintenance
virilizing dose: 100 mg/m^2/dose
twice a month.
SUBCUTANEOUS (PELLETS)
Adults, adolescents. 150-450 mg
q3-6mo.
TRANSDERMAL (PATCH
[TESTODERM])
Adults, Elderly. Start therapy with
6 mg/day patch. Apply patch to
scrotal skin.
TRANSDERMAL (PATCH
[TESTODERM TTS])
Adults, Elderly. Apply TTS patch to
arm, back, or upper buttocks.
TRANDERMAL (PATCH
[ANDRODERM])
Adults, Elderly. Start therapy with
5 mg/day patch applied at night.
Apply patch to abdomen, back,
thighs, or upper arms.
TRANSDERMAL (GEL
[ANDROGEL])
Adults, Elderly. Initial dose of 5 mg
delivers 50 mg testosterone and is
applied once daily to the abdomen,
shoulders, or upper arms. May
increase to 7.5 g, then to 10 g, if
necessary.
TRANSDERMAL (GEL [TESTIM])
Adults, Elderly. Initial dose of 5 g
delivers 50 mg testosterone and is
applied once a day to the shoulders
or upper arms. May increase to 10 g.
BUCCAL SYSTEM (STRIANT)
Adults, Elderly. 30 mg q12hr.

▸ **Delayed puberty**
IM
Adults. 50-200 mg q2-4wk.
Adolescents. 40-50 mg/m^2/dose
every month for 6 mo.
SUBCUTANEOUS (PELLETS)
Adults, Adolescents. 150-450 mg
q3-6mo.
▸ **Breast carcinoma**
IM (AQUEOUS)
Adults. 50-100 mg 3 times a week.
IM (CYPIONATE OR ETHANATE)
Adults. 200-400 mg q2-4wk.
IM (PROPIONATE)
Adults. 50-100 mg 3 times a week.

CONTRAINDICATIONS
Cardiac impairment, hypercalcemia,
pregnancy, prostate or breast cancer
in males, severe hepatic or renal
disease

INTERACTIONS
Drug
Hepatotoxic medications: May
increase the risk of hepatotoxicity.
Oral anticoagulants: May increase
the effects of oral anticoagulants.
Herbal
None known.
Food
None known.

DIAGNOSTIC TEST EFFECTS
May increase blood Hgb level and
Hct, as well as serum LDL, alkaline
phosphatase, bilirubin, calcium,
potassium, sodium, and AST
(SGOT) levels. May decrease serum
HDL level.

SIDE EFFECTS
Frequent
Gynecomastia, acne
Females: Hirsutism, amenorrhea or
other menstrual irregularities, deepening of voice, clitoral enlargement
that may not be reversible when drug
is discontinued

T

Occasional

Edema, nausea, insomnia, oligospermia, priapism, male-pattern baldness, bladder irritability, hypercalcemia (in immobilized patients or those with breast cancer), hypercholesterolemia, inflammation and pain at IM injection site

Transdermal: Pruritus, erythema, skin irritation

Rare

Polycythemia (with high dosage), hypersensitivity

SERIOUS REACTIONS

• Peliosis hepatitis (presence of blood-filled cysts in parenchyma of liver), hepatic neoplasms, and hepatocellular carcinoma have been associated with prolonged high-dose therapy.

• Anaphylactic reactions occur rarely.

PRECAUTIONS & CONSIDERATIONS

Caution is warranted with diabetes and hepatic or renal impairment. Testosterone use is contraindicated during breast-feeding. Use testosterone with caution in children because its safety and efficacy have not been established. Testosterone use in the elderly may increase the risk of hyperplasia or stimulate growth of occult prostate carcinoma. Avoid taking any other medications, including OTC drugs, without first consulting the physician. Consume a diet high in calories and protein; food may be better tolerated if small, frequent meals are eaten.

Notify the physician of weight gain of 5 lbs or more per week, acne, nausea, vomiting, or foot swelling. Females should report deepening of voice, hoarseness, or menstrual irregularities; males should report difficulty urinating, frequent erections, or gynecomastia. Blood Hgb and Hct, B/P, intake and output, weight, serum cholesterol, electrolyte levels, and liver function test should be monitored. Hand or wrist X-rays should be obtained when using the drug in prepubertal children.

Storage

Keep teriparatide refrigerated, minimizing the time out of the refrigerator. Don't freeze the drug; discard if it becomes frozen.

Administration

For IM use, inject testosterone deep into the gluteal muscle. Do not give testosterone IV. Warming and shaking redissolves crystals that may form in long-acting preparations. A wet needle may cause the solution to become cloudy; this does not affect potency.

Apply Testoderm to clean, dry scrotal skin that has been dry-shaved for optimal skin contact. Apply Testoderm TTS to the arm, back, or upper buttocks. Apply Androderm to clean, dry skin on the back, abdomen, upper arms, or thighs. Don't apply it to the scrotum, bony prominences, such as the shoulder; or oily, damaged, or irritated skin. Don't apply Androderm to the same site for 7 days.

Apply the transdermal gel to clean, dry, intact skin of shoulder or upper arm, preferably in the morning. Androgel may also be applied to the abdomen. Open the packet, squeeze the entire contents into the palm of the hand, and apply at once to the affected site. Allow the gel to dry. Don't apply the gel to the genital areas.

Apply Striant to the gum area above the incisor tooth, alternating sides of the mouth with each application. Striant is not affected by consumption of alcohol or food, gum chewing, or tooth brushing. Remove Striant product before placing the new one.

Tetracaine
tet′ra-cane
(AK-T Caine, Cepacol, Viractin, Pontocaine, Opticaine)
Do not confuse with procaine, lidocaine.

CATEGORY AND SCHEDULE
Pregnancy Risk Category: C

CLASSIFICATION
Anesthetics, local, spinal

MECHANISM OF ACTION
Tetracaine causes a reversible blockade of nerve conduction by decreasing nerve membrance permeability to sodium. *Therapeutic Effect:* Local anesthetic.

PHARMACOKINETICS
Systemic absorption of tetracaine is variable. Metabolized by plasma pseudocholinesterasis. Excreted in the urine.

AVAILABILITY
Solution for injection: 0.2%, 0.3%, 1%, 2% (Pontocaine)
Cream: 1%
Ointment: 0.5%

INDICATIONS AND DOSAGES
▸ **Anesthetize lower abdomen**
SPINAL
Adults. 3-4 ml (9-12 mg) of a 0.3% solution
▸ **Anesthetize perineum**
SPINAL
Adults. 1-2 ml (3-6 mg) of a 0.3% solution
▸ **Anesthetize upper abdomen**
SPINAL
Adults. 5 ml (15 mg) of a 0.3% solution

▸ **Obstetric anesthesia, low spinal (saddle block) anesthesia**
SPINAL
Adults. 1-2 ml (2-14 mg) of a 0.2% solution
▸ **Anesthesia of the perineum**
INTRATHECAL
Adults. 0.5 ml (5 mg) as a 1% solution, diluted with equal amount of CSF or 10% dextrose injection.
▸ **Anesthesia of the perineum and lower extremeties**
INTRATHECAL
Adults. 1 ml (10 mg) as a 1% solution, diluted with equal amount of CSF or 10% dextrose injection.
▸ **Anesthesia up to the costal margin**
INTRATHECAL
Adults. 1.5-2 ml (15-20 mg) as a 1% solution, diluted with equal amount of CSF.
▸ **Topical anesthesia**
TOPICAL
Adults. Apply to the affected areas as needed. Maximum dosage is 28 g per 24 hours.
Children. Apply to the affected areas as needed. Maximum dosage is 7 g in a 24-hour period.
▸ **Topical anesthesia of nose and throat, abolish laryngeal and esophageal reflexes prior to diagnostic procedure**
TOPICAL
Adults. Direct application of a 0.25% or 0.5% topical solution or by oral inhalation of a nebulized 0.5% solution. Total dose should not exceed 20 mg.
▸ **Mild pain, burning and/or pruritis associated with herpes labialis (cold sores or fever blisters)**
TOPICAL
Adults and children 2 yr and older. Apply to the affected area no more than 3-4 times a day.
▸ **Ophthalmic anesthesia**
TOPICAL
Adults. 1-2 drops of a 0.5% solution.

T

CONTRAINDICATIONS

Hypersensitivity, to esther local anesthetics, sulfites, PABA, infection or inflammation at the injection site, bacteremia, platelet abnormalities, thrombocytopenia, increased bleeding time, uncontrolled coagulopathy, or anticoagulant therapy, sulfonamide therapy.

INTERACTIONS

Drug

Local anesthetics: The toxic effects are additive.

Cholinesterase inhibitors: Local anesthetics can antagonize the effects of these medications.

Neuromuscular blockers: Local anesthetics prolong and enhance the effects of these medications.

Anihypertensives, nitrates, vasodilators: Additive hypotensive effects.

Opiate agonists: May lead to increased depression of the CNS

Class IA and III antiarrhythmics, macrolide and ketolide antibiotics, quinolone antibiotics, alfuzosin, arsenic trioxide, astemizole, beta agonists, amoxapine, bepridil, cisapride, chloroquine, clozapine, cyclobenzaprine, dolasetron, droperidol, flecainide, halofantrine, haloperidol, halogenated anesthetics, levomethadyl, maprotiline, methadone, octreotide, palonosetron, pentamidine, chlorpromazine, fluphenazine, mesoridazine, pimozide, probucol, propafenone, risperidone, sertindole, tacrolimus, terfenadine, vardenafil, ziprasidone: May increase the risk of cardiotoxicity, including QT prolongation.

MAOIs: Increased risk of hypotension.

Herbal

None known.

Food

None known.

DIAGNOSTIC TEST EFFECTS

None known.

💧 IV Compatibilities

Water, physiologic saline solution, dextrose solution, CSF

SIDE EFFECTS

Frequent

Burning, stinging, or tenderness, skin rash, itching, redness, or inflammation, numbness or tingling of the face or mouth, pain at the injection site, sensitivity to light, swelling of the eye or eyelid, watering or the eyes, acute ocular pain and ocular irritation (burning, stinging, or redness)

Occasional

Paresthesias, weakness and paralysis of lower extremity, hypotension, high or total spinal block, urinary retention or incontinence, fecal incontinence, headache, back pain, septic meningitis, meningismus, arachnoiditis, shivering cranial nerve palsies due to traction on nerves from loss of CSF, and loss of perineal sensation and sexual function

Rare

Anxiety, restlessness, difficulty breathing shortness of breath, dizziness, drowsiness, lightheadedness, nausea, vomiting, seizures (convulsions), slow, irregular heartbeat (palpitations), swelling of the face or mouth, skin rash, itching (hives), tremors, visual impairment.

SERIOUS REACTIONS

• Tetracaine induced CNS toxicity usually presents with symptoms of a CNS stimulation such as anxiety, apprehension, restlessness, nervousness, disorientation, confusion, dizziness, tinnitus, blurred vision, tremor, and/or seizures.

Subsequently, depressive symptoms may occur including drowsiness, respiratory arrest, or coma.

- Depression or cardiac excitability and contractility may cause AV block, ventricular arrhythmias, or cardiac arrest. Symptoms of local anesthetic CNS toxicity, such as dizziness, tongue numbness, visual impairment or disturbances, and muscular twitching appear to occur before cardiotoxic effects. Cardiotoxic effects include angina, QT prolongation, PR prolongation, atrial fibrillation, sinus bradycardia, hypotension, palpitations, and cardiovascular collapse. Maternal seizures and cardiovascular collapse may occur following paracervical block in early pregnancy due to rapid systemic absorption.

! Tetracaine is more likely than any other topical anesthetic to cause contact reactions including skin rash (unspecified), mucous membrane irritation, erythema, pruritis, urticaria, burning, stinging, edema, or tenderness.

! During labor and obstetric delivery, local anesthetics can cause varying degrees of maternal, fetal, and neonatal toxicities. Fetal heart rate should be monitored continuously because fetal bradycardia may occur in patients receiving tetracaine anesthesia and may be associated with fetal acidosis. Maternal hypotension can result from regional anesthesia; patient position can alleviate this problem. Spinal tetracaine may cause decreased uterine contractility or maternal expulsion efforts and alter the forces of parturition.

PRECAUTIONS & CONSIDERATIONS

Caution is warranted with heart or liver disease, myasthenia gravis, and history of drug allergies. Be aware that it is unknown if tetracaine crosses the placenta or is distributed in the breast milk. There are no age-related precautions noted in children or the elderly.

Administration

To apply eye drops, wash hands first. To avoid contamination, do not touch the dropper tip or let it touch the eye or any other surface. Tilt head back, gaze upward and pull down the lower eyelid to make a pouch. Place dropper directly over eye and administer the prescribed number of drops. Look downward and gently close eye for 1 to 2 minutes. Place one finger at the corner of the eye near the nose and apply gentle pressure. This will prevent the medication from draining away from the eye. Try not to blink initially and do not rub the eye. Do not rinse the dropper. Replace cap after use. If using another kind of eye drop, wait at least five minutes before applying other medications. Administer eye drops before eye ointments, to allow the eye drops to enter the eye. The usual dosage is 1 or 2 drops in the affected eye before the procedure.

After applying to the eye, do not rub or wipe the eye until the anesthetic has worn off and feeling in the eye returns. Doing so may cause injury or damage to the eye. The effects of tetracaine last for about 20 minutes. However, if more than one dose is applied, the effects may last longer. If tetracaine is in contact with fingers, it may cause a rash with dryness and cracking of the skin. If you touch your eye after this medicine has been applied, wash your hands as soon as possible.

Tetracycline
tet-ra-sye'kleen
(Apo-Tetra [CAN], Latycin [AUS],
Mysteclin [AUS], Novotetra
[CAN], Nu-Tetra [CAN], Sumycin,
Tetrex [AUS])

CATEGORY AND SCHEDULE
Pregnancy Risk Category: D
(B with topical form)

CLASSIFICATION
Anti-infectives, ophthalmic,
topical, antibiotics, tetracyclines,
dermatologics

MECHANISM OF ACTION
A tetracycline antibiotic that inhibits
bacterial protein synthesis by binding to ribosomes. *Therapeutic Effect:*
Bacteriostatic.

PHARMACOKINETICS
Readily absorbed from the GI tract.
Protein binding: 30%-60%. Widely
distributed. Excreted in urine; eliminated in feces through biliary system.
Not removed by hemodialysis. **Half-
life:** 6-11 hr (increased in impaired
renal function).

AVAILABILITY
Capsules: 250 mg, 500 mg.
Oral Suspension: 125 mg/5 ml.
Tablets: 250 mg, 500 mg.
Topical Solution. 2.2 mg/ml.
Topical Ointment: 3%.

INDICATIONS AND DOSAGES
▸ **Inflammatory acne vulgaris, Lyme
disease, mycoplasmal disease,
Legionella infections, Rocky
Mountain spotted fever, chlamydial
infections in patients with gonorrhea**
PO
Adults, Elderly. 250-500 mg q6-12hr.

Children 8 yr and older. 25-50 mg/
kg/day in 4 divided doses. Maximum:
3 g/day.
▸ ***Helicobacter pylori* infections**
PO
Adults, Elderly. 500 mg 2-4 times a
day (in combination).
TOPICAL
Adults, Elderly. Apply twice a day
(once in the morning, once in the
evening).
▸ **Dosage in renal impairment**
Dosage interval is modified based
on creatinine clearance.

Creatinine Clearance	Dosage Interval
50-80 ml/min	Usual dose q8-12hr
10-50 ml/min	Usual dose q12-24hr
Less than 10 ml/min	Usual dose q24hr

CONTRAINDICATIONS
Children 8 years and younger,
hypersensitivity to tetracyclines or
sulfites

INTERACTIONS
Drug
Carbamazepine, phenytoin:
May decrease tetracycline blood
concentration.
Cholestyramine, colestipol:
May decrease tetracycline
absorption.
Oral contraceptives: May decrease
the effects of oral contraceptives.
Herbal
St. John's wort: May increase the
risk of photosensitivity.
Food
Dairy products: Inhibit tetracycline
absorption.

DIAGNOSTIC TEST EFFECTS
May increase BUN and serum alkaline phosphatase, amylase, bilirubin,
AST (SGOT), and ALT (SGPT)
levels.

SIDE EFFECTS
Frequent
Dizziness, lightheadedness, diarrhea, nausea, vomiting, abdominal cramps, possibly severe photosensitivity
Topical: Dry, scaly skin; stinging or burning sensation
Occasional
Pigmentation of skin or mucous membranes, rectal or genital pruritus, stomatitis
Topical: Pain, redness, swelling, or other skin irritation.

SERIOUS REACTIONS
• Superinfection (especially fungal), anaphylaxis, and benign intracranial hypertension may occur.
• Bulging fontanelles occur rarely in infants.

PRECAUTIONS & CONSIDERATIONS
Caution is warranted with those who can't avoid sun or ultraviolet exposure because such exposure may produce a severe photosensitivity reaction. Tetracycline readily crosses the placenta and is distributed in breast milk. Women in the last half of pregnancy should avoid using tetracycline because it may inhibit skeletal growth of the fetus. Tetracycline use is not recommended for children 8 years and younger because it may cause permanent discoloration of teeth or enamel hypoplasia and may inhibit skeletal growth. No age-related precautions have been noted in the elderly.

History of allergies, especially to tetracyclines or sulfites, should be determined before drug therapy. Pattern of daily bowel activity, stool consistency, food intake and tolerance, skin for rash should be assessed. Be alert for signs and symptoms of superinfection, such as anal or genital pruritus, diarrhea, and ulceration or changes of the oral mucosa

or tongue. B/P and LOC should be monitored because of the potential for increased intracranial pressure.
Administration
! Space drug doses evenly around the clock. Take capsules and tablets with a full glass of water 1 hour before or 2 hours after a meal.

For topical use, cleanse the area gently before application. Because of the drug's potential for staining skin, wear gloves during application and apply the drug only to the affected area.

Tetrahydrozoline Hydrochloride
tet-ra-hi-droz'o-leen
(Visine, Tyzine)

CATEGORY AND SCHEDULE
Pregnancy Risk Category: C

CLASSIFICATION
Decongestants, nasal, ophthalmics

MECHANISM OF ACTION
A vasoconstrictor that stimulates alpha-adrenergic receptors in sympathetic nervous system. Constricts arterioles. *Therapeutic Effect:* Reduces redness, irritation, and congestion.

PHARMACOKINETICS
May be systemically absorbed. Metabolic, elimination rates unknown.

AVAILABILITY
Nasal Solution: 0.05%, 0.1% (Tyzine).
Ophthalmic Solution: 0.05% (Visine).

INDICATIONS AND DOSAGES
▸ **Relief of itching, minor irritation and to control hyperemia with superficial corneal vascularity**
OPHTHALMIC
Adults, Elderly, Children. 1-2 drops 2-4 times/day.
▸ **Relief of nasal congestion of rhinitis, the common cold, sinusitis, hay fever, or other allergies; reduces swelling and improves visualization for surgery or diagnostic procedures; opens obstructed eustachian ostia with ear inflammation**
INTRANASAL
Adults, Elderly, Children older than 6 yr. 2-4 drops (0.1% solution) to each nostril q4-6hr (no sooner than q3hr).
Children 2-6 yr. 2-3 drops (0.05% solution) to each nostril q4-6hr (no sooner than q3hr).

CONTRAINDICATIONS
Children less than 2 years of age, the 0.1% nasal solution is contraindicated in children less than 6 years of age, angle closure glaucoma or other serious eye diseases, hypersensitivity to tetrahydrozyline or any component of the formulation

INTERACTIONS
Drug
Maprotiline, tricyclic antidepressants: May increase pressor effects.
MAOIs: May cause severe hypertensive reaction.
Herbal
Ma huang: May increase CNS stimulation.
Food
None known.

DIAGNOSTIC TEST EFFECTS
None known.

SIDE EFFECTS
Occasional
Intranasal: Transient burning, stinging, sneezing, dryness of mucosa
Ophthalmic: Irritation, blurred vision, mydriasis
Systemic sympathomimetic effects may occur with either route: headache, hypertension, weakness, sweating, palpitations, tremors. Prolonged use may result in rebound congestion

SERIOUS REACTIONS
• Overdosage may result in CNS depression with drowsiness, decreased body temperature, bradycardia, hypotension, coma, and apnea.

PRECAUTIONS & CONSIDERATIONS
Caution is warranted with cardiac disease, hyperthyroidism, hypertension, diabetes mellitus, cerebral arteriosclerosis, bronchial asthma, and concurrent use of MAOIs. Be aware that safety in pregnancy and lactation has not been established. Safety and efficacy have not been established in children less than 2 years of age. There are no age-related precautions noted in the elderly.
Storage
Store at room temperature.
Administration
For ophthalmic use, first tilt head backward and look up. Place finger on lower eyelid and pull out until a pocket is formed between eye and lower lid. Hold dropper above pocket and place correct number of drops into pocket. Close eye gently. Apply gentle finger pressure to lacrimal sac (bridge of the nose, inside corner of the eye) for 1-2 minutes. Remove excess solution around eye with tissue. Discontinue and consult physician immediately if ocular pain or visual changes occur or if condition worsens or continues for more than 72 hours.

For intranasal use, drops should be administered while in lateral, head-low position or reclining with head tilted back as far as possible. Maintain same position for 5 minutes. Then add drops to other nostril. Dropper containers should be used by only one person. Tips of dispensers or droppers should be rinsed well with hot water after use. Discontinue and consult physician if rebound congestion occurs.

Thalidomide
thal-e-doe-mide
(Thalomid)

CATEGORY AND SCHEDULE
Pregnancy Risk Category: X

CLASSIFICATION
Immunomodulators, tumor necrosis factor modulators

MECHANISM OF ACTION
An immunomodulator whose exact mechanism is unknown. Has sedative, anti-inflammatory, and immunosuppressive activity, which may be due to selective inhibition of the production of tumor necrosis factor-alpha. *Therapeutic Effect:* Improves muscle wasting in HIV patients; reduces local and systemic effects of leprosy.

AVAILABILITY
Capsules: 50 mg.

INDICATIONS AND DOSAGES
▶ **AIDS-related muscle wasting**
PO
Adults. 100-300 mg a day.
▶ **Leprosy**
PO
Adults, Elderly. Initially, 100-300 mg/day as single bedtime

dose, at least 1 hr after the evening meal. Continue until active reaction subsides, then reduce dose q2-4 wk in 50-mg increments.

OFF-LABEL USES
Treatment of Crohn's disease, recurrent aphthous ulcers in HIV patients, wasting syndrome associated with HIV or cancer

CONTRAINDICATIONS
Neutropenia, peripheral neuropathy; pregnancy, sensitivity to thalidomide

INTERACTIONS
Drug
Alcohol, other CNS depressants: May increase sedative effects.
Medications associated with peripheral neuropathy (such as isoniazid, lithium, metronidazole, phenytoin): May increase peripheral neuropathy.
Medications that decrease effectiveness of hormonal contraceptives (such as carbamazepine, protease inhibitors, rifampin): May decrease the effectiveness of the contraceptive; patient must use two other methods of contraception.
Herbal
None known.
Food
None known.

DIAGNOSTIC TEST EFFECTS
None known.

SIDE EFFECTS
Frequent
Somnolence, dizziness, mood changes, constipation, dry mouth, peripheral neuropathy
Occasional
Increased appetite, weight gain, headache, loss of libido, edema of face and limbs, nausea, alopecia, dry skin, rash, hypothyroidism

SERIOUS REACTIONS
• Neutropenia, peripheral neuropathy, and thromboembolism occur rarely.

PRECAUTIONS & CONSIDERATIONS
Caution is warranted with history of seizures. Thalidomide is contraindicated in pregnant women. Females of childbearing age should perform a pregnancy test within 24 hours before beginning thalidomide therapy, and then every 2 to 4 weeks. Avoid consuming alcohol or using other drugs that cause drowsiness during thalidomide therapy. Also, avoid tasks that require mental alertness or motor skills until response to the drug has been established.

Notify the physician if symptoms of peripheral neuropathy occur. HIV viral load, nerve conduction studies, and WBC count should be monitored.

Administration
Administer thalidomide with water at least 1 hour after the evening meal and, if possible, at bedtime because of the risk of developing somnolence.

Theophylline
thee-off´i-lin
(Aerobin [GERMANY]; Aerodyne Retard [AUSTRIA]; Afonilum Forte [GERMANY]; Afonilum Mite [GERMANY]; Afonilum Retard [GERMANY]; Almarion [THAILAND]; Armophylline [France]; Asmasalon [PHILIPPINES]; Asperal-T [Belgium]; Austyn [KOREA]; Bronchoretard [GERMANY]; Bronsolvan [Indonesia]; Cronasma [GERMANY]; Deo-Q Syrup [KOREA]; Ditenaten [GERMANY]; Elixofilina [MEXICO, PERU]; Elixophyllin; Euphylong [ISRAEL, HONG KONG]; Euphylong Retardkaps [GERMANY]; Euphylong SR [PHILIPPINES]; Godafilin [SPAIN]; Lasma [ISRAEL, ENGLAND]; Nefoben [ARGENTINA]; Neobiphyllin [CHINA]; Neulin SA [SOUTH AFRICA]; Neulin-SR [TAIWAN]; Nuelin [PUERTO RICO, COSTA RICA, DENMARK, DOMINICAN REPUBLIC, EL SALVADOR, FINLAND, HONDURAS, MALAYSIA, NORWAY, PANAMA, PHILIPPINES]; Nuelin SA [SOUTH AFRICA, ISRAEL, COSTA RICA, DOMINICAN REPUBLIC, EL SALVADOR, GUATEMALA, HONDURAS, PANAMA]; Nuelin SR [ISRAEL, AUSTRALIA, HONG KONG, MALAYSIA, THAILAND]; Pharphylline [NETHERLANDS]; Phylobid [SOUTH AFRICA, INDIA]; Protheo [CHINA]; Pulmidur [AUSTRIA, GERMANY]; Slo-Bid Gyrocaps; Quibron-T; Quibron T SR [US, CANADA, INDONESIA]; Slo-Theo [HONG KONG]; Solosin [GERMANY]; Somofillina [ITALY]; Teobid [COLOMBIA]; Teoclear [KOREA]; Teoclear LA [ARGENTINA]; Teofilina Retard [COLOMBIA]; Teolixir [SPAIN]; Teolong [MEXICO];

Teosona [ARGENTINA]; Theo-2
[BELGIUM]; Theo-24; Theo-Bros
[GREECE]; Theochron; Theo-Dur;
Theolair; Theolair SR; Theolair S
[PERU]; Theolan [KOREA, TAIWAN];
Theolin [SINGAPORE]; Theolin SR
[SINGAPORE]; Theolong [JAPAN];
Theomax [SPAIN]; Theon
[SWITZERLAND]; Theo PA [INDIA];
Theoplus [BULGARIA, SINGAPORE,
SPAIN]; Theoplus Retard [AUSTRIA,
GREECE]; Theospirex Retard
[AUSTRIA, SWITZERLAND];
Theostat LP [FRANCE]; Theotard
[ISRAEL]; Theo-Time; Theotrim
[ISRAEL]; Theovent LA [HONG
KONG]; Theo von CT [GERMANY];
Tiodilax [ARGENTINA]; T-Phyl;
Truxophyllin; Tyrex [PERU];
Unicontin-400 Continus [INDIA];
Uni-Dur; Unifyl Retard
[SWITZERLAND]; Uniphyl;
Uniphyl CR [KOREA]; Uniphyllin
[TAIWAN]; UniphyllinContinus
[SOUTH AFRICA]; Xanthium
[SINGAPORE]; Xantivent
[SWITZERLAND])

CATEGORY AND SCHEDULE
Pregnancy risk category: C

CLASSIFICATION
Bronchodilators, xanthine
derivatives

MECHANISM OF ACTION
An antiasthmatic medication with
two distinct actions in the airways of
patients with reversible obstruction;
smooth muscle relaxation and
suppression of the response of
airways to stimuli. Mechanisms of
action are not known with certainty.
It is known theophylline increases
force of contraction of diaphragmatic
muscles by enhancing calcium
uptake through adenosine-mediated
channels. *Therapeutic Effect:* Causes
bronchodilation and decreased
airway reactivity.

PHARMACOKINETICS
The pharmacokinetics of theophylline
vary widely among similar patients
and cannot be predicted by age, sex,
body weight or other demographic
characteristics. Rapidly and
completely absorbed after oral administration in solution or immediate-
release solid oral dosage form.
Distributed freely into fat-free
tissues. Extensively metabolized in
liver. **Half-life:** 4-8 hr.

AVAILABILITY
Capsule, Extended Release: 100 mg
(Slo-Bid Gyrocaps); 125 mg; 200 mg
(Slo-Bid Gyrocaps); 300 mg (Slo-Bid
Gyrocaps)
Elixir: 80 mg/15 ml (Elixophyllin)
Solution, Intravenous: 40 mg/100 ml,
80 mg/100 ml, 160 mg/100 ml,
200 mg/100 ml, 200 mg/50 ml,
320 mg/100 ml, 400 mg/100 ml
Solution, Oral: 80 mg/15 ml
(Truxophyllin)
Tablet: 100 mg
Tablet, Extended Release: 100 mg
(Theo-Dur, Theochron, Theo-Time);
200 mg (Theo-Dur, Theochron,
Theo-Time); 300 mg (Theo-Dur,
Theochron, Theo-Time); 400 mg
(Uni-Dur); 450 mg (Theochron)

INDICATIONS AND DOSAGES
▸ Chronic asthma/lung diseases
PO
Adults. Acute symptoms: 5 mg/kg
as a loading dose, maintenance
3 mg/kg every 8 hours (non-smokers),
3 mg/kg every 6 hours (smokers),
2 mg/kg every 8 hours (older patients),
1-2 mg/kg every 12 hours (CHF);
IV 5 mg/kg load over 20 minutes,

maintenance 0.2 mg/kg/hr
(CHF, elderly), 0.43 mg/kg/hr
(non-smokers), 0.7 mg/kg/hr
(young adult smokers).

Slow titration: initial dose
16 mg/kg/day or 400 mg daily,
whichever is less, doses divided
every 6-8 hours

Dosage adjustment after serum theophylline measurement: Serum level
5-10 mcg/ml, maintain dose by 25%,
recheck level in 3 days. Serum
level 10-20 mcg/ml, maintain
dosage if tolerated, recheck level
every 6-12 months. Serum level
20-25 mcg/ml, decrease dose by
10%, recheck level in 3 days. Serum
level 25-30 mcg/ml, skip next dose,
decrease dose by 25%, recheck level
in 3 days. Serum level >30 mcg/ml,
skip next 2 doses, decrease dose by
50%, recheck level in 3 days.

Children 9-16 yr: 5 mg/kg as a
loading dose, maintenance 3 mg/kg
every 6 hours; IV 5 mg/kg load over
20 minutes, maintenance 0.7 mg/
kg/hr.

Children 1-9 yr: 5 mg/kg as a
loading dose, maintenance 4 mg/kg
every 6 hours; IV 5 mg/kg load over
20 minutes, maintenance 0.8 mg/
kg/hr.

Infants: [(0.2 X age in weeks) +5]
X kg = 24-hour dose in mg; divide
into every 8-hour dosing (6 weeks
to 6 months), every 6-hour dosing
(6-12 months); IV 5 mg/kg load over
20 minutes, maintenance dose in
mg/kg/hr [(0.0008 X age in
weeks) + 0.21]

OFF-LABEL USES
Apnea, bradycardia of prematurity

CONTRAINDICATIONS
Hypersensitivity to theophylline or
any component of the formulation,
active peptic ulcer disease, underlying
seizure disorders unless receiving

appropriate anti-convulsant
medication.

INTERACTIONS
Drug
**Adenosine, diazepam, flurazepam,
lorazepam, midazolam:** May
decrease therapeutic effect at adenosine receptors.
**Alcohol, allopurinol, cimetidine,
ciprofloxacin, clarithromycin,
disulfiram, erythromycin, enoxacin,
estrogen, fluvoxamine, interferon
alpha-A, methotrexate, mexiletine,
pentoxifylline, propafenone, propranolol, thiabendazole, ticlopidine,
troleandomycin, verapamil:** May
decrease theophylline clearance.
**Aminoglutethimide, carbamazepine,
isoproterenol, moricizinel, phenobarbital, phenytoin, rifampin,
sulfinpyrazone:** May increase
theophylline clearance.
Ephedrine: May cause synergistic
CNS effects.
Halothane: May cause ventricular
arrhythmia.
Ketamine: May decrease seizure
threshold.
Lithium: May increase lithium
clearance.
Herbal
Capsicum: May increase absorption
and effect.
Ipriflavone, St. John's wort: May
decrease metabolism of theophylline.
Food
High-fat content meals:
May decrease theophylline
absorption.
Charbroiled foods: May increase
elimination of theophylline.
**Caffeine, dietary protein, and
carbohydrates:** May increase the
activity and side effects caused by
theophylline. Large amounts should
be avoided. Low-carbohydrate, high-protein diets, charbroiled beef, and
large amounts of cruciferous

vegetables (broccoli, Brussels sprouts, cabbage, and cauliflower) can reduce theophylline activity.

DIAGNOSTIC TEST EFFECTS
None known.

SIDE EFFECTS
Anxiety, dizziness, headache, insomnia, lightheadedness, muscle twitching, restlessness, seizures, dysrhythmias, fluid retention with tachycardia, hypotension, palpitations, pounding heartbeat, sinus tachycardia, anorexia, bitter taste, diarrhea, dyspepsia, gastroesophageal reflux, nausea, vomiting, urinary frequency, increased respiratory rate, flushing, urticaria

SERIOUS REACTIONS
• Severe toxicity from theophylline overdose is a relatively rare event.

PRECAUTIONS & CONSIDERATIONS
Caution is warranted with peptic ulcer, hyperthyroidism, seizure disorders, hypertension, and cardiac arrhythmias (excluding bradyarrhythmias). Be aware that dose adjustments must be made for those who smoke. Be aware that theophylline crosses the placenta and is distributed in breast milk. A dose reduction should be used when starting theophylline in the elderly. Avoid excessive amounts of caffeine as well as extremes in dietary protein and carbohydrates. Charbroiled foods may increase elimination and reduce the half-life.

Nervousness, restlessness, and increased heart rate may occur during theophylline therapy. Signs and symptoms of theophylline toxicity are persistent, repetitive vomiting and serum theophylline level should be drawn and dose should be withheld.

Administration
Take this medication with a full glass of water on an empty stomach, at least 1 hour before or 2 hours after a meal. Do not chew or crush the extended-release tablets; swallow them whole. Extended-release capsules may be swallowed whole or opened and the contents mixed with soft food and swallowed without chewing.

Thiabendazole
thye-a-ben'da-zole
(Mintezol)

CATEGORY AND SCHEDULE
Pregnancy Risk Category: C

CLASSIFICATION
Antihelmintics

MECHANISM OF ACTION
An antihelmintic agent that inhibits helminth-specific mitochondrial fumarate reductase. *Therapeutic Effect:* Suppresses parasite production.

PHARMACOKINETICS
Rapidly and well absorbed from the gastrointestinal (GI) tract. Rapidly metabolized in liver. Primarily excreted in urine; partially eliminated in feces. Removed **Half-life:** 1.2 hr.

AVAILABILITY
Suspension: 500 mg/5 ml (Mintezol).
Tablets: 500 mg (Mintezol).

INDICATIONS AND DOSAGES
Dose is based on patient's body weight

▸ **Cutaneous lava migrans (creeping eruption)**
PO
Adults, Elderly, Children.
50 mg/kg/day q12hr for 2 days.
Maximum: 3 g/day.

▸ **Intestinal roundworms**
PO
Adults, Elderly, Children.
50 mg/kg/day q12hr for 2 days.
Maximum: 3 g/day.

▸ **Strongloidiasis (thread worms)**
PO
Adults, Elderly, Children.
50 mg/kg/day q12hr for 2 days.
Maximum: 3 g/day.

▸ **Trichinosis**
PO
Adults, Elderly, Children.
50 mg/kg/day q12hr for 2-4 days.
Maximum: 3 g/day.

▸ **Visceral larva migrans**
PO
Adults, Elderly, Children.
50 mg/kg/day q12hr for 7 days.
Maximum: 3 g/day.

OFF-LABEL USES

Angiostrongyliasis, capillaria infestations, dracunculus infestations, pediculosis capitis, tinea infections

CONTRAINDICATIONS

Prophylactic treatment of pinworm infestation, hypersensitivity to thiabendazole or its components

INTERACTIONS

Drug
Theophylline, other xanthines:
May increase levels of theophylline or other xanthinges.
Herbal
None known.
Food
None known.

DIAGNOSTIC TEST EFFECTS

None known.

SIDE EFFECTS

Occasional
Dizziness, drowsiness, nausea, vomiting, diarrhea
Rare
Erythema multiform, liver damage

SERIOUS REACTIONS

• Overdose includes symptoms of altered mental status and visual problems.
• Erythema multiform, liver damage, and Stevens-Johnsons syndrome occur rarely.

PRECAUTIONS & CONSIDERATIONS

Caution is necessary with malnutrition or anemia, mixed helminthic infections, liver and renal dysfunction. Thiabendazole is not for prophylactic use, and it is not suitable for treatment of mixed infections with ascaris. It is unknown if thiabendazole crosses the placenta and is distributed in breast milk. There are no age-related precautions noted in children or the elderly. Urine may be red-brown or dark during drug therapy. Thiabendazole may also cause drowsiness. Tasks requiring mental alertness or motor skills should be avoided.
Administration
Dose should be based on weight:
  Adults: 1 g for 100 lb body wt.
         1.25 g for 125 lb body wt.
         1.5 g for 150 lb body wt.
  Children: 0.25 g for 30 lb body wt.
         0.5 g for 50 lb body wt.
         0.75 g for 75 lb body wt.
         1 g for 100 lb body wt.
Chew tablets before swallowing.
Take with meals or milk to minimize gastrointestinal (GI) irritation.

Thiamine (Vitamin B₁)
thy'a-min
(Beta-Sol [AUS], Betaxin [CAN], Thiamilate)

CATEGORY AND SCHEDULE
Pregnancy Risk Category: A (C if used in doses above recommended daily allowance)
OTC (tablets)

CLASSIFICATION
Vitamins/minerals

MECHANISM OF ACTION
A water-soluble vitamin that combines with adenosine triphosphate in the liver, kidneys, and leukocytes to form thiamine diphosphate, a coenzyme that is necessary for carbohydrate metabolism. *Therapeutic Effect:* Prevents and reverses thiamine deficiency.

PHARMACOKINETICS
Readily absorbed from the GI tract, primarily in duodenum, after IM administration. Widely distributed. Metabolized in the liver. Primarily excreted in urine.

AVAILABILITY
Tablets: 50 mg, 100 mg, 250 mg, 500 mg.
Injection: 100 mg/ml.

INDICATIONS AND DOSAGES
▸ **Dietary supplement**
PO
Adults, Elderly. 1-2 mg/day.
Children. 0.5-1 mg/day.
Infants. 0.3-0.5 mg/day.

▸ **Thiamine deficiency**
PO
Adults, Elderly. 5-30 mg/day, as a single dose or in 3 divided doses, for 1 mo.
Children. 10-50 mg/day in 3 divided doses.
▸ **Thiamine deficiency in patients who are critically ill or have malabsorption syndrome**
IV, IM
Adults, Elderly. 5-100 mg, 3 times a day.
Children. 10-25 mg/day.
▸ **Metabolic disorders**
PO
Adults, Elderly, Children. 10-20 mg/day; increased up to 4 g/day in divided doses.

CONTRAINDICATIONS
None known.

INTERACTIONS
Drug
None known.
Herbal
None known.
Food
None known.

DIAGNOSTIC TEST EFFECTS
None known.
▒ **IV Compatibilities**
Famotidine (Pepcid), multivitamins

SIDE EFFECTS
Frequent
Pain, induration, and tenderness at IM injection site

SERIOUS REACTIONS
• IV administration may result in a rare, severe hypersensitivity reaction marked by a feeling of warmth, pruritus, urticaria, weakness, diaphoresis, nausea, restlessness, tightness in throat, angioedema, cyanosis,

pulmonary edema, GI tract bleeding, and cardiovascular collapse.

PRECAUTIONS & CONSIDERATIONS

Caution is warranted with Wernicke's encephalopathy. Thiamine crosses the placenta; it is unknown if it's excreted in breast milk. No age-related precautions have been noted in children or the elderly. Consuming foods rich in thiamine, including legumes, nuts, organ meats, pork, rice bran, seeds, wheat germ, whole grain and enriched cereals, and yeast, is encouraged.

Urine may appear bright yellow during therapy. Before and during treatment, signs and symptoms of thiamine deficiency, including peripheral neuropathy, ataxia, hyporeflexia, muscle weakness, nystagmus, ophthalmoplegia, confusion, peripheral edema, bounding arterial pulse, and tachycardia, should be assessed.

Administration

! IM and IV administration routes are used only in acutely ill patients and those who are unresponsive to the PO route, such as those with malabsorption syndrome. The IM route is preferred over the IV route. The solution may be given by IV push or may be added to most IV solutions and given as an IV infusion.

IM injection may cause discomfort.

Thiethylperazine
thye-eth-il-per′azeen
(Torecan)
Do not confuse with thioridazine.

CATEGORY AND SCHEDULE
Pregnancy Risk Category: X

CLASSIFICATION
Antiemetics/antivertigo, phenothiazines

MECHANISM OF ACTION
A piperazine phenothiazine that acts centrally to block dopamine receptors in chemoreceptor trigger zone (CTZ) in central nervous system (CNS). *Therapeutic Effect:* Relieves nausea and vomiting.

AVAILABILITY
Injection: 5 mg/ml (Torecan).
Tablets: 10 mg (Torecan).

INDICATIONS AND DOSAGES
▸ **Nausea or vomiting**
PO/RECTAL/IM
Adults, Elderly. 10 mg 1-3 times/day.

CONTRAINDICATIONS
Comatose states, severe CNS depression, pregnancy, hypersensitivity to phenothiazines

INTERACTIONS
Drug
Alcohol, CNS depressants: May increase respiratory depression and the hypotensive effects of thiethylperazine.
Epinephrine: May block alpha-adrenergic effects of epinephrine causing hypotension and tachycardia.
Extrapyramidal symptom-producing medications: Increased

risk of extrapyramidal symptoms (EPS).
Levodopa: May decrease the effects of levodopa.
Quinidine: May increase cardiac effects.
Herbal
None known.
Food
None known.

DIAGNOSTIC TEST EFFECTS
None known.

SIDE EFFECTS
Frequent
Drowsiness, dizziness
Occasional
Blurred vision, decreased color/night vision, fever, headache, orthostatic hypotension, rash, ringing in ears, constipation, dry mouth, decreased sweating.

SERIOUS REACTIONS
• Extrapyramidal symptoms manifested as torticollis (neck muscle spasm), oculogyric crisis (rolling back of eyes), and akathisia (motor restlessness, anxiety) occur rarely.

PRECAUTIONS & CONSIDERATIONS
Caution should be used with dehydration, high fever, and electrolyte imbalance. Be aware that thiethylperazine is contraindicated in pregnant women. It is unknown if thiethylperazine is distributed in breast milk. Safety and efficacy have not been established in children. Caution should be used in the elderly because they are more susceptible to anticholinergic effects, such as dry mouth, extrapyramidal symptoms (EPS), orthostatic hypotension, and sedative effects; a lower thiethylperazine dosage may be recommended.
Storage
Store at room temperature.

Administration
Inject IM deeply into large muscle mass. Lie down and remain at least 1 hour after administratin. Relief from nausea and vomiting usually occurs within 30 minutes of drug administration.
Take oral tablets with food or a full glass of water or milk to reduce GI upset.
To insert suppositories, first remove foil wrapper and moisten the suppository with cold water. Lie down on side and use finger to push the suppository well up into the rectum. If the suppository is too soft to insert, chill it in the refrigerator for 30 minutes or run cold water over it before removing the foil wrapper. Wash hands with soap and water.

Thioridazine
thye-or-rid′a-zeen
(Aldazine [AUS], Apo-Thioridazine [CAN], Mellaril, Melleril [AUS], Thioridazine Intensol)
Do not confuse thioridazine with thiothixene or Thorazine, or Mellaril with Mebaral.

CATEGORY AND SCHEDULE
Pregnancy Risk Category: C

CLASSIFICATION
Antipsychotics, phenothiazines

MECHANISM OF ACTION
A phenothiazine that blocks dopamine at postsynaptic receptor sites. Possesses strong anticholinergic and sedative effects. *Therapeutic Effect:* Suppresses behavioral response in

psychosis; reduces locomotor activity and aggressiveness.

AVAILABILITY

Oral Solution (Concentrate [Thioridazine Intensol]): 30 mg/ml. *Tablets (Melleril):* 10 mg, 15 mg, 25 mg, 50 mg, 100 mg, 150 mg, 200 mg.

INDICATIONS AND DOSAGES
▶ **Psychosis**
PO
Adults, Elderly, Children 12 yr and older. Initially, 25-100 mg 3 times a day; dosage increased gradually. Maximum: 800 mg/day.
Children 2-11 yr. Initially, 0.5 mg/ kg/day in 2-3 divided doses. Maximum: 3 mg/kg/day.

OFF-LABEL USES
Treatment of behavioral problems in children, dementia, depressive neurosis

CONTRAINDICATIONS
Angle-closure glaucoma, blood dyscrasias, cardiac arrhythmias, cardiac or hepatic impairment, concurrent use of drugs that prolong QT interval, severe CNS depression

INTERACTIONS
Drug
Alcohol, other CNS depressants: May increase respiratory depression and the hypotensive effects of thioridazine.
Antithyroid agents: May increase the risk of agranulocytosis.
Extrapyramidal symptom-producing medications: May increase the risk of extrapyramidal symptoms.
Hypotension-producing agents: May increase hypotension.
Levodopa: May decrease the effects of levodopa.

Lithium: May decrease the absorption of thioridazine and produce adverse neurologic effects.
MAOIs, tricyclic antidepressants: May increase the anticholinergic and sedative effects of thioridazine.
Herbal
None known.
Food
None known.

DIAGNOSTIC TEST EFFECTS
May cause EKG changes. Therapeutic serum level is 0.2-2.6 mcg/ml; toxic serum level is not established.

SIDE EFFECTS
Occasional
Drowsiness during early therapy, dry mouth, blurred vision, lethargy, constipation or diarrhea, nasal congestion, peripheral edema, urine retention
Rare
Ocular changes, altered skin pigmentation (in those taking high doses for prolonged periods), photosensitivity, darkening of urine

SERIOUS REACTIONS
• Prolonged QT interval may produce torsades de pointes, a form of ventricular tachycardia, and sudden death.

PRECAUTIONS & CONSIDERATIONS
Caution is warranted with benign prostatic hypertrophy, decreased GI motility, seizures, urinary retention, and visual problems. Urine may darken and drowsiness and dizziness may occur but generally subsides with continued therapy. Alcohol, tasks requiring mental alertness or motor skills, and exposure to artificial light and sunlight should be avoided. B/P, CBC, EKG, serum potassium level, and liver function test results, including serum alkaline

phosphatase, bilirubin, AST (SGOT), and ALT (SGPT) levels, should be monitored. Extrapyramidal symptoms should be assessed.

Administration

Know that the therapeutic serum level for thioridazine is 0.2 to 2.6 mcg/ml, and the toxic serum level is not established. Avoid skin contact with the oral solution because it can cause contact dermatitis. Full therapeutic effect may take up to 6 weeks to appear. Do not abruptly discontinue the drug after long-term use.

Thiothixene

thye-oh-thix′een
(Navane)
Do not confuse thiothixene with thioridazine.

CATEGORY AND SCHEDULE
Pregnancy Risk Category: C

CLASSIFICATION
Antipsychotics

MECHANISM OF ACTION
An antipsychotic that blocks postsynaptic dopamine receptor sites in brain. Has alpha-adrenergic blocking effects, and depresses the release of hypothalamic and hypophyseal hormones. *Therapeutic Effect:* Suppresses psychotic behavior.

PHARMACOKINETICS
Well absorbed from the GI tract after IM administration. Widely distributed. Metabolized in the liver. Primarily excreted in urine. Unknown if removed by hemodialysis. **Half-life:** 34 hr.

AVAILABILITY
Capsules: 1 mg, 2 mg, 5 mg, 10 mg, 20 mg.
Oral Concentrate: 5 mg/ml.
Injection: 5 mg of thiothixene and 59.6 mg of mannitol per ml when reconstituted with 2.2 ml of sterile water for injection.

INDICATIONS AND DOSAGES
▸ **Psychosis**
PO
Adults, Elderly, Children older than 12 yr. Initially, 2 mg 3 times a day. Maximum: 60 mg/day.
IM
Adults, Elderly, Children older than 12 yr. Initially, 4 mg 2-4 times a day. Maximum: 30 mg/day.

CONTRAINDICATIONS
Blood dyscrasias, circulatory collapse, CNS depression, coma, history of seizures

INTERACTIONS
Drug
Alcohol, other CNS depressants: May increase CNS and respiratory depression and the hypotensive effects of thiothixene.
Extrapyramidal symptom-producing medications: May increase the risk of extrapyramidal symptoms.
Levodopa: May inhibit the effects of levodopa.
Quinidine: May increase cardiac effects.
Herbal
Kava kava, St. John's wort, valerian: May increase CNS depression.
Food
None known.

DIAGNOSTIC TEST EFFECTS
May decrease serum uric acid level.

T

SIDE EFFECTS
Expected
Hypotension, dizziness, syncope (occur frequently after first injection, occasionally after subsequent injections, and rarely with oral form)
Frequent
Transient drowsiness, dry mouth, constipation, blurred vision, nasal congestion
Occasional
Diarrhea, peripheral edema, urine retention, nausea
Rare
Ocular changes, altered skin pigmentation (in those taking high doses for prolonged periods), photosensitivity

SERIOUS REACTIONS
• The most common extrapyramidal reaction is akathisia, characterized by motor restlessness and anxiety. Akinesia, marked by rigidity, tremor, increased salivation, masklike facial expression, and reduced voluntary movements, occurs less frequently. Dystonias, including torticollis, opisthotonos, and oculogyric crisis, occur rarely.
• Tardive dyskinesia, characterized by tongue protrusion, puffing of the cheeks, and chewing or puckering of the mouth, occurs rarely but may be irreversible. Elderly female patients have a greater risk of developing this reaction.
• Grand mal seizures may occur in epileptic patients, especially those receiving the drug by IM administration.
• Neuroleptic malignant syndrome occurs rarely.

PRECAUTIONS & CONSIDERATIONS
Caution is warranted with alcohol withdrawal, severe cardiovascular disorders, glaucoma, benign prostatic hyperplasia, and exposure to extreme heat. Thiothixene crosses the placenta and is distributed in breast milk. Children are more prone to develop extrapyramidal and neuromuscular symptoms, especially dystonias. The elderly are more prone to anticholinergic effects (such as dry mouth), extrapyramidal symptoms, orthostatic hypotension, and increased sedation.

Drowsiness and dizziness may occur but generally subsides with continued therapy. Alcohol, tasks requiring mental alertness or motor skills, and exposure to artificial light and sunlight should be avoided. Notify the physician if fluid retention, fever, or visual disturbances occur. Pattern of daily bowel activity and stool consistency, B/P, and signs of extrapyramidal reactions should be assessed.
Administration
Take thiothixene without regard to food. Avoid skin contact with the oral solution because it can cause contact dermatitis. The drug's full therapeutic effect may take up to 6 weeks to appear.

For IM use, reconstitute drug with 2.2 ml of sterile water.

Thyroid
thye'roid
(Armour Thyroid, Nature-Thyroid NT, Westhyroid)

CATEGORY AND SCHEDULE
Pregnancy Risk Category: A

CLASSIFICATION
Hormones/hormone modifiers, thyroid agents

MECHANISM OF ACTION
A natural hormone derived from animal sources, usually beef or pork, that is involved in normal metabolism, growth, and development, especially the central nervous system (CNS) of infants. Possesses catabolic and anabolic effects. Provides both levothyroxine and liothyronine hormones. *Therapeutic Effect:* Increases basal metabolic rate, enhances gluconeogenesis, stimulates protein synthesis.

PHARMACOKINETICS
Partially absorbed from the gastrointestinal (GI) tract. Protein binding: 99%. Widely distributed. Metabolized in liver to active, liothyronine (T_3), and inactive, reverse triiodothyronine (rT_3), metabolites. Eliminated by biliary excretion. **Half-life:** 2-7 days.

AVAILABILITY
Capsules: 15 mg, 30 mg, 60 mg, 90 mg, 120 mg, 180 mg, 240 mg.
Tablets: 30 mg, 32.5 mg, 60 mg, 65 mg, 120 mg, 130 mg, 180 mg, 15 mg, 30 mg, 60 mg, 90 mg, 120 mg, 180 mg, 240 mg, 300 mg (Armour Thyroid).
32.4 mg, 64.8 mg, 129.6 mg, 194.4 mg (Nature-Thyroid NT, Westhyroid).

INDICATIONS AND DOSAGES
▶ **Hypothyroidism**
PO
Adults, Elderly. Initially, 15-30 mg. May increase by 15 mg increments q2-4wk. Maintenance: 60-120 mcg/day. Use 15 mg in patients with cardiovascular disease or myxedema.
Children 12 yr and older. 90 mg/day.
Children 6-12 yr. 60-90 mg/day.
Children older than 1-5 yr. 45-60 mg/day.

Children older than 6-12 mo. 30-45 mg/day.
Children 3 mo. and younger. 15-30 mg/day.

CONTRAINDICATIONS
Uncontrolled adrenal cortical insufficiency, untreated thyrotoxicosis, treatment of obesity, uncontrolled angina, uncontrolled hypertension, uncontrolled myocardial infarction, and hypersensitivity to any component of the formulations

INTERACTIONS
Drug
Cholestyramine, colestipol: May decrease absorption of thyroid hormones.
Estrogens, oral contraceptives: May decrease effects of thyroid hormones.
Insulin, oral hypoglycemics: May decrease effects of insulin and oral hypoglycemics.
Oral anticoagulants: May increase hypoprothrombinemic effects of oral anticoagulants
Tricyclic antidepressants: May increase risk of toxicity of both drugs.
Herbal
Bugleweed: May decrease effects of thyroid hormones.
Food
None known.

SIDE EFFECTS
Rare
Dry skin, GI intolerance, skin rash, hives, severe headache

SERIOUS REACTIONS
• Excessive dosage produces signs and symptoms of hyperthyroidism including weight loss, palpitations, increased appetite, tremors, nervousness, tachycardia, hypertension,

T

headache, insomnia, and menstrual irregularities.
• Cardiac arrhythmias occur rarely.

PRECAUTIONS & CONSIDERATIONS

Caution is warranted with angina pectoris, hypertension, or other cardiovascular disease as well as adrenal insufficiency, cardiovascular disease, coronary artery disease, diabetes insipidus, and diabetes mellitus. Thyroid hormone does not cross the placenta and is minimally excreted in breast milk. There are no age-related precautions noted in children. Be aware that thyroid hormone should be used cautiously in neonates in interpreting thyroid function tests. The elderly may be more sensitive to thyroid effects. Individualized dosages are recommended for this population. Signs of nervousness or tremors should be reported.

Administration

The following are equivalent doses between the thyroid preparations: thyroid 65 mg, thyroglobulin 65 mg, Thyroid Strong 43 mg, levothyroxine 0.1 mg, liothyronine 25 mcg, and liotrix 50 to 60 mcg of levothyroxine and 12.5 to 15 mcg of liothyronine.

Begin therapy with small doses and increase the dosage gradually, as prescribed. Take at the same time each day to maintain hormone levels. Take on an empty stomach.

Tiagabine
ti-ah-ga′bean
(Gabitril)

CATEGORY AND SCHEDULE
Pregnancy Risk Category: C

CLASSIFICATION
Anticonvulsants

MECHANISM OF ACTION
An anticonvulsant that enhances the activity of gamma-aminobutyric acid, the major inhibitory neurotransmitter in the CNS. *Therapeutic Effect:* Inhibits seizures.

AVAILABILITY
Tablets: 2 mg, 4 mg, 12 mg, 16 mg.

INDICATIONS AND DOSAGES
▶ **Adjunctive treatment of partial seizures**
PO
Adults, Elderly. Initially, 4 mg once a day. May increase by 4-8 mg/day at weekly intervals. Maximum: 56 mg/day.
Children 12-18 yr. Initially, 4 mg once a day. May increase by 4 mg at week 2 and by 4-8 mg at weekly intervals thereafter. Maximum: 32 mg/day.

CONTRAINDICATIONS
None known.

INTERACTIONS
Drug
Carbamazepine, phenobarbital, phenytoin: May increase tiagabine clearance.
Valproic acid: May alter the effects of valproic acid.

Herbal
None known.
Food
None known.

DIAGNOSTIC TEST EFFECTS
None known.

SIDE EFFECTS
Frequent (34%-20%)
Dizziness, asthenia, somnolence, nervousness, confusion, headache, infection, tremor
Occasional
Nausea, diarrhea, abdominal pain, impaired concentration

SERIOUS REACTIONS
• Overdose is characterized by agitation, confusion, hostility, and weakness. Full recovery occurs within 24 hours.

PRECAUTIONS & CONSIDERATIONS
Caution is warranted with hepatic impairment and in those who take other CNS depressants concurrently. Dizziness may occur, so change positions slowly—from recumbent to sitting position before standing, and alcohol and tasks requiring mental alertness or motor skills should be avoided. History of the seizure disorder, including the duration, frequency, and intensity of seizures, should be reviewed before and during therapy. CBCs and blood chemistry tests to assess hepatic and renal function should be performed before and during treatment.
Administration
Tiagabine should be taken with food.

Ticarcillin
tie-car-sill'in
(Ticar)

CATEGORY AND SCHEDULE
Pregnancy Risk Category: B

CLASSIFICATION
Antibiotics, penicillins

MECHANISM OF ACTION
Binds to bacterial cell wall, inhibiting bacterial cell wall synthesis. *Therapeutic Effect:* Causes cell lysis, death. Bactericidal.

PHARMACOKINETICS
Well absorbed. Widely distributed. Protein binding: 45%-60%. Minimal metabolism in liver. Primarily excreted unchanged in urine. Moderately dialyzable. **Half-life:** 1.2 hr (half-life is increased in those with impaired renal function).

AVAILABILITY
Powder for Reconstitution: 1g, 3 g, 20 g (Ticar).

INDICATIONS AND DOSAGES
▶ **Septicemia; skin and skin-structure, bone, joint, and lower respiratory tract infections; and endometriosis**
IV
Adults, Elderly, Children over 40 kg. 200-300 mg/kg/day q4-6hr or 3 g q4hr or 4 g q6hr. Maximum: 18 g/day.
Children and infants under 40 kg. 200-300 mg/kg/day q4-6hr. Maximum: 18 g/day.
Neonates over 2000 g. 75 mg/kg IV q8hr under 7 days old; 100 mg/kg IV q8hr over 7 old.
Neonates under 2000 g. 75 mg/kg IV q12hr under 7 days old; 75 mg/kg q8hr over 7 days old.

T

▸ **Urinary tract infection (UTI), complicated**
IV
Adults, Elderly, Children over 40 kg.
150-200 mg/kg/day divided q4-6hr or 3 g q6hr.
Children under 40 kg. 150-200 mg/kg/day in divided doses q6-8hr.
▸ **Urinary tract infection (UTI), uncomplicated**
IV/IM
Adults, Elderly, Children over 40 kg.
1 g q6hr.
Children under 40 kg. 50-100 mg/kg/day in divided doses q6-8hr.
▸ **Dosage in renal impairment**

Creatinine Clearance	Dosage Interval
30-60 ml/min	2 g q4hr
10-30 ml/min	2 g q8hr
Less than 10 ml/min	2 g q12hr

CONTRAINDICATIONS
Hypersensitivity to any penicillin

INTERACTIONS
Drug
Anticoagulants, heparin, NSAIDs, thrombolytics: May increase the risk of hemorrhage with high dosages of ticarcillin.
Probenecid: May increase ticarcillin blood concentration and risk of toxicity.
Herbal
None known.
Food
None known.

DIAGNOSTIC TEST EFFECTS
May cause positive Coombs' test. May increase bleeding time, serum alkaline phosphatase, serum bilirubin, serum creatinine, serum LDH, SGOT (AST), and SGPT (ALT) levels. May decrease serum potassium, sodium, and uric acid levels.

▦ IV INCOMPATIBILITIES
Amphotericin B complex (Abelcet, AmBisome, Amphotec), vancomycin (Vancocin)
▽ IV Compatibilities
Diltiazem (Cardizem), heparin, insulin, morphine, propofol (Diprivan)

SIDE EFFECTS
Frequent
Phlebitis, thrombophlebitis with IV dose, rash, urticaria, pruritus, smell or taste disturbances
Occasional
Nausea, diarrhea, vomiting
Rare
Headache, fatigue, hallucinations, bleeding, or bruising

SERIOUS REACTIONS
• Overdosage may produce seizures and neurologic reactions.
• Superinfections, including potentially fatal antibiotic-associated colitis, may result from bacterial imbalance.
• Severe hypersensitivity reactions, including anaphylaxis, occur rarely.

PRECAUTIONS & CONSIDERATIONS
Caution is warranted with a history of allergies, especially to cephalosporins, and renal impairment. Be aware that ticarcillin readily crosses the placenta, appears in amniotic fluid and cord blood, and is distributed in breast milk in low concentrations. Ticarcillin use in infants may lead to allergic sensitization, candidiasis, diarrhea, and skin rash.

Be aware that the safety and efficacy of this drug have not been established in children younger than 3 months. Age-related renal impairment may require dosage adjustment in the elderly.

Notify the physician if severe diarrhea, a rash or itching, or any other unusual sign or symptom occurs.

Storage

After reconstitution for IM injection, ticarcillin solution retains potency for 12 hours at room temperature or 24 hours if refrigerated. After reconstitution for IV administration, solutions in concentrations of 10 to 50 mg/ml retain most of their potency for 48 to 72 hours at room temperature or 14 days if refrigerated or 30 days when frozen.

Administration

Ticarcillin is generally given IV. IM injection is only for the treatment of uncomplicated urinary tract infections.

For direct intravenous use of ticarcillin, add at least 4 ml of D_5W, 0.9% NaCl, or lactated Ringers injection to each 1 g vial. Each gram of ticarcillin may be further diluted if desired. The resulting solution should be administered as slowly as possible to avoid vein irritation.

For intermittent infusions of ticarcillin, administer over 30 minutes to 2 hour periods in adults. For neonates, administer over a 10- to 20-minute period. Because of the potential for hypersensitivity reactions such as anaphylaxis, start initial dose at a few drops per minute, increase slowly to ordered rate; monitor the patient the first 10 to 15 minutes, then check the patient every 10 minutes.

For IM injection of ticarcillin, add 2 ml of sterile water for injection, 1% lidocaine hydrochloride injection (without epinephrine), or sodium chloride injection to each 1 g vial to provide a concentration of 1 g per 2.6 ml.

Ticarcillin Disodium/ Clavulanate Potassium

tyekar-sill'in klav'yoo-la-nate
(Timentin)

CATEGORY AND SCHEDULE

Pregnancy Risk Category: B

CLASSIFICATION

Antibiotics, penicillins

MECHANISM OF ACTION

Ticarcillin binds to bacterial cell walls, inhibiting cell wall synthesis. Clavulanate inhibits the action of bacterial beta-lactamase. *Therapeutic Effect:* Ticarcillin is bactericidal in susceptible organisms. Clavulanate protects ticarcillin from enzymatic degradation.

PHARMACOKINETICS

Widely distributed. Protein binding: ticarcillin 45%-60%, clavulanate 9%-30%. Minimally metabolized in the liver. Primarily excreted unchanged in urine. Removed by hemodialysis. **Half-life:** 1-1.2 hr (increased in impaired renal function).

AVAILABILITY

Powder for Injection: 3.1 g.
Premixed Solution for Infusion: 3.1 g/100 ml.

INDICATIONS AND DOSAGES

▸ **Skin and skin structure, bone, joint, and lower respiratory tract infections; septicemia; endometriosis**
IV
Adults, Elderly. 3.1 g (3 g ticarcillin) q4-6hr. Maximum: 18-24 g/day.
Children 3 mo and older.
200-300 mg (as ticarcillin) q4-6hr.

T

▶ **UTIs**
IV
Adults, Elderly. 3.1 g q6-8hr.
▶ **Dosage in renal impairment**
Dosage interval is modified based on creatinine clearance.

Creatinine Clearance	Dosage Interval
10-30 ml/min	Usual dose q8hr
Less than 10 ml/min	Usual dose q12hr

CONTRAINDICATIONS
Hypersensitivity to any penicillin

INTERACTIONS
Drug
Anticoagulants, heparin, NSAIDs, thrombolytics: May increase the risk of hemorrhage with high dosages of ticarcillin.
Probenecid: May increase ticarcillin blood concentration and risk of toxicity.
Herbal
None known.
Food
None known.

DIAGNOSTIC TEST EFFECTS
May increase bleeding time and serum alkaline phosphatase, bilirubin, creatinine, sLDH, AST (SGOT), and ALT (SGPT) levels. May decrease serum potassium, sodium, and uric acid levels. May cause a positive Coombs' test.

▨ IV INCOMPATIBILITIES
Amphotericin B complex (Abelcet, AmBisome, Amphotec), vancomycin (Vancocin)
▨ IV Compatibilities
Diltiazem (Cardizem), heparin, insulin, morphine, propofol (Diprivan)

SIDE EFFECTS
Frequent
Phlebitis or thrombophlebitis (with IV dose), rash, urticaria, pruritus, altered smell or taste
Occasional
Nausea, diarrhea, vomiting
Rare
Headache, fatigue, hallucinations, bleeding, or ecchymosis

SERIOUS REACTIONS
* Overdosage may produce seizures and other neurologic reactions.
* Antibiotic-associated colitis and other superinfections may result from bacterial imbalance.
* Severe hypersensitivity reactions, including anaphylaxis, occur rarely.

PRECAUTIONS & CONSIDERATIONS
Caution is warranted with renal impairment or a history of allergies, especially to cephalosporins. Ticarcillin readily crosses the placenta, appears in cord blood and amniotic fluid, and is distributed in breast milk in low concentrations. Ticarcillin may lead to allergic sensitization, candidiasis, diarrhea, and skin rash in infants. The safety and efficacy of ticarcillin have not been established in children younger than 3 months. Age-related renal impairment may require dosage adjustment in the elderly.

History of allergies, especially to cephalosporins or penicillins, should be determined before giving the drug. Withhold and promptly notify the physician if rash or diarrhea occurs. Severe diarrhea with abdominal pain, blood or mucus in stool, and fever may indicate antibiotic-associated colitis. Signs and symptoms of superinfection, including anal or genital pruritus, black hairy tongue, diarrhea, increased fever, sore throat, ulceration or changes of oral mucosa, and vomiting should be monitored. Food tolerance, intake and output, renal function tests, urinalysis, and the injection sites should be assessed.

Storage

The solution normally appears colorless to pale yellow; a darker color indicates a loss of potency. The reconstituted IV infusion (piggyback) is stable for 24 hours at room temperature and 3 days if refrigerated. Discard the solution if a precipitate forms.

Administration

This drug is available in ready-to-use containers. For IV infusion (piggyback), reconstitute each 3.1-g vial with 13 ml sterile water for injection or 0.9% NaCl to provide a concentration of 200 mg ticarcillin and 6.7 mg clavulanic acid per milliliter. Shake the vial to assist reconstitution. Further dilute with 50 to 100 ml D_5W or 0.9% NaCl. Infuse the drug over 30 minutes. Because of the potential for hypersensitivity reactions such as anaphylaxis, start the initial dose at a few drops per minute, and then increase it slowly to the ordered rate. Stay with the patient for the first 10 to 15 minutes during the initial dose; then check every 10 minutes during the infusion for signs and symptoms of hypersensitivity or anaphylaxis.

Ticlopidine
tye-klo′pa-deen
(Apo-Ticlopidine [CAN], Ticlid, Tilodene [AUS])

CATEGORY AND SCHEDULE
Pregnancy Risk Category: B

CLASSIFICATION
Platelet inhibitors

MECHANISM OF ACTION

An aggregation inhibitor that inhibits the release of adenosine diphosphate from activated platelets, which prevents fibrinogen from binding to glycoprotein IIb/IIIa receptors on the surface of activated platelets. *Therapeutic Effect:* Inhibits platelet aggregation and thrombus formation.

AVAILABILITY

Tablets: 250 mg.

INDICATIONS AND DOSAGES
▶ **Prevention of stroke**
PO
Adults, Elderly. 250 mg twice a day.

OFF-LABEL USES

Treatment of intermittent claudication, sickle cell disease, subarachnoid hemorrhage

CONTRAINDICATIONS

Active pathologic bleeding, such as bleeding peptic ulcer and intracranial bleeding, hematopoietic disorders, including neutropenia and thrombocytopenia; presence of hemostatic disorder; severe hepatic impairment

INTERACTIONS
Drug
Aspirin, heparin, oral anticoagulants, thrombolytics: May increase

the risk of bleeding with these drugs.
Herbal
None known.
Food
None known.

DIAGNOSTIC TEST EFFECTS

May increase serum cholesterol, serum alkaline phosphatase, bilirubin, triglyceride, AST (SGOT), and ALT (SGPT) levels. May prolong bleeding time. May decrease neutrophil and platelet counts.

SIDE EFFECTS

Frequent (13%-5%)
Diarrhea, nausea, dyspepsia, including heartburn, indigestion, GI discomfort, and bloating
Rare (2%-1%)
Vomiting, flatulence, pruritus, dizziness

SERIOUS REACTIONS

• Neutropenia occurs in approximately 2% of patients.
• Thrombotic thrombocytopenia purpura, agranulocytosis, hepatitis, cholestatic jaundice, and tinnitus occur rarely.

PRECAUTIONS & CONSIDERATIONS

Caution is warranted with an increased risk of bleeding and severe hepatic or renal disease. Safety and efficacy of ticlopidine in children have not been established. No age-related precautions have been noted in the elderly.

Laboratory studies, particularly hepatic enzyme tests and CBC, should be obtained. Pattern of daily bowel activity and stool consistency, B/P for hypotension, and skin for rash, should be monitored.
Administration
Take ticlopidine with food or just after meals to increase bioavailability

and decrease GI discomfort. Ticlopidine should be discontinued 10-14 days before surgery if antiplatelet effect is not desired.

Tiludronate
ti-loo'dro-nate
(Skelid)

CATEGORY AND SCHEDULE
Pregnancy Risk Category: C

CLASSIFICATION
Bisphosphonates

MECHANISM OF ACTION

A calcium regulator that inhibits functioning osteoclasts through disruption of cytoskeletal ring structure and inhibition of osteoclastic proton pump. *Therapeutic Effect:* Inhibits bone resorption.

AVAILABILITY

Tablets: 200 mg.

INDICATIONS AND DOSAGES

▶ **Paget's disease**
PO
Adults, Elderly. 400 mg once a day for 3 mo. Must take with 6-8 ounces plain water. Do not give within 2 hr of food intake. Avoid giving aspirin, calcium supplements, mineral supplements, or antacids within 2 hr of tiludronate administration.

CONTRAINDICATIONS

GI disease, such as dysphagia and gastric ulcer, impaired renal function.

INTERACTIONS
Drug
Antacids containing aluminum or magnesium, calcium, salicylates: May interfere with the absorption of tiludronate.
Herbal
None known.
Food
None known.

DIAGNOSTIC TEST EFFECTS
None known.

SIDE EFFECTS
Frequent (9%-6%)
Nausea, diarrhea, generalized body pain, back pain, headache
Occasional
Rash, dyspepsia, vomiting, rhinitis, sinusitis, dizziness

PRECAUTIONS & CONSIDERATIONS
Caution is warranted with hyperparathyroidism, hypocalcemia, and vitamin D deficiency. Because there are no adequate and well-controlled studies in pregnant women, it is unknown if tiludronate causes fetal harm or is excreted in breast milk. Safety and efficacy of tiludronate have not been established in children. No age-related precautions have been noted in the elderly. Serum calcium, serum alkaline phosphatase, osteocalcin, and urinary hydroxyproline levels should be adjusted to assess the effectiveness of tiludronate.
Administration
Take tiludronate at least 2 hours before or after beverages, food, other medications, calcium or other mineral supplements, and vitamin D. Take with 6 to 8 ounces of plain water (not mineral water).

Timolol
tim′oh-lole
(Apo-Timol [CAN], Apo-Timop [CAN], Betimol, Blocadren, Gen-Timolol [CAN], Istadol, Optimol [AUS], PMS-Timolol [CAN], Tenopt [AUS], Timoptic, Timoptic OccuDose, Timoptic XE, Timoptol [AUS], Timoptol XE [AUS])
Do not confuse timolol with atenolol, or Timoptic with Viroptic.

CATEGORY AND SCHEDULE
Pregnancy Risk Category: C (D if used in second or third trimester)

CLASSIFICATION
Antiadrenergics, beta blocking, ophthalmics

MECHANISM OF ACTION
An antihypertensive, antimigraine, and antiglaucoma agent that blocks beta$_1$- and beta$_2$-adrenergic receptors. *Therapeutic Effect:* Reduces intraocular pressure (IOP) by reducing aqueous humor production, lowers B/P, slows the heart rate, and decreases myocardial contractility.

PHARMACOKINETICS

Route	Onset	Peak	Duration
PO	15-45 min	0.5-2.5 hr	4 hr
Ophthalmic	30 min	1-2 hr	12-24 hr

Well absorbed from the GI tract. Protein binding: 10%. Minimal absorption after ophthalmic administration. Metabolized in the liver. Primarily excreted in urine.

Not removed by hemodialysis.
Half-life: 4 hr. Systemic absorption may occur with ophthalmic administration.

AVAILABILITY
Tablets (Blocadren): 5 mg, 10 mg, 20 mg.
Ophthalmic Gel (Timoptic-XE): 0.25%, 0.5%.
Ophthalmic Solution (Betimol, Timoptic, Timoptic OccuDose): 0.25%, 0.5%.

INDICATIONS AND DOSAGES
▸ **Mild to moderate hypertension**
PO
Adults, Elderly. Initially, 10 mg twice a day, alone or in combination with other therapy. Gradually increase at intervals of not less than 1 wk. Maintenance: 20-60 mg/day in 2 divided doses.
▸ **Reduction of cardiovascular mortality in definite or suspected acute MI**
PO
Adults, Elderly. 10 mg twice a day, beginning 1-4 wk after infarction.
▸ **Migraine prevention**
PO
Adults, Elderly. Initially, 10 mg twice a day. Range: 10-30 mg/day.
▸ **Reduction of IOP in open-angle glaucoma, aphakic glaucoma, ocular hypertension, and secondary glaucoma**
OPHTHALMIC
Adults, Elderly, Children. 1 drop of 0.25% solution in affected eye(s) twice a day. May be increased to 1 drop of 0.5% solution in affected eye(s) twice a day. When IOP is controlled, dosage may be reduced to 1 drop once a day. If patient is switched to timolol from another antiglaucoma agent, administer concurrently for 1 day. Discontinue other agent on following day.

▸ **Ophthalmic**
Adults, Elderly. Timoptic XE: 1 drop/day Istalol: Apply once daily.

OFF-LABEL USES
Systemic: Treatment of anxiety, cardiac arrhythmias, chronic angina pectoris, hypertrophic cardiomyopathy, migraine, pheochromocytoma, thyrotoxicosis, tremors
Ophthalmic: To decrease IOP in acute or chronic angle-closure glaucoma, treatment of angle-closure glaucoma during and after iridectomy, malignant glaucoma, secondary glaucoma

CONTRAINDICATIONS
Bronchial asthma, cardiogenic shock, CHF unless secondary to tachyarrhythmias, COPD, patients receiving MAOI therapy, second- or third-degree heart block, sinus bradycardia, uncontrolled cardiac failure

INTERACTIONS
Drug
Diuretics, other antihypertensives: May increase hypotensive effect.
Insulin, oral hypoglycemics: May mask symptoms of hypoglycemia and prolong hypoglycemic effects of these drugs.
NSAIDs: May decrease antihypertensive effect.
Sympathomimetics, xanthines: May mutually inhibit effects.
Herbal
None known.
Food
None known.

DIAGNOSTIC TEST EFFECTS
May increase antinuclear antibody titer and BUN, serum LDH, serum lipoprotein, serum alkaline phosphatase, serum bilirubin, serum creatinine, serum potassium, serum uric

acid, AST (SGOT), ALT (SGPT), and serum triglyceride levels.

SIDE EFFECTS

Frequent
Diminished sexual function, drowsiness, difficulty sleeping, unusual tiredness or weakness
Ophthalmic: Eye irritation, visual disturbances
Occasional
Depression, cold hands or feet, diarrhea, constipation, anxiety, nasal congestion, nausea, vomiting, bradycardia, bronchospasm
Rare
Altered taste, dry eyes, itching, numbness of fingers, toes, or scalp

SERIOUS REACTIONS

• Overdose may produce profound bradycardia, hypotension, and bronchospasm.
• Abrupt withdrawal may result in diaphoresis, palpitations, headache, and tremors.
• Timolol administration may precipitate CHF and MI in patients with cardiac disease; thyroid storm in those with thyrotoxicosis; and peripheral ischemia in those with existing peripheral vascular disease.
• Hypoglycemia may occur in patients with previously controlled diabetes.
• Ophthalmic overdose may produce bradycardia, hypotension, bronchospasm, and acute cardiac failure.

PRECAUTIONS & CONSIDERATIONS

Caution is warranted with hyperthyroidism, impaired hepatic or renal function, and inadequate cardiac function. Precautions apply to both oral and ophthalmic administration because of the possible systemic absorption of ophthalmic timolol. Timolol is distributed in breast milk and is not for use in breast-feeding women because of the potential for serious adverse effects in the breast-fed infant. Timolol use should be avoided in pregnant women after the first trimester because it may result in low-birth-weight infants. The drug may also produce apnea, bradycardia, hypoglycemia, or hypothermia during childbirth. The safety and efficacy of timolol have not been established in children. In the elderly, age-related peripheral vascular disease increases susceptibility to decreased peripheral circulation. Be aware that salt and alcohol intake should be restricted. Nasal decongestants or OTC cold preparations (stimulants) should not be used without physician approval. Tasks that require mental alertness or motor skills should be avoided.

Notify the physician of excessive fatigue, prolonged dizziness or headache, or shortness of breath. Pattern of daily bowel activity and stool consistency, EKG for arrhythmias (particularly premature ventricular contractions), B/P, heart rate, IOP (with ophthalmic preparation), and liver and renal function test results should be monitored during treatment. If pulse rate is 60 beats/minute or lower or systolic B/P is less than 90 mm Hg, withhold the medication and contact the physician.

Administration
Take timolol without regard to meals. Tablets may be crushed. Do not abruptly discontinue timolol. Compliance is essential to control angina, arrhythmias, glaucoma, and hypertension.
! When administering ophthalmic gel, invert container and shake once before each use.
For ophthalmic administration, place a gloved finger on the lower eyelid and pull it out until pocket is formed between the eye and lower lid. Hold the dropper above the pocket and

T

place the prescribed number of drops or amount of prescribed gel into pocket. Close eyes gently so that medication will not be squeezed out of the sac. Apply gentle digital pressure to the lacrimal sac at the inner canthus for 1 minute after installation to lessen the risk of systemic absorption.

Tinidazole
ty-ni′da-zole
(Tindamax)

CATEGORY AND SCHEDULE
Pregnancy Risk Category: C

CLASSIFICATION
Antiprotozoals

MECHANISM OF ACTION
A nitroimidazole derivative that is converted to the active metabolite by reduction of cell extracts of *Trichomonas*. The active metabolite causes DNA damage in pathogens. *Therapeutic Effect:* Produces antiprotozoal effect.

PHARMACOKINETICS
Rapidly and completely absorbed. Protein binding: 12%. Distributed in all body tissues and fluids; crosses blood-brain barrier. Significantly metabolized. Primarily excreted in urine; partially eliminated in feces. **Half-life:** 12-14 hr.

AVAILABILITY
Tablets: 250 mg, 500 mg.

INDICATIONS AND DOSAGES
▸ **Intestinal amebiasis**

PO
Adults, Elderly. 2 g/day for 3 days.
Children 3 yr and older. 50 mg/kg/day (up to 2 g) for 3 days.
▸ **Amebic hepatic abscess**
PO
Adults, Elderly. 2 g/day for 3-5 days.
Children 3 yr and older. 50 mg/kg/day (up to 2 g) for 3-5 days.
▸ **Giardiasis**
PO
Adults, Elderly. 2 g as a single dose.
Children 3 yr and older. 50 mg/kg (up to 2 g) as a single dose.
▸ **Trichomoniasis**
PO
Adults, Elderly. 2 g as a single dose.

CONTRAINDICATIONS
First trimester of pregnancy, hypersensitivity to nitroimidazole derivatives

INTERACTIONS
Drug
Alcohol: May cause a disulfiram-type reaction.
Cholestyramine, oxytetracycline: May decrease the effectiveness of tinidazole; separate dosage times.
Cimetidine, fosphenytoin, keto-conazole, phenobarbital, rifampin: Decreases the metabolism of tinidazole.
Cyclosporine, fluorouracil, lithium, phenytoin (IV), tacrolimus: May increase blood levels of these drugs.
Disulfiram: May increase the risk of psychotic reactions (separate dose by 2 weeks).
Oral anticoagulants: Increase the risk of bleeding.
Herbal
None known.
Food
None known.

DIAGNOSTIC TEST EFFECTS
May increase serum LDH, triglyceride, AST (SGOT), and ALT (SGPT) levels.

SIDE EFFECTS
Occasional (4%-2%)
Metallic or bitter taste, nausea, weakness, fatigue, or malaise
Rare (less than 2%)
Epigastric distress, anorexia, vomiting, headache, dizziness, red-brown or darkened urine

SERIOUS REACTIONS
• Peripheral neuropathy, characterized by paresthesia, is usually reversible if tinidazole treatment is stopped as soon as neurologic symptoms appear.
• Superinfection, hypersensitivity reaction, and seizures occur rarely.

PRECAUTIONS & CONSIDERATIONS
Caution is warranted with blood dyscrasia, candidiasis (may present more prominent symptoms during tinidazole therapy), central nervous system disease (risk of seizure or peripheral neuropathy), liver impairment, and concurrent treatment with related agents such as metronidazole. Tinidazole crosses the placenta and is distributed in breast milk. Safety and efficacy of tinidazole have not established in children younger than 3 years. There are no age-related precautions noted in the elderly. Avoid alcohol while taking tinidazole and for at least 3 days after discontinuing the medication.
Storage
Store at room temperature.
Administration
Score tablets may be crushed. Take with regard to meals or snack to minimize GI irritation. Do not miss a dose and complete the full length of treatment.

Tinzaparin
tin-za-pair'in
(Innohep)

CATEGORY AND SCHEDULE
Pregnancy Risk Category: B

CLASSIFICATION
Anticoagulants

MECHANISM OF ACTION
A low-molecular-weight heparin that inhibits factor Xa. Causes less inactivation of thrombin, inhibition of platelets, and bleeding than standard heparin. Does not significantly influence bleeding time, PT, aPTT.
Therapeutic Effect: Produces anticoagulation.

PHARMACOKINETICS
Well absorbed after subcutaneous administration. Primarily eliminated in urine. **Half-life:** 3-4 hr.

AVAILABILITY
Injection: 20,000 anti-Xa international units/ml.

INDICATIONS AND DOSAGES
▸ **Deep vein thrombosis**
SUBCUTANEOUS
Adults, Elderly. 175 anti-Xa international units/kg once a day. Continue for at least 6 days and until patient is sufficiently anticoagulated with warfarin (International Normalizing Ratio [INR] of 2 or more for 2 consecutive days).

CONTRAINDICATIONS
Active major bleeding, concurrent heparin therapy, hypersensitivity to heparin or pork products,

thrombocytopenia associated with positive in vitro test for antiplatelet antibody

INTERACTIONS
Drug
Anticoagulants, platelet inhibitors: May increase the risk of bleeding.
Herbal
Ginkgo biloba: May increase the risk of bleeding.
Food
None known.

DIAGNOSTIC TEST EFFECTS
Increases (reversible) LDH, serum alkaline phosphatase, AST (SGOT), and ALT (SGPT) levels.

SIDE EFFECTS
Frequent (16%)
Injection site reaction, such as inflammation, oozing, nodules, and skin necrosis
Rare (less than 2%)
Nausea, asthenia, constipation, epistaxis

SERIOUS REACTIONS
• Overdose may lead to bleeding complications ranging from local ecchymoses to major hemorrhage. Antidote: Dose of protamine sulfate (1% solution) should be equal to dose of tinzaparin injected. One mg protamine sulfate neutralizes 100 units of tinzaparin. A second dose of 0.5 mg tinzaparin per 1 mg protamine sulfate may be given if aPTT tested 2-4 hours after the initial infusion remains prolonged.

PRECAUTIONS & CONSIDERATIONS
Caution is warranted with conditions associated with increased risk of hemorrhage, history of recent GI ulceration and hemorrhage, history of heparin-induced thrombocytopenia, impaired renal function, uncontrolled arterial hypertension, and in the elderly. Tinzaparin should be used with caution in pregnant women, particularly during the last trimester and immediately postpartum because it increases the risk of maternal hemorrhage. It is unknown if tinzaparin is excreted in breast milk. Safety and efficacy of tinzaparin have not been established in children. The elderly may be more susceptible to bleeding.

Notify the physician of chest pain, injection site reaction, such as inflammation, nodules, oozing, numbness, pain, swelling or tingling of joints, unusual bleeding, or bruising. PT, INR, and CBC, including platelet count, should be monitored before and during therapy. Be aware of signs of bleeding, including bleeding at injection or surgical sites or from gums, blood in stool, bruising, hematuria, and petechiae.
Storage
Store at room temperature.
Administration
! Do not mix with other injections or infusions. Do not give IM.
Administer tinzaparin by subcutaneous route only.

The parenteral form normally appears clear and colorless to pale yellow. Lie down before administering by deep subcutaneous injection.

Tioconazole
tyo-con'a-zole
(Gynecure [CAN], Monistat-1,
Trosyd [CAN], Vagistat)

CATEGORY AND SCHEDULE
Pregnancy Risk Category: C

CLASSIFICATION
Antifungals, topical,
dermatologics

MECHANISM OF ACTION
An imidazole derivative that inhibits
synthesis of ergosterol (vital component of fungal cell formation).
Therapeutic Effect: Damaging fungal
cell membrane. Fungistatic.

PHARMACOKINETICS
Negliglble absorption from vaginal
application.

AVAILABILITY
Vaginal Ointment: 6.5% (Monistat-1,
Vagistat).

INDICATIONS AND DOSAGES
▸ **Vulvovaginal candidiasis**
INTRAVAGINAL
Adults, Elderly. 1 applicatorful
just before bedtime as a single
dose.

CONTRAINDICATIONS
Hypersensitivity to tioconazole
or other imidazole antifungal
agents

INTERACTIONS
Drug
None known.
Herbal
None known.
Food
None known.

DIAGNOSTIC TEST EFFECTS
None known.

SIDE EFFECTS
Frequent (25%)
Headache
Occasional (6%-1%)
Burning, itching
Rare (less than 1%)
Irritation, vaginal pain, dysuria,
dryness of vaginal secretions, vulvar
edema/swelling

SERIOUS REACTIONS
• None reported.

PRECAUTIONS & CONSIDERATIONS
Caution is warranted with diabetes
and HIV or AIDS infection. It is
unknown if tioconazole is distributed
in breast milk. Safety and efficacy
have not been established in children.
There are no age-related precautions
noted in the elderly. Separate personal
items that come in contact with
affected areas.
Storage
Store at room temperature.
Administration
Insert applicatorful high into vagina
just before bedtime. Contact physician if itching or burning continues.
Be aware that tioconazole base
may interact with latex or rubber.
Condoms or diaphragms should
not be used within 72 hours of
administration.

T

Tiopronin
tye-o-pro'nin
Thiola

CATEGORY AND SCHEDULE
Pregnancy Risk Category: C

CLASSIFICATION
Cystine depleting agents

MECHANISM OF ACTION
A sulfhydryl compound with similar properties to those of penicillamine and glutathione that undergoes thiol-disulfide exchange with cysteine to form tiopronin-cysteine, a mixed disulfide. This disulfide is water soluble, unlike cysteine, and does not crystallize in the kidneys. May break disulfide bonds present in bronchial secretions and break the mucus complexes. *Therapeutic Effect:* Decreases cysteine excretion.

PHARMACOKINETICS
Moderately absorbed from the gastrointestinal (GI) tract. Primarily excreted in urine. Following oral administration, up to 48% of dose appears in urine during the first 4 hours and up to 78% by 72 hours. **Half-life:** 53 hr.

AVAILABILITY
Tablets: 100 mg (Thiola).

INDICATIONS AND DOSAGES
▸ **Crystinuria**
PO
Adults, Elderly. Initially, 800 mg in 3 divided doses. Adjust and maintain crystine concentration below its solubility limit (usually less than 250 mg/l).
Children 9 yr and older. 15 mg/kg/day in 3 divided doses. Adjust and maintain crystine concentration below its solubility limit (usually less than 250 mg/l).

OFF-LABEL USES
Cataracts, epilepsy, hepatitis, rheumatoid arthritis

CONTRAINDICATIONS
History of agranulocytosis, aplastic anemia, or thrombocytopenia while on tiopronin, pregnancy and lactation, hypersensitivity to tiopronin or its components

INTERACTIONS
Drug
None known.
Herbal
None known.
Food
Sodium: May increase cystine in urine.

DIAGNOSTIC TEST EFFECTS
None known.

▦ IV INCOMPATIBILITIES
None known.
▯ **IV Compatibilities**
None known.

SIDE EFFECTS
Frequent
Pain, swelling, tenderness of skin, rash, hives, itching, oral ulcers
Occasional
GI upset, taste or smell impairment, bloody or cloudy urine, chills, difficulty in breathing, high blood pressure, hoarseness, joint pain, swelling of feet or lower legs, tenderness of glands
Rare
Chest pain, cough, difficulty in chewing, talking, swallowing, double vision, general feeling of discomfort, illness, weakness, muscle weakness,

spitting up blood, swelling of lymph glands

SERIOUS REACTIONS
• Hematologic abnormalities, including myelosuppression, unusual bleeding, drug fever, renal complications, and lupus erythematous-like reaction including fever, arthralgia, and lymphadenopathy rarely occur.

PRECAUTIONS & CONSIDERATIONS
Caution is warranted with history of penicillamine exposure; serious adverse reactions are more likely to occur. It is unknown if tiopronin crosses the placenta or is distributed in breast milk. Safety and efficacy of tiopronin have not been established in children less than 9 years old. There are no age-related precautions noted in the elderly. Drastic dietary changes especially in sodium should be avoided. Fluid intake should be increased to maintain urine pH at a normal range of 6.5-7.
Administration
Take tiopronin on an empty stomach.

Tiotropium
ty-oh'tro-pee-um
(Spiriva)

CATEGORY AND SCHEDULE
Pregnancy Risk Category: C

CLASSIFICATION
Anticholinergics, bronchodilators

MECHANISM OF ACTION
An anticholinergic that binds to recombinant human muscarinic receptors at the smooth muscle,

resulting in long-acting bronchial smooth-muscle relaxation.
Therapeutic Effect: Relieves bronchospasm.

PHARMACOKINETICS

Route	Onset	Peak	Duration
Inhalation	N/A	N/A	24-36 hr

Binds extensively to tissue. Protein binding: 72%. Metabolized by oxidation. Excreted in urine.
Half-life: 5-6 days

AVAILABILITY
Powder for Inhalation:
18 mcg/capsule (in blister packs containing 6 capsules with inhaler).

INDICATIONS AND DOSAGES
▸ COPD
INHALATION
Adults, Elderly. 18 mcg (1 capsule)/day via *HandiHaler* inhalation device.

CONTRAINDICATIONS
History of hypersensitivity to atropine or its derivatives, including ipratropium

INTERACTIONS
Drug
Ipratropium: Concurrent administration with this drug is not recommended.
Herbal
None known.
Food
None known.

DIAGNOSTIC TEST EFFECTS
None known.

SIDE EFFECTS
Frequent (16%-6%)
Dry mouth, sinusitis, pharyngitis, dyspepsia, UTI, rhinitis

T

Occasional (5%-4%)
Abdominal pain, peripheral edema, constipation, epistaxis, vomiting, myalgia, rash, oral candidiasis

SERIOUS REACTIONS
• Angina pectoris, depression, and flulike symptoms occur rarely.

PRECAUTIONS & CONSIDERATIONS
Caution is warranted with angle-closure glaucoma, benign prostatic hyperplasia, and bladder neck obstruction. It is unknown if tiotropium is distributed in breast milk. The safety and efficacy of tiotropium have not been established in children. The elderly are more likely to experience constipation, dry mouth, and UTI. Drink plenty of fluids to decrease the thickness of lung secretions. Avoid excessive use of caffeinated products, such as chocolate, cocoa, cola, coffee, and tea.

Pulse rate and quality, respiratory rate, depth, rhythm and type, ABG levels, and clinical improvement should be monitored. Fingernails and lips should be assessed for cyanosis, including a blue or dusky color in light-skinned patients and a gray color in dark-skinned patients, which are signs of hypoxemia.

Storage
Store tiotropium capsules at room temperature. Protect them from extreme temperatures and moisture. Don't store capsules in the HandiHaler device.

Administration
For inhalation, open the HandiHaler dustcap by pulling it up; then open the mouthpiece. Place the capsule in the center chamber and firmly close the mouthpiece until you hear a click, leaving the dustcap open. Use only 1 capsule for inhalation at a time. Holding the HandiHaler device with the mouthpiece up, press the piercing button completely once and then release it. Exhale completely before inhaling slowly and deeply, at a rate sufficient to hear the capsule vibrate. Hold breath for as long as is comfortable and then exhale slowly. Repeat this process a second time to ensure the full dose is received. Rinse mouth with water immediately after inhalation to prevent mouth and throat dryness and oral candidiasis.

Tirofiban
tye-roe-fye′ban
(Aggrastat)
Do not confuse Aggrastat with Aggrenox.

CATEGORY AND SCHEDULE
Pregnancy Risk Category: B

CLASSIFICATION
Platelet inhibitors

MECHANISM OF ACTION
An antiplatelet and antithrombotic agent that binds to platelet receptor glycoprotein IIb/IIIa, preventing binding of fibrinogen. *Therapeutic Effect:* Inhibits platelet aggregation and thrombus formation.

PHARMACOKINETICS
Poorly bound to plasma proteins; unbound fraction in plasma: 35%. Limited metabolism. Primarily eliminated in the urine (65%) and, to a lesser amount, in the feces. Removed by hemodialysis. **Half-life:** 2 hr. Clearance is significantly decreased in severe renal impairment (creatinine clearance less than 30 ml/min).

AVAILABILITY

Injection Premix: 12.5 mg/250 ml, 25 mg/500 ml (50 mcg/ml).
Vial: 250 mcg/ml.

INDICATIONS AND DOSAGES

▸ **Inhibition of platelet aggregation**
IV
Adults, Elderly. Initially, 0.4 mcg/kg/min for 30 min; then continue at 0.1 mcg/kg/min through procedure and for 12-24 hr after procedure.
▸ **Severe renal insufficiency (creatinine clearance less than 30 ml/min)**
Adults, Elderly. Half the usual rate of infusion.

CONTRAINDICATIONS

Active internal bleeding or a history of bleeding diathesis within previous 30 days, arteriovenous malformation or aneurysm, history of intracranial hemorrhage, history of thrombocytopenia after prior exposure to tirofiban, intracranial neoplasm, major surgical procedure within previous 30 days, severe hypertension, stroke

INTERACTIONS

Drug
Drugs that affect hemostasis (such as aspirin, heparin, NSAIDs, and warfarin): May increase the risk of bleeding
Herbal
None known.
Food
None known.

DIAGNOSTIC TEST EFFECTS

Decreases Hct, Hgb, and platelet count.

▩ IV INCOMPATIBILITIES

Do not mix with other medications.

SIDE EFFECTS

Occasional (6%-3%)
Pelvis pain, bradycardia, dizziness, leg pain

Rare (2%-1%)
Edema and swelling, vasovagal reaction, diaphoresis, nausea, fever, headache

SERIOUS REACTIONS

• Signs and symptoms of overdose include generally minor mucocutaneous bleeding and bleeding at the femoral artery access site.
• Thrombocytopenia occurs rarely.

PRECAUTIONS & CONSIDERATIONS

Caution is warranted with hemorrhagic retinopathy, platelet counts less than 150,000/mm^3, renal impairment, and those who are also receiving drugs affecting hemostasis, such as warfarin. It is unknown if tirofiban is distributed in breast milk. Safety and efficacy of tirofiban have not been established in children. There is an increased risk of bleeding in the elderly. Use tirofiban with caution in this population. Be aware that it may take longer to stop bleeding during tirofiban therapy.

Notify the physician of any unusual bleeding or before a surgery or new drugs are prescribed. aPTT should be monitored 6 hours after the beginning of the heparin infusion. Heparin dosage should be adjusted to maintain aPTT at approximately 2 times control. NG tube and urinary catheter should be avoided, if possible.

Storage
Store at room temperature and protect from light. Use only clear solution. Discard unused solution 24 hours after start of infusion.

Administration
! Heparin and tirofiban can be administered through the same IV line.

For injection for solution (250 mcg/ml), withdraw and discard 100 ml from a 500-ml bag of 0.9% NaCl or D$_5$W and replace this volume with 100 ml of tirofiban drawn from two 50-ml vials, or withdraw and discard 50 ml from a 250-ml bag and replace with 50 ml of tirofiban drawn from one 50-ml vial to achieve a final concentration of 50 mcg/ml. Mix injection for solution (250 mcg/ml) well before administration. For injection (50 mcg/ml) premix in 500-ml IntraVia container, tear off the dust cover to open the IntraVia container. Check the IntraVia container for leaks by squeezing the inner bag firmly; if a leak is found or if the solution is not clear, discard the solution. Do not add other drugs or remove injection (50 mcg/ml) premix solution directly from the bag with a syringe. Do not use plastic containers in series connections because doing so may result in air embolism caused by drawing air from the first container that holds no solution. For loading dose, give 0.4 mcg/kg/min for 30 minutes. For maintenance infusion, give 0.1 mcg/kg/min.

Tizanidine
tye-zan'i-deen
(Zanaflex)

CATEGORY AND SCHEDULE
Pregnancy Risk Category: C

CLASSIFICATION
Adrenergic agonists, musculoskeletal agents, relaxants, skeletal muscle

---

MECHANISM OF ACTION
A skeletal muscle relaxant that increases presynaptic inhibition of spinal motor neurons mediated by alpha$_2$-adrenergic agonists, reducing facilitation to postsynaptic motor neurons. *Therapeutic Effect:* Reduces muscle spasticity.

PHARMACOKINETICS

Route	Onset	Peak	Duration
PO	N/A	1-2 hr	3-6 hr

Metabolized in the liver. **Half-life**: 4-8 hr.

AVAILABILITY
Tablets: 2 mg, 4 mg.

INDICATIONS AND DOSAGES
▸ **Muscle spasticity**
PO
Adults, Elderly. Initially 2-4 mg, gradually increased in 2- to 4-mg increments and repeated q6-8hr. Maximum: 3 doses/day or 36 mg/24 hr.

OFF-LABEL USES
Spasticity associated with multiple sclerosis or spinal cord injury

CONTRAINDICATIONS
None known.

INTERACTIONS
Drug
Alcohol, other CNS depressants: May increase CNS depressant effects.
Antihypertensives: May increase tizanidine's hypotensive potential.
Oral contraceptives: May reduce tizanidine clearance.
Phenytoin: May increase serum levels and risk of toxicity of phenytoin.
Herbal
None known.
Food
None known.

DIAGNOSTIC TEST EFFECTS

May increase serum alkaline phosphatase, AST (SGOT), and ALT (SGPT) levels.

SIDE EFFECTS

Frequent (49%-41%)
Dry mouth, somnolence, asthenia
Occasional (16%-4%)
Dizziness, UTI, constipation
Rare (3%)
Nervousness, amblyopia, pharyngitis, rhinitis, vomiting, urinary frequency

SERIOUS REACTIONS

• Hypotension (a reduction in either diastolic or systolic B/P) may be associated with bradycardia, orthostatic hypotension and, rarely, syncope. The risk of hypotension increases as dosage increases; B/P may decrease within 1 hour after administration.

PRECAUTIONS & CONSIDERATIONS

Caution is warranted with hypotension and cardiac, hepatic, or renal disease. The safety and efficacy of tizanidine have not been established in children. In the elderly, age-related renal impairment may warrant cautious use.

Low blood pressure, impaired coordination, and sedation may occur. Avoid alcohol, CNS depressants, and tasks that require mental alertness or motor skills. Change positions slowly to prevent dizziness. Baseline serum alkaline phosphatase and total bilirubin levels should be obtained. Therapeutic response, such as decreased stiffness, tenderness, and intensity of skeletal muscle pain and improved mobility, should be assessed.

Administration

Do not abruptly discontinue the medication.

Tobramycin Sulfate

toe-bra-mye'sin
(AK-Tob, Apo-Tobramycin
[CAN], Nebcin, PMS-
Tobramycin, TOBI, Tobrex)

CATEGORY AND SCHEDULE

Pregnancy Risk Category: C
(B, ophthalmic form)

CLASSIFICATION

Antibiotics, aminoglycosides

MECHANISM OF ACTION

An aminoglycoside antibiotic that irreversibly binds to protein on bacterial ribosomes. *Therapeutic Effect:* Interferes with protein synthesis of susceptible microorganisms.

PHARMACOKINETICS

Rapid, complete absorption after IM administration. Protein binding: 30%. Widely distributed (doesn't cross the blood-brain barrier; low concentrations in CSF. Excreted unchanged in urine. Removed by hemodialysis. **Half-life:** 2-4 hr (increased in impaired renal function and neonates; decreased in cystic fibrosis and febrile or burn patients).

AVAILABILITY

Injection Solution (Nebcin):
10 mg/ml, 40 mg/ml.
Injection Powder for Reconstitution (Nebcin): 1.2 g.
Ophthalmic Ointment (Tobrex): 0.3%.
Ophthalmic Solution (AKTob, Tobrex): 0.3%.
Nebulization Solution (TOBI):
60 mg/ml.

INDICATIONS AND DOSAGES

‣ **Skin and skin structure, bone, joint, respiratory tract, postoperative,**

T

intra-abdominal, and burn wound infections; complicated UTIs; septicemia; meningitis
IV, IM
Adults, Elderly. 3-6 mg/kg/day in 3 divided doses or 4-6.6 mg/kg once a day.

▸ **Superficial eye infections, including blepharitis, conjunctivitis, keratitis, and corneal ulcers**
OPHTHALMIC OINTMENT
Adults, Elderly. Usual dosage, apply a thin strip to conjunctiva q8-12hr (q3-4hr for severe infections).
OPHTHALMIC SOLUTION
Adults, Elderly. Usual dosage, 1-2 drops in affected eye q4hr (2 drops/hr for severe infections).

▸ **Bronchopulmonary infections in patients with cystic fibrosis**
INHALATION SOLUTION
Adults. Usual dosage, 60-80 mg twice a day for 28 days, then off for 28 days.
Children. 40-80 mg 2-3 times/day.

▸ **Dosage in renal impairment**
Dosage and frequency are modified based on the degree of renal impairment and the serum drug concentration. After a loading dose of 1-2 mg/kg, the maintenance dose and frequency are based on serum creatinine levels and creatinine clearance.

CONTRAINDICATIONS

Hypersensitivity to tobramycin, other aminoglycosides (cross-sensitivity), and their components

INTERACTIONS

Drug
Nephrotoxic medications, other aminoglycosides, ototoxic medications: May increase the risk of nephrotoxicity and ototoxicity.
Neuromuscular blockers: May increase neuromuscular blockade.

Herbal
None known.
Food
None known.

DIAGNOSTIC TEST EFFECTS

May increase serum bilirubin, BUN, serum creatinine, serum LDH, SGOT (AST), and SGPT (ALT) levels. May decrease serum calcium, magnesium, potassium, and sodium concentrations. Therapeutic peak serum level is 5-20 mcg/ml; therapeutic trough serum level is 0.5-2 mcg/ml. Toxic peak serum level is greater than 20 mcg/ml; toxic trough serum level is greater than 2 mcg/ml.

▨ IV INCOMPATIBILITIES

Amphotericin B complex (Abelcet, AmBisome, Amphotec), heparin, hetastarch (Hespan), indomethacin (Indocin), propofol (Diprivan), sargramostim (Leukine, Prokine)

▨ IV Compatibilities

Amiodarone (Cordarone), calcium gluconate, diltiazem (Cardizem), furosemide (Lasix), hydromorphone (Dilaudid), insulin, magnesium sulfate, midazolam (Versed), morphine, theophylline

SIDE EFFECTS

Occasional
IM: Pain, induration
IV: Phlebitis, thrombophlebitis
Topical: Hypersensitivity reaction (fever, pruritus, rash, urticaria)
Ophthalmic: Tearing, itching, redness, eyelid swelling
Rare
Hypotension, nausea, vomiting

SERIOUS REACTIONS

• Nephrotoxicity (as evidenced by increased BUN and serum creatinine levels and decreased creatinine clearance) may be reversible if the drug is stopped at the first sign of nephro-toxic symptoms.

• Irreversible ototoxicity (manifested as tinnitus, dizziness, ringing or roaring in ears, and hearing loss) and neurotoxicity (manifested as headache, dizziness, lethargy, tremor, and visual disturbances) occur occasionally. The risk of these reactions increases with higher dosages or prolonged therapy and when the solution is applied directly to the mucosa.

• Superinfections, particularly fungal infections, may result from bacterial imbalance with any administration route.

• Anaphylaxis may occur.

PRECAUTIONS & CONSIDERATIONS

Caution is warranted with concomitant use of neuromuscular blockers and in those with impaired renal function or auditory or vestibular impairment. Tobramycin readily crosses the placenta and is distributed in breast milk. Tobramycin may cause fetal nephrotoxicity. The ophthalmic form should not be used in breast-feeding mothers and only when specifically indicated in pregnant women. Immature renal function in neonates and premature infants may increase the risk of toxicity. Age-related renal impairment may require a dosage adjustment in elderly patients.

Determine the patient's history of allergies, especially to aminoglycosides, sulfites, and parabens (for topical and ophthalmic routes), before giving the drug. Establish the baseline hearing acuity before beginning therapy. Intake and output and urinalysis results, as appropriate, should be monitored. To maintain adequate hydration, encourage the patient to drink fluids. Monitor urinalysis results for casts, RBCs,

WBCs, and decreased specific gravity. Be alert for ototoxic and neurotoxic side effects. If giving ophthalmic tobramycin, monitor the patient's eye for burning, itching, redness, eyelid swelling and tearing. If giving topical tobramycin, monitor for itching and redness. Be alert for signs and symptoms of superinfection, particularly changes in the oral mucosa, diarrhea, and genital or anal pruritus. Monitor peak and trough serum drug levels.

Storage

Store ophthalmic preparation and solution vials for injection at room temperature. Solutions may be discolored by light or air, but discoloration doesn't affect drug potency.

Administration

! Space parenteral doses evenly around the clock. Be aware that dosages are based on ideal body weight. Expect to monitor peak and trough serum drug levels. The therapeutic peak serum level is 5 to 20 mcg/ml, and the therapeutic trough level is 0.5 to 2 mcg/ml; the toxic peak serum level is greater than 20 mcg/ml, and the toxic trough level is greater than 2 mcg/ml.

For IV use, dilute with 50 to 200 ml of D_5W or 0.9% NaCl. The amount of diluent for infant and children dosages depends on individual needs. Infuse over 20 to 60 minutes.

For IM use, to minimize injection site discomfort, administer the IM injection slowly and deep into the gluteus maximus rather than the lateral aspect of the thigh.

For ophthalmic use, place a gloved finger on the lower eyelid, and pull it out until a pocket is formed between the eye and lower lid. Hold the dropper above the pocket and place the correct number of drops (or 1/4 to 1/2 inch of ointment) into the pocket. Close the eye gently.

After administering ophthalmic solution, apply digital pressure to the lacrimal sac for 1 to 2 minutes to minimize drainage into the nose and throat, thereby reducing the risk of systemic effects. After applying ophthalmic ointment, close the eye for 1 to 2 minutes. Roll the eyeball to increase the drug's contact with the eye. Use a tissue to remove excess solution or ointment around the eye.

Tocainide
toe-kay'nide
(Tonocard)

CATEGORY AND SCHEDULE
Pregnancy Risk Category: C

CLASSIFICATION
Antiarrhythmics, class IB

MECHANISM OF ACTION
An amide-type local anesthetic that shortens the action potential duration and decreases the effective refractory period and automaticity in the His-Purkinje system of the myocardium by blocking sodium transport across myocardial cell membranes.
Therapeutic Effect: Suppresses ventricular arrhythmias.

AVAILABILITY
Tablets: 400 mg, 600 mg.

INDICATIONS AND DOSAGES
▸ **Suppression and prevention of ventricular arrhythmias**
PO
Adults, Elderly. Initially, 400 mg q8hr. Maintenance: 1.2-1.8 g/day in divided doses q8hr. Maximum: 2400 mg/day.

CONTRAINDICATIONS
Hypersensitivity to local anesthetics, second- or third-degree AV block

INTERACTIONS
Drug
Beta-adrenergic blockers: May increase pulmonary wedge pressure and decrease cardiac index.
Other antiarrhythmics: May increase risk of adverse cardiac effects.
Herbal
None known.
Food
None known.

DIAGNOSTIC TEST EFFECTS
None known.

SIDE EFFECTS
Tocainide is generally well tolerated.
Frequent (10%-3%)
Minor, transient lightheadedness, dizziness, nausea, paraesthesia, rash, tremor
Occasional (3%-1%)
Clammy skin, night sweats, myalgia
Rare (less than 1%)
Restlessness, nervousness, disorientation, mood changes, ataxia (muscular incoordination), visual disturbances

SERIOUS REACTIONS
• High dosage may produce bradycardia or tachycardia, hypotension, palpitations, increased ventricular arrhythmias, premature ventricular contractions (PVCs), chest pain, and exacerbation of CHF.

PRECAUTIONS & CONSIDERATIONS
Caution is warranted with bone marrow failure, CHF, hepatic and renal impairment, and pre-existing arrhythmias.

Notify the physician of any CNS disturbances, including disorientation, incoordination, mood changes, and restlessness or any signs and symptoms of CHF, including distended neck veins, dyspnea (particularly on exertion or lying down), night cough, and peripheral edema. Tasks that require mental alertness or motor skills should be avoided until response to the drug has been established. EKG and pulse rate for quality and irregularity should be monitored at baseline and periodically during therapy. Fluid status, electrolytes, hands for tremor, skin for rash or clamminess, intake and output, and weight should also be assessed.

Administration

! When giving tocainide to those receiving IV lidocaine, give single 600-mg dose 6 hours before cessation of lidocaine and repeat in 6 hours, as prescribed. Then give standard tocainide maintenance doses. Tocainide's therapeutic serum level is 4 to 10 mcg/ml; its toxic level has not been established.

Tolazamide

tole-az′a-mide
(Tolinase)
Do not confuse with tolbu-tamide, tocainide, or tolazine.

CATEGORY AND SCHEDULE
Pregnancy Risk Category: D

CLASSIFICATION
Antidiabetic agents, sulfonyl-ureas, first generation

MECHANISM OF ACTION
A first-generation sulfonylurea that promotes release of insulin from beta cells of pancreas.

Therapeutic Effect: Lowers blood glucose concentration.

PHARMACOKINETICS
Well absorbed from the gastrointestinal (GI) tract. Extensively metabolized in liver to five metabolites, three which are active. Primarily excreted in urine. Unknown if removed by hemodialysis. **Half-life:** 7 hr.

AVAILABILITY
Tablets: 100 mg, 250 mg, 500 mg; 100 mg, 250 mg (Tolinase).

INDICATIONS AND DOSAGES
▶ **Diabetes mellitus**
PO
Adults, Elderly. Initially, 100-250 mg once a day, with breakfast or first main meal. Maintenance: 100-1000 mg once a day. May increase by increments of 100-250 mg weekly, based on blood glucose response. May increase by 100-250 mg/day at weekly intervals. Maximum: 1000 mg/day. Doses more than 500 mg/day should be given in 2 divided doses with meals.

OFF-LABEL USES
None known.

CONTRAINDICATIONS
Diabetic complications, such as ketosis, acidosis, and diabetic coma, sole therapy for type 1 diabetes mellitus, hypersensitivity to tolazamide or its components

INTERACTIONS
Drug
Beta-blockers: May increase hypoglycemic effect and mask signs of hypoglycemia.
Cimetidine, fluoroquinolones, fluconazole, MAOIs, quinidine,

T

ranitidine, large doses of
salicylates: May increase effects of
tolazamide.
Corticosteroids, lithium, thiazide
diuretics: May decrease effects of
tolazamide.
Oral anticoagulants: May increase
effects of oral anticoagulants.
Herbal
Bitter melon, fenugreek, ginseng,
glucomannan, glucosamine,
gymnema extracts, licorice,
psyllium, St. John's wort: May
increase risk of hypoglycemia.
Food
None known.

DIAGNOSTIC TEST EFFECTS
May increase BUN, LDH concentrations, serum alkaline phosphatase,
creatinine, and SGOT (AST) levels.

▓ IV INCOMPATIBILITIES
None known.
▓ IV Compatibilities
None known.

SIDE EFFECTS
Frequent
Altered taste sensation, dizziness,
drowsiness, weight gain, constipation, diarrhea, heartburn, nausea,
vomiting, stomach fullness,
headache
Occasional
Increased sensitivity of skin to
sunlight, peeling of skin, itching,
rash

SERIOUS REACTIONS
• Severe hypoglycemia may occur
due to overdosage and insufficient
food intake, especially with
increased glucose demands.
• GI hemorrhage, cholestatic
hepatic jaundice, leukopenia, thrombocytopenia, pancytopenia, agranulocytosis and aplastic or hemolytic
anemia occurs rarely.

PRECAUTIONS & CONSIDERATIONS
Caution is necessary with hypoglycemia or loss of glycemic control
due to secondary failure. Replace
with insulin if necessary if stress
from fever, infection, trauma, or
surgery has occurred. Tolazamide
use is not recommended during
pregnancy. It is unknown if tolazamide is distributed in breast milk.
Safety and efficacy of tolazamide
have not been established in children. Be aware that hypoglycemia
may be difficult to recognize in the
elderly patients.
   Signs and symptoms of hypoglycemia, such as anxiety, cool,
wet skin, diplopia, dizziness,
headache, hunger, numbness in
mouth, tachycardia, and tremors, or
hyperglycemia, including deep, rapid
breathing, dim vision, fatigue, nausea,
polydipsia, polyphagia, polyuria, and
vomiting may occur during treatment.
Candy, sugar packets, or other sugar
supplements should be carried for
immediate response to hypoglycemia.
Sunscreen and protective eyewear
should be worn to prevent the effects
of light sensitivity.
Administration
Take tolazamide with breakfast or
first main meal. Divide into 2 doses
if taking more than 500 mg/day.

Tolbutamide

tole-byoo′ta-mide
(Apo-Tolbutamide [CAN],
Orinase, Orinase Diagnostic,
Rastinon [AUS], Tol-Tab)
**Do not confuse with
tolazamide, tocainide,
or tolazine.**

CATEGORY AND SCHEDULE
Pregnancy Risk Category: C

CLASSIFICATION
Antidiabetic agents, sulfonylureas, first generation

MECHANISM OF ACTION
A first-generation sulfonylurea that
promotes the release of insulin from
beta cells of pancreas. *Therapeutic
Effect:* Lowers blood glucose
concentration.

PHARMACOKINETICS

Route	Onset	Peak	Duration
PO	1 hr	5-8 hr	12-24 hr
IV	N/A	30-45 min	90-181 min

Well absorbed from the gastrointestinal (GI) tract. Protein binding: 80%-
99%. Extensively metabolized in
liver to 2 inactive metabolites,
primarily via oxidation. Excreted in
urine. Removed by hemodialysis.
Half-life: 4.5-6.5 hr.

AVAILABILITY
Tablets: 500 mg (Orinase, Tol-Tab).
Injection, Powder for Reconstitution:
1 g (Orinase Diagnostic).

INDICATIONS AND DOSAGES
▸ **Diabetes mellitus**
PO
Adults. Initially, 1 g daily, with
breakfast or first main meal, or in
divided doses. Maintenance:
0.25-3 g once a day. After dose of
2 g is reached, dosage should be
increased in increments of up to
2 mg q1-2wk, based on blood
glucose response. Maximum:
3 g/day.
▸ **Endocrine tumor diagnosis**
IV
Adults. 1 g infused over 2-3 minutes.

CONTRAINDICATIONS
Diabetic ketoacidosis with or
without coma, sole therapy for
type 1 diabetes mellitus, use in
children, hypersensitivity to tolbutamide or any component of its
formulation

INTERACTIONS
Drug
Beta-blockers: May increase the
hypoglycemic effect and mask signs
of hypoglycemia.
**Cimetidine, fluoroquinolones,
fluconazole, MAOIs, quinidine,
ranitidine, large doses of salicylates:** May increase the effects of
tolbutamide.
**Corticosteroids, lithium, thiazide
diuretics:** May decrease the effects
of tolbutamide.
Oral anticoagulants: May increase
the effects of oral anticoagulants.
Fosphenytoin, phenytoin: May
increase the risk of phenytoin
toxicity.
Rifampin: May decrease effectiveness of tolbutamide.
Sertraline: May decrease the clearance of tolbutamide.
Herbal
**Bitter melon, fenugreek, ginseng,
glucomannan, glucosamine,
gymnema extracts, licorice,
psyllium, St. John's wort:** May
increase the risk of hypoglycemia.
Food
None known.

T

DIAGNOSTIC TEST EFFECTS
May increase BUN, LDH concentrations, serum alkaline phosphatase, creatinine, and SGOT (AST) levels.

SIDE EFFECTS
Frequent
Increased sensitivity of skin to sunlight, peeling of skin, itching, rash, dizziness, drowsiness, weight gain, constipation, diarrhea, heartburn, nausea, headache, pain at injection site
Occasional
Altered taste sensation, constipation, vomiting, stomach fullness

SERIOUS REACTIONS
• Severe hypoglycemia may occur because of overdosage or insufficient food intake, especially with increased glucose demands.
• Cardiovascular mortality has been reported higher in patients treated with tolbutamide.
• GI hemorrhage, cholestatic hepatic jaundice, leukopenia, thrombocytopenia, pancytopenia, agranulocytosis and aplastic or hemolytic anemia occurs rarely.

PRECAUTIONS & CONSIDERATIONS
Caution is warranted with adrenal or pituitary insufficiency, hypoglycemic reactions, loss of glycemic control due to secondary failure, and impaired liver function. Replacement with insulin may be necessary during stress due to infection, fever, trauma, or surgery. It is unknown if tolbutamide is distributed in breast milk. Safety and efficacy of this drug have not been established in children. Hypoglycemia may be difficult to recognize in the elderly. Age-related renal impairment may increase sensitivity to glucose-lowering in the elderly.

Signs and symptoms of hypoglycemia, such as anxiety, cool, wet skin, diplopia, dizziness, headache, hunger, numbness in mouth, tachycardia, and tremors, or hyperglycemia, including deep, rapid breathing, dim vision, fatigue, nausea, polydipsia, polyphagia, polyuria, and vomiting may occur during treatment. Candy, sugar packets, or other sugar supplements should be carried for immediate response to hypoglycemia. Sunscreen and protective eyewear should be worn to prevent the effects of light sensitivity.

Administration
Take oral tolbutamide with breakfast or first main meal or in divided doses.

Give IV tolbutamide 1 g over 2-3 minutes. Reconstitute tolbutamide with 20 ml of diluent provided in an ampoule in tolbutamide package.

Tolcapone
toll′ka-pone
(Tasmar)

CATEGORY AND SCHEDULE
Pregnancy Risk Category: C

CLASSIFICATION
Antiparkinson agents, dopaminergics

MECHANISM OF ACTION
An antiparkinson agent that inhibits the enzyme catechol-*O*-methyltransferase (COMT), potentiating dopamine activity and increasing the duration of action of levodopa. *Therapeutic Effect:* Relieves signs and symptoms of Parkinson's disease.

PHARMACOKINETICS
Rapidly absorbed after PO administration. Protein binding: 99%. Metabolized in the liver. Eliminated primarily in urine (60%) and, to a lesser extent, in feces (40%). Unknown if removed by hemodialysis. **Half-life:** 2-3 hr.

AVAILABILITY
Tablets: 100 mg, 200 mg.

INDICATIONS AND DOSAGES
▸ **Adjunctive treatment of Parkinson's disease**
PO
Adults, Elderly. Initially, 100-200 mg 3 times a day concomitantly with each dose of carbidopa and levodopa. Maximum: 600 mg/day.

CONTRAINDICATIONS
None known.

INTERACTIONS
Drug
Levodopa: Increases the duration of action of this drug.
Herbal
None known.
Food
All foods: Decrease tolcapone bioavailability by 10%-20% if given within 1 hour before or 2 hour after drug administration.

DIAGNOSTIC TEST EFFECTS
May increase AST (SGOT) and ALT (SGPT) levels.

SIDE EFFECTS
! Frequency of side effects increases with dosage. The following effects are based on a 200-mg dose.
Frequent (35%-16%)
Nausea, insomnia, somnolence, anorexia, diarrhea, muscle cramps, orthostatic hypotension, excessive dreaming

Occasional (11%-4%)
Headache, vomiting, confusion, hallucinations, constipation, diaphoresis, bright yellow urine, dry eyes, abdominal pain, dizziness, flatulence
Rare (3%-2%)
Dyspepsia, neck pain, hypotension, fatigue, chest discomfort

SERIOUS REACTIONS
• Upper respiratory tract infection and UTI occur in 7%-5% of patients.
• Too-rapid withdrawal from therapy may produce withdrawal-emergent hyperpyrexia, characterized by fever, muscular rigidity, and altered LOC.
• Dyskinesia and dystonia occur frequently.

PRECAUTIONS & CONSIDERATIONS
Caution is warranted with baseline hypotension, severe hepatic or renal impairment, a history of hallucinations and orthostatic hypotension. Notify the physician if the female is planning to become pregnant. It is unknown if tolcapone is distributed in breast milk. Tolcapone is not used in children. The elderly are at increased risk for hallucinations. Typically, hallucinations in the elderly occur within the first 2 weeks of therapy.

Dizziness, drowsiness, and nausea may occur initially but will diminish or disappear with continued treatment. Alcohol and tasks that require mental alertness or motor skills should be avoided. Change positions slowly to prevent orthostatic hypotension. Also, urine may turn bright yellow. Notify the physician if dark urine, falls, fatigue, itching, loss of appetite, persistent nausea, yellowing of the skin and sclera of the eyes, or abnormal contractions of the head, neck, or trunk occurs. Baseline vital signs should be assessed at baseline.

T

AST (SGOT) and ALT (SGPT) levels should be monitored every 2 weeks for the first year, every 4 weeks for the next 6 months, and every 8 weeks thereafter. Relief of symptoms, such as improvement of masklike facial expression, muscular rigidity, shuffling gait, and resting tremors of the hands and head should also be assessed during treatment.

Administration

! Always administer tolcapone with carbidopa and levodopa. Expect to discontinue tolcapone if ALT and AST levels exceed the upper limits of normal or signs and symptoms of hepatic failure develop.

Take tolcapone without regard to food.

Tolmetin
tole'met-in
(Novo-Tolmetin [CAN], Tolectin, Tolectin DS)

CATEGORY AND SCHEDULE
Pregnancy Risk Category: C, D if used in third trimester or near delivery

CLASSIFICATION
Analgesics, non-narcotic, non-steroidal anti-inflammatory drugs

MECHANISM OF ACTION
A nonsteroidal anti-inflammatory that produces analgesic and anti-inflammatory effect by inhibiting prostaglandin synthesis. *Therapeutic Effect:* Reduces inflammatory response and intensity of pain stimulus reaching sensory nerve endings.

PHARMACOKINETICS
Rapidly absorbed from the gastrointestinal (GI) tract. Metabolized in liver. Excreted in urine. Minimally removed by hemodialysis. **Half-life:** 5 hr.

AVAILABILITY
Tablets: 200 mg, 600 mg (Tolectin).
Capsules: 400 mg (Tolectin DS).

INDICATIONS AND DOSAGES
▶ **Rheumatoid arthritis, osteoarthritis**
PO
Adults, Elderly. Initially, 400 mg 3 times/day (including 1 dose upon arising, 1 dose at bedtime). Adjust dose at 1-2 wk intervals. Maintenance: 600-1800 mg/day in 3-4 divided doses.
▶ **Juvenile rheumatoid arthritis**
PO
Children more than 2 yr. Initially, 20 mg/kg/day in 3-4 divided doses. Maintenance: 15-30 mg/kg/day in 3-4 divided doses.

OFF-LABEL USES
Treatment of ankylosing spondylitis, psoriatic arthritis

CONTRAINDICATIONS
Severely incapacitated, bedridden, wheelchair bound, hypersensitivity to aspirin or other NSAIDs

INTERACTIONS
Drug
Antacids: May decrease concentrations of tolmetin.
Antihypertensives, diuretics: May decrease the effects of antihypertensives and diuretics.
Aspirin, salicylates: May increase the risk of GI bleeding and side effects.
Bone marrow depressants: May increase the risk of hematologic reactions.

Heparin, oral anticoagulants, thrombolytics: May increase the effects of heparin, oral anticoagulants and thrombolytics.
Lithium: May increase the blood concentration and risk of toxicity of lithium.
Methotrexate: May increase the risk of toxicity of methotrexate.
Probenecid: May increase tolmetin blood concentration.
Herbal
Ginkgo biloba: May increase the risk of bleeding.
Feverfew: May decrease the effects of feverfew.
Food
None known.

DIAGNOSTIC TEST EFFECTS
May increase BUN, potassium, liver function tests. May decrease Hgb, Hct. May prolong bleeding time.

SIDE EFFECTS
Occasional
Nausea, vomiting, diarrhea, abdominal cramping, dyspepsia (heartburn, indigestion, epigastric pain), flatulence, dizziness, headache, weight decrease or increase
Rare
Constipation, anorexia, rash, pruritus

SERIOUS REACTIONS
• Peptic ulcer, GI bleeding, gastritis, and severe hepatic reaction (cholestasis, jaundice) occur rarely.
• Nephrotoxicity (dysuria, hematuria, proteinuria, nephrotic syndrome) and severe hypersensitivity reaction (fever, chills, bronchospasm) occur rarely.

PRECAUTIONS & CONSIDERATIONS
Caution is warranted with impaired renal function, impaired cardiac function, coagulation disorders, and history of upper GI disease. Be aware that tolmetin crosses the placenta. It is unknown if the drug is distributed in breast milk. Be aware that tolmetin use should be avoided during the last trimester of pregnancy as the drug may adversely affect the fetal cardiovascular system causing premature closure of ductus arteriosus. Safety and efficacy of tolmetin have not been established in children less than 2 years of age. Be aware that GI bleeding or ulceration is more likely to cause serious adverse effects in the elderly. Age-related renal impairment may increase the risk of liver or renal toxicity and a reduced dosage is recommended in the elderly. Avoid alcohol and aspirin during tolmetin therapy as these substances increase the risk of GI bleeding.
Storage
Store at room temperature.
Administration
Take with food, milk, or antacids if GI distress occurs. Therapeutic effect is noted in 1-3 weeks.

Tolnaftate
tole-naf´tate
(Absorbine Jr. Antifungal, Aftate Antifungal, Fungi-Guard, Pitrex [CAN], Tinactin Antifungal, Tunactin Antifungal Jock Itch, Tinaderm, Ting)

CATEGORY AND SCHEDULE
Pregnancy Risk Category: B
OTC (aerosol liquid, aerosol powder, cream, gel, powder, solution)

CLASSIFICATION
Carbamothioic acid derivative, antifungal

MECHANISM OF ACTION
An antifungal that distorts hyphae and stunts mycelial growth in susceptible fungi. *Therapeutic Effect:* Results in fungal cell death.

AVAILABILITY
Aerosol, liquid, topical: 1 % (Aftate, Tinactin Antifungal, Ting).
Aerosol, powder, topical: 1% (Aftate, Tinactin Antifungal, Tinactin Antifungal Jock Itch, Ting).
Cream: 1% (Fungi-Guard, Tinactin Antifungal, Tinactin Antifungal Jock Itch).
Gel: 1% (Absorbine Jr. Antifungal).
Powder: 1% (Tinactin Antifungal).
Solution, topical: 1% (Absorbine Jr. Antifungal, Tinaderm).

INDICATIONS AND DOSAGES
▸ **Tinea pedis, tinea cruris, tinea corporis**
TOPICAL
Adults, Elderly, Children 2 yr and older. Spray aerosol or apply 1-3 drops of solution or a small amount of cream, gel, or powder 2 times daily for 2-4 wk.

OFF-LABEL USES
Onchomycosis

CONTRAINDICATIONS
Nail and scalp infections, hypersensitivity to tolnaftate or any component of its formulation

INTERACTIONS
Drug
None known.
Herbal
None known.
Food
None known.

DIAGNOSTIC TEST EFFECTS
None known.

SIDE EFFECTS
Rare
Irritation, burning, pruritus, contact dermatitis

SERIOUS REACTIONS
• None known.

PRECAUTIONS & CONSIDERATIONS
It is unknown if tolnaftate is excreted in breast milk. There are no age-related precautions noted in children. Age-related renal impairment may require dosage adjustment in the elderly. Affected areas should be kept clean and dry. Light clothing should be worn to promote ventilation as well as ventilated shoes and shoes and socks should be changed at least once a day.
Administration
Apply and rub gently into the affected and surrounding area. Wash hands before and after applying tolnaftate to the skin. Topical therapy may be used for up to 4 weeks for tinea pedis or tinea corporis, and up to 2 weeks for tinea cruris.

Tolterodine
tol-tare'oh-deen
(Detrol, Detrol LA)

CATEGORY AND SCHEDULE
Pregnancy Risk Category: C

CLASSIFICATION
Anticholinergics, relaxants, urinary tract

MECHANISM OF ACTION
An antispasmodic that exhibits potent antimuscarinic activity by interceding via cholinergic

muscarinic receptors, thereby inhibiting urinary bladder contraction. *Therapeutic Effect:* Decreases urinary frequency, urgency.

PHARMACOKINETICS
Rapidly and well absorbed after PO administration. Protein binding: 96%. Extensively metabolized in the liver to active metabolite. Primarily excreted in urine. Unknown if removed by hemodialysis. **Half-life:** 1.9-3.7 hr.

AVAILABILITY
Tablets (Detrol): 1 mg, 2 mg.
Capsules (Extended-Release [Detrol LA]): 2 mg, 4 mg.

INDICATIONS AND DOSAGES
▸ **Overactive bladder**
PO
Adults, Elderly. 1-2 mg twice a day.
▸ **Dosage in severe renal or hepatic impairment**
PO
Adults, Elderly. 1 mg twice a day.
PO (EXTENDED-RELEASE)
Adults, Elderly. 2-4 mg once a day.

CONTRAINDICATIONS
Uncontrolled angle-closure glaucoma, urine retention

INTERACTIONS
Drug
Clarithromycin, erythromycin, itraconazole, ketoconazole, miconazole: May increase tolterodine blood concentration.
Fluoxetine: May inhibit tolterodine metabolism.
Herbal
None known.
Food
None known.

DIAGNOSTIC TEST EFFECTS
None known.

SIDE EFFECTS
Frequent (40%)
Dry mouth
Occasional (11%-4%)
Headache, dizziness, fatigue, constipation, dyspepsia (heartburn, indigestion, epigastric discomfort), upper respiratory tract infection, UTI, dry eyes, abnormal vision (accommodation problems), nausea, diarrhea
Rare (3%)
Somnolence, chest or back pain, arthralgia, rash, weight gain, dry skin

SERIOUS REACTIONS
• Overdose can result in severe anticholinergic effects, including abdominal cramps, facial warmth, excessive salivation or lacrimation, diaphoresis, pallor, urinary urgency, blurred vision, and prolonged QT interval.

PRECAUTIONS & CONSIDERATIONS
Caution is warranted with renal impairment, clinically significant bladder outflow obstruction (increases risk of urine retention), GI obstructive disorders such as pyloric stenosis (increases risk of gastric retention), and treated angle-closure glaucoma. It is unknown if tolterodine is distributed in breast milk. However, breast-feeding is not recommended. The safety and efficacy of this drug have not been established in children. No age-related precautions have been noted in the elderly.

Blurred vision, GI upset, constipation, and dry eyes and mouth may occur. Notify the physician of a change in vision. Incontinence and residual urine in the bladder should be determined.
Administration
Take tolterodine without regard to food.

T

Topiramate
toe-peer′a-mate
(Topamax)
**Do not confuse with
Toprol XL.**

CATEGORY AND SCHEDULE
Pregnancy Risk Category: C

CLASSIFICATION
Anticonvulsants

MECHANISM OF ACTION
An anticonvulsant that blocks repetitive, sustained firing of neurons by enhancing the ability of gamma-aminobutyric acid to induce an influx of chloride ions into the neurons; may also block sodium channels. *Therapeutic Effect:* Decreases seizure activity.

PHARMACOKINETICS
Rapidly absorbed after PO administration. Protein binding: 13%-17%. Not extensively metabolized. Primarily excreted unchanged in urine. Removed by hemodialysis. **Half-life:** 21 hr.

AVAILABILITY
Capsules (Sprinkle): 15 mg, 25 mg.
Tablets: 25 mg, 50 mg, 100 mg, 200 mg.

INDICATIONS AND DOSAGES
▶ **Adjunctive treatment of partial seizures, Lennox-Gastant syndrome**
PO
Adults, Elderly, Children older than 17 yr. Initially, 25-50 mg for 1 wk. May increase by 25-50 mg/day at weekly intervals. Maximum: 1600 mg/day.
Children 2-16 yr. Initially, 1-3 mg/kg/day to maximum of 25 mg.

May increase by 1-3 mg/kg/day at weekly intervals. Maintenance: 5-9 mg/kg/day in 2 divided doses.
▶ **Tonic-clonic seizures**
PO
Adults, Elderly, Children. Dosage is individualized and titrated.
▶ **Migraine prevention**
PO
Adults, Elderly. 100 mg/day in 2 divided doses.
▶ **Dosage in renal impairment**
Expect to reduce drug dosage by 50% in patients with tonic-clonic seizures who have a creatinine clearance of less than 70 ml/min.

OFF-LABEL USES
Prevention of migraine headaches, treatment of alcohol dependence

CONTRAINDICATIONS
None known.

INTERACTIONS
Drug
Alcohol, other CNS depressants: May increase CNS depression.
Carbamazepine, phenytoin, valproic acid: May decrease topiramate blood concentration.
Carbonic anhydrase inhibitors: May increase the risk of renal calculi.
Oral contraceptives: May decrease the effectiveness of oral contraceptives.
Herbal
None known.
Food
None known.

DIAGNOSTIC TEST EFFECTS
None known.

SIDE EFFECTS
Frequent (30%-10%)
Somnolence, dizziness, ataxia, nervousness, nystagmus, diplopia, paresthesia, nausea, tremor

Occasional (9%-3%)
Confusion, breast pain, dysmenorrhea, dyspepsia, depression, asthenia, pharyngitis, weight loss, anorexia, rash, musculoskeletal pain, abdominal pain, difficulty with coordination, sinusitis, agitation, flu-like symptoms
Rare (3%-2%)
Mood disturbances, such as irritability and depression; dry mouth; aggressive behavior

SERIOUS REACTIONS

• Psychomotor slowing, impaired concentration, language problems (such as word-finding difficulties), and memory disturbances occur occasionally. These reactions are generally mild to moderate but may be severe enough to require discontinuation of drug therapy.

PRECAUTIONS & CONSIDERATIONS

Caution is warranted with impaired hepatic adrenal function, predisposition to renal calculi, and hypersensitivity to topiramate. It is unknown if topiramate is distributed in breast milk. Be aware that topiramate decreases oral contraceptive effectiveness and an alternative means of contraception should be used during therapy. No age-related precautions have been noted in children older than 2 years. In the elderly, age-related renal impairment may require dosage adjustment.

Drowsiness and dizziness may occur, so alcohol and tasks requiring mental alertness or motor skills should be avoided. Notify the physician of blurred vision or other visual changes. Seizure disorder, including the onset, duration, frequency, intensity, and type of seizures, should be assessed before and during treatment. Renal function, including BUN and serum creatinine levels, should also be monitored. Adequate hydration should be maintained to decrease the risk of kidney stones.
Administration
Don't break tablets because they have a bitter taste. Take topiramate without regard to food. Capsules may be swallowed whole or contents sprinkled on a teaspoonful of soft food and swallowed immediately. They should not be chewed. Do not abruptly discontinue topiramate because this may precipitate seizures. Strict maintenance of drug therapy is essential for seizure control.

Topotecan
toe-poe-tee′kan
(Hycamtin)

CATEGORY AND SCHEDULE
Pregnancy Risk Category: D

CLASSIFICATION
Antineoplastics, topoisomerase inhibitors

MECHANISM OF ACTION
A DNA topoisomerase inhibitor that interacts with topoisomerase I, an enzyme that allows DNA replication by producing reversible single-strand breaks in DNA that relieve torsional strain. Topotecan prevents religation of the DNA strand, resulting in damage to double-strand DNA and cell death. *Therapeutic Effect:* Kills cancer cells.

PHARMACOKINETICS
Hydrolyzed to active form after IV administration. Protein binding: 35%. Excreted in urine. **Half-life:** 2-3 hr (increased in impaired renal function).

AVAILABILITY
Powder for Injection: 4 mg (single-dose vial).

INDICATIONS AND DOSAGES
▶ **Ovarian carcinoma, small-cell lung cancer**
IV
Adults, Elderly. 1.5 mg/m²/day over 30 min for 5 consecutive days, beginning on day 1 of a 21-day course. Minimum of four courses recommended. If severe neutropenia (neutrophil count less than 1500/mm²) occurs during treatment, reduce dose for subsequent courses by 0.25 mg/m², or administer filgrastim (G-CSF) no sooner than 24 hr after the last dose of topotecan.
▶ **Dosage in renal impairment**
No dosage adjustment is necessary in patients with mild renal impairment (creatinine clearance of 40-60 ml/min). For moderate renal impairment (creatinine clearance of 20-39 ml/min), give 0.75 mg/m².

OFF-LABEL USES
Treatment of solid tumors including osteosarcoma, neuroblastoma, pediatric leukemia, rhabdomyosarcoma

CONTRAINDICATIONS
Baseline neutrophil count less than 1500 cells/mm³, breast-feeding, pregnancy, severe myelosuppression

INTERACTIONS
Drug
Cisplatin: May increase the severity of myelosuppression.
Live-virus vaccines: May potentiate virus replication, increase vaccine side effects, and decrease the patient's antibody response to the vaccine.
Other bone marrow depressants: May increase the risk of myelosuppression.
Herbal
None known.
Food
None known.

DIAGNOSTIC TEST EFFECTS
May increase serum bilirubin, AST (SGOT), and ALT (SGPT) levels. May decrease RBC, leukocyte, neutrophil, and platelet counts.

🩸 IV INCOMPATIBILITIES
Dexamethasone (Decadron), 5-fluorouracil, mitomycin (Mutamycin)
💉 IV Compatibilities
Carboplatin (Paraplatin), cisplatin (Platinol AQ), cyclophosphamide (Cytoxan), doxorubicin (Adriamycin), etoposide (VePesid), gemcitabine (Gemzar), granisetron (Kytril), ondansetron (Zofran), paclitaxel (Taxol), vincristine (Oncovin)

SIDE EFFECTS
Frequent
Nausea (77%); vomiting (58%); diarrhea, total alopecia (42%); headache (21%); dyspnea (21%)
Occasional
Paraesthesia (9%) constipation, abdominal pain (3%)
Rare
Anorexia, malaise, arthralgia, asthenia, myalgia

SERIOUS REACTIONS
• Severe neutropenia (neutrophil count less than 500 cells/mm³) occurs in 60% of patients, usually during the first course of therapy. The neutrophil nadir usually occurs at a median of 11 days after starting therapy.
• Thrombocytopenia (platelet count less than 25,000/mm³) occurs in 26% of patients, and severe anemia (RBC count less than 8 g/dl) occurs in 40% of patients. The platelet and RBC nadirs usually occur at a median of 15 days after starting the first course of therapy.

PRECAUTIONS & CONSIDERATIONS

Caution is warranted with hepatic and renal impairment and mild myelosuppression.

Because of the risk of fetal harm, pregnant women should not take topotecan, especially in the first trimester. It is unknown if topotecan is distributed in breast milk; however, breast-feeding is not recommended. The safety and efficacy of topotecan have not been established in children. In the elderly, age-related renal impairment may require dosage adjustment. Vaccinations and coming in contact with crowds and people with known infections should be avoided.

CBC, especially blood Hgb levels, and platelet count should be assessed before each topotecan dose. Know that myelosuppression may precipitate life-threatening anemia, hemorrhage, and infection. If platelet count drops, minimize trauma (for example, by avoiding IM or rectal drug administration and by gently repositioning the person). Premedicate with antiemetics, if ordered, on the day of treatment, starting at least 30 minutes before topotecan administration. Electrolyte levels, hydration status, and intake and output should also be monitored because diarrhea and vomiting are common side effects of topotecan.

Storage

Store vials at room temperature in original cartons. Reconstituted vials diluted for infusion are stable at room temperature in ambient lighting for up to 24 hours.

Administration

! As prescribed, do not give topotecan if baseline neutrophil count is less than 1500 cells/mm^3 and platelet count is less than 100,000/mm^3.

Reconstitute each 4-mg vial with 4 ml sterile water for injection.

Further dilute with 50 to 100 ml 0.9% NaCl or D$_5$W. Administer the drug by IV infusion over 30 minutes. Be aware that extravasation is associated with only mild local reactions, such as ecchymosis and erythema.

Toremifene
(Fareston)

CATEGORY AND SCHEDULE
Pregnancy Risk Category: D

CLASSIFICATION
Antineoplastics, antiestrogens, estrogen receptor modulators, selective, hormones/hormone modifiers

MECHANISM OF ACTION
A nonsteroidal antiestrogen and antineoplastic agent that binds to estrogen receptors on tumors, producing a complex that decreases DNA synthesis and inhibits estrogen effects. *Therapeutic Effect:* Blocks growth-stimulating effects of estrogen in breast cancer.

PHARMACOKINETICS
Well absorbed after PO administration. Metabolized in the liver. Eliminated in feces. **Half-life:** Approximately 5 days.

AVAILABILITY
Tablets: 60 mg.

INDICATIONS AND DOSAGES
▶ **Breast cancer**
PO
Adults. 60 mg/day until disease progression is observed.

OFF-LABEL USES
Treatment of desmoid tumors, endometrial carcinoma

CONTRAINDICATIONS
History of thromboembolic disease

INTERACTIONS
Drug
Carbamazepine, phenobarbital, phenytoin: May decrease toremifene blood concentration.
Warfarin: May increase PT.
Herbal
None known.
Food
None known.

DIAGNOSTIC TEST EFFECTS
May increase serum alkaline phosphatase, bilirubin, calcium, and AST (SGOT) levels.

SIDE EFFECTS
Frequent
Hot flashes (35%); diaphoresis (20%); nausea (14%); vaginal discharge (13%); dizziness, dry eyes (9%)
Occasional (5%-2%)
Edema, vomiting, vaginal bleeding
Rare
Fatigue, depression, lethargy, anorexia

SERIOUS REACTIONS
• Ocular toxicity (cataracts, glaucoma, decreased visual acuity) and hypercalcemia may occur.

PRECAUTIONS & CONSIDERATIONS
Caution is warranted with preexisting endometrial hyperplasia, leukopenia, and thrombocytopenia. Toremifene use should be avoided during pregnancy because this drug may cause fetal harm. Nonhormonal methods of contraception should be used during treatment. It's unknown if toremifene is distributed in breast milk; however, breast-feeding is not recommended. Toremifene is not prescribed for children; the safety and efficacy of this drug in children have not been established. No age-related precautions have been noted in the elderly.

Initial flare-up of symptoms, including bone pain and hot flashes, may occur but will subside with continued therapy. Notify the physician if nausea and vomiting, leg cramps, shortness of breath, weakness, weight gain, or vaginal bleeding, discharge, or itching, occur. Estrogen receptor assay test should be performed before starting therapy. CBC and serum calcium levels should be monitored before and periodically during toremifene therapy. Be aware of signs and symptoms of hypercalcemia, including constipation, deep bone or flank pain, excessive thirst, hypotonicity of muscles, increased urine output, nausea and vomiting, and renal calculi.
Administration
Take oral toremifene without regard to food.

Torsemide
tor′se-mide
(Demadex)
Do not confuse torsemide with furosemide.

CATEGORY AND SCHEDULE
Pregnancy Risk Category: B

CLASSIFICATION
Diuretics, loop

MECHANISM OF ACTION
A loop diuretic that enhances excretion of sodium, chloride, potassium,

and water at the ascending limb of the loop of Henle; also reduces plasma and extracellular fluid volume. *Therapeutic Effect:* Produces diuresis; lowers B/P.

PHARMACOKINETICS

Route	Onset	Peak	Duration
PO	1 hr	1-2 hr	6-8 hr
IV	10 min	1 hr	6-8 hr

Rapidly and well absorbed from the GI tract. Protein binding: 97%-99%. Metabolized in the liver. Primarily excreted in urine. Not removed by hemodialysis. **Half-life:** 3.3 hr.

AVAILABILITY
Tablets: 5 mg, 10 mg, 20 mg, 100 mg. *Injection:* 10 mg/ml.

INDICATIONS AND DOSAGES
▶ **Hypertension**
PO
Adults, Elderly. Initially, 5 mg/day. May increase to 10 mg/day if no response in 4-6 wk. If no response, additional antihypertensive added.
▶ **CHF**
PO, IV
Adults, Elderly. Initially, 10-20 mg/day. May increase by approximately doubling dose until desired therapeutic effect is attained. Doses greater than 200 mg have not been adequately studied.
▶ **Chronic renal failure**
PO, IV
Adults, Elderly. Initially, 20 mg/day. May increase by approximately doubling dose until desired therapeutic effect is attained. Doses greater than 200 mg have not been adequately studied.
▶ **Hepatic cirrhosis**
PO, IV
Adults, Elderly. Initially, 5 mg/day given with aldosterone antagonist or potassium-sparing diuretic. May increase by approximately doubling dose until desired therapeutic effect is attained. Doses greater than 40 mg have not been adequately studied.

CONTRAINDICATIONS
Anuria, hepatic coma, severe electrolyte depletion

INTERACTIONS
Drug
Amphotericin B, nephrotoxic medications, ototoxic medications: May increase the risk of nephrotoxicity and ototoxicity.
Anticoagulants, heparin, thrombolytics: May decrease the effects of these drugs.
Digoxin: May increase the risk of digoxin toxicity associated with torsemide-induced hypokalemia.
Lithium: May increase the risk of lithium toxicity.
NSAIDs, probenecid: May decrease the diuretic effect of torsemide.
Other antihypertensives: May increase the risk of hypotension.
Other hypokalemia-causing medications: May increase the risk of hypokalemia.
Herbal
None known.
Food
None known.

DIAGNOSTIC TEST EFFECTS
May increase BUN, serum creatinine, and serum uric acid levels. May decrease serum calcium, chloride, magnesium, potassium, and sodium levels.

▓ IV INCOMPATIBILITIES
Don't mix torsemide with any other medications except for milrinone (Primacor).

T

💧**IV Compatibilities**
Milrinone (Primacor)

SIDE EFFECTS
Frequent (10%-4%)
Headache, dizziness, rhinitis
Occasional (3%-1%)
Asthenia, insomnia, nervousness,
diarrhea, constipation, nausea,
dyspepsia, edema, EKG changes,
pharyngitis, cough, arthralgia,
myalgia
Rare (less than 1%)
Syncope, hypotension, arrhythmias

SERIOUS REACTIONS
• Ototoxicity may occur with high
doses or a too-rapid IV administration.
• Overdose produces acute,
profound water loss; volume and
electrolyte depletion; dehydration;
decreased blood volume; and circulatory collapse.

PRECAUTIONS & CONSIDERATIONS
Caution is warranted with ascites,
hepatic cirrhosis, renal impairment,
systemic lupus erythematosus,
history of ventricular arrhythmias,
hypersensitivity to sulfonamides,
with cardiac patients and in the
elderly. It is unknown if torsemide is
excreted in breast milk. The safety
and efficacy of this drug have not
been established in children. No age-
related precautions have been noted
in the elderly. Consuming foods high
in potassium such as apricots,
bananas, legumes, meat, orange
juice, raisins, whole grains, including cereals, and white and sweet
potatoes, is encouraged. Avoid
taking other medications, including
OTC drugs, without first consulting
the physician.
An increase in the frequency and
volume of urination may occur.
Notify the physician of cramps,
dizziness, an irregular heartbeat,
muscle weakness, nausea, or hearing
abnormalities. Blood pressure (B/P),
vital signs, electrolytes, intake and
output, and weight should be monitored before and during treatment. Be
aware of signs of electrolyte disturbances such as hypokalemia or
hyponatremia. Hypokalemia may
cause arrhythmias, altered mental
status, muscle cramps, asthenia, and
tremor. Know that less potassium is
lost with torsemide than with
furosemide.
Storage
Store torsemide at room temperature.
Administration
Take torsemide with food to avoid
GI upset, preferably with breakfast
to prevent nocturia.
❗ Flush IV line with 0.9% NaCl before
and after torsemide administration.
Torsemide may be given undiluted
as IV push over 2 minutes. For
continuous IV infusion, dilute with
0.9% or 0.45% NaCl or D_5W and
infuse over 24 hours. Administer IV
push slowly because too-rapid
administration may cause ototoxicity.

Tositumomab and Iodine 131 I-Tositumomab
toe-sit-two′mo-mab
(Bexxar)

CATEGORY AND SCHEDULE
Pregnancy Risk Category: X

CLASSIFICATION
Antineoplastics, monoclonal
antibodies, radiopharmaceuticals

MECHANISM OF ACTION
A monoclonal antibody composed
of an antibody conjoined with a

radiolabeled antitumor antibody. The antibody portion binds specifically to the CD20 antigen, which is found on pre-B and B lymphocytes and on more than 90% of B-cell non-Hodgkin lymphomas resulting in formation of a complex. *Therapeutic Effect:* Induces cytotoxicity associated with ionizing radiation from the radioisotope. Depletes circulating CD20-positive cells.

PHARMACOKINETICS

Elimination of iodine 131 (^{131}I) occurs by decay and excretion in urine. **Half-life:** 8 days. Patients with high tumor burden, splenomegaly, or bone marrow involvement have a faster clearance, shorter half-life, and larger volume of distribution.

AVAILABILITY

Kit (dosimetric): (Bexxar) tositumomab 225 mg/16.1 ml (2 vials), tositumomab 35 mg/2.5 ml (1 vial), and iodine^{131} tositumomab 0.1 mg/ml (1 vial).
Kit (therapeutic): (Bexxar) tositumomab 225 mg/16.1 ml (2 vials), tositumomab 35 mg/2.5 ml (1 vial), and iodine^{131} tositumomab 1.1 mg/ml (1 or 2 vials).

INDICATIONS AND DOSAGES
▸ **Non-Hodgkin's lymphoma**
IV
Adults, Elderly. Dosage contains 4 components. Day 0: tositumomab 450 mg/50 NaCl over 60 min. Then iodine^{131} tositumomab 35 mg in 30 ml NaCl over 20 min. Day 7: tositumomab 450 mg/50 NaCl over 60 min. Then, iodine^{131} tositumomab to deliver 65-75 cGy total body irradiation and tositumomab 35 mg over 20 min.

CONTRAINDICATIONS

Hypersensitivity to murine proteins

INTERACTIONS
Drug
Anticoagulants, medications that interfere with platelet function: Increase the risk of bleeding and hemorrhage.
Herbal
None known.
Food
None known.

DIAGNOSTIC TEST EFFECTS

May decrease blood Hct and Hgb levels, platelet and WBC counts, and thyroid-stimulating hormone level.

SIDE EFFECTS
Frequent (46%-18%)
Asthenia, fever, nausea, cough, chills
Occasional (17%-10%)
Rash, headache, abdominal pain, vomiting, anorexia, myalgia, diarrhea, pharyngitis, arthralgia, rhinitis, pruritus
Rare (9%-5%)
Peripheral edema, diaphoresis, constipation, dyspepsia, back pain, hypotension, vasodilation, dizziness, somnolence

SERIOUS REACTIONS

- Infusion toxicity, characterized by fever, rigors, diaphoresis, hypotension, dyspnea, and nausea, may occur during or within 48 hours of the infusion.
- Severe, prolonged myelosuppression, characterized by neutropenia, anemia, and thrombocytopenia, occurs in 71% of patients.
- Sepsis occurs in 45% of patients.
- Hemorrhage occurs in 12% of patients.
- Myelodysplastic syndrome occurs in 8% of patients.

T

PRECAUTIONS & CONSIDERATIONS
Caution is warranted with active systemic infection,

immunosuppression, and impaired renal function. The use of the ^{131}I-tositumomab component is contraindicated during pregnancy and causes severe, possibly irreversible hypothyroidism in neonates. Because ^{131}I is excreted in breast milk, breast-feeding is not recommended. The safety and efficacy of this drug have not been established in children. The elderly (older than 65 years) have exhibited a lower overall response rate to the drug. They've also had a lower incidence, but longer duration, of severe hematologic toxicity. Immunizations during therapy and contact with those who have recently received a live-virus vaccine should be avoided.

Notify the physician if bruising, fever, signs of local infection, sore throat, or unusual bleeding from any site occurs. CBC should be obtained before beginning therapy and at least weekly after administration for at least 10 weeks. Laboratory values should be monitored for evidence of severe and prolonged anemia, neutropenia, and thrombocytopenia. Know that time to nadir is 4 to 7 weeks and the duration of cytopenias (predominantly grade 3 and 4 thrombocytopenia and grade 3 and 4 neutropenia) is approximately 30 days. Signs and symptoms for hematologic toxicity (including excessive fatigue and weakness, chills, fever, ecchymosis, and unusual bleeding from any site) and hypothyroidism (including fatigue, sensitivity to cold, unexplained weight gain, and constipation) should be assessed.

Storage

Refrigerate tositumomab vials before dilution. Protect from strong light. After dilution, tositumomab solution is stable for 24 hours if refrigerated and 8 hours at room temperature.

Discard any unused portion left in the vial. Do not shake.

Administration

! Pretreat by administering diphenhydramine 50 mg and acetaminophen 650-1000 mg 1 hour before administering tositumomab; followed by acetaminophen 650-1000 mg every 4 hours for 2 doses, then every 4 hours as needed. Full recovery from hematologic toxicities is not a requirement for giving the second dose. Be aware that the regimen consists of 4 components given in 2 separate steps: the dosimetric step, followed 7 to 14 days later by the therapeutic step. During the infusion, use IV tubing with an in-line 0.22 micron filter, and use the same tubing for both the dosimetric and therapeutic steps because changing the filter results in drug loss. Plan to reduce the infusion rate by 50% for mild to moderate infusion toxicity and to interrupt the infusion for severe infusion toxicity. Expect to resume therapy at 50% of the infusion rate when toxic reactions have resolved.

! Administer a thyroid protective agent such as potassium iodide, as prescribed, beginning 24 hours before administration of the ^{131}I-tositumomab dosimetric step and continuing for 2 weeks after administration of the therapeutic step. Remember that reconstitution amounts and rates of administration are the same for both the dosimetric and therapeutic steps.

Use strict aseptic technique in preparing the drug to protect the patient from infection. Follow radiation safety protocols. Reconstitute 450 mg tositumomab in 50 ml 0.9% NaCl. Reconstitute 450 mg tositumomab in 50 ml 0.9% NaCl. Infuse tositumomab over 60 minutes. Keep ^{131}I-tositumomab frozen until thawing it before drug administration. Thawed ^{131}I-tositumomab doses are stable for 8 hours if refrigerated. Discard any unused portion. Reconstitute ^{131}I-tositumomab in 30 ml 0.9% NaCl. Infuse ^{131}I-tositumomab over 20 minutes.

Tramadol
tray′mah-doal
(Tramal [AUS], Tramal SR [AUS], Ultram, Zydol [AUS])
Do not confuse tramadol with Toradol, or Ultram with Ultane.

CATEGORY AND SCHEDULE
Pregnancy Risk Category: C

CLASSIFICATION
Analgesics, narcotic-like

MECHANISM OF ACTION
An analgesic that binds to mu-opioid receptors and inhibits reuptake of norepinephrine and serotonin. Reduces the intensity of pain stimuli reaching sensory nerve endings. *Therapeutic Effect:* Alters the perception of and emotional response to pain.

PHARMACOKINETICS

Route	Onset	Peak	Duration
PO	Less than 1 hr	2-3 hr	4-6 hr

Rapidly and almost completely absorbed after PO administration. Protein binding: 20%. Extensively metabolized in the liver to active metabolite (reduced in patients with advanced cirrhosis). Primarily excreted in urine. Minimally removed by hemodialysis. **Half-life:** 6-7 hr.

AVAILABILITY
Tablets: 50 mg.

INDICATIONS AND DOSAGES
▸ **Moderate to moderately severe pain**
PO
Adults, Elderly. 50-100 mg q4-6hr. Maximum: 400 mg/day for patients younger than 75 yr; 300 mg/day for patients older than 75 yr.
▸ **Dosage in renal impairment**
For patients with creatinine clearance of less than 30 ml/min, increase dosing interval to q12hr. Maximum: 200 mg/day.
▸ **Dosage in hepatic impairment**
Dosage is decreased to 50 mg q12hr.

CONTRAINDICATIONS
Acute alcohol intoxication; concurrent use of centrally acting analgesics, hypnotics, opioids, or psychotropic drugs

INTERACTIONS
Drug
Alcohol, other CNS depressants: May increase CNS or respiratory depression and hypotension.
Carbamazepine: Decreases tramadol blood concentration.
MAOIs: Increase tramadol blood concentration.
Herbal
None known.
Food
None known.

DIAGNOSTIC TEST EFFECTS
May increase serum creatinine, AST (SGOT), and ALT (SGPT) hepatic levels. May decrease blood Hgb level. May cause proteinuria.

SIDE EFFECTS
Frequent (25%-15%)
Dizziness or vertigo, nausea, constipation, headache, somnolence

T

Occasional (10%-5%)
Vomiting, pruritus, CNS stimulation (such as nervousness, anxiety, agitation, tremor, euphoria, mood swings, and hallucinations), asthenia, diaphoresis, dyspepsia, dry mouth, diarrhea
Rare (less than 5%)
Malaise, vasodilation, anorexia, flatulence, rash, blurred vision, urine retention or urinary frequency, menopausal symptoms

SERIOUS REACTIONS
• Overdose results in respiratory depression and seizures.
• Tramadol may have a prolonged duration of action and cumulative effect in patients with hepatic or renal impairment.

PRECAUTIONS & CONSIDERATIONS
Extreme caution should be used with acute abdominal conditions, hepatic or renal impairment, increased intracranial pressure, opioid dependence, and a sensitivity to opioids. Tramadol crosses the placenta and is distributed in breast milk. The safety and efficacy of tramadol have not been established in children. Age-related renal impairment may require a dosage adjustment in the elderly. Alcohol and OTC drugs, such as analgesics and sedatives, should be avoided.
Blurred vision, dizziness, and drowsiness may occur, so tasks requiring mental alertness or motor skills should be avoided. Notify the physician of any chest pain, difficulty breathing, excessive sedation, muscle weakness, palpitations, seizures, severe constipation, or tremors. CBC and liver and renal function studies should be obtained before therapy. B/P, pulse rate, pattern of daily bowel activity and stool consistency, bladder for urine

retention, and therapeutic response should be monitored during tramadol use.
Administration
! Be aware that dialysis patients can receive their regular dose on the day of dialysis.
Take tramadol without regard to food.

Trandolapril
tran-doe'la-pril
(Gopten [AUS], Mavik, Odrik [AUS])
Do not confuse with tramadol.

CATEGORY AND SCHEDULE
Pregnancy Risk Category: C (D if used in second or third trimester)

CLASSIFICATION
Angiotensin converting enzyme inhibitors

MECHANISM OF ACTION
An ACE inhibitor that suppresses the renin-angiotensin-aldosterone system and prevents the conversion of angiotensin I to angiotensin II, a potent vasoconstrictor; may also inhibit angiotensin II at local vascular and renal sites. Decreases plasma angiotensin II, increases plasma renin activity, and decreases aldosterone secretion. *Therapeutic Effect:* Reduces peripheral arterial resistance and pulmonary capillary wedge pressure; improves cardiac output and exercise tolerance.

PHARMACOKINETICS
Slowly absorbed from the GI tract. Protein binding: 80%. Metabolized

in the liver and GI mucosa to active metabolite. Primarily excreted in urine. Removed by hemodialysis.
Half-life: 24 hr.

AVAILABILITY
Tablets: 1 mg, 2 mg, 4 mg.

INDICATIONS AND DOSAGES
▶ **Hypertension (without diuretic)**
PO
Adults, Elderly. Initially, 1 mg once a day in nonblack patients, 2 mg once a day in black patients. Adjust dosage at least at 7-day intervals. Maintenance: 2-4 mg/day. Maximum: 8 mg/day.
▶ **CHF**
PO
Adults, Elderly. Initially, 0.5-1 mg, titrated to target dose of 4 mg/day.

CONTRAINDICATIONS
History of angioedema from previous treatment with ACE inhibitors

INTERACTIONS
Drug
Alcohol, antihypertensives, diuretics: May increase the effects of trandolapril.
Lithium: May increase lithium blood concentration and risk of lithium toxicity.
NSAIDs: May decrease the effects of trandolapril.
Potassium-sparing diuretics, potassium supplements: May cause hyperkalemia.
Herbal
None known.
Food
None known.

DIAGNOSTIC TEST EFFECTS
May increase BUN, serum alkaline phosphatase, serum bilirubin, serum creatinine, serum potassium, AST (SGOT), and ALT (SGPT) levels.

May decrease serum sodium levels. May cause positive antinuclear antibody titer.

SIDE EFFECTS
Frequent (35%-23%)
Dizziness, cough
Occasional (11%-3%)
Hypotension, dyspepsia (heartburn, epigastric pain, indigestion), syncope, asthenia (loss of strength), tinnitus
Rare (less than 1%)
Palpitations, insomnia, drowsiness, nausea, vomiting, constipation, flushed skin

SERIOUS REACTIONS
• Excessive hypotension (first-dose syncope) may occur in patients with CHF and in those who are severely salt or volume depleted.
• Angioedema and hyperkalemia occur rarely.
• Agranulocytosis and neutropenia may be noted in those with collagen vascular disease, including scleroderma and systemic lupus erythematosus, and impaired renal function.
• Nephrotic syndrome may be noted in those with history of renal disease.

PRECAUTIONS & CONSIDERATIONS
Caution is warranted with CHF, collagen vascular disease, hyperkalemia, hypovolemia, renal impairment, and renal stenosis. Trandolapril crosses the placenta, is distributed in breast milk, and may cause fetal or neonatal morbidity or mortality. Safety and efficacy of trandolapril have not been established in children. No age-related precautions have been noted in the elderly.

Dizziness and light-headedness may occur. Tasks that require mental alertness or motor skills should be avoided. Notify the physician if chest pain, cough, diarrhea, difficulty swallowing, fever, palpitations, sore throat, swelling of the face, or vomiting occur. Be alert to fluctuations in B/P. If an excessive reduction in B/P occurs, place the person in the supine position with legs elevated. CBC and blood chemistry should be obtained before beginning trandolapril therapy, then every 2 weeks for the next 3 months, and periodically thereafter in patients with autoimmune disease, or renal impairment, and in those who are taking drugs that affect immune response or leukocyte count. Crackles and wheezing should be assessed in persons with CHF. BUN, serum creatinine, and serum potassium levels, WBC count, urinalysis, intake and output, and pattern of daily bowel activity and stool consistency should also be monitored.

Administration
Take trandolapril without regard to food. Crush tablets as necessary.

Tranylcypromine
tran-ill-sip′roe-meen
(Parnate)

CATEGORY AND SCHEDULE
Pregnancy Risk Category: C

CLASSIFICATION
Antidepressants, monoamine oxidase inhibitors

MECHANISM OF ACTION
An MAOI that inhibits the activity of the enzyme monoamine oxidase at CNS storage sites, leading to increased levels of the neurotransmitters epinephrine, norepinephrine, serotonin, and dopamine at neuronal receptor sites. *Therapeutic Effect:* Relieves depression.

AVAILABILITY
Tablets: 10 mg.

INDICATIONS AND DOSAGES
▶ **Depression refractory to or intolerant of other therapy**
PO
Adults, Elderly. Initially, 10 mg twice a day. May increase by 10 mg/day at 1- to 3-wk intervals up to 60 mg/day in divided doses.

CONTRAINDICATIONS
CHF, children younger than 16 years, pheochromocytoma, severe hepatic or renal impairment, uncontrolled hypertension

INTERACTIONS
Drug
Alcohol, other CNS depressants: May increase CNS depressant effects.
Buspirone: May increase B/P.
Caffeine-containing medications: May increase the risk of cardiac arrhythmias and hypertension.
Carbamazepine, cyclobenzaprine, maprotiline, other MAOIs: May precipitate hypertensive crisis.
Dopamine, tryptophan: May cause sudden, severe hypertension.
Fluoxetine, trazodone, tricyclic antidepressants: May cause serotonin syndrome and neuroleptic malignant syndrome.
Insulin, oral antidiabetics: May increase the effects of these drugs.
Meperidine, other opioid analgesics: May produce diaphoresis, immediate excitation, rigidity, and severe hypertension or hypotension, sometimes leading to severe

respiratory distress, vascular collapse, seizures, coma, and death.
Herbal
None known.
Food
Caffeine, chocolate, tyramine-containing foods (such as aged cheese): May cause sudden, severe hypertension.

DIAGNOSTIC TEST EFFECTS
None known.

SIDE EFFECTS
Frequent
Orthostatic hypotension, restlessness, GI upset, insomnia, dizziness, lethargy, weakness, dry mouth, peripheral edema
Occasional
Flushing, diaphoresis, rash, urinary frequency, increased appetite, transient impotence
Rare
Visual disturbances

SERIOUS REACTIONS
• Hypertensive crisis occurs rarely and is marked by severe hypertension, occipital headache radiating frontally, neck stiffness or soreness, nausea, vomiting, diaphoresis, fever or chills, clammy skin, dilated pupils, palpitations, tachycardia or bradycardia, and constricting chest pain.

PRECAUTIONS & CONSIDERATIONS
Caution is warranted with cardiac arrhythmias, frequent or severe headaches, hypertension, suicidal tendencies, and within several hours of ingestion of contraindicated substance, such as tyramine-containing food. Foods that require bacteria or molds for their preparation or preservation (such as yogurt and aged cheese), foods containing tyramine (such as avocados, bananas, broad beans, meat tenderizers, liver,

smoked or pickled meats and fish, papayas, figs, raisins, sour cream, soy sauce, beer, wine, and yeast extracts), and excessive amounts of caffeine-containing foods or beverages (including chocolate, coffee, and tea) should be avoided.

Dizziness may occur, so change positions slowly, and alcohol and tasks that require mental alertness or motor skills should be avoided. Notify the physician if headache or neck soreness or stiffness occurs. If hypertensive crisis occurs, phentolamine 5-10 mg IV should be administered. B/P, temperature, and weight should be assessed.

Administration
! Make sure at least 14 days elapse between the use of tranylcypromine and a selective serotonin reuptake inhibitor.

Take the second daily dose no later than 4 PM to avoid insomnia. Depression may start to lift during the first week of therapy and the drug's full therapeutic benefit will occur within 3 weeks.

Trastuzumab
tras-too´-ze-mab
(Herceptin)

CATEGORY AND SCHEDULE
Pregnancy Risk Category: B

CLASSIFICATION
Antineoplastics, monoclonal antibodies

MECHANISM OF ACTION
Binds to the HER-2 protein, which is overexpressed in 25%-30% of primary breast cancers, thereby inhibiting proliferation of tumor cells.

Therapeutic Effect: Inhibits the growth of tumor cells and mediates antibody-dependent cellular cytotoxicity.

PHARMACOKINETICS
Half-life: 5.8 days (range: 1-32 days).

AVAILABILITY
Injection, Powder for Reconstitution: 440 mg.

INDICATIONS AND DOSAGES
▸ **Breast cancer**
IV
Adults, Elderly. Initially, 4 mg/kg as a 30-90-min infusion, then 2 mg/kg weekly as a 30-min infusion.

CONTRAINDICATIONS
Pre-existing cardiac disease

INTERACTIONS
Drug
Cyclophosphamide, doxorubicin, epirubicin: May increase the risk of cardiac dysfunction.
Herbal
None known.
Food
None known.

DIAGNOSTIC TEST EFFECTS
None known.

▨ IV INCOMPATIBILITIES
Don't mix trastuzumab with any other medications or with D_5W.

SIDE EFFECTS
Frequent (greater than 20%)
Pain, asthenia, fever, chills, headache, abdominal pain, back pain, infection, nausea, diarrhea, vomiting, cough, dyspnea
Occasional (15%-5%)
Tachycardia, CHF, flu-like symptoms, anorexia, edema, bone pain, arthralgia, insomnia, dizziness, paresthesia, depression, rhinitis, pharyngitis, sinusitis
Rare (less than 5%)
Allergic reaction, anemia, leukopenia, neuropathy, herpes simplex

SERIOUS REACTIONS
- Cardiomyopathy, ventricular dysfunction, and CHF occur rarely.
- Pancytopenia may occur.

PRECAUTIONS & CONSIDERATIONS
Caution should be used in those who have previously received cardiotoxic drug therapy or radiation therapy to the chest wall and in those with a known hypersensitivity to the drug. It is unknown if trastuzumab is distributed in breast milk. The safety and efficacy of trastuzumab have not been established in children. Age-related cardiac dysfunction may require cautious use in the elderly. Vaccinations and coming in contact with crowds, people with known infections, and anyone who has recently received an oral polio vaccine should be avoided.

Notify the physician of nausea and vomiting, abdominal pain, back pain, chills, and fever. Left ventricular function and baseline EKG and multigated acquisition (MUGA) scan should be obtained before starting therapy. CBC should be monitored before and periodically during therapy. Signs and symptoms of deteriorating cardiac function should also be assessed.
Storage
Refrigerate unopened vials. After reconstitution of the vial with bacteriostatic water for injection, the solution is stable for 28 days if refrigerated. After reconstitution of the vial with sterile water for injection without a preservative, use the solution immediately; discard unused portions.

Administration
! Don't give trastuzumab by IV push or IV bolus. Do not use dextrose solutions for reconstitution.

Reconstitute the vial with 20 ml bacteriostatic water for injection (with benzyl alcohol) to yield a concentration of 21 mg/ml. If the patient is hypersensitive to benzyl alcohol, use sterile water for injection. Add the calculated dose from the vial to an IV solution of 250 ml 0.9% NaCl (do not use D_5W). Gently mix contents in bag. The reconstituted IV solution normally appears colorless to pale yellow. IV solution reconstituted in 0.9% NaCl is stable for up to 24 hours if refrigerated. Give loading dose (4 mg/kg) over 90 minutes. Give maintenance infusion (2 mg/kg) over 30 minutes.

Trazodone
tray′zoe-done
(Apo-Trazodone [CAN], Desyrel, Novo-Trazodone [CAN], PMS-Trazodone [CAN])
Do not confuse Desyrel with Delsym or Zestril.

CATEGORY AND SCHEDULE
Pregnancy Risk Category: C

CLASSIFICATION
Antidepressants, miscellaneous

MECHANISM OF ACTION
An antidepressant that blocks the reuptake of serotonin at neuronal presynaptic membranes, increasing its availability at postsynaptic receptor sites. *Therapeutic Effect:* Relieves depression.

PHARMACOKINETICS
Well absorbed from the GI tract. Protein binding: 85%-95%. Metabolized in the liver. Primarily excreted in urine. Unknown if removed by hemodialysis. **Half-life:** 5-9 hr.

AVAILABILITY
Tablets: 50 mg, 100 mg, 150 mg, 300 mg.

INDICATIONS AND DOSAGES
▸ Depression
PO
Adults. Initially, 150 mg/day in equally divided doses. Increase by 50 mg/day at 3- to 4-day intervals until therapeutic response is achieved. Maximum: 600 mg/day.
Elderly. Initially, 25-50 mg at bedtime. May increase by 25-50 mg every 3-7 days. Range: 75-150 mg/day.
Children 6-18 yr. Initially, 1.5-2 mg/kg/day in divided doses. May increase gradually to 6 mg/kg/day in 3 divided doses.

OFF-LABEL USES
Treatment of neurogenic pain

CONTRAINDICATIONS
None known.

INTERACTIONS
Drug
Alcohol, CNS depression-producing medications: May increase CNS depression.
Antihypertensives: May increase the effects of antihypertensives.
Digoxin, phenytoin: May increase the blood concentration of these drugs.
Indinavir, ketoconazole, ritonavir: May increase the blood concentration and toxicity of trazodone.

T

Herbal
St. John's wort: May increase the adverse effects of trazodone.
Food
None known.

DIAGNOSTIC TEST EFFECTS
May decrease serum WBC and neutrophil counts.

SIDE EFFECTS
Frequent (9%-3%)
Somnolence, dry mouth, light-headedness, dizziness, headache, blurred vision, nausea, vomiting
Occasional (3%-1%)
Nervousness, fatigue, constipation, generalized aches and pains, mild hypotension
Rare
Photosensitivity reaction

SERIOUS REACTIONS
• Priapism, diminished or improved libido, retrograde ejaculation, and impotence occur rarely.
• Trazodone appears to be less cardiotoxic than other antidepressants, although arrhythmias may occur in patients with pre-existing cardiac disease.

PRECAUTIONS & CONSIDERATIONS
Caution is warranted with arrhythmias and cardiac disease. Trazodone crosses the placenta and is minimally distributed in breast milk. The safety and efficacy of trazodone have not been established in children younger than 6 years. Lower dosages are recommended for the elderly, who are more likely to experience hypotensive or sedative effects.

Anticholinergic and sedative effects may occur, so avoid alcohol and tasks that require mental alertness or motor skills. Tolerance usually develops to these side effects. Notify the physician if a painful, prolonged penile erection occurs. CBC, neutrophil and WBC counts, and liver and renal function tests should be assessed during therapy. EKG should also be obtained to assess for arrhythmias.
Administration
Take trazodone shortly after a meal or snack to reduce the risk of dizziness or lightheadedness. Crush tablets, as needed.

Treprostinil
treh-prost'in-ill
(Remodulin)

CATEGORY AND SCHEDULE
Pregnancy Risk Category: B

CLASSIFICATION
Platelet inhibitors, prostaglandins, vasodilators

MECHANISM OF ACTION
An antiplatelet that directly dilates pulmonary and systemic arterial vascular beds, inhibiting platelet aggregation. *Therapeutic Effect:* Reduces symptoms of pulmonary arterial hypertension associated with exercise.

PHARMACOKINETICS
Rapidly, completely absorbed after subcutaneous infusion; 91% bound to plasma protein. Metabolized by the liver. Excreted mainly in the urine with a lesser amount eliminated in the feces. **Half-life:** 2-4 hr.

AVAILABILITY
Injection: 1 mg/ml, 2.5 mg/ml, 5 mg/ml, 10 mg/ml.

INDICATIONS AND DOSAGES
▶ **Pulmonary arterial hypertension**
CONTINUOUS SUBCUTANEOUS INFUSION
Adults, Elderly. Initially, 1.25 ng/kg/min. Reduce infusion rate to 0.625 ng/kg/min if initial dose cannot be tolerated. Increase infusion rate in increments of no more than 1.25 ng/kg/min per week for the first 4 wk and then no more than 2.5 ng/kg/min per week for the duration of infusion.
▶ **Hepatic impairment (mild to moderate)**
Adults, Elderly. Decrease the initial dose to 0.625 ng/kg/min based on ideal body weight and increase cautiously.

CONTRAINDICATIONS
None known.

INTERACTIONS
Drug
Anticoagulants, aspirin, heparin, thrombolytics: May increase the risk of bleeding.
Drugs that alter B/P, including antihypertensive agents, diuretics, vasodilators: Reduced B/P caused by treprostinil may be exacerbated by these drugs.
Herbal
None known.
Food
None known.

DIAGNOSTIC TEST EFFECTS
None known.

SIDE EFFECTS
Frequent
Infusion site pain, erythema, induration, rash
Occasional
Headache, diarrhea, jaw pain, vasodilation, nausea

Rare
Dizziness, hypotension, pruritus, edema

SERIOUS REACTIONS
• Abrupt withdrawal or sudden large reductions in dosage may result in worsening of pulmonary arterial hypertension symptoms.

PRECAUTIONS & CONSIDERATIONS
Caution is warranted with liver or renal impairment and in the elderly. It is unknown if treprostinil is distributed in breast milk. Safety and efficacy of treprostinil have not been established in children. In the elderly, age-related decreased cardiac, hepatic, and renal function as well as concurrent disease or other drug therapy may require dosage adjustment. Consider dosage selection carefully in the elderly, because of the increased incidence of diminished organ function. Notify the physician of signs of increased pulmonary artery pressure, such as dyspnea, cough, or chest pain.
Storage
Store at room temperature and administer without further dilution. Do not use a single vial for longer than 14 days after initial use.
Administration
Give as a continuous subcutaneous infusion via a subcutaneous catheter, using an infusion pump designed for subcutaneous drug delivery. Calculate the infusion rate using the following formula: Infusion rate (ml/hr) = Dose (ng/kg/min) multiplied by Weight (kg) multiplied by (0.00006/treprostinil dosage strength concentration [mg/ml]). To avoid potential interruptions in drug delivery, provide the patient with immediate access to a backup infusion pump and spare subcutaneous infusion sets. Abrupt withdrawal or sudden large reductions

in dosage may result in worsening of pulmonary arterial hypertension symptoms.

Tretinoin
tret′i-noyn
(Altinac, Avita, Renova, Retin-A, Retin-A Micro, Vesanoid)

CATEGORY AND SCHEDULE
Pregnancy Risk Category: D (oral), C (topical)

CLASSIFICATION
Antineoplastics, retinoids, dermatologics, keratolytics

MECHANISM OF ACTION
A retinoid that decreases cohesiveness of follicular epithelial cells. Increases turnover of follicular epithelial cells. Bacterial skincounts are not altered. Transdermal: Exerts its effects on growth and differentiation of epithelial cells. Antineoplastic: Induces maturation, decreases proliferation of acute promyelocytic leukemia (APL) cells. *Therapeutic Effect:* Causes expulsion of blackheads; alleviates fine wrinkles, hyperpigmentation; causes repopulation of bone marrow and blood by normal hematopoietic cells.

PHARMACOKINETICS
Topical: Minimally absorbed. Oral: Well absorbed following oral administration. Protein binding: 95%. Metabolized in liver. Primarily excreted in urine, minimal excretion in feces. **Half-life:** 0.5-2 hr.

AVAILABILITY
Capsules: 10 mg (Vesanoid).

Cream: 0.025% (Altinac, Avita, Retin-A), 0.02% (Renova), 0.05% (Altinac, Renova, Retin-A), 0.1 % (Altinac, Retin-A).
Gel: 0.01% (Retin-A), 0.025% (Avita, Retin-A), 0.04% (Retin-A Micro), 0.1% (Retin-A Micro).
Topical Liquid: 0.05% (Retin-A).

INDICATIONS AND DOSAGES
▶ **Acne**
TOPICAL
Adults. Apply once daily at bedtime.
TRANSDERMAL
Adults. Apply to face once daily at bedtime.
▶ **Acute promyelocytic leukemia**
PO
Adults. 45 mg/m^2/day given as two evenly divided doses until complete remission is documented. Discontinue therapy 30 days after complete remission or after 90 days of treatment, whichever comes first.

OFF-LABEL USES
Treatment of disorders of keratinization, including photo-aged skin, liver spots

CONTRAINDICATIONS
Sensitivity to parabens (used as preservative in gelatin capsule)

INTERACTIONS
Drug
Topical
Keratolytic agents (e.g., sulfur, benzoyl peroxide, salicylic acid), medicated soaps, shampoos, astringents, spice or lime cologne, permanent wave solutions, hair depilatories: May increase skin irritation.
Photosensitive medication (thiazides, tetracyclines, fluoroquinolones, phenothiazines, sulfonamides): May augment phototoxicity.

PO
Ketoconazole: May increase
tretinoin concentration.
Herbal
Vitamin A: May increase risk of
vitamin A toxicity.
Food
None known.

DIAGNOSTIC TEST EFFECTS
PO: Leukocytosis occurs
commonly (40%). May elevate
liver function tests, cholesterol,
triglycerides.

SIDE EFFECTS
Expected
Topical
Temporary change in pigmentation,
photosensitivity, local inflammatory
reactions (peeling, dry skin, stinging,
erythema, pruritus) are to be
expected and are reversible with
discontinuation of tretinoin
Frequent
PO
Headache, fever, dry skin/oral
mucosa, bone pain, nausea, vomiting, rash
Occasional
PO
Mucositis, earache or feeling of
fullness in ears, flushing, pruritus,
increased sweating, visual disturbances, hypo/hypertension, dizziness, anxiety, insomnia, alopecia,
skin changes
Rare
PO
Change in visual acuity, temporary
hearing loss

SERIOUS REACTIONS
PO
• Retinoic acid syndrome (fever,
dyspnea, weight gain, abnormal
chest auscultatory findings, episodic
hypotension) occurs commonly as
does leukocytosis.

• Syndrome generally occurs during
first month of therapy (sometimes
occurs following first dose).
• Pseudo tumor cerebri may be
noted, especially in children
(headache, nausea, vomiting, visual
disturbances).
• Possible tumorigenic potential
when combined with ultraviolet
radiation.
Topical
• Possible tumorigenic potential
when combined with ultraviolet
radiation.

PRECAUTIONS & CONSIDERATIONS
Caution should be used with elevated
cholesterol and/or triglycerides and
considerable sun exposure in their
occupation or hypersensitivity to
sun. Be aware that tretinoin should
be avoided in pregnant women. Be
aware that it is unknown if tretinoin
is distributed in breast milk; exercise
caution in nursing mother. Tretinoin
may have a teratogenic and embryotoxic effect.
   All women of childbearing potential should be warned of risk to fetus
if pregnancy occurs. Two reliable
forms of contraceptives should be
used concurrently during therapy
and for 1 month after discontinuation of therapy, even in infertile,
premenopausal women. A pregnancy
test should be obtained within 1 week
prior to institution of therapy. Liver
function tests and cholesterol and
triglyceride levels should be monitored before and during therapy.
Avoid exposure to sunlight or
sunbeds; sunscreens and protective
clothing should be used. Affected
areas should also be protected from
wind, cold. If skin is already
sunburned, do not use until fully
recovered. Keep tretinoin away from
eyes, mouth, angles of nose, and
mucous membranes. Do not use

T

medicated, drying, or abrasive soaps; wash face no more than 2-3 times/day with bland soap. Avoid use of preparations containing alcohol, menthol, spice, or lime such as shaving lotions, astringents, and perfume. Mild redness, peeling are expected; decrease frequency or discontinue medication if excessive reaction occurs. Non-medicated cosmetics may be used; however, cosmetics must be removed before tretinoin application.

Storage
Store at room temperature.

Administration
Take oral tretinoin with food. Do not crush or break capsule.

For topical administration, thoroughly cleanse area before applying tretinoin. Lightly cover only the affected area. Liquid may be applied with fingertip, gauze, or cotton, taking care to avoid running onto unaffected skin. Keep medication away from eyes, mouth, angles of nose, mucous membranes. Wash hands immediately after application. Improvement noted during first 24 weeks of therapy. Therapeutic results noted in 2-3 weeks; optimal results in 6 weeks.

Triamterene
try-am′ter-een
(Dyrenium)
Do not confuse triamterene with trimipramine.

CATEGORY AND SCHEDULE
Pregnancy Risk Category: C
(D if used in pregnancy-induced hypertension)

CLASSIFICATION
Diuretics, potassium sparing

MECHANISM OF ACTION
A potassium-sparing diuretic that inhibits sodium, potassium, ATPase. Interferes with sodium and potassium exchange in distal tubule, cortical collecting tubule, and collecting duct. Increases sodium and decreases potassium excretion. Also increases magnesium, decreases calcium loss. *Therapeutic Effect:* Produces diuresis and lowers B/P.

PHARMACOKINETICS

Route	Onset	Peak	Duration
PO	2-4 hr	N/A	7-9 hr

Incompletely absorbed from the GI tract. Widely distributed. Metabolized in the liver. Primarily eliminated in feces via biliary route. **Half-life:** 1.5-2.5 hr (increased in renal impairment).

AVAILABILITY
Capsules: 50 mg, 100 mg.

INDICATIONS AND DOSAGES
▸ **Edema, hypertension**
PO
Adults, Elderly. 25-100 mg/day as a single dose or in 2 divided doses. Maximum: 300 mg/day.

Children. 2-4 mg/kg/day as a single dose or in 2 divided doses. Maximum: 6 mg/kg/day or 300 mg/day.

OFF-LABEL USES
Treatment adjunct for hypertension, prevention and treatment of hypokalemia

CONTRAINDICATIONS
Drug-induced or pre-existing hyperkalemia, progressive or severe renal disease, severe hepatic disease

INTERACTIONS
Drug
ACE inhibitors (such as captopril), potassium-containing medications, potassium supplements: May increase the risk of hyperkalemia.
Anticoagulants, heparin: May decrease the effects of these drugs.
Lithium: May decrease the clearance and increase the risk of toxicity of lithium.
NSAIDs: May decrease the antihypertensive effect of triamterene.
Herbal
None known.
Food
None known.

DIAGNOSTIC TEST EFFECTS
May increase urinary calcium excretion; BUN and blood glucose levels; and serum calcium, creatinine, potassium, magnesium, and uric acid levels. May decrease serum sodium levels.

SIDE EFFECTS
Occasional
Fatigue, nausea, diarrhea, abdominal pain, leg cramps, headache
Rare
Anorexia, asthenia, rash, dizziness

SERIOUS REACTIONS
• Triamterene use may result in hyponatremia (somnolence, dry mouth, increased thirst, lack of energy) or severe hyperkalemia (irritability, anxiety, heaviness of legs, paresthesia, hypotension, bradycardia, EKG changes [tented T waves, widening QRS complex, ST segment depression]).
• Agranulocytosis, nephrolithiasis, and thrombocytopenia occur rarely.

PRECAUTIONS & CONSIDERATIONS
Caution is warranted with diabetes mellitus, history of renal calculi, hepatic or renal impairment and concurrent use of potassium-sparing diuretics or potassium supplements. Triamterene crosses the placenta and is distributed in breast milk. Breastfeeding is not recommended for patients taking this drug. The safety and efficacy of this drug have not been established in children. The elderly may be at increased risk for developing hyperkalemia. Avoid consuming salt substitutes and foods high in potassium.

An increase in the frequency and volume of urination may occur. Notify the physician of dry mouth, fever, headache, nausea and vomiting, persistent or severe weakness, sore throat, or unusual bleeding or bruising blood pressure (B/P), vital signs, electrolytes, intake and output, and weight should be monitored before and during treatment. Be aware of signs of electrolyte disturbances such as hypokalemia or hyponatremia. Hypokalemia may cause arrhythmias, altered mental status, muscle cramps, asthenia, and tremor.
Administration
Take triamterene with food if GI disturbances occur. Do not crush or break capsules. Therapeutic effect takes several days to begin and can last for several days after the drug is discontinued.

T

Triazolam

trye-ay'zoe-lam
(Apo-Triazo [CAN], Halcion)
**Do not confuse Halcion with
Haldol or Healon.**

CATEGORY AND SCHEDULE
Pregnancy Risk Category: X
Controlled Substance
Schedule: IV

CLASSIFICATION
Benzodiazepines,
sedatives/hypnotics

MECHANISM OF ACTION
A benzodiazepine that enhances the
action of the inhibitory neurotransmitter gamma-aminobutyric acid,
resulting in CNS depression.
Therapeutic Effect: Induces sleep.

AVAILABILITY
Tablets: 0.125 mg, 0.25 mg.

INDICATIONS AND DOSAGES
▸ **Insomnia**
PO
Adults, Children older than 18 yr.
0.125-0.5 mg at bedtime.
Elderly. 0.0625-0.125 mg at
bedtime.

CONTRAINDICATIONS
Angle-closure glaucoma; CNS
depression; pregnancy or breast-
feeding; severe, uncontrolled pain;
sleep apnea

INTERACTIONS
Drug
Alcohol, other CNS depressants:
May increase CNS depression.
Herbal
Kava kava, valerian: May increase
CNS depression.

Food
Grapefruit, grapefruit juice: May
alter the absorption of triazolam.

DIAGNOSTIC TEST EFFECTS
None known.

SIDE EFFECTS
Frequent
Somnolence, sedation, dry mouth,
headache, dizziness, nervousness,
light-headedness, incoordination,
nausea, rebound insomnia (may
occur for 1-2 nights after drug is
discontinued)
Occasional
Euphoria, tachycardia, abdominal
cramps, visual disturbances
Rare
Paradoxical CNS excitement or restlessness (particularly in elderly or
debilitated patients)

SERIOUS REACTIONS
• Abrupt or too-rapid withdrawal
may result in pronounced restlessness, irritability, insomnia, hand
tremors, abdominal or muscle
cramps, vomiting, diaphoresis, and
seizures.
• Overdose results in somnolence,
confusion, diminished reflexes,
respiratory depression, and
coma.

PRECAUTIONS & CONSIDERATIONS
Caution is warranted in persons
with a potential for drug abuse.
Pregnancy should be determined
before therapy begins. Drowsiness
may occur. Avoid alcohol, CNS
depressants, and tasks that require
mental alertness or motor skills.
Smoking should also be avoided
because it can reduce the drug's
effectiveness. Cardiovascular,
mental, and respiratory status and
hepatic function should be monitored throughout therapy.

Administration

Take triazolam without regard to food. Crush tablets as needed. Don't administer the drug with grapefruit juice.

Trientine
trye-en'teen
(Syprine)

CATEGORY AND SCHEDULE
Pregnancy Risk Category: C

CLASSIFICATION
Antidotes, chelators

MECHANISM OF ACTION
An oral chelating agent that foms complexes by binding metal ions particularly copper. *Therapeutic Effect:* Binds to copper and induces cupruresis.

PHARMACOKINETICS
None reported.

AVAILABILITY
Capsules: 250 mg (Syprine).

INDICATIONS AND DOSAGES
▶ **Wilson's disease**
PO
Adults, Elderly. 750-1250 mg/day in 2-4 divided doses. Maximum: 2 g/day.
Children 12 yr and older. 500-750 mg/day in 2-4 divided doses. Maximum: 1500 mg/day.

CONTRAINDICATIONS
Hypersensitivity to trientine or its components

INTERACTIONS
Drug
Iron preparations: May decrease absorption of both drugs.
Herbal
None known.
Food
None known.

DIAGNOSTIC TEST EFFECTS
None known.

SIDE EFFECTS
Occasional
Contact dermatitis, dystonia, muscular spasm, myasthenia gravis

SERIOUS REACTIONS
• Iron deficiency anemia and systemic lupus erythematosus rarely occur.

PRECAUTIONS & CONSIDERATIONS
Caution is necessary with cystinuria, rheumatoid arthritis, and biliary cirrhosis.
It is unknown if trientine is distributed in breast milk. Safety and efficacy of trientine have not been established in children younger than 12 years old. There are no age-related precautions noted in the elderly. Serum-free copper level and copper analysis should be obtained every 6-12 months. Adequate fluid intake should be maintained.
Storage
Store trientine bottles in the refrigerator.
Administration
Be aware that trientine is second-line therapy for people intolerant of penicillamine. Do not open or chew capsules. Take 1 hour before or 2 hours after meals. Long-term maintenance dose should be determined at 6-12 month intervals.

T

Trifluridine
trye-flure'i-deen
(Viroptic)
Do not confuse with Zostrix.

CATEGORY AND SCHEDULE
Pregnancy Risk Category: C

CLASSIFICATION
Antivirals, ophthalmics

MECHANISM OF ACTION
An antiviral agent that incorporates into DNS causing increased rate of mutation and errors in protein formation. *Therapeutic Effect:* Prevents viral replication.

PHARMACOKINETICS
Intraocular solution is undetectable in serum. **Half-life:** 12 min.

AVAILABILITY
Ophthalmic solution: 1% (Viroptic).

INDICATIONS AND DOSAGES
▸ **Herpes simplex virus ocular infections**
OPHTHALMIC
Adults, Elderly, Children older than 6 yr. 1 drop onto cornea q2hr while awake. Maximum: 9 drops/day. Continue until corneal ulcer has completely reepithelialized; then, 1 drop q4hr while awake (minimum: 5 drops/day) for an additional 7 days.

CONTRAINDICATIONS
Hypersensitivity to trifluridine or any component of the formulation

INTERACTIONS
Drug
None known.

Herbal
None known.
Food
None known.

DIAGNOSTIC TEST EFFECTS
None known.

SIDE EFFECTS
Frequent
Transient stinging or burning with instillation
Occasional
Edema of eyelid
Rare
Hypersensitivity reaction

SERIOUS REACTIONS
• Ocular toxicity may occur if used longer than 21 days.

PRECAUTIONS & CONSIDERATIONS
Be aware that trifluridine use should not exceed 21 days due to the potential for ocular toxicity. It may cause transient irritation of the conjunctiva and cornea. Be aware that trifluridine is not recommended during pregnancy or lactation due to mutagenic effects in vitro. Safety and efficacy have not been established in children less than 6 years of age. There are no age-related precautions noted in the elderly.

If no improvement occurs after 7 days or complete healing after 14, contact the physician. Report any itching, swelling, redness, or increased irritation.
Storage
Refrigerate trifluridine; avoid freezing.
Administration
For ophthalmic use, do not touch applicator tip to any surface. Place finger on lower eyelid and pull out until pocket is formed between eye and lower lid. Hold dropper above pocket and place prescribed number

of drops in pocket. Close eyes gently so medication will not be squeezed out of sac. Apply gentle finger pressure to the lacrimal sac at inner canthus for 1 min following installation (lessens risk of systemic absorption).

Trihexyphenidyl
trye-hex-ee-fen'i-dill
(Artane, Apo-Trihex [CAN])

CATEGORY AND SCHEDULE
Pregnancy Risk Category: C

CLASSIFICATION
Anticholinergics, antiparkinson agents

MECHANISM OF ACTION
An anticholinergic agent that blocks central cholinergic receptors (aids in balancing cholinergic and dopaminergic activity). *Therapeutic Effect:* Decreases salivation, relaxes smooth muscle.

PHARMACOKINETICS
Well absorbed from gastrointestinal (GI) tract. Primarily excreted in urine. **Half-life:** 3.3-4.1 hr.

AVAILABILITY
Elixer: 2 mg/5 ml (Artane).
Tablets: 2 mg, 5 mg (Artane).

INDICATIONS AND DOSAGES
▶ **Parkinsonism**
PO
Adults, Elderly. Initially, 1 mg on first day. May increase by 2 mg/day at 3-5 day intervals up to 6-10 mg/day

(12-15 mg/day in patients with postencephalitic parkinsonism).
▶ **Drug-induced extrapyramidal symptoms**
PO
Adults, Elderly. Initially, 1 mg/day. Range: 5-15 mg/day.

CONTRAINDICATIONS
Angle closure glaucoma, GI obstruction, paralytic ileus, intestinal atony, severe ulcerative colitis, prostatic hypertrophy, myasthenia gravis, megacolon, hypersensitivity to trihexyphenidyl or any component of the formulation

INTERACTIONS
Drug
Alcohol, CNS depressants: May increase sedative effect.
Amantadine, anticholinergics, MAOIs: May increase anticholinergic effects.
Antacids, antidiarrheals: May decrease absorption and effects of trihexyphenidyl.
Herbal
None known.
Food
None known.

DIAGNOSTIC TEST EFFECTS
None known.

SIDE EFFECTS
Elderly (more than 60 yr) tend to develop mental confusion, disorientation, agitation, psychotic-like symptoms
Frequent
Drowsiness, dry mouth
Occasional
Blurred vision, urinary retention, constipation, dizziness, headache, muscle cramps
Rare
Seizures, depression, rash

T

SERIOUS REACTIONS
• Hypersensitivity reaction (eczema, pruritus, rash, cardiac disturbances, photosensitivity) may occur.
• Overdosage may vary from CNS depression (sedation, apnea, cardiovascular collapse, death) to severe paradoxical reaction (hallucinations, tremor, seizures).

PRECAUTIONS & CONSIDERATIONS
Caution is warranted with treated open-angle glaucoma, autonomic neuropathy, pulmonary disease, esophageal reflux, hiatal hernia, heart disease, hyperthyroidism, and hypertension. It is unknown if trihexyphenidyl crosses the placenta or is distributed in breast milk. Safety and efficacy have not been established in children. The elderly are more sensitive to the effects of trihexyphenidyl as well as anxiety, confusion, and nervousness.

Dry mouth, drowsiness, and dizziness are expected side effects of this drug. Avoid alcohol and do not drive, use machinery, or engage in other activities that require mental acuity if dizziness or blurred vision occurs.

Storage
Store at room temperature.

Administration
Be aware not to use sustained-release capsules for initial therapy. Once stabilized, may switch, on mg-for-mg basis, giving in 3 daily doses and with food. High doses may be divided into 4 doses, at meal times and at bedtime.

Trimethobenzamide
trye-meth-oh-ben'za-mide
(Tigan)

CATEGORY AND SCHEDULE
Pregnancy Risk Category: C

CLASSIFICATION
Anticholinergics, antiemetics/antivertigo

MECHANISM OF ACTION
An anticholinergic that acts at the chemoreceptor trigger zone in the medulla oblongata. *Therapeutic Effect:* Relieves nausea and vomiting.

PHARMACOKINETICS

Route	Onset	Peak	Duration
PO	10-40 min	N/A	3-4 hr
IM	15-30 min	N/A	2-3 hr

Partially absorbed from the GI tract. Distributed primarily to the liver. Metabolic fate unknown. Excreted in urine. **Half-life:** 7-9 hr.

AVAILABILITY
Capsules: 100 mg, 300 mg.
Injection: 100 mg/ml.
Suppositories: 100 mg, 200 mg.

INDICATIONS AND DOSAGES
▸ Nausea and vomiting
PO
Adults, Elderly. 300 mg 3-4 times a day.
Children weighing 30-100 lb. 100-200 mg 3-4 times a day.
IM
Adults, Elderly. 200 mg 3-4 times a day.
RECTAL
Adults, Elderly. 200 mg 3-4 times a day.

Children weighing 30-100 lb.
100-200 mg 3-4 times a day.
Children weighing less than 30 lb.
100 mg 3-4 times a day.

CONTRAINDICATIONS

Hypersensitivity to benzocaine or
similar local anesthetics; use of
parenteral form in children or
suppositories in premature infants or
neonates

INTERACTIONS
Drug
CNS depressants: May increase
CNS depression.
Herbal
None known.
Food
None known.

DIAGNOSTIC TEST EFFECTS
None known.

SIDE EFFECTS
Frequent
Somnolence
Occasional
Blurred vision, diarrhea, dizziness,
headache, muscle cramps
Rare
Rash, seizures, depression,
opisthotonos, parkinsonian
syndrome, Reye's syndrome (marked
by vomiting, seizures)

SERIOUS REACTIONS
• A hypersensitivity reaction, manifested as extrapyramidal symptoms
such as muscle rigidity and allergic
skin reactions, occurs rarely.
• Children may experience paradoxical reactions, marked by restlessness,
insomnia, euphoria, nervousness,
and tremor.
• Overdose may produce CNS
depression (manifested as sedation,
apnea, cardiovascular collapse, and
death) or severe paradoxical reactions

(such as hallucinations, tremor, and
seizures).

PRECAUTIONS & CONSIDERATIONS
Caution is warranted with dehydration, electrolyte imbalances, high
fever, and the debilitated or elderly.
It is unknown if trimethobenzamide
crosses the placenta or is distributed
in breast milk. No age-related precautions have been noted in children or
the elderly. Don't administer the
parenteral form to children or the
suppositories to neonates. Tasks that
require mental alertness or motor
skills should be avoided until response
to the drug has been established.

Drowsiness may occur. Notify the
physician of headache, visual disturbances, restlessness, or involuntary
muscle movements. B/P, intake and
output, vomitus, and skin for hydration status should be assessed.
Administration
! The elderly (older than 60 years)
are at increased risk for developing
agitation, disorientation, confusion,
and psychotic-like symptoms. Don't
administer trimethobenzamide by the
IV route because it produces severe
hypotension.

Take oral trimethobenzamide
without regard to food. Don't crush,
open, or break the capsules.

For IM use, inject the drug deep
into a large muscle mass, usually the
upper outer gluteus maximus.

For rectal use, if the suppository
is too soft, refrigerate it for 30 minutes
or run cold water over the foil wrapper. Moisten the suppository with
cold water before inserting it well
into the rectum.

T

Trimethoprim
trye-meth′oh-prim
(Apo-Tremethoprim [CAN],
Primsol, Proloprim)

CATEGORY AND SCHEDULE
Pregnancy Risk Category: C

CLASSIFICATION
Antibiotics, folate antagonists

MECHANISM OF ACTION
A folate antagonist that blocks
bacterial biosynthesis of nucleic
acids and proteins by interfering
with the metabolism of folinic acid.
Therapeutic Effect: Bacteriostatic.

PHARMACOKINETICS
Rapidly and completely absorbed
from the GI tract. Protein binding:
42%-46%. Widely distributed,
including to CSF. Metabolized in the
liver. Primarily excreted in urine.
Moderately removed by hemodialysis. **Half-life:** 8-10 hr (increased in
impaired renal function and
newborns; decreased in children).

AVAILABILITY
Oral Solution (Primsol): 50 mg/5 ml.
Tablets (Proloprim): 100 mg, 200 mg.

INDICATIONS AND DOSAGES
▸ **Acute, uncomplicated UTI**
PO
*Adults, Elderly, Children 12 yr and
older.* 100 mg q12hr or 200 mg
once a day for 10 days.
Children younger than 12 yr.
4-6 mg/kg/day in 2 divided doses for
10 days.
▸ **Dosage in renal impairment**
Dosage and frequency are modified
based on creatinine clearance.

Creatinine Clearance	Dosage Interval
Greater than 30 ml/min	No change
15-29 ml/min	50 mg q12hr

OFF-LABEL USES
Prevention of bacterial UTIs, treat-
ment of pneumonia caused by
Pneumocystis carinii

CONTRAINDICATIONS
Infants younger than 2 months,
megaloblastic anemia due to folic
acid deficiency

INTERACTIONS
Drug
**Folate antagonists (including
methotrexate):** May increase the
risk of megaloblastic anemia.
Herbal
None known.
Food
None known.

DIAGNOSTIC TEST EFFECTS
May increase BUN and serum biliru-
bin, creatinine, AST (SGOT), and
ALT (SGPT) levels.

SIDE EFFECTS
Occasional
Nausea, vomiting, diarrhea,
decreased appetite, abdominal
cramps, headache
Rare
Hypersensitivity reaction (pruritus,
rash), methemoglobinemia (bluish
fingernails, lips, or skin; fever; pale
skin; sore throat; unusual tiredness),
photosensitivity

SERIOUS REACTIONS
• Stevens-Johnson syndrome,
erythema multiforme, exfoliative
dermatitis, and anaphylaxis occur
rarely.

• Hematologic toxicity (thrombocytopenia, neutropenia, leukopenia, megaloblastic anemia) is more likely to occur in elderly, debilitated, or alcoholic patients; in patients with impaired renal function; and in those receiving prolonged high dosage.

PRECAUTIONS & CONSIDERATIONS

Caution is warranted with impaired hepatic or renal function or folic acid deficiency. Trimethoprim readily crosses the placenta and is distributed in breast milk. The safety and efficacy of trimethoprim have not been established in children. No age-related precautions have been noted in the elderly, but they may have an increased incidence of thrombocytopenia. Avoid sun and ultraviolet light.

Report bleeding, bruising, skin discoloration, fever, pallor, rash, sore throat, and tiredness. Hematology and renal function tests should be assessed before and during therapy.

Administration

Space doses evenly around the clock to maintain a constant drug level in urine. Take trimethoprim without regard to food (or with food if stomach upset occurs). Space drug doses evenly around the clock and complete the full course of trimethoprim therapy, which usually lasts 10-14 days.

Trimetrexate
try-meh-trex-ate
(Neutrexin)
Do not confuse with Amicar.

CATEGORY AND SCHEDULE
Pregnancy Risk Category: D

CLASSIFICATION
Antibiotics, folate antagonists, antiprotozoals

MECHANISM OF ACTION
A folate antagonist that inhibits the enzyme dihydrofolate reductase (DHFR). *Therapeutic Effect:* Disrupts purine, DNA, RNA, protein synthesis, with consequent cell death.

PHARMACOKINETICS
Following IV administration, distributed readily into ascitic fluid. Metabolized in liver. Eliminated in urine. **Half-life:** 11-20 hr.

AVAILABILITY
Powder for Injection: 25 mg (Neutrexin).

INDICATIONS AND DOSAGES
▶ **Pneumocystis carinii pneumonia (PCP)**
IV INFUSION
Adults. Trimetrexate: 45 mg/m^2 once daily over 60-90 min. Leucovorin: 20 mg/m^2 over 5-10 min q6hr for total daily dose of 80 mg/m^2, or orally as 4 doses of 20 mg/m^2 spaced equally throughout the day. Round up the oral dose to the next higher 25-mg increment. Recommended course of therapy: 21 days trimetrexate, 24 days leucovorin.

T

OFF-LABEL USES

Treatment of non-small cell lung, prostate, and colorectal cancer

CONTRAINDICATIONS

Clinically significant hypersensitivity to trimetrexate, leucovorin, or methotrexate

INTERACTIONS

Drug

Erythromycin, rifampin, rifabutin, ketoconazole, fluconazole, acetaminophen: May alter timetrexate plasma concentration.
Cimetidine: May reduce trimetrexate metabolism.
Clotrimazole, ketoconazole, miconazole: May inhibit trimetrexate metabolism.
Herbal
None known.
Food
None known.

DIAGNOSTIC TEST EFFECTS

May increase SGOT (AST), SGPT (ALT), alkaline phosphatase, bilirubin, BUN, serum creatinine. May decrease Hgb, Hct, leukocytes, platelet counts.

IV INCOMPATIBILITIES

Foscarnet (Foscavir), indomethacin (Indocin)

SIDE EFFECTS

Occasional
Fever, rash, pruritus, nausea, vomiting, confusion
Rare
Fatigue

SERIOUS REACTIONS

* Trimetrexate given without concurrent leucovorin may result in serious or fatal hematologic, hepatic, and/or renal complications, including bone marrow suppression, oral and GI mucosal ulceration, and renal and hepatic dysfunction.
* In event of overdose, stop trimetrexate and give leucovorin 40 mg/m^2 q6hr for 3 days.
* Anaphylaxis occurs rarely.

PRECAUTIONS & CONSIDERATIONS

Caution is warranted with fertility impairment and hematologic, renal or hepatic impairment. It is unknown if trimetrexate crosses the placenta or is distributed in breast milk. Trimetrexate may cause fetal harm. Safety and efficacy have not been established in children or the elderly. Leucovorin therapy must extend for 72 hours past the last dose of trimetrexate. To allow for full therapeutic effect of trimetrexate to occur, zidovudine treatment should be discontinued during trimetrexate therapy.

Neutrophil count, platelet count, liver function tests (SGOT, SGPT, alkaline phosphatase), and renal values (serum creatinine, BUN) for development of serious toxicities should be monitored. Unusual bleeding or bruising, black tarry stools, blood in urine or stools, pinpoint red spots on skin should be reported.

Storage
Store vials for parenteral use at room temperature. After reconstitution, solution is stable under refrigeration or at room temperature for up to 24 hours. Do not freeze reconstituted solution. Discard unused portion after 24 hr.

Administration
Be aware that even though trimetrexate and leucovorin are given concurrently, they must be administered separately or precipitate will occur instantly; flush IV line thoroughly with 10 ml D$_5$W between infusions. Dilute leucovorin according to leucovorin instructions and give over

5-10 min q6hr. Be aware that in event of hematologic, renal, hepatic toxicities, doses of trimetrexate and leucovorin should be modified.

Be aware if solution comes in contact with skin or mucosa, wash with soap and water immediately. Use proper cytoxic disposal technique. Do not reconstitute with solution containing either chloride ion or leucovorin, since precipitate occurs instantly. Reconstituted solution appears as pale greenish yellow. Inspect for particulate matter. Discard if cloudiness or precipitate is present.

Reconstitute each 25-mg vial with 2 ml D_5W or sterile water for injection to provide concentration of 12.5 mg/ml. Complete dissolution should occur within 30 seconds. Filter the reconstituted solution prior to further dilution. Further dilute with D_5W to yield a final concentration of 0.25-2 mg/ml. Give diluted solution by IV infusion over 60-90 minutes. Flush IV line thoroughly with at least 10 ml D_5W before and after administering trimetrexate.

Trimipramine

trye-mih-prah-meen
(Apo-Trimip [CAN],
Novo-Tripramine [CAN],
Nu-Trimipramine [CAN],
Rhotrimine [CAN], Surmontil)
**Do not confuse with
desipramine.**

CATEGORY AND SCHEDULE

Pregnancy Risk Category: D

CLASSIFICATION

Antidepressants, tricyclic

MECHANISM OF ACTION

A tricyclic antibulimic, anticataplectic, antidepressant, antinarcoleptic, antineuralgic, antineuritic, and antipanic agent that blocks the reuptake of neurotransmitters, such as norepinephrine and serotonin, at presynaptic membranes, increasing their concentration at postsynaptic receptor sites. May demonstrate less autonomic toxicity than other tricyclic antidepressants. *Therapeutic Effect:* Results in antidepressant effect. Anticholinergic effect controls nocturnal enuresis.

PHARMACOKINETICS

Rapidly, completely absorbed after PO administration, and not affected by food. Protein binding: 95%. Metabolized in liver (significant first-pass effect). Primarily excreted in urine. Not removed by hemodialysis. **Half-life:** 16-40 hr.

AVAILABILITY

Capsules: 25 mg, 50 mg, 100 mg (Surmontil).

INDICATIONS AND DOSAGES
▸ **Depression**
PO
Adults. 50-150 mg/day at bedtime. Maximum: 200 mg/day for outpatients, 300 mg/day for inpatients.
Elderly. Initially, 25 mg/day at bedtime. May increase by 25 mg q3-7 days. Maximum: 100 mg/day.

CONTRAINDICATIONS

Acute recovery period after myocardial infarction (MI), within 14 days of MAOI ingestion, hypersensitivity to trimipramine or any component of the formulation

INTERACTIONS
Drug
Alcohol, central nervous system (CNS) depressants: May increase CNS and respiratory depression and the hypotensive effects of trimipramine.

Anticoagulants: May increase risk of bleeding.

Antipsychotics (amisulpride, haloperidol, risperidone, sertindole, quetiapine, sultopride, zotepine): May increase the cardiac effects (QT prolongation, torsades de pointes, cardiac arrest).

Antithyroid agents: May increase the risk of agranulocytosis.

Amprenavir, atazanavir: May increase serum concentrations and risk of toxicity of trimipramine.

Atomoxetine: May increase plasma concentrations of atomoxetine.

Barbiturates: May decrease trimipramine serum concentrations and possible additive adverse effects.

Baclofen: May increase the risk of memory loss and/or muscle tone.

Cimetidine: May increase trimipramine blood concentration and risk of toxicity.

Cisapride: May increase the cardiac effects.

Class 1, 1A, and III antiarrhythmic agents: May increase the cardiac effects.

Clonidine, guanadrel: May decrease the effects of clonidine and guanadrel.

Cotrimoxazole, fluconazole: May increase the cardiac effects.

Duloxetine, fluoxetine, paroxetine, sertraline: May increase serum concentrations and risk of toxicity.

Estrogens: May increase the antidepressant effectiveness and risk of tricyclic toxicity.

Gatifloxacin, gemifloxacin, grepafloxacin, sparfloxacin,

telithromycin: May increase the cardiac effects.

Halofantrine, halothane: May increase the cardiac effects.

MAOIs: May increase the risk of hyperpyrexia, hypertensive crisis, and seizures.

Phenothiazines: May increase anticholinergic and sedative effects of trimipramine.

Phenytoin: May decrease trimipramine blood concentration.

Quinidine: May increase the risk of trimipramine toxicity.

Sympathomimetics: May increase the cardiac effects.

Vasopressin: May increase the cardiac effects.

Zolmitriptan: May increase the cardiac effects.
Herbal
Ginkgo biloba: May decrease seizure threshold.

St. John's wort: May have additive effect.

DIAGNOSTIC TEST EFFECTS
May alter blood glucose levels and EKG readings.

SIDE EFFECTS
Frequent
Drowsiness, fatigue, dry mouth, blurred vision, constipation, delayed micturition, postural hypotension, diaphoresis, disturbed concentration, increased appetite, urinary retention, photosensitivity.
Occasional
Gastrointestinal (GI) disturbances, such as nausea, and a metallic taste sensation.
Rare
Paradoxical reaction, marked by agitation, restlessness, nightmares, insomnia, extrapyramidal symptoms, particularly fine hand tremors.

SERIOUS REACTIONS
- High dosage may produce cardio-vascular effects, such as severe postural hypotension, dizziness, tachycardia, palpitations, arrhythmias, and seizures. High dosage may also result in altered temperature regulation, including hyperpyrexia or hypothermia.
- Abrupt withdrawal from prolonged therapy may produce headache, malaise, nausea, vomiting, and vivid dreams.

PRECAUTIONS & CONSIDERATIONS
Caution is warranted with cardiac disease, diabetes mellitus, glaucoma, hiatal hernia, history of seizures, history or urinary obstruction or retention, hyperthyroidism, increased intraocular pressure (IOP), liver disease, prostatic hypertrophy, renal disease, and schizophrenia. It is unknown if trimipramine crosses the placenta or is distributed in breast milk. Be aware that trimipramine is not recommended in children younger than 18 years. Dose reduction may be required in the elderly.

Tolerance usually develops to anticholinergic effects, postural hypotension, and sedative effects during therapy. Avoid tasks that require mental alertness or motor skills until response to trimipramine is established.

Administration
Take with food or milk if GI distress occurs.

Trioxsalen
trye-ox'a-len
(Trisoralen)

CATEGORY AND SCHEDULE
Pregnancy Risk Category: C

CLASSIFICATION
Photosensitizers, psoralens

MECHANISM OF ACTION
A member of the family of psoralens that induces the process of melano-genesis by a mechanism that is not known. *Therapeutic Effect:* Enhances pigmentation.

PHARMACOKINETICS
Rapidly absorbed from the gastrointestinal (GI) tract. **Half-life:** 2 hr. (Skin sensitivity to light remains for 8-12 hr.)

AVAILABILITY
Tablets: 5 mg (Trisoralen).

INDICATIONS AND DOSAGES
▸ Pigmentation
PO
Adults, Elderly, Children 12 yr and older. 10 mg/day 2 hr before exposure to UVA light or sun exposure.
▸ Vitiligo
PO
Adults, Elderly, Children 12 yr and older. 10 mg/day 2-4 hr before exposure to UVA light.

OFF-LABEL USES
Polymorphous light eruption, psoriasis, sunlight sensitivity

CONTRAINDICATIONS
Concomitant disease states associated with photosensitivity

T

(acute lupus erythematosus, porphyria, leukoderma of infectious origin), concomitant use of preparations with any internal or external photosensitizing capacity, children under 12 years old, hypersensitivity to trioxsalen or any component of the formulation

INTERACTIONS
Drug
None known.
Herbal
None known.
Food
Furocoumarin foods: May increase risk of severe burns.

SIDE EFFECTS
Occasional
Gastric discomfort, photosensitivity, pruritus

SERIOUS REACTIONS
• Overdose or overexposure may result in serious blistering and burning.

PRECAUTIONS & CONSIDERATIONS
Caution is warranted with albinism, hydroa, leukoderma of infectious origin, lupus erythematosus, polymorphic light eruptions, porphyria, xeroderma pigmentosum, aphakia, severe cardiovascular disease, cataracts, and skin cancer. It is unknown if trioxsalen crosses the placenta or is distributed in breast milk. Safety and efficacy have not been determined in children younger than 12 years old. There are no age-related precautions noted in the elderly. Furocoumarin containing foods such as carrots, celery, limes, figs, mustard, parsley, parsnips, which contain natural psoralens should be avoided because it will increase the risk of severe burns and blistering. Direct and indirect

sunlight should be avoided for 8 hours after therapy. If sunlight cannot be avoided, protective clothing and/or sunscreens should be worn.

If burning, blistering, or intractable pruritus occurs, trioxsalen should be discontinued.
Administration
Therapy with trioxsalen should not exceed 14 days nor should the dosage be increased. Take with food or milk to reduce gastric discomfort.

Triptorelin Pamoate
trip'toe-rel-in
(Trelstar Depot, Trelstar LA)

CATEGORY AND SCHEDULE
Pregnancy Risk Category: X

CLASSIFICATION
Antineoplastics, hormones/hormone modifiers, gonadotropin-releasing hormone analogs

MECHANISM OF ACTION
A gonadotropin-releasing hormone (GnRH) analogue and antineoplastic agent that inhibits gonadotropin hormone secretion through a negative feedback mechanism. Circulating levels of luteinizing hormone, follicle-stimulating hormone, testosterone, and estradiol rise initially, then subside with continued therapy. *Therapeutic Effect:* Suppresses growth of abnormal prostate tissue.

AVAILABILITY
Powder for Injection (Trelstar Depot): 3.75 mg.
Powder for Injection (Trelstar LA): 11.25 mg.

INDICATIONS AND DOSAGES
▸ **Prostate cancer**
IM
Adults, Elderly. 3.75 mg once
q28 days (Trelstar Depot). 11.25 mg
q84 days (Trelstar LA).

CONTRAINDICATIONS
Hypersensitivity to luteinizing
hormone-releasing hormone
(LHRH) or LHRH agonists

INTERACTIONS
Drug
Hyperprolactinemic drugs:
Reduce the number of pituitary
gonadotropin-releasing hormone
(GnRH) receptors.
Herbal
None known.
Food
None known.

DIAGNOSTIC TEST EFFECTS
May alter serum pituitary-gonadal
function test results. May cause transient increase in serum testosterone
levels, usually during first week of
treatment.

SIDE EFFECTS
Frequent (greater than 5%)
Hot flashes, skeletal pain, headache,
impotence
Occasional (5%-2%)
Insomnia, vomiting, leg pain,
fatigue
Rare (less than 2%)
Dizziness, emotional lability, diar-
rhea, urine retention, UTIs, anemia,
pruritus

SERIOUS REACTIONS
• Bladder outlet obstruction,
skeletal pain, hematuria,
and spinal cord compression
(with weakness or paralysis
of the lower extremities) may
occur.

Women who are or may be pregnant
shouldn't use this drug. Pregnancy
should be determined before beginning triptorelin therapy. It is
unknown if triptorelin is excreted in
breast milk. The safety and efficacy
of triptorelin have not been established in children. No age-related
precautions have been noted in
the elderly.

Blood in urine, increased skeletal
pain, and urine retention may occur
initially, but these symptoms usually
subside within 1 week. Notify the
physician if difficulty breathing,
infection at the injection site, numbness of the arms or legs, breast pain
or swelling, persistent nausea or
vomiting, or rapid heartbeat develop.
Prostatic acid phosphatase (PAP),
prostate-specific antigen (PSA), and
serum testosterone levels should be
obtained periodically during therapy.
Serum testosterone and PAP levels
should increase during the first week
of therapy. The testosterone level
should then decrease to baseline
level or less within 2 weeks, and the
PAP level should decrease within
4 weeks.

A worsening of signs and symptoms of prostatic cancer, especially
during the first week of therapy, due
to a transient increase in testosterone
level should be carefully assessed.
Administration
Administer under the supervision of
a physician. Do not miss monthly
injections.

Trospium
trose'pee-um
(Sanctura)

CATEGORY AND SCHEDULE
Pregnancy Risk Category: C

CLASSIFICATION
Anticholinergics, relaxants,
urinary tract

MECHANISM OF ACTION
An anticholinergic that antagonizes
the effect of acetylcholine on
muscarinic receptors, producing
parasympatholytic action.
Therapeutic Effect: Reduces smooth
muscle tone in the bladder.

PHARMACOKINETICS
Minimally absorbed after PO administration. Protein binding: 50%-85%.
Distributed in plasma. Excreted
mainly in feces and, to a lesser
extent, in urine. **Half life:** 20 hr.

AVAILABILITY
Tablets: 20 mg.

INDICATIONS AND DOSAGES
▸ **Overactive bladder**
PO
Adults. 20 mg 2 times/day.
Elderly (75 yr and older). Titrate
dosage down to 20 mg once a day,
based on tolerance.
▸ **Dosage in renal impairment**
For patients with creatinine clearance
less than 30 ml/min, dosage reduced
to 20 mg once a day at bedtime.

CONTRAINDICATIONS
Decreased GI motility, gastric retention, uncontrolled angle-closure
glaucoma, urine retention

INTERACTIONS
Drug
Other anticholinergic agents:
Increases the severity and frequency
of side effects and may alter the
absorption of other drugs because of
anticholinergic effects on GI motility.
**Digoxin, metformin, morphine,
pancuronium, procainamide, teno-
fovir, vancomycin:** May increase
trospium blood concentration.
Herbal
None known.
Food
High-fat meal: May reduce
trospium absorption.

DIAGNOSTIC TEST EFFECTS
None known.

SIDE EFFECTS
Frequent (20%)
Dry mouth
Occasional (10%-4%)
Constipation, headache
Rare (less than 2%)
Fatigue, upper abdominal pain,
dyspepsia, flatulence, dry eyes,
urine retention

SERIOUS REACTIONS
• Overdose may result in severe
anticholinergic effects, such as
abdominal pain, nausea and vomiting, confusion, depression, diaphoresis, facial flushing, hypertension,
hypotension, respiratory depression,
irritability, lacrimation, nervousness,
and restlessness.
• Supraventricular tachycardia and
hallucinations occur rarely.

PRECAUTIONS & CONSIDERATIONS
Caution is warranted with renal or
hepatic impairment, intestinal atony,
obstructive GI disorders, significant
bladder obstruction, ulcerative colitis, myasthenia gravis, and angle-
closure glaucoma. It is unknown if

trospium crosses the placenta or is distributed in breast milk. The safety and efficacy of trospium have not been established in children.

The elderly (age 75 and older) have a higher incidence of constipation, dry mouth, dyspepsia, urine retention, and UTI.

Notify the physician of increased salivation or sweating, an irregular heartbeat, nausea and vomiting, or severe abdominal pain. Intake and output, pattern of daily bowel activity and stool consistency, and symptomatic relief should be assessed.

Storage
Store trospium at room temperature.

Administration
Don't break or crush the tablets. Take the drug at least 1 hour before meals or on an empty stomach. Do not take trospium with high-fat meals because it may reduce absorption.

Trovafloxacin/
Alatrofloxacin
troh-va-flocks-ah-sin
(Trovan)

CATEGORY AND SCHEDULE
Pregnancy Risk Category: C

CLASSIFICATION
Antibiotics, quinolones

MECHANISM OF ACTION
A fluoroquinolone that inhibits the DNA enzyme gyrase in susceptible microorganisms, interfering with bacterial DNA replication and repair. *Therapeutic Effect:* Produces bactericidal activity.

PHARMACOKINETICS
Well absorbed from the gastrointestinal (GI) tract. Protein binding: 76%. Widely distributed including cerebrospinal fluid (CSF). Metabolized in liver by conjugation. Excreted in feces. Not removed by hemodialysis. **Half-life:** 9-13 hr.

AVAILABILITY
Tablets: 100 mg, 200 mg (Trovan).
Injection: 200 mg/40 ml,
300 mg/60 ml (Trovan).

INDICATIONS AND DOSAGES
▸ **Pneumonia**
PO/IV
Adults, Elderly. 200 mg q24hr for 7-14 days.
▸ **Skin and skin-structure infections**
PO/IV
Adults, Elderly. 200 mg q24hr for 10-14 days.
▸ **Gynecologic infections**
IV
Adults, Elderly. 300 mg q24hr for 7-14 days.
PO
Adults, Elderly. 100 mg q24hr for 7-14 days.
▸ **Abdominal infection**
Adults, Elderly. 300 mg q24hr for 7-14 days.
▸ **Bronchitis**
PO
Adults, Elderly. 100 q24hr for 7-10 days.

CONTRAINDICATIONS
History of hypersensitivity to other fluoroquinolones

INTERACTIONS
Drug
Antacids, iron preparations, sucralfate: Decrease trovafloxacin absorption.
Antidiabetic agents: May increase changes in blood glucose and

T

increase risk of hypo/hyperglycemia.
Corticosteroids: May increase risk of tendon rupture

Herbal
Dandelion: May decrease trovafloxacin effectiveness.
Fennel seed: May decrease bioavailability of trovafloxacin and result in treatment failure.

Food
None known.

DIAGNOSTIC TEST EFFECTS
May alter blood glucose levels.

SIDE EFFECTS
Occasional
Diarrhea, dizziness, drowsiness, headache, lightheadedness, vaginal pain and discharge

Rare
Confusion, hallucinations, restlessness, seizures, tremors, rapid heartbeat, shortness of breath, abdominal pain, dark urine, fatigue, loss of appetite, nausea, vomiting, jaundice, pain at injection site, stomach cramps, diarrhea, tendon rupture, increased sensitivity of skin to sunlight

SERIOUS REACTIONS
• Pseudomembranous colitis as evidenced by severe abdominal pain and cramps, and severe watery diarrhea, and fever, may occur.
• Superinfection manifested as genital or anal pruritus, ulceration or changes in oral mucosa, and moderate to severe diarrhea, may occur.
• Hypersensitivity reactions, including photosensitivity as evidenced by rash, pruritus, blistering, swelling, and the sensation of the skin burning have occurred in patients receiving fluoroquinolone therapy.

PRECAUTIONS & CONSIDERATIONS
Caution is warranted with mild to moderate cirrhosis, exposure to

sunlight, symptomatic pancreatitis, glucose 6-phosphate dehydrogenase deficiency, and suspected central nervous system (CNS) disorders. Be aware that trovafloxacin has been associated with serious liver injury. Use exceeding 2 weeks is associated with a greater risk of injury. Obtain history of hypersensitivity to trovafloxacin and quinolones before beginning drug therapy as well as baseline liver function tests. Trovafloxacin is excreted in breast milk, and rovafloxacin use should be avoided during pregnancy. The safety and efficacy of trovafloxacin have not been established in children younger than 18 years of age. There are no age-related precautions noted in the elderly.

Be alert for superinfection such as genital/anal pruritus, ulceration or changes in oral mucosa, moderate to severe diarrhea, and new or increased fever. Avoid excessive sunlight/artificial ultraviolet light (reaction may occur up to several weeks after stopping therapy). Do not take antacids (aluminum, magnesium), sucralfate, iron, and multivitamin preparations with zinc within 2 hours of trovafloxacin administration as these drugs significantly reduce trovafloxacin absorption. Avoid tasks that require mental alertness or motor skills until response to the drug is established. Notify physician if chest pain, difficulty breathing, palpitations, persistent diarrhea, swelling, or tendon pain occurs.

Storage
Store tablets and vials at room temperature. After diluted, solution is stable for 7 days when refrigerated or up to 3 days at room temperature.

Administration
Be aware that initial therapy with trovafloxacin should be started in an

inpatient setting. Therapy should not exceed 14 days.

Take oral trovafloxacin without regard to food.

For IV use, trovafloxacin should not be diluted with 0.9% NaCl or Lactated Ringers.

A solution equivalent to a final concentration of 1 to 2 mg/ml should be prepared with 5% Dextrose, 0.45% NaCl, 5% Dextrose and 0.45% NaCl, 0.45% NaCl, 5% Dextrose and 0.3% NaCl, or Lactated Ringer's and 5% Dextrose. Administer as an infusion over 60 minutes. Do not administer rapidly or as an undiluted bolus.

T

Undecylenic Acid

un-de-sye-len'ik
(Caldesene Medicated Powder, Cruex Antifungal Cream, Cruex Antifungal Powder, Cruex Antifungal Spray Powder, Decylenes Powder, Desenex Antifungal Cream, Desenex Antifungal Liquid, Desenex Antifungal Ointment, Desenex Antifungal Penetrating Foam, Desenex Antifungal Powder, Desenex Antifungal Spray Powder, Godochom Solution)

CATEGORY AND SCHEDULE

Pregnancy Risk Category: NR
OTC

CLASSIFICATION

Antifungals, topical, dermatologics

MECHANISM OF ACTION

An antifungal whose mechanism of action is not well understood. *Therapeutic Effect:* Fungistatic.

AVAILABILITY

Aerosol powder: 10% (Cruex Antifungal Spray Powder, Desenex Antifungal Spray Powder).
Aerosol foam: 10% (Desenex Antifungal Penetrating Foam).
Cream: 20% (Cruex Antifungal Cream, Desenex Antifungal Cream).
Solution, topical: 10% (Desenex Antifungal Liquid), 25% (Gordochom Solution).
Ointment: 20% (Desenex Antifungal Ointment).
Powder: 10% (Caldesene Medicated Powder, Cruex Antifungal Powder, Decylenes Powder), 19% (Desenex Antifungal Powder).

INDICATIONS AND DOSAGES

▸ Tinea pedis, tinea corporis
TOPICAL
Adults, Children 2 yr and older.
Apply 2 times/day to affected area for 4 wk.

CONTRAINDICATIONS

Hypersensitivity to undecylenic acid or any component of its formulation

INTERACTIONS

Drug
None known.
Herbal
None known.
Food
None known.

DIAGNOSTIC TEST EFFECTS

None known.

SIDE EFFECTS

Occasional
Skin irritation, rash

SERIOUS REACTIONS

• Hypersensitivity reactions characterized by rash, facial swelling, pruritus, and a sensation of warmth occur.

PRECAUTIONS & CONSIDERATIONS

Caution should be used in children younger than 2 years old and with diabetes mellitus. There are no precautions noted in pregnant women. Safety and efficacy of undecylenic acid has not been established in children younger than 2 years. There are no age-related precautions noted in the elderly. Skin should be kept clean and dry. Light clothing should be worn to promote ventilation. Affected area should not be covered with occlusive dressing. The physician should be notified if skin irritation occurs.

Administration
Topical therapy should not be used on scalp or nails. Apply and rub gently into the affected and surrounding area.

Ursodiol
your-soo'dee-ol
(Actigall, Urso)

CATEGORY AND SCHEDULE
Pregnancy Risk Category: B

CLASSIFICATION
Gallstone solubilizers

MECHANISM OF ACTION
A gallstone solubilizing agent that suppresses hepatic synthesis and secretion of cholesterol; inhibits intestinal absorption of cholesterol. *Therapeutic Effect:* Changes the bile of patients with gallstones from precipitating (capable of forming crystals) to cholesterol solubilizing (capable of being dissolved).

AVAILABILITY
Capsules: 300 mg.
Tablets: 250 mg.

INDICATIONS AND DOSAGES
▶ **Dissolution of radiolucent, noncalcified gallstones when cholecystectomy is not recommended; treatment of biliary cirrhosis**
PO
Adults, Elderly. 8-10 mg/kg/day in 2-3 divided doses. Treatment may require months. Obtain ultrasound image of gallbladder at 6-mo intervals for first year. If gallstones have dissolved, continue therapy and repeat ultrasound within 1-3 mo.

▶ **Prevention of gallstones**
PO
Adults, Elderly. 300 mg twice a day.

OFF-LABEL USES
Treatment of alcoholic cirrhosis, biliary atresia, chronic hepatitis, gallstone formation, sclerosing cholangitis, prophylaxis of liver transplant rejection

CONTRAINDICATIONS
Allergy to bile acids, calcified cholesterol stones, chronic hepatic disease, radiolucent bile pigment stones, radiopaque stones

INTERACTIONS
Drug
Aluminum-containing antacids, cholestyramine: May decrease the absorption and effects of ursodiol.
Estrogens, oral contraceptives: May decrease the effects of ursodiol.
Herbal
None known.
Food
None known.

DIAGNOSTIC TEST EFFECTS
May alter liver function test results.

SIDE EFFECTS
Occasional
Diarrhea

SERIOUS REACTIONS
• None significant.

U

PRECAUTIONS & CONSIDERATIONS
It is unknown if tegaserod is distributed in breast milk. Safety and efficacy of tegaserod have not been established in children. No age-related precautions have been noted in the elderly.
  Blood serum chemistry values, including BUN, serum alkaline

phosphatase, bilirubin, creatinine, AST (SGOT), and ALT (SGPT) levels, should be obtained before the start of ursodiol therapy, 1 and 3 months after therapy begins, and every 6 months thereafter, to assess hepatic function.

Administration

Take with meals or a snack because the drug dissolves more readily in the presence of bile acid and pancreatic juice. Ursodiol therapy requires months. Avoid taking antacids within hours of taking ursodiol

Valacyclovir
val-a-sye´kloe-ver
(Valtrex)

CATEGORY AND SCHEDULE
Pregnancy Risk Category: B

CLASSIFICATION
Antivirals

MECHANISM OF ACTION
A virustatic antiviral that is converted to acyclovir triphosphate, becoming part of the viral DNA chain. *Therapeutic Effect:* Interferes with DNA synthesis and replication of herpes simplex virus and varicella- zoster virus.

PHARMACOKINETICS
Rapidly absorbed after PO administration. Protein binding: 13%-18%. Rapidly converted by hydrolysis to the active compound acyclovir. Widely distributed to tissues and body fluids (including CSF). Primarily eliminated in urine. Removed by hemodialysis. **Half-life:** 2.5-3.3 hr (increased in impaired renal function).

AVAILABILITY
Caplets: 500 mg, 1000 mg.

INDICATIONS AND DOSAGES
▸ **Herpes zoster (shingles)**
PO
Adults, Elderly. 1 g 3 times a day for 7 days.
▸ **Herpes simplex (cold sores)**
PO
Adults, Elderly. 2 g twice a day for 1 day.

▸ **Initial episode of genital herpes**
PO
Adults, Elderly. 1 g twice a day for 10 days.
▸ **Recurrent episodes of genital herpes**
PO
Adults, Elderly. 500 mg twice a day for 3 days.
▸ **Prevention of genital herpes**
PO
Adults, Elderly. 500-1000 mg/day.
▸ **Dosage in renal impairment**
Dosage and frequency are modified based on creatinine clearance.

Creatinine Clearance	Herpes Zoster	Genital Herpes
50 ml/min or higher	1 g q8hr	500 mg q12hr
30-49 ml/min	1 g q12hr	500 mg q12hr
10-29 ml/min	1 g q24hr	500 mg q24hr
Less than 10 ml/min	500 mg q24hr	500 mg q24hr

OFF-LABEL USES
To reduce the risk of heterosexual transmission of genital herpes

CONTRAINDICATIONS
Hypersensitivity to or intolerance of acyclovir, valacyclovir, or their components

INTERACTIONS
Drug
Cimetidine, probenecid: May increase acyclovir blood concentration.
Herbal
None known.
Food
None known.

DIAGNOSTIC TEST EFFECTS
None known.

V

SIDE EFFECTS
Frequent
Herpes zoster (17%-10%): Nausea, headache
Genital herpes (17%): Headache
Occasional
Herpes zoster (7%-3%): Vomiting, diarrhea, constipation (50 yr or older), asthenia, dizziness (50 yr and older)
Genital herpes (8%-3%): Nausea, diarrhea, dizziness
Rare
Herpes zoster (3%-1%): Abdominal pain, anorexia
Genital herpes (3%-1%): Asthenia, abdominal pain

SERIOUS REACTIONS
• None known.

PRECAUTIONS & CONSIDERATIONS
Caution is warranted with advanced HIV infection, bone marrow or renal transplantation, concurrent use of nephrotoxic agents, dehydration, fluid or electrolyte imbalance, neurologic abnormalities, and renal or liver impairment. Be aware that valacyclovir may cross the placenta and be distributed in breast milk. The safety and efficacy of this drug have not been established in children. In the elderly, age-related renal impairment may require dosage adjustment. Do not touch lesions with fingers to avoid spreading infection to new sites. Avoid sexual intercourse during the duration of lesions to prevent infecting partner.

Tissue cultures should be obtained from those with herpes simplex and herpes zoster before giving the first dose of valacyclovir. Therapy may proceed before test results are known. Complete blood count (CBC), liver or renal function tests, and urinalysis should be monitored. Maintain adequate fluids. Fingernails should be kept short and hands clean. Pap smears should be done at least annually due to increased risk of cervical cancer in women with genital herpes.

Administration
❗ Be aware that therapy should be initiated at the first sign of shingles and that valacyclovir is most effective within 48 hours of the onset of zoster rash.

Give oral valacyclovir without regard to meals. Do not crush or break tablets. Continue therapy for the full length of treatment and evenly space doses around the clock.

Valdecoxib
val-de-cocks′ib
(Bextra)

CATEGORY AND SCHEDULE
Pregnancy Risk Category: B
(D if used in third trimester or near delivery)

CLASSIFICATION
Analgesics, non-narcotic, COX-2 inhibitors, nonsteroidal anti-inflammatory drugs

MECHANISM OF ACTION
An NSAID that inhibits cyclo-oxygenase-2, the enzyme responsible for producing prostaglandins, which cause pain and inflammation. *Therapeutic Effect:* Reduces inflammatory response and intensity of pain.

PHARMACOKINETICS
Rapidly and almost completely absorbed from the GI tract. Widely distributed. Extensively metabolized in the liver. Primarily eliminated in urine. **Half-life:** 8-11 hr.

AVAILABILITY
Tablets: 10 mg, 20 mg.

INDICATIONS AND DOSAGES
▶ **Osteoarthritis, rheumatoid arthritis**
PO
Adults, Elderly. 10 mg once a day.
▶ **Primary dysmenorrhea**
PO
Adults, Elderly. 20 mg twice a day.

CONTRAINDICATIONS
Hypersensitivity to aspirin or
NSAIDs, severe hepatic or renal
impairment

INTERACTIONS
Drug
Anticoagulants: May increase the
effects of anticoagulants.
Aspirin, other salicylates: May
increase the risk of GI side effects
such as bleeding.
Dextromethorphan: May increase
the plasma level of dextromethorphan.
Fluconazole, ketoconazole: May
increase the plasma concentration of
valdecoxib.
Herbal
None known.
Food
None known.

DIAGNOSTIC TEST EFFECTS
May increase BUN and serum creatinine levels and liver function test
results.

SIDE EFFECTS
Frequent (8%-4%)
Headache
Occasional (3%-2%)
Dizziness
Rare (less than 2%)
Dyspepsia, nausea, diarrhea, sinusitis,
peripheral edema

SERIOUS REACTIONS
• None known.

PRECAUTIONS & CONSIDERATIONS
Be aware that there is an increased
cardiovascular risk and an increased
rate of a rare, serious skin reaction.
Caution is warranted with smokers,
alcoholism, moderate hepatic impairment, concurrent use of anticoagulants or steroids, and the elderly.
Valdecoxib is excreted in breast
milk. Valdecoxib should not be used
during the third trimester of pregnancy because it may cause adverse
effects in the fetus, such as premature
closure of the ductus arteriosus. The
safety and efficacy of valdecoxib
have not been established in children
younger than 18 years. The elderly
are more likely to experience adverse
reactions than those who are younger.
Avoid alcohol and aspirin during
therapy because these substances
increase the risk of GI bleeding. Tasks
that require mental alertness or
motor skills should also be avoided.
  BUN, serum creatinine levels, and
liver function test results should be
assessed during therapy. Therapeutic
response, such as decreased pain,
stiffness, swelling, and tenderness,
improved grip strength, and increased
joint mobility, should be evaluated.
Administration
Do not crush or break film-coated
tablets. Take valdecoxib without
regard to food.

V

Valganciclovir

val-gan-sye′kloh-veer
(Valcyte)

CATEGORY AND SCHEDULE
Pregnancy Risk Category: C

CLASSIFICATION
Antivirals

MECHANISM OF ACTION
A synthetic nucleoside that competes with viral DNA esterases and is incorporated directly into growing viral DNA chains. *Therapeutic Effect:* Interferes with DNA synthesis and viral replication.

PHARMACOKINETICS
Well absorbed and rapidly converted to ganciclovir by intestinal and hepatic enzymes. Widely distributed. Slowly metabolized intracellularly. Primarily excreted unchanged in urine. Removed by hemodialysis. **Half-life:** 18 hr (increased in impaired renal function).

AVAILABILITY
Tablets: 450 mg.

INDICATIONS AND DOSAGES
▶ **Cytomegalovirus (CMV) retinitis in patients with normal renal function**
PO
Adults. Initially, 900 mg (two 450-mg tablets) twice a day for 21 days. Maintenance: 900 mg once a day.
▶ **Prevention of CMV after transplant**
PO
Adults, Elderly. 900 mg once a day beginning within 10 days of transplant and continuing until 100 days post-transplant.

▶ **Dosage in renal impairment**
Dosage and frequency are modified based on creatinine clearance.

Creatinine Clearance	Induction Dosage	Maintenance Dosage
60 ml/min or more	900 mg twice/day	900 mg once/day
40-59 ml/min	450 mg twice/day	450 mg once/day
25-39 ml/min	450 mg once/day	450 mg q2 days
10-24 ml/min	450 mg q2 days	450 mg twice/week

CONTRAINDICATIONS
Hypersensitivity to acyclovir or ganciclovir

INTERACTIONS
Drug
Amphotericin B, cyclosporine: May increase the risk of nephrotoxicity.
Bone marrow depressants: May increase bone marrow depression.
Imipenem and cilastatin: May increase the risk of seizures.
Probenecid: Decreases renal clearance of valganciclovir.
Zidovudine (AZT): May increase the risk of hematologic toxicity.
Herbal
None known.
Food
All foods: Maximize drug bioavailability.

DIAGNOSTIC TEST EFFECTS
May decrease blood Hct and Hgb levels, serum creatinine level, platelet count, and WBC count

SIDE EFFECTS
Frequent (16%-9%)
Diarrhea, neutropenia, headache
Occasional (8%-3%)
Nausea, anemia, thrombocytopenia

Rare (less than 3%)
Insomnia, paraesthesia, vomiting, abdominal pain, fever

SERIOUS REACTIONS
• Hematologic toxicity, including severe neutropenia (most common), anemia, and thrombocytopenia, may occur.
• Retinal detachment occurs rarely.
• An overdose may result in renal toxicity.
• Valganciclovir may decrease sperm production and fertility.

PRECAUTIONS & CONSIDERATIONS
Extreme caution should be used in children because of long-term carcinogenicity and risk of reproductive toxicity. Caution should also be used with history of cytopenic reactions to other drugs, preexisting cytopenias, and renal impairment and in the elderly who are at a greater risk of renal impairment. Valganciclovir should not be used during pregnancy because of the drug's mutagenic potential. Effective contraception should be used during therapy because of the drug's mutagenic potential. Female patients taking valganciclovir should avoid breast-feeding. Breast-feeding may be resumed no sooner than 72 hours after the last dose of valganciclovir. Be aware that the safety and efficacy of this drug have not been established in children younger than 12 years of age. In the elderly, age-related renal impairment may require dosage adjustment.
Blood chemistry, hematologic baselines, and serum creatinine levels should be evaluated. Intake and output should be monitored, and ensure that the patient maintains adequate hydration (minimum 1500 ml/24 hours). Ophthalmologic exams should

be obtained every 4 to 6 weeks during treatment. Valganciclovir may temporarily or permanently inhibit sperm production in males; valganciclovir may temporarily or permanently suppress fertility in females.
Administration
Do not break or crush tablets (potentially carcinogenic). Avoid contact with skin. Wash skin with soap and water if contact occurs. Give valganciclovir with food.

Valproic Acid/ Valproate Sodium/ Divalproex Sodium
(Depakene) (Deopacon) (Depakote, Depakote ER, Depakote Sprinkle)

CATEGORY AND SCHEDULE
Pregnancy Risk Category: D

CLASSIFICATION
Anticonvulsants

MECHANISM OF ACTION
An anticonvulsant, antimanic, and antimigraine agent that directly increases concentration of the inhibitory neurotransmitter gamma-aminobutyric acid. *Therapeutic Effect:* Reduces seizure activity.

PHARMACOKINETICS
Well absorbed from the GI tract. Protein binding: 80%-90%. Metabolized in the liver. Primarily excreted in urine. Not removed by hemodialysis. **Half-life:** 6-16 hr (may be increased in hepatic impairment, the elderly, and children younger than 18 mo).

V

AVAILABILITY
Capsules (Depakene): 250 mg.
Syrup (Depakene): 250 mg/5 ml.
Tablets (Delayed-Release [Depakote]): 125 mg, 250 mg, 500 mg.
Tablets (Extended-Release [Depakote ER]): 500 mg.
Capsules Sprinkles (Depakote Sprinkle): 125 mg.
Injection (Depacon): 100 mg/ml.

INDICATIONS AND DOSAGES
▶ **Seizures**
PO
Adults, Elderly, Children 10 yr and older. Initially, 10-15 mg/kg/day in 1-3 divided doses. May increase by 5-10 mg/kg/day at weekly intervals up to 30-60 mg/kg/day. Usual adult dosage: 1000-2500 mg/day.
IV
Adults, Elderly, Children. Same as oral dose but given q6hr.
▶ **Manic episodes**
PO
Adults, Elderly. Initially, 750 mg/day in divided doses. Maximum: 60 mg/kg/day.
▶ **Prevention of migraine headaches**
PO (EXTENDED-RELEASE TABLETS)
Adults, Elderly. Initially, 500 mg/day for 7 days. May increase up to 1000 mg/day.
PO (DELAYED-RELEASE TABLETS)
Adults, Elderly. Initially, 250 mg twice a day. May increase up to 1000 mg/day.

OFF-LABEL USES
Treatment of myoclonic, simple partial, and tonic-clonic seizures

CONTRAINDICATIONS
Active hepatic disease

INTERACTIONS
Drug
Alcohol, other CNS depressants: May increase CNS depressant effects.
Amitriptyline, primidone: May increase the blood concentration of these drugs.
Anticoagulants, heparin, platelet aggregation inhibitors, thrombolytics: May increase the risk of bleeding.
Carbamazepine: May decrease valproic acid blood concentration.
Hepatotoxic medications: May increase the risk of hepatotoxicity.
Phenytoin: May increase the risk of phenytoin toxicity and decrease the effects of valproic acid.
Herbal
None known.
Food
None known.

DIAGNOSTIC TEST EFFECTS
May increase serum LDH, bilirubin, AST (SGOT), and ALT (SGPT) levels. Therapeutic serum level is 50-100 mcg/ml; toxic serum level is greater than 100 mcg/ml.

▓ IV INCOMPATIBILITIES
Do not mix valproic acid with any other medications.

SIDE EFFECTS
Frequent
Epilepsy: Abdominal pain, irregular menses, diarrhea, transient alopecia, indigestion, nausea, vomiting, tremors, weight gain or loss
Mania (22%-19%): Nausea, somnolence
Occasional
Epilepsy: Constipation, dizziness, drowsiness, headache, skin rash, unusual excitement, restlessness
Mania (12%-6%): Asthenia, abdominal pain, dyspepsia (heartburn, indigestion, epigastric distress), rash

Rare

Epilepsy: Mood changes, diplopia, nystagmus, spots before eyes, unusual bleeding or ecchymosis

SERIOUS REACTIONS

- Hepatotoxicity may occur, particularly in the first 6 months of valproic acid therapy. It may be preceded by loss of seizure control, malaise, weakness, lethargy, anorexia, and vomiting rather than abnormal serum liver function test results.
- Blood dyscrasias may occur.

PRECAUTIONS & CONSIDERATIONS

Caution is warranted with bleeding abnormalities and a history of hepatic disease. Valproic acid crosses the placenta and is distributed in breast milk. Children younger than 2 years are at increased risk for hepatotoxicity. Lower dosages are recommended for the elderly, although no age-related precautions have been noted for this age-group.

Drowsiness and dizziness may occur, so alcohol and tasks requiring mental alertness or motor skills should be avoided. Notify the physician of abdominal pain, altered mental status, bleeding, easy bruising, lethargy, loss of appetite, nausea, vomiting, weakness, or yellowing of skin. Seizure disorder, including the onset, duration, frequency, intensity, and type of seizures, should be assessed before and during treatment. CBC and serum alkaline phosphatase, ammonia, bilirubin, AST (SGOT), and ALT (SGPT) levels should also be monitored. CBC and platelet count should be obtained before beginning valproic acid therapy, 2 weeks later, and again 2 weeks after the maintenance dose has been established.

Storage

Store vials at room temperature. Diluted solutions are stable for 24 hours; discard unused portion.

Administration

! Regular-release and delayed-release formulations are given in 2-4 divided doses daily; extended-release formulations are given once a day.

Take oral valproic acid without regard to food. Don't take it with carbonated drinks. Capsule contents may be sprinkled on applesauce and given immediately; however, don't break, chew, or crush the sprinkle beads. Give delayed-release or extended-release tablets whole. Do not abruptly discontinue valproic acid after long-term use because this may precipitate seizure. Strict maintenance of drug therapy is essential for seizure control.

For IV use, dilute each single dose with at least 50 ml D_5W, 0.9% NaCl, or Lactated Ringer's solution. Infuse over 5-10 minutes. Don't exceed an infusion rate of 3 mg/kg/minute (5-minute infusion) or 1.5 mg/kg/minute (10-minute infusion). Too-rapid infusion increases the likelihood of side effects. Be aware that the therapeutic serum drug level is 50-100 mcg/ml, and the toxic serum level is greater than 100 mcg/ml.

V

Valsartan
val-sar′tan
(Diovan)
Do not confuse with Valstan.

CATEGORY AND SCHEDULE
Pregnancy Risk Category: C
(D if used in second or third trimester)

CLASSIFICATION
Angiotensin II receptor antagonists

MECHANISM OF ACTION
An angiotensin II receptor, type AT_1, antagonist that blocks vasoconstrictor and aldosterone-secreting effects of angiotensin II, inhibiting the binding of angiotensin II to the AT_1 receptors. *Therapeutic Effect:* Causes vasodilation, decreases peripheral resistance, and decreases B/P.

PHARMACOKINETICS
Poorly absorbed after PO administration. Food decreases peak plasma concentration. Protein binding: 95%. Metabolized in the liver. Recovered primarily in feces and, to a lesser extent, in urine. Unknown if removed by hemodialysis. **Half-life:** 6 hr.

AVAILABILITY
Tablets: 40 mg, 80 mg, 160 mg, 320 mg.

INDICATIONS AND DOSAGES
▸ **Hypertension**
PO
Adults, Elderly. Initially, 80-160 mg/day in patients who are not volume depleted. May increase up to a Maximum: 320 mg/day.

▸ **CHF**
PO
Adults, Elderly. Initially, 40 mg twice a day. May increase up to 160 mg twice a day. Maximum: 320 mg/day.

CONTRAINDICATIONS
Bilateral renal artery stenosis, biliary cirrhosis or obstruction, hypoaldosteronism, severe hepatic impairment

INTERACTIONS
Drug
Diuretics: Produces additive hypotensive effects.
Herbal
None known.
Food
Decreases peak plasma concentration of valsartan.

DIAGNOSTIC TEST EFFECTS
May increase AST (SGOT), ALT (SGPT), and serum bilirubin, creatinine, and potassium levels. May decrease blood Hgb and Hct levels.

SIDE EFFECTS
Rare (2%-1%)
Insomnia, fatigue, heartburn, abdominal pain, dizziness, headache, diarrhea, nausea, vomiting, arthralgia, edema

SERIOUS REACTIONS
• Overdosage may manifest as hypotension and tachycardia. Bradycardia occurs less often.
• Viral infection and upper respiratory tract infection (cough, pharyngitis, sinusitis, rhinitis) occur rarely.

PRECAUTIONS & CONSIDERATIONS
Caution is warranted with coronary artery disease, mild to moderate hepatic impairment, unilateral renal artery stenosis, and those receiving potassium-sparing diuretics or potassium supplements. For those with

severe CHF, signs and symptoms of impaired renal function, which may develop during valsartan therapy, should be monitored. It is unknown if valsartan is distributed in breast milk; it may cause fetal harm. Females should avoid valsartan during the second and third trimester. Safety and efficacy of valsartan have not been established in children. No age-related precautions have been noted in the elderly.

Dizziness may occur. Tasks that require mental alertness or motor skills should be avoided. Notify the physician if fever or sore throat occurs. Apical pulse and B/P should be assessed immediately before each olmesartan dose, and regularly throughout therapy. Be alert to fluctuations in apical pulse and B/P. If an excessive reduction in B/P occurs, place the person in the supine position with feet slightly elevated and notify the physician. Serum electrolyte levels, liver and renal function tests, urinalysis, and pulse rate should be assessed. Maintain adequate hydration; exercising outside during hot weather should be avoided in order to decrease the risk of dehydration and hypotension.

Administration
! Valsartan may be given concurrently with other antihypertensives. If B/P is not controlled by valsartan alone, expect to administer a diuretic, as prescribed.

Take valsartan without regard to meals.

Vancomycin
van-koe-mye′sin
(Vancocin, Vancocin CP [AUS], Vancocin HCL Pulvules [AUS])

CATEGORY AND SCHEDULE
Pregnancy Risk Category: B

CLASSIFICATION
Antibiotics, glycopeptides

MECHANISM OF ACTION
A tricyclic glycopeptide antibiotic that binds to bacterial cell walls, altering cell membrane permeability and inhibiting RNA synthesis. *Therapeutic Effect:* Bactericidal.

PHARMACOKINETICS
PO: Poorly absorbed from the GI tract. Primarily eliminated in feces. Parenteral: Widely distributed. Protein binding: 55%. Primarily excreted unchanged in urine. Not removed by hemodialysis. **Half-life:** 4-11 hr (increased in impaired renal function).

AVAILABILITY
Capsules: 125 mg, 250 mg.
Powder for Oral Suspension (Vancocin): 1 g (provides 250 mg/5 ml after mixing).
Powder for Injection: 500 mg, 1 g.
Infusion (Premix): 500 mg/100 ml, 1 g/200 ml.

INDICATIONS AND DOSAGES
▸ **Treatment of bone, respiratory tract, skin and soft-tissue infections, endocarditis, peritonitis, and septicemia; prevention of bacterial endocarditis in those at risk (if penicillin is contraindicated) when undergoing biliary, dental, GI, GU, or**

respiratory surgery or invasive procedures
IV
Adults, Elderly. 500 mg q6hr or 1 g q12hr.
Children older than 1 mo.
40 mg/kg/day in divided doses q6-8hr.
Maximum: 3-4 g/day.
Neonates. Initially, 15 mg/kg, then 10 mg/kg q8-12hr.
▸ **Staphylococcal enterocolitis, antibiotic-associated pseudomembranous colitis caused by** *Clostridium difficile*
PO
Adults, Elderly. 0.5-2 g/day in 3-4 divided doses for 7-10 days.
Children. 40 mg/kg/day in 3-4 divided doses for 7-10 days.
Maximum: 2 g/day.
Dosage in renal impairment
After a loading dose, subsequent dosages and frequency are modified based on creatinine clearance, the severity of the infection, and the serum concentration of the drug.

OFF-LABEL USES
Treatment of brain abscess, perioperative infections, staphylococcal or streptococcal meningitis

CONTRAINDICATIONS
None known.

INTERACTIONS
Drug
Aminoglycosides, amphotericin B, aspirin, bumetanide, carmustine, cisplatin, cyclosporine, ethacrynic acid, furosemide, streptozocin:
May increase the risk of ototoxicity and nephrotoxicity of parenteral vancomycin.
Cholestyramine, colestipol: May decrease the effects of oral vancomycin.
Herbal
None known.

Food
None known.

DIAGNOSTIC TEST EFFECTS
May increase BUN level.
Therapeutic peak serum level is 20-40 mcg/ml; therapeutic trough serum level is 5-15 mcg/ml. Toxic peak serum level is greater than 40 mcg/ml; toxic trough serum level is greater than 15 mcg/ml.

🦠 IV INCOMPATIBILITIES
Albumin, amphotericin B complex (Abelcet, AmBisome, Amphotec), aztreonam (Azactam), cefazolin (Ancef), cefepime (Maxipime), cefotaxime (Claforan), cefotetan (Cefotan), cefoxitin (Mefoxin), ceftazidime (Fortaz), ceftriaxone (Rocephin), cefuroxime (Zinacef), foscarnet (Foscavir), heparin, idarubicin (Idamycin), nafcillin (Nafcil), piperacillin and tazobactam (Zosyn), ticarcillin and clavulanate (Timentin)
💧 IV Compatibilities
Amiodarone (Cordarone), calcium gluconate, diltiazem (Cardizem), hydromorphone (Dilaudid), insulin, lorazepam (Ativan), magnesium sulfate, midazolam (Versed), morphine, potassium chloride, propofol (Diprivan)

SIDE EFFECTS
Frequent
PO: Bitter or unpleasant taste, nausea, vomiting, mouth irritation (with oral solution)
Rare
Parenteral: Phlebitis, thrombophlebitis, or pain at peripheral IV site; dizziness; vertigo; tinnitus; chills; fever; rash; necrosis with extravasation
PO: Rash.

SERIOUS REACTIONS
• Nephrotoxicity and ototoxicity may occur.

- 'Red-neck' syndrome (redness on face, neck, arms, and back; chills; fever; tachycardia; nausea or vomiting; pruritus; rash; unpleasant taste) may result from too-rapid injection.

PRECAUTIONS & CONSIDERATIONS

Caution is warranted with pre-existing hearing impairment or renal dysfunction and in those taking other ototoxic or nephrotoxic medications concurrently. Vancomycin crosses the placenta; it is unknown if it's distributed in breast milk. Close monitoring of serum drug levels is recommended in premature neonates and young infants. Age-related renal impairment may increase the risk of ototoxicity and nephrotoxicity in the elderly. Dosage adjustment is recommended.

Notify the physician if rash, tinnitus, or signs and symptoms of nephrotoxicity occur. Laboratory tests are an important part of therapy. Know that the vancomycin therapeutic peak serum level is 20 to 40 mcg/ml, and the trough level is 5 to 15 mcg/ml. The toxic peak serum level is greater than 40 mcg/ml, and the trough level is greater than 15 mcg/ml. Skin for rash, intake and output, renal function, balance and hearing acuity, and the IV site should be assessed during vancomycin therapy.

Storage

The refrigerated oral solution is stable for 2 weeks. After reconstitution, the IV solution may be refrigerated and should be used within 14 days.

Administration

Be aware that vancomycin is usually not given for systemic infections because it's poorly absorbed from the GI tract; however, some patients with colitis may absorb the drug effectively. Reconstitute powder for oral solution as appropriate and administer it orally or by NG tube.

Don't use powder for oral solution for IV administration.

! Give vancomycin by intermittent IV infusion (piggyback) or continuous IV infusion. Don't give by IV push because this may result in exaggerated hypotension. For intermittent IV infusion (piggyback), reconstitute each 500-mg or 1-g vial with 10 ml or 20 ml, respectively, of sterile water for injection to provide a concentration of 50 mg/ml. Further dilute to a final concentration of no more than 5 mg/ml. Discard the solution if a precipitate forms. Administer the solution over 60 minutes or more. Monitor the patient's B/P closely during the infusion. ADD-Vantage vials should not be used in neonates, infants, and children requiring less than a 500-mg dose.

Vardenafil

(Levitra)
Do not confuse Levitra with Lexiva.

CATEGORY AND SCHEDULE

Pregnancy Risk Category: not applicable

CLASSIFICATION

Impotence agents, phosphodiesterase inhibitors

MECHANISM OF ACTION

An erectile dysfunction agent that inhibits phosphodiesterase type 5, the enzyme responsible for degrading cyclic guanosine monophosphate in the corpus cavernosum of the penis, resulting in smooth muscle relaxation and increased blood flow. *Therapeutic Effect:* Facilitates an erection.

V

PHARMACOKINETICS

Rapidly absorbed after PO administration. Extensive tissue distribution. Protein binding: 95%. Metabolized in the liver. Excreted primarily in feces; a lesser amount eliminated in urine. Drug has no effect on penile blood flow without sexual stimulation. **Half-life:** 4-5 hr.

AVAILABILITY

Tablets: 2.5 mg, 5 mg, 10 mg, 20 mg.

INDICATIONS AND DOSAGES

▶ **Erectile dysfunction**
PO
Adults. 10 mg approximately 1 hr before sexual activity. Dose may be increased to 20 mg or decreased to 5 mg, based on patient tolerance. Maximum dosing frequency is once daily.
Elderly (older than 65 yr). 5 mg.
▶ **Dosage in moderate hepatic impairment**
PO
For patients with Child-Pugh class B hepatic impairment, dosage is 5 mg 60 min before sexual activity.
▶ **Dosage with concurrent ritonavir**
PO
Adults. 2.5 mg in a 72-hr period.
▶ **Dosage with concurrent ketoconazole or itraconazole (at 400 mg/day), or indinavir**
PO
Adults. 2.5 mg in a 24-hour period.
▶ **Dosage with concurrent ketoconazole or itraconazole (at 200 mg/day), or erythromycin**
PO
Adults. 5 mg in a 24-hr period.

CONTRAINDICATIONS

Concurrent use of alpha-adrenergic blockers, sodium nitroprusside, or nitrates in any form

INTERACTIONS

Drug
Alpha-adrenergic blockers, nitrates: Potentiates the hypotensive effects of these drugs.
Erythromycin, indinavir, itraconazole, ketoconazole, ritonavir: May increase vardenafil blood concentration.
Herbal
None known.
Food
High-fat meals: Delay drug's maximum effectiveness.

DIAGNOSTIC TEST EFFECTS

None known.

SIDE EFFECTS

Occasional
Headache, flushing, rhinitis, indigestion
Rare (less than 2%)
Dizziness, changes in color vision, blurred vision

SERIOUS REACTIONS

• Prolonged erections (lasting over 4 hours) and priapism (painful erections lasting over 6 hours) occur rarely.

PRECAUTIONS & CONSIDERATIONS

Caution is warranted with an anatomic deformity of the penis, cardiac, hepatic or renal impairment, and conditions that increase the risk of priapism, including leukemia, multiple myeloma, and sickle cell anemia. No age-related precautions have been noted in the elderly, but their initial dose should be 5 mg. Be aware vardenafil is not effective without sexual stimulation. Avoid using nitrate drugs and alpha-adrenergic blockers concurrently with vardenafil. Seek treatment immediately if an erection lasts longer than 4 hours.

Administration
Take vardenafil approximately
1 hour before sexual activity. Don't
crush or break film-coated tablets.
High-fat meals delay the drug's
maximum effectiveness.

Vasopressin
vay-soe-press'in
(Pitressin, Pressyn [CAN])
**Do not confuse Pitressin with
Pitocin.**

CATEGORY AND SCHEDULE
Pregnancy Risk Category: B

CLASSIFICATION
Antidiuretics, hormones/
hormone modifiers

MECHANISM OF ACTION
A posterior pituitary hormone
that increases reabsorption of water
by the renal tubules. Increases
water permeability at the distal
tubule and collecting duct.
Directly stimulates smooth muscle
in the GI tract. *Therapeutic Effect:*
Causes peristalsis and
vasoconstriction.

PHARMACOKINETICS

Route	Onset	Peak	Duration
IV	N/A	N/A	0.5-1 hr

IM/
  sub-
  cutaneous
	1-2 hr	N/A	2-8 hr

Distributed throughout extracellular
fluid. Metabolized in the liver and
kidney. Primarily excreted in urine.
Half-life: 10-20 min.

AVAILABILITY
Injection: 20 units/ml.

INDICATIONS AND DOSAGES
▸ **Cardiac arrest**
IV
Adults, Elderly. 40 units as a
one-time bolus.
▸ **Diabetes insipidus**
IV INFUSION
Adults, Children. 0.5 mUnits/kg/hr.
May double dose q30min.
Maximum: 10 mUnits/kg/hr.
IM, SUBCUTANEOUS
Adults, Elderly. 5-10 units 2-4 times
a day. Range: 5-60 unit/day.
Children. 2.5-10 units, 2-4 times
a day.
▸ **Abdominal distention, intestinal
paresis**
IM
Adults, Elderly. Initially, 5 units.
Subsequent doses, 10 units q3-4hr.
▸ **GI hemorrhage**
IV INFUSION
Adults, Elderly. Initially,
0.2-0.4 unit/min progressively
increased to 0.9 unit/min.
Children. 0.002-0.005 unit/kg/min.
Titrate as needed. Maximum:
0.01 unit/kg/min.
▸ **Vasodilatory shock**
IV
Adults, Elderly. Initially,
0.04-0.1 unit/min. Titrate to desired
effect.

OFF-LABEL USES
Adjunct in treatment of acute,
massive hemorrhage

CONTRAINDICATIONS
None known.

INTERACTIONS
Drug
**Alcohol, demeclocycline, lithium,
norepinephrine:** May decrease the
effects of vasopressin.

Carbamazepine, chlorpropamide, clofibrate: May increase the effects of vasopressin.
Herbal
None known.
Food
None known.

DIAGNOSTIC TEST EFFECTS
None known.

▦ IV INCOMPATIBILITIES
Amphotericin B complex (Abelcet, AmBisome, Amphotec), diazepam (Valium), etomidate (Amidate), furosemide (Lasix), thiopentothal
▣ IV Compatibilities
Dobutamine (Dobutrex), dopamine (Intropin), heparin, lorazepam (Ativan), midazolam (Versed), milrinone (Primacor), verapamil (Calan, Isoptin).

SIDE EFFECTS
Frequent
Pain at injection site (with vasopressin tannate)
Occasional
Abdominal cramps, nausea, vomiting, diarrhea, dizziness, diaphoresis, pale skin, circumoral pallor, tremors, headache, eructation, flatulence
Rare
Chest pain; confusion; allergic reaction, including rash or hives, pruritus, wheezing or difficulty breathing, facial and peripheral edema; sterile abscess (with vasopressin tannate)

SERIOUS REACTIONS
• Anaphylaxis, MI, and water intoxication have occurred.
• The elderly and very young are at higher risk for water intoxication.

PRECAUTIONS & CONSIDERATIONS
Caution is warranted with arteriosclerosis, asthma, cardiac disease, goiter with cardiac complications, migraine, nephritis, renal disease, seizures, and vascular disease. Vasopressin should be used cautiously in breast-feeding women. Vasopressin should be used cautiously in children and the elderly because of the risk of water intoxication and hyponatremia in these age-groups.

Notify the physician of chest pain, headache, shortness of breath, or other symptoms. B/P, serum electrolyte levels, pulse rate, urine specific gravity, intake and output, and weight should be monitored before and during therapy. Be alert for early signs of water intoxication, such as somnolence, headache, and listlessness.
Storage
Store at room temperature.
Administration
❗ May administer intranasally on cotton pledgets, or by nasal spray; individualize dosage.

For IV use, dilute with D_5W or 0.9% NaCl to concentration of 0.1 to 1 unit/ml. Give as IV infusion.

For IM or subcutaneous, give with 1 to 2 glasses of water to reduce side effects.

Venlafaxine
ven-la-fax′een
(Effexor, Effexor XR)

CATEGORY AND SCHEDULE
Pregnancy Risk Category: C

CLASSIFICATION
Antidepressants, miscellaneous

MECHANISM OF ACTION
A phenethylamine derivative that potentiates CNS neurotransmitter

activity by inhibiting the reuptake of serotonin, norepinephrine and, to a lesser degree, dopamine. *Therapeutic Effect:* Relieves depression.

PHARMACOKINETICS
Well absorbed from the GI tract. Protein binding: 25%-30%. Metabolized in the liver to active metabolite. Primarily excreted in urine. Not removed by hemodialysis. **Half-life:** 3-7 hr; metabolite, 9-13 hr (increased in hepatic or renal impairment).

AVAILABILITY
Capsules (Extended-Release [Effexor XL]): 37.5 mg, 75 mg, 150 mg.
Tablets (Effexor): 25 mg, 37.5 mg, 50 mg, 75 mg, 100 mg.

INDICATIONS AND DOSAGES
▸ **Depression**
PO
Adults, Elderly. Initially, 75 mg/day in 2-3 divided doses with food. May increase by 75 mg/day at intervals of 4 days or longer. Maximum: 375 mg/day in 3 divided doses.
PO (EXTENDED-RELEASE)
Adults, Elderly. 75 mg/day as a single dose with food. May increase by 75 mg/day at intervals of 4 days or longer. Maximum: 225 mg/day.
▸ **Anxiety disorder**
PO (EXTENDED-RELEASE)
Adults. 37.5-225 mg/day.
▸ **Dosage in renal and hepatic impairment**
Expect to decrease venlafaxine dosage by 50% in patients with moderate hepatic impairment, 25% in patients with mild to moderate renal impairment, and 50% in patients on dialysis (withhold dose until completion of dialysis).

OFF-LABEL USES
Prevention of relapses of depression; treatment of attention-deficit hyperactivity disorder, autism, chronic fatigue syndrome, obsessive-compulsive disorder

CONTRAINDICATIONS
Use within 14 days of MAOIs

INTERACTIONS
Drug
MAOIs: May cause neuroleptic malignant syndrome, autonomic instability (including rapid fluctuations of vital signs), extreme agitation, hyperthermia, mental status changes, myoclonus, rigidity, and coma.
Herbal
St. John's wort: May increase the sedative-hypnotic effect of venlafaxine.
Food
None known.

DIAGNOSTIC TEST EFFECTS
May increase BUN level and serum alkaline phosphatase, bilirubin, cholesterol, uric acid, AST (SGOT), and ALT (SGPT) levels. May decrease serum phosphate and sodium levels. May alter blood glucose and serum potassium levels.

SIDE EFFECTS
Frequent (greater than 20%)
Nausea, somnolence, headache, dry mouth
Occasional (20%-10%)
Dizziness, insomnia, constipation, diaphoresis, nervousness, asthenia, ejaculatory disturbance, anorexia
Rare (less than 10%)
Anxiety, blurred vision, diarrhea, vomiting, tremor, abnormal dreams, impotence

V

SERIOUS REACTIONS

* A sustained increase in diastolic B/P of 10-15 mm Hg occurs occasionally.

PRECAUTIONS & CONSIDERATIONS

Caution is warranted with suicidal tendencies and those with abnormal platelet function, CHF, volume depletion, hyperthyroidism, mania, angle-closure glaucoma, hepatic and renal impairment, and seizure disorder. Notify the physician if pregnant or planning to become pregnant. It is unknown if venlafaxine is excreted in breast milk. The safety and efficacy of venlafaxine have not been established in children. No age-related precautions have been noted in the elderly.

Drowsiness, dizziness, and light-headedness may occur, so avoid alcohol and tasks that require mental alertness or motor skills. B/P, pulse rate, and weight should be assessed during therapy.

Administration

! When discontinuing venlafaxine, plan to taper the dosage slowly over 2 weeks. Allow at least 14 days to elapse before switching from an MAOI to venlafaxine and at least 7 days to elapse before switching from venlafaxine to an MAOI.

Take venlafaxine with food or milk if the patient experiences GI distress. Crush scored tablets if needed. Do not break, open, or crush extended-release capsules.

Verapamil

ver-ap′a-mill

(Anpec [AUS], Apo-Verap [CAN], Calan, Calan SR, Chronovera [CAN], Cordilox SR [AUS], Covera-HS, Isoptin SR, Novo-Veramil [CAN], Novo-Veramil SR [CAN], Veracaps SR [AUS], Verahexal [AUS], Verelan, Verelan PM)

Do not confuse Isoptin with Intropin, or Verelan with Virilon, Vivarin, or Voltaren.

CATEGORY AND SCHEDULE

Pregnancy Risk Category: C

CLASSIFICATION

Antiarrhythmics, class IV, calcium channel blockers

MECHANISM OF ACTION

A calcium channel blocker and antianginal, antiarrhythmic, and antihypertensive agent that inhibits calcium ion entry across cardiac and vascular smooth-muscle cell membranes. This action causes the dilation of coronary arteries, peripheral arteries, and arterioles. *Therapeutic Effect:* Decreases heart rate and myocardial contractility and slows SA and AV conduction. Decreases total peripheral vascular resistance by vasodilation.

PHARMACOKINETICS

Route	Onset	Peak	Duration
PO	30 min	1-2 hr	6-8 hr
PO (extended-release)	30 min	N/A	N/A
IV	1-2 min	3-5 min	10-60 min

Well absorbed from the GI tract. Protein binding: 90% (60% in neonates). Undergoes first-pass metabolism in the liver to active metabolite. Primarily excreted in urine. Not removed by hemodialysis. **Half-life:** 2-8 hr.

AVAILABILITY
Caplet (Calan SR): 120 mg, 180 mg, 240 mg.
Capsules (Extended-Release [Verelan PM]): 100 mg, 200 mg, 300 mg.
Capsules (Sustained-Release [Verelan]): 120 mg, 180 mg, 240 mg, 360 mg.
Tablets (Calan): 40 mg, 80 mg, 120 mg.
Tablets (Sustained-Release [Isoptin SR]): 120 mg, 180 mg, 240 mg.
Injection: 2.5 mg/ml.

INDICATIONS AND DOSAGES
▸ **Supraventricular tachyarrhythmias, temporary control of rapid ventricular rate with atrial fibrillation or flutter**
IV
Adults, Elderly. Initially, 5-10 mg; repeat in 30 min with 10-mg dose.
Children 1 to 15 yr. 0.1 mg/kg. May repeat in 30 min up to a maximum second dose of 10 mg. Not recommended in children younger than 1 yr.
▸ **Arrhythmias, including prevention of recurrent paroxysmal supraventricular tachycardia and control of ventricular resting rate in chronic atrial fibrillation or flutter (with digoxin)**
PO
Adults, Elderly. 240-480 mg/day in 3-4 divided doses.
▸ **Vasospastic angina (Prinzmetal's variant), unstable (crescendo or preinfarction) angina, chronic stable (effort-associated) angina**
PO
Adults. Initially, 80-120 mg 3 times a day. For elderly patients and those with hepatic dysfunction, 40 mg 3 times a day. Titrate to optimal dose. Maintenance: 240-480 mg/day in 3-4 divided doses.
PO (COVERA-HS)
Adults, Elderly. 180-480 mg/day at bedtime.
▸ **Hypertension**
PO
Adults, Elderly. Initially, 40-80 mg 3 times a day. Maintenance: 480 mg or less a day.
PO (COVERA-HS)
Adults, Elderly. 180-480 mg/day at bedtime.
PO (EXTENDED-RELEASE)
Adults, Elderly. 120-240 mg/day. May give 480 mg or less a day in 2 divided doses.
PO (VERELAN PM)
Adults, Elderly. 100-300 mg/day.

OFF-LABEL USES
Treatment of hypertrophic cardiomyopathy, vascular headaches

CONTRAINDICATIONS
Atrial fibrillation or flutter and an accessory bypass tract, cardiogenic shock, heart block, sinus bradycardia, ventricular tachycardia

INTERACTIONS
Drug
Beta blockers: May have additive effect.
Carbamazepine, quinidine, theophylline: May increase verapamil blood concentration and risk of toxicity.
Digoxin: May increase digoxin blood concentration.
Disopyramide: May increase negative inotropic effect.

V

Procainamide, quinidine: May increase risk of QT-interval prolongation.
Herbal
None known.
Food
Grapefruit, grapefruit juice: May increase verapamil blood concentration.

DIAGNOSTIC TEST EFFECTS
EKG waveform may show increased PR interval. Therapeutic serum level is 0.08-0.3 mcg/ml.

▨ IV INCOMPATIBILITIES
Amphotericin B complex (Abelcet, AmBisome, Amphotec), nafcillin (Nafcil), propofol (Diprivan), sodium bicarbonate
▨ IV Compatibilities
Amiodarone (Cordarone), calcium chloride, calcium gluconate, dexamethasone (Decadron), digoxin (Lanoxin), dobutamine (Dobutrex), dopamine (Intropin), furosemide (Lasix), heparin, hydromorphone (Dilaudid), lidocaine, magnesium sulfate, metoclopramide (Reglan), milrinone (Primacor), morphine, multivitamins, nitroglycerin, norepinephrine (Levophed), potassium chloride, potassium phosphate, procainamide (Pronestyl), propranolol (Inderal)

SIDE EFFECTS
Frequent (7%)
Constipation
Occasional (4%-2%)
Dizziness, light-headedness, headache, asthenia (loss of strength, energy), nausea, peripheral edema, hypotension
Rare (less than 1%)
Bradycardia, dermatitis or rash

SERIOUS REACTIONS
• Rapid ventricular rate in atrial flutter or fibrillation, marked hypotension, extreme bradycardia, CHF, asystole, and second- and third-degree AV block occur rarely.

PRECAUTIONS & CONSIDERATIONS
Caution is warranted with CHF, hepatic or renal impairment, sick sinus syndrome and in those concurrently receiving beta blockers or digoxin. Verapamil crosses the placenta and is distributed in breast milk. Breast-feeding is not recommended for patients taking this drug. No age-related precautions have been noted in children. In the elderly, age-related renal impairment may require cautious use. Grapefruit juice, which may increase verapamil blood concentration, should be avoided. Alcohol and tasks that require alertness and motor skills should also be avoided.

Be aware that EKG should be monitored for changes, particularly PR-interval prolongation. Notify the physician of significant PR-interval or other EKG changes. B/P, pulse, and stool consistency and frequency should be assessed. The onset, type (sharp, dull, or squeezing), radiation, location, intensity, and duration of anginal pain and its precipitating factors, such as exertion and emotional stress should be recorded. Be aware that concurrent administration of sublingual nitroglycerin therapy may be used for relief of anginal pain.
Storage
Store at room temperature.
Administration
Take tablets that are not sustained-release with or without food. Sustained-release form should be given on an empty stomach. Swallow extended-release or

sustained-released preparations whole and without chewing or crushing. If needed, open sustained-release capsules and sprinkle contents on applesauce. Swallow the applesauce immediately, without chewing. Do not abruptly discontinue verapamil. Compliance is essential to control anginal pain.

For IV use, give undiluted, if desired. Administer IV push over more than 2 minutes for adults and children and over more than 3 minutes for the elderly. Continuous EKG monitoring during IV injection is required for children and recommended for adults.

Monitor EKG for asystole, extreme bradycardia, heart block, PR-interval prolongation, and rapid ventricular rates. Notify the physician of significant EKG changes. Monitor B/P every 5-10 minutes, or as ordered. Keep the patient in a recumbent position for at least 1 hour after IV administration. Keep in mind that the therapeutic serum level for verapamil is 0.08 to 0.3 mcg/ml.

Vitamin A
vight'ah-myn A
(Aquasol A, Palmitate A)
Do not confuse Aquasol A with Anusol.

CATEGORY AND SCHEDULE
Pregnancy Risk Category: A (X if used in doses above recommended daily allowance)

CLASSIFICATION
Vitamins/minerals

MECHANISM OF ACTION
A fat-soluble vitamin that may act as a cofactor in biochemical reactions.

Therapeutic Effect: Is essential for normal function of retina, visual adaptation to darkness, bone growth, testicular and ovarian function, and embryonic development; preserves integrity of epithelial cells.

PHARMACOKINETICS
Rapidly absorbed from the GI tract if bile salts, pancreatic lipase, protein, and dietary fat are present. Transported in blood to the liver, where it's metabolized; stored in parenchymal hepatic cells, then transported in plasma as retinol, as needed. Excreted primarily in bile and, to a lesser extent, in urine.

AVAILABILITY
Capsules: 10,000 units, 25,000 units.
Injection (Aquasol A):
50,000 units/ml.
Tablets (Palmitate A): 5000 units, 15,000 units.

INDICATIONS AND DOSAGES
▶ **Severe vitamin A deficiency**
PO
Adults, Elderly, Children 8 yr and older. 500,000 units/day for 3 days; then 50,000 units/day for 14 days, then 10,000-20,000 units/day for 2 mo.
Children 1-8 yr. 5000 units/kg/day for 5 days, then 5000-10,000 units/day for 2 mo.
Children younger than 1 yr. 5000-10,000 units/day for 2 mo.
IM
Adults, Elderly, Children 8 yr and older. 100,000 units/day for 3 days; then 50,000 units/day for 14 days.
Children 1-8 yr. 17,500-35,000 units/day for 10 days.
Children younger than 1 yr. 7500-15,000 units/day.
▶ **Malabsorption syndrome**
PO
Adults, Elderly, Children 8 yr and older. 10,000-50,000 units/day.

V

▸ **Dietary supplement**
PO
Adults, Elderly. 4000-5000 units/day.
Children 7-10 yr. 3300-
3500 units/day.
Children 4-6 yr. 2500 units/day.
Children 6 mo-3 yr. 1500-
2000 units/day.
Neonates younger than 5 mo.
1500 units/day.

CONTRAINDICATIONS
Hypervitaminosis A

INTERACTIONS
Drug
**Cholestyramine, colestipol,
mineral oil:** May decrease the
absorption of vitamin A.
Isotretinoin: May increase the risk
of toxicity.
Herbal
None known.
Food
None known.

DIAGNOSTIC TEST EFFECTS
May increase BUN and serum
cholesterol, calcium, and triglyceride
levels. May decrease blood erythrocyte and leukocyte counts.

SIDE EFFECTS
None known.

SERIOUS REACTIONS
• Chronic overdose produces
malaise, nausea, vomiting, drying or
cracking of skin or lips, inflammation of tongue or gums, irritability,
alopecia, and night sweats.
• Bulging fontanelles have occurred
in infants.

PRECAUTIONS & CONSIDERATIONS
Caution is warranted with renal
impairment. Vitamin A crosses
the placenta and is distributed in
breast milk. Use caution when
administering high doses of vitamin
A to children and the elderly.
Consuming foods rich in vitamin A,
including cod, halibut, tuna, and
shark, is encouraged, naturally occurring vitamin A is found only in animal
sources. Avoid taking cholestyramine
(Questran), colestipol, and mineral
oil during vitamin A therapy.
  Urine may appear bright yellow
during therapy. Before and during
treatment, assess for signs and symptoms of vitamin A deficiency, including night blindness, dry and brittle
nails, alopecia, and drying of corneas.
Be alert for symptoms of overdose
when receiving prolonged administration of more than 25,000 units/day.
The therapeutic serum vitamin A
level is 80 to 300 units/ml.
Administration
❗ IM administration is used only in
acutely ill patients or patients unresponsive to the oral route, such as
those with malabsorption syndrome.
  Do not crush, open, or break
capsules. Take vitamin A without
regard to food.
  For adults, an IM injection dose
of 1 ml (50,000 units) may be given
in the deltoid muscle; a dose greater
than 1 ml should be given in a large
muscle mass, such as the gluteus
maximus muscle. The anterolateral
thigh is the preferred site for infants
younger than 7 months.

Vitamin D (Cholecalciferol, Vitamin D3; Ergocalciferol, Vitamin D2)

vight′ah-myn D
(Calciferol, Drisdol, Ostoforet
[CAN])

CATEGORY AND SCHEDULE

Pregnancy Risk Category: A
(D if used in doses above recommended daily allowance)

CLASSIFICATION

Vitamins

MECHANISM OF ACTION

A fat-soluble vitamin that stimulates calcium and phosphate absorption from small intestine, promotes secretion of calcium from bone to blood, and promotes resorption of phosphate in renal tubules; also acts on bone cells to stimulate skeletal growth and on parathyroid gland to suppress hormone synthesis and secretion. *Therapeutic Effect:* Essential for absorption and utilization of calcium and phosphate and normal bone calcification. Reduces parathyroid hormone level. Improves phosphorus and calcium homeostasis in chronic renal failure.

PHARMACOKINETICS

Readily absorbed from small intestine. Concentrated primarily in liver and fat deposits. Activated in the liver and kidneys. Eliminated by biliary system; excreted in urine.
Half-life: 19-48 hr for ergocalciferol.

AVAILABILITY

Capsules (Drisdol): 50,000 units (1.25 mg).

Injection (Calciferol):
500,000 units/ml (12.5 mg).
Oral Liquid Drops (Calciferol, Drisdol): 8000 units/ml.

INDICATIONS AND DOSAGES

! Oral dosing is preferred. Administer the drug IM only in patients with GI, hepatic, or biliary disease associated with malabsorption of vitamin D.
▸ **Dietary supplement**
PO
Adults, Elderly, Children. 10 mcg (400 units)/day.
Neonates. 10-20 mcg (400-800 units)/day.
▸ **Renal failure**
PO
Adults, Elderly. 0.5 mg/day.
Children. 0.1-1 mg/day.
▸ **Hypoparathyroidism**
PO
Adults, Elderly. 625 mcg-5 mg/day (with calcium supplements).
Children. 1.25-5 mg/day (with calcium supplements).
▸ **Nutritional rickets, osteomalacia**
PO
Adults, Elderly, Children. 25-125 mcg/day for 8-12 wk.
Adults, Elderly (with malabsorption syndrome). 250-7500 mcg/day.
Children (with malabsorption syndrome). 250-625 mcg/day.
▸ **Vitamin D-dependent rickets**
PO
Adults, Elderly. 250 mcg-1.5 mg/day.
Children. 75-125 mcg/day.
Maximum: 1500 mcg/day.
▸ **Vitamin D-resistant rickets**
PO
Adults, Elderly. 250-1500 mcg/day (with phosphate supplements).
Children. Initially 1000-2000 mcg/day (with phosphate supplements). May increase in 250- to 600-mcg increments q3-4mo.

V

CONTRAINDICATIONS

Hypercalcemia, malabsorption syndrome, vitamin D toxicity

INTERACTIONS
Drug

Aluminum-containing antacids (long-term use): May increase aluminum blood concentration and risk of aluminum bone toxicity.
Calcium-containing preparations, thiazide diuretics: May increase the risk of hypercalcemia.
Magnesium-containing antacids: May increase magnesium blood concentration.
Mineral oil: Excessive use of mineral oil decreases vitamin D absorption.
Herbal
None known.
Food
None known.

DIAGNOSTIC TEST EFFECTS

May increase serum cholesterol, calcium, magnesium, and phosphate levels. May decrease serum alkaline phosphatase level.

SIDE EFFECTS
None known.

SERIOUS REACTIONS

• Early signs and symptoms of overdose are weakness, headache, somnolence, nausea, vomiting, dry mouth, constipation, muscle and bone pain, and metallic taste.
• Later signs and symptoms of overdose include polyuria, polydipsia, anorexia, weight loss, nocturia, photophobia, rhinorrhea, pruritus, disorientation, hallucinations, hyperthermia, hypertension, and cardiac arrhythmias.

PRECAUTIONS & CONSIDERATIONS

Caution is warranted with coronary artery disease, renal calculi, and renal impairment. It is unknown if vitamin D crosses the placenta or is distributed in breast milk. Children may be more sensitive to the effects of vitamin D. No age-related precautions have been noted in the elderly. Avoid taking mineral oil. Those receiving chronic renal dialysis should not take magnesium-containing antacids during vitamin D therapy. Consuming foods rich in vitamin D, including milk, eggs, leafy vegetables, margarine, meats, and vegetable oils and shortening, is encouraged.

BUN and serum alkaline phosphatase, calcium, creatinine, magnesium, phosphate, and urinary calcium levels should be monitored.
Administration
! Be aware that 1 mcg of vitamin D = 40 units.
Begin vitamin D therapy at the lowest possible dosage. Take vitamin D without regard to food. Swallow the capsules whole and avoid crushing, chewing, or opening them.

Vitamin E
vight'ah-myn E
(Aqua Gem E, Aquasol E, E-Gems, Key-E, Key-E Kaps)
Do not confuse Aquasol E with Anusol.

CATEGORY AND SCHEDULE
Pregnancy Risk Category: A
(C if used in doses above recommended daily allowance)
OTC

CLASSIFICATION
Vitamins/minerals

MECHANISM OF ACTION
An antioxidant that prevents oxidation of vitamins A and C, protects fatty acids from attack by free radicals, and protects RBCs from hemolysis by oxidizing agents. *Therapeutic Effect:* Prevents and treats vitamin E deficiency.

PHARMACOKINETICS
Variably absorbed from the GI tract (requires bile salts, dietary fat, and normal pancreatic function). Primarily concentrated in adipose tissue. Metabolized in the liver. Primarily eliminated by biliary system.

AVAILABILITY
Capsules (E-Gems): 100 units, 600 units, 800 units, 1000 units, 1200 units.
Capsules (Aqua-Gem E, Key-E Kaps): 200 units, 400 units.
Tablets (Key-E): 100 units, 200 units, 400 units, 800 units.

INDICATIONS AND DOSAGES
▶ **Vitamin E deficiency**
PO
Adults, Elderly. 60-75 units/day.
Children. 1 unit/kg/day.

OFF-LABEL USES
To decrease severity of tardive dyskinesia

CONTRAINDICATIONS
None known.

INTERACTIONS
Drug
Cholestyramine, colestipol, mineral oil: May decrease the absorption of vitamin E.
Iron (large doses): May increase vitamin E requirements.
Herbal
None known.

Food
None known.

DIAGNOSTIC TEST EFFECTS
None known.

SIDE EFFECTS
None known.

SERIOUS REACTIONS
• Chronic overdose may produce fatigue, weakness, nausea, headache, blurred vision, flatulence, and diarrhea.

PRECAUTIONS & CONSIDERATIONS
Vitamin E use may impair the hematologic response with iron deficiency anemia. It is unknown if vitamin E crosses the placenta or is distributed in breast milk. No age-related precautions have been noted with normal dosages in children or the elderly. Consuming foods high in vitamin E, including eggs, meats, milk, leafy vegetables, margarine, and vegetable oils and shortening, is encouraged.

Notify the physician of signs and symptoms of toxicity including blurred vision, diarrhea, nausea, dizziness, flu-like symptoms, or headache.
Administration
Don't crush, open, or break capsules or tablets. Take vitamin E without regard to food.

V

Voriconazole
vohr-ee-con'ah-zole
(Vfend)

CATEGORY AND SCHEDULE
Pregnancy Risk Category: D

CLASSIFICATION
Antifungals

MECHANISM OF ACTION
A triazole derivative that inhibits the synthesis of ergosterol, a vital component of fungal cell wall formation. *Therapeutic Effect:* Damages fungal cell wall membrane.

PHARMACOKINETICS
Rapidly and completely absorbed after PO administration. Widely distributed. Protein binding: 98%. Metabolized in the liver. Primarily excreted as a metabolite in urine. **Half-life:** 6 hr.

AVAILABILITY
Tablets: 50 mg, 200 mg.
Injection Powder for Reconstitution: 200 mg.
Powder for Oral Suspension: 200 mg/5 ml.

INDICATIONS AND DOSAGES
▸ **Invasive aspergillosis, other serious fungal infections caused by *Scedosporium apiospermum* and *Fusarium* species**
PO
Adults, Elderly weighing 40 kg and more. Initially, 400 mg q12hr for 2 doses on day 1. Maintenance: 200 mg q12hr.
Adults, Elderly weighing less than 40 kg. Initially, 200 mg q12hr for 2 doses on day 1.

Maintenance: 100 mg q12hr (may increase to 150 mg q12hr).
▸ **Usual parenteral dosage**
IV
Adults, Elderly, Children. Initially, 6 mg/kg/dose q12hr for 2 doses, then 4 mg/kg/dose q12hr (may decrease to 3 mg/kg/dose if patient is unable to tolerate 4 mg/kg/dose).
▸ **Esophageal candidiasis**
PO
Adults, Elderly weighing 40 kg and more. 200 mg q12hr for minimum of 14 days, then at least 7 days following resolution of symptoms.
Adults, Elderly weighing less than 40 kg. 100 mg q12hr for minimum 14 days, then at least 7 days following resolution of symptoms.

CONTRAINDICATIONS
Concurrent administration of carbamazepine; ergot alkaloids; pimozide or quinidine (may cause prolonged QT interval or torsades de pointes); rifabutin; rifampin; or sirolimus

INTERACTIONS
Drug
Cyclosporine, omeprazole, phenytoin, rifabutin, sirolimus, tacrilimus, warfarin: May increase plasma concentrations of these drugs.
Phenytoin, rifabutin, rifampin: May decrease voriconazole plasma concentration.
Herbal
None known.
Food
None known.

DIAGNOSTIC TEST EFFECTS
May increase serum alkaline phosphatase and SGPT (ALT) levels.

▓ IV INCOMPATIBILITIES
Don't mix voriconazole with any other medications.

SIDE EFFECTS
Frequent (20%-5%)
Abnormal vision, fever, nausea, rash, vomiting
Occasional (5%-2%)
Headache, chills, hallucinations, photophobia, tachycardia, hypertension

SERIOUS REACTIONS
* Hepatotoxicity occurs rarely.

PRECAUTIONS & CONSIDERATIONS
Caution should be used with hypersensitivity to other antifungal agents or impaired renal or liver function. Be aware that voriconazole may cause fetal harm. Use effective contraception during voriconazole treatment. Be aware that the safety and efficacy of voriconazole have not been established in children younger than 12 years. There are no age-related precautions noted in the elderly.

Expect to monitor liver and renal function test results. Evaluate and monitor visual function, including color perception, visual acuity, and visual field, for drug therapy lasting longer than 28 days. Avoid driving at night because voriconazole may cause visual changes, such as blurred vision or photophobia. Avoid performing hazardous tasks if changes in vision occur. Avoid direct sunlight.

Storage
Store powder for injection at room temperature. Use reconstituted solution immediately. Do not use reconstituted solution after 24 hours when refrigerated.

Administration
Give oral voriconazole 1 hour before or 1 hour after a meal.

Reconstitute 200-mg vial with 19 ml sterile water for injection to provide a concentration of 10 mg/ml. Further dilute with 0.9% NaCl or D_5W to provide a concentration of 5 mg/ml or less. Infuse over 1 to 2 hours at a concentration of 5 mg/ml or less.

V

Warfarin
war′far-in
(Apo-Warfarin [CAN], Coumadin,
Gen-Warfarin [CAN], Jantoven,
Marevan [AUS], Tar-Warfarin
[CAN])
**Do not confuse Coumadin with
Kemadrin.**

CATEGORY AND SCHEDULE
Pregnancy Risk Category: D

CLASSIFICATION
Anticoagulants

MECHANISM OF ACTION
A coumarin derivative that interferes
with hepatic synthesis of vitamin
K-dependent clotting factors,
resulting in depletion of coagulation
factors II, VII, IX, and X.
Therapeutic Effect: Prevents further
extension of formed existing clot;
prevents new clot formation or
secondary thromboembolic
complications.

PHARMACOKINETICS

Route	Onset	Peak	Duration
PO	1.5-3 days	5-7 days	N/A

Well absorbed from the GI tract.
Metabolized in the liver. Primarily
excreted in urine. Not removed
by hemodialysis. **Half-life:** 1.5-
2.5 days.

AVAILABILITY
Tablets (Coumadin, Jantoven): 1 mg,
2 mg, 2.5 mg, 3 mg, 4 mg, 5 mg,
6 mg, 7.5 mg, 10 mg.
Injection (Coumadin): 5-mg vial.

INDICATIONS AND DOSAGES
▶ **Anticoagulant**
PO
Adults, Elderly. Initially, 5-15 mg/day
for 2-5 days; then adjust based on
International Normalized Ratio
(INR). Maintenance: 2-10 mg/day.
Children. Initially, 0.1-0.2 mg/kg
(maximum 10 mg). Maintenance:
0.05-0.34 mg/kg/day.
▶ **Usual elderly dosage (maintenance)**
PO, IV
Elderly. 2-5 mg/day.

OFF-LABEL USES
Prevention of recurrent cerebral
embolism, myocardial reinfarction;
treatment adjunct in transient
ischemic attacks

CONTRAINDICATIONS
Neurosurgical procedures, open
wounds, pregnancy, severe hypertension, severe hepatic or renal damage,
uncontrolled bleeding, ulcers

INTERACTIONS
Drug
**Acetaminophen, allopurinol,
amiodarone, anabolic steroids,
androgens, aspirin, cefamandole,
cefoperazone, chloral hydrate,
chloramphenicol, cimetidine, clofibrate, danazol, dextrothyroxine,
diflunisal, disulfiram, erythromycin, fenoprofen, gemfibrozil,
indomethacin, methimazole,
metronidazole, oral hypoglycemics,
phenytoin, plicamycin, propylthiouracil, quinidine, salicylates,
sulfinpyrazone, sulfonamides,
sulindac:** Warfarin increases the
effects of these drugs.
Alcohol: May enhance warfarin's
anticoagulant effect.
**Barbiturates, carbamazepine,
cholestyramine, colestipol,
estramustine, estrogens,
griseofulvin, primidone,**

rifampin, vitamin K: Warfarin decreases the effects of these drugs.
Herbal
American ginseng, St. John's wort: May decrease the effectiveness of warfarin.
Feverfew, garlic, ginkgo biloba, ginseng, glucosamine-chondroitin: May increase the risk of bleeding.
Food
None known.

DIAGNOSTIC TEST EFFECTS
None known.

SIDE EFFECTS
Occasional
GI distress, such as nausea, anorexia, abdominal cramps, diarrhea
Rare
Hypersensitivity reaction, including dermatitis and urticaria, especially in those sensitive to aspirin

SERIOUS REACTIONS
• Bleeding complications ranging from local ecchymoses to major hemorrhage may occur. Drug should be discontinued immediately and vitamin K or phytonadione administered. Mild hemorrhage: 2.5-10 mg PO, IM, or IV. Severe hemorrhage: 10-15 mg IV and repeated q4hr, as necessary.
• Hepatotoxicity, blood dyscrasias, necrosis, vasculitis, and local thrombosis occur rarely.

PRECAUTIONS & CONSIDERATIONS
Caution is warranted with risk for hemorrhage and in those with active tuberculosis, diabetes, gangrene, heparin-induced thrombocytopenia, or necrosis. Warfarin use is contraindicated in pregnancy because it causes fetal and neonatal hemorrhage and intrauterine death. Warfarin crosses the placenta and is distributed in breast milk. Children are more susceptible to the effects of warfarin. In the elderly, there is an increased risk of hemorrhage; a lower drug dosage is recommended. Other medications, including OTC drugs, should be avoided. An electric razor and soft toothbrush should be used to prevent bleeding during therapy. Avoid alcohol, drastic dietary changes, and salicylates.

Urine may become red-orange. Notify the physician before having dental work or surgery. Notify the physician of abdominal or back pain, gingival bleeding, black stool, bleeding, brown, dark or red urine, coffee ground vomitus, or red-speckled mucus from cough. INR should be determined before administration and daily after therapy begins. When INR is stabilized, INR determinations should be followed every 4 to 6 weeks. Pulse, Hct, platelet count, AST (SGOT) and ALT (SGPT) levels, and stool and urine cultures for occult blood, regardless of administration route, should be monitored.
Storage
Store at room temperature and protect from light. Don't refrigerate. Use reconstituted solution within 4 hours; discard unused portion.
Administration
! Remember that warfarin dosage is highly individualized and is based on PT and INR.

Crush scored tablets as needed. Give oral warfarin without regard to food. If GI upset occurs, give with food. Take warfarin exactly as prescribed. Do not take or discontinue other medications without physician approval. Do not change from one brand of warfarin to another.

For IV use, to reconstitute, add 2.7 ml sterile water for injection to 5-mg vial to produce a 2 mg of warfarin per ml of solution.

W

Xylometazoline

zye-loe-met-az'oh-leen
(Otrivin Measured-Dose Pump
with Moisturizers, Otrivin Nasal
Drops, Otrivin Nasal Spray,
Otrivin Nasal Spray with
Eucalyptol, Otrivin Nasal Spray
with Moisturizers, Otrivin
Pediatric Nasal Drops, Otrivin
Pediatric Nasal Spray, Otrivin
With Measured-Dose Pump)

CATEGORY AND SCHEDULE
Pregnancy Risk Category: C

CLASSIFICATION
Decongestant, imidazoline
derivative

MECHANISM OF ACTION
A sympathomimetic that directly
acts on alpha-adrenergic receptors
in arterioles of the nasal mucosa to
produce vasoconstriction resulting
in decreased blood flow. *Therapeutic
Effect:* Decreased nasal
congestion.

PHARMACOKINETICS
Onset of action occurs within
5-10 minutes for a duration of
action of 5-6 hours. Well absorbed
through nasal mucosa. May also
be systemically absorbed from
both nasal mucosa and gastrointestinal (GI) tract. **Half-life:**
Unknown.

AVAILABILITY
Nasal Drops: 0.05% (Otrivin
Pediatric Nasal Drops), 0.1%
(Otrivin Nasal Drops).
Nasal Spray: 0.1% (Otrivin Nasal
Spray).

INDICATIONS AND DOSAGES
▸ Rhinitis
INTRANASAL
*Adults, Elderly, Children 12 yr
and older.* 1-3 drops (0.1%) in
each nostril q8-10hr or 1 to 2 sprays
(0.1%) in each nostril q8-10hr.
Maximum: 3 doses/day.
Children 2-12 yr. 2 or 3
drops (0.05%) in each nostril
q8-10hr.

CONTRAINDICATIONS
Narrow-angle glaucoma,
rhinitis sicca, children under
6 years, hypersensitivity to
xylometazoline or other adrenergic
agents

INTERACTIONS
Drug
MAOIs: May increase risk of
hypertensive crisis.
**Maprotiline, tricyclic antidepres-
sants:** May increase effects of
xylometazoline.
Herbal
None known.
Food
None known.

DIAGNOSTIC TEST EFFECTS
None known.

SIDE EFFECTS
Occasional
Nasal: Burning, stinging, drying
nasal mucosa, sneezing, rebound
congestion

SERIOUS REACTIONS
• Large doses may produce
tachycardia, palpitations, lightheadedness, nausea, and
vomiting.
• Overdosage in patients older than
60 years of age may produce hallucinations, CNS depression, and
seizures.

PRECAUTIONS & CONSIDERATIONS

Caution is warranted with cardiovascular disease, diabetes mellitus, hypertension, pheochromocytoma, prostatic enlargement, and thyroid disease. It is unknown if xylometazoline crosses the placenta or is distributed in breast milk. Safety and efficacy of xylometazoline have not been established in children younger than 2 years of age. Age-related prostatic hypertrophy may require dosage adjustment in the elderly.

Fast, irregular and pounding heartbeat, headache, insomnia, light-headedness, nausea, nervousness, and trembling can occur if xylometazoline is systemically absorbed. If used too frequently, rebound effects can occur. Xylometzoline should not be used longer than 72 hours.

Administration

Instill 1-3 drops in each nostril every 8-10 hours. Do not use for longer than 3 to 5 days due to the risk of rebound congestion.

X

Yohimbine

yoe-him′ been
(Actibine, Aphrodyne, Dayto-Himbin, PMS-Yohimbine [CAN], Yocon, Yohimbe, Yohimex, Yovital)

CATEGORY AND SCHEDULE

Pregnancy Risk Category: N/A

CLASSIFICATION

Antiadrenergics, alpha blocking, impotence agents

MECHANISM OF ACTION

An herb that produces genital blood vessel dilation, improves nerve impulse transmission to genital area. Increases penile blood flow, central sympathetic excitation impulses to genital tissues. *Therapeutic Effect:* Improves sexual vigor, affects impotence.

PHARMACOKINETICS

Rapidly absorbed. Extensive metabolism in liver and kidneys. Minimal excretion in urine as unchanged drug. **Half-life:** 36 min.

AVAILABILITY

Tablets: 5 mg (Actibine), 5.4 mg (Aphrodyne, Dayto-Himbin, Yocon, Yovital, Yohimex).

INDICATIONS AND DOSAGES

▸ **Impotence**
PO
Adults, Elderly. 5.4 mg 3 times/day.
▸ **Orthostatic hypotension**
PO
Adults, Elderly. 12.5 mg/day.

OFF-LABEL USES

Treatment of SSRI-induced sexual dysfunction, weight loss, sympa-thicolytic and mydriatic, aphrodisiac

CONTRAINDICATIONS

Renal disease, hypersensitivity to yohimbine or any component of the formulation

INTERACTIONS
Drug

Antidiabetics, antihypertensives: May interfere with the effects of these drugs.
Clonidine: May antagonize the effects of clonidine.
MAOIs, linezolid, sympathomimet-ics, tricyclic antidepressants: Has additive effects with these drugs.
Herbal
Ephedra: May increase the risk of hypertensive crises.
Ginkgo biloba, St. John's wort: May have additive therapeutic and adverse effects.
Food
Caffeine-containing products (such as coffee, tea, and chocolate), tyramine-containing foods (such as aged cheese and chianti wine): May increase the risk of hyperten-sive crises.

DIAGNOSTIC TEST EFFECTS

None known.

SIDE EFFECTS

Excitement, tremors, insomnia, anxi-ety, hypertension, tachycardia, dizzi-ness, headache, irritability, salivation, dilated pupils, nausea, vomiting, hypersensitivity reaction

SERIOUS REACTIONS

• Paralysis, severe hypotension, irreg-ular heartbeats, and cardiac failure may occur. Overdose can be fatal.

PRECAUTIONS & CONSIDERATIONS

Caution is warranted with anxiety, diabetes mellitus, hypertension, post-traumatic stress disorder, and schizophrenia. Yohimbine is generally not used in females. Its use is contraindicated in breast-feeding and pregnant women. Safety and efficacy of yohimbine have not been established in children. Age-related liver and renal impairment may require discontinuation of yohimbine in the elderly. Over-the-counter drugs should be avoided without first consulting with the physician.

Administration

Reduce dose if side effects occur. May reduce to ½ tablet 3 times a day followed by gradual increases to 1 tablet 3 times a day.

Y

Zafirlukast
za-feer'loo-kast
(Accolate)
**Do not confuse Accolate with
Accupril or Aclovate.**

CATEGORY AND SCHEDULE
Pregnancy Risk Category: B

CLASSIFICATION
Leukotriene antagonists/
inhibitors

MECHANISM OF ACTION
An antiasthmic that binds to
leukotriene receptors, inhibiting
bronchoconstriction due to
sulfur dioxide, cold air, and
specific antigens, such as
grass, cat dander, and ragweed.
Therapeutic Effect: Reduces airway
edema and smooth muscle
constriction; alters cellular activity
associated with the inflammatory
process.

PHARMACOKINETICS
Rapidly absorbed after PO
administration (food reduces
absorption). Protein binding: 99%.
Extensively metabolized in the
liver. Primarily excreted in feces.
Unknown if removed by
hemodialysis. **Half-life:** 10 hr.

AVAILABILITY
Tablets: 10 mg, 20 mg.

INDICATIONS AND DOSAGES
▶ **Bronchial asthma**
PO
*Adults, Elderly, Children 12 yr and
older.* 20 mg twice a day.
Children 5-11 yr. 10 mg twice
a day.

CONTRAINDICATIONS
None known.

INTERACTIONS
Drug
Aspirin: Increases zafirlukast blood
concentration.
Erythromycin, theophylline:
Decreases zafirlukast blood concen-
tration.
Warfarin: Increases PT.
Herbal
None known.
Food
None known.

DIAGNOSTIC TEST EFFECTS
May increase ALT (SGPT) level.

SIDE EFFECTS
Frequent (13%)
Headache
Occasional (3%)
Nausea, diarrhea
Rare (less than 3%)
Generalized pain, asthenia, myalgia,
fever, dyspepsia, vomiting,
dizziness

SERIOUS REACTIONS
• Concurrent administration of
inhaled corticosteroids increases
the risk of upper respiratory tract
infection.

PRECAUTIONS & CONSIDERATIONS
Caution is warranted with impaired
hepatic function. Zafirlukast is
distributed in breast milk. It is not
recommended for breast-feeding
women. The safety and efficacy of
this drug have not been established
in children younger than 5 years. No
age-related precautions have been
noted in the elderly. Be aware zafirlukast is not intended to treat acute
asthma episodes. Drink plenty of
fluids to decrease the thickness of
lung secretions.

Liver function, pulse rate and quality as well as respiratory depth, rate, rhythm, and type should be monitored. Fingernails and lips for cyanosis, manifested as a blue or dusky color in light-skinned patients and a gray color in dark-skinned patients, should also be assessed. Notify the physician if abdominal pain, nausea, flu-like symptoms, jaundice, or worsening of asthma occurs.

Administration

Take zafirlukast 1 hour before or 2 hours after meals. Don't crush or break tablets. Take zafirlukast as prescribed, even during symptom-free periods. Do not alter the dosage or abruptly discontinue other asthma medications.

Zalcitabine (DDC)

zal-site′a-been
(Hivid)

CATEGORY AND SCHEDULE
Pregnancy Risk Category: C

CLASSIFICATION
Antivirals, nucleoside reverse transcriptase inhibitors

MECHANISM OF ACTION
A nucleoside reverse transcriptase inhibitor that inhibits viral DNA synthesis. *Therapeutic Effect:* Prevents replication of HIV-1.

PHARMACOKINETICS
Readily absorbed from the GI tract (absorption decreased by food). Protein binding: 4%. Undergoes phosphorylation intracellularly to the active metabolite. Primarily excreted in urine. Removed by hemodialysis. **Half-life:** 1-3 hr; metabolite,

2.6-10 hr (increased in impaired renal function).

AVAILABILITY
Tablets: 0.375 mg, 0.75 mg.

INDICATIONS AND DOSAGES
▶ **HIV infection (in combination with other antiretrovirals)**
PO
Adults, Children 13 yr and older.
0.75 mg q8hr.
Children younger than 13 yr.
0.01 mg/kg q8hr. Range: 0.005-0.01 mg/kg q8hr.
▶ **Dosage in renal impairment**
Dosage and frequency are modified based on creatinine clearance.

Creatinine Clearance	Dose
10-40 ml/min	0.75 mg q12hr
Less than 10 ml/min	0.75 mg q24hr

CONTRAINDICATIONS
Moderate or severe peripheral neuropathy

INTERACTIONS
Drug
Medications associated with peripheral neuropathy (including cisplatin, disulfiram, phenytoin, vincristine): May increase the risk of neuropathy.
Medications causing pancreatitis (including IV pentamidine): May increase the risk of pancreatitis.
Herbal
None known.
Food
None known.

DIAGNOSTIC TEST EFFECTS
May increase serum alkaline phosphatase, amylase, bilirubin, lipase, AST (SGOT), ALT (SGPT), and triglyceride levels. May decrease

Z

serum calcium, magnesium, and phosphate levels. May alter blood glucose and sodium levels.

SIDE EFFECTS
Frequent (28%-11%)
Peripheral neuropathy, fever, fatigue, headache, rash
Occasional (10%-5%)
Diarrhea, abdominal pain, oral ulcers, cough, pruritus, myalgia, weight loss, nausea, vomiting
Rare (4%-1%)
Nasal discharge, dysphagia, depression, night sweats, confusion

SERIOUS REACTIONS
• Peripheral neuropathy (characterized by numbness, tingling, burning, and pain in the lower extremities) occurs in 17% to 31% of patients. These symptoms may be followed by sharp, shooting pain and progress to a severe, continuous, burning pain that may be irreversible if the drug is not discontinued in time.
• Pancreatitis, leukopenia, neutropenia, eosinophilia, and thrombocytopenia occur rarely.

PRECAUTIONS & CONSIDERATIONS
! Extreme caution should be used with preexisting neuropathy and low CD4 cell counts because of an increased risk of developing peripheral neuropathy. Caution is also warranted with a history of alcohol abuse, diabetes, liver disease, peripheral neuropathy, renal impairment, and weight loss. Be aware that it is unknown if zalcitabine crosses the placenta or is distributed in breast milk. Breast-feeding is not recommended in this population because of the possibility of HIV transmission. There are no age-related precautions in children younger than 6 months. In children, dosages are not established. In the elderly, age-related

renal impairment may require dosage adjustment. Zalcitabine is not a cure for HIV, nor does it reduce transmission of the disease, opportunistic illnesses associated with advanced HIV infection may occur.
! Although rare, assess for impending, potentially fatal pancreatitis as evidenced by abdominal pain, increasing serum amylase levels, nausea, rising triglyceride levels, and vomiting. If these signs or symptoms, particularly abdominal pain, occur withhold the drug and immediately notify the physician. Expect to monitor complete blood count (CBC), serum amylase, and serum triglyceride levels before and during therapy. Assess for signs and symptoms of a therapeutic response to drug therapy, including decreased fatigue, increased energy, and weight gain.
Administration
Zalcitabine is best taken on an empty stomach because food decreases drug absorption.
May take with food to decrease GI distress. Space doses evenly around the clock.

Zaleplon
zal′e-plon
(Sonata, Stamoc [CAN])

CATEGORY AND SCHEDULE
Pregnancy Risk Category: C

CLASSIFICATION
Sedatives/hypnotics

MECHANISM OF ACTION
A nonbenzodiazepine that enhances the action of the inhibitory neurotransmitter gamma-aminobutyric acid. *Therapeutic Effect:* Induces sleep.

AVAILABILITY
Capsules: 5 mg, 10 mg.

INDICATIONS AND DOSAGES
▶ **Insomnia**
PO
Adults. 10 mg at bedtime. Range:
5-20 mg.
Elderly. 5 mg at bedtime.

CONTRAINDICATIONS
Severe hepatic impairment

INTERACTIONS
Drug
Alcohol, other CNS depressants:
May increase CNS depression.
Cimetidine: May increase the effect
of zaleplon.
Rifampin: Decreases the zaleplon
blood concentration.
Herbal
None known.
Food
High-fat, heavy meals: May delay
onset of sleep by approximately
2 hours.

DIAGNOSTIC TEST EFFECTS
None known.

SIDE EFFECTS
Expected
Somnolence, sedation, mild rebound
insomnia (on first night after drug is
discontinued)
Frequent (28%-7%)
Nausea, headache, myalgia, dizziness
Occasional (5%-3%)
Abdominal pain, asthenia, dyspep-
sia, eye pain, paresthesia
Rare (2%)
Tremors, amnesia, hyperacusis (acute
sense of hearing), fever, dysmenorrhea

SERIOUS REACTIONS
• Zaleplon may produce altered
concentration, behavior changes, and
impaired memory.

• Taking the drug while up and
about may result in adverse CNS
effects, such as hallucinations,
impaired coordination, dizziness,
and light-headedness.
• Overdose results in somnolence,
confusion, diminished reflexes, and
coma.

PRECAUTIONS & CONSIDERATIONS
Caution is warranted with mild to
moderate hepatic impairment, signs
or symptoms of depression, and a
hypersensitivity to aspirin (may
cause an allergic-type reaction).
Drowsiness may occur. Avoid
alcohol, CNS depressants, and tasks
that require mental alertness or
motor skills. Disturbed sleep may
occur for 1 or 2 nights after
discontinuing the drug.
Administration
If desired, open zaleplon capsules
and mix the contents with food.
Avoid taking this drug with or
immediately after a high-fat meal to
avoid delayed absorption.

Zanamivir
za-na′mi-veer
(Relenza)

CATEGORY AND SCHEDULE
Pregnancy Risk Category: B

CLASSIFICATION
Antivirals

MECHANISM OF ACTION
An antiviral that appears to inhibit
the influenza virus enzyme
neuraminidase, which is essential for
viral replication. *Therapeutic Effect:*
Prevents viral release from infected
cells.

Z

AVAILABILITY
Powder for Inhalation: 5 mg/blister.

INDICATIONS AND DOSAGES
▸ **Influenza virus**
INHALATION
Adults, Elderly, Children 7 yr and older. 2 inhalations (one 5-mg blister per inhalation for a total dose of 10 mg) twice a day (approximately 12 hr apart) for 5 days.
▸ **Prevention of influenza virus**
INHALATION
Adults, Elderly. 2 inhalations once a day for the duration of the exposure period.

CONTRAINDICATIONS
None known.

INTERACTIONS
Drug
None known.
Herbal
None known.
Food
None known.

DIAGNOSTIC TEST EFFECTS
May increase serum CK level and liver function test results.

SIDE EFFECTS
Occasional (3%-2%)
Diarrhea, sinusitis, nausea, bronchitis, cough, dizziness, headache
Rare (less than 1.5%)
Malaise, fatigue, fever, abdominal pain, myalgia, arthralgia, urticaria

SERIOUS REACTIONS
• Neutropenia may occur.
• Bronchospasm may occur in those with a history of COPD or bronchial asthma.

PRECAUTIONS & CONSIDERATIONS
Caution should be used with asthma and COPD. Be aware that persons requiring an inhaled bronchodilator at the same time as zanamivir should receive the bronchodilator before zanamivir. Pattern of daily bowel activity and stool consistency should be assessed. Dizziness may occur. Avoid contact with those who are at high risk for influenza.
Storage
Store at room temperature.
Administration
Using the Diskhaler device provided, exhale completely; then, holding the mouthpiece 1 inch away from lips, inhale and hold breath as long as possible before exhaling. Rinse mouth with water immediately after inhalation to prevent mouth and throat dryness. Continue treatment for the full 5-day course and evenly space doses around the clock.

Ziconotide
zi-koe′no-tide
(Prialt)

CATEGORY AND SCHEDULE
Pregnancy Risk Category: C

CLASSIFICATION
Analgesics, non-narcotic

MECHANISM OF ACTION
A synthetic peptide that selectively binds to N-type voltage-sensitive calcium channels located on afferent nerves in the spinal cord. This binding is thought to block N-type calcium channels. *Therapeutic Effect:* Blocks excitatory neurotransmitter release, reducing sensitivity to painful stimuli.

AVAILABILITY
Solution: 25-mcg/ml (20-ml), 100-mcg/ml (1-ml, 2-ml, 5-ml) vials.

INDICATIONS AND DOSAGES
▶ **Pain control**
INTRATHECAL
Adults, Elderly. Initially,
2.4 mcg/day (0.1 mcg/hour). May
titrate to maximum of 19.2 mcg/day
(0.8 mcg/hr).

CONTRAINDICATIONS
History of psychosis, presence of
infection at the injection site, uncontrolled bleeding, or spinal canal
obstruction that impairs CSF circulation, IV administration

INTERACTIONS
Drug
Other CNS depressants: May
enhance the adverse and toxic effects
of these drugs.
Herbal
None known.
Food
None known.

DIAGNOSTIC TEST EFFECTS
May increase serum kinase levels.

SIDE EFFECTS
Frequent (47%-11%)
Dizziness, nausea, somnolence,
weakness, diarrhea, confusion,
ataxia, headache, vomiting, gait
disturbance, memory impairment,
hypertonia
Occasional (10%-7%)
Anorexia, visual disturbances, anxiety,
urinary retention, speech disorder,
aphasia, nystagmus, paresthesia, fever,
hallucinations, nervousness, vertigo
Rare
Insomnia, dry skin, constipation,
arthralgia, myalgia, tremor

SERIOUS REACTIONS
• Atrial fibrillation, cerebral vascular accident, seizures, kidney failure
(acute), myoclonus, and psychosis
occurs rarely.

PRECAUTIONS & CONSIDERATIONS
Ziconotide should be used cautiously
in the elderly because they are
at increased risk of developing
confusion.
Administration
For intrathecal use, administer
ziconotide only with a Medtronic
SynchroMed EL or SynchroMed II
Infusion System, or the Simms
Deltec Cadd Micro External
Microinfusion Device and Catheter.
Refer to the manufacturer's manuals
for instructions for initial filling and
refilling of the reservoir.

Zidovudine
zyde-o'vue-deen
(Apo-Zidovudine [CAN], AZT,
Novo-AZT [CAN], Retrovir)
**Do not confuse the combina-
tion drug Combivir with
Combivent or Retrovir with
ritonavir.**

CATEGORY AND SCHEDULE
Pregnancy Risk Category: C

CLASSIFICATION
Antivirals, nucleoside reverse
transcriptase inhibitors

MECHANISM OF ACTION
A nucleoside reverse transcriptase
inhibitor that interferes with viral
RNA-dependent DNA polymerase,
an enzyme necessary for viral HIV
replication. *Therapeutic Effect:*
Interferes with HIV replication, slowing the progression of HIV infection.

PHARMACOKINETICS
Rapidly and completely absorbed
from the GI tract. Protein binding:
25%-38%. Undergoes first-pass

metabolism in the liver. Crosses the blood-brain barrier and is widely distributed, including to CSF. Primarily excreted in urine. Minimal removal by hemodialysis. **Half-life:** 0.8-1.2 hr (increased in impaired renal function).

AVAILABILITY
Capsules: 100 mg.
Syrup: 50 mg/5 ml.
Tablets: 300 mg.
Injection: 10 mg/ml.

INDICATIONS AND DOSAGES
▸ **HIV infection**
PO
Adults, Elderly, Children older than 12 yr. 200 mg q8hr or 300 mg q12hr.
Children 12 yr and younger. 160 mg/m^2/dose q8hr. Range: 90-180 mg/m^2/dose q6-8hr.
Neonates. 2 mg/kg/dose q6hr.
IV
Adults, Elderly, Children older than 12 yr. 1-2 mg/kg/dose q4hr.
Children 12 yr and younger. 120 mg/m^2/dose q6hr.
Neonates. 1.5 mg/kg/dose q6hr.

OFF-LABEL USES
Prophylaxis in health care workers at risk of acquiring HIV after occupational exposure

CONTRAINDICATIONS
Life-threatening allergic reactions to zidovudine or its components

INTERACTIONS
Drug
Bone marrow depressants, ganciclovir: May increase myelosuppression.
Clarithromycin: May decrease zidovudine blood concentration.
Probenecid: May increase zidovudine blood concentrations and the risk of zidovudine toxicity.

Herbal
None known.
Food
None known.

DIAGNOSTIC TEST EFFECTS
May increase mean corpuscular volume.

▦ IV INCOMPATIBILITIES
None known.
🮲 IV Compatibilities
Dexamethasone (Decadron), dobutamine (Dobutrex), dopamine (Intropin), heparin, lorazepam (Ativan), morphine, potassium chloride

SIDE EFFECTS
Expected (46%-42%)
Nausea, headache
Frequent (20%-16%)
Abdominal pain, asthenia, rash, fever, acne
Occasional (12%-8%)
Diarrhea, anorexia, malaise, myalgia, somnolence
Rare (6%-5%)
Dizziness, paresthesia, vomiting, insomnia, dyspnea, altered taste

SERIOUS REACTIONS
• Serious reactions include anemia, which occurs most commonly after 4-6 weeks of therapy, and granulocytopenia; both effects are more likely to occur in patients who have a low Hgb level or granulocyte count before beginning therapy.
• Neurotoxicity (as evidenced by ataxia, fatigue, lethargy, nystagmus, and seizures) may occur.

PRECAUTIONS & CONSIDERATIONS
Caution is warranted with bone marrow compromise, decreased liver blood flow, and renal and liver dysfunction. Be aware that it is unknown if zidovudine crosses the

placenta or is distributed in breast milk. Be aware that it is unknown if fetal harm or effects on fertility can occur from use of this drug. There are no age-related precautions noted in children. There is no information on the effects of this drug's use in the elderly. Zidovudine does not cure HIV or AIDS, but acts to reduce symptoms and slow or arrest disease progression. Be aware that the person should not receive drugs that are cytotoxic, myelosuppressive, or nephrotoxic, because these drugs may increase the risk of zidovudine toxicity.

Expect to obtain specimens for viral diagnostic tests before starting therapy. Therapy may begin before results are obtained. Check hematology reports to establish an accurate baseline. Monitor CD4 cell count, complete blood count (CBC), Hgb levels, HIV RNA plasma levels, mean corpuscular volume (MCV), and reticulocyte count. Assess for rash, bleeding, dizziness, headache, insomnia, pattern of daily bowel activity and stool consistency, and signs and symptoms of opportunistic infections, such as chills, cough, fever, and myalgia. Report bleeding from gums, nose, or rectum to the physician immediately. Dental work should be done before therapy or after blood counts return to normal, which is often weeks after therapy has stopped.

Storage
Keep capsules in a cool, dry place. Protect from light. After dilution, IV solution is stable for 24 hours at room temperature; 48 hours if refrigerated. Do not use if particulate matter is present or discoloration occurs.

Administration
Food or milk does not affect GI absorption of oral zidovudine.

Space doses evenly around the clock. Take the medication in an upright position to prevent esophageal ulceration.

Must dilute before IV administration. Remove calculated dose from vial and add to D_5W to provide a concentration no greater than 4 mg/ml. Infuse over 1 hour.

Zileuton
zye-lew-ton
(Zyflo)
Do not confuse Zyban.

CATEGORY AND SCHEDULE
Pregnancy Risk Category: C

CLASSIFICATION
Leukotriene antagonists/inhibitors

MECHANISM OF ACTION
A leukotriene inhibitor that inhibits the enzyme responsible for producing inflammatory response. Prevents formation of leukotrienes (leukotrienes induce bronchoconstriction response, enhances vascular permeability, stimulates mucus secretion). *Therapeutic Effect:* Prevents airway edema, smooth muscle contraction, and the inflammatory process, relieving signs and symptoms of bronchial asthma.

PHARMACOKINETICS
Rapidly absorbed from gastrointestinal (GI) tract. Protein binding: 93%. Metabolized in liver. Primarily excreted in urine. Unknown if

Z

removed by hemodialysis. **Half-life:** 2.1-2.5 hr.

AVAILABILITY
Tablets: 600 mg (Zyflo).

INDICATIONS AND DOSAGES
▸ **Bronchial asthma**
PO
Adults, Elderly, Children 12 yr and older. 600 mg 4 times/day. Total daily dosage: 2400 mg.

CONTRAINDICATIONS
Active liver disease, impaired liver function, hypersensitivity to zileuton or any component of the formulation

INTERACTIONS
Drug
Beta blockers: May increase effects of beta blockers.
Cyclosporine, calcium channel blockers, theophylline: May increase concentration/toxicity of these drugs.
Warfarin: May increase PT in those receiving warfarin.

DIAGNOSTIC TEST EFFECTS
May increase liver transaminase, SGOT (ALT).

SIDE EFFECTS
Frequent
Headache
Occasional
Dyspepsia, nausea, abdominal pain, asthenia (loss of strength), myalgia
Rare
Conjunctivitis, constipation, dizziness, flatulence, insomnia

SERIOUS REACTIONS
• Liver dysfunction occurs rarely and may be manifested as right upper quadrant pain, nausea, fatigue, lethargy, pruritus, jaundice or flulike symptoms.

PRECAUTIONS & CONSIDERATIONS
Caution should be used with history of alcoholism. It is unknown if zileuton crosses the placenta or is distributed in breast milk. Zileuton use is not recommended in breast-feeding women. Safety and efficacy of this drug have not been established in children younger than 12 years of age. There are no age-related precautions noted in the elderly.

Zileuton is not for the treatment of acute asthma episodes. Increase fluid intake to decrease the viscosity of lung secretions.
Storage
Store at room temperature.
Administration
Take without food. Do not alter the dosage or abruptly discontinue the medication.

Zinc Oxide/Zinc Sulfate
zink ox'ide zink sul'fate
(Balmex, Desitin) (Orazinc)

CATEGORY AND SCHEDULE
Pregnancy Risk Category: C

CLASSIFICATION
Chelating agent, ophthalmic astringent, trace element

MECHANISM OF ACTION
A mineral that acts as a co-factor for enzymes that are important for protein and carbohydrate metabolism. Therapeutic Effect: Zinc oxide acts as a mild astringent and skin protectant.

Zinc sulfate helps maintain normal growth and tissue repair as well as skin hydration.

AVAILABILITY
Zinc Oxide
Ointment: 10%, 20%, 40%.
Zinc Sulfate
Capsules: 110 mg, 220 mg.
Tablets: 110 mg.
Injection: 1 mg/ml.

INDICATIONS AND DOSAGES
▶ **Mild skin irritations and abrasions (such as chapped skin, diaper rash)**
TOPICAL (OXIDE)
Adults, Elderly, Children. Apply as needed.
▶ **Treatment and prevention of zinc deficiency, wound healing.**
PO (SULFATE)
Adults, Elderly. 220 mg 3 times a day.

CONTRAINDICATIONS
None known.

INTERACTIONS
Drug
H blockers (such as famotidine): May decrease zinc absorption.
Quinolones (such as ciprofloxacin, tetracycline): May decrease the absorption of these drugs.
Herbals
None known.
Food
Coffee, dairy products: May decrease zinc absorption.

DIAGNOSTIC TEST EFFECTS
None known.

SIDE EFFECTS
None known.

SERIOUS REACTIONS
• None known.

PRECAUTIONS & CONSIDERATIONS
Don't exceed the prescribed dosage. Excessive zinc intake can cause impaired leukocyte function, a reduction in HDL levels, and vomiting. Coffee and dairy products may decrease the absorption of oral zinc sulfate capsules and tablets.
   Skin integrity should be monitored for signs of improvement. Notify the physician if the skin condition doesn't improve after 7 days of treatment.
Administration
Take oral zinc sulfate with food.
   For topical use, apply zinc oxide after cleaning and drying the affected area. Zinc oxide is for external use only. Avoid use in the eyes.

Ziprasidone
zye-pray′za-done
(Geodon)

CATEGORY AND SCHEDULE
Pregnancy Risk Category: C

CLASSIFICATION
Antipsychotics

MECHANISM OF ACTION
A piperazine derivative that antagonizes alpha-adrenergic, dopamine, histamine, and serotonin receptors; also inhibits reuptake of serotonin and norepinephrine. *Therapeutic Effect:* Diminishes symptoms of schizophrenia and depression.

PHARMACOKINETICS
Well absorbed after PO administration. Food increases bioavailability. Protein binding: 99%. Extensively metabolized in the liver. Not removed by hemodialysis. **Half-life:** 7 hr.

Z

AVAILABILITY
Capsules: 20 mg, 40 mg, 60 mg, 80 mg.
Injection: 20 mg/ml.

INDICATIONS AND DOSAGES
▸ **Schizophrenia**
PO
Adults, Elderly. Initially, 20 mg twice a day with food. Titrate at intervals of no less than 2 days. Maximum: 80 mg twice a day.
IM
Adults, Elderly. 10 mg q2hr or 20 mg q4hr. Maximum: 40 mg/day.
▸ **Bipolar mania**
PO
Adults, Elderly. 40 mg 2 times/day.

CONTRAINDICATIONS
Conditions that prolong the QT interval, such as congenital long QT syndrome

INTERACTIONS
Drug
Alcohol, other CNS depressants: May increase CNS depression.
Carbamazepine: May decrease ziprasidone blood concentration.
Ketoconazole: May increase ziprasidone blood concentration.
Herbal
None known.
Food
All foods: Enhance the bioavailability of ziprasidone.

DIAGNOSTIC TEST EFFECTS
May prolong the QT interval.

SIDE EFFECTS
Frequent (30%-16%)
Headache, somnolence, dizziness
Occasional
Rash, orthostatic hypotension, weight gain, restlessness, constipation, dyspepsia

SERIOUS REACTIONS
• Prolongation of QT interval may produce torsades de pointes, a form of ventricular tachycardia. Patients with bradycardia, hypokalemia, or hypomagnesemia are at increased risk.

PRECAUTIONS & CONSIDERATIONS
Caution is warranted with bradycardia, hypokalemia, and hypomagnesemia because of a greater risk for developing torsades de pointes or atypical ventricular tachycardia. It is unknown if ziprasidone crosses the placenta or is distributed in breast milk. The safety and efficacy of ziprasidone have not been established in children. No age-related precautions have been noted in the elderly.

Drowsiness may occur, so tasks that require mental alertness or motor skills should be avoided. EKG and blood chemistries to check for magnesium and potassium levels should be obtained before beginning therapy and routinely thereafter.
Storage
Store vials at room temperature, and protect them from light. The reconstituted solution is stable for 24 hours at room temperature or 7 days refrigerated.
Administration
Take ziprasidone with food to increase its bioavailability.

For IM use, reconstitute each vial with 1.2 ml sterile water for injection to provide a concentration of 20 mg/ml.

Zoledronic Acid
zole-eh-drone'ick
(Zometa)

CATEGORY AND SCHEDULE
Pregnancy Risk Category: C

CLASSIFICATION
Bisphosphonates

MECHANISM OF ACTION
A bisphosphonate that inhibits the resorption of mineralized bone and cartilage; inhibits increased osteoclastic activity and skeletal calcium release induced by stimulatory factors produced by tumors. *Therapeutic Effect:* Increases urinary calcium and phosphorus excretion; decreases serum calcium and phosphorus levels.

AVAILABILITY
Injection Powder for Reconstitution: 4 mg.
Injection Solution: 4 mg/5 ml.

INDICATIONS AND DOSAGES
▸ **Hypercalcemia**
IV INFUSION
Adults, Elderly. 4 mg IV infusion given over no less than 15 min. Retreatment may be considered, but at least 7 days should elapse to allow for full response to initial dose.
▸ **Multiple myeloma**
IV
Adults, Elderly. 4 mg q3-4wk.

CONTRAINDICATIONS
Hypersensitivity to other bisphosphonates, including alendronate, etidronate, pamidronate, risedronate, and tiludronate

INTERACTIONS
Drug
Calcium-containing medications, vitamin D: May antagonize the effects of zoledronic acid in treatment of hypercalcemia.
Herbal
None known.
Food
None known.

DIAGNOSTIC TEST EFFECTS
May decrease serum magnesium, calcium, and phosphate levels.

▩ IV INCOMPATIBILITIES
Do not mix with other medications.

SIDE EFFECTS
Frequent (44%-26%)
Fever, nausea, vomiting, constipation
Occasional (15%-10%)
Hypotension, anxiety, insomnia, flu-like symptoms (fever, chills, bone pain, myalgia, and arthralgia), nausea, vomiting, constipation
Rare
Conjunctivitis

SERIOUS REACTIONS
• Renal toxicity may occur if IV infusion is administered in less than 15 minutes.

PRECAUTIONS & CONSIDERATIONS
Caution is warranted with history of aspirin-sensitive asthma or hypoparathyroidism, renal impairment, and risk of hypocalcemia. Because there are no adequate and well-controlled studies in pregnant women, it is unknown if zoledronic acid causes fetal harm or is excreted in breast milk. Safety and efficacy of zoledronic acid have not been established in children. Age-related renal impairment may require cautious use or dosage adjustment in the elderly. Avoid drugs containing calcium and

Z

vitamin D, such as antacids, because they might antagonize the effects of zoledronic acid.

Notify the physician of fever. CBC, Hgb, Hct, renal function test results, intake and output, and serum electrolytes, including serum calcium, magnesium, and phosphate levels should be established. Be aware that adequate hydration should be maintained before administering zoledronic acid.

Storage
Store at room temperature. If not used immediately, reconstituted solution should be refrigerated; time from reconstitution to end of administration should not exceed 24 hours

Administration
Reconstitute 4-mg vial with 5 ml sterile water for injection. Allow drug to dissolve before withdrawing. Further dilute with 100 ml 0.9% NaCl or D_5W. Adequate hydration is essential during zoledronic acid administration. Administer as an IV infusion over not less than 15 minutes. Infusing over less than 15 minutes increases the risk of renal function deterioration.

Zolmitriptan
zohl-mih-trip′tan
(Zomig, Zomig Rapimelt [CAN], Zomig-ZMT)

CATEGORY AND SCHEDULE
Pregnancy Risk Category: C

CLASSIFICATION
Serotonin receptor agonists

MECHANISM OF ACTION
A serotonin receptor agonist that binds selectively to vascular receptors, producing a vasoconstrictive effect on cranial blood vessels. *Therapeutic Effect:* Relieves migraine headache.

PHARMACOKINETICS
Rapidly but incompletely absorbed after PO administration. Protein binding: 15%. Undergoes first-pass metabolism in the liver to active metabolite. Eliminated primarily in urine (60%) and, to a lesser extent, in feces (30%). **Half-life:** 3 hr.

AVAILABILITY
Tablets (Zomig): 2.5 mg, 5 mg.
Tablets (Orally Disintegrating [Zomig-ZMT]): 2.5 mg, 5 mg.
Nasal Spray (Zomig): 5 mg/0.1 ml.

INDICATIONS AND DOSAGES
▶ **Acute migraine attack**
PO
Adults, Elderly, Children older than 18 yr. Initially, 2.5 mg or less. If headache returns, may repeat dose in 2 hr. Maximum: 10 mg/24 hr.
INTRANASAL
Adults, Elderly. 5 mg. May repeat in 2 hr. Maximum: 10 mg/24 hr.

CONTRAINDICATIONS
Arrhythmias associated with conduction disorders, basilar or hemiplegic migraine, coronary artery disease, ischemic heart disease (including angina pectoris, history of MI, silent ischemia, and Prinzmetal's angina), uncontrolled hypertension, use within 24 hr of ergotamine-containing preparations or another serotonin receptor agonist, use within 14 days of MAOIs, Wolff-Parkinson-White syndrome

INTERACTIONS
Drug
Ergotamine-containing medications: May produce a vasospastic reaction.

Fluoxetine, fluvoxamine, paroxetine, sertraline: May produce hyperreflexia, incoordination, and weakness.
MAOIs: May dramatically increase plasma concentration of zolmitriptan.
Oral contraceptives: Decrease zolmitriptan clearance and volume of distribution.
Herbal
None known.
Food
None known.

DIAGNOSTIC TEST EFFECTS
None known.

SIDE EFFECTS
Frequent (8%-6%)
Oral: Dizziness; tingling; neck, throat, or jaw pressure; somnolence
Nasal: Altered taste, paraesthesia
Occasional (5%-3%)
Oral: Warm or hot sensation, asthenia, chest pressure
Nasal: Nausea, somnolence, nasal discomfort, dizziness, asthenia, dry mouth
Rare (2%-1%)
Diaphoresis, myalgia, paresthesia

SERIOUS REACTIONS
• Cardiac reactions (including ischemia, coronary artery vasospasm, and MI) and noncardiac vasospasm-related reactions (such as hemorrhage and CVA) occur rarely, particularly in patients with hypertension, diabetes, or a strong family history of coronary artery disease; obese patients; smokers; males older than 40 years; and postmenopausal women.

PRECAUTIONS & CONSIDERATIONS
Caution is warranted with controlled hypertension, a history of CVA, mild to moderate hepatic or renal impairment, and cardiovascular risk factors.

It is unknown if zolmitriptan is distributed in breast milk. The safety and efficacy of zolmitriptan have not been established in children younger than 12 years. No age-related precautions have been noted in the elderly. Tasks that require mental alertness or motor skills should be avoided.

Dizziness may occur. Notify the physician immediately if blood in urine or stool, chest pain, palpitations, easy bruising, numbness or pain in the arms or legs, throat tightness, or swelling of the eyelids, face, or lips occurs. B/P and hepatic function should be assessed. Migraines and associated symptoms, including nausea and vomiting, photophobia, and phonophobia (sound sensitivity) should be assessed before and during treatment.

Administration
Take oral zolmitriptan without regard to food.

For nasal use, blow nose gently to clear nasal passages. With the head upright, close one of the nostrils with an index finger and breathe gently through the mouth. Insert the nozzle about ½ inch into the open nostril. Close mouth, then take a breath through the nose while depressing the plunger and releasing the spray. Remove the nozzle from the nose, and gently breathe in through the nose and out through the mouth for 15-20 seconds. Do not breathe in deeply.

Z

Zolpidem

zole-pi′dem

(Ambien, Stilnox [AUS])

Do not confuse Ambien with Amen.

CATEGORY AND SCHEDULE

Pregnancy Risk Category: B

Controlled Substance

Schedule: IV

CLASSIFICATION

Sedatives/hypnotics

MECHANISM OF ACTION

A nonbenzodiazepine that enhances the action of the inhibitory neurotransmitter gamma-aminobutyric acid. *Therapeutic Effect:* Induces sleep and improves sleep quality.

PHARMACOKINETICS

Route	Onset	Peak	Duration
PO	30 min	N/A	6-8 hr

Rapidly absorbed from the GI tract. Protein binding: 92%. Metabolized in the liver; excreted in urine. Not removed by hemodialysis. **Half-life:** 1.4-4.5 hr (increased in hepatic impairment).

AVAILABILITY

Tablets: 5 mg, 10 mg.

INDICATIONS AND DOSAGES

▸ Insomnia

PO

Adults. 10 mg at bedtime.

Elderly, Debilitated. 5 mg at bedtime.

CONTRAINDICATIONS

None known.

INTERACTIONS

Drug

Alcohol, other CNS depressants: May increase CNS depression.

Herbal

None known.

Food

None known.

DIAGNOSTIC TEST EFFECTS

None known.

SIDE EFFECTS

Occasional (7%)

Headache

Rare (less than 2%)

Dizziness, nausea, diarrhea, muscle pain

SERIOUS REACTIONS

• Overdose may produce severe ataxia, bradycardia, altered vision (such as diplopia), severe drowsiness, nausea and vomiting, difficulty breathing, and unconsciousness.

• Abrupt withdrawal of the drug after long-term use may produce asthenia, facial flushing, diaphoresis, vomiting, and tremor.

• Drug tolerance or dependence may occur with prolonged, high-dose therapy.

PRECAUTIONS & CONSIDERATIONS

Caution is warranted with depression, hepatic impairment, and a history of drug dependence. It is unknown if zolpidem crosses the placenta or is distributed in breast milk. The safety and efficacy of zolpidem have not been established in children. In the elderly, age-related hepatic impairment and an increased susceptibility to falls or confusion may require a dosage adjustment. Be aware that this drug may cause dependence or tolerance with prolonged use.

Drowsiness may occur. Avoid alcohol, CNS depressants, and tasks that require mental alertness or motor skills. B/P, pulse rate, and respiratory rate, rhythm, and depth should be assessed immediately before administering zolpidem. Therapeutic response, such as decrease in the number of nocturnal awakenings and an increased duration of sleep, should be monitored.

Administration

For faster sleep onset, take zolpidem on an empty stomach. Do not abruptly discontinue the drug after long-term use.

Zonisamide
zoh-nis′a-mide
(Zonegran)

CATEGORY AND SCHEDULE
Pregnancy Risk Category: C

CLASSIFICATION
Anticonvulsants

MECHANISM OF ACTION
A succinimide that may stabilize neuronal membranes and suppress neuronal hypersynchronization by blocking sodium and calcium channels. *Therapeutic Effect:* Reduces seizure activity.

PHARMACOKINETICS
Well absorbed after PO administration. Extensively bound to RBCs. Protein binding: 40%. Primarily excreted in urine. **Half-life:** 63 hr (plasma), 105 hr (RBCs).

AVAILABILITY
Capsules: 25 mg, 50 mg, 100 mg.

INDICATIONS AND DOSAGES
▸ **Partial seizures**
PO
Adults, Elderly, Children older than 16 yr. Initially, 100 mg/day for 2 wk. May increase by 100 mg/day at intervals of 2 wk or longer. Range: 100-600 mg/day.

OFF-LABEL USES
Treatment of obesity, weight loss

CONTRAINDICATIONS
Allergy to sulfonamides

INTERACTIONS
Drug
Alcohol, other CNS depressants: May increase zonisamide's sedative effect.
Carbamazepine, phenobarbital, phenytoin, valproic acid: May increase the metabolism and decrease the effect of zonisamide.
Herbal
None known.
Food
None known.

DIAGNOSTIC TEST EFFECTS
May increase BUN and serum creatinine levels.

SIDE EFFECTS
Frequent (17%-9%)
Somnolence, dizziness, anorexia, headache, agitation, irritability, nausea
Occasional (8%-5%)
Fatigue, ataxia, confusion, depression, impaired memory or concentration, insomnia, abdominal pain, diplopia, diarrhea, speech difficulty
Rare (4%-3%)
Paresthesia, nystagmus, anxiety, rash, dyspepsia, weight loss

Z

SERIOUS REACTIONS

• Overdose is characterized by bradycardia, hypotension, respiratory depression, and coma.
• Leukopenia, anemia, and thrombocytopenia occur rarely.

PRECAUTIONS & CONSIDERATIONS

Caution is warranted with renal impairment. It is unknown if zonisamide is distributed in breast milk. The safety and efficacy of this drug have not been established in children younger than 16 years. Lower dosages are recommended for the elderly, although no age-related precautions have been noted for this age-group.

Drowsiness and dizziness may occur, so alcohol and tasks requiring mental alertness or motor skills should be avoided. Notify the physician of abdominal or back pain, blood in urine, easy bruising, fever, rash, sore throat, or ulcers in the mouth. Seizure disorder, including the onset, duration, frequency, intensity, and type of seizures, should be assessed before and during treatment. CBC and blood chemistry tests to assess renal and hepatic function should be performed before and periodically during therapy.

Administration

Take zonisamide without regard to food. Swallow the capsules whole. Don't take this drug if allergic to sulfonamides. Do not abruptly discontinue zonisamide after long-term use because this may precipitate seizures. Strict maintenance of drug therapy is essential for seizure control.

Appendixes

Appendix A
Anesthetics: General

Appendix B
Anesthetics: Local

Appendix C
Controlled Drugs (United States)

Appendix D
Cultural Aspects of Drug Therapy

Appendix E
Drugs of Abuse

Appendix F
English-to-Spanish Drug Phrases
    Translator

Appendix G
FDA Pregnancy Categories

Appendix H
Normal Laboratory Values

Appendix I
Signs and Symptoms of Electrolyte
    Imbalance

Appendix J
Techniques of Medication
    Administration

Appendix K
Insulins Table

Appendix L
Medication Math

Appendix M
Error-Prone Drug Name
    Abbreviations

APPENDIXES

APPENDIX A
Anesthetics: General

Uses	Action
IV anesthetic agents are used to induce general anesthesia. The general anesthetic state consists of unconsciousness, amnesia, analgesia, immobility, and attenuation of autonomic responses to noxious stimuli. *Volatile inhalation agents* produce all the components of the anesthetic state but are administered through the lungs via an anesthesia machine. Agents for use include desflurane, enflurane, halothane, isoflurane, and sevoflurane. They're used in practice to maintain general anesthesia.	*IV anesthetic agents* act on the gamma-aminobutyric acid (GABA) receptor complex to produce central nervous system (CNS) depression. GABA is the primary inhibitory neurotransmitter in the CNS. Ketamine produces dissociation between the thalamus and the limbic system. *Volatile inhalation agents* aren't fully understood, but may disrupt neuronal transmission throughout the CNS. These agents may either block excitatory or enhance inhibitory transmission through axons or synapses.

Anesthetics: General

Name	Availability	Uses	Dosage Range	Side Effects
Etomidate (Amidate)	I: 2 mg/ml	IV induction	0.2-0.6 mg/kg	Myoclonus, pain on injection, nausea, vomiting, respiratory depression
Ketamine (Ketalar)	I: 10 mg/ml, 50 mg/ml, 100 mg/ml	Analgesia, sedation, IV induction	1-4.5 mg/kg	Delirium, euphoria, nausea, vomiting
Methohexital (Brevital)	Powder for injection: 500 mg	IV induction, sedation	50-120 mg	Cardiovascular depression, myoclonus, nausea, vomiting, respiratory depression
Midazolam (Versed)	I: 1 mg/ml, 5 mg/ml	Anxiolytic, amnesic, sedation	1-5 mg titrated slowly	Respiratory depression
Propofol (Diprivan)	I: 10 mg/ml	Sedation IV induction Maintenance	0.5 mg/kg 2-2.5 mg/kg 100-200 mcg/kg/min	Cardiovascular depression, delirium, euphoria, pain on injection, respiratory depression
Thiopental (Pentothal)	Powder for injection: 2.5% (25 mg/ml)	IV induction	Titrate vs. pt response. **Average:** 50-75 mg	Cardiovascular depression, nausea, vomiting, respiratory depression

I, Injection; *IV,* intravenous; *pt,* patient. (From *Mosby's 2006 Drug Consult for Nurses.* St. Louis, 2006, Mosby.)

APPENDIX B
Anesthetics: Local

Uses	Action
Local anesthetics suppress pain by blocking impulses along axons. Suppression of pain does not cause generalized depression of the entire nervous system. Local anesthetics may be given topically and by injection (local infiltration, peripheral nerve block [axillary], IV regional [bier block], epidural, and spinal).	Most local anesthetics fall into one of two groups: esters or amides. Both provide anesthesia and analgesia by reversibly binding to and blocking sodium (Na) channels. This slows the rate of depolarization of the nerve action potential, thus propagation of the electrical impulses needed for nerve conduction is prevented.

Anesthetics: Local

Name	Uses	Onset (min)	Duration (hr)	Side Effects*
ESTERS **Chloroprocaine** (Nesacaine)	Local infiltrate Nerve block Spinal	6-12	0.25-0.5	Excitation (e.g., seizures) followed by decreased level of consciousness (drowsiness to unconsciousness), bradycardia, heart block, decreased myocardial contractile force, hypotension, hypersensitivity reaction
Procaine (Novocain)	Local infiltrate Nerve block Spinal	2-5	0.25-1	Same as above
Tetracaine	Topical Spinal	15	2-3	Same as above
AMIDES **Bupivacaine** (Marcaine, Sensorcaine)	Local infiltrate Nerve block Epidural Spinal	5	2-4	Same as above

Continued

Name	Uses	Onset (min)	Duration (hr)	Side Effects*
Etidocaine (Duranest)	Local infiltrate Nerve block Epidural	3-5	5-10	Same as above
Levobupi- vacaine (Chirocaine)	Nerve block Epidural	—	—	Same as above
Lidocaine	Local infiltrate Nerve block Spinal Epidural Topical IV regional	300	0.5-1	Same as above
Mepivacaine (Carbocaine, Polocaine)	Local infiltrate Nerve block Epidural	300	0.75-1.5	Same as above
Ropivacaine (Naropin)	Local infiltrate Nerve block Epidural Spinal	200	2-6	Same as above

*Most side effects are manifestations of excessive plasma concentrations.
Fast, Less than 1 hour; *moderate,* 1-3 hours; *long,* 3-12 hours. (From *Mosby's 2006 Drug Consult for Nurses.* St. Louis, 2006, Mosby.)

CONTROLLED DRUGS (UNITED STATES)

Schedule I: Medications having no legal medical use. These substances may be used for research purposes with proper registration (e.g., heroin, LSD).

Schedule II: Medications having a legitimate medical use but are characterized by a very high abuse potential and/or potential for severe physical and psychic dependency. Emergency telephone orders for limited quantities of these drugs are authorized, but the prescriber must provide a written, signed prescription order (e.g., morphine, amphetamines).

Schedule III: Medications having significant abuse potential (less than Schedule II). Telephone orders are permitted (e.g., opiates in combination with other substances such as acetaminophen).

Schedule IV: Medications having a low abuse potential. Telephone orders are permitted (e.g., benzodiazepines, propoxyphene).

Schedule V: Medications having the lowest abuse potential of the controlled substances. Some Schedule V products may be available without a prescription (e.g., certain cough preparations containing limited amounts of an opiate).

(From *Mosby's 2006 Drug Consult for Nurses.* St. Louis, 2006, Mosby.)

CULTURAL ASPECTS OF DRUG THERAPY

The term *ethnopharmacology* was first used to describe the study of medicinal plants used by indigenous cultures. More recently, it is being used as a reference to the action and effects of drugs in people from diverse racial, ethnic, and cultural backgrounds. Although there are insufficient data from investigations involving people from diverse backgrounds that would provide reliable information on ethnic-specific responses to all medications, there is growing evidence that modifications in dosages are needed for some members of racial and ethnic groups. There are wide variations in the perception of side effects by patients from diverse cultural backgrounds. These differences may be related to metabolic differences that result in higher or lower levels of the drug, individual differences in the amount of body fat, or cultural differences in the way individuals perceive the meaning of side effects and toxicity. Nurses and other health care providers need to be aware that variations can occur with side effects, adverse reactions, and toxicity so that patients from diverse cultural backgrounds can be monitored.

Some cultural differences in response to medications include the following:

African Americans: Generally, African Americans are less responsive to beta-blockers (e.g., propranolol [Inderal]) and angiotensin-converting enzyme (ACE) inhibitors (e.g., enalapril [Vasotec]).

Asian Americans: On average, Asian Americans have a lower percentage of body fat, so dosage adjustments must be made for fat-soluble vitamins and other drugs (e.g., vitamin K used to reverse the anticoagulant effect of warfarin).

Hispanic Americans: Hispanic Americans may require lower dosages and may experience a higher incidence of side effects with the tricyclic antidepressants (e.g., amitryptyline).

Native Americans: Alaskan Eskimos may suffer prolonged muscle paralysis with the use of succinylcholine when administered during surgery.

There has been a desire to exert more responsibility over one's health and, as a result, a resurgence of self-care practices. These practices are often influenced by folk remedies and the use of medicinal plants. In the United States, there are several major ethnic population subgroups (white, black, Hispanic, Asian, and Native Americans). Each of these ethnic groups has a wide range of practices that influence beliefs and interventions related to health and illness. At any given time, in any group, treatment may consist of the use of traditional herbal therapy, a combination of ritual and prayer with medicinal plants, customary dietary and environmental practices, or the use of Western medical practices.

AFRICAN AMERICANS

Many African Americans carry the traditional health beliefs of their African heritage. Health denotes harmony with nature of the body, mind, and spirit, whereas illness is seen as disharmony that results from natural causes or divine punishment. Common practices to the art of healing include treatments with herbals and rituals known empirically to restore health. Specific forms of healing include using home remedies, obtaining medical advice from a physician, and seeking spiritual healing.

Examples of healing practices include the use of hot baths and warm compresses for rheumatism, the use of herbal teas for respiratory illnesses, and the use of kitchen condiments in folk remedies. Lemon, vinegar, honey, saltpeter, alum, salt, baking soda, and Epsom salt are common kitchen ingredients used. Goldenrod, peppermint, sassafras, parsley, yarrow, and rabbit tobacco are a few of the herbals used.

HISPANIC AMERICANS

The use of folk healers, medicinal herbs, magic, and religious rituals and ceremonies are included in the rich and varied customs of Hispanic Americans. This ethnic group believes that God is responsible for allowing health or illness to occur. Wellness may be viewed as good luck, a reward for good behavior, or a blessing from God. Praying, using herbals and spices, wearing religious objects such as medals, and maintaining a balance in diet and physical activity are methods considered appropriate in preventing evil or poor health.

Hispanic ethnopharmacology is more complementary to Western medical practices. After the illness is identified, appropriate treatment may consist of home remedies (e.g., use of vegetables and herbs), use of over-the-counter patent medicines, and use of physician-prescribed medications.

ASIAN AMERICANS

For Asian Americans, harmony with nature is essential for physical and spiritual well-being. Universal balance depends on harmony among the elemental forces: fire, water, wood, earth, and metal. Regulating these universal elements are two forces that maintain physical and spiritual harmony in the body: the *yin* and the *yang*. Practices shared by most Asian cultures include meditation, special nutritional programs, herbology, and martial arts. Therapeutic options available to the traditional Chinese physicians include prescribing herbs, meditation, exercise, nutritional changes, or acupuncture.

NATIVE AMERICANS

The theme of total harmony with nature is fundamental to traditional Native American beliefs about health. It is dependent on maintaining a state of equilibrium among the physical body, the mind, and the environment. Health practices reflect this holistic approach. The method of healing is determined traditionally by the medicine man, who diagnoses the ailment and recommends the appropriate intervention.

Treatment may include heat, herbs, sweat baths, massage, exercise, diet changes, or other interventions performed in a curing ceremony.

EUROPEAN AMERICANS

Europeans often use home treatments as the front-line interventions. Traditional remedies practiced are based on the magical or empirically validated experience of ancestors. These cures are often practiced in combination with religious rituals or spiritual ceremonies.

Household products, herbal teas, and patent medicines are familiar preparations used in home treatments (e.g., salt water gargle for sore throat).

(Adapted from *Mosby's 2006 Drug Consult for Nurses*. St. Louis, 2006, Mosby.)

DRUGS OF ABUSE

Name (Brand)	Class	Signs and Symptoms	Treatment
Acid (see LSD)			
Adam (see MDMA)			
Amphetamine (Adderall, Dexedrine)	Stimulant	Tachycardia, hypertension, diaphoresis, agitation, headache, seizures, dehydration, hypokalemia, lactic acidosis. Severe overdose: hyperthermia, dysrhythmia, shock, rhabdomyolysis, liver necrosis, acute renal failure.	Control agitation, reverse hyperthermia, support hemodynamic function. **Antidote:** No specific antidote.
Angel dust (see phencyclidine)			
Apache (see fentanyl)			
Barbiturates (Nembutal, Seconal)	Depressant	Hypotension, hypothermia, apnea, nystagmus, ataxia, hyporeflexia, somnolence, stupor, coma.	Airway management, decontamination, supportive care. **Antidote:** No specific antidote.
Barbs (see barbiturates)			
Benzodiazepines (Xanax, Valium, Librium, Halcion)	Depressant	Respiratory depression, hypothermia, hypotension, nystagmus, miosis, diplopia, bradycardia, nausea, vomiting, impaired speech and coordination, amnesia, ataxia, somnolence, confusion, depressed deep tendon reflexes.	**Antidote:** Flumazenil (Romazicon) is a specific antidote
Black tar (see heroin)			
Horse (see heroin)			
Boomers (see LSD)			
Buttons (see mescaline)			

Cactus (see mescaline)			
Candy (see benzodiazepines)			
China girl (see fentanyl)			
China white (see heroin)			
Cocaine	Stimulant	Hypertension, tachycardia, mild hyperthermia, mydriasis, pallor, diaphoresis, psychosis, paranoid delusions, mania, agitation, seizures.	Control agitation, seizures, hyperthermia, support hemodynamic function. **Antidote:** No specific antidote.
Codeine	Opioid	Miosis, respiratory depression, decreased mental status, hypotension, cardiac dysrhythmia, hypoxia, bronchoconstriction, constipation, decreased intestinal motility, ileus, lethargy, coma.	Airway management, hemodynamic support. **Antidote:** Naloxone, nalmefene.
Coke (see cocaine)			
Crank (see amphetamine)			
Crank (see heroin)			
Crystal (see amphetamine)			
Crystal meth (see methamphetamine)			
Cubes (see LSD)			
Downers (see benzodiazepines)			
Ecstasy (see MDMA)			

Continued

(Adapted from *Mosby's 2006 Drug Consult for Nurses*. St. Louis, 2006, Mosby.)

Name (Brand)	Class	Signs and Symptoms	Treatment
Fentanyl (Sublimaze)	Opioid	Miosis, respiratory depression, decreased mental status, hypotension, cardiac dysrhythmia, hypoxia, bronchoconstriction, constipation, decreased intestinal motility, ileus, lethargy, coma.	Airway management, hemodynamic support. **Antidote:** Naloxone, nalmefene.
Flunitrazepam (Rohypnol)	Depressant	Drowsiness, slurred speech, impaired judgment and motor skills, hypothermia, hypotension, bradycardia, diplopia, blurred vision, nystagmus, respiratory depression, nausea, constipation, depression, lethargy, headache, ataxia, coma, amnesia, incoordination, tremors, vertigo.	Supportive care, airway control. **Antidote:** Flumazenil (Romazicon).
Forget me pill (see flunitrazepam)			
GHB (gamma-hydroxybutyrate)	CNS depressant	Dose-related CNS depression, amnesia, hypotonia, drowsiness, dizziness, euphoria. Other effects: bradycardia, hypotension, hypersalivation, vomiting, hypothermia. Higher dosages: Cheyne-Stokes respiration, seizures, coma, death. Users become highly agitated.	Supportive care. Severe intoxication may require airway support, including intubation. **Antidote:** No specific antidote.
Gib (see GHB)			
Goodfellas (see fentanyl)			
Grass (see marijuana)			
Hashish (see marijuana)			
Heroin	Opioid	Miosis, coma, apnea, pulmonary edema, bradycardia, hypotension, pinpoint pupils, CNS depression, seizures.	Airway management. **Antidote:** Naloxone, nalmefene.

Ice (see amphetamine)			
Ketamine (Ketalar)	Anesthetic	Feeling of dissociation from one's self (sense of floating over one's body), visual hallucinations, lack of coordination, hypertension, tachycardia, palpitations, respiratory depression, apnea, confusion, negativism, hostility, delirium, reduced awareness.	Supportive care, esp. respiratory and cardiac function. **Antidote:** No specific antidote.
Keets (see ketamine)			
Kit-kat (see ketamine)			
Liquid ecstasy (see GHB)			
Liquid X (see GHB)			
LSD	Hallucinogen	Diaphoresis, mydriasis, dizziness, twitching, flushing, hyperreflexia, hypertension, psychosis, behavioral changes, emotional lability, euphoria or dysphoria, paranoia, vomiting, diarrhea, anorexia, restlessness, incoordination, tremors, ataxia.	Airway management, control activity associated with hallucinations, psychosis, panic reaction. **Antidote:** No specific antidote.
Ludes (see methaqualone)			
Magic mushroom (see psilocybin)			
Marijuana	Cannabinoid	Increased appetite, reduced motility, constipation, urinary retention, seizures, euphoria, somnolence, heightened awareness, relaxation, altered time perception, short-term memory loss, poor concentration, mood alterations, disorientation, decreased strength, ataxia, slurred speech, respiratory depression, coma.	Airway management, supportive care. **Antidote:** No specific antidote.

Continued

Name (Brand)	Class	Signs and Symptoms	Treatment
MDMA (Methylene dioxymethamphetamine)	Stimulant	Euphoria, intimacy, closeness to others, loss of appetite, tachycardia, jaw tension, bruxism, diaphoresis.	Antidote: No specific antidote.
Mescaline	Hallucinogen	Diaphoresis, mydriasis, dizziness, twitching, flushing, hyperreflexia, hypertension, psychosis, behavioral changes, emotional instability, euphoria or dysphoria, paranoia, vomiting, diarrhea, anorexia, restlessness, incoordination, tremors, ataxia.	Airway management, control activity associated with hallucinations, psychosis, panic reaction. Antidote: No specific antidote.
Meth (see methamphetamine)			
Methamphetamine (Desoxyn)	Stimulant	Hypertension, hyperthermia, hyperpyrexia, agitation, hyperactivity, fasciculation, seizures, coma, tachycardia, dysrhythmias, pale skin, diaphoresis, restlessness, talkativeness, insomnia, headache, coma, delusions, paranoia, aggressive behavior, visual, tactile, or auditory hallucinations.	Airway control, hyperthermia, seizures, dysrhythmias. Antidote: No specific antidote.
Methaqualone (Quaalude)	Depressant	Slurred speech, impaired judgment and motor skills, hypothermia, hypotension, bradycardia, diplopia, blurred vision, nystagmus, mydriasis, respiratory depression, depression, lethargy, headache, ataxia, coma, amnesia, incoordination, hypertonicity, myoclonus, tremors, vertigo.	Airway management, supportive care. Antidote: No specific antidote.
Methylphenidate (Ritalin) Seizures	Stimulant	Agitation, hypertension, tachycardia, hyperthermia, mydriasis, dry mouth, nausea, vomiting, anorexia, abdominal pain, agitation, hyperactivity, insomnia, euphoria, dizziness, paranoid ideation, social withdrawal, delirium, hallucinations, psychosis, tremors, seizures.	Control agitation, hyperthermia, seizures, support hemodynamic function. Antidote: No specific antidote.

Miss Emma (see morphine)		
Mister blue (see morphine)		
Morphine (MS-Contin, Roxanol)	Opioid	Miosis, respiratory depression, decreased mental status, hypotension, cardiac dysrhythmia, hypoxia, bronchoconstriction, constipation, decreased intestinal motility, ileus, lethargy, coma.	Airway management, hemodynamic support. **Antidote:** Naloxone, nalmefene.
Oxy (see oxycodone)		
Oxycodone (OxyContin)	Opioid	Miosis, respiratory depression, decreased mental status, hypotension, cardiac dysrhythmia, hypoxia, bronchoconstriction, constipation, decreased intestinal motility, ileus, lethargy, coma.	Airway management, hemodynamic support. **Antidote:** Naloxone, nalmefene
OxyContin (see oxycodone)		
Peace pill (see phencyclidine)		
Phencyclidine (PCP)	Hallucinogen	Nystagmus, hypertension, tachycardia, agitation, hallucinations, violent behavior, impaired judgment, delusions, psychosis.	Support blood pressure, manage airway, control agitation. **Antidote:** No specific antidote.
Phennies (see barbiturates)		
Pot (see marijuana)		
Propoxyphene (Darvon)	Depressant	Respiratory depression, seizures, cardiac toxicity, miosis, dysrhythmias, nausea, vomiting, anorexia, abdominal pain, constipation, drowsiness, coma, confusion, hallucinations.	Maintain airway, seizures, cardiac toxicity. **Antidote:** Naloxone.

Continued

Name (Brand)	Class	Signs and Symptoms	Treatment
Psilocybin	Hallucinogen	Diaphoresis, mydriasis, dizziness, twitching, flushing, hyperreflexia, hypertension, psychosis, behavioral changes, emotional lability, euphoria or dysphoria, paranoia, vomiting, diarrhea, anorexia, restlessness, incoordination, tremors, ataxia.	Manage airway, control activity associated with hallucinations, psychosis, panic reaction. **Antidote:** No specific antidote.
Purple passion (see psilocybin)			
Quay (see methaqualone)			
Reefer (see marijuana)			
Rock (see cocaine)			
Rocket fuel (see phencyclidine)			
Roofies (see flunitrazepam)			
Rope (see flunitrazepam)			
Rophies (see flunitrazepam)			
Salty water (see GHB)			
Schoolboy (see codeine)			
Scoop (see GHB)			
Snow (see cocaine)			
Special K (see ketamine)			

Speed (see amphetamine)		
STP (see MDMA)		
Super acid (see ketamine)		
Super K (see ketamine)		
Tranks (see benzodiazepines)		
Uppers (see amphetamine)		
White girl (see cocaine)		
Yellow jackets (see barbiturates)		
Yellow sunshine (see LSD)		

"CLUB DRUG" WEB SITES
www.drugfreeamerica.org
Partnership for a Drug-Free America
www.clubdrugs.org
Consumer-oriented site sponsored by the National Institute on Drug Abuse
www.health.org
Substance Abuse and Mental Health Services Administration
www.projectghb.org
Independent site devoted to risks and dangers of GHB use
www.nida.nih.gov National Institute on Drug Abuse
www.dea.gov
Drug Enforcement Administration
www.whitehousedrugpolicy.org
Office of National Drug Control Policy
(From *Mosby's 2006 Drug Consult for Nurses*. St. Louis, 2006, Mosby.)

ENGLISH-TO-SPANISH DRUG PHRASES TRANSLATOR
Taking the Medication History

Are you allergic to any medications? (If yes:)
¿Es alérgico a algún medicamento? (sì:)
(Ehs ah-lehr-hee-koh ah ahl-goon meh-dee-kah-mehn-toh) (see:)
—Which medications are you allergic to?
¿A cuál medicamento es alérgico?
(ah koo-ahl meh-dee-kah-mehn-toh ehs ah-lehr-hee-koh)
—What happens when you develop an allergic reaction?
¿Qué le pasa cuando desarrolla una reacción alérgica?
(Keh leh pah-sah koo-ahn-doh deh-sah-roh-yah oo-nah reh-ahk-see-ohn
ah-lehr-hee-kah)
—What did you do to relieve or stop the allergic reaction?
¿Qué hizo para aliviar o detener la reacción alérgica?
(Keh ee-soh pah-rah ah-lee-bee-ahr oh deh-teh-nehr lah reh-ahk-see-ohn
ah-lehr-hee-kah)
Do you take any over-the-counter, prescription, or herbal medications?
(If yes:)
¿Toma medicamentos sin receta, con receta, o naturistas (hierbas medicinales)?
(sì:)
(Toh-mah meh-dee-kah-mehn-tohs seen reh-seh-tah, kohn reh-seh-tah, oh
nah-too-rees-tahs [ee-ehr-bahs meh-dee-see-nah-lehs]) (see:)
—Why do you take each medication?
¿Porqué toma cada medicamento?
(Pohr-keh toh-mah kah-dah meh-dee-kah-mehn-toh)
—What is the dosage for each medication?
¿Cuál es la dosis de cada medicamento?
(Koo-ahl ehs lah doh-sees deh kah-dah meh-dee-kah-mehn-toh)
—How often do you take each medication?
¿Con qué frequencia toma cada medicamento?
(Kohn keh freh-koo-ehn-see-ah toh-mah kah-dah meh-dee-kah-mehn-toh)
    Once a day? ¿Una vez por dìa; diariamente?
    (Oo-nah behs pohr dee-ah; dee-ah-ree-ah-mehn-teh)
    Twice a day? ¿Dos veces por dìa?
    (dohs beh-sehs pohr dee-ah)
    Three times a day? ¿Tres veces por dìa?
    (Trehs beh-sehs pohr dee-ah)
    Four times a day? ¿Cuatro veces por dìa?
    (Koo-ah-troh beh-sehs pohr-dee-ah)
    Every other day? ¿Cada tercer dìa?
    (Kah-dah tehr-sehr dee-ah)
    Once a week? ¿Una vez por semana?
    (Oo-nah behs pohr seh-mah-nah)
How does each medication make you feel?
¿Como le hace sentir cada medicamento?
(Koh-moh leh ah-seh sehn-teer kah-dah meh-dee-kah-mehn-toh)
—Does the medication make you feel better?
¿Le hace sentir mejor el medicamento?

(Heh ah-seh sehn-teer meh-hohr ehl meh-dee-kah-mehn-toh)
—Does the medication make you feel the same or unchanged?
¿Le hace sentir igual o sin cambio el medicamento?
(Leh ah-seh sehn-teer ee-goo-ahl oh seen kam-bee-oh ehl meh-dee-kah-mehn-toh)
—Does the medication make you feel worse? (If yes:)
¿Se siente peor con el medicamento? (si:)
(Seh see-ehn teh peh-ohr kohn ehl meh-dee-kah-mehn-toh) (see:)
What do you do to make yourself feel better?
¿Qué hace para sentirse mejor?
(Keh ah-seh pah-rah sehn-teer-seh meh-hohr)

(From *Mosby's 2006 Drug Consult for Nurses*. St. Louis, 2006, Mosby.)

PREPARING FOR TREATMENT TO MEDICATION THERAPY
Medication Purpose

English	Spanish	Pronunciation
This medication will help relieve:	**Este medicamento le ayudará a aliviar:**	**(Ehs-teh meh-dee-kah-mehn-toh leh ah-yoo-dah-rah ah ah-lee-bee-ahr)**
abdominal gas	gases intestinales	(gah-sehs een-tehs-tee-nah-lehs)
abdominal pain	dolor intestinal; dolor en el abdomen	(doh-lohr een-tehs-tee-nahl; doh-lohr eh ehl ahb-doh-mehn)
chest congestion	congestión del pecho	(kohn-hehs-tee-ohn dehl peh-choh)
chest pain	dolor del pecho	(doh-lohr dehl peh-choh)
constipation	constipación; estreñimiento	(Kohns-tee-pah-see-ohn; ehs-treh-nyee-mee-ehn-toh)
cough	tos	(tohs)
headache	dolor de cabeza	(doh-lohr-deh kah-beh-sah)
muscle aches and pains	achaques musculares y dolores	(ah-chah-kehs moos-koo-lah-rehs ee doh-loh-rehs)
pain	dolor	(doh-lohr)
This medication will prevent:	**Este medicamento prevendrá:**	**(Ehs-teh meh-dee-kah-mehn-toh preh-behn-drah)**
blood clots	coágulos de sangre	(koh-ah-goo-lohs deh sahn-greh)
constipation	constipación; estreñimiento	(Kohns-tee-pah-see-ohn; ehs-treh-nyee-mee-ehn-toh)
contraception	contracepción; embarazo	(kohn-trah-sehp-see-ohn; ehm-bah-rah-soh)
diarrhea	diarrea	(dee-ah-reh-ah)
infection	infección	(een-fehk-see-ohn)
seizures	convulciónes; ataque epiléptico	(kohn-bool-see-ohn-ehs; ah-tah-keh eh-pee-lehp-tee-koh)
shortness of breath	respiración corta; falta de aliento	(rehs-pee-rah-see-ohn kohr-tah; fahl-tah deh ah-lee-ehn-toh)
wheezing	el resollar; la respiración ruidosa, sibilante	(ehl reh-soh-yahr; lah rehs-pee-rah-see-ohn roo-ee-doh-sah, see-bee-lahn-teh)
This medication will increase your:	**Este medicamento aumentará su:**	**(Ehs-teh meh-dee-kah-mehn-toh ah-oo-mehn-tah-rah soo:)**
ability to fight infections	habilidad a combatir infecciones	(ah-bee-lee-dahd ah kohm-bah-teer een-fehk-see-oh-nehs)
appetite	apetito	(ah-peh-tee-toh)
blood iron levels	nivel de hierro en la sangre	(nee-behl deh ee-eh-roh ehn lah sahn-greh)
blood sugar	azúcar en la sangre	(ah-soo-kahr ehn lah sahn-greh)
heart rate	pulso; latido	(pool-soh; lah-tee-doh)

English	Spanish	Pronunciation
red blood cell count	cuenta de células rojas	(koo-ehn-tah deh seh-loo-lahs roh-hahs)
thyroid hormone levels	niveles de hormona tiroide	(nee-beh-lehs deh ohr-moh-nah tee-roh-ee-deh)
urine volume	volumen de orina	(boh-loo-mehn deh oh-ree-nah)

This medication will decrease your: / **Este medicamento reducirá su:** (Ehs-teh meh-dee-kah-mehn-toh reh-doo-see-rah soo:)

English	Spanish	Pronunciation
anxiety	ansiedad	(ahn-see-eh-dahd)
blood cholesterol level	nivel de colesterol en la sangre	(nee-behl deh koh-lehs-the-rohl ehn lah sahn-greh)
blood lipid level	nivel de lipido en la sangre	(nee-behl deh lee-pee-doh ehn lah sahn-greh)
blood pressure	presión arterial; de sangre	(preh-see-ohn ahr teh-ree-ahl; deh sahn-greh)
blood sugar level	nivel de azúcar en la sangre	(nee-behl deh ah-soo-kahr ehn lah sahn-greh)
heart rate	pulso; latido	(pool-soh; lah-tee-doh)
stomach acid	ácido en el estómago	(ah-see-doh ehn ehl ehs-toh-mah-goh)
thyroid hormone levels	niveles de hormona tiroide	(nee-beh-lehs deh ohr-moh-nah tee-roh-ee-deh)
weight	peso	(peh-soh)

This medication will treat: / **Este medicamento sirve para:** (Ehs-teh meh-dee-kah-mehn-toh seer-beh pah-rah)

English	Spanish	Pronunciation
cancer of your ___	cancer de su ___	(kahn-sehr deh soo)
depression	depresión	(deh-preh-see-ohn)
HIV infection	infección de VIH	(een-fehk-see-ohn deh beh ee ah-cheh)
inflammation	inflamación	(een-flah-mah-see-ohn)
swelling	hinchazón	(een-chah-sohn)
the infection in your ___	la infección en su ___	(lah een-fehk-see-ohn ehn soo)
your abnormal heart rhythm	su ritmo anormal de corazón	(soo reet-moh ah-nohr-mahl deh koh-rah-sohn)
your allergy to ___	su alergia a ___	(soo eh-lehr-hee-ah ah)
your rash	su erupción; sarpullido	(soo eh-roop-see-ohn; sahr-poo-yee-doh)

ADMINISTERING MEDICATION

Swallow this medication with water or juice.
Tragüe este medicamento con agua o jugo
(Trah-geh ehs-teh meh dee-kah-mehn-toh kohn ah-goo-ah oh hoo-goh)
If you cannot swallow the medication whole, I can crush it and put it in food.
Si no puede tragar el medicamento entero puedo aplastarlo (triturarlo) y ponerlo en el alimento.
(See noh poo-eh-deh trah-gahr ehl meh-dee-kah-mehn-toh ehn-teh-roh poo-eh-doh ah-plahs-tahr-loh [tree-too-rahr-loh] ee poh-nehr-loh ehn ehl ah lee-mehn-toh)
I need to mix this medication with water or juice before you drink it.
Necesito mezclar este medicamento en agua o jugo antes de que lo tome.
(Neh-seh-see-toh mehs-klahr ehs-teh meh-dee-kah-mehn-toh ehn ah-goo-ah oh hoo-goh ahn-tehs deh keh loh toh-meh)
Do not chew this medication. Swallow it whole.
No mastique este medicamento. Tragüelo entero.
(Noh mahs-tee-keh ehs-teh meh-dee-kah-mehn-toh. Trah-geh-loh ehn-teh-roh)
Gargle with this medication and then swallow it.
Haga gargaras con este medicamento y luego tragüelo.
(Ah-gah gahr-gah-rahs koh ehs-teh meh-dee-kah-mehn-toh ee loo-eh-goh trah-geh-loh)
Place this medication under your tongue and let it dissolve.
Ponga este medicamento bajo la lengua y deje que se disuelva
(Pohn-gah ehs-teh meh-dee-kah-mehn-toh bah-hoh lah lehn-goo-ah ee deh-heh keh seh dee-soo-ehl-bah)
I would like to give this injection in your:
Quiero aplicar esta injección en su:
(Kee-eh-roh ah-plee-kahr ehs-tah een-yehk-see-ohn ehn soo:)
—abdomen
abdomen
(ahb-doh-mehn)
—arm
brazo
(brah-soh)
—buttocks
nalga
(nahl-gah)
—hip
cadera
(kah-deh-rah)
—thigh
muslo
(moos-loh)
I will give you this medication through your intravenous line.
Le daré este medicamento por el tubo de suero intravenoso.
(Leh dah-reh ehs-teh meh-dee-kah-mehn-toh pohr ehl too-boh deh soo-eh-roh een-trah-beh-noh-soh)

Let me know if you feel burning or pain at the intravenous site.
Digame si siente ardor o dolor en el sitio del suero intravenoso.
(Dee-gah-meh see see-ehn-teh ahr-dohr oh doh-lohr ehn ehl see-tee-oh dehl
soo-eh-roh een-trah-beh-noh-soh)
I need to insert this suppository into your rectum (or vagina).
Necesito meter este supositorio en el recto (o vagina).
(Neh-seh-see-toh meh-tehr ehs-teh soo-poh-see-toh-ree-oh ehn ehl rehk-toh
[oh bah-hee-nah])
I need to put this medication into each ear; left ear; right ear.
Necesito poner este medicamento en cada oreja; oreja izquierda; oreja
derecha.
(Neh-seh-see-toh poh-nehr ehs-teh meh-dee-kah-mehn-toh ehn kah-dah
oh-reh-hah; oh-reh-hah ees-kee-ehr-dah; -oh-reh-hah deh-reh-chah)
I need to put this medication into each eye; left eye; right eye.
Necesito poner este medicamento en cada ojo; ojo izquierdo; ojo derecho.
(Neh-seh-see-toh poh-nehr ehs-teh meh-dee-kah-mehn-toh ehn kah-dah oh-
hoh; oh-hoh ees-kee-ehr-doh; oh-hoh deh-reh-choh)

PREPARING FOR DISCHARGE
The generic name for this medication is _____.
El nombre genérico (sin marca) de este medicamento es _____.
(Ehl nohn-breh heh-neh-ree-koh [seen mahr-kah] deh ehs-teh meh-dee-kah-
mehn-toh ehs)
The trade name for this medication is _____.
El nombre comercial de este medicamento es _____.
(Ehs nohm-breh koh-mehr-see-ahl deh ehs-teh meh-dee-kah-mehn-toh ehs)
Take the medication exactly as prescribed.
Tome el medicamento exactamente como se receta.
(Toh-meh ehl meh-dee-kah-mehn-toh ehx-ahk-tah-mehn-teh koh-moh seh
reh-seh-tah)
You can safely break a scored tablet in half.
Puede partir por la mitad la tableta que tiene una muesca (marca).
(Poo-eh-deh pahr-teer pohr lah mee-tahd lah tah-bleh-tah keh tee-eh-neh
oo-nah moo-ehs-kah [mahr-kah])
Do not crush or chew enteric-coated, extended-release, or sustained-release
tablets or capsules.
No aplaste (triture) o mastique una tableta con capa entérica, de acción
prolongada o de mantenimiento.
(Noh ah-plahs-teh [tree-too-reh] oh mahs-tee-keh oo-nah tah-bleh-tah
kohn-kah-pah ehn-teh-ree-kah, deh ahk-see-ohn proh-lohn-gah-dah oh deh
mahn-teh-nee-mee-ehn-toh)
If you miss a dose:
Si pierde una dosis:
(See pee-ehr-deh oo-nah doh-sees:)
    —take it as soon as you remember it.
    tómela tan pronto se acuerde.
    (toh-meh-lah tahn prohn-toh seh ah-koo-ehr-deh)

—wait until the next dose.

espere hasta la siguiente dosis.

(ehs-peh-reh ahs-tah lah see-ghee-ehn-teh doh-sees)

—do not double the next dose.

No doble la siguiente dosis.

(noh doh-bleh lah see-ghee-ehn-teh doh-sees)

—contact your physician.

llame a su médico.

(yah-meh ah soo meh-dee-koh)

Do not stop taking your medication without first speaking with your physician.

No deje de tomar su medicamento sin hablar primero con su médico.

(Noh deh-heh deh toh-mahr soo meh-dee-kah-ehn-toh seen ah-blahr
pree-meh-roh kohn soo meh-dee-koh)

Do not drink alcohol while taking this medication.

No tome alcohol cuando tome este medicamento.

(Noh toh-meh ahl-kohl koo-ahn-doh toh-meh ehs-teh meh-dee-kah-
mehn-toh)

Do not drive or operate machinery while taking this medication.

No maneje o use maquinaria cuando toma este medicamento.

(Noh mah-neh-heh oh oo-seh mah-kee-nah-ree-ah koo-ahn-doh toh-mah
ehs-teh meh-dee-kah-mehn-toh)

Notify your physician right away if you experience a dangerous side effect.

Llame a su médico inmediatamente si tiene efectos secundarios peligrosos.

(Llah-meh ah soo meh-dee-koh een-meh-dee-ah-tah-mehn-teh see tee-eh-neh
eh-fehk-tohs seh-koon-dah-ree-ohs peh-lee-groh-sohs)

Check with your physician before taking any over-the-counter medications.

Cheque con su médico antes de tomar medicamentos sin receta.

(Cheh-keh kohn soo meh-dee-koh ahn-tehs deh toh-mahr meh-dee-kah-mehn-
tohs seen reh-seh-tah)

Notify your physician if you are pregnant or are planning to become pregnant
while taking this medication.

Dígale a su médico si está embarazada o planea el embarazo cuando toma
este medicamento.

(Dee-gah-leh ah soo meh-dee-koh see ehs-tah ehm-bah-rah-sah-dah oh
plah-neh-ah ehl ehm-bah-rah-soh koo-ahn-doh toh-mah ehs-teh meh-dee-kah-
mehn-toh)

Notify your physician if you are breast-feeding while taking this medication.

Dígale a su médico si está amamantando (dando de pecho) cuando toma este
medicamento.

(Dee-gah-leh ah soo meh-dee-koh see ehs-tah ah-mah-mahn-tahn-doh [dahn-
doh deh peh-choh] koo-ahn-doh toh-mah ehs-teh meh-dee-kah-mehn-toh)

Refill your prescription right away, unless you don't need it anymore.

Rellene su receta inmediatamente, a menos que no la necesite.

(Reh-yeh-neh soo reh-seh-tah een-meh-dee-ah-tah-mehn-teh, ah meh-nohs
keh noh lah neh-seh-see-teh)

PROPER MEDICATION STORAGE

Discard expired medications because they may become dangerous or ineffective.
Tire los medicamentos con fecha vencida (caducados) porque pueden ser
peligrosos o inefectivos.
(Tee-reh lohs meh-dee-kah-mehn-tohs kohn feh-chah behn-see-dah [kah-doo-kah-
dohs] pohr-keh poo-eh-dehn sehr peh-lee-groh-sohs oh een-eh-fehk-tee-bohs)
Keep all medications out of the reach of children at all times.
Guarde todos los medicamentos fuera del alcance de los niños todo el tiempo.
(Goo-ahr-deh toh-dohs lohs meh-dee-kah-mehn-tohs foo-eh-rah dehl
ahl-kahn-seh deh lohs nee-nyohs toh-doh ehl tee-ehm-poh)
Store the medication:
Almacene (guarde) el medicamento:
(Ahl-mah-seh-neh [goo-ahr-deh] ehl meh-dee-kah-mehn-toh:)
   —in its original container.
   en su empaque original.
   (ehn-soo ehm-pah-keh oh-ree-hee-nahl)
   —in a cool, dry place.
   en un lugar fresco y seco.
   (ehn oon loo-gahr frehs-koh ee seh-koh)
   —away from heat.
   lejos del calor.
   (leh-hohs dehl kah-lohr)
   —at room temperature.
   a temperatura ambiente
   (ah tehm-peh-rah-too-rah ahm-bee-ehn-teh)
   —out of direct sunlight.
   fuera de la luz directa del sol.
   (foo-eh-rah deh lah loos dee-rehk-tah dehl sohl)
   —in the refrigerator.
   en el refrigerador.
   (ehn ehl reh-free-heh-rah-dohr)

English	Spanish	Pronunciation
Selected Drug Classes	**Clasificación de Drogas Selectas (Medicamentos Selectos)**	**(Klah see-fee-kah-see-ohn deh droh-gahs seh-lehk-tahs [Meh-dee-kah-mehn-tohs Seh-lehk-tohs])**
Analgesic (narcotic, non-narcotic)	Analgésico (narcótico, no narcótico)	(Ah-nahl-heh-see-koh [nahr-koh-tee-koh, noh nahr-koh-tee-koh])
Antacid	Antácido	(Ahn-tee-ah-see-doh)
Antianginal	Antianginoso	(Ahn-tee-ahn-hee-noh-soh)
Antianxiety	Ansiolitico	(Ahn-see-oh-lee-tee-koh)
Antiarrhythmic	Antiarritmico	(Ahn-tee-ah-reet-mee-koh)
Antibiotic	Antibiótico	(Ahn-tee-bee-oh-tee-koh)
Anticoagulant	Anticoagulante	(Ahn-tee-koh-ah-goo-lahn-teh)
Anticonvulsant	Anticonvulsivo	(Ahn-tee-kohn-bool-see-boh)
Antidepressant	Antidepresivo	(Ahn-tee-deh-preh-see-boh)
Antidiarrheal	Antidiarréicos	(Ahn-tee-dee-ah-reh-ee-kohs)
Antifungal	Antimicótico	(Ahn-tee-mee-koh-tee-koh)
Antihistamine	Antihistaminico	(Ahn-tee-ees-tah-mee-nee-koh)
Antihyperlipemic	Antiperlipémico	(Ahn-tee-ee-pehr-lee-peh-mee-koh)
Antihypertensive	Antihipertensivo	(Ahn-tee-ee-pehr-tehn-see-boh)
Anti-inflammatory	Antiinflamatorio; Contra la inflamación	(Ahn-tee-een-flah-mah-toh-ree-oh; kohn-trah lah een-flah- mah-see-ohn)
Antimigraine	Antimigrañoso	(Ahn-tee-mee-grah-nyoh-soh)
Antiparkinsonian	Contra el Parkinson	(Kohn-trah ehl Pahr-keen-sohn)
Antipsychotic	Medicamentos sicóticos	(Meh-dee-kah-mehn-tohs see-koh-tee-kohs)
Antipyretic	Antitérmicos	(Ahn-tee-tehr-mee-kohs)
Antiseptic	Antiséptico	(Ahn-tee-sehp-tee-koh)
Antispasmodic	Antiespasmódic	(Ahn-tee-ehs-pahs-moh-dee-koh)
Antithyroid	Antitiroideos	(Ahn-tee-tee-roh-ee-deh-ohs)
Antituberculosis	Antifímicos	(Ahn-tee-fee-mee-kohs)
Antitussive	Antitusígenos	(Ahn-tee-too-see-heh-nohs)
Antiviral	Antivirales	(Ahn-tee-bee-rah-lehs)
Appetite suppressant	Antisupresivos del apetito	(Ahn-tee-soo-preh-see-bohs dehl ah-peh-tee-toh)
Appetite stimulant	Estimulantes del apetito	(Ehs-tee-moo-lahn-tehs dehl ah-peh-tee-toh)
Bronchodilator	Bronquoliticos	(Brohn-kee-oh-lee-tee-kohs)

Cancer chemotherapy	Quimioterapia de Cancer	(Kee-mee-oh teh-rah-pee-ah deh kahn-sehr)
Decongestant	Anticongestivo	(Ahn-tee-kohn-hehs-tee-boh)
Digestant	Digestible	(Dee-hehs-tee-bleh)
Diuretic	Diurético	(Dee-oo-reh-tee-koh)
Emetic	Emético	(Eh-meh-tee-koh)
Fertility	Inductor de la Ovulación	(Een-doohk-tohr deh lah Oh-boo-lah-see-ohn)
Herbal	Medicamentos Naturales; Hierbas Medicinales	(Meh-dee-kah-mehn-tohs Nah-too-rah-lehs, Ee-ehr-bhas Meh-dee-see-nah-lehs)
Hypnotic	Hipnótico	(Eep-noh-tee-koh)
Insulin	Insulina	(Een-soo-lee-nah)
Laxative	Laxante	(Lahx-ahn-teh)
Mineral	Mineral	(Mee-neh-rahl)
Muscle relaxant	Relajante Muscular	(Reh-lah-hahn-teh Moos-koo-lahr)
Oral contraceptive	Anticonceptivos Orales	(Ahn-tee-kohn-sehp-tee-bohs Oh-rah-lehs)
Oral hypoglycemic	Hipoglicémico Oral	(Ee-poh-glee-seh-mee-koh Oh-rahl)
Sedative	Sedantes	(She-dahn-tehs)
Steroid	Esteroide	(Ehs-teh-roh-ee-deh)
Thyroid Hormone	Tiroideos, Hormona Tiroide	(Tee-roh-ee-deh-ohs, Ohr-moh-nah Tee-roh-ee-deh)
Vaccine	Vacuna	(Bah-koo-nah)
Administration Routes	**Modo de Uso**	**(Moh-doh deh Oo-soh)**
By mouth	Oral	(Oh-rahl)
Intradermal	Intradermica	(Een-trah-dehr-mee-kah)
Intramuscular	Intramuscular	(Een-trah-moos-koo-lahr)
Intravenous	Intravenosa	(Een-trah-beh-noh-sah)
Nasal	Nasal	(Nah-sahl)
Oral	Oral	(Oh-rahl)
Otic	Ótica	(Oh-tee-kah)
Patch	Parche	(Pahr-cheh)
Rectal	Rectal	(Rehk-tahl)

Continued

English	Spanish	Pronunciation
Subcutaneous	Subcutanea	(Soob-koo-tah-neh-ah)
Sublingual	Sublingual	(Soob-leen-goo-ahl)
Topical	Topical, Local	(Toh-pee-kahl, Loh-kahl)
Vaginal	Vaginal	(Bah-hee-nahl)
Drug Preparations	**Presentación del Medicamento**	**(Preh-sehn-tah-see-ohn dehl Meh-dee-kah-mehn-toh)**
Capsule	Cápsula	(Kahp-soo-lah)
Cream	Crema	(Kreh-mah)
Drops	Gotas	(Goh-tahs)
Elixir	Elixir, Jarabe	(Eh-leex-eer, Hah-rah-beh)
Fluid	Líquido	(Lee-kee-doh)
Gel	Gel, Jalea	(Hehl, Hah-leh-ah)
Inhaler	Inhalador*	(Een-ah-lah-dohr)
Injection	Inyección	(Een-yehk-see-ohn)
Liquid	Líquido	(Lee-kee-doh)
Lotion	Loción	(Loh-see-ohn)
Lozenge	Trocisco, pastilla	(Troh-sees-koh, Pahs-tee-yah)
Ointment	Ungüento	(Oon-goo-ehn-toh)
Pill	Píldora, Pastilla	(Peel-doh-rah, Pahs-tee-yah)
Powder	Polvo	(Pohl-boh)
Spray	Spray	(Sp-rah-ee)
Suppository	Supositorio	(Soo-poh-see-toh-ree-oh)
Syrup	Jarabe	(Hah-rah-beh)
Tablet	Tableta	(Tah-bleh-tah)
Administration Frequency	**Frecuencia de la Administración**	**(Freh-koo-ehn-see-ah deh lah Ahd-mee-nees-trah-see-ohn)**
Once a day	Una vez por día; diariamente	(Oo-nah behs pohr dee-ah; dee-ah-ree-ah-mehn-teh)
Twice a day	Dos veces por día	(Dohs beh-sehs pohr dee-ah)
Three times a day	Tres veces por día	(Trehs beh-sehs pohr dee-ah)
Four times a day	Cuatro veces por día	(Koo-ah-troh beh-sehs pohr dee-ah)

English	Spanish	Pronunciation
Every other day	Cada tercer día	(Kah-dah tehr-sehr dee-ah)
Once a week	Una vez por semana	(Oo-nah behs pohr seh-mah-nah)
Every 4 hours	Cada cuatro horas	(Kah-dah koo-ah-troh oh-rahs)
Every 6 hours	Cada seis horas	(Kah-dah she-ees oh-rahs)
Every 8 hours	Cada ocho horas	(Kah-dah oh-choh oh-rahs)
Every 12 hours	Cada doce horas	(Kah-dah doh-seh oh-rahs)
In the morning	En la mañana	(Ehn lah mah-nyah-nah)
In the afternoon	En la tarde	(Ehn lah tahr-deh)
In the evening	En la noche	(Ehn lah noh-cheh)
Before bedtime	Antes de acostarse	(Ahn-tehs deh ah-kohs-tahr-seh)
Before meals	Antes de la comida; Antes del alimento	(Ahn-tehs dehl lah koh-mee-dah; Ahn-tehs dehl ah-lee-mehn-toh)
With meals	Con los alimentos; Con la comida	(Kohn lohs ah-lee-mehn-tohs; Kohn lah koh-mee-dah)
After meals	Después de los alimentos, Después de la comida	(Dehs-poo-ehs deh lohs ah-lee-mehn-tohs; Dehs-poo-ehs deh lah koh-mee-dah)
Only when you need it	Solo cuando la necesite	(Soh-loh koo-ahn-doh lah neh-seh-see-teh)
When you have (pain)	Cuando tiene (dolor)	(Koo-ahn-doh tee-eh-neh) (doh-lohr)
50 Common Side Effects	**Cincuenta Efectos Secundarios Comúnes**	**(Seen-koo-ehn-tah Eh-fehk-tohs Seh-koon-dah-ree-ohs Koh-moo-nehs)**
Abdominal cramps	Retorcijón abdominal	(Reh-tohr-see-hohn ahb-doh-mee-nahl)
Abdominal pain	Dolor abdominal	(Doh-lohr ahb-doh-mee-nahl)
Abdominal swelling	Inflamación abdominal	(Een-flah-mah-see-ohn ahb-doh-mee-nahl)
Anxiety	Ansiedad	(Ahn-see-eh-dahd)
Blood in the stool	Sangre en el excremento	(Sahn-greh ehn ehl ehx-kreh-mehn-toh)
Blood in the urine	Sangre en la orina	(Sahn-greh ehn la oh-ree-nah)
Bone pain	Dolor de hueso*	(Doh-lohr deh oo-eh-soh)
Chest pain	Dolor de pecho	(Doh-lohr deh peh-choh)
Chest pounding	Palpitación; latidos fuertes o en el pecho	(Pahl-pee-tah-see-ohn; lah-tee-dohs foo-ehr-tehs ehnehl peh-choh)

*The **h** is silent.

Continued

English	Spanish	Pronunciation
Chills	Escalofrío	(Ehs-kah-loh-free-oh)
Confusion	Confusión	(Kohn-foo-see-ohn)
Constipation	Constipación, estreñimiento	(Kohns-tee-pah-see-ohn, ehs-treh-nyee-mee-ehn-toh)
Cough	Tos	(Tohs)
Mental depression	Depresión mental	(Deh-preh-see-ohn mehn-tahl)
Diarrhea	Diarrea	(Dee-ah-reh-ah)
Difficult urination	Dificultad al orinar	(Dee-fee-kool-tahd ahl oh-ree-nahr)
Difficulty breathing	Dificultad al respirar	(Dee-fee-kool-tahd ahl rehs-pee-rahr)
Difficulty sleeping	Dificultad al dormir	(Dee-fee-kool-tahd ahl dohr-meer)
Dizziness	Mareos; vahídos	(Mah-reh-ohs; bah-ee-dohs)
Dry mouth	Boca seca	(Boh-kah seh-kah)
Easy bruising	Fragilidad capilar; le salen moretones con facilidad	(Frah-hee-lee-dahd kah-pee-lahr; leh sah-lehn moh-reh-toh-nehs kohn fah-see-lee-dahd)
Faintness	Desvanecimiento; sintió un vahido	(Dehs-bah-neh-see-mee-ehn-toh; seen-tee-oh oon bah-ee-doh)
Fatigue	Fatiga, cansancio	(Fah-tee-gah, kahn-sahn-see-oh)
Fever	Fiebre	(Fee-eh-breh)
Frequent urination	Orina frecuente	(Oh-ree-nah freh-koo-ehn-teh)
Headache	Dolor de cabeza	(Doh-lohr deh kah-beh-sah)
Impotence	Impotencia	(Eem-poh-tehn-see-ah)
Increased appetite	Aumento en el apetito	(Ah-oo-mehn-toh ehn ehl ah-peh-tee-toh)
Increased gas	Flatulencia	(Flah-too-lehn-see-ah)
Increased perspiration	Aumento en el sudor	(Ah-oo-mehn-toh ehn ehl soo-dohr)
Indigestion	Indigestión	(En-dee-hehs-tee-ohn)
Itching	Comezón	(Koh-meh-sohn)
Loss of appetite	Pérdida en el apetito	(Pehr-dee-dah ehn ehl ah-peh-tee-toh)
Menstrual changes	Cambios en la menstruación; cambio en el ciclo menstrual	(Kahm-bee-ohs ehn la mehns-truh-ah-see-ohn; Kahm-bee-oh ehn ehl see-kloh mehns-truh-ahl)
Mood changes	Cambio en el humor; cambio en la disposición	(Kahm-bee-oh ehn ehl oo-mohr, Kahm-bee-oh ehn lah dees-poh-see-see-ohn)

Muscle pain	Dolores musculares	(Doh-loh-rehs moos-koo-lah-rehs)
Muscle aches	Achaques musculares	(Ah-chah-kehs moos-koo-lah-rehs)
Muscle cramps	Calambre muscular	(Kah-lahm-breh moos-koo-lahr)
Nasal congestion	Congestión nasal	(Kohn-hehs-tee-ohn nah-ahl)
Nausea	Nausea	(Nah-oo-seh-ah)
Ringing in the ears	Zumbido en los oidos	(Soom-bee-doh ehn lohs oh-ee-dohs)
Skin rash	Erupción en la piel	(Eh-roop-see-ohn ehn lah pee-ehl)
Swelling on the hands, legs, or feet	Hinchazón en las manos, piernas, o pies	(Een-chah-sohn ehn lahs mah-nohs, pee-ehr-nahs, oh pee-ehs)
Vaginal bleeding	Sangrado vaginal	(Sahn-grah-doh bah-hee-nahl)
Vision changes	Cambios en la visión; cambios en la vista	(Kahm-bee-ohs ehn lah bee-see-ohn; cahm-bee-ohs ehn lah bees-tah)
Vomiting	Vomitando	(Boh-mee-tahn-doh)
Weakness	Debilidad	(Deh-bee-lee-dahd)
Weight gain	Aumento de peso	(Ah-oo-mehn-toh deh peh-soh)
Weight loss	Pérdida de peso	(Pehr-dee-day deh peh-soh)
Wheezing	Resollar; respiración sibilante	(Reh-soh-yahr; rehs-pee-rah-see-ohn see-bee-lahn-teh)

(From *Mosby's 2006 Drug Consult for Nurses.* St. Louis, 2006, Mosby.)

FDA PREGNANCY CATEGORIES

! Medications should be used during pregnancy only if clearly needed.

A: Adequate and well-controlled studies have failed to show a risk to the fetus in the first trimester of pregnancy (also, no evidence of risk has been seen in later trimesters). Possibility of fetal harm appears remote.

B: Animal reproduction studies have failed to show a risk to the fetus and there are no adequate/well-controlled studies in pregnant women.

C: Animal reproduction studies have shown an adverse effect on the fetus and there are no adequate/well-controlled studies in humans. However, the benefits may warrant use of the drug in pregnant women despite potential risks.

D: There is positive evidence of human fetal risk based on data from investigational or marketing experience or from studies in humans, but the potential benefits may warrant use of the drug despite potential risks (e.g., use in life-threatening situations in which other medications cannot be used or are ineffective).

X: Animal or human studies have shown fetal abnormalities and/or there is evidence of human fetal risk based on adverse reaction data from investigational or marketing experience where the risks in using the medication clearly outweigh potential benefits.

(From *Mosby's 2006 Drug Consult for Nurses.* St. Louis, 2006, Mosby.)

NORMAL LABORATORY VALUES
Hematology/Coagulation

Test	Specimen	Normal Range
Activated partial thromboplastin time (aPTT)	Whole blood	25-35 sec
Erythrocyte count (RBC count)	Whole blood	M: 4.3-5.7 million cells/mm³ F: 3.8-5.1 million cells/mm³
Hematocrit (HCT, Hct)	Whole blood	M: 39%-49% F: 35%-45%
Hemoglobin (Hb, Hgb)	Whole blood	M: 13.5-17.5 g/dl F: 12.0-16.0 g/dl
Leukocyte count (WBC count)	Whole blood	4.5-11.0 thousand cells/mm³
Leukocyte differential count	Whole blood	
Basophils		0%-0.75%
Eosinophils		1%-3%
Lymphocytes		23%-33%
Monocytes		3%-7%
Neutrophils—bands		3%-5%
Neutrophils—segmented		54%-62%
Mean corpuscular hemoglobin (MCH)	Whole blood	26-34 pg/cell
Mean corpuscular hemoglobin concentration (MCHC)	Whole blood	31%-37% Hb/cell
Mean corpuscular volume (MCV)	Whole blood	80-100 fL
Partial thromboplastin time (PTT)	Whole blood	60-85 sec
Platelet count (thrombocyte count)	Whole blood	150-450 thousand/mm³
Prothrombin time (PT)	Whole blood	11-13.5 sec
RBC count (see Erythrocyte count)		

(From *Mosby's 2006 Drug Consult for Nurses*. St. Louis, 2006, Mosby.)

Continued

Clinical Chemistry
(Serum Plasma/Urine)

Test	Specimen	Normal Range
Alanine aminotransferase (ALT, SGPT)	Serum	0-55 units/L
Albumin	Serum	3.5-5 g/dl
Alkaline phosphatase	Serum	M: 53-128 units/L
		F: 42-98 units/L
Anion gap	Plasma or serum	5-14 mEq/L
Aspartate aminotransferase (AST, SGOT)	Serum	0-50 units/L
Bilirubin (conjugated direct)	Serum	0-0.4 mg/dl
Bilirubin (total)	Serum	0.2-1.2 mg/dl
Calcium (total)	Serum	8.4-10.2 mg/dl
Carbon dioxide (CO_2) total	Plasma or serum	20-34 mEq/L
Chloride	Plasma or serum	96-112 mEq/L
Cholesterol (total)	Plasma or serum	Less than 200 mg/dl
C-Reactive protein	Serum	68-8200 ng/ml
Creatine kinase (CK)	Serum	M: 38-174 units/L
		F: 26-140 units/L
Creatine kinase isoenzymes	Serum	Fraction of total: Less than 0.04-0.06
Creatinine	Plasma or serum	M: 0.7-1.3 mg/dl F: 0.6-1.1 mg/dl
Creatinine clearance	Plasma or serum and urine	M: 90-139 ml/min/1.73 m^2
		F: 80-125 ml/min/1.73 m^2
Free thyroxine index (FTI)	Serum	1.1-4.8
Glucose	Serum	Adults: 70-105 mg/dl; older than 60 yr:
		80-115 mg/dl
Hemoglobin A_{1c}	Whole blood	5.6%-7.5% of total Hgb
Homovanillic acid (HVA)	Urine, 24 hr	1.4-8.8 mg/day
17-Hydroxycorticosteroids (17-OHCS)	Urine, 24 hr	M: 3-10 mg/day F: 2-8 mg/day
Iron	Serum	M: 65-175 mcg/dl
		F: 50-170 mcg/dl

Iron-binding capacity, total (TIBC)	Serum	250-450 mcg/dl
Lactate dehydrogenase (LDH)	Serum	0-250 units/L
Magnesium	Serum	1.3-2.3 mg/dl
Oxygen (PO$_2$)	Whole blood, arterial	83-100 mm Hg
Oxygen saturation	Whole blood, arterial	95%-98%
pH	Whole blood, arterial	7.35-7.45
Phosphorus, inorganic	Serum	2.7-4.5 mg/dl
Potassium	Serum	3.5-5.1 mEq/L
Protein (total)	Serum	6-8.5 g/dl
Sodium	Plasma or serum	136-146 mEq/L
Specific gravity	Urine	1.002-1.030
Thyrotropin (hTSH)	Plasma or serum	2-10 mU/ml
Thyroxine (T$_4$) total	Serum	5-12 mcg/dl
Triglycerides (TG)	Serum, after 12-hr fast	20-190 mg/dl
Triiodothyronine resin uptake test (T$_3$RU)	Serum	22%-37%
Urea nitrogen	Plasma or serum	7-25 mg/dl
Urea nitrogen/creatinine ratio	Serum	12/1-20/1
Uric acid	Serum	M: 3.5-7.2 mg/dl
		F: 2.6-6 mg/dl
Vanillylmandelic acid (VMA)	Urine, 24 hr	2-7 mg/day

SIGNS AND SYMPTOMS OF ELECTROLYTE IMBALANCE
HYPOGLYCEMIA (excessive insulin)
Tremors, cold/clammy skin, mental confusion, rapid/shallow respirations, unusual fatigue, hunger, drowsiness, anxiety, headache, muscular incoordination, paresthesia of tongue/mouth/lips, hallucination, increased pulse/blood pressure, tachycardia, seizures, coma.

HYPERGLYCEMIA (insufficient insulin)
Hot/flushed/dry skin, fruity breath odor, excessive urination (polyuria), excessive thirst (polydipsia), acute fatigue, air hunger, deep/labored respirations, mental changes, restlessness, nausea, polyphagia (excessive appetite).

HYPOKALEMIA (potassium level less than 3.5 mEq/L)
Weakness/paresthesia of extremities, muscle cramps, nausea, vomiting, diarrhea, hypoactive bowel sounds, absent bowel sounds (paralytic ileus), abdominal distention, weak/irregular pulse, postural hypotension, difficulty breathing, disorientation, irritability.

HYPERKALEMIA (potassium level greater than 5.0 mEq/L)
Diarrhea, muscle weakness, heaviness of legs, paresthesia of tongue/hands/feet, slow/irregular pulse, decreased blood pressure, abdominal cramps, oliguria/anuria, respiratory difficulty, cardiac abnormalities.

HYPONATREMIA (sodium level less than 130 mEq/L)
Abdominal cramping, nausea, vomiting, diarrhea, cold/clammy skin, poor skin turgor, tremulousness, muscle weakness, leg cramps, increased pulse rate, irritability, apprehension, hypotension, headache.

HYPERNATREMIA (sodium level greater than 150 mEq/L)
Hot/flushed/dry skin, dry mucous membranes, fever, extreme thirst, dry/rough/red tongue, edema, restlessness, postural hypotension, oliguria.

HYPOCALCEMIA (calcium level less than 8.4 mg/dl)
Circumoral/peripheral numbness and tingling, muscle twitching; Chvostek's sign (facial muscle spasm; test by tapping of facial nerve anterior to earlobe, just below zygomatic arch), muscle cramping, Trousseau's sign (carpopedal spasm), seizures, arrhythmias.

HYPERCALCEMIA (calcium level greater than 10.2 mg/dl)
Muscle hypotonicity, incoordination, anorexia, constipation, confusion, impaired memory, slurred speech, lethargy, acute psychotic behavior, deep bone pain, flank pain.

(From *Mosby's 2006 Drug Consult for Nurses.* St. Louis, 2006, Mosby.)

TECHNIQUES OF MEDICATION ADMINISTRATION

Ophthalmic

Eye Drops

1. Wash hands.
2. Instruct patient to lie down or tilt head backward and look up.
3. Gently pull lower eyelid down until a pocket (pouch) is formed between eye and lower lid (conjunctival sac).
4. Hold dropper above pocket. Without touching tip of eye dropper to eyelid or conjunctival sac, place prescribed number of drops into the center pocket (placing drops directly onto eye may cause a sudden squeezing of eyelid, with subsequent loss of solution). Continue to hold the eyelid for a moment after the drops are applied (allows medication to distribute along entire conjunctival sac).
5. Instruct patient to close eyes gently so that medication is not squeezed out of sac.
6. Apply gentle finger pressure to the lacrimal sac at the inner canthus (bridge of the nose, inside corner of the eye) for 1-2 min (promotes absorption, minimizes drainage into nose and throat, lessens risk of systemic absorption).
7. Remove excess solution around eye with a tissue.
8. Wash hands immediately to remove medication on hands. Never rinse eye dropper.

Eye Ointment

1. Wash hands.
2. Instruct patient to lie down or tilt head backward and look up.
3. Gently pull lower eyelid down until a pocket (pouch) is formed between eye and lower lid (conjunctival sac).
4. Hold applicator tube above pocket. Without touching the applicator tip to eyelid or conjunctival sac, place prescribed amount of ointment ($1/4$-$1/2$ inch) into the center pocket (placing ointment directly onto eye may cause discomfort).
5. Instruct patient to close eye for 1-2 min, rolling eyeball in all directions (increases contact area of drug to eye).
6. Inform patient of temporary blurring of vision. If possible, apply ointment just before bedtime.
7. Wash hands immediately to remove medication on hands. Never rinse tube applicator.

Otic

1. Ear drops should be at body temperature (wrap hand around bottle to warm contents). Body temperature instillation prevents startling of patient.
2. Instruct patient to lie down with head turned so affected ear is upright (allows medication to drip into ear).
3. Instill prescribed number of drops toward the canal wall, not directly on eardrum.
4. To promote correct placement of ear drops, pull the auricle down and posterior in children and pull the auricle up and posterior in adults.

Nasal
Nose Drops and Sprays
1. Instruct patient to blow nose to clear nasal passages as much as possible.
2. Tilt head slightly forward if instilling nasal spray, slightly backward if instilling nasal drops.
3. Insert spray tip into 1 nostril, pointing toward inflamed nasal passages, away from nasal septum.
4. Spray or drop medication into 1 nostril while holding other nostril closed and concurrently inspire through nose to permit medication as high into nasal passages as possible.
5. Discard unused nasal solution after 3 mo.

Inhalation
Aerosol (Multidose Inhalers)
1. Shake container well before each use.
2. Exhale slowly and as completely as possible through the mouth.
3. Place mouthpiece fully into mouth, holding inhaler upright, and close lips fully around mouthpiece.
4. Inhale deeply and slowly through the mouth while depressing the top of the canister with the middle finger.
5. Hold breath as long as possible before exhaling slowly and gently.
6. When 2 puffs are prescribed, wait 2 min and shake container again before inhaling a second puff (allows for deeper bronchial penetration).
7. Rinse mouth with water immediately after inhalation (prevents mouth and throat dryness).

Sublingual
1. Administer while seated.
2. Dissolve sublingual tablet under tongue (do not chew or swallow tablet).
3. Do not swallow saliva until tablet is dissolved.

Topical
1. Gently cleanse area prior to application.
2. Use occlusive dressings only as ordered.
3. Without touching applicator tip to skin, apply sparingly; gently rub into area thoroughly unless ordered otherwise.
4. When using aerosol, spray area for 3 sec from 15-cm distance; avoid inhalation.

Transdermal
1. Apply transdermal patch to clean, dry, hairless skin on upper arm or body (not below knee or elbow).
2. Rotate sites (prevents skin irritation).
3. Do not trim patch to adjust dose.

Rectal
1. Instruct patient to lie in left lateral Sims position.
2. Moisten suppository with cold water or water-soluble lubricant.
3. Instruct patient to slowly exhale (relaxes anal sphincter) while inserting suppository well up into rectum.
4. Inform patient as to length of time (20-30 min) before desire for defecation occurs or less than 60 min for systemic absorption to occur, depending on purpose for suppository.

Subcutaneous

1. Use 25- to 27-gauge, ½- to ⅝-inch needle; 1-3 ml. Angle of insertion depends on body size: 90-degree if patient is obese. If patient is very thin, gather the skin at the area of needle insertion and administer also at a 90-degree angle. A 45-degree angle may be used in a patient with average weight.
2. Cleanse area to be injected with circular motion.
3. Avoid areas of bony prominence, major nerves, blood vessels.
4. Aspirate syringe before injecting (to avoid intra-arterial administration), except insulin, heparin.
5. Inject slowly; remove needle quickly.

IM
Injection Sites

1. Use the dorsogluteal (upper outer quadrant) site if volume to be injected is 1-3 ml. Use 18- to 23-gauge, 1.25- to 3-inch needle. Needle should be long enough to reach the middle of the muscle.
2. Do not use this site in children <2 yr or in those who are emaciated. Patient should be in prone position.
3. Using 90-degree angle, flatten the skin area using the middle and index fingers and inject between them.

1. Use the ventrogluteal site if volume to be injected is 1-5 ml. Use 20- to 23-gauge, 1.25- to 2.5-inch needle. Needle should be long enough to reach the middle of the muscle.
2. This is the preferred site for adults, children >7 mo. Patient should be in supine lateral position.
3. Using 90-degree angle, flatten the skin area using the middle and index fingers and inject between them.

1. Use the deltoid site if volume to be injected is 0.5-1 ml. Use 23- to 25-gauge, ⅛- to ½-inch needle. Needle should be long enough to reach the middle of the muscle.
2. Patient may be in prone, sitting, supine, or standing position.
3. Using 90-degree angle or angled slightly toward acromion, flatten the skin area using the thumb and index finger and inject between them.

1. Anterolateral thigh is site of choice for infants and children <7 mo. Use 22- to 25-gauge, ⅝- to 1-inch needle.
2. Patient may be in supine or sitting position.
3. Using 90-degree angle, flatten the skin area using the thumb and index finger and inject between them.

Z-Track Technique

1. Draw up medication with one needle, and use new needle for injection (minimizes skin staining).
2. Administer deep IM in upper outer quadrant of buttock only (dorsogluteal site).
3. Displace the skin lateral to the injection site before inserting the needle.
4. Withdraw the needle before releasing the skin.

IV

1. Medication may be given as direct IV, intermittent (piggyback), or continuous infusion.
2. Ensure that medication is compatible with solution being infused (see IV compatibility chart in this drug handbook).
3. Do not use if precipitate is present or discoloration occurs.
4. Check IV site frequently for correct infusion rate, evidence of infiltration, extravasation.

Intravenous medications are administered by the following:

1. Continuous infusing solution.
2. Piggyback (intermittent infusion).
3. Volume control setup (medication contained in a chamber between the IV solution bag and the patient).
4. Bolus dose (a single dose of medication given through an infusion line or heparin lock). Sometimes this is referred to as an IV push.

Adding medication to a newly prescribed IV bag:

1. Remove the plastic cover from the IV bag.
2. Cleanse rubber port with an alcohol swab.
3. Insert the needle into the center of the rubber port.
4. Inject the medication.
5. Withdraw the syringe from the port.
6. Gently rotate the container to mix the solution.
7. Label the IV including the date, time, medication, and dosage. It should be placed so it is easily read when hanging.
8. Spike the IV tubing and prime the tubing.

Hanging an IV piggyback (IVPB):

1. When using the piggyback method, lower the primary bag at least 6 inches below the piggyback bag.
2. Set the pump as a secondary infusion when entering the rate of infusion and volume to be infused.
3. Most piggyback medications contain 50-100 cc and usually infuse in 20-60 min, although larger-volume bags will take longer.

Administering IV medications through a volume control setup (Buretrol):

1. Insert the spike of the volume control set (Buretrol, Soluset, Pediatrol) into the primary solution container.
2. Open the upper clamp on the volume control set and allow sufficient fluid into volume control chamber.
3. Fill the volume control device with 30 cc of fluid by opening the clamp between the primary solution and the volume control device.

Administering an IV bolus dose:

1. If an existing IV is infusing, stop the infusion by pinching the tubing above the port.
2. Insert the needle into the port and aspirate to observe for a blood return.
3. If the IV is infusing properly with no signs of infiltration or inflammation, it should be patent.

4. Blood indicates that the intravenous line is in the vein.
5. Inject the medication at the prescribed rate.
6. Remove the needle and regulate the IV as prescribed.

(Modified from *Mosby's 2006 Drug Consult for Nurses.* St. Louis, 2006, Mosby.)

COMMONLY PRESCRIBED INSULINS FOR INSULIN-DEPENDENT DIABETES MELLITUS (IDDM)

Generic	Trade	Human/Animal	Length of Action
Insulin injection	Regular Iletin I	Beef or pork	Rapid
	Regular Iletin II	Purified pork	Rapid
	Novolin R	Human	Rapid
Isophane insulin	NPH Iletin I	Beef or pork	Intermediate
	Humulin N	Human	Intermediate
Isophane insulin suspension and insulin injection	Humulin 70/30	Human	Intermediate
Isophane insulin suspension and insulin injection	Humulin 50/50	Human	Intermediate
Insulin zinc suspension	Lente L	Purified pork	Intermediate
	Humulin L	Human	Intermediate
Insulin zinc suspension; extended lente	Humulin Ultralente	Human	Long acting
Insulin analog injection	Humalog	Human	Rapid
Insulin glargine	Lantus	Human	Long acting

(From Hopper T: *Mosby's Pharmacy Technician: Principles & Practice.* St. Louis, 2004, Saunders.)

MEDICATION MATH
Calculation of Doses

Frequently, dosages ordered do not correspond exactly to what is available and must be calculated.

Ratio/proportion: A patient is to receive 65 mg of a medication. It is available as 80 mg × 2 ml.

What volume (ml) needs to be administered to the patient?

STEP 1: Set up ratio.

$$\frac{80 \text{ mg}}{2 \text{ ml}} = \frac{65}{x \text{ (ml)}}$$

STEP 2: Cross multiply and divide each side by the number with x to determine volume to be administered.

$$(80 \text{ mg}) (x \text{ ml}) = (65 \text{ mg}) (2 \text{ ml})$$
$$80x = 130$$
$$x = 130/80 \text{ or } 6625 \text{ ml}$$

Calculations in micrograms/kilogram per minute (mcg/kg/min):

A 63-year-old patient (weight 165 lbs) is to receive medication A at a rate of 8 mcg/kg/min. Given a solution containing medication A in a concentration of 500 mg/250ml, at what rate (ml/hr) would you infuse this medication?

STEP 1: Convert to same units. In this problem the dose is expressed in mcg/kg; therefore convert weight to kg (2.2 lbs = 1 kg) and drug concentration to mcg/ml (1 mg = 1000 mcg).

165 lb divided by 2.2 = 75 kg

$$\frac{500 \text{ mg}}{250 \text{ ml}} = 2 \text{ mg/ml} = 2000 \text{ mcg/ml}$$

STEP 2: Number of mcg/hr.

75 kg × 8 mcg/kg/min = 600 mcg/min or 36,000 mcg/hr

STEP 3: Number of ml/hr.

36,000 mcg/hr divided by 2000 mcg/ml = 18 ml/hr

(From *Mosby's 2006 Drug Consult for Nurses.* St. Louis, 2006, Mosby.)

ERROR-PRONE DRUG NAME ABBREVIATIONS

Drug Name Abbreviations	Intended Meaning	Misinterpretation	Correction
ARA A	Vidarabine	Mistaken as cytarabine (ARA C)	Use complete drug name
AZT	Zidovudine (Retrovir)	Mistaken as azathioprine or aztreonam	Use complete drug name
CPZ	Compazine (prochlorperazine)	Mistaken as chlorpromazine	Use complete drug name
DPT	Demerol-Phenergan-Thorazine	Mistaken as diphtheria-pertussis-tetanus (vaccine)	Use complete drug name
DTO	Diluted tincture of opium, or deodorized tincture of opium (Paregoric)	Mistaken as tincture of opium	Use complete drug name
HCl	Hydrochloric acid or hydrochloride	Mistaken as potassium chloride ("H" is misinterpreted as "K")	Use complete drug name unless expressed as salt of a drug
HCT	Hydrocortisone	Mistaken as hydrochlorothiazide	Use complete drug name
HCTZ	Hydrochlorothiazide	Mistaken as hydrocortisone (seen as HCT250 mg)	Use complete drug name
MgSO4**	Magnesium sulfate	Mistaken as morphine sulfate	Use complete drug name
MS, MSO4**	Morphine sulfate	Mistaken as magnesium sulfate	Use complete drug name
MTX	Methotrexate	Mistaken as mitoxantrone	Use complete drug name
PCA	Procainamide	Mistaken as Patient Controlled Analgesia	Use complete drug name
PTU	Propylthiouracil	Mistaken as mercaptopurine	Use complete drug name
T3	Tylenol with codeine No. 3	Mistaken as liothyronine	Use complete drug name
TAC	Triamcinolone	Mistaken as tetracaine, Adrenalin, cocaine	Use complete drug name
TNK	TNKase	Mistaken as "TPA"	Use complete drug name
ZnSO4	Zinc sulfate	Mistaken as morphine sulfate	Use complete drug name

**Identified drug name abbreviations above are also included on Joint Commission's "minimum list" of dangerous abbreviations, acronyms, and symbols that must be included on an organization's "Do Not Use" list, effective January 1, 2004. An updated list of frequently asked questions about this Joint Commission requirement can be found on their website at *www.jcaho.org*. (From *Mosby's Nursing PDQ for Medication Safety*. St. Louis, 2005, Mosby.)

Abortifacient Any treatment or substance that facilitates loss (abortion) of a fetus

Absorption The passage of nutrients from food, liquids, and medicines across the barriers that separate the body from the environment, such as skin, lungs, gut

Accommodation The changes that occur in the ocular lens to allow it to focus to various distances

ACE Angiotensin converting enzyme; important target for the treatment of cardiovascular problems

Acidification The conversion to an acid environment

Acidosis The increase of acid content of the blood resulting from the accumulation of acid (H^+) or loss of bicarbonate (HCO_3^-) and CO_2; the pH of blood is lowered

Acoustic nerve The eighth cranial nerve; carries sensory information about hearing and equilibrium to the various parts of the brain including the cerebellum and medulla

Acquired immunity Immunity that has been acquired through exposure to an antigen or infectious agent; vs. passive immunity

Acute A symptom or condition that appears suddenly and lasts for a short period

Adaptogen A substance with a non-specific action that casues improved resistance to physical and mental stress

Addison's disease Condition resulting in a decrease in the adrenocortical hormones, mineralocorticoids and glucocorticoids, that causes symptoms including muscle weakness and weight loss

Adenoma An abnormal growth of glandular epithelial tissue

Adjuvant A substance added to a mixture, to preserve the activity of the active ingredient in a predictable way

Adrenalin The hormone that binds to adrenergic receptors, causes the fight or flight response, also known in the US as epinephrine

Adrenergic Relating to a class of drugs (alpha & beta) found mainly in the autonomic sympathetic nervous system that bind to receptors like epinephrine and beta-blockers

Adverse effect Those side effects on the body that are not intended as the principal therapeutic effect of the drug; vs. pharmacologic effect

Aerobic Organisms that need oxygen to survive; vs. anaerobic

Afferent The direction of neuronal impulse from the body toward the central nervous system (CNS)

Agonist A substance that binds and activates a membrane receptor

AIDS Acquired immunodeficiency syndrome, a condition of a gradually weakened immune system

Alcoholic extract Soluble fraction of plant material obtained after extraction with ethanol

Alkaloid A chemical substance containing nitrogen as part of a herterocyclic ring structure; often highly active as a drug

Allergen A substance that triggers an allergic reaction

Allopathy A medical system that uses substances to cause an effect different or counter to those caused by the condition under treatment

GLOSSARY

*Some definitions from Hopper T: *Mosby's Pharmacy Technician. Principles and Practice.* St. Louis, 2004, Saunders.

Alopecia Loss of hair

Alkalosis The decrease of acid in the blood resulting from the accumulation of alkali or reduction of acid content; the pH of blood is raised

Alligation A method of determining the needed amounts of two different concentrations to prepare a needed concentration

Amenorrhea Absence or suppression of menses

Amino acids Macromolecules that chemically form the building blocks of proteins

Anabolism To build up; the constructive phase of metabolism

Anaerobic Organisms that live in the absence of oxygen

Analeptic A substance that stimulates the central nervous system

Analgesic A drug that reduces the perception of pain; categories include opioids and narcotics

Anaphylactic shock A severe allergic reaction that causes blood pressure to decrease rapidly, the heart to go into ventricular tachycardia, and airways to close; a medical emergency that will cause death if not treated immediately

Androgen Male sex hormones related from the cholesterol family

Anemia A deficiency of circulating red blood cells; a symptom of disease, not a disease

Anesthetic A substance that causes localized or general loss of sensation

Angina pectoris Severe pain in the chest, usually due to compromised oxygen/blood flow

Antacid An agent that promotes decreased production or increased neutralization of hydrochloric acid produced by the stomach; categories include H_2 blockers, proton pump inhibitors, and absorptives

Antagonist Inhibitor at membrane receptors; blocks the activity of an endogenious ligand

Anthelmintic A substance that kills or expels intestinal worms

Antiarrhythmic The class of agents that rebalance irregular muscular contractions of the heart; categories include beta blockers and calcium channel blockers

Antibiotics Chemical agents used to stop microorganism growth or replication; generally refers to agents used to treat infections caused by bacteria and parasites

Antibiotic spectrum The variety of microbes that a particular antibiotic can treat. Broad-spectrum agents can treat many different types of organisms, whereas narrow-spectrum agents treat only a select few.

Antibodies Proteins contained within plasma cells that neutralize or destroy antigens; also known as immunoglobulins

Anticoagulant A substance that prevents blood from clotting

Anticonvulsant Agents that reduce or counter seizures/convulsions or abnormal electrical firing of brain signals

Antidepressants Agents that counter a clinical state of depression characterized by anhedonia, mood disturbance, loss of productivity

Antidote A substance that counteracts poisoning

Antiemetic An agent that counters nausea and vomiting

Antigen The marker on cell surfaces that marks the cell as a "self-cell"; stimulates the production of antibodies

Antihistamine A substance that improves allergic symptoms by blocking the action of histamine

Antihypertensive A substance that reduces blood pressure

Anti-inflammatory A substance that causes symptomatic relief by reducing swelling, redness, and pain

Antimicrobials Chemical agents produced by scientists to prevent growth of or kill microorganisms

Antimycotic Antifungal agent

Antineoplastic An agent used to prevent the development, proliferation, or growth of neoplastic cells; a medication used in treatment of abnormal cells

Antioxidant A substance that is able to protect cells or counteract the damage caused by oxidation and oxygen-free radicals

Antipruritic A drug that relieves, or prevents, itching, usually an antihistamine or an anti-inflammatory drug

Antipsychotic Drugs that manage a variety of psychiatric conditions, including schizophrenia, delirium/dementia, agitation, paranoia, and mania

Antipyretic A substance that alleviates fever

Antiseptic A substance that slows or stops infection, growth of microorganisms on surfaces such as skin

Antispasmodic A substance that reduces muscular spasms and tension

Antitussive A drug that can decrease the coughing reflex of the central nervous system (CNS) and reduces the urge to cough

Anuria The inability to urinate

Anxiety Feelings of apprehension, dread, and fear, with characteristics including tension, restlessness, tachycardia, dyspnea, and a sense of hopelessness; symptoms of fear not caused by any danger or threat

APAP N-acetyl-para-amino-phenol; also known generically as acetaminophen or paracetamol

Aperitif A drink that stimulates the appetite

Apnea Cessation of breathing

Apothecary Latin term for pharmacist

Appendicitis Inflammation of the appendix

Aqueous extract Soluble fraction of plant material obtained after extraction with water

Aqueous humor Lymph-type fluid that is found in both anterior and posterior chambers of the eye

Aromatherapy The medicinal use of aroma substances by inhalation, bath, massage

Arrhythmia Any variation from the normal rhythm of the heart, either in rate, regularity, flow of impulse; treated with drugs that slow, speed, or change the rate of conductance of the electricity in the heart

Arteriosclerosis Accumulation of fatty deposits in the blood vessels causing them to narrow and harden, resulting in heart disease or strokes

Artery A vessel that carries oxygenated blood from the heart to the tissues of the body

Arthritis Inflammation of joints

ASA Acetylsalicylic acid; aspirin

Aseptic technique The procedures used to eliminate the possibility of a drug becoming contaminated with microbes or particles

Asthenia Diminishing strength and energy

Asthma A condition in which narrowing of the airways impedes breathing

Astringent Substance (often tannins) that reacts with proteins in wounds, on the surface of cells or membranes, resulting in a protective layer and causing contraction

Ataxia Loss of muscle coordination

Atherosclerosis Changes in arterial walls that lead to arteriosclerosis

Attenuated An altered or weakened live vaccine made from the disease organism that the vaccine protects against

Auditory canal A 1-inch tube that runs from the opening of the external ear to the eardrum, or middle ear

Auditory ossicles The set of three small bony structures in the ear: malleus, incus, and stapes

Autoimmune disease A condition in which a person's tissues are attacked by his/her immune system; abnormal antigen-antibody reaction

Autonomic Literally, self-controlling or involuntary

Autonomic nervous system (ANS) Division of the nervous system that controls the involuntary body functions, such as heart muscle, smooth muscles and glands; comprises the sympathetic and parasympathetic divisions; as opposed to the voluntary nervous system

Auxiliary label An adhesive label that is attached to a container with specific instructions or information pertaining to the medication inside

Avitaminosis Vitamin deficiency

Axon The part of a nerve cell that conducts impulses away from the cell body

Ayurveda A lifestyle-based holistic medical system originating in India 5000 years ago, with a pharmacopoeia of herbs, metals, and inorganic elements; massage; acupuncture; yoga; nutrition; focusing on rejuvenation, self-healing, and detoxification

Bacteria Uni-cellular organisms

Bactericidal Agents that kill bacteria

Bacteriostatic Agents that prevent the growth of bacteria but do not kill them

Benign A nonmalignant growth of tumor cells; not recurrent; favorable for recovery

Benign prostatic hypertrophy Nonmalignant enlargement of prostate gland resulting from proliferation of both stroma and gland elements; properly called benign prostatic hyperplasia

Beta-carotene An orange plant pigment that is converted in the body to vitamin A

Binary fission The method of reproduction by which a single cell divides into two separate cells

Biology The study of life

Biopsy A procedure in which a piece of tissue is removed from a patient for examination and diagnosis, to take a sample of the whole

Bipolar disorder Mood disorder in which patient alternates between excessive phases of manic and depressive episodes; formerly known as manic-depressive

Blister pack Container usually made of plastic that holds a single-dose tablet or capsule

Blood-brain barrier A barrier formed by special characteristics of capillaries in the brain to prevent certain chemicals from moving into the brain

Blood urea nitrogen (BUN) A laboratory test that measures the nitrogen waste in blood in the form of urea

Bradycardia Slow beating of the heart; in adults, less than 60 beats per minute

Bradykinins A 9-amino acid peptide, made from kininogen by blood elements in the inflammatory pathway, is a potent vasodilator, causes pain, contraction, and inflammatory reactions in tissues

Brand/trade name Trademark of a drug or device registered by the originating manufacturing company

Bronchitis Inflammation of the mucous membranes of the bronchial tubes in the lungs

Bronchodilator A substance that reduces bronchial muscle spasm and opens the airway, used for asthma

Bulk compounding A larger quantity of medication that can fill a large order at one time or several smaller orders in the future

Bulk forming Fiber used as a stimulant to the intestines or to cause a feeling of fullness to decrease appetite

Cachexia Weight loss due to chronic illness or prolonged emotional stress

Calibration Determination of the accuracy of an instrument or measuring device against a standard

Cancer A general term used to describe malignant and abnormally invasive growth of cells, known as neoplasms

Candidiasis Infection with the fungus Candida albicans or related species, also called a yeast infection and treated with anti-fungals

Capillary A *minute* blood vessel that connects the ends of the smallest arteries (arterioles) to the smallest veins (venules), where exchanges of nutrients and wastes, O_2 and CO_2 can occur; blood vessels at cellular level

Carbohydrates Chemical substances that include sugars, glycogen, starches, and cellulose; composed of carbon, hydrogen, and oxygen molecules

Carcinogen A substance or chemical that can increase the risk of developing cancer

Carcinoma Malignant growth of epithelial cells

Carminative A substance that reduces flatulence, or intestinal gas

Catabolism To break down; the destructive phase of metabolism

Catalyst A molecule that allows chemical reactions to take place rapidly but is not altered in the reaction

Cataract Loss of transparency of the lens of the eye

Cell body The main part of a neuron, or nerve cell, from which axons and dendrites extend

Cerebrospinal fluid (CSF) A fluid that fills the ventricles of the brain and the spaces of the brain or spinal cord and the arachnoid layer of the meninges

Cervical The region from the base of the skull to the upper chest or thorax

Chemotherapy The treatment of a disease with toxic chemical substances to slow the disease process or to kill cells

Chiropractic A therapy system that uses manual manipulation of the joints and muscles to relieve organ and muscle dysfunction

Chloasma Hyperpigmentation of skin, limited or confined to a certain area

Chronic obstructive pulmonary disease (COPD) A disease process where the lungs have decreased ability for gas exchange; types include emphysema and chronic bronchitis

Chyme Food of a soupy acidic consistency as it passes from mixing with stomach enzymes into the small intestine

Clinical pharmacist Pharmacist who directly monitors patient medications and health in inpatient, ambulatory, and some community settings

Clinical trial The development of new drugs constists of 4 phases: 1. preclinical studies and early clinical studies with non-humans, 2. clinical studies of larger scope looking at safety in humans 3. human studies with more patients looking for efficacy of the drug, 4. large-scale human studies looking for efficacy and safety

CNS Central nervous system

Coagulate To solidify or change from a fluid state to a more solid state

Code blue A coded message to indicate an emergency in a hospital situation, usually cardiopulmonary arrest

Coenzyme A compound that activates an enzyme

Cofactor Usually a vitamin, mineral, or molecule that must be present for other factors to be active in a chemical reaction

Colic Abdominal pains, caused by muscle contraction of an abdominal organ, and usually accompanied by nausea, vomiting, and perspiration

Commission E Recommendations of a group of German experts in the 1990s regarding the usefulness and efficacy of plant drugs

Communication The ability to express oneself in such a way that one is readily and clearly understood

Competency The capability or proficiency to perform a function

Compounding The act of mixing, reconstituting, and packaging a drug

Condyloma Warts of the genital-anal region, usually caused by virus of the Papilloma group

Cones Photoreceptors responsible for perceiving color (daylight vision) in the retina of the eye, actually an extension of brain cells

Confidentiality To keep privileged information from being disclosed without the patient's consent

Congestive heart failure (CHF) Accumulation of blood in the circulatory system due to the heart's inability to pump efficiently

Conjunctiva The mucous membranes of the eyes and eyelids, can get inflamed to cause pinkeye

Constipation Decreased bowel movements leading to prolonged passage time of feces/stools that are often thus dry and hard

Continuing Education (CE) Professional education beyond the basic technical level, usually required for license maintenance and renewal

Cornea The transparent tissue covering the anterior portion of the eye

Corpus luteum A group of cells in the ovary that secrete estrogen and progesterone and have released an egg

Cough reflex An automated response in the throat when stimulated to clear air passages of foreign substances and mucus by a forceful expiration

Cream A hydrophilic base

Cretinism Condition in which the development of the brain and body is inhibited by congenital lack of thyroid hormones

Crohn's disease Chronic inflammation of the intestinal tract

Cushing's disease Syndrome in which an increase in secretions of the adrenal cortex create symptoms such as a moon face and deposits of fat on the upper back (buffalo hump)

Cyclooxygenase Enzymes that catalyze prostaglandin and other inflammation chemical biosynthesis, inhibited by COX inhibitors, aspirin, and similar agents

Cycloplegia Paralysis of the ciliary muscle in the eye

Cystic fibrosis An inherited disorder that causes production of very thick mucus in the respiratory tract due to impaired chloride ion flow; affects the pancreas and sweat glands; patient experiences difficulty breathing and frequent respiratory infections, eventually leading to severe scarring and death

Cystitis Inflammation of the urinary bladder, possibly caused by a bacterial infection

Cytotoxic A substance that is toxic to cells

Debride To remove dead or damaged tissue

Decoction Watery extract obtained by boiling, used in making plant medicines

Decongestants Drugs that reduce swelling of the mucous membranes by constricting dilated blood vessels; reduced blood flow to nasal tissues reduces nasal congestion and opens air passages

Dementia Loss of individually acquired mental skills; Alzheimer's disease is a severe form

Dendrite The part of a neuron that branches out to receive and bring impulses to the cell body

Deoxyribonucleic acid (DNA) The complex nucleic acids that are base for genetic continuance

Depot An area of the body where a substance can accumulate or be stored for later distribution

Depression A mental state characterized by sadness; changes in sleep, appetite, and sex drive; feelings of loss and grief; hopelessness; and may include suicidal thoughts; associated with low concentrations of dopamine, noradrenaline, or serotonin

Dermatitis Inflammation of the skin associated with itching and burning

Desquamation A normal process of shedding the top layer of the skin, also known as exfoliation

Diabetes mellitus Chronic abnormally high blood sugar levels caused by improper function of the pancreas

Diagnosis A doctor's assessment of the cause of a condition

Dialysis The passage of a solute through a semipermeable membrane to remove toxic materials and to maintain fluid, electrolyte, and pH of the body system; often used to describe treatment of the blood when the kidneys no longer function in end-stage renal disease (ESRD)

Diaphoretic A substance that increases sweating

Diarrhea Watery, loose stools, abnormal to the patient's usual frequency

Dietary supplement A substance that is marketed and sold as a non-food, non-drug item but not as a therapeutic agent, often includes vitamins, minerals, herbs, and medicines from non-allopathic medical systems

Digestion The mechanical, chemical, and enzymatic action of breaking food into molecules that can be absorbed and then used in metabolism

Diuresis The secretion and passage of large amounts of urine from the body

Diuretic An agent that increases urine output, diuresis

DNA Deoxyribonucleic acid, the biomolecules in the cells of most living things that store genetic information

Dogma A code of beliefs based on tradition rather than fact

GLOSSARY

Dromotropic An agent that alters the beating of a cell

Dropsy Outdated term for hydrops

Drug Enforcement Agency (DEA) Federal agency within the Department of Justice that regulates the misuse of controlled substances

Dysentery Inflammation of the colon; often caused by bacteria (shigella) or viruses, accompanied by pain and severe diarrhea

Dysmenorrhea Painful menstruation

Dyspepsia Indigestion

Dystonia Symptoms that include twisting, repeated jerking movements, and/or abnormal posture

Dysuria Painful urination

Eczema Inflammation of the skin with redness, itching, and oozing vesicular lesions; sometimes associated with a triad with gut problems and ear infections, and relieved by changing diet, assessing allergies, and cleaning environment

Edema A local or generalized condition in which body tissues retain an excessive amount of tissue fluid outside of the blood vessels

Efferent The conduction of electrical impulses away from the CNS toward the body

Electrolytes Charged elements, composed of cations (molecules having net positive charges) and anions (molecules having net negative charges)

Elixir A base solution that is a mixture, emulsion, or suspension of alcohol and water

Emesis Vomiting

Endometriosis Condition where tissue resembling endometrium is found outside the uterine cavity, usually in the pelvic area

Endometrium The mucus membrane lining of the uterus, where a fertilized egg implants to form a placenta and embryo

Endorphins Peptides made by the body with actions similar to morphine

Enteritis Inflammation of the intestines

Enzyme A protein that speeds up a chemical reaction by reducing the amount of energy required to initiate a reaction; also called a biological catalyst

Epilepsy A chronic brain condition characterized by seizures and loss of consciousness

Erythema Redness of the skin resulting from capillary dilation

Essential oil Mixture of volatile terpenoids responsible for the taste and smell of many plants, especially spices, the basic ingredients used in aromatherapy

Estrogen A family of related compounds serving as female sex hormones

Ethics The values and morals that are used within a profession

Eustachian tube A tubular structure within the middle ear that connects to the nasopharynx (throat)

Euthyroid Normal functioning thyroid gland

Excretion Elimination of waste products through stools, urine, sweat, and breath

Exophthalmos Abnormal protrusion or prominence of the eyeball, usually due to increased thyroid hormone, also called proptosis

Expectorant Chemical that causes the removal of mucous secretions from the respiratory system; loosens and thins sputum and bronchial secretions for ease of removal through coughing

Extract A concentrated preparation in semi-liquid, solid, or dry

GLOSSARY

powder of the soluble fraction of plant material

Extrapyramidal Associated with functional effects outside of the pyramidal tracts controlling motor activities and posture, coordination, support, and walking; symptoms of taking antipsychotic medications that include parkinsonism, dystonia, and tremors

Euthyroid Normal functioning thyroid gland

FDA Food and Drug Administration

Facts and Comparisons Reference book found in most pharmacies containing detailed information on all medications

Facultative anaerobe A microorganism that can live with or without oxygen

Fallopian tubes Narrow passage tube connecting an ovary with the uterus

Fat-soluble Drugs that are absorbed into the body's fat layer

Fat-soluble vitamin Vitamin that is soluble in fat, and therefore is stored in body fat; vitamins A, D, E, and K are fat-soluble

Fertilization The process by which the sperm unites with the ovum to create a new life

Floor stock Supplies kept on hand in different units of a hospital

Food and Drug Administration (FDA) Federal agency within the Department of Health and Human Services that regulates the manufacture and safeguarding of medications

Formulary A list of preferred drugs to be stocked by the pharmacy; also a list of drugs covered by an insurance company

Fungicide An agent that kills fungus

Gametes Sex cells of reproduction: ova and sperm

Gastritis Inflammation of the stomach lining

Gauge The size of the needle opening; smaller gauge numbers indicate larger openings

Generic name Name assigned to a medication by the FDA; nonproprietary name of a drug

Globulin A protein that is insoluble in water; immune globulins protect against diseases

Glucose Simple six-carbon sugar; one of the basic building blocks of energy used by the body

Goiter Condition in which the thyroid is enlarged, commonly from a lack of iodine known as simple goiter, or because of a tumor, known as toxic goiter

Government insurance Includes Medicaid and Medicare

Gram The basic unit of mass (weight) of the metric system, equal to the weight of a cubic centimeter (cc) or a milliliter (ml) of water

Gram-negative bacteria Bacteria that are unable to keep crystal violet stain when washed in acid alcohol, due to a phospholipid outer membrane that prevents staining; named after Dr. HCJ Gram

Gram-positive bacteria Bacteria that are able to keep crystal violet stain when washed in acid alcohol, due to a thick peptidoglycan that holds stain

Graves' disease Hyperplasia/hypersecretion of thyroid causing exophthalmos, diffuse goiter, and skin changes, usually autoimmune in origin

Hallucinogen A substance that induces the perception of objects that are not actually present

Health Insurance Portability and Accountability Act of 1996 (HIPAA) Federal act designed to protect patients' rights by having them explicitly sign agreements to who views their medical information

Heartburn Uncomfortable burning sensation in the chest, rising toward the throat, due to the return of stomach acid into the esophagus, located just next to the heart

Helminth Multicellular worm

Hematuria Blood in the urine

Hemoglobin The iron-containing molecule that carries oxygen to and carbon dioxide from body tissues and that gives red blood cells their color

Hemolysis Disruption of red blood cells

Hemorrhage Profuse bleeding

Hemorrhoids Known commonly as piles, painful and swollen anal veins

Hemostatic A substance or procedure that reduces or stops bleeding

Hepatitis Inflammation of the liver

Hepatotoxic Toxic to the liver

Herb A plant that is used for its medicinal properties

Herpes simplex Localized permanent recurring infection on the lips or genitalia, caused by the herpes virus

Histamine A chemical produced by mast cells, a type of white blood cells, and released during inflammation reactions that interacts with tissues to produce itching, vasodilation, and decreased blood pressure as part of an allergic reaction

HIV Human immunodeficiency virus; associated with AIDS

HMO Health Maintenance Organization

Hodgkin's Disease A cancer of lymph cells (lymphoma) that originates in one lymph node and later spreads to other organs

Homeopathy An empiric and energetic holistic system of therapy based on the belief that medicinal remedies causing specific symptoms can be used to treat an illness that manifests the same symptoms

Homeostasis The equilibrium pertaining to the balance of the body with respect to fluid levels, pH level, and chemicals

Horizontal flow hood Environment for the preparation of sterile products that uses air originating from the back of the hood moving forward across the hood out into the room

Hormone Chemical substances produced and secreted into the bloodstream or duct by an endocrine gland, resulting in physiologic responses at specific target tissues elsewhere in the body

Household system A system of measurement commonly used for weight, volume, and length in the United States

HPLC High performance liquid chromatography; a technique used to analyze chemical compounds and extracts

Hydrophilic Literally, water loving; any substance that easily dissolves into water

Hydrophobic Literally, water avoiding; any substance that does not go into or mix in water

Hyperalimentation Parenteral nutrition for patients who are unable to eat solids or liquids

Hypercalcemia Unusually high concentration of calcium in the blood

Hyperemia Abnormal blood accumulation in a localized part of the body

Hyperglycemia Abnormally high glucose content circulating in the bloodstream

Hyperlipidemia Characterized by high lipid values in the blood, triglycerides >160 mg/dl, and cholesterol >200 mg/dl

Hyperplasia Abnormal increase in the growth of an organ, due to cells dividing and increasing in number

Hypertension High blood pressure, >140/90 mm Hg

Hypertonic solution Abnormally high salt levels having a higher osmotic pressure than blood or another body fluid

Hypertrophy Abnormal increase in the size of an organ, with cell numbers remaining constant

Hypervitaminosis A disorder caused by the accumulation of too many vitamins in the body; more common with fat-soluble vitamins

Hypnotic A substance that induces sleep

Hypocalcemia Low concentration of calcium in the blood

Hypoglycemia Abnormally low glucose content circulating in the bloodstream

Hypoplasia Incomplete or under-development of an organ or tissue

Hypothermia Low body temperature

Hypotension Low blood pressure with values under 105/60 mm Hg

Icterus Jaundice, yellowish discoloration of body organs such as skin and eyes due to bile pigments from the liver not being metabolized properly

Immunity Protection of the body through resistance to infection via factors in the immune system, the immune response of the body, or from agents such as vaccinations

in utero In the uterus, before birth

in vitro In the laboratory or test tube

in vivo In a living animal or human

Inert ingredient An ingredient that has little or no effect on body functions

Inflammation Localized swelling, redness, pain, and heat, usually as a result of an infection or injury

Influenza An acute and highly contagious respiratory tract infection caused by one of many influenza viruses that infect mucus membranes of the respiratory tract

Infusion Refers to a preparation that is made by adding boiling water to the required amount of drug, which is allowed to steep for 5-10 minutes before it is strained. Such a preparation is often loosely referred to as 'tea'; vs. maceration

Ingestion The act of taking in food or liquid

Inhibit To stop or hold back; to keep a reaction from taking place

Inotropic A substance that affects the force or energy of contraction of muscles

Inpatient A hospitalized patient

Inpatient pharmacy A pharmacy in a hospital or institutional setting

Insomnia Difficulty falling or staying asleep

Insulin A hormone of the pancreas that controls the level of glucose in the blood

Intrinsic factor A naturally-produced protein that is necessary for the absorption of vitamin B_{12}

Invasive The tendency for a tumor or mass to move into tissues and/or organs in close proximity

Ion channel Membrane proteins that can form water-containing pores so that mineral ions can enter or leave cells

Jaundice Yellowish discoloration of body organs such as skin and eyes due to bile pigments from the liver not being metabolized properly

Kcal Kilocalorie; a measurement of energy or heat expended or used up in a chemical activity; the amount of heat needed to change the temperature of 1 kg of water one degree Celsius

Keratolytic A drug that causes shedding of the outer layer of the skin

Labyrinth A system of cavities or canals; in the inner ear, the bony maze composed of the vestibular utricle, saccule, cochlea, and 3 semicircular canals

Lactation Production and secretion of milk by female mammary glands

Laminar flow hood Environment for the preparation of sterile products

Laxative A substance that loosens stool forming in the bowels

Legend drug Drug that requires a prescription for dispensing

Leucopenia Low white blood cell count

Leukemia A progressive disease marked by malignancy of the blood-forming cells found in the hemopoietic tissues, organs, and bloodstream, causing the circulation of abnormal blood cells

Leukorrhea Vaginal discharge of white or yellowish fluid

Ligand A substance that binds to a receptor

Liniment Ointment for topical application

Lipids Fats and fatty acids; substances soluble in non-polar solvents and insoluble in water

Lipid-lowering A substance that lowers triglyceride or cholesterol levels in blood

Lipophilic A substance soluble in oil or a non-polar solvent

Lumbar Pertaining to the loins; the region of the sides of the back that includes the area between the ribs and the pelvis; the area around the waist

Lymphoma A term used to describe a malignant disorder of lymphoid tissue

Maceration Refers to a preparation that is made by adding cold water to the required amount of drug or plant material, which is allowed to soak at room temperature for 6-8 hours before it is strained; vs. infusion

Macro Large

Malaria A parasitic disease caused by Plasmodium parasites; transmitted to humans by mosquitoes

Malignant An invasive and destructive pattern of rapid, abnormal cell growth; often fatal

Mania A form of psychosis characterized by uncontrolled and excessive excitement, elevated mood, and exalted feelings

MAO The enzyme monoamine oxidase, catalyses the removal of amine groups from dopamine and norepinephrine

MAO inhibitor Inhibitor of monoamine oxidase that degrades the neurotransmitters epinephrine, norepinephrine, dopamine, and serotonin

MAR Medication administration record

Mastitis Inflammation of the breast

Mastodynia Pain in swollen female breasts

Materia medica Listing of the various materials from plants, animals, or minerals that are used in medical and healing systems

Melanoma A malignant tumor/neoplasm of the pigment-producing cells of skin and mucosa; may metastasize to other organs

Menopause Permanent cessation of menstruation due to decreased production of female sex hormones; a natural phenomenon around age 50 in which the woman completes her reproductive phase of her life

Menorrhagia Abnormally severe menstruation

Metabolism The physical and chemical changes that take place within an organism

Metastasis The movement or spread of cancerous cells through the body to organs in distant areas

Meter Basic measurement of length in the metric system

Metered dose inhaler (MDI) A dispenser for supplying medications to the lungs through inhalation

Micro Small

Microbial Refers to minute living organisms visible with a microscope, fungi, protozoa, and bacteria

Microbiology The study of microscopic organisms

Microgram One one-thousandth of a milligram; metric unit of measure; 10^{-6} grams

Microtubules Linear tubular structure of cells essential for cell division and transport process in the cell

Micturition Urination

Migraine Recurrent condition of severe pain in the head often accompanied by symptoms such as nausea and visual disturbances

Milligram One one-thousandth of a gram; metric unit of measure; 10^{-3} grams

Mineralocorticoid The steroids of the adrenal cortex, primarily aldosterone, which regulates salt metabolism

Miosis Contraction of the pupil resulting in less light going into the eye

Mitochondrion Important compartment of eukaryotic cells; site of

the Krebs cycle and respiration chain, production of ATP; have their own DNA

Mitosis Cellular reproduction that creates two identical daughter cells from the parent cell's DNA

Molecular biosynthesis The making of chemical compounds within a living organism

Monoamine oxidase (MAO) An enzyme (includes MAO-A and MAO-B) found in the nerve terminals, the neurons, and liver cells; inactivates chemicals such as tyramine, catecholamines, serotonin, and certain medications

Monograph Medication information sheet that includes side effects, dosage forms, indications, and other important information; must be provided by the manufacturer to FDA

Morals Ethics; honorable beliefs

Morphology Appearance, including shape, size, structure, and stain characteristics of organisms; study of organisms without studying the function

Mortar and pestle A bowl and rounded knob used to grind substances into fine powder

Mucilage A solution of viscous/slimy substances usually polysaccharides, that form a protective layer over inflamed mucosal tissues

Mucolytic Substance that dissolves mucous, such as in the bronchus

Mucosa Mucous tissue layer on the inside of the respiratory, gastrointestinal tract

Mucus Clear, viscous secretion formed by mucous membranes

Multiple sclerosis Disorder of the central nervous system caused by a destruction of the myelin around axons in the brain and spinal cord, leading to various neurological symptoms

Mutagenic A substance that induces genetic mutations

Myalgia Non-localized muscle pain

Muscarinic Relating to acetylcholine receptor type and cholinergic function of parasympathetic and autonomic nervous system, including decrease in heart rate, dilation of arterioles, increase in gut motility and stimulation of glands

Mutation An unexpected change in the molecular structure within the DNA, sometimes causing a permanent change in expression of proteins in cells

Mycosis Fungal disease

Mydriasis Dilation of the pupil resulting in more light going into the eye

Myopia Nearsightedness

Myxedema Condition associated with the a decrease in overall thyroid function in adults; also known as hypothyroidism

Narcotic A substance that produces insensibility or stupor, combined with a sense of well-being

National Association of Boards of Pharmacy (NABP) National organization for members of state boards of pharmacy

Naturopathy A holistic system of healing that emphasizes the body's inherent power of regaining balance and harmony

Necrosis Death of cells or tissue

Negative feedback A self-regulating mechanism in which the output of a system has input or control on the process; a factor within a system that causes a corrective action to return the system to normal range

Neoplasm An abnormal tissue growth

Nephritis Kidney inflammation

Nerve terminal The end portion of the neuron where nerve impulses cause chemical to be released; these neurochemicals cross a small space, the synaptic cleft, to carry the impulse to another neuron

Neuralgia Severe pain along nerve ends

Neuron The functional unit of the nervous system, which included the cell body, dendrites, axon, and terminals

Neurosis Mental illness arising from stress or anxiety in the patient's environment without loss of contact with reality; phobias can be listed in this category; vs. psychosis

Neurotransmitter Signal compounds in synapses of neurons that help to convert an electric signal into a chemical response; important neurotransmitters are acetylcholine, epinephrine, norepinephrine, dopamine, serotonin, histamine, glycine, GABA, glutamate, endorphins and peptides

Nicotinic Relating to acetylcholine receptor subtype and cholinergic function of autonomic nervous system, especially at ganglion and neuromuscular junction, causing skeletal muscle changes and widespread organ regulation

NKDA No known drug allergy

NKFA No known food allergy

Nocturia Nightly urge to urinate

Nonproductive cough Cough that does not produce mucous secretions from respiratory tract

Normal flora Microorganisms that reside harmlessly in the body and do not cause disease but may aid the host organism

Nosocomial infection An infection acquired while hospitalized

NSAIDs Nonsteroidal anti-inflammatory drugs

Nucleic acid The molecule bases contained within deoxyribonucleic acid (DNA)

Nutritional supplement A preparation that supplies additional nutrients or active compounds to the body that may not be obtained by the normal diet

Ointment A semisolid hydrophobic medicinal preparation used topically

On-call A medication to be administered when directed, usually for preanesthesia

Oncogene A previously normal gene that may be adversely affected by infection, such as a retrovirus, which causes a mutation and may produce cancer

Oocyte or ova The female reproductive germ cell

Ophthalmic Pertaining to the eye

Orbit The rotation of electrons around the nucleus; the bone casing of the eye

Organic Term used for products grown and processed without use of artificial chemicals, such as hormones, pesticides, or plastic derivatives, wild-harvested materials usually qualify

Osteoporosis Condition associated with the decrease of bone mass and the softening of the bones, resulting in the increased possibility of bone fractures

OTC Over-the-counter; a drug sold without prescription in the US, non-legend medications

Otic Pertaining to the ear

Otitis Inflammation of the ear

Outpatient pharmacy Pharmacies that serve patients in their communities; pharmacies that are not in inpatient facilities

Oxytocic Speeding up of parturition, or birth

Oxytocin A pituitary gland hormone that stimulates lactation, induces uterine contractions and labor

Paget's disease Condition affecting older adults in which the density of the bones decreases, resulting in softening and weakening

Palliative Brings relief but does not cure

PAR Periodic automatic replacement

Parasite Organism that uses a host for nourishment and reproduction without benefiting host

Parasympathetic nervous system Division of the autonomic nervous system that functions during restful situations; "breed or feed" part of ANS, slows heart rate, increases intestinal smooth muscle and gland activity, relaxes sphincter muscles

Parenteral Medication administered by routes outside the gut or enteric system, common routes include subcutaneous, intravenous, or intramuscular injection

Parkinson's disease A progressive neurological disease caused by degeneration of the substantia nigra and a reduction of dopamine concentrations, marked by lack of muscular coordination and mental deterioration, manifesting in unnaturally slow or rigid movements

Passive immunity Resistance that has been acquired through a transfer of antibodies from outside the body, from mother to child, from animal contact, or from vaccinations

Pathogen A micro-organism that may cause disease

Peptic ulcer An ulcerative condition of the lower esophagus, stomach, or duodenum, often resulting from the bacterium *Helicobacter pylori* (*H pylori*)

Peptidoglycan The substance that comprises bacterial cell walls, thicker in gram-positive than in gram-negative microbes

Periodontitis Inflammation of the area around a tooth

Peripheral nervous system (PNS) The division of the nervous system outside the brain and spinal cord

Peripheral parenteral Injection of a medication into the veins located on the periphery of the body system, in arms or legs, instead of a central vein or artery

Peristalsis The contraction and relaxation of the tubular muscles of the esophagus and intestines that move food substances from the mouth to the anus; waves of involuntary contraction in the digestive system

Pharmacist Person who dispenses drugs and counsels patients about drugs

Pharmacodynamics The study of how medicinal substances work in the body, whether they bind to a receptor

Pharmacognosy The study of herbal drugs, their identification, properties and uses

Pharmacokinetics The study of how medicinal substances are absorbed, moved, distributed, metabolized, and excreted

Pharmacology The study of the nature, properties and uses of drugs and their effects on the body; includes the study of both endogenous and synthesized active compounds

Pharmacopoeia An official and authoritative book or publication listing all the various drugs that may be used

Phlegm Catarrhal secretion or sputum

Phosphodiesterase Important enzyme of signal transduction, inactivates cAMP or cGMP

Phospholipids Phosphorylated lipids that are the building blocks of cell membranes

Photosensitization Increased sensitivity to sunlight

Physician's Desk Reference (PDR) Reference book of medications

Phytotherapy Application of plant drugs or products derived from plants to cure diseases or to relieve symptoms

Placebo Drug preparation without active ingredient that cannot be distinguished from the original drug; used as an inert compound to control clinical studies

Placebo effect An improvement of a health condition that cannot be ascribed to the treatment used

PMS Premenstrual syndrome, now called premenstrual dysphoric disorder, PMDD; usually occurs a few days before menstruation with symptoms of fear, irritability, changing mood, insomnia, headache, swollen breasts, abdominal pain, edema, decreased libido; thought to be due to changing sex hormone levels causing hypoglycemia and endogenous opioid release

POS Point of sale

Poultice A semisolid mass of plant materials in oil or water applied to the skin

PPO Preferred Provider Organization

Pre-op A drug ordered to be given before surgery or preoperatively

PRN Pro re nata (latin); take as needed

Prodrug A substance that is converted to its active form within the body

Productive cough Cough that expectorates mucous secretions from respiratory tract

Professionalism Conforming to principles of conduct (work ethics)

as accepted by others in the profession

Prophylaxis Treatment given before an event to prevent the event from happening

Prostaglandins A group of physiologically active substances in the cell membrane of tissues that cause stimulation of muscles and numerous other metabolic effects; released during cell damage and promoting the inflammation process, including pain, swelling, heat

Prostate A gland at the base of the male bladder that secretes a fluid that forms a part of semen, stimulating sperm motility

Protectant A substance that acts as a barrier between the skin and an irritant

Protocol A set of standards and guidelines within which a facility works

Proton A subatomic particle of an atom that holds a positive charge, the hydrogen ion H^+

Protozoa Kingdom Protista; unicellular organisms that are usually parasites

Pruritis Itching

Psoriasis Skin condition caused by an enhanced growth of dermal cells, resulting in the production of excess skin or dandruff

Psychosis A mental illness characterized by loss of contact with reality

Psychotherapeutic Relating to classes of drugs or agents that affect the mind and brain; categories include tricyclic antidepressants, SSRIs, phenothiazines

Psychotropic A substance that affects the mind or mood

Pyretic A substance that induces fever

Recall When a drug or device must be returned to the manufacturer

due to failure to meet FDA standards

Receptor Protein often attached to a cell membrane, that has a binding site for another molecule called a ligand, important for signal transduction in cells

Reconstitution To mix a liquid and a powder to form a suspension or solution

Remission The span of time during which a disease, such as cancer, is not spreading; this may be permanent or temporary

Resorption Uptake of a substance through the skin or a mucous membrane

Rheumatism General term referring to painful joints

Rhinitis Inflammation of the mucosal lining of the nose; runny nose

ROA Route of administration

Rods Photoreceptors that respond to dim light and are responsible for black and white color (night vision)

RTS Return to stock

Rx Latin for "recipe," commonly used to mean "prescription," legend drug, prescription drug

Sarcoma A malignant, neoplastic growth arising from connective tissue

Saturated fat Fats with fatty acids saturated with hydrogen, therefore without double bonds, such as animal fats, coconut oil; more easily taken up by the body and therefore unfavorable

Schizophrenia A group of mental disorders characterized by inappropriate emotions and unrealistic thinking

Script A prescription

Sedative-hypnotics Substances that calm down the nerves and decrease activity and excitement, used to induce sleep; tranquilizer

Semen The fluid in which the seeds of an organism can stay and travel for a short period of time

Shaman Medicine person who holds a high place of honor in a tribe and emphasizes spiritual connection

Sig Medication directions written in pharmacy terms on a prescription

Sitz-bath An immersion bath used for medicinal purposes

Solute The ingredient that is dissolved into a solution

Solution A water base in which the ingredient(s) dissolves completely

Solvent The greater part of a solution; what the ingredient is dissolved into

Somatic The motor neurons that control voluntary actions of the skeletal muscles

Soporific A substance that induces or promotes sleep

Spasm Involuntary contraction of muscles

Species Latin origin meaning "kind" or type; used to differentiate one biologic item from another

Sputum Fluid coughed up from the lungs and bronchial tissues

Spondylitis Inflammation of vertebrae

STAT order A medication order that must be filled as soon as possible, usually within 5 to 15 minutes

Steroid Messenger chemical produced by the body that helps fight inflammation and pain

Sunscreen A substance that protects the skin from ultraviolet (UV) light, which causes sunburns; skin protectant factor (SPF) rates effectiveness

Suspension A solution is which the powder does not dissolve into the base and must be shaken before using

Symbiotic A close relationship between two species, in which both can benefit

Sympathetic nervous system Division of the autonomic nervous system that functions during stressful situations; "fight or flight" part of ANS, accelerates the heart rate, constricts blood vessels, and raises blood pressure; mediated by alpha- and beta-adrenergic receptors

Sympathomimetic Resembling the adrenergic effects of the sympathetic nervous system

Synapse The space between which neurons are connected with each other or with target tissues via neurotransmitters as a way of converting electrical into chemical signals

Synergistic The phenomenon that the combined effect of two or more substances is greater than the sum of their individual effects

Synthesis The formation of components within a body system

Synthetic Medication made in a laboratory or factory

Syrup A sugar-based liquid solution intended to ease oral administration of a drug

Systemic Affecting the entire body rather than individual body parts

Tachycardia Fast beating of the heart; in adults, more than 100 beats per minute

Tardive dyskinesia Unwanted side effects of taking dopamine blockers that include slow, rhythmical involuntary movements that are either generalized or specific to one muscle group

Taxonomy The science of classification and nomenclature of organisms

TCM Traditional Chinese Medicine; one of the oldest therapeutic systems of mankind still in use

Tea An infusion made by pouring boiling water over a measured quantity of dried plant material and leaving it for a while to steep; vs. maceration

Teratogenic A substance that causes abnormal growth in an embryo

Testosterone The male sex hormone

Therapeutic Curative, treatment that is effective

Thoracic Related to the chest or thorax

Thrombin An enzyme that is converted in coagulating blood from prothrombin, that then reacts with fibrinogen, converting it into fibrin, which is then essential in the formation of blood clots. Tested by performing a prothrombin time (PT) or partial thromboplastin time (PTT) blood test

Thrombolytic Medication used to break up a thrombus or blood clot

Thrush A fungal infection of mucous membranes marked by white patches, caused by *Candida spp.*

Thyroxine Known as T_4; contains four ions of iodine

Tincture A base solution of alcohol

Tinnitus Ringing noise in the ear

Tisane An herbal tea often made from flowers that is not as strong as an infusion

Tonic A substance that maintains or restores health and vigor, usually taken over a lengthy period

Topical application External application, on the skin

Total parenteral nutrition (TPN) Large-volume intravenous (IV) nutrition administered through the central vein (subclavian vein) allowing for a higher concentration of solutions

Tourette's syndrome A neurologic disorder characterized by multiple motor tics, lack of muscle coordination, and involuntary purposeless movements that are often accompanied by grunts and barks

Toxicology Science that studies toxins and their effects in humans or animals

Toxoid A toxin that has been rendered harmless but still invokes an antigenic response

Trace elements Chemical elements that are needed by the body in very small amounts

Trade name Brand name drug; the company that first applies for a patent on the chemical structure of a medication or generic name is allowed to name the product with a patented name

Transporter A membrane protein that catalyzes the transport of a molecule from one side of a biomembrane to the other side

Triiodothyronine Known as T3; contains three ions of iodine

Tuberculosis A bacterial disease caused by *Mycobacterium tuberculosis* that affects the lungs and later other organs, often chronic and fatal if not treated long-term

Tumor An abnormal growth of tissue, can be benign or malignant

Tympanic membrane A membranous skin that separates the external ear from the middle ear

Ulcer A lesion on the skin or a mucous membrane; a lesion on the mucosal lining of the stomach or intestines that causes burning pain, bleeding, and maldigestion

Unit dose A single dose of a drug delivered in one time period

Universal precautions A set of standards that lowers the possibility of contamination; used to prepare medications and to avoid infections

Unsaturated fat fats with fatty acids with double bonds between the carbon atoms instead of hydrogens, such as olive oil and canola oil; less easily taken up by the body and therefore favorable; vs. saturated fat

Urinary calculi Concrete formations of salts, usually stones, in the tubes below the kidney where urine flows

Urticaria A skin eruption of itching wheals

Vaccine Toxoids or attenuated viral components that are given to create a response from the body that results in immunity

Varicose veins Abnormally distended veins, usually seen in the outer thighs

Vasoconstrictor A substance that causes narrowing of the blood vessels

Vasodilation Widening of the blood vessels that allows for increased blood flow

Vector A carrier, especially one who transfers an infective agent from one host to another without getting the disease; for example, a mosquito bite transfers malaria from the mosquito's saliva without the mosquito having the disease

Vein A vessel that carries deoxygenated blood to or toward the heart

Vertical flow hood Environment for preparation of chemotherapy treatments that uses air originating from the roof of the hood moving downward that is captured in a vent located on the floor of the hood

Vertigo Sensation of instability

Villus A projection from the surface of a mucous membrane; in the gastric tract, these projections increase the surface area for absorption of nutrients and liquids in the small intestines

Virology The study of viruses

Virus Infectious complex of macromolecules that contain their genetic information either as DNA or RNA; replicates by using the host's cell parts, including deoxyribonucleic acid (DNA), ribosomes, and proteins to form new viral particles

Viscosity The thickness of a solution or fluid (e.g., corn syrup is very viscous)

Vitamin An organic substance that occurs in many foods and is necessary in trace amounts for the normal metabolic functioning of the human body; water-soluble vitamins B and C are not readily stored by the body but continually excreted in the urine and must be constantly replaced; see fat-soluble vitamin

Volatile oil Various terpenoids that evaporate easily, usually add taste and smell to plants

Volume The amount of substance enclosed within a container

Vomit The expulsion of matter from the stomach via the mouth

Wild-crafting The collection of medicinal material from natural plant populations in a sustainable way

Worker's compensation A government-required and enforced coverage for workers injured on the job

Yeast Simple eukaryotic cells belonging to the fungus kingdom; Candida spp. commonly infect human vulnerable mucous membranes

Index

Lorcet 10/650, 664.
See also Hydrocodone
Lorcet Plus, 663. See also Hydrocodone
Lorcet-HD, 663. See also Hydrocodone
Loroxide. See Benzoyl peroxide
Lortab, 663. See also Hydrocodone
Lortab 5/500, 663. See also Hydrocodone
Lortab 7.5/500, 663.
See also Hydrocodone
Lortab 10/500, 664.
See also Hydrocodone
Losartan, 819-820
Losec [CAN]. See Omeprazole
Lotensin. See Benazepril
Lotrel. See Lovastatin
Lotrimin, 344. See also Clotrimazole
Lotrimin AF, 344. See also Clotrimazole
Lotrimin-AF, 908. See also Miconazole
Lotronex. See Alosetron
Lovan [AUS]. See Fluoxetine
Lovastatin, 821-822
drug interactions
bosentan, 185
cyclosporine, 366
erythromycin, 517
gemfibrozil, 620
itraconazole, 753
ketoconazole, 760
niacin, 981
telithromycin, 1330
Lovenox. See Enoxaparin
Lovir [AUS]. See Acyclovir
Low spinal (saddle block) anesthesia,
1349
Lower abdominal procedures: anesthesia
for, 1349
hyperbaric spinal, 200
Lower back pain, 844
Lower extremity procedures: anesthesia
for, 1349
hyperbaric spinal, 200
Lower respiratory tract infections, 79, 82,
246, 811, 1016, 1034, 1369, 1371
anaerobic, 904
severe, 1234
Lower urinary tract hypermotility, 683
Lowsium Plus. See Magaldrate
Loxapac [CAN]. See Loxapine
Loxapine, 822-823
drug interactions
cabergoline, 209
pergolide, 1100
Loxitane, 822. See also Loxapine
Lozide [CAN]. See Indapamide
Lozol. See Indapamide

L.P.V. [AUS]. See Penicillin V potassium
LSD, 1499
Lubrication, general, 157
Lucrin [AUS]. See Leuprolide
Lucrin Depot Inj [AUS]. See Leuprolide
Ludes. See Methaqualone
Ludiomil, 834. See also Maprotiline
Lufyllin, 475. See also Dyphylline
Lugol's solution. See also Potassium
iodide
availability, 1154
indications and dosages, 1154, 1155
Luminal. See also Phenobarbital
IV incompatibilities
ephedrine, 496
oxytetracycline, 1054
Lunesta. See Eszopiclone
Lung cancer
non-small cell, 618-619
small-cell, 545-546, 1402
Lung disease, chronic, 1357-1358
LupiCare Dandruff, 1255, 1256.
See also Salicylic acid
LupiCare II, 1255. See also Salicylic acid
LupiCare Psoriasis, 1255, 1256.
See also Salicylic acid
Lupron. See also Leuprolide
availability, 783
indications and dosages, 783-784
precautions & considerations, 784-785
Lupron Depot. See also Leuprolide
availability, 783
indications and dosages, 783
precautions & considerations, 784, 785
Lupron Depot-Ped, 783.
See also Leuprolide
Lupus erythematosus, 679
Luride. See Sodium fluoride
Lustra, 676. See also Hydroquinone
Lustra-AF, 676. See also Hydroquinone
Luvox. See Fluvoxamine
Luxiq, 166. See also Betamethasone
Lyme disease, 277, 1352
early, 279
Lymphocyte immune globulin N,
823-825
Lymphogranuloma venereum, 467
Lymphoma
cutaneous T-cell, 881
refractory, 172
follicular, 719
non-Hodgkin's, 1407
induction of remission in, 370
maintenance of remission in, 370
Lysodren. See Mitotane